CURRENT THERAPY IN SPORTS MEDICINE-2

Surgical Titles in the Current Therapy Series

Callaham:
Current Therapy in Emergency Medicine
Cameron:
Current Surgical Therapy
Charles, Glover:
Current Therapy in Obstetrics
Ernst, Stanley:
Current Therapy in Vascular Surgery
Fazio:
Current Therapy in Colon and Rectal Surgery
Foley, Payne:
Current Therapy of Pain
Garcia, Mastroianni, Amelar, Dubin:
Current Therapy of Infertility
Garcia, Mikuta, Rosenblum:
Current Therapy in Surgical Gynecology
Gates:
Current Therapy in Otolaryngology—Head and Neck Surgery
Grillo, Austen, Wilkins, Mathisen, Vlahakes:
Current Therapy in Cardiothoracic Surgery
Jay:
Current Therapy in Podiatric Surgery
Long:
Current Therapy in Neurological Surgery
Marsh:
Current Therapy in Plastic and Reconstructive Surgery
Parrillo:
Current Therapy in Critical Care Medicine
Resnick, Kursh:
Current Therapy in Genitourinary Surgery
Rogers:
Current Practice in Anesthesiology
Spaeth, Katz:
Current Therapy in Ophthalmic Surgery
Trunkey, Lewis:
Current Therapy of Trauma
Torg, Welsh, Shephard:
Current Therapy in Sports Medicine

CURRENT THERAPY IN SPORTS MEDICINE-2

JOSEPH S. TORG, M.D.

Professor of Orthopaedic Surgery
University of Pennsylvania
Director
University of Pennsylvania Sports Medicine Center
Philadelphia, Pennsylvania

R. PETER WELSH, M.B., CH.B., F.R.C.S.(C), F.A.C.S.

Assistant Professor of Surgery
University of Toronto Faculty of Medicine
Deputy Chief of Surgery
Orthopaedic and Arthritic Hospital
Toronto, Ontario

ROY J. SHEPHARD, M.D. (LOND), PH.D.

Director
School of Physical and Health Education
Professor of Applied Physiology
University of Toronto Faculty of Medicine
Toronto, Ontario

B.C. DECKER INC. • Toronto • Philadelphia

Publisher

B.C. Decker Inc
3228 South Service Road
Burlington, Ontario L7N 3H8

B.C. Decker Inc
320 Walnut Street
Suite 400
Philadelphia, Pennsylvania 19106

Sales and Distribution

United States and Puerto Rico
The C.V. Mosby Company
11830 Westline Industrial Drive
Saint Louis, Missouri 63146

Canada
McAinsh & Co. Ltd.
2760 Old Leslie Street
Willowdale, Ontario M2K 2X5

Australia
McGraw-Hill Book Company Australia Pty. Ltd.
4 Barcoo Street
Roseville East 2069
New South Wales, Australia

Brazil
Editora McGraw-Hill do Brasil, Ltda.
Rua Tabapua, 1.105, Itaim-Bibi
Sao Paulo, S.P. Brasil

Colombia
Interamericana/McGraw-Hill de Colombia, S.A.
Apartado Aereo 81078
Bogota, D.E. Colombia

Europe
McGraw-Hill Book Company GmbH
Lademannbogen 136
D-2000 Hamburg 63
West Germany

France
MEDSI/McGraw-Hill
6, avenue Daniel Lesueur
75007 Paris, France

Hong Kong and China
McGraw-Hill Book Company
Suite 618, Ocean Centre
5 Canton Road
Tsimshatsui, Kowloon
Hong Kong

India
Tata McGraw-Hill Publishing Company, Ltd.
12/4 Asaf Ali Road, 3rd Floor
New Delhi 110002, India

Indonesia
P.O. Box 122/JAT
Jakarta, 1300 Indonesia

Italy
McGraw-Hill Libri Italia, s.r.l.
Piazza Emilia, 5
1-20129 Milano MI
Italy

Japan
Igaku-Shoin Ltd.
Tokyo International P.O. Box 5063
1-28-36 Hongo, Bunkyo-ku,
Tokyo 113, Japan

Korea
C.P.O. Box 10583
Seoul, Korea

Malaysia
No. 8 Jalan SS 7/6B
Kelana Jaya
47301 Petaling Jaya
Selangor, Malaysia

Mexico
Interamericana/McGraw-Hill de Mexico, S.A. de C.V.
Cedro 512, Colonia Atlampa
(Apartado Postal 26370)
06450 Mexico, D.F., Mexico

New Zealand
McGraw-Hill Book Co. New Zealand Ltd.
5 Joval Place, Wiri
Manukau City, New Zealand

Panama
Editorial McGraw-Hill Latinoamericana, S.A.
Apartado Postal 2036
Zona Libre de Colon
Colon, Republica de Panama

Portugal
Editora McGraw-Hill de Portugal, Ltda.
Rua Rosa Damasceno 11A–B
1900 Lisboa, Portugal

South Africa
Libriger Book Distributors
Warehouse Number 8
"Die Ou Looiery"
Tannery Road
Hamilton, Bloemfontein 9300

Southeast Asia
McGraw-Hill Book Co.
348 Jalan Boon Lay
Jurong, Singapore 2261

Spain
McGraw-Hill/Interamericana de Espana, S.A.
Manuel Ferrero, 13
28020 Madrid, Spain

Taiwan
P.O. Box 87–601
Taipei, Taiwan

Thailand
632/5 Phaholyothin Road
Sapan Kwai
Bangkok 10400
Thailand

United Kingdom, Middle East and Africa
McGraw-Hill Book Company (U.K.) Ltd.
Shoppenhangers Road
Maidenhead, Berkshire
SL6 2QL England

Venezuela
McGraw-Hill/Interamericana, C.A.
2da. calle Bello Monte
(entre avenida Casanova y Sabana Grande)
Apartado Aereo 50785
Caracas 1050, Venezuela

NOTICE

The authors and publisher have made every effort to ensure that the patient care recommended herein, including choice of drugs and drug dosages, is in accord with the accepted standards and practices at the time of publication. However, since research and regulation constantly change clinical standards, the reader is urged to check the product information sheet included in the package of each drug, which includes recommended doses, warnings, and contraindications. This is particularly important with new or infrequently used drugs.

Current Therapy in Sports Medicine – 2

ISBN 1–55664–009–9

Library of Congress catalog card number: 85–643454

10 9 8 7 6 5 4 3 2 1

CONTRIBUTORS

FRED L. ALLMAN, Jr., M.D.

Orthopaedic Consultant, Georgia Tech and Atlanta Public Schools; Director, Sports Medicine Clinic, PC Atlanta, Georgia

Overuse Injury in the Throwing Sports

A. AMENDOLA, M.D.

Resident, University of Western Ontario; Chief Resident, Department of Orthopaedics, University Hospital, London, Ontario

Chronic Exertional Compartment Syndrome

JAMES R. ANDREWS, M.D.

Clinical Professor of Orthopaedics and Sports Medicine, University of Virginia Medical School, Charlottesville, Virginia; Orthopaedic Surgeon, Alabama Sports Medicine and Orthopaedic Center, Birmingham, Alabama

Principles of Shoulder Arthroscopy

DAVID L. ANDERS, M.D.

Assistant Professor, Department of Internal Medicine, Medical College of Georgia; Educational Coordinator for Medicine, University Hospital, Augusta, Georgia

Exercise in the Secondary Prevention of Ischemic Heart Disease

FREDERICK C. BALDUINI, M.D.

Assistant Clinical Professor of Orthopaedics, University of Pennsylvania; Staff, Graduate Hospital, Hospital of the University of Pennsylvania, and Presbyterian Hospital, Philadelphia, Pennsylvania

Synthetic Ligamentous Replacement

STEVEN N. BLAIR, P.E.D.

Director of Epidemiology, Institute for Aerobics Research, Dallas, Texas

Exercise in the Primary Prevention of Ischemic Heart Disease

JAMES P. BRADLEY, M.D.

Clinical Instructor, Department of Orthopaedics, University of Pittsburgh; Oakland Orthopaedics, Pittsburgh, Pennsylvania

Ulnar Neuritis and Ulnar Collateral Ligament Instabilities in Overarm Throwers

ROBERT L. BRAND, M.D.

Assistant Clinical Professor of Surgery and Orthopaedics, Medical College of Georgia; Team Physician, Augusta College, Augusta, Georgia

Operative Management of Ligamentous Injuries

DAVID E. BROWN, M.D.

Assistant Professor of Orthopaedic Surgery, University of Nebraska Medical Center; Associate Team Physician, University of Nebraska, Omaha, Nebraska

Patellar Dislocation, Subluxation, and the Elmslie-Trillat Procedure

DAVID R. BROWN, Ph.D.

Professor of Psychology, Miami University, Miami, Ohio

Hypnosis

LEONARD A. BRUNO, M.D.

Clinical Associate Professor of Surgery, Temple University School of Medicine; Chief, Department of Neurosurgery, Germantown Hospital, Philadelphia, Pennsylvania

Head Injuries

CHARLES R. BULL, M.D., B.Sc.(Med), F.R.C.S.(C), F.A.C.S., F.I.C.S.

Consulting Surgeon, Humber Hospital and Orthopaedic and Arthritic Hospital; Chief Medical Officer, Team Canada (Hockey); Director, Alan Eagleson Sports Clinic, York University; Director, Fitness Institute Clinics, Toronto, Ontario, Canada

Orthotic Devices: Indications

Soft Tissue Injury to the Hip and Thigh

BERNARD R. CAHILL, M.D.

Clinical Professor of Orthopaedics, Peoria School of Medicine; Medical Director, Great Plains Sports Medical Foundation, Peoria, Illinois

Atraumatic Osteolysis of the Distal Clavicle

JOHN C. CAMERON, M.D., F.R.C.S.(C)

Director, Athletic Injuries Clinic, and Lecturer, University of Toronto Faculty of Medicine; Staff Orthopaedic Surgeon, Toronto, Ontario, Canada

Osteochondritis Dissecans, Osteochondral Fractures, and Osteoarthritis

JOHN D. CANTWELL, M.D.

Clinical Associate Professor of Medicine, Medical College of Georgia, Augusta; Director of the Preventive Medical Center, Cardiac Rehabilitation, and Internal Medicine Residency Training Program, Georgia Baptist Medical Center, Atlanta, Georgia

Exercise in the Secondary Prevention of Ischemic Heart Disease

WILLIAM G. CARSON, Jr., M.D.

Assistant Clinical Professor of Orthopaedics, University of South Florida; Director, the Sports Medicine Clinic of Tampa, Tampa, Florida
Arthroscopy of the Elbow

S.C. CHEN, M.B., B.S., B.A.(Tech), F.R.C.S., L.R.C.P.

Consultant Orthopaedic Surgeon, Enfield Group of Hospitals, Chase Farm Hospital, Enfield, Middlesex, England
Patellar Pain Syndrome: Instability and Lateral Retinacular Release

BERNARD G. COSTELLO, M.D., F.R.C.S.(C)

Assistant Professor of Orthopaedic Surgery, McGill University; Senior Orthopaedic Surgeon, Royal Victoria Hospital, Montreal, Quebec, Canada
Ligament Instability

EDWARD V. CRAIG, M.D.

Associate Professor of Orthopaedic Surgery, University of Minnesota Hospital; Consultant, Veterans' Administration Hospital, Minneapolis, Minnesota
Sonographic Evaluation of the Rotator Cuff

GORDON CUMMING, M.D., B.Sc.(Med), F.R.C.P.C.

Professor, Department of Pediatrics, University of Manitoba; Children's Hospital of Winnipeg, Health Sciences Center, Winnipeg; Director and Vice President, Great West Life Assurance Company, Winnipeg, Manitoba, Canada
Exercise Therapy in Pediatric Cardiology

MURRAY K. DALINKA, M.D.

Professor, Department of Radiology and Orthopaedic Surgery, Hospital of the University of Pennsylvania, Philadelphia, Pennsylvania
Magnetic Resonance Imaging of the Shoulder

MAURO G. Di PASQUALE, B.Sc., M.D.

Medical Consultant, International Power-Lifting Federation, Toronto, Ontario, Canada
Anabolic Steroids to Enhance Performance
Anabolic Steroids and Injury Treatment

ROD K. DISHMAN, Ph.D.

Associate Professor, College of Education, University of Georgia; Director, Behavioral Fitness Laboratory, University of Georgia, Athens, Georgia
Physical Activity in Medical Care

THOMAS J. DOUBT, Ph.D.

Head, Exercise Physiology Group, Diving Medicine Department, Naval Medical Research Institute, Bethesda, Maryland
Hazards of Cold Water

LEITH G. DOUGLAS, M.D., F.R.C.S.(C), F.A.C.S.

Assistant Professor, Department of Surgery, University of Toronto; Plastic Surgeon, The Wellesley Hospital; Team Plastic Surgeon, Toronto Maple Leafs Hockey Club, Toronto, Ontario, Canada
Facial Injuries

I.W.D. DYMOND, M.B., B.Ch., F.R.C.S.(Ed), F.C.S.(SA) (Orth), M.Med.

Surgeon, Morningside Clinic, Morningside, South Africa
Isolated Fracture of the Ulnar Shaft

MICHAEL EASTERBROOK, M.D., F.R.C.S.(C.), F.A.C.S.

Associate Professor, Department of Ophthalmology, University of Toronto, Toronto, Ontario, Canada; Chairman, Task Force, Canadian Standards Association Committee on Eye Protection in Racquet Sports; Consultant, Canadian, United States, and International Squash Racquets Associations, Canadian and American Racquetball Associations, and Canadian Badminton Association
Eye Protectors in Racquet Sports

HARVARD ELLMAN, M.D.

Associate Clinical Professor, Division of Orthopaedic Surgery, University of California at Los Angeles, Los Angeles, California
Arthroscopic Subacromial Decompression

EDWARD FINK, M.D.

Clinical Fellow of the Orthopaedic and Arthritic Hospital, Toronto, Ontario, Canada
Injuries to the Acromioclavicular Joint
Impingement Syndrome

KENNETH D. FITCH, M.D., F.A.C.S.M.

Medical Consultant, Department of Human Movement and Recreation, University of Western Australia; Physician and Head, Sports Injuries Clinic, Royal Perth Rehabilitation Hospital, Nedlands, Australia
Exercise-Induced Bronchial Obstruction

T.J.R. FRANCIS, Surgeon Commander, Royal Navy

Exchange Medical Officer, Diving Medicine Department, Naval Medical Research Institute, Bethesda, Maryland; Senior Specialist, Occupational Medicine, British Royal Navy
Hazards of Cold Water

THOMAS A. GENNARELLI, M.D.

Associate Professor of Neurosurgery, University of Pennsylvania School of Medicine, Philadelphia, Pennsylvania
Head Injuries

ROGER M. GLASER, Ph.D., F.A.C.S.M.

Professor of Physiology and Biophysics, Wright State University School of Medicine; Senior Research Health Scientist, Veterans Administration Medical Center; Director of Clinical Studies, Rehabilitation Institute of Ohio, Miami Valley Hospital, Dayton, Ohio

Spinal Cord Injuries and Neuromuscular Stimulation Exercise

NORMAN GLEDHILL, Ph.D., F.A.C.S.(C)

Professor and Chairman, Department of Physical Education, Recreation and Athletics, York University, Downsview, Ontario, Canada

Blood Doping and Performance

JACK GOODMAN, Ph.D.

Assistant Professor, School of Physical and Health Education, University of Toronto; Research Fellow, Cardiopulmonary and Nuclear Cardiology Laboratory, The Toronto Hospital, Toronto, Ontario, Canada

Exercise Rehabilitation for Coronary Artery Bypass Graft Patients

NEIL F. GORDON, M.B., B.Ch., Ph.D.

Director of Exercise Physiology, Institute for Aerobics Research, Dallas, Texas

Exercise in the Primary Prevention of Ischemic Heart Disease

VOJTECH HAINER, M.D., Ph.D.

Associate Professor, and Head, Obesitology Unit, IVth Internal Clinic, Medical School, Charles University, Prague, Czechoslovakia

Exercise in Growing and Adult Obese Individuals

G.D. HARPUR, M.D., C.C.F.P.

Assistant Clinical Professor, Department of Family Medicine, University of Western Ontario, London, Ontario; Medical Director, Tobermory Hyperbaric Facility, Tobermory, Ontario, Canada

Emergency Treatment of Diving Injuries

HAMILTON HALL, M.D., F.R.C.S.(C)

Associate Professor, Department of Surgery, University of Toronto; Staff Orthopaedic Surgeon, Orthopaedic and Arthritic Hospital and Women's College Hospital; Orthopaedic Consultant to the National Ballet of Canada; Medical Director, Canadian Back Institute, Toronto, Ontario, Canada

Conservative Back Care

RICHARD J. HAWKINS, M.D., F.R.C.S.(C)

Professor, Department of Surgery, Division of Orthopaedics, University of Western Ontario, London, Ontario, Canada

Rotator Cuff Tears

NETA A. HODGE, Pharm.D.

Clinical Pharmacist

Athletic Injuries and the Use of Medication

BRUCE R. HUFFER, M.D.

Private Orthopaedic Practice, Orthopaedic and Fracture Clinic, San Jose, California

Disorders Affecting Tendon Structures

M.E. HUNT, B.Sc.(P.T.)

Lecturer, Department of Rehabilitation Medicine, University of Toronto Faculty of Medicine, Toronto, Ontario, Canada

Physiotherapy in Sports Medicine

CHRISTINE HUTTON, M.B., Ch.B.

Registrar, Auckland Hospital, Auckland, New Zealand

Periarticular Overuse Syndromes

Patellofemoral Arthralgia, Patellar Instability, and Chondromalacia Patella

WENDY C. JEROME, Ph.D.

Professor, School of Human Movement, Laurentian University of Sudbury, Sudbury, Ontario, Canada

Anxiety and Depression: Exercise for Mood Enhancement

FRANK W. JOBE, M.D.

Clinical Professor, Department of Orthopaedics, University of Southern California, Los Angeles; Associate, Kerlan-Jobe Orthopaedic Clinic; Medical Director, Biomechanics Laboratory, Centinela Hospital Medical Center, Inglewood, California

Ulnar Neuritis and Ulnar Collateral Ligament Instabilities in Overarm Throwers

NORMAN L. JONES, M.D., F.R.C.P., F.R.C.P.(C)

Professor of Medicine, McMaster University; Director, Ambrose Cardiorespiratory Unit, Chedoke-McMaster Hospitals, Hamilton, Ontario, Canada

Exercise in Chronic Airway Obstruction

GARY KAMEN, Ph.D., F.A.C.S.M.

Associate Professor, Departments of Physical Therapy and Health Sciences, and Associate Research Professor, Neuromuscular Research Center, Boston University, Boston, Massachusetts

Neuromuscular Physiology

ELIEZER KAMON, Ph.D.

Professor of Physiology and Applied Economics, Pennsylvania State University, University Park, Pennsylvania

Exercise Prescription for Heart Disease

FRIEDRICH W. KEMMER, M.D.

Associate Professor of Internal Medicine, Department of Medicine, Division of Nephrology, Henrich Heine Universität Düsseldorf, Düsseldorf, West Germany
Exercise in Diabetic Patients

HAN C.G. KEMPER, M.D., Ph.D.

Professor in Health Science, Faculty of Human Movement Sciences, and Working Group of Physical Exercise and Health, Vrye Universiteit and Universiteit van Amsterdam, Amsterdam, The Netherlands
Exercise and Training in Childhood and Adolescence

SANFORD S. KUNKEL, M.D.

Orthopaedic Surgeon, Orthopaedics Indianapolis Inc., Indianapolis, Indiana
Rotator Cuff Tears

M.T. LUCKING, M.D., M.R.C.S., L.R.C.P.

Advisor, British Amateur Athletic Board, Birmingham, England
Control of Drug Abuse

IAN MACNAB, M.B., Ch.B., F.R.C.S., F.R.C.S.(C)

Professor of Surgery, University of Toronto Faculty of Medicine; Division of Orthopaedics, The Wellesley Hospital, Toronto, Ontario, Canada
Backache

DAVID C. MANN, M.D.

Assistant Professor, Division of Orthopaedics, University of Wisconsin School of Medicine, Madison, Wisconsin
Spinal Deformity and Sports

FRANK C. McCUE III, M.D.

Alfred R. Shands Professor of Orthopaedic Surgery and Plastic Surgery of the Hand, and Director, Division of Sports Medicine and Hand Surgery, and Team Physician, Department of Athletics, University of Virginia, Charlottesville, Virginia
Coach's Finger

JOHN A. McCULLOCH, M.D., F.R.C.S.(C)

Professor of Orthopaedics, Northeastern Ohio Universities College of Medicine, Rootstown, Ohio
Ruptured Lumbar Discs (Herniated Nucleus Pulposus)

J. SIMON McGRAIL, M.D., M.S., F.R.C.S.(C)

Professor of Otolaryngology, University of Toronto Faculty of Medicine; Chief, ENT Department, Wellesley Hospital; Physician, Toronto Maple Leafs (Hockey) and Team Canada (Hockey), Toronto, Ontario, Canada
Ear, Nose, and Throat Injuries

RENA A. MENDELSON, M.S., D.Sc.

Professor and Director, School of Nutrition, Consumer and Family Studies, Ryerson Polytechnical Institute, Toronto, Ontario, Canada
Vitamins and Exercise

LYLE J. MICHELI, M.D.

Assistant Professor, Clinical Orthopaedics, Harvard Medical School; Director, Division of Sports Medicine, Children's Hospital, Boston, Massachusetts
Spinal Deformities

ROLF MOCELLIN, M.D.

Professor, Department of Pediatric Cardiology, Universitats-Kinderklinik, Freiburg, West Germany
Exercise Testing in Pediatric Cardiology

ALAN R. MORTON, M.Sc., Ed.D., F.A.C.S.M.

Associate Professor, Department of Human Movement and Recreation Studies, University of Western Australia, Nedlands, West Australia
Exercise-Induced Bronchial Obstruction

PATRICIA A. NIXON, Ph.D.

Research Assistant Professor of Pediatrics, University of Pittsburgh School of Medicine; Exercise Physiologist, Department of Pediatrics, Children's Hospital of Pittsburgh, Pittsburgh, Pennsylvania
Exercise in Cystic Fibrosis

TIMOTHY DAVID NOAKES, M.B., Ch.B., M.D., F.A.C.S.M.

Associate Professor and Director, MRC/UCT Bioenergetics of Exercise Research Unit, Department of Physiology, University of Cape Town Medical School, Cape Town, South Africa
Fluid and Mineral Needs

FRANK NOFTALL, M.D., F.R.C.S.(C)

Assistant Clinical Professor of Surgery, Memorial University of Newfoundland; Staff Orthopaedic Surgeon, Health Sciences Centre, General Hospital and St. Clare's Mercy Hospital, St. John's, Newfoundland, Canada
Patellofemoral Dysfunction

JOHN H. OLIVER, M.D., F.R.C.S.(C)

Clinical Lecturer, Department of Orthopaedics, McGill University Faculty of Medicine, Montreal, Quebec, Canada
Stress Fracture of the Lower Exremity

DAVID M. ORENSTEIN, M.D.

Associate Professor of Pediatrics, University of Pittsburgh School of Medicine; Associate Professor of Instruction and Learning (Exercise Physiology), School of Education, University of Pittsburgh; Director, Department of Pulmonology, and Cystic Fibrosis Center, Children's Hospital of Pittsburgh, Pittsburgh, Pennsylvania
Exercise in Cystic Fibrosis

A. LEE OSTERMAN, M.D.

Associate Professor, Orthopaedics and Hand Surgery, Hospital of the University of Pennsylvania, Philadelphia, Pennsylvania
Wrist Arthroscopy

JANA PAŘÍZKOVÁ, M.D., Ph.D., D.Sc.

Senior Research Officer, Research Institute for Physical Education, Charles University, Prague, Czechoslovakia
Exercise in Growing and Adult Obese Individuals

ROBERT C. PASHBY, M.D., F.R.C.S.(C)

Assistant Professor of Ophthalmology, University of Toronto Faculty of Medicine; Active Staff, Department of Ophthalmology, Toronto General Hospital and the Hospital for Sick Children, Toronto, Ontario, Canada
Ocular Injuries

THOMAS J. PASHBY

Emeritus Associate Professor of Ophthalmology, University of Toronto Faculty of Medicine; Honorary Consultant, Department of Ophthalmology, The Hospital for Sick Children, Toronto, Ontario, Canada
Ocular Injuries

HELENE PAVLOV, M.D.

Clinical Professor of Radiology, Cornell Medical College; Hospital for Special Surgery, New York, New York
Haglund's Syndrome

MICHAEL J. PLYLEY, Ph.D.

Associate Professor, School of Physical and Health Education, Departments of Community Health and Physiology, University of Toronto, Toronto, Ontario, Canada
Physiologic Principles of Exercise Testing

JERILYNN C. PRIOR, M.D., F.R.C.P.(C)

Associate Professor of Medicine, Division of Endocrinology, University of British Columbia Faculty of Medicine; Active Endocrinology Staff, Vancouver General Hospital, Vancouver, British Columbia, Canada
Reproductive Changes in the Athlete

MICHAEL R. REDLER, M.D.

Fellow in Hand Surgery and Sports Medicine, Department of Orthopaedics and Rehabilitation, University of Virginia, Charlottesville, Virginia
Coach's Finger

DAVID COLLINSON REID, M.D., M.C.S.P., F.R.C.S.(C), M.Ch.(Orth)

Professor of Orthopaedic Surgery, Adjunct Professor of Rehabilitation Medicine, and Honorary Professor of Physical Education, University of Alberta; Director, Glen Sather University of Alberta, Sports Medicine Clinic, Edmonton, Alberta, Canada
Selected Lesions Around the Talus

THOMAS REILLY, B.A., Dip.P.E., M.Sc., Ph.D., M.I.Biol., F.Erg.S.

Professor of Sports Science, Centre for Sport and Exercise Sciences, School of Health Sciences, Liverpool Polytechnic, Liverpool, England
Time Zone Shift and Sleep Deprivation Problems

CECIL H. RORABECK, M.D., F.R.C.S.(C)

Professor, Orthopaedic Surgery, University of Western Ontario; Chief, Division of Orthopaedic Surgery, University Hospital, London, Ontario, Canada
Chronic Exertional Compartment Syndrome

CARTER R. ROWE, M.D.

Associate Professor of Orthopaedic Surgery (Emeritus), Harvard Medical School; Senior Orthopaedic Surgeon, Massachusetts General Hospital, Boston, Massachusetts
Anterior Glenohumeral Subluxation/Dislocation: The Bankart Procedure

G. JAMES SAMMARCO, M.D., F.A.C.S.

Clinical Professor of Orthopaedic Surgery, University of Cincinnati; Director of Foot and Ankle Fellowship, Cincinnati, Ohio
Soft Tissue Injuries

DAVID J. SANDERSON, B.Sc., M.Sc., Ph.D.

Assistant Professor, School of Physical Education, University of British Columbia, Vancouver, British Columbia, Canada
Biomechanics in Sports Medicine

ALEXANDER A. SAPEGA, M.D.

Assistant Professor of Orthopaedic Surgery, and Attending Surgeon, University of Pennsylvania School of Medicine; Chief of Sports Medicine Service, Philadelphia Veterans' Administration Hospital, Philadelphia, Pennsylvania
Arthroscopically Assisted Reconstruction of the Anterior Cruciate Ligament

SCOTT P. SCHEMMEL, M.D.

Former Fellow, Alabama Sports Medicine and Orthopaedic Center, Birmingham, Alabama; Staff Orthopaedic Surgeon, Seindler Orthopaedic Clinic, Iowa City, Iowa
Principles of Shoulder Arthroscopy

MONA M. SHANGOLD, M.D.

Assistant Professor of Obstetrics and Gynecology, Georgetown University School of Medicine; Director, Sports Gynecology Center, Georgetown University Hospital, Washington, D.C.
Special Concerns of the Female Athlete

ROY J. SHEPHARD, M.D.(Lond), Ph.D., D.P.E., F.A.C.S.M.

Director, School of Physical and Health Education, and Professor of Applied Physiology, Department of Preventive Medicine and Biostatistics, University of Toronto Faculty of Medicine; Consultant, Toronto Rehabilitation Centre, and Gage Research Institute, Toronto Western Hospital, Toronto, Ontario, Canada
Physiologic Responses to Exercise
Exercise and Preventive Medicine

KENNETH H. SIDNEY, Ph.D.

Associate Professor, School of Human Movement, Laurentian University, Sudbury, Ontario, Canada
Anxiety and Depression: Exercise for Mood Enhancement

FRANCES SILVERMAN, B.Sc., M.Sc., Ph.D.

Assistant Professor, University of Toronto, Toronto, Ontario, Canada
Air Pollution and Exercise

CHRISTOPHER W. SIWEK, M.D.

Attending Orthopaedic Surgeon, Susan B. Allen Memorial Hospital, El Dorado, Kansas
Quadriceps and Patellar Tendon Ruptures

GEORGE A. SNOOK, M.D., F.A.C.S.

Chief of Orthopaedics, Cooley Dickinson Hospital, Northampton; Consultant, University of Massachusetts, Amherst, Massachusetts
Lateral Ankle Reconstruction for Chronic Instability

R. SUKE, M.D., C.C.F.P., B.Eng.

Assistant Clinical Professor, Department of Family Medicine, McMaster University, Hamilton, Ontario, Canada
Emergency Treatment of Diving Injuries

JOHN M. SULLIVAN, M.B., Ch.B., F.R.A.C.S.

Orthopaedic Surgeon, Waikato Hospital, Hamilton, New Zealand
Rupture of the Achilles Tendon

JOHN R. SUTTON, M.D., F.R.A.C.P., F.R.C.P.(C)

Professor, Department of Medicine, McMaster University; Consultant, Intensive and Coronary Care Units, McMaster University Medical Centre, Hamilton, Ontario, Canada
Exercise at High Altitudes

SUSAN M. TARLO, M.B., B.S., M.R.C.P.(UK), F.R.C.P.(C)

Assistant Professor, University of Toronto; Staff Physician, Respiratory Division, Toronto General Hospital; Staff Physician, Gage Research Institute, Toronto, Ontario, Canada
Air Pollution and Exercise

PETER M. TIIDUS, M.Sc.

Senior Tutor and Undergraduate Coordinator, School of Physical and Health Education, University of Toronto, Toronto, Ontario, Canada
Dietary Protein Requirements for the Athlete
Exercise and Muscle Soreness

JOSEPH S. TORG, M.D.

Professor of Orthopaedic Surgery, University of Pennsylvania; Director, University of Pennsylvania Sports Medicine Center, Philadelphia, Pennsylvania
Injuries to the Cervical Spine
Orthotic Devices: Fabrications
Plantar Fasciitis
Stress Fractures of the Tarsal Navicular
Head Injuries
Fractures of the Base of the Fifth Metatarsal Distal to the Tuberosity: The Jones Fracture
Cervical Spinal Stenosis with Cord Neurapraxia and Transient Quadriplegia
A Modified Bristow-Helfet-May Procedure for the Recurrent Dislocation and Subluxation of the Shoulder
Haglund's Syndrome

ELLY TREPMAN, M.D.

Clinical Fellow in Orthopaedic Surgery, Harvard Medical School; Fellow in Sports Medicine, Children's Hospital, Boston, Massachusetts
Spinal Deformities

ROBERT BRUCE URCH, M.Sc., C.A.C.P.T.(P)

Charge Technician, Gage Research Institute, Toronto, Ontario, Canada
Air Pollution and Exercise

WALTER P. VAN HELDER, M.D., M.Eng., Ph.D.

Assistant Professor of Sports Medicine and Surgery, School of Physical and Health Education, University of Toronto Faculty of Medicine; Staff Physician, Department of Emergency Medicine, Toronto Western Hospital, Toronto, Ontario, Canada
Cardiopulmonary Physiology

JOSEPH J. VEGSO, M.S., A.T., C.

Director of Athletic Training and Educational Programs, The Sports Medicine Institute/Phoenix Orthopaedic Surgeons, Ltd., Glendale, Arizona
Principles of Stretching
Nonoperative Management of Ankle Injuries
Principles of Strength Training

JESUS VILLEGAS, M.D.

Research Assistant, Institute for Aerobics Research, Dallas, Texas
Exercise in the Primary Prevention of Ischemic Heart Disease

J. PETER WELSH, M.B., Ch.B., F.R.C.S.(C), F.A.C.S.

Assistant Professor, Department of Surgery, University of Toronto; Deputy Chief of Surgery, The Orthopaedic and Arthritic Hospital, Toronto, Ontario, Canada

Injuries to the Acromioclavicular Joint

Injury to the Anterior Cruciate Ligament

Metatarsalgia and Other Common Problems

Patellofemoral Arthralgia, Patellar Instability, and Chondromalacia Patella

Disorders Affecting Tendon Structures

Periarticular Overuse Syndromes

FRANKLIN D. WILSON, M.D.

Clinical Associate Professor, Indiana University Medical Center, Indianapolis; Orthopaedic Consultant, Taylor University, Upton, and Anderson University, Anderson; Orthopaedic Surgeon, Capital Orthopaedics P.C., Indianapolis, Indiana

Valgus Extension Overload in Pitching Elbow

C. STEWART WRIGHT, M.D., F.R.C.S.(C)

Lecturer, University of Toronto Faculty of Medicine; Staff Orthopaedic Surgeon, Orthopaedic and Arthritic Hospital and Sunnybrook Medical Centre, Toronto, Ontario, Canada

Overuse Syndromes

Tendon Injuries in the Hand and Wrist

Fractures and Dislocations in the Hand and Wrist

DAVID YOUNG, B.Sc., M.D., M.Sc., F.R.C.S.(C)

Professor and Chairman, Discipline of Obstetrics and Gynecology, Memorial University of Newfoundland; Chief, Obstetrics and Gynecology, Grace General Hospital, St. John's, Newfoundland, Canada

Exercise and Pregnancy

MICHAEL B. ZLATKIN, M.D., F.R.C.P.(C)

Assistant Professor, Department of Radiology, Hospital of the University of Pennsylvania, Philadelphia, Pennsylvania

Magnetic Resonance Imaging of the Shoulder

PREFACE

Sports medicine as a discipline has matured, and the care of the athlete occupies an important place in the delivery of health care. With fitness and health the concern of all, competitive and recreational athletes present their physicians, trainers, therapists, and coaches with an assortment of problems and disorders to diagnose and manage.

Participation in sports inevitably means that injuries will be sustained. Many maladies were previously neglected or considered of little medical importance because no gross pathologic process was readily identifiable, but must now be considered; for example, myofascial strains of the lumbar spine or overuse syndromes of the shoulder and elbow or the knee, foot, and ankle are now recognized as having substantial socioeconomic importance affecting performance both in the work place and on the sports field.

This second volume brings together several areas of advancement, matching an up-to-date account of exercise physiology and applied sports medicine with details of the many maladies peculiar to the sports discipline. There is an emphasis on prevention and training as well as on current management procedures, and the scope of the work is, we feel, quite unique. Environmental factors such as heat, cold, and altitude are discussed, as well as sex, age, and concomitant medical problems ranging from diabetes to blood-doping, emphasizing the impact of these influences on athletic performance.

The scope of the original work has been expanded considerably in this second edition. The influence of a new co-editor, Dr. Joseph Torg, is strongly seen, and the addition of numerous illustrations and detailed reading material greatly enhances the value of this book. New techniques such as arthroscopy of the shoulder, wrist, and elbow and arthroscope-assisted knee ligament surgery are presented in detail, making this indeed an account of current therapy in sports medicine.

New authors have been selected for their acknowledged expertise in each of the topic areas. An international group of contributors has addressed current management concepts in a clear and informative manner. We are most appreciative of their succinct contributions.

The present volume is directed particularly to those involved in the coaching, training, and treatment of athletes, including orthopaedists, physical medicine specialists, team physicians, trainers, physiotherapists, and physical educators. More than this, however, the scope of the work is such that it should provide an invaluable addition to the library of the family practitioner, who is now dealing more and more with athletes of all ages. This edition presents a concise update covering a vast number of topics that may be met in day-to-day practice in the management of the sportsman and sportswoman.

Joseph S. Torg
R. Peter Welsh
Roy J. Shephard

Toronto, 1989

CONTENTS

ELBOW

FOREARM, WRIST, AND HAND

REHABILITATION

PHYSIOLOGIC AND MEDICAL ASPECTS

PHYSIOLOGIC RESPONSES TO EXERCISE

ROY J. SHEPHARD, M.D., Ph.D., D.P.E.

In the context of an examination for exercise or sport, the physician is often asked about the influence of increased physical activity upon body functions, and the implications for future health. It may thus be helpful to review some of the main physiologic responses to both acute and chronic exercise, and to consider ways in which these responses may contribute to an improvement of health.

ACUTE DISEASE

The reported incidence of acute disease can be affected by an altered perception of health, an altered exposure to disease, or an altered immune response.

Perceived Health

An improvement of mood state can lead to an improvement of perceived health. The physiologic basis is sometimes a mechanical arousal through an increased traffic of nerve impulses in the reticular formation of the brain (induced by stimulation of proprioceptors), and sometimes a secretion of arousing hormones (including the catecholamines and the endorphins). In terms of both perceived health and physical performance, each individual has an optimal level of arousal; this optimum is higher for extraverts than for introverts. The dose of exercise must thus be gauged to bring each person to the peak of her or his arousal curve.

The secretion of catecholamines is not normally increased unless the exercise is quite intense or there is associated emotional excitement (e.g., much more catecholamine is secreted during a hockey game than during an equivalent intensity of exercise on a cycle ergometer). The addictive, morphine-like beta-endorphins are secreted only during sustained and very vigorous exercise, and are unlikely to be implicated in the mood changes associated with ordinary "exercise for health" programs.

Disease Exposure

Disease exposure depends on contact with pathogens and their efficient removal from the body. Most forms of exercise make the skin hot, sweaty, and softer. It thus becomes readily penetrated by viruses, fungi, and staphylococci, which unfortunately may accumulate in poorly drained and cleaned shower areas.

Swimming likewise softens the skin and increases exposure to specific bacteria, viruses, and parasites, particularly if a pool is crowded and the water is warm and generally contaminated.

Other forms of vigorous exercise cause a switch from nasal to oronasal breathing, with the inspiration of large volumes of air via the mouth. If this air is cold or polluted with chemicals such as sulfur dioxide, the activity of the tracheal cilia is temporarily suppressed, with a decrease in the rate of elimination of small particles, including bacteria and viruses.

Finally, vigorous exercise causes a redistribution of blood flow to the working muscles and the associated spinal neurons. It may thus carry circulating bacteria or viruses to vulnerable tissues; e.g., exercise is said to cause a localization of anterior poliomyelitis to the active anterior horn cells.

Immune Response

There has been much study of immune responses to exercise in the last few years, although unfortunately the exercise protocols have not been well controlled, the timing of any blood sampling has varied widely, and sometimes the experimental situation has been complicated by either acute competitive stress or psychological reactions to more chronic problems of "overtraining."

The current consensus seems to be that moderate exercise has little effect on the immune system, but that very strenuous and stressful activity can cause a temporary inhibition of immune function, with the possibility of a transient increase in susceptibility to disease. If an athlete undertakes repeated and prolonged bouts of exercise, to the point of overtraining, the suppression of immune function becomes more marked. Analysis of data is complicated, because a single bout of strenuous exercise leads to an increase in lymphocyte count, but a decrease in the proportion of cells that respond to mitogen stimulation. Moreover, if the individual is well trained but not overtrained, there may be an enhanced mitogenic response to a given bout of exercise. Finally, because the acute exercise-induced changes in lymphocyte count and activity are transient in nature, they may have little impact on susceptibility to disease.

Nevertheless, the more long-term changes of immune function have practical significance for those attending top-level athletes; if such individuals are overtrained, they may succumb to infection. Lymphocyte responses are also attracting attention as a possible method of detecting the onset of overtraining.

CHRONIC DISEASE

Regular exercise affects most of the major systems of the body, and many of these changes have implications for the onset of clinically recognizable disease.

Cardiovascular System

The most obvious effect of training is a decrease in heart rate, both at rest and at any given intensity of submaximal exercise. The main basis of this bradycardia is probably a central increase of parasympathetic nerve activity, since a larger dose of atropine is required to induce a vagal block after training. However, there may also be a local increase of acetylcholine production within cardiac tissue, and during fixed-intensity exercise the trained individual has a lesser secretion of catecholamines, possibly with some change in the number or sensitivity of catecholamine-binding sites in the myocardium. The training-induced decrease in heart rate lengthens the diastolic portion of the cardiac cycle, which is the interval during which most of the coronary perfusion occurs; this change in itself does much to correct myocardial ischemia.

After training the stroke volume is increased in rest and light exercise and is better maintained in heavy exercise. This reflects not only better oxygenation of the heart muscle, but also (1) an increase of venous tone and of total blood volume, both changes contributing to a greater preloading of the heart; (2) an increase of myocardial contractility, increasing the fraction of the ventricular contents that is expelled at each beat; and (3) some decrease in blood pressure and thus afterloading of the ventricle.

To a first approximation, the work rate of the heart is proportional to the double product (systolic pressure times heart rate; this simple formula assumes a constancy of heart size, stroke volume, and myocardial contractility). Thus, if training decreases both systolic pressure and heart rate for a given external effort, there is a substantial decrease in the cardiac work rate and a much lesser likelihood that exercise will induce significant myocardial ischemia (with a corresponding decrease in the risk of angina, myocardial infarction, ventricular fibrillation, and sudden death).

Very prolonged and vigorous activity appears to be necessary to induce hypertrophy of the cardiac muscle. As with skeletal muscle, an overload is needed to increase protein synthesis, and there may also be genetically determined interindividual differences in the susceptibility to such training. Ventricular hypertrophy decreases the intramural tension at any given blood pressure, and in the short term it thus decreases the risk of myocardial ischemia. However, it is less certain that the enlarged heart muscle is an advantage if it persists after training has ceased, and indeed some authors suggest that former athletes have an increased risk of myocardial ischemia owing to their greater heart size. Local improvements of coronary vascular supply have been described in some experimental animals after prolonged training; however, it is less clear that such responses occur in humans, perhaps because less exercise is normally undertaken.

Most reports suggest that a small but statistically significant decrease in resting blood pressure is induced by regular exercise, although there are some possible artifacts, including habituation to the testing laboratory and an improved fit of the measuring cuff as subcutaneous fat is lost. At any given intensity of submaximal exercise the blood pressure tends to be lower after training, in part because fewer catecholamines are produced and in part because the skeletal muscles are stronger. However, the increase of myocardial contractility may allow a person to reach a higher blood pressure during maximal effort. The lowering of blood pressure in submaximal effort should reduce the risk of both heart attacks and cerebrovascular accidents.

Respiratory System

Although regular exercise increases peak performance in patients with many forms of chronic respiratory disease, the physiologic changes of respiratory function induced by regular training are limited. There is commonly a small increase of vital capacity, possibly because the chest muscles are strengthened; greater thoracic strength allows a small increase in the compression of the rib cage and a greater expulsion of blood from the pulmonary vessels. Because training induces an increase in pulmonary blood volume, there may be a small increase in pulmonary diffusing capacity. However, there is no evidence that regular exercise can regenerate lung tissue that has been destroyed by chronic chest disease; any benefit of exercise in such conditions must be attributed to (1) an increase in the mechanical efficiency of physical activity, with a lesser oxygen consumption by both the leg and the chest muscles; (2) a strengthening of the leg muscles, with a lesser production of anaerobic metabolites, and thus a lower respiratory minute volume for a given intensity of exercise; (3) encouragement of mucus expectoration; and (4) psychological factors, including a breaking of the vicious cycle of dyspnea, fear of exercise, muscular weakness, and greater dyspnea.

The oronasal breathing that develops at a ventilation of 30 to 40 liters per minute causes some of the inspirate to bypass the normal scrubbing, warming, and humidifying function of the nose, so that a person with "twitchy" airways becomes more vulnerable to bronchospasm during and immediately after exercise. However, exercise-induced bronchospasm can be prevented in most people by previous administration of cromolyn sodium. If the air is cold and dry, some form of mask that warms and humidifies the inspired air is also helpful.

Skeletal Muscles

At one time, experts in preventive medicine recommended pure endurance exercise, such as jogging, and some authors specifically rejected any forms of exercise that were directed to a strengthening of the skeletal muscles. In those who concentrate on endurance events, such as marathon runners, muscles in parts of the body that are not used during performance may actually show some weakening. It is also known that the rise in blood pressure induced by muscle contraction is proportional to the fraction of maximal voluntary force that is exerted. Thus, in circumstances in which a weakened muscle must be used, endurance performers show a greater rise in blood pressure than their peers. Muscle loss is particularly likely to occur if the athlete is worried about becoming too fat—an obsession seen in some distance runners and more commonly in gymnasts and ballet dancers. In essence, food intake does not match energy expenditures, and since athletes already have only limited reserves of fat, the required energy is found by a breakdown of body proteins.

Conversely, if the muscles are strengthened by isometric or heavy isotonic exercise, the rise in blood pressure during subsequent exercise is lessened, with a reduced risk of cardiac problems and joint injuries. The essential principle of muscle-building activity is overload, which encourages the synthesis of new muscle protein; there is an increase of fiber cross-section and possibly some splitting of fibers, but no appearance of new fibers (at least in the adult). In the early phases of training the gains of strength outpace the increase in muscle dimensions. This reflects neural adjustments. By an increased synchronization of neural impulses and perhaps by calling on a larger fraction of the total neuron pool or reducing voluntary inhibition of the contraction, a greater force is developed for a given muscle mass. Eventually, there may be small increases in the local capillary supply to trained muscles, with increases in collateral blood flow; both of these changes help the person who has a tendency toward peripheral vascular disease.

Two early arguments against strength training were that the added muscle mass increased cardiac work, and that the training regimen might in itself precipitate a heart attack. Certainly a heavy person must perform more work when displacing body mass, but if the limb muscles have been strengthened, body movement can probably be accomplished with a lesser rise in blood pressure (which is the main determinant of cardiac work rate). If an isometric contraction is held for a long period, the blood pressure rises progressively until the person is exhausted. However, it appears possible to induce gains of muscle strength by much briefer contractions; if adequate rest intervals are allowed between contractions, anaerobic metabolites can be dispersed and a major rise in blood pressure can be avoided.

Skeletal System

Prolonged physical inactivity (e.g., a period of enforced bed rest or the adoption of a very sedentary lifestyle) leads to a progressive loss of calcium from the major bones of the body. Conversely, if there is an increase in weightbearing activity, the bone mineral content is increased; in athletes who exercise particularly hard, it may be possible to see a local strengthening of the bone architecture. There have also been reports that the hydroxyproline content of the bone matrix is increased by regular exercise.

Training programs also increase the strength of tendons and ligaments, so that more force is required to rupture them or to tear them from their bony attachments. The synthesis of collagen is increased, the hydroxyproline content of the tendon rises, and an increase of collagen turnover reduces the number of cross-linkages between individual collagen fibrils, thus making the tendinous structures less brittle.

The immediate effect of physical activity is to decrease the water content and thus the thickness of articular cartilage; however, the long-term effect on cartilage is to increase both its thickness and its resistance to compression, thereby reducing the dangers of tears and subsequent osteoarthritis.

Metabolic Effects

The harmful effects of obesity have long been recognized. In essence, humans obey Newton's laws of thermodynamics; they are not able to generate energy de novo, so that an accumulation of fat must represent an inappropriate balance between energy intake in the form of food and energy expenditure in the form of exercise. Despite obese individuals' pleas to the contrary, observation shows that they consume more food than do people of normal body mass, while taking less exercise in an essentially similar situation. Moderate obesity, e.g., a 10-kg excess of body fat, may have been accumulated through a very small energy imbalance, perhaps a 1 percent excess of food or a 1 percent reduction of physical activity, sustained over many years. Unfortunately a difference of this order is very difficult to measure and impossible for the individual to perceive. A further possible factor affecting energy balance is an interindividual difference in the completeness of food absorption. A choice of refined carbohydrates such as sugar encourages a complete absorption of food, whereas the fat–rich meat diet preferred by many athletes is absorbed more poorly; moreover, regular vigorous exercise increases intestinal motility, thereby reducing food absorption.

Progress in correcting obesity may be disappointing, whether the attempt is based on dieting or exercising. One problem is that in an obese person a large part of the total daily energy expenditure is attributable to resting metabolism, and if a negative energy balance is created by dieting or an increase of physical activity, the body compensates for this (at least in part) by a change of about 15 percent in the resting metabolic demand. Exercise is an important component of a reducing regimen from several points of view. An acute bout of exercise raises blood sugar and thus suppresses appetite, at least temporarily. Physical activity may also induce a sustained increase in resting metabolism (although this issue is still vigorously debated). Finally, an exercise recommendation is positive, pleasant advice that helps to elevate the mood of the patient (whereas dieting alone tends to induce depression). The objective of a "reducing regimen" is to lose excess fat rather than to reduce total body mass; sometimes the fat loss may be greater than simple weighing would suggest, since exercise helps to conserve lean tissue and may even increase the lean mass in parts of the body that have been exercised. Very vigorous exercise tends to burn carbohydrate, and the patient is exhausted before any large total amount of energy has been consumed. Moderate exercise (at 50 to 60 percent of maximal oxygen intake) is thus the best type of exercise to recommend to the obese person; if such activity can be sustained over 20 minutes or more per session, there will be a progressive secretion of fat-mobilizing hormones. A person who is grossly obese may find it difficult to undertake sufficient physical activity to ensure the required fat loss within a reasonable daily exercise time. It is thus common practice to supplement an increase of energy expenditure (perhaps 2 megajoules, 500 kcal, per day) with a similar decrease of food intake.

Exercise apparently has little influence on total serum cholesterol if the body mass is held constant. There are two problems related to attempts to reduce blood cholesterol levels. First, the body can alter the amounts of cholesterol excreted via the bile and reabsorbed from the intestines; second, the body has a relatively large capacity to synthesize cholesterol from the normal building blocks of metabolism, acetoacetyl CoA and acetyl CoA. Thus, if the energy intake is excessive, a part of the excess energy is converted to cholesterol. On a low-cholesterol diet, hepatic synthesis can reach 800 to 1,000 mg per day.

For reasons that are still not completely understood, prolonged exercise (for instance, jogging 18 to 20 km per week) can nevertheless increase the proportion of cholesterol that is in the useful, scavenging high-density lipoprotein (HDL) fraction, while decreasing the undesirable low-density lipoprotein (LDL) fraction. The specific subfraction that increases is HDL_2, with an associated increase of the apoprotein A-I, but not of A-II. Biochemical changes probably include an increase in the activity of the enzyme lecithin-cholesterol acyltransferase (LCAT), which is capable of esterifying the cholesterol and thus allowing the formation of high-density particles; these particles then pass to the liver, where they inhibit endogenous cholesterol synthesis. There may also be an increase in the number or sensitivity of extrahepatic LDL receptors, facilitating the extrahepatic clearance of cholesterol.

In high-risk patients with substantially elevated cholesterol values, a lowering of serum cholesterol has been shown to reduce the incidence of cardiac events, although the impact on total mortality is less clear-cut; possibly, the cell membranes become accustomed to operating in a high-cholesterol environment and react adversely to a change. There is a strong possibility that induction of a similar absolute change in serum cholesterol levels could have a beneficial effect on individuals with more normal concentrations of serum lipids, although this has yet to be demonstrated experimentally.

Interactions between regular exercise and insulin sensitivity are complex. For the young adult, there are those who debate the value of exercise as a specific treatment, while still recommending it to prevent subsequent complications such as ischemic heart disease. There is more general agreement that in the older person with maturity-onset diabetes, regular exercise can lower resting blood sugar and increase insulin sensitivity, reducing the need for insulin injections and in some cases eliminating the need for insulin treatment. However, it is less clearly established that the glucose tolerance curve can be normalized by exercise, even in persons with the maturity-onset form of diabetes.

Central Nervous System

Some reports have suggested that regular physical activity improves intellectual performance in young children and slows the deterioration of neural function in senior citizens.

In young children a higher academic performance recorded on school report cards has been linked to an enhancement of body awareness, including a more accurate perception of body dimensions, a better appreciation of the vertical, and finger recognition; these findings support the classical French concept of a linkage between psychomotor development and intellectual attainment.

In older people it has been speculated that exercise may help performance by periodically raising the systemic blood pressure and thus increasing brain perfusion. However, physical activity may also act less directly, by increasing an individual's arousal and thus awareness of surroundings, or merely by increasing a patient's interest in life. Irrespective of mechanisms, the training-induced gains in functions such as reaction time are substantial and of practical importance to the individual concerned.

CONCLUSION

Habitual exercise induces changes in various body systems that intuitively seem to have a positive value for health. Such changes are important from two points of view. First, it is difficult to design conclusive epidemiologic proof of the health value of regular moderate physical activity. However, it becomes more reasonable to accept suggestive epidemiologic evidence when the physiologist or biochemist can outline a plausible mechanism whereby benefit could be derived. Moreover, through an understanding of the mechanism of benefit, it becomes possible to tailor the exercise prescription so that the health-giving effects of exercise can be maximized and any side effects held to a minimum.

For many functional gains, the desirable form of physical activity is moderate endurance effort; e.g., 30-minute exercise sessions held to an intensity of 60 to 70 percent of maximal oxygen intake, just below the anaerobic threshold. However, there is increasing evidence that some of the gains we have discussed can be obtained at quite moderate intensities of effort (e.g., by fast walking) provided that this is carried out regularly and for a substantial time per session. The optimal exercise prescription also encourages the development of muscle strength and flexibility. Plainly, it is not possible to equate good health simply with high scores on a single measure of fitness such as maximal oxygen intake; account must be taken of multiple variables. Finally, the effort expended may have greater practical significance than the score attained (since the latter can be strongly influenced by inheritance).

SUGGESTED READING

Dustman RE, Ruhling RO, Russell EM, et al. Aerobic exercise and improved neuropsychological function of older individuals. Neurobiol Aging 1984; 5:35–42.

Haskell WL. The influence of exercise on the concentration of triglyceride and cholesterol in plasma. Exerc Sport Sci Rev 1984; 12:205–244.

Herzlich C. Health and illness. London: Academic Press, 1973.

Kavanagh T. A cold weather "jogging mask" for angina patients. Can Med Assoc J 1970; 103:1290–1291.

Keast D, Cameron K, Morton AR. Exercise and the immune response. Sports Med 1988; 5:248–267.

Lind AR, McNicol GW. Muscular factors which determine the cardiovascular responses to sustained and rhythmic exercise. Can Med Assoc J 1967; 96:706–712.

Martens R. Arousal and motor performance. Exerc Sport Sci Rev 1974; 2:155–188.

Niinimaa V, Cole P, Mintz S, Shephard RJ. The switching point from nasal to oro-nasal breathing. Respir Physiol 1980; 42:61–71.

Shephard RJ. The determination of body composition in biological anthropology. London: Cambridge University Press, 1989.

Shephard RJ. Endurance fitness. 2nd ed. Toronto: University of Toronto Press, 1977.

Shephard RJ. Physiology and biochemistry of exercise. New York: Praeger, 1982.

Shephard RJ. Physical activity and growth. Chicago: Year Book, 1982.

Shephard RJ. Biochemistry of exercise. Springfield, IL: Charles C Thomas, 1983.

Shephard RJ. Cardiovascular aspects of sports medicine. In: Teitz C, ed. The scientific foundations of sports medicine. Toronto: BC Decker, 1989:27.

Smith EL, Smith PE, Ensign CJ, Shea MM. Bone involution decrease in exercising middle-aged women. Calcif Tissue Int 1984; 36 (Suppl. I):S129–S138.

Tipton C. Exercise, training and hypertension. Exerc Sport Sci Rev 1984; 12:245–306.

EXERCISE AND PREVENTIVE MEDICINE

ROY J. SHEPHARD, M.D., Ph.D., D.P.E.

There is still scope for an increase in the number of physicians prescribing exercise as a form of preventive medicine, despite increasingly strong arguments in favor of such a recommendation. The arguments are marshaled here with a prime focus on the prevention of ischemic heart disease and other atherosclerotic disorders.

EXERCISE AND HEART DISEASE

The Cardiac Epidemic

Strong interest in the possible preventive value of physical activity was sparked by a "cardiac epidemic." Morris noted from an analysis of death certificates in England and Wales that there had been a marked increase in the cardiac death rate from 1931 to 1948. This was attributable largely to acute rather than chronic cardiovascular disease.

Other authors described similar cardiac epidemics in the United States and Canada. Moreover, Anderson and Halliday showed by both a reanalysis of Canadian death certificates and a separation of cases of sudden death that the trend toward an increase of cardiac deaths could not be attributed to any shift of diagnostic "fashion."

Many hypotheses were advanced to account for the cardiac epidemic, but one popular explanation was that there had been a decline of physical activity in Western society, associated with the widespread ownership of cars, mechanization of industry, and the sedentary leisure encouraged by television. In retrospect, such influences may have been significant in North American communities, but they can hardly explain the observations made by Morris. From 1931 to 1939 England was in the grip of a severe economic depression, with more than 2 million unemployed. Few people could afford cars; from 1939 to 1945 there were the added privations of war, with little except black-market gasoline for a wealthy few. Over this same period British factories received little capital investment, and for the most part industries continued to operate with antiquated machinery that had been installed in the early part of the Industrial Revolution. Television broadcasting admittedly was initiated in 1936, but few British people were able to afford the luxury of a television set until the mid-1950s.

Despite the faulty nature of the basic hypothesis concerning the cardiac epidemic, Morris's paper sparked some fascinating epidemiologic research that provided evidence for the preventive value of both occupational and leisure activity.

Occupational Activity

Epidemiologists quickly recognized that daily work provided a steady source of interindividual differences in personal energy expenditures. Studies thus compared the incidence of ischemic heart disease between men employed in nominally active and sedentary occupations.

Morris and colleagues were interested by the London Transport bus system, which in the early 1950s employed both drivers and "conductors." The former sat in the padded comfort of a leather chair steering the bus through the busy London traffic, while the latter had the responsibility of climbing to the upper deck of the bus twice in every mile in order to check the tickets of passengers; a total of some 190 ascents of the staircase were made per work shift. At first inspection this seemed the ideal epidemiologic comparison; the two groups had similar salaries and socioeconomic status and they ate at the same canteens that were provided at all major bus termini. Morris was thus gratified to find that the coronary heart disease mortality rate was only 46 percent as high in the conductors as in the drivers; likewise, the incidence of myocardial infarction was only 53 percent as high, and the total incidence of coronary heart disease was only 70 percent as high in the conductors. The coronary pathology seen in conductors dying of other conditions was also 57 to 68 percent of that seen in those drivers who died of intercurrent disease. However, the incidence of angina in the conductors was 198 percent of that found in the drivers, possibly because the greater energy demands of ticket selling brought to light cardiac problems that were being overlooked in the drivers. The major criticism of the London Transport study was that the occupation (driver or conductor) was initially self-selected. In a later paper, "The epidemiology of uniforms," Morris and associates demonstrated that the type of person who sought work as a driver was initially fatter and had a higher serum cholesterol level than the individual who began work as a conductor. At recruitment, the drivers thus had a greater risk of ischemic heart disease than the conductors.

Unfortunately, occupation is usually largely self-selected. However, there are exceptions. Brunner compared office and field workers in the Jewish kibbutzim. Here the type of employment was determined by the kibbutz committee, and nutrition and socioeconomic status were closely comparable for both classes of worker. It thus seemed reasonable to attribute a threefold intercategory difference in the incidence of coronary heart disease mortality to the preventive value of vigorous farm work.

Likewise, Paffenbarger argued that union regulations forced all San Francisco longshoremen to begin working as heavy manual laborers without the opportunity for self-selection. Paffenbarger's study of this population was more sophisticated than some of its predecessors. An attempt was made to control, in a crude multivariate fashion, for other risk factors (including smoking habits and blood pressure). Paffenbarger further argued that since the protective effect of vigorous exercise was seen with respect to sudden death, it was unlikely that his findings could be attributed to the seeking of lighter work by sick members of the labor force.

Although the Californian longshoremen study provides strong evidence of the preventive value of vigorous occupational activity, it now has mainly historical interest (at least in North America). The energy costs of dockwork have dropped dramatically with containerization, and most other modern industries show a similar decrease of physical demands, to the point that if physical activity has health value, it must be sought through deliberate leisure programs rather than the selection of a "heavy" occupation.

Leisure Activity

Both Morris and Paffenbarger made prospective surveys examining the health value of leisure activity. Their studies provide the most conclusive evidence available on the preventive value of regular exercise; they will thus be described in some detail.

Morris and colleagues examined 17,000 executive-grade civil servants, using a simple questionnaire to assess their activity habits at entry to the survey. They reasoned that their sample was reasonably homogeneous from a socioeconomic point of view, and argued that because the individuals under study had much experience in the completion of forms, these would provide reliable information on personal daily activity patterns. All members of the group were initially free of symptomatic ischemic heart disease, so Morris and associates reasoned that it was unlikely that their activity habits had been predetermined by disease. The data suggested that there was substantial protection against a first clinical attack of myocardial infarction among those who participated in various forms of voluntary physical activity, including (1) the climbing of more than 450 stairs per day; (2) taking more than 5 minutes per day of active recreation, keeping fit, or "vigorous getting about" (near-maximal effort); and (3) engaging in more than 30 minutes per day of "heavy" leisure activity (more than 31 kJ per minute). Among possible confounding factors, the active half of Morris's sample contained somewhat fewer smokers (26 percent versus 32 percent), more individuals with a systemic blood pressure greater than 150/90 mm Hg, and fewer people with a serum cholesterol level of more than 6.4 mmol per liter. However, the active and inactive subgroups were comparable with respect to height, body mass, and skinfold thicknesses. The added energy expenditure in those who were apparently protected against heart attacks was about 750 kJ per day.

Paffenbarger and colleagues examined 16,936 Harvard alumni in an analogous type of prospective study. Substantial protection against ischemic heart disease (an attack rate of 1.00 relative to a standard figure of 1.64) was associated with an additional leisure energy expenditure of 8,000 kJ per week. Moreover, the age-adjusted cardiac fatality rate showed a steep downward gradient with additional energy expenditure over the range from 2,000 to 10,000 kJ per week, although no further advantage was associated with a higher energy expenditure than this. Multivariate analysis showed that protection was associated with energy expenditures independently of such variables as smoking habits, blood pressure, Quetelet index, early parental death, or participation in sports while at university. Participation in strenuous sports alone yielded a protection ratio of 1.00 to 1.38, but significant protection was also associated with walking at least 1 mile per day (a ratio of 1.00 to 1.26) and the climbing of only 50 stairs per day (a ratio of 1.00 to 1.25). Moreover, in partial answer to the criticism of self-selection, Paffenbarger and colleagues pointed out that university athletes who subsequently became inactive apparently lost their protection, while those who became active after leaving the university developed protection against heart disease. The end result from an optimal dose of exercise seemed to be a 2-year extension of lifespan, although a fair part of the additional lifespan was occupied by the active leisure.

Paffenbarger finally calculated the potential impact on community health of an exercise intervention relative to other forms of health education such as the encouragement of smoking cessation or the control of hypertension. Although the control of hypertension had a somewhat greater impact on prognosis for the individual, Paffenbarger suggested that in terms of community health this was compensated by the fact that inactivity was more prevalent than hypertension among well-educated individuals in the United States. There remain several difficulties when carrying out this type of calculation. First, while the prevalence of hypertension is fairly clearly established, we do not know a great deal about current activity patterns in the community, nor is it altogether clear what intensity and duration of activity are needed to provide cardiovascular protection. Finally, there is little information on the short- and long-term success of educational programs designed to increase physical activity; as with smoking, it is likely that the short-term community response will be marred by a high rate of recidivism, but there may be a more long-term trend toward acceptance of exercise advice.

Other surveys of leisure activity and cardiovascular health have generally confirmed the observations made by Morris and Paffenbarger, although many have been criticized because of a limited reliability of activity estimates, a positive correlation between a high social class and participation in active leisure, and correlations between a physically active lifestyle and other positive forms of health behavior. Montoye noted in the Tecumseh survey that hypertension and a favorable lipid profile were most prevalent in the sedentary members of the community, while Williams and associates found that individuals with a high-density lipoprotein (HDL) cholesterol level were more easily persuaded to become involved in a long-distance jogging program. In the Seven Country study, Keys found no association between a combined index of occupational and leisure activity and various measures of cardiac disease; however, this reflects a method of statistical analysis that assigned most of the available variance to blood pressure and serum lipids, variables that are known to be influenced by physical activity. On the other hand, the Framingham study noted that over 24 years of prospective observation, an active lifestyle reduced the incidence of both coronary disease and myocardial infarction by a factor of 3.0 in men and 2.5 in women; while there was no evidence that activity influenced the incidence of peripheral arterial disease, atherothrombotic brain infarctions were also less common in active people. Garcia-Palmieri and associates applied the Framingham activity index in an 8.5-year prospective study of Puerto Ricans; again, an inverse association between exercise and the risk of ischemic heart disease was observed. In the Oslo study, the risk of ischemic heart disease was found to be lower in those who had active leisure pursuits than in those who were active at work but sedentary at home; however, the interpretation of this observation was complicated by socioeconomic differences between the active and sedentary occupational groups. In Holland, Magnus and associates found that the victims of ischemic heart disease were less active than controls, although benefit could not be related to the dose or intensity of exercise, and no advantage was apparently gained from seasonal or occasional bouts of physical activity. Observations in Finland suggested that a low level of physical activity increased the overall risk of death, but did not increase the 2-year incidence of either myocardial infarction or stroke. Some other community studies have found benefits from exercise and/or fitness, including the Western Collaborative study, a survey of public safety officers in Los Angeles, the Health Insurance Plan of New York, and two prospective studies in Denmark. Even the supposedly negative Gothenburg study demonstrated a trend toward inactive leisure in those who subsequently developed ischemic heart disease.

A Causal Association?

Epidemiologist Bradford Hill noted nine criteria that together suggested that an association between two variables was causal in nature. In the case of exercise and the prevention of heart disease, the association is only moderately strong, a 50 to 100 percent improvement of prognosis for active individuals. However, the advantage is relatively *consistent* from one study to another, and a number of both occupational and leisure studies have spanned the long latent period linking inactivity with atherosclerosis, demonstrating an appropriate *temporal relationship.* Paffenbarger's data further indicated a nice *biologic gradient* with the dose of exercise, and there have been many *plausible hypotheses* as to why exercise should help in controlling the disease.

However, there is a lack of *specificity* in the association; some sedentary people remain free of the disease, and other active people have a heart attack at an early age. This reflects in part the slow and silent nature of the disease process; some sedentary people remain free of symptoms despite extensive atherosclerosis, while other people become active after extensive lesions have developed. Further, atherosclerosis is a multifactorial disease, and some people have a high risk because of a congenital disorder of lipid metabolism, despite vigorous exercise. Finally, there may be an optimal dose of exercise that is exceeded by the occasional enthusiast, with adverse consequences.

Moreover, there is some lack of *coherence* in the explanation: for example, angina is increased in active persons, and unaccustomed vigorous exercise may precipitate rather than prevent a heart attack. *Experimental verification* is difficult because exercise cannot be administered in a randomized, double-blind fashion; the necessary sample size for a conclusive controlled experiment would be very large because of a high drop-out rate, and exercise might change other facets of lifestyle. Finally, we have yet to identify compounds that are produced during exercise and that exert an *analogous* protective effect if administered independently of physical activity.

Despite lack of conclusive proof of the causal nature of the association, the evidence is sufficiently strong to recommend regular moderate exercise as good preventive medicine for our patients; it is likely both to reduce the incidence of heart attacks and to extend lifespan.

PREVENTION OF OTHER DISORDERS

There have been suggestions that regular exercise may prevent a number of other disorders; there may be an improvement of overall lifestyle, gains in perceived health and mood state, a decreased risk of certain complications of obesity such as hypertension, maturity-onset diabetes, and cholecystitis, a strengthening of cartilage, ligaments, and bone structure, and a decreased incidence of certain forms of malignancy. However, partly because these conditions have less clear end points than a heart attack or sudden death, the proof of benefit is weaker than for ischemic heart disease.

Overall Lifestyle

While there is some "clustering" of good lifestyle habits, the reported association between exercise and other variables such as abstinence from smoking has sometimes been less than might be imagined. This may reflect the nature of the questions used to define "exercise"; when the emphasis has been on health-related exercise, the association of such activity with other good habits has been closer.

In a controlled study of an employee fitness program, we observed that males who were regular attenders at the exercise classes showed a reduction of some 2 years in their "appraised age" as determined by the Canadian Health Hazard Appraisal instrument; this was due to such changes as a lesser consumption of cigarettes and alcohol, a reduction of obesity, and some decrease in systemic blood pressure.

Perceived Health

A large fraction of consultations in the average physician's office reflect a deterioration of perceived health rather than any clear-cut organic disorder.

Any patient lives on a health continuum that ranges from positive health to perceived illness. A deterioration of mood state can displace the individual's condition toward perceived illness, so that a medical consultation is requested; conversely, if regular exercise improves mood state, the demand for medical services diminishes. Some evidence of an effect of this sort was seen in a controlled study in Toronto; in the year after introduction of an employee fitness program, personnel at the experimental company decreased their demands for both hospital care and medical consultations.

Mood State

Many patients claim that they exercise because it makes them "feel better." However, it is surprisingly difficult to demonstrate an improvement of mood state by the formal paper-and-pencil tests of the clinical psychologist. One difficulty in obtaining proof of a change in mood is that most of the available questionnaires have been devised for disturbed patients. An average sample of sedentary people thus begins an experiment with very normal scores. Exercise has had more obvious benefit in situations in which patients were initially depressed; for example, exercise has helped to correct the depression that commonly accompanies an acute myocardial infarction.

Complications of Obesity

Many clinical trials have demonstrated that regular endurance exercise induces a small but clinically valuable 5 to 10 mm Hg decrease in resting blood pressure; an increase of physical activity is thus a useful adjunct to other simple forms of therapy in individuals with borderline hypertension.

Studies of populations undergoing acculturation to a sedentary lifestyle have suggested that a decrease of physical activity is associated with a rising incidence of type II diabetes. There have also been suggestions that increased activity can restore insulin sensitivity and lower fasting blood glucose in type II diabetes, although the improvement in glucose tolerance has been more disappointing. The main argument in favor of exercise for the diabetes prone person seems to be the prevention of associated cardiovascular disease, although the presence of silent cardiovascular disease is also a strong argument for caution in exercise prescription.

Prolonged endurance exercise, to the equivalent of 18 to 20 km of jogging per week, induces a small increase of HDL cholesterol, with a corresponding decrease in the risk of both atherosclerotic disease and gallbladder disease.

Musculoskeletal Problems

In the early stages of training, an overzealous approach to exercise can cause an alarming incidence of musculoskeletal injuries, including muscle pulls and tendon tears, but regular exercise has a favorable long-term influence on the musculoskeletal system. A strengthening of the muscles reduces the strains withstood by both ligaments and cartilage. Regular exercise also strengthens the ligaments and thickens articular cartilage, while weightbearing activity increases bone density. All these changes reduce the likelihood of injury for a given imposed combination of forces.

Malignancy

The overall effect of exercise on malignancy is small. Indeed, some studies have suggested that athletes may show a small increase in the number of deaths from certain forms of malignancy.

However, when individual types of tumor are distinguished, there is evidence that gastrointestinal tumors are less common in athletes than in sedentary persons. A study of women who were athletes at university has suggested further that breast and cervical cancers are less common than expected in this sample, possibly as a result of exercise-induced changes in estrogen levels. However, as in many studies of former athletes, no proof was offered that the women concerned had subsequently persisted with their sport, nor indeed was it shown conclusively that they had engaged in more physical activity than their peers while at university.

DISADVANTAGES OF EXERCISE

As with any other form of preventive medicine, it is finally necessary to weigh the benefits of regular physical exercise critically against its disadvantages. Possible objections to physical activity prescription include the costs, musculoskeletal problems, and exercise-induced deaths.

Costs

If all the adult population were to engage regularly in vigorous physical activity, communities might incur substantial costs for the provision of necessary programs and facilities. However, such costs can be held to a minimum by an exercise prescription that emphasizes building the activity into the normal day; suitable recommendations include fast walking while carrying moderate weights and the replacement of electrical devices by muscle-powered equipment.

Many patients find the time commitment of regular exercise to be a serious disincentive, and this is a further argument in favor of building the required activity into the normal day. It is then much less likely to be forgotten and is perceived as taking less of the person's time.

If rigorous demands are made for medical clearance and subsequent supervision of exercise candidates, this again can generate heavy program costs. Medical examination is important for those contemplating high-level sports performance, but if a person is symptom free, Canadian experience suggests that a simple questionnaire may provide an adequate preliminary clearance for those planning a moderate, health-giving increase of daily exercise. Further, our experience with an employee fitness program provides no evidence that regular moderate activity increases the demand for either orthopaedic or electrocardiographic services.

Musculoskeletal Problems

Some exercise programs involving middle-aged adults have produced injury rates as high as 50 percent. Such problems seem related to (1) failure to consider the individual's history, (2) lack of an adequate warm-up, and (3) overvigorous progression.

If there is a clinical history of recent joint disorders, the exercise program should be designed to minimize the stress on the affected joint while strengthening the surrounding muscles. Sometimes it may be sufficient to replace the heavy impact stress of jogging by a less demanding exercise such as fast walking, but in other patients it may be desirable to switch to a weight-supported type of activity such as swimming or calisthenics in a swimming pool.

The likelihood of musculoskeletal injury is further reduced if a daily routine begins with 5 to 10 minutes of gentle stretching exercises. Sudden bouncing and twisting movements should be avoided, since these are particularly likely to cause injury.

Finally, the rate of progression of an exercise prescription should be consistent with the individual's initial condition. The total amount and intensity of exercise prescribed for any given session should not leave the person more than pleasantly tired the next day. If such simple precautions are observed, there is no evidence that orthopaedic claims are increased by participation in an exercise program.

Exercise-related Deaths

If a person undertakes sudden, vigorous, and unaccustomed exercise, there is a five- to tenfold increase in the chances of cardiac death while the activity is continuing. The risk is much less with exercise that is well matched to the patient's physical condition, but any type of exercise leads to some statistical increase of acute cardiac risk.

Nevertheless, if one considers the total likelihood of death over a 24-hour period, the increase of cardiac risk during a work-out is more than offset by the decreased risk that the regular exerciser encounters in the periods between bouts of physical activity.

Top athletes occasionally may die from hypo- and hyperthermia, drowning, various problems of underwater exploration, the pulmonary edema of high altitudes, and mechanical injury during competition. However, such hazards are unlikely to be encountered by the ordinary person who engages in a modest increase of health-giving physical activity.

OVERALL RECOMMENDATION

The recommendation to participate in regular moderate exercise is a simple and positive piece of advice that the physician can offer to all patients. If the prescription is not overly ambitious, there is little evidence that harm will result, and the likelihood of clinical disease (particularly ischemic heart disease) will be substantially reduced, with a corresponding increase in both the quantity and the quality of the patient's life. Although the extension of lifespan is welcome, the gain in life quality remains the argument that will convince most patients to increase their physical activity.

SUGGESTED READING

Anderson TW, Halliday ML. The male epidemic: 50 years of ischaemic heart disease. Public Health (Lond) 1979; 93:163–172.

Brunner D. Studies in preventive cardiology. Coronary heart disease—epidemiology and rehabilitation. Jaffa: Government Hospital, Donolo, 1973.

Haskell WL. The influence of exercise on the concentration of triglyceride and cholesterol in human plasma. Exerc Sport Sci Rev 1984; 12:205–244.
Herzlich C. Health and illness. London: Academic Press, 1973.
Kemmer FW. Exercise and diabetes. In: Torg J, Welsh P, Shephard RJ, eds. Current therapy in sports medicine-2. Toronto: BC Decker, 1989.
Morgan WP, Goldston SE. Exercise and mental health. Washington, DC: Hemisphere Publications, 1987.
Morris JN. Recent history of coronary disease. Lancet 1951; 1:1–7.
Morris JN, Everitt MG, Pollard RL, Chave SP, Semmence AM. Vigorous exercise in leisure time. Protection against coronary heart disease. Lancet 1980; 2:1207–1210.
Morris JN, Heady JA, Raffle PA. Physique of London busmen: epidemiology of uniforms. Lancet 1956; 2:569–570.
Morris JN, Heady J, Raffle P, Roberts C, Parks J. Coronary heart disease and physical activity of work. Lancet 1953; 2:1053–1057, 1111–1120.
Paffenbarger R. Physical activity and fatal heart attack: protection or selection? In: Amsterdam EA, Wilmore JH, deMaria AN, eds. Exercise in cardiovascular health and disease. New York: Yorke Books, 1977.
Paffenbarger RS, Hyde RT, Wing AL, Hsieh CC. Physical activity, all-cause mortality and longevity of college alumni. N Engl J Med 1986; 314:605–613.
Shephard RJ. Ischaemic heart disease and exercise. London: Croom Helm, 1981.
Shephard RJ. Exercise in coronary heart disease. Sports Med 1985; 3:26–49.
Shephard RJ. The value of exercise in preventive medicine. In: Evered D, Whelan J, eds. The value of preventive medicine. London: Pitman, 1985.
Shephard RJ. The economic benefits of enhanced fitness. Champaign, IL: Human Kinetics, 1986.
Shephard RJ. Exercise and malignancy. Sports Med 1986; 3:235–241.
Shephard RJ. Corey P, Cox M. Health hazard appraisal—the influence of an employee fitness programme. Can J Public Health 1982; 73:183–187.
Siscovick D, LaPorte RE, Newman JM. The disease specific benefits and risks of physical activity and exercise. Public Health Rep 1985; 100:180–188.
Tipton C. Exercise, training and hypertension. Exerc Sport Sci Rev 1984; 12:245–306.

EXERCISE AND TRAINING IN CHILDHOOD AND ADOLESCENCE

HAN C.G. KEMPER, M.D., Ph.D.

Children are generally thought to be naturally physically active. In recent years, however, the physical activity of youngsters has been a subject of great concern to health officials. Up to a generation ago, physical activity was a natural part of life for most children. This is no longer so, and one may well ask whether the child or the adolescent now gets the physical activity required for healthy development. In many ways, the lifestyle of children and adolescents starts to resemble that of adults. The necessity for physical activity has been greatly reduced, owing to mechanization and automatization of work and leisure. Currently, physical activity depends on such factors as body build, physical fitness, the amount and use of free time, and the accessibility of recreational and sports facilities.

Hypoactivity is a direct or indirect cause of many pediatric diseases. In arthritis, cerebral palsy, cystic fibrosis, severe cyanotic heart disease, obesity, and scoliosis, hypoactivity is inherent in the disease and is a direct result of it. Children with bronchial asthma, diabetes mellitus, epilepsy, noncyanotic heart diseases, and hemophilia can be active, but often they are not. Restrictions reflect overprotection by the parents or an uneducated attitude of teachers and health practitioners, or both.

Physical inactivity is an important risk factor for coronary heart disease. Atherosclerosis starts soon after birth. It is often suggested that a sufficient amount and intensity of regular physical activity could decelerate this process. However, an epidemiologic prospective study, comparing a large number of physically active children with a randomized group of less active children over a long period, has never yet been conducted and apparently cannot be carried out. There is unfortunately no possibility of a double-blind study in which physical activity can be measured.

One way out of this dilemma is to measure habitual physical activity on a longitudinal basis and to group individuals according to activity patterns.

In the course of development, there are critical periods that determine whether individuals will later lead a physically active life:

1. Childhood (ages 4 to 12), when they first attend school.
2. Adolescence (ages 13 to 19), when they enter secondary school, with restriction of free time by homework, a shift from bicycles to motorcycles at ages 15 to 16, and a further change to automobiles at ages 18 to 19.

This chapter surveys the short- and long-term effects of exercise in children, the exercise programs that can be used to test children and adolescents, and the possibilities for assessing habitual physical activity.

SHORT-TERM EFFECTS OF EXERCISE

For mechanical energy to be released at the myofibrillar level, adenosine triphosphate (ATP) must be split. Because this high-energy compound is available only in small quantities, there is a need for reinforcement of ATP, supplied by anaerobic sources (creatine phosphate [CP] and lactic acid system) and aerobic sources (oxygen transport system).

Muscle contractions cannot be sustained from anaerobic sources for longer than 1 minute. In contrast, muscle contractions utilizing aerobic sources can last minutes or even hours, unless there is a shortage of substrate (particularly glycogen).

Most activities utilize both aerobic and anaerobic sources, but are roughly subdivided into low power–long duration (aerobic) activities such as long distance running, swimming, skating, cycling, and skiing; and high power–short duration (anaerobic) activities such as sprinting, jumping, and throwing.

It is still argued whether children and adolescents are characteristically aerobic or anaerobic performers relative to adults.

Anaerobic Performances

Short-term power output, even when standardized for body size (body mass or active muscle mass), is distinctly lower in children than in young adults. There are no large differences in the level of ATP and CP, but a lower glycolytic rate is suggested by lower lactate concentrations in blood and muscle.

Aerobic Performances

The most commonly used index of maximal aerobic power is the maximal oxygen intake ($\dot{V}O_2$max), the highest volume of O_2 that can be consumed by the body per unit of time.

Figure 1 illustrates a concomitant increase of $\dot{V}O_2$max with age in both boys and girls. Until the age of 12 years, values grow equally in both sexes. Although the $\dot{V}O_2$max of boys keeps increasing until the age of about 18 years, it hardly develops beyond the age of 14 years in girls. In relative terms, $\dot{V}O_2$max is expressed per kilogram of body mass ($\dot{V}O_2$max/body mass) (Fig. 2). There is hardly any age-dependent change in boys, but the relative $\dot{V}O_2$max declines in girls, reflecting a decrease in body fitness and a relative decrease of lean body mass.

An alternative and more theoretical approach is based on the scaling theory. It is assumed that body segments retain fairly constant proportions during childhood and adolescence. Linear dimensions are related to stature (L), surfaces have areas that are related to L^2, and volumes to L^3. Muscle forces should be scaled to L^2 (since they are proportional to cross-sectional area), while lung or heart volume and work are proportional to L^3.

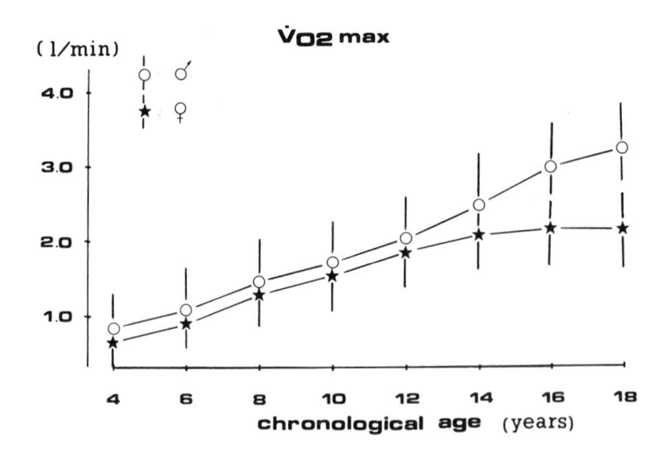

Figure 1 Mean and standard deviation of maximal aerobic power of boys and girls in relation to chronologic age. (Data from Saris WHM, 1982 and Kemper HCG, 1985.)

Power, which is work/time, should be scaled to L^2, while time is proportional to L and $\dot{V}O_2$max (volume/time) is proportional to L^2. If we relate $\dot{V}O_2$max to body height squared, values for children are lower than in healthy young adults. Experimentally, longitudinal studies show height exponents of from 2.25 to 3.0 in boys and 2.0 in girls.

If the theoretical expression $\dot{V}O_2$max/L^2 is correct, the changes with age suggest that in girls the state of the aerobic system remains relatively constant, while in boys one sees an increase over and above that expected from increasing body size (Fig. 3).

Differing longitudinal trends between the sexes may reflect differences in habitual physical activity. Although boys and girls were active for similar

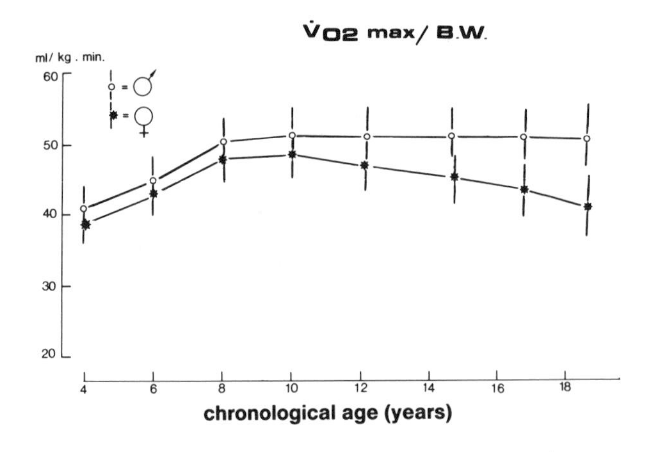

Figure 2 Maximal aerobic power of boys and girls per kilogram of body mass ($\dot{V}O_2$/kg) in relation to chronologic age. (Data as in Figure 1.)

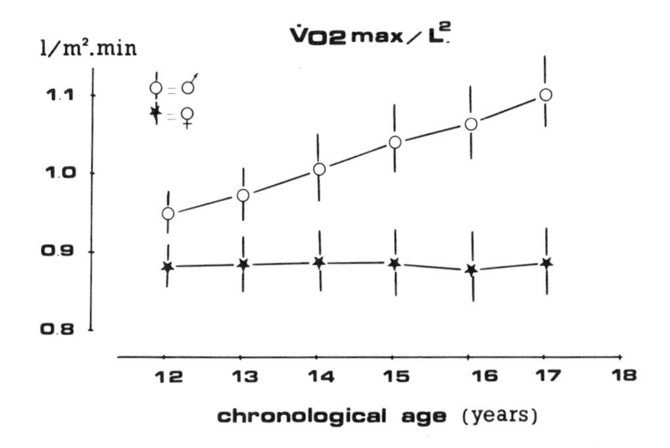

Figure 3 Developmental curves (mean and standard error) of $\dot{V}O_2max/L^2$ in a group of Dutch teenagers (boys and girls versus chronologic age). (Data from Kemper HCG, Verschuur R, 1987)

times, the boys participated in more intensive activities.

Mechanical Efficiency (ME). During cycle ergometry, the ratio between external mechanical work and the chemical energy utilized is similar in children, adolescents, and adults (with a mean value of about 25 percent). In contrast, the ME during walking and running is about 20 percent lower in children. Davies demonstrated that when children were loaded with external weights, they ran more efficiently than without. This is probably because at a certain running speed the children with a higher body mass had frequencies of leg movements that matched the forces necessary to produce economic conversion of chemical energy to mechanical work. Perhaps because children are less capable of anaerobic exercise than adults, they make faster O_2 uptake adjustments at the onset of exercise.

LONG-TERM EFFECTS OF EXERCISE

If exercise is repeated over weeks and months, it induces the morphologic and functional changes of "training."

Research on the training of children faces many methodologic problems. Changes due to growth, development, and maturation can also influence the results. Control groups must be included in the design, but they can very seldom be assigned randomly.

Owing to the above constraints, most studies of training in childhood are correlative and not causative.

Training Principles

Changes are specific to the training stimulus. Aerobic, endurance-like activities induce systemic effects (e.g., hypertrophy and dilatation of the right ventricle) and improvements of oxidative capacity in active muscles (including increases of aerobic enzymes and capillary density).

Anaerobic, short-term–high-power activities induce different effects, such as muscle hypertrophy (increases of myofibrils and connective, tendinous, and ligamentous tissue) and adaptations in the nervous system (e.g., recruitment patterns and synchronization of motor units).

Training is based on two general principles:

1. Recognition of the major energy system used to perform a given activity.
2. Overload throughout training.

All training programs must be specific to the energy system(s) predominantly used during (sports) performances (Table 1).

The overload principle implies that the exercise resistance is near maximal and that it is increased gradually as the child's performance capacity improves. The amount of training can be characterized by its intensity, duration, and frequency.

The intensity of an activity is determined by the metabolic demands ($\dot{V}O_2$), the strain on the cardiovascular system (heart rate), or in the case of strength training by the weight to be lifted. Although intensity is often described in absolute terms, in children and adolescents it should be described in relation to the maximal capability of the individual. There is no training effect below a certain threshold. For young adults, the threshold of aerobic power is about 65 percent of $\dot{V}O_2$max or 75 percent of maximal heart rate, while for strength training the threshold is about 70 percent of maximal voluntary isometric contraction (Fmax). When dynamic tasks are involved, the maximal number of repetitions of muscle contractions can be used, the so-called repetition maximum (RM). If the RM of a dynamic task appears to be below 10, it can be assumed that this equals an isometric force of over 70 percent of Fmax.

In order to maintain overload, a program must be progressive.

TABLE 1 Predominant Energy Systems Used in Various Sports Events, Expressed as a Percentage of Total Energy Consumption

Type of Activity	*Phosphate System (%)*	*Lactic Acid System (%)*	*Oxygen Transport System (%)*
100 m running 400 m skating	98	2	0
100 m swimming 1,500 m skating	90	10	0
10 km running 800 m swimming	0	10	90

There is no optimal frequency of training, because frequency interacts with the intensity and the duration of training sessions. In therapeutic and fitness programs it is generally recommended that individuals should not train more than three times a week.

The duration of training sessions for children should be at least 30 minutes but not longer than 1 hour. The minimal duration of 30 minutes allows a 10-minute warm-up at the beginning and a 5-minute cool-down at the end of the session. The maximum of 60 minutes avoids a middle part of the session when the training threshold must be exceeded by a child who is already fatigued and losing attention.

Training Methods

Muscle Training

Muscular strength may be defined as the force or tension a muscle can exert against a resistance during a single maximal effort. Because there are three basic kinds of muscle contractions: (1) isometric, (2) miometric (or concentric), and (3) pliometric (or eccentric), there are also three types of muscle training.

There is no simple optimal program to develop strength. Specificity is important. The best program thus involves the same muscle contractions as in the performance. The newest method is isokinetic training: the device permits the development of maximal muscular tension throughout the full range of joint movement (while the speed can be kept constant). This is an advantage over dynamic weight training, in which this is never the case.

Programs to improve strength consist mainly of high loads and low repetitions. In contrast, muscular endurance (the ability to perform repeated contractions over an extended period) are developed by frequent repetitions at low loads. Strength training seems more effective in postpubescent than in prepubescent boys, possibly because of the low levels of androgens in prepubescent boys.

General Conditioning

Much of the improvement in sports performances over the past century can be attributed not only to early selection and to increased participation rates, but also to the refinement of training methods. Apart from well-known continuous endurance training programs involving running, bicycling, and swimming, interval training has been introduced. Interval methods are characterized by the intensity and duration of loading, the length of recovery periods, and the number of repetitions. There are three main types: interval sprint training, interval tempo training, and interval duration training (Table 2).

Interval sprint training is directed mainly to increasing the capacity of the phosphate system (ATP and CP); the intensity is high and the duration of loading and recovery are short. To allow replenishment of the phosphate battery, a relatively long recovery period is needed. For an efficient loading of the lactic acid system, loading must be extended to 1 or 2 minutes, with recovery periods between 2 and 4 minutes. Interval duration training uses the longest loading periods in order to involve the oxygen transport system, although the ratio of loading to recovery period is the smallest (1:1).

TABLE 2 Guidelines for Interval Training Methods

	Interval Sprint Training	*Interval Tempo Training*	*Interval Duration Training*
Energy system mainly involved	Phosphate	Lactic Acid	Oxygen
Duration of load (sec)	10–30	30–120	120–300
Duration of recovery (sec)	30–90	60–240	120–310
Ratio load: recovery	1:3	1:2	1:1
Number of repetitions	25–30	10–20	3–5

Interval training is an excellent system that can be used for athletes in any sport as well as nonathletes interested in general fitness and rehabilitation. The alternating periods of load and recovery are more tailored to children's behavior than continuous loading, which is boring and takes more training time than interval training.

Anaerobic training increases ATP, CP, glycogen, and phosphofructokinase levels in the muscles of children.

The aerobic trainability of children is less than expected. Most training studies have reported improving performances, but before the age of peak height velocity (in girls around 12 and in boys around 13 years of age) the maximal aerobic power often does not improve significantly. Possible explanations for the improvement in endurance performance without a concomitant increase in $\dot{V}O_2max$ include an improvement of mechanical efficiency, an improvement in anaerobic capacity, and a relatively high level of habitual activity.

PEDIATRIC EXERCISE TESTING

This section considers how to test anaerobic and aerobic power and how to apply data in the prevention, diagnosis, and therapy of childhood diseases.

Field Performance Tests

If no laboratory equipment is available and a large number of children have to be tested in a short time, so-called physical fitness tests are used. Choice of tests is based mostly on face validity and/or statistic validity. The relationship with physiologic variables is generally disappointing. For instance, simple running tests of aerobic endurance are much affected by motivation, previous experience of the test, and environmental factors such as weather and floor surface. Thus, the 12-minute run or the 20-meter progressive shuttle run shows very low coefficients of correlation with $\dot{V}O_2$max measurements ($r = 0.4$ and 0.7), indicating that at best 50 percent of the total variance can be explained by $\dot{V}O_2$max. Other performance tests all have a certain skill character and therefore are not limited by one prime physiologic function. Bearing these limitations in mind, the use of standardized tests for measuring physical fitness and presenting normative data can nevertheless be stimulating for physical education and sport.

Laboratory Tests for Aerobic and Anaerobic Power

In children who have a fair degree of coordination anaerobic power can be assessed by vertical jumps, stair running, or short-term cycle ergometer tests.

Aerobic power can be measured on a cycle ergometer or a motor-driven treadmill. In young children the treadmill is the best choice because (1) all children can learn to run on it, (2) more muscle mass is involved than during cycling, and (3) premature termination of the exercise test due to local muscle fatigue is avoided. Very young and mentally retarded children cannot always keep in pace with the metronome on a mechanically braked cycle ergometer. Furthermore, younger children require special cycles with reduced dimensions.

The exercise protocol for determining $\dot{V}O_2$max involves increasing treadmill inclination and speed every 1 to 3 minutes until the child can no longer maintain the activity despite strong encouragement. The Bruce protocol (Table 3) is feasible for 4- to 18-year-old boys and girls.

Success in reaching a true $\dot{V}O_2$max can be evaluated from the increase of $\dot{V}O_2$ in the last stage relative to the previous stage. In adults, the increase should be less than 150 ml; however, this criterion is met in only 50 percent of boys and girls. Secondary criteria include (1) reaching 95 percent of the age-predicted maximal heart rate (200 beats per minute minus age in years), and (2) a respiratory gas exchange ratio ($\dot{V}CO_2/\dot{V}O_2$) of more than 1.00.

TABLE 3 Bruce Treadmill Protocol for Measurement of $\dot{V}O_2$max

Stage	*Treadmill Speed (km/hr)*	*Treadmill Inclination (%)*	*Stage Duration (min)*
1	2.7	10	3
2	4.0	12	3
3	5.5	14	3
4	6.6	16	3
5	8.0	18	3
6	8.8	20	3
7	9.7	22	3

Indirect measurements of $\dot{V}O_2$max appear to be very unreliable. Although the heart rate is easily monitored, it cannot be used to predict $\dot{V}O_2$max in children. Even more than in adults, the linear relationship between heart rate and external work rate is influenced by environmental factors (particularly temperature), emotional factors, and mechanical efficiency. Using a single submaximal exercise and the Astrand-Ryhming nomogram, $\dot{V}O_2$max can be over- or underestimated by more than 15 percent.

Pediatric Exercise Testing

Bar-Or summarized the clinical value of exercise testing:

1. The physical working capacity of the child is evaluated in relation to activities they can sustain (e.g., the walk to school) or in prescribing the intensity of remedial activities.
2. Specific pathophysiologic characteristics are evaluated better than at rest, when the functional demands are lower (e.g., ischemic changes in the electrocardiogram or exercise-induced asthma).
3. The adequacy of drug medication such as insulin is assessed at different activity levels.
4. The risk of future chronic diseases such as hypertension is predicted.
5. Children who have lost confidence in their ability to exercise (e.g., those who are overweight) are motivated for further exercise.

MEASUREMENT OF PHYSICAL ACTIVITY

To evaluate the contribution of exercise to the health and fitness of children, it is necessary not only to perform exercise tests but also to assess their daily physical activity pattern. Physical activities provide fun and excitement, while games and sports also help the development of personal and social attributes. From a physiologic point of view, physical activities are measured in terms of energy expenditure. The method adopted should fulfill at least three criteria:

1. Minimal interference with normal daily activity.
2. It should be applicable over a continuous period of 24 hours, in order to include school and leisure activities.
3. It should be valid with respect to the gold standard (measurement of energy expenditure).

Available methods (Table 4) include (1) measurements of oxygen uptake, heart rate, and body movements; and (2) observation of the intensity, duration, and frequency of movements.

TABLE 4 Characteristics of Various Methods of Physical Activity Measurement

	Criteria		
	Social Acceptability	*Applicability Over 24 Hr*	*Validity Relative to $\dot{V}O_2$ Measurement*
Measurement methods			
Oxygen uptake	x	x	xxx
Heart rate	xx	xx	xx
Movement counter	xxx	xxx	x
Observational methods			
Diary	xx	xx	xx
Questionnaire	xx	xxx	x

Rating scale: xxx = "best"; x = "worst."

Most of the daily physical activity of youth is dynamic and aerobic, involving a large proportion of the total muscle mass (e.g., walking, jumping, and running) with durations of more than 2 to 3 minutes. To determine energy expenditures in real life, indirect, noninvasive methods have been developed.

Measurement Methods

For measurement of oxygen uptake, a portable Douglas bag provides valid information on the intensity of simple activities. The energy expenditure can be calculated, since 1 liter of oxygen is about equal to 5 kcal or 21 kJ. This method is valid and reliable, but not very suitable when assessing the daily physical activity pattern. Measurement of heart rate (HR) is a good alternative. At intensities above 30 to 40 percent of $\dot{V}O_2$max, the increase of cardiac output is entirely due to an increase in HR, and there is thus a linear relationship between $\dot{V}O_2$ and HR. However, the same $\dot{V}O_2$ elicits different heart rates in different individuals, since HR is also dependent on age and training level. The HR–$\dot{V}O_2$ relationship must therefore be determined for each individual separately. Rapid development of microelectronics has reduced both the price and the size of instruments; some now take the form of a wrist watch!

Body movements can be registered by:

1. Pedometers. These are attached to the person's waistband, and measure vertical displacements of the center of gravity of the body.
2. Actometers. These are essentially self-winding wristwatches from which the escape mechanism has been removed. The rotor is connected directly to the dial. They can be worn at the ankle or thigh.
3. Stepcounters. These are built into the shoe. They measure the frequency and force applied with each step.
4. Accelerometers. These are small electronic motion sensors that measure the intensity of movements.

Body movement counters are the least valid with respect to $\dot{V}O_2$ measurements, but their applicability remains high because of their small size and low cost.

Observational Methods

A direct analysis of motion in time can be administered using a prestructured diary with previously defined activity categories and a clear timetable. The cooperation of the individual is essential; this imposes a large burden on the child during the day.

A recall questionnaire makes retrospective observations over a period varying from 1 day to 1 year. The accuracy of the answers decreases with increasing time lag, as a result of memory bias. Moreover, many individuals overestimate the intensity and duration of their previous physical activity. In balancing accuracy against the representativeness of both activity behavior (which day and how many days are selected) and the population, the questionnaire method remains an alternative approach for epidemiologic research.

Table 4 gives an overview of the methods of physical activity measurement. There is no simple indication of the best method. Probably direct measurements in a small sample over a short time should be combined with indirect observations over an extended period, using a larger sample.

SUGGESTED READING

Acheson KJ, Campbell IT, Edholm OG, Miller DS, Stock MN. The measurement of daily energy expenditure—an evaluation of some techniques. Am J Clin Nutr 1980; 33:1155–1164.
American Alliance for Health, Physical Education, Recreation and Dance. Lifetime health related physical fitness, test manual. Reston, VA: AAHPERD, 1980.
Astrand PO. Experimental studies of physical working capacity in relation to sex and age. Copenhagen: Munksgaard, 1952.
Astrand PO, Rodahl K. Textbook of work physiology. Physiological bases of exercise. 3rd ed. New York: McGraw-Hill, 1986.
Bar-Or O. Pediatric sports medicine for the practitioner. New York: Springer, 1983.

Binkhorst RA, Kemper HCG, Saris WHM. Children and exercise. XI. International series on sport sciences. Vol 15. Champaign, IL: Human Kinetics, 1985.
Bradfield RB. Assessment of typical daily energy expenditure. Am J Clin Nutr 1971; 24:1140–1154.
Council of Europe. Handbook for the EUROFIT Tests of physical fitness. Strasbourg: Council of Europe, 1988.
Davies CTM. Metabolic cost of exercise and physical performance in children with some observations on external loading. Eur J Appl Physiol 1980; 45:95–102.
Davies CTM, Barnes C, Godfrey S. Body composition and maximal exercise performance in children. Hum Biol 1972; 44:195–214.
Davies CTM, Rennie D. Human power output. Nature 1968; 217:770.
Edholm OG. The assessment of habitual activity. In: Evang K, Lange Andersen K, eds. Physical activity in health and disease. Oslo: Universitetsforlaget, 1966; 187.
Eriksson BO. Physical training, oxygen supply and muscle metabolism in 11–15 year old boys. Acta Physiol Scand (Suppl) 1972; 384:1–48.
Fox EL, Mathews DK. The physiological basis of physical education and athletics. Philadelphia: WB Saunders, 1981.
Godfrey S. Exercise testing in children: application in health and disease. London: WB Saunders, 1974.
Inbar O, Bar-Or O. Anaerobic characteristics of male children and adolescents. Med Sci Sports Exerc 1986; 18:264–269.
Kemper HCG. Growth, health and fitness of teenagers. Longitudinal research in international perspective. Med Sports Sci. Vol 20. Basel: Karger, 1985.
Kemper HCG, Verschuur R. Effect of 5 versus 3 lessons a week physical education program upon the physical development of 12- and 13-year-old schoolboys. J Sports Med Phys Fitness 1976; 16:319–326.
Kemper HCG, Verschuur R. Longitudinal study of maximal aerobic power in teenagers. Ann Hum Biol 1987; 14:435–444.
Kobayashi K, Kitamure M, Miura M, et al. Aerobic power as related to body growth and training in Japanese boys: a longitudinal study. J Appl Physiol 1978; 44:666–672.
Krahenbuhl GS, Skinner JS, Kohrt WM. Developmental aspects of maximal aerobic power in children. Exerc Sport Sci Rev 1985; 13:503–538.
Lange Andersen K, Masironi R, Rutenfranz J, et al. Habitual physical activity and health. WHO Regional Publications, European series No. 6. Copenhagen: WHO, 1978.
Lange Andersen K, Shephard RJ, Denolin H, Varnauskas E, Masironi R. Fundamentals of exercise testing. Geneva: WHO, 1971.
La Porte RE, Kuller LH, Kupfer DJ, et al. An objective measure of physical activity for epidemiologic research. Am J Epidemiol 1979; 109:158–168.
Macek M, Vavra J. The adjustment of oxygen uptake at the onset of exercise: a comparison between prepubertal boys and young adults. Int J Sports Med 1980; 1:75–77.
Masironi R, Denolin H. Physical activity in disease, prevention and treatment. Padua: Piccin, 1985.
Mechelen W van, Hlobil H, Kemper HCG. Validation of two running tests as estimates of maximal aerobic power in children. Eur J Appl Physiol 1986; 55:503–506.
Mirwald RL, Bailey DA. Longitudinal comparison of aerobic power and heart rate responses at submaximal and maximal workloads in active and inactive boys age 8 to 16 years. In: Borms J, Hauspie R, Sand A, Suzanne C, Hebbelinck M, eds. Human growth and development. New York: Plenum, 1984:561.
Mirwald RL, Bailey DA. Maximal aerobic power, a longitudinal analysis. London: Sports Dynamics, 1986.
Mirwald RL, Bailey DA, Cameron N, Rasmussen PL. Longitudinal comparison of aerobic power in active and inactive boys aged 7.0 to 17.0 years. Ann Hum Biol 1981; 8:405–414.
Montoye HJ. Estimation of habitual physical activity by questionnaire and interview. Am J Clin Nutr 1971; 24:1113–1118.
Montoye HJ, Wasburn R, Servais S, et al. Estimation of energy expenditure by a portable accelerometer. Med Sci Sport Exerc 1983; 15:403–407.
Montoye HJ. Risk indicators for cardiovascular disease in relation to physical activity in youth. In: Binkhorst RA, Kemper HCG, Saris WHM, eds. Children and exercise XI. International series on sport sciences. Vol 15. Champaign, IL: Human Kinetics, 1985:3.
Rutenfranz J, Berndt I, Knauth P. Daily physical activity, investigated by time budget studies and physical performance capacity of schoolboys. In: Borms J, Hebbelinck M, eds. Children and exercise. Acta Paediatr Belg (Suppl) 1974; 28:79–86.
Rutenfranz J, Seliger V, Andersen KL, et al. Differences in maximal aerobic power related to the daily physical activity in childhood. In: Borg G, ed. Physical work and effort. London: Pergamon, 1975:279.
Sargeant AJ. Short-term muscle power in children and adolescents. In: Bar-Or O, ed. Advances in pediatric sport sciences. Vol III. Biological issues. Champaign, IL: Human Kinetics, 1989.
Sargeant AJ, Dolan P. Optimal velocity for maximal short-term power output in cycling. Int J Sports Med 1984; 5:124–125.
Saris WHM. Aerobic power and daily physical activity in children with special reference to methods and cardiovascular risk indicators. Thesis, Nijmegen University, Krips Repro Meppel, 1982.
Saris WHM, Binkhorst RA. The use of pedometer and actometer in studying daily physical activity in man. Eur J Appl Physiol 1977; 37:219–235.
Schmidt-Nielsen. Scaling, why is animal size so important. Cambridge: Cambridge University Press, 1984.
Shephard KJ. Physical activity and growth. Chicago: Year Book, 1982.
Sprynarova S. Longitudinal study of the influence of different physical activity programs on functional capacity of boys from 11–18 years. Acta Paediatr Belg (Suppl) 1974; 28:204–213.
Strømme SB, Frey H, Harlem OK, et al. Physical activity and health, summary and main conclusions. Scand J Soc Med (Suppl) 1982; 29:9–37.
Verschuur R. Daily physical activity and health, longitudinal changes during the teenage period. Thesis, Universiteit van Amsterdam. Haarlem: de Vrieseborch, 1987.
Verschuur R, Kemper HCG. Adjustment of pedometers to make them more valid in assessing running. Int J Sports Med 1980; 1:87–89.
Vrijens J. Muscle strength development in the pre- and postpubescent age. Med Sport Sci, 1978; 11: 152–158.

REPRODUCTIVE CHANGES IN THE ATHLETE

JERILYNN C. PRIOR, M.D., F.R.C.P. (C)

The term "athletic amenorrhea," although commonly used in lay and medical writing, is inappropriate. It has never been proved that exercise by itself causes a 6-month loss of periods (the definition of amenorrhea). However, hypothalamic reproductive changes do occur during athletic training in both men and women. Factors associated with reproductive changes in women athletes will be reviewed briefly as a necessary background to subsequent treatment recommendations.

The first factor that often affects the reproductive system of athletes is immaturity. Athletes are usually young and have started some sort of exercise program at, or prior to, menarche. Reproductive changes occur in most normal young women during the process of maturation. In a population of nonexercising young women, regular menstrual cycles of normal luteal length usually do not occur for 10 years after the first menstrual flow. It is not unexpected, then, that cycle irregularity and lack of normal ovulation are present and more prevalent in *exercising* teenagers. For example, 79 percent of teenage entrants to an Australian professional ballet school experienced changes in their menstrual cycle.

The second factor causing reproductive change in the athlete is exercise itself. Prospective studies of women with normal ovulatory cycles show changes with increasing exercise. Before any menstrual cycle changes occur, premenstrual breast and fluid symptoms decrease. With increasing exercise, the menstrual cycle changes to short luteal phase cycles (less than 10 days from egg release until the start of the next period) and to anovulatory cycles (cycles with no egg release). These exercising women have no weight loss and maintain normal menstrual cycle intervals (21 to 36 days).

The characteristic pattern of menstrual cycle alteration with exercise shows changes developing during the initial or any subsequent *intensification* of exercise. Acute increases in exercise intensity and duration are more likely to change the menstrual cycle than slow or gradual ones. Once an increase in activity level is stabilized, the menstrual cycle returns to normal. Neuroendocrine studies suggest that the reproductive adaptation to exercise takes place in the hypothalamus.

Weight loss (with or without low body fat) is the third contributor to reproductive change in the athlete. Because all aerobic training programs demand energy expenditure, and since some sports require low body mass for performance (long distance running, broad jump) or for aesthetic reasons (ballet, gymnastics), loss of weight is common during training. It is difficult to separate the effects of weight change from those related to exercise per se. The best example of the effect of weight loss is a prospective training study of sedentary college-age women who ran 16 km (10 miles) per day by the second exercise cycle. One of 12 women (6 percent) randomized to a weight maintenance program had delayed menstrual flow, in contrast to 12 of 16 women (75 percent) in the weight loss program who ran the same distance.

Emotional stress is the final factor that may alter reproduction and is also associated with exercise. Since humans cannot be experimentally subjected to major psychological stress, there are few prospective data quantitatively relating emotions to reproductive change. One study showed that menstrual cycle patterns of women away from home differed from those still living with their parents. In another study, students had more changes in the luteal phase during the nursing school academic year than during the summer break. Athletes are often away from home for training, coaching, or competition. Racing is stressful. So is dealing with coaching or sporting authorities. Added worries about athletic success, school, or money may also concern most athletes.

In summary, at least four factors often work together in the athlete to cause reproductive changes. The young age at which many athletes begin training may delay the normal maturation of the reproductive system. Exercise, by itself, both acutely and chronically, can produce changes in neurotransmitters and subsequently in hormones and reproduction. The final two factors commonly associated with athletic endeavor are weight loss and emotional stress. The approach to treatment of the athlete with reproductive alteration follows from the above understanding of the causes of these changes and the control of reproduction.

This approach to therapy for reproductive change in the athlete also assumes that barrier methods of contraception, which will not further suppress reproduction, can and will be used. A list of contraceptive options for the athlete and their respective virtues is shown in Table 1.

INITIAL TREATMENT PHASE: STABILIZATION

It follows very logically that the first approach to treatment of athletes is to search for and identify the contributing factors. It is important to know the age and maturity of the athletes at the time when intensive training was begun. It is necessary to understand the pattern of training, how rapidly exercise intensity was increased, and whether weight loss also occurred. Finally, the person treating athletes

TABLE 1 Options for Contraception for the Athlete

Methods	*Positive Effects*	*Negative Effects*
Oral contraceptives	Decreased negative bone balance Predictable cycles Decreased risk of breast or endometrial cancer Less dysmenorrhea	Increased risk of thrombosis (heart attack and stroke) Suppression of hypothalamic system Tendency to increase % fat Lowering of maximal aerobic performance
Barrier methods plus contraceptive jelly	No suppression of hypothalamic system No side effects	May be inconvenient
IUD	No suppression of hypothalamus	Risk of pelvic infection Menometrorrhagia Dysmenorrhea
Rhythm	No suppression of hypothalamus	Increased risk of pregnancy
Abstinence	?	?

Republished with permission from Prior JC, Vigna Y. Gonadal steroids in athletic women. Contraception, complications and performance. Sports Med 1985; 2:287–295.

must understand them well enough for the emotional impact of recent life events (including athletic endeavor) to become clear.

Athletes will be taught how youth, exercise, weight loss, and emotional stress may work together to cause adaptive reproductive system changes. They learn to record exercise, weight, and reproductive change (with tools such as the daily symptom diary and basal temperature record) so that they are active participants in the therapy. A scheme for treatment is shown in Figure 1.

Obviously, if an amenorrheic woman is sexually active, pregnancy must be excluded. If a young woman is 16 years old and has never had a menstrual flow (primary amenorrhea), an ovarian cause for lack of flow (premature ovarian failure) can be excluded by a normal serum follicle-stimulating hormone (FSH) level. With the above two exceptions, no other hormonal evaluations need be made initially.

Stabilization of the exercise program is the first and often the only necessary therapy. The training need not be stopped; it must simply be kept at the same or a slightly lower level of intensity for approximately 3 months. Weight gain of 1 to 2 kg often takes place when the training level is no longer increasing. If not, restoration of excess weight loss can be encouraged by asking athletes to eat one or two additional servings per day of complex carbohydrate foods such as cereals, rice, or pasta.

SECOND PHASE: EVALUATION AND COUNSELING

After 3 months of stable exercise, the athlete's records show the success of exercise stabilization and weight gain. Often the first period has occurred or the first ovulation (as indicated by premenstrual breast enlargement or tenderness with or without fluid symptoms). Ovulatory cycles can be confirmed by a progesterone level in the week before the flow of 5 ng per deciliter, or 19 nmol per liter.

If there have been no signs of hormonal recovery, two possibilities exist: (1) the exercise-nutrition changes did not happen or (2) some additional suppressors of reproduction, unrelated to exercise, are present. If the exercise has not been modified, or if more weight loss has occurred, athletes may fear decreased performance, may be afraid of becoming fat, or may worry about losing control if they make the suggested changes.

If the exercise is stabilized and some weight has been regained, but no recovery of the reproductive system is present, a low or normal serum prolactin level must be demonstrated to exclude a prolactin-producing pituitary tumor. Also, signs of androgen excess such as increased acne and facial hair may indicate that increases in testosterone are interfering with normal reproduction. If signs of androgen excess are present and/or the testosterone level is above normal, spironolactone (a mild diuretic with antiandrogenic properties) may be prescribed. The usual dose is 100 to 200 mg per day. The drug eliminates acne in 1 to 3 months and excess hair in 1 to 3 years. It has no nonallergic side effects when prescribed in conjunction with cyclic medroxyprogesterone (Provera) taken 10 mg per day during days 16 to 25 of the menstrual cycle (assuming the first day of flow is day 1) or for 10 days per month if no flow appears.

Emotional stress is the most common block to reproductive recovery. Anorexia must be ruled out. If present, it must be treated with behavioral psychological methods. The lack of physiologic maturation and the total emotional commitment to sport may create fear of adulthood and the unknown nonsporting world. Consistent, positive, and patient support is necessary before recovery can occur, no matter how much the exercise is reduced or how much weight is gained.

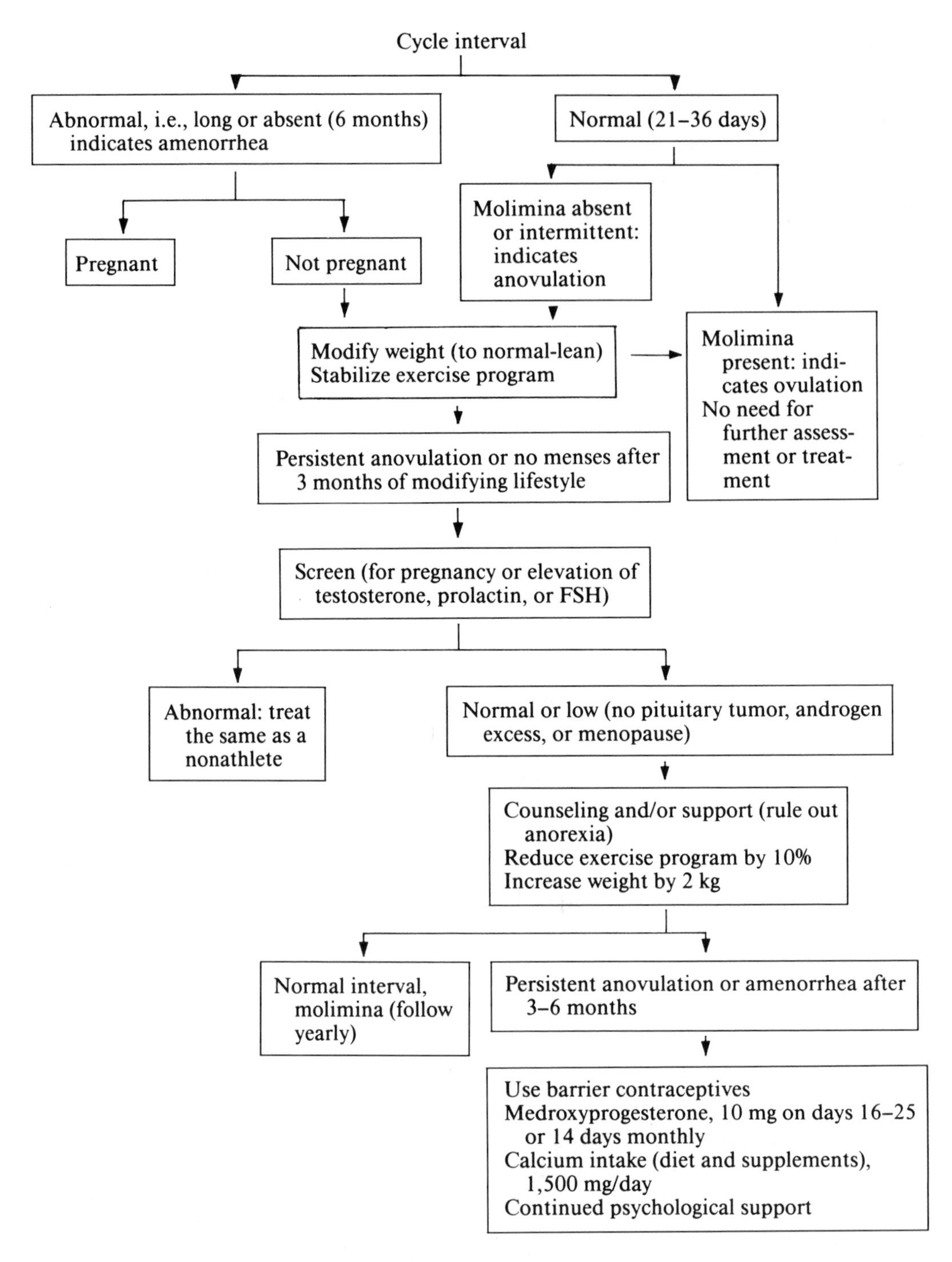

Figure 1 A stepwise therapeutic approach to reproductive changes in athletic women. (From Prior JC. Exercise in women. Med N America, Fall 1987, 16–23. Reprinted with permission.)

THIRD PHASE: TREATMENT

If it appears that the reproductive changes have persisted for years and that they will not readily recover with the aforementioned steps, some intervention may be needed.

Bone loss and risk of osteoporosis are the most serious concerns. An epidemiologic study of women who were active in college sports compared with matched college alumnae who were not does not suggest that the active women had more fractures after age 45 than their controls. It is prudent, however, to assess the spinal bone mineral (using dual photon absorptiometry or some other low-radiation, quantitative method rather than x-ray) if an athlete has had no periods, infrequent periods, or lack of ovulation for more than 2 years.

Treatment to prevent (further) bone loss includes a diet that maintains a normal lean mass (probably more than 5 kilojoules [1,200 calories] per day) and has adequate calcium (more than 3 dairy servings a day or supplements to achieve 700 to 1,000 mg per day of elemental calcium), and administration of cyclic medroxyprogesterone, 10 mg per day during days 16 to 25 of the cycle or for 10 days per month. Preliminary data, now being tested in a double-blind clinical trial, suggest that this treatment will increase bone by approximately 8 percent in the first year.

Infertility can be approached in the same way as outlined above, except that no medications should be taken other than progesterone vaginal suppositories (25 mg twice a day during days 16 to 25 of the cycle) in place of medroxyprogesterone.

Irregular flow, heavy bleeding, or spotting are rare in athletic as opposed to nonathletic anovulatory women and risk of endometrial cancer are probably low. (Estrogen, as indicated by flow, in the absence of progesterone, is the endometrial cancer risk state.) Anovulatory cycles (as documented by lack of cyclic breast and fluid symptoms, a low premenstrual serum progesterone level, or both) and bleeding problems can be treated effectively by cyclic medroxyprogesterone, as described above. Vaginal dryness (which rarely is a problem except in women who have had years of amenorrhea) can be treated with lubricants before intercourse, or if severe with a small amount of estrogen cream applied with the fingertip to the mucosal-labial junction once or twice a week.

The treatment program just outlined differs from many other regimens for the athlete with reproductive change. If the full maturation of the hypothalamus is sought, if the exercise-related changes are known to be adaptive, and if no emotional problem is interfering with recovery, this approach works. It appears more logical to use this approach than to treat with suppressive doses of gonadal steroids or with the oral contraceptive pill (the purpose of which is to suppress ovulation). The full understanding and cooperation of the athlete herself determines the outcome of the program.

This treatment plan for the athlete with reproductive changes assumes that these changes are reversible and are caused by numerous factors in addition to exercise. Young age (and therefore reproductive immaturity), low nutritional reserves (decreased fat weight), intense emotional stress, changes in home environment, and high energy output (exercise training and competition) often occur in the athlete. Together, these factors produce the reproductive changes that have been attributed to exercise.

When therapy appears appropriate, cyclic medroxyprogesterone, 10 mg per day for 10 days each month, may prevent bone loss and stimulate a return to cyclic menstruation. If amenorrhea has persisted for years, assessment of trabecular bone density (with dual photon absorptiometry) is indicated. Contraception for the athlete should not further suppress the central control of reproduction. Therefore, barrier methods, rather than the oral contraceptive pill, are preferable.

SUGGESTED READING

Abraham SF, Beaumont PJV, Fraser IS, Llwellyn-Jones D. Body weight, exercise and menstrual status among ballet dancers in training. Br J Obstet Gynecol 1982; 89:507–510.

Bullen BA, Skrinar GS, Beitins IZ, et al. Induction of menstrual disorders by strenuous exercise in untrained women. N Engl J Med 1985; 312:1349–1353.

Cumming DC, Yang JC, Rebar RW, Yen SSC. Treatment of hirsutism with spironolactone. JAMA 1982; 247:1295–1298.

Metcalf MG, Skidmore OS, Lowry GF, Mackenzie JA. Incidence of ovulation in the years after menarche. J Endocrinol 1983; 97:213–219.

Nagata I, Kato K, Seki K, Furuya K. Ovulatory disturbances. J Adolesc Health Care 1986; 7:1–5.

Prior JC. Exercise in women. Med N America, Fall, 1987, 16–23.

Prior JC. Medroxyprogesterone increases trabecular bone density in women with menstrual disorders. Endocrine Society (abstr), 1987. 69th Annual Abstracts and Program, No. 560.

Prior JC. Physical exercise and the neuroendocrine control of reproduction. Baillieres Clin Endocrinol Metab 1987; 1:299–317.

Prior JC, Cameron K, Ho Yuen B, Thomas J. Menstrual cycle changes with marathon training: anovulation and short luteal phase. Can J Appl Sport Sci 1982; 7:173–177.

Prior JC, Ho Yuen B, Clement P, Bowie L, Thomas J. Reversible luteal phase changes and infertility associated with marathon training. Lancet 1982; 1:209–270.

Prior JC, Vigna Y. Gonadal steroids in athletic women. Contraception, complications and performance. Sports Med 1985; 2:287–295.

Prior JC, Vigna Y, Sciarretta D, Alojado N, Schulzer M. Conditioning exercise decreases premenstrual symptoms: a prospective, controlled 6-month trial. Fertil Steril 1987; 47:402–408.

Vollman RF. Major problems in obstetrics and gynecology. Vol 7. 1977:121.

Wyshak G, Frisch RE, Albright TE, Albright NL, Schiff I. Bone fractures among former college athletes compared with nonathletes in the menopausal and post-menopausal years. Obstet Gynecol 1987; 69:121–126.

EXERCISE IN GROWING AND ADULT OBESE INDIVIDUALS

JANA PAŘÍZKOVÁ, M.D., D.Sc.
VOJTĚCH HAINER, M.D., Ph.D.

The prevalence of obesity varies considerably with age. Studies in Czechoslovakia have shown that obesity is relatively rare in children of preschool age compared with those of younger school age and adolescents; its frequency becomes high in adults, but decreases again in those of advanced age. International comparisons of the frequency of obesity in the various age categories have been difficult up to now, because the criteria for obesity have not yet been precisely defined. The Royal College of Physicians and the World Health Organization have agreed inter alia on the introduction of the body mass index* and of the waist-to-hip ratio, in addition to other somatic indices such as the thickness of triceps and biceps skinfolds, as simple and generally acceptable measures of obesity. Nevertheless, the percentage of depot fat remains the main characteristic used in the diagnosis of obesity, which may be defined as an excessive accumulation of fat relative to muscle mass.

Clinical studies in the Czechoslovakian population have shown that simple obesity without primary hormonal or metabolic deviations is the most frequently encountered type of obesity. Overeating, a low level of habitual activity, and a resultant energy imbalance, along with a genetic predisposition, seem to play the essential role in the pathogenesis of this type of obesity.

In preschool children the level of spontaneous physical activity is usually very high. In a longitudinal pedometer study, preschool children covered a distance of 98 km in 1 week, but after entering primary school, the same children covered an average weekly distance of only 52 km. This reduction of physical activity was observed not only on weekdays, but also during weekends. The increased prevalence of obesity in school-age children can be attributed in part to this decrease of physical activity.

Measurements made in 5,092 boys and girls before they entered primary school (average age 6.4 years) showed that about 3 percent were overweight and obese, while 4 to 5 percent were underweight and lean, relative to growth grids for the Czechoslovakian population. The body mass index of obese boys and girls averaged slightly over 20, compared with the standard value of 15 for this age and the figure of 12 to 13 observed in underweight children. The circumferences of the arms, chest, abdomen, and thighs were significantly higher in the obese children. As regards physical performance, only the standing broad jump was shorter in obese than in nonobese children. The dynamic performance, as evaluated by a 20-m dash and skill tests, was the same in all preschool children, whether normal, overweight, or underweight.

The prevalence of obesity among the *younger school-age and adolescent children* of Czechoslovakia is estimated at 10 to 15 percent, relative to the growth grids mentioned above. Obesity at this age is characterized by a significant change of body composition; not only is there an excessive deposition of body fat, but there is also an increase in the absolute lean body mass. However, one commonly used clinical index of muscle mass, the creatinine coefficient, is lower in the obese. Aerobic power, as expressed by the maximal oxygen intake ($\dot{V}O_2max$ [$ml \cdot kg^{-1} \cdot min^{-1}$]) is also low in obese children and adolescents. On the other hand, the oxygen cost of submaximal workload $\dot{V}O_2$ ($ml \cdot kg^{-1} \cdot min^{-1}$) is higher than in normal or asthenic children, with a lower mechanical efficiency, especially when the workload includes the transfer of the child's own body mass. The results of physical performance tests are mostly poorer in the obese child, with the exception of measures of muscle strength. In adolescents, also, primary hormonal disturbances are extremely rare, indicating that overeating and lack of exercise are the main causes of obesity at this age.

REDUCING THERAPY

A reduction of food intake (to about 4,200 kJ per day) decreased body mass and body fat content in obese children, but at the same time the growth in stature was slowed. Therefore, a combination of an exercise-induced increase of energy output along with a monitoring of diet was adopted as therapy. Children aged 8 to 15 years with milder degrees of obesity were treated in an outpatient department for obese children and during summer camps that lasted for 7 weeks. The diet provided 7,100 kJ per day, with a reduced proportion of fats and carbohydrates, 1.5 liters of all liquids (only pure water was freely available), and an increased intake of fiber. The main component of therapy was a program of organized exercise, supervised by physical education instructors. Gymnastics, track-and-field disciplines, swimming, and suitable sport games were included in a daily program for 6 hours per day. Touristic excursions were made at least once a week; walks of 1½ to 2 hours duration were required after dinner every day. When the children claimed fatigue, dancing was substituted; this was always accepted with great enthusiasm.

After 7 weeks of attendance at the summer camps, children lost 11 to 14 percent of their initial

---

* Body mass index (BMI) = $\frac{\text{weight kg}}{\text{height m}^2}$.

body mass; densitometry indicated that this was largely due to a reduction of excess fat. In this selected subgroup of boys who were 10 to 12 years old, significant reduction of body mass, BMI, and body fat were accompanied by an increased percentage of lean body mass, despite a slight reduction in its absolute amount. The absolute body fat content decreased by an average of 25 to 28 percent of the initial value. The $\dot{V}O_2max$ ($ml \cdot kg^{-1} \cdot min^{-1}$) was increased significantly (Table 1), being achieved after a longer duration and higher velocity of treadmill running (before weight reduction: maximal velocity 11.21 ± 0.48 km per hour, duration 3.42 ± 0.34 minute; after weight reduction: maximal velocity 11.78 ± 0.63 km per hour, duration 4.57 ± 0.78 minute).

Another longitudinal study of obese boys and girls attending a summer therapeutic camp showed that the reduction of body mass, BMI, and depot fat was linked to an improvement of functional indices, with a decrease of $\dot{V}O_2$ ($ml \cdot kg^{-1} \cdot min^{-1}$) when performing a fixed submaximal workload on a cycle ergometer (one-sixth of the maximal work rate; Table 2). The economy of work is improved and the mechanical efficiency is increased after the trimming of excessive body fat by exercise. This facilitates an increase of spontaneous physical activity, which is generally low in obese children. This is due, inter alia, to the greater strain that exercise imposes upon these children. Vital capacity and physical performance test scores also improved as obesity was corrected. The serum cholesterol decreased significantly in boys, as well as the concentration of free fatty acids (FFA). The reaction of FFA to maximal work indicates that their release and utilization during muscular work was enhanced after the period of adaptation to an increased work rate and weight loss.

TABLE 1 Changes of Body Composition, Body Mass Index (BMI), and Aerobic Power in Seven Obese Boys Before and After Exercise Reducing Therapy

Reduction Therapy	*Before*		*After*	
	$\bar{x}$	*SD*	$\bar{x}$	*SD*
Height (cm)	153.7	5.3	153.9	5.3*
Body mass (kg)	57.3	5.3	50.7	4.7*
Body mass index	24.2	1.2	21.4	1.2*
Fat (%)	30.1	2.4	24.2	3.4*
$\dot{V}O_2max$ ($ml \cdot kg^{-1} \cdot min^{-1}$)	38.8	3.2	40.7	3.4*

*$p < 0.001$.

For more severe cases of childhood obesity, complex spa therapy was organized. Children aged 8 to 15 years attended the spa for 2 months and frequented its school. Their food intake with the exception of proteins was reduced by about 25 to 33 percent relative to the recommended dietary allowances (RDA) for a given age group, never exceeding 7,530 kJ per day. Exercise therapy was adjusted according to the degree of obesity. At the beginning of treatment the children exercised only while lying on the back or abdomen, or in a sitting position. At first, only very easy gymnastic exercises were applied, but gradually more demanding ones were introduced with the aim of strengthening the muscles of the abdomen, back, and buttocks. Adequate breathing was also encouraged. Various individually prescribed exercises in the standing position were later introduced for a limited period, so as not to overload the lower extremities. Exercises to correct body posture and flat feet were also prescribed. Children exercised in small groups of six to eight, two to three times per day, for sessions of 10 to 15 minutes. As therapy continued, some track-and-field disciplines and sport games were introduced, along with walks of up to 6 km per day. Twice a week the children exercised in a hyperthermic swimming pool, and once a week they swam and exercised in a pool heated to 27° C.

The above-mentioned spa therapy resulted in a weight loss of about 10 to 12 percent of the initial value, and the absolute amount of depot fat decreased significantly by 28 to 30 percent.* Vital capacity increased, and scores for the Kraus-Weber test improved significantly. The creatinine index showed a significant increase in a subsample of both boys (n = 32, before weight reduction 16.17 ± 4.04,

* Calculated from 10 skinfolds.

TABLE 2 Changes of Body Composition and Functional Indices in Obese Boys and Girls Before and After Exercise Reducing Therapy

Reduction Therapy	*Boys (n = 18)*				*Girls (n = 15)*			
	Before		*After*		*Before*		*After*	
	$\bar{x}$	*SE*	$\bar{x}$	*SE*	$\bar{x}$	*SE*	$\bar{x}$	*SE*
Body mass (kg)	65.8	3.3	58.5	2.8	70.3	2.9	63.1	2.4
Body mass index	27.7	1.3	23.8	1.4	28.9	1.2	25.7	1.2
Fat (%)	31.4	2.4	25.2	2.1	31.9	3.1	27.1	3.2
$\dot{V}O_2$ ($ml \cdot kgBM^{-1} \cdot min^{-1}$)	11.6	0.2	9.7	0.4	10.2	2.0	9.7	2.0
$\dot{V}O_2$ ($ml \cdot kgLBM^{-1} \cdot min^{-1}$)	17.2	0.3	12.9	0.06	15.4	1.0	13.3	0.2
Vital capacity (L)	2.94	0.11	3.07	0.12	2.64	0.12	2.83	0.13

All differences significant—$p < 0.001$.
BM = body mass, LBM = lean body mass.

after 19.98 ± 4.25) and girls (n = 50, before 15.62 ± 3.57, after 18.19 ± 4.38). The arm muscle circumferences also increased significantly in all children. Along with that, the overall body posture and foot arch posture improved after reduction of body mass.

Generally, treatment in both summer camps and spa proved to be beneficial; results were always better in boys than in girls, which may reflect natural pubertal trends for the development of functional capacity and fatness, respectively. The preservation of the beneficial results of treatment varied individually, apparently depending on the regularity with which children attended the outpatient department for obese children over the school year. The motivation of the children and their parents was a decisive factor guaranteeing positive morphologic, functional, biochemical, metabolic, and psychological consequences of the exercise therapy.

Clinical studies of adult obesity show differences in response to reducing therapy, depending on the distribution of subcutaneous fat. In simple obesity the distribution of subcutaneous fat (expressed by the ratio of the sum of skinfolds on the trunk to that on the extremities) is the same as in normal women; this type of obesity is easier to treat than the "spider-like" form, in which disproportionately more fat is deposited on the trunk, and some metabolic disturbances occur.

A complex regimen for adults with gross uncomplicated obesity was developed by the VIth Medical Department of the Medical School, Charles University. A formula diet of 1,555 kJ per day (Table 3) is combined with a regimen of regular exercise. The latter includes 30-min sessions of aerobic gymnastics, 15-min bouts of cycling on a cycle ergometer three times per day (with individual modifications), and 2 hours of walking at an intensity sufficient to increase the heart rate up to 130 beats per minute. Obese patients spent 4 weeks in the obesity unit and lost 9 to 10 percent of their initial body mass. There were significant sex-linked differences in morphologic indices both before and after reduction therapy: height, body mass, BMI, and waist-to-hip ratio were all significantly higher in men, despite the fact that the percentage of fat* and the thickness of the triceps skinfold were significantly greater in women. Only the subscapular skinfold did not differ between the two sexes (Table 4).

TABLE 3 Composition of Low-Energy Diet (Dairy Research Institute, Prague)

Protein	36.0 g
Carbohydrate	50.0 g
Fat	3.0 g
Fiber	5.6 g
Energy content	1,555 kJ (372 kcal)
Vitamins	recommended daily allowance
Sodium	39.1 mmol
Potassium	48.6 mmol
Chloride	56.4 mmol
Calcium	31.0 mmol
Phosphorus	32.3 mmol
Magnesium	14.4 mmol

After participation in reducing therapy, body mass, BMI, the percentage of depot fat and the thickness of individual skinfolds all decreased significantly. However, the waist-to-hip ratio did not change. The absolute amount of body fat decreased by 18 to 23 percent, but most patients remained overweight (see Table 4). The estimation of body composition from skinfold readings indicated, much as did densitometry in massively obese children, that the loss of body fat was accompanied by some loss of lean body mass. This conclusion was supported by the finding of a decrease in resting metabolic rate (RMR) in both sexes (average before reduction of body mass 5.45 ± 1.13 kJ per minute, after 4.44 ± 1.38 kJ per minute, $p < 0.01$). The nitrogen balance measured in 32 patients was negative only at the beginning of therapy; during the last week it again became positive (Table 5).

The absence of stressful side effects from the prescribed regimen was shown by a lack of change in cortisol, growth hormone (GH), and prolactin concentrations (PRL—measured by usual procedures including radioimmunoassay) during treatment at

* Calculated from 10 skinfolds.

TABLE 4 Morphological Data Before and After Treatment of the Obese

	Females (n = 28)				*Males (n = 12)*			
	Before		*After*		*Before*		*After*	
	$\bar{x}$	*SD*	$\bar{x}$	*SD*	$\bar{x}$	*SD*	$\bar{x}$	*SD*
Age (yr)	38.9	7.3	—	—	36.6	11.9	—	—
Height (cm)	166.0	7.7	—	—	174.3	5.3	—	—
Body mass (kg)	102.0	15.5	92.3	15.0*	126.5	17.0	115.2	13.3*
Body mass index	37.0	4.5	33.4	4.2*	41.9	7.8	38.3	7.8*
Fat (%)	34.9*	3.2	30.5	3.4*	28.9	2.3	26.1	2.8*
Skinfolds*								
Triceps (mm)	31.7	9.4	24.5	6.5*	22.5	11.0	17.6	8.3*
Subscapular	40.6	9.4	31.3	9.1*	43.7	11.6	34.4	11.9*
Waist/hip ratio	0.87	0.07	0.86	0.07	1.03	0.06	1.03	0.07

* Measured by modified Best caliper (Pařízková, 1977). The Harpenden caliper cannot be used in extremely obese patients.

TABLE 5 "Catabolic" Nitrogen Excretion During Reducing Therapy in 32 Obese Patients

	Days of Treatment				
	1	*7*	*14*	*21*	*28*
Catabolic N (g/24 hr)					
$\bar{x}$	11.6	11.7	12.4	6.3*	5.1†
SD	6.2	7.3	10.1	4.3	3.1
Nitrogen balance (g/24 hr)	−5.84	−5.95	−6.68	−0.51	+0.69

* $p < 0.01$ (vs. day "1").
† $p < 0.001$ (vs. day "1").

the obesity unit. A statistically insignificant decline of serum cortisol concentrations observed at the end of therapy may have helped to prevent protein loss with adaptation to the prescribed regimen. Serum concentrations of thyroxine (T_4) and thyroid-stimulating hormone (TSH) did not change; however, triiodothyronine (T_3) decreased slightly but significantly (Table 6). The reduction of RMR, although higher than expected on the basis of weight loss, cannot be attributed to a low T_3 syndrome; the decrease was too small (up to 17 percent) and was not accompanied by any simultaneous decline in a peripheral index of thyroid function (the Achilles tendon reflex time). The daily consumption of 50 g of carbohydrates may have helped to prevent a more marked fall in T_3 production. Therefore, the decrease of RMR should be attributed to other energy-sparing mechanisms, including a decrease of beta-adrenergic and dopaminergic activity. Administration of theophylline derivatives with thermogenic properties prevented the fall of RMR during the second part of the weight reduction regimen. Physical activity may have counterbalanced the energy-conserving metabolic adaptation to dieting in our patients. There were no significant changes of serum testosterone concentration, although there was some tendency to a moderate rise during the fourth week of the reducing therapy.

Weight reduction also had a beneficial influence on arterial blood pressure; both systolic and diastolic pressures decreased significantly in all obese patients after reduction of their body mass (Table 7). The decrease was especially marked in those patients who were originally hypertensive (average systolic readings before 162.1 ± 11.5, after 131.1 ± 9.7 mm Hg; diastolic readings before 102.5 ± 3.6, after 88.6 ± 9.0 mm Hg, $p < 0.001$). The concentrations of serum cholesterol and triacylglycerols were significantly reduced after weight loss, while high density lipoprotein (HDL) cholesterol and the ratio of HDL cholesterol to total cholesterol were unaffected (see Table 7). Blood glucose concentrations decreased only slightly (before 5.24 ± 2.0, after weight reduction 4.68 ± 1.8 mmol per liter).

TABLE 6 Serum Concentrations of Selected Hormones Before and After Reducing Therapy in 32 Obese Patients

	Before Therapy		After Therapy	
Hormone	$\bar{x}$	*SD*	$\bar{x}$	*SD*
Cortisol (nmol/L)	432	249	325	247
GH (mU/L)	1.42	0.94	1.35	1.66
PRL (mU/L)	415	344	538	464
T_4 (nmol/L)	136	27	125	32
T_3 (nmol/L)	1.73	0.61	1.45	0.33
TSH (mU/L)	2.50	1.55	3.20	2.05*
IRI (mU/L)	17.3	2.0	10.5	5.6*
Urinary G-peptide (μg/24 hr)	28.1	24.8	12.1	14.2

* $p < 0.05$.

TABLE 7 Blood Pressures and Blood Lipid Levels of 40 Obese Patients Before and After Reducing Therapy

	Before Therapy		After Therapy	
Variable	$\bar{x}$	*SD*	$\bar{x}$	*SD*
Systolic pressure (mm Hg)	143	16	126	11*
Diastolic pressure (mm Hg)	89	9	82	9†
Total cholesterol (TC) (mmol/L)	6.11	1.55	5.07	1.44‡
HDL cholesterol	1.43	0.27	1.33	0.33
HDL-C/TC ratio	0.245	0.07	0.279	0.11
Triacylglycerols (mmol/L)	2.04	1.55	1.36	0.61‡

* $p < 0.001$.
† $p < 0.001$.
‡ $p < 0.05$.

After termination of treatment in the obesity unit, patients were regularly followed up once a month in groups of six to nine individuals. Measurements of body mass and waist-to-hip ratio along with psychological interventions fostered competition in conserving weight reduction, while allowing an exchange of individual experiences of dieting, exercise, and a general change of lifestyle. A study in 91 obese patients who had reduced their body weight by 4-week intermittent periods of starvation showed a clear relationship between the regularity of such check-ups and the extent of weight decrements. Moderately obese women were successfully treated by an 18-day program of diet and exercise in recreational centers, supervised by medical doctors and qualified physical education instructors.

At any age, a combination of exercise therapy with an adequately reduced diet monitored by outpatient departments, medically supervised summer camps or spas, and obesity clinics and centers is effective and beneficial. However, therapy is more difficult and the results are less permanent in older patients with more severe obesity. Some massively obese adults were able to restore a part of their weight even during the clinical therapy, indicating a rapid adaptation to the reduced energy intake and the exercise-induced increase of energy output, which in their case could not be of sufficient intensity to counter metabolic changes. Exercise tolerance also decreases with increasing age and fatness. Therefore, early prevention of obesity by weight watching and physical fitness development from early childhood remain the main preventive measures against both obesity and accompanying health problems.

SUGGESTED READING

Epstein LH, Wing RR, Koeske R, Valoski A. Effects of diet plus exercise on weight change in parents and children. J Consult Clin Psychol 1984; 52:429–437.

Hainer V, Kunešová M, Pařízková J, et al. Low energy diet in the treatment of obesity. Čs Gastroenterol, in press, 1988.

Hainer V, Šonka J, Kunešová M, et al. Low energy diet and physical exercise in the treatment of obesity (in Czech). Čas Lék Čes, in press, 1988.

Hainer V, Žák A, Malec B, et al. The effect of weight reduction on the hypothalamohypophyseal function and serum lipids level in obese patients (in Czech). Čas Lék Čes 1982; 121:837–843.

Hejda S, Ošancová K. Problems in a country with a high prevalence of obesity. Proceedings of 26th Symposium of the Group of European Nutritionists, Bibliotheca Nutr Dieta. Basel: S Karger, in press.

Malkovská M, Čeněk A, Růžičková H. The importance of physical exercise in reduction therapy of obese children in spa (in Czech). Rehabilitácia 1973; 6:147–159.

Pařízková J. Total body fat and skinfold thickness in children. Metabolism, 1961; 10:794–807.

Pařízková J. Body fat and physical fitness. The Hague: Martinus Nijhoff BV/Medical Division, 1977.

Pařízková J. Physical training in weight reduction of obese adolescents. Ann Clin Res 1982; (14 Suppl) 34:63–68.

Pařízková J, Adamec A, Berdychová J, et al. Growth, fitness and nutrition in preschool children. Prague: Charles University, 1984.

Prokopec M. The trend of development of children population in ČSR over the last 30 years (in Czech). Čsl Hygiena 1986; 31:541–557.

Royal College of Physicians: Obesity. A report of the Royal College of Physicians. JR Coll Phys 1983; 17:1–58.

Skamenová B, Pařízková J. Assessment of disproportional (spider-like) and diffuse type of obesity by measurement of the total and subcutaneous body fat (in Czech). Čas Lék Čes 1963; 102:142–146.

Šonka J. New trends in obesitology. Prague: Acta Univ Carol Med, in press, 1988.

Spaulding SW, Chopra IJ, Sherwin RS, Lyall SS. Effect of caloric restriction and dietary composition on serum T_3 and reverse T_3 in man. J Clin Endocrinol Metab 1976; 42:197–200.

Šprynarová Š, Pařízková J. Changes in the aerobic capacity and body composition in obese boys after reduction. J Appl Physiol 1965; 20:934–937.

Talbot NB. Measurement of obesity by the creatinine coefficient. J Dis Child 1938; 55:42–50.

Tremblay A, Fontaine E, Poehlman ET, et al. The effect of exercise training on resting metabolic rate in lean and moderately obese individuals. Int J Obes 1986; 10:511–517.

World Health Organization. Energy and protein requirements. Report of a Joint FAO/WHO/UNU Expert Consultation. Tech Rep Ser 724. Geneva, 1985.

World Health Organization. Consultation on the epidemiology of obesity. Warsaw, 21–23 October, 1987. Regional Office for Europe, World Health Organization.

EXERCISE IN CYSTIC FIBROSIS

DAVID M. ORENSTEIN, M.D.
PATRICIA A. NIXON, Ph.D.

Cystic fibrosis (CF) is the most common life-shortening inherited disease in white populations, occurring in approximately one of 2,000 live births. Although there is no cure for the disease, advances in treatment have increased the median age of survival from 10.6 years in 1966 to 26.5 years in 1986. The basic defect in CF seems to be related to the inability of the chloride ion to pass through various epithelia. This defect in turn leads to the production of sweat that is very high in chloride and sodium, and mucus that is abnormally thick and viscous. In the pancreas the mucus blocks the ducts, leading to maldigestion, malabsorption, and malnutrition. In the lungs the mucus causes bronchiolar obstruction, which in the absence of treatment leads to infection and eventually fibrosis, with a progressive loss of pulmonary function. It is the pulmonary involvement that accounts for more than 90 percent of the morbidity and mortality.

Treatment is directed at both digestive and respiratory problems. The digestion of dietary fats and proteins is enhanced with pancreatic enzyme supplements. Antibiotics are prescribed to fight pulmonary bacterial infection, and various physical means, such as chest physical therapy and postural drainage, are employed to prevent or relieve bronchiolar obstruction.

Exercise intolerance and exertional dyspnea are common complaints of patients with CF, and such complaints worsen as the disease progresses. In general, exercise tolerance is directly related to pulmonary function. Patients with mild lung disease have better exercise tolerance than those with severe disease. Although this relationship holds true for groups of patients, it is not possible to predict exercise tolerance for an individual from the results of pulmonary function tests. For example, as shown in Figure 1, disease severity (indicated by the ratio of residual volume to total lung capacity [RV/TLC]), is directly and significantly related to exercise tolerance (measured by peak oxygen intake [$\dot{V}O_2$]) for the total group. However, the variability in peak $\dot{V}O_2$ among individuals with a given RV/TLC ratio is quite wide.

Exercise intolerance appears to be related to ventilatory rather than cardiac limitations. Patients with CF meet the increased metabolic demands of exercise by employing a large respiratory minute ventilation ($\dot{V}_E$) to compensate for an increased dead space. In people with normal lungs, the $\dot{V}_E$ during exhaustive work seldom exceeds 60 to 70 percent of maximal voluntary ventilation (MVV). However, in patients with CF, the $\dot{V}_E$ during maximal exercise may approach or even exceed the resting MVV, which suggests that all of the ventilatory capacity is employed, leaving no reserve. The exaggerated $\dot{V}_E$ may further impair exercise performance by requiring oxygen to be shunted away from exercising muscles to ventilatory muscles in order to meet the increased metabolic cost of breathing.

In most patients with CF, proper gas exchange is maintained by increased $\dot{V}_E$ and improved ventilation-perfusion ($\dot{V}/\dot{Q}$) matching. However, some patients with severe disease may be unable to maintain $\dot{V}/\dot{Q}$ or adequate alveolar ventilation, and they develop oxyhemoglobin desaturation and carbon dioxide retention. Some patients experience oxyhemoglobin desaturation without carbon dioxide retention, presumably because of altered $\dot{V}/\dot{Q}$ matching. Whether oxyhemoglobin desaturation itself limits exercise tolerance is not known.

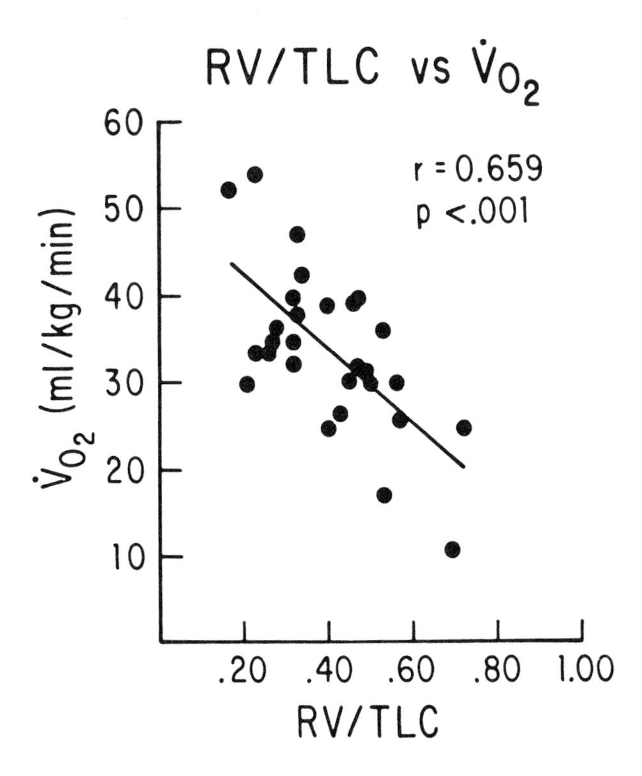

Figure 1 Peak oxygen uptake ($\dot{V}O_2$) plotted against residual volume (RV) divided by total lung capacity (TLC) for 28 patients with cystic fibrosis. Higher RV/TLC ratios indicate greater air trapping, and therefore represent worse bronchiolar obstruction.

Cardiovascular factors do not appear to limit exercise capacity in most patients with CF. Most patients can reach age-predicted levels of maximal heart rate, with a normal cardiac output. However, in sicker individuals, an impaired ventilatory capacity may limit exercise before the cardiovascular system is maximally stressed, resulting in a peak m heart rate that is below age-predicted levels. In some patients, radionuclide studies show evidence of right ventricular dysfunction and (more rarely) left ventricular dysfunction. For the most part, these cardiovascular limitations are less important than the ventilatory limitations in impairing exercise performance.

EXERCISE TESTING IN CYSTIC FIBROSIS

Exercise tests can provide important information about the patient's pulmonary function and reserve that cannot be obtained from standard pulmonary function tests. Specific objectives of exercise testing in CF include the following:

1. Evaluation of disease severity.
2. Measurement of aerobic fitness (peak oxygen intake) and functional exercise capacity.
3. Examination of cardiorespiratory responses to exercise.
4. Provision of a basis for prescribing exercise within safe limits.
5. Assessment of changes that occur with treatment intervention (e.g., medications, chest physical therapy, exercise training) or with progression of disease.

Safety Precautions

Exercise testing may not be indicated for all patients, particularly those at a late stage in the disease, with cor pulmonale and overt right ventricular failure.

Exercise testing during an acute pulmonary exacerbation may not be appropriate, depending on the objectives of testing. With an acute infection, the exercise tolerance is reduced and therefore not representative of the patient's "normal" exercise capacity. However, exercise testing during an infection provides specific information about the patient's current exercise tolerance, as well as the response to treatment of the infection.

Hundreds of patients with CF, including many with severe pulmonary involvement, have been tested with no untoward effects. Nevertheless, we recommend that standard safety precautions be observed. Testing should be conducted by personnel trained in cardiopulmonary resuscitation and emergency procedures. The laboratory should also be equipped with emergency equipment and drugs.

Maximal Incremental Tests

The particular testing protocol and the exercise device to be used (e.g., a treadmill or cycle ergometer) depend on the objectives of the tests as well as the experience and preference of the laboratory. Functional exercise capacity and aerobic fitness are best evaluated by a progressive maximal exercise test, such as the Godfrey protocol, which is performed on a cycle ergometer. The test starts at zero resistance and varying increments are applied each minute, depending on the person's height. The test ends when the patient can no longer maintain the prescribed pedaling frequency.

Protocols that adjust the work rate according to body mass may also be used.

With the maximal exercise test, it is important to verify that the patient has made a maximal effort. This verification can be made by examining the heart rate (HR), $\dot{V}_E$, and/or the respiratory exchange ratio ($\dot{V}co_2/\dot{V}o_2$) attained at the highest work rate. The peak HR should reach age-predicted maximal levels ($\pm$ 10 beats per minute), unless it is limited by ventilatory factors as reflected in a peak $\dot{V}_E$ that exceeds 70 percent of the resting MVV. The peak respiratory exchange ratio (RER) should exceed 1.1.

In rare cases, intolerable dyspnea may cause the patient to stop exercising before other variables reach maximal levels.

Maximal exercise tests are often very difficult for patients, who may experience hard coughing spells and shortness of breath. Sicker patients may be fatigued for hours after a maximal test. Discretion should thus be used to determine whether the information to be gained from a maximal effort warrants the fatigue and discomfort that will be suffered by the patient.

Observations to Be Made During the Test

During the exercise test, the following observations provide optimal information about the cardiorespiratory responses to exercise: power output, $\dot{V}_E$, $\dot{V}o_2$, carbon dioxide production ($\dot{V}co_2$), end-tidal carbon dioxide tension ($PetCO_2$), oxygen saturation (SaO_2), RER, and HR. The electrocardiogram (ECG) should be monitored continuously, and the blood pressure is also measured periodically throughout the test. Oxygen saturation should be monitored continuously and can be measured noninvasively, using an ear oximeter. If SaO_2 falls, the work intensity (HR) at which this occurs should be noted for use in prescribing safe exercise.

In the absence of metabolic equipment, the measurements of oxygen saturation, power output, blood pressure, and heart rate (with continuous monitoring of the ECG) can provide sufficient information about the patient's exercise tolerance.

Criteria for Terminating the Test

The exercise test should be terminated for any of the following reasons:

1. If the patient is unable to maintain the prescribed pedaling rate on the cycle ergometer, or is unable to keep up with the speed of the treadmill.
2. If the patient asks for the test to be terminated because of extreme discomfort of any kind.
3. If the oxygen saturation drops below 80 percent. (This criterion is precautionary; we have never observed any irreversible ill effects from short-term hypoxemia in this setting.)
4. If any life-threatening ECG abnormalities appear.
5. If the systolic blood pressure exceeds 250 mm Hg, or decreases, or fails to increase, with an increased power output.
6. If the diastolic blood pressure exceeds 120 mm Hg.

More detailed criteria for terminating an exercise test are presented in the American College of Sports Medicine's *Guidelines for Graded Exercise Testing and Exercise Prescription.* In our own experience with the CF population, most tests are terminated because a maximal effort has been reached. We have never been forced to stop a test because of cardiovascular abnormalities.

Interpretation of Test Results

Peak power output and oxygen intake are often normal in patients mildly affected with CF, but these values decrease substantially as the disease progresses. The trend for decreasing peak oxygen intake with progressive pulmonary deterioration is evident. Furthermore, as in the normal population, the peak oxygen intake of female patients is lower than that of male patients. A high $\dot{V}_E$ is commonly observed, the peak $\dot{V}_E$ approaching or even exceeding the MVV. The ventilatory equivalent for oxygen ($\dot{V}_E/\dot{V}o_2$) is often elevated, suggesting that $\dot{V}_E$ is increased primarily to compensate for increased dead space. The oxygen intake may be greater at any given submaximal work rate, owing to the added oxygen cost of breathing.

The peak heart rate may reach normal age-predicted levels (220 minus age in years) in patients with mild disease, but may drop well below age-predicted levels in severely affected patients. The heart rate at submaximal work rates is often higher than normal, because of deconditioning, hypoxemia, the increased work of breathing, or any combination of these factors.

Like most normal individuals, patients with CF are able to exercise beyond their anaerobic threshold, i.e., at power outputs in which the oxygen supply is insufficient to meet energy requirements, and aerobic metabolism must be supplemented by anaerobic metabolism. Therefore, the respiratory exchange ratio (RER = $\dot{V}CO_2/\dot{V}O_2$) reaches levels between 1.1 and 1.3 in most patients who exercise to the point of exhaustion.

In most patients with CF, normal arterial levels of oxygen and carbon dioxide are maintained throughout exercise. However, in patients with severely diminished pulmonary function, oxyhemoglobin desaturation may occur, with or without carbon dioxide retention. It is probably important to identify both these patients and the work rate and heart rate at which they desaturate. As demonstrated in Figure 2, patients with a 1-second forced expiratory volume (FEV_1) less than 50 percent of forced vital capacity (FVC) are more likely to exhibit oxygen desaturation than patients with an FEV_1 greater than 50 percent of FVC. However, even in patients with pronounced airway obstruction, it is clear that oxyhemoglobin saturation often stays the same or even increases with exercise.

Benefits of Exercise Training

Few well-controlled studies have addressed the effects of exercise training upon patients with CF. However, several published studies suggest that such patients may benefit from exercise training programs in several ways: (1) they can increase ventilatory muscle endurance; (2) they can become more fit, with a higher peak $\dot{V}O_2$ and a lower heart rate during submaximal work. It is unclear whether exercise programs can improve pulmonary function in patients with CF; some studies indicate improvement and others indicate no change.

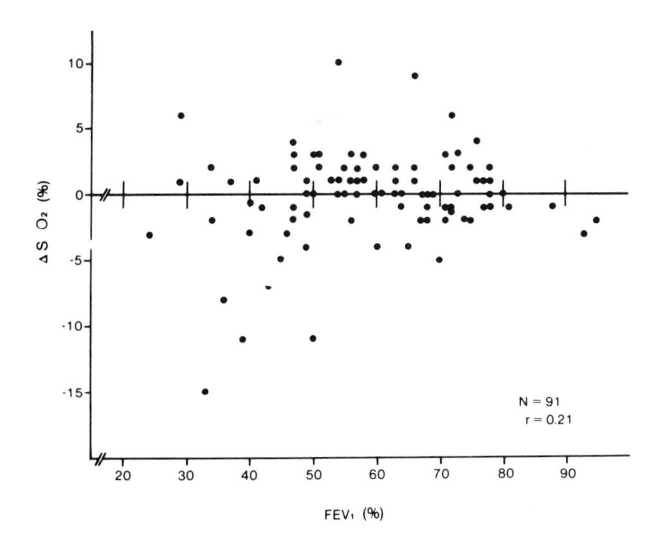

Figure 2 Changes in oxyhemoglobin saturation (SaO_2) with exercise plotted against FEV_1/FVC. (From Henke KG, Orenstein DM. Oxygen saturation during exercise in cystic fibrosis. Am Rev Respir Dis 1984; 129:708–711.)

There is some evidence that exercise may be as effective as chest physical therapy (postural drainage and percussion) for clearing mucus and maintaining pulmonary function. However, we feel that stronger evidence is needed before chest physical therapy is discontinued or replaced by exercise as the method of enhancing mucus clearance.

EXERCISE PRESCRIPTION

The large majority of children, adolescents, and adults with CF can exercise safely and enjoyably, with no restrictions. They do not require any specific exercise prescription and can be expected to reap the same psychosocial and physical benefits from sport and exercise participation as their unaffected peers. Some may even achieve exceptional athletic success, as for example the three Norwegian teenagers who completed the New York City Marathon in 1984. In some cases in which disease severity or an excess of caution on the part of parents, teachers, coaches, or even physicians have dictated a sedentary existence, an exercise prescription may be necessary.

The aerobic exercise conditioning program should be individually prescribed, based on the exercise test results. The program should take into account the modality, intensity, duration, and frequency of exercise.

Modality

To promote an increase in exercise tolerance and cardiorespiratory fitness, endurance activities that involve rhythmic contraction of large muscle groups should be selected for training, such as walking, jogging, cycling, or swimming. As with any exercise treatment for any group of people, the activity should be one that the patient enjoys, in order to promote compliance.

Intensity

The intensity of exercise should take into consideration the peak exercise tolerance of the patient and any maladaptive responses that occurred during the exercise test. In general, exercise may be prescribed at a level that elicits a heart rate between 70 and 85 percent of the patient's peak heart rate. Exercise in this range has been shown to be well tolerated and effective in increasing the cardiorespiratory fitness of patients with CF.

In patients who demonstrate abnormal responses such as extreme oxygen desaturation, intolerable dyspnea, or ECG abnormalities during the test, the exercise intensity should be limited to a heart rate at least 10 beats below that at which these responses occur.

Duration

Initially, the conditioning period of each exercise session should be about 10 minutes. As the patient's functional capacity improves, this can be increased gradually to 20 to 30 minutes. We have found an increase of 1 to 2 minutes per session each week is well tolerated by patients with CF. If the weekly increase is not tolerated, there is no rush in reaching the goal of 20- to 30-minute sessions, since we are trying to establish a life-long exercise habit. The extra time should make little difference in reaching the ultimate goal, particularly if it encourages patient compliance.

Each exercise session should include a 5- to 10-minute warm-up period before and a 5- to 10-minute cool-down period after the conditioning session. The warm-up period should consist of stretching exercises to warm the skeletal muscles, and low-intensity aerobic exercise (such as walking or cycling) to increase the heart rate gradually from resting levels to near the target heart rate range. The cool-down should include low-intensity walking to avoid venous pooling, and stretching to alleviate muscle tightness.

Frequency

In general, the exercise should be carried out three to five times a week, in order to accomplish a conditioning response. More frequent training is not beneficial in the normal population and may even increase the risk of a musculoskeletal injury, particularly with weightbearing activities.

The benefits of a specific aerobic conditioning program compared with generally increased levels of habitual activity accomplished through lifestyle changes (such as walking up steps rather than elevators, and getting off the bus several stops earlier) have not been studied.

SPECIAL CONSIDERATIONS

Oxygen Supplementation

Exercise should be prescribed cautiously for persons who exhibit significant decreases in oxygen saturation during the exercise test. Supplemental oxygen improves exercise tolerance and oxygenation in adult patients with chronic obstructive pulmonary disease. In patients with CF, it reduces minute ventilation and heart rate during exercise. However, the effect of oxygen supplementation on the oxygen saturation during exercise has yet to be examined in this population.

Exercise in the Heat

In spite of abnormally high concentrations of sodium and chloride in their sweat, patients with CF exhibit normal thermoregulation during exercise.

Similar thermoregulatory changes and acclimation were observed in patients with CF and normal control subjects in response to 70 minutes of cycle exercise in the heat on 8 consecutive days. Rectal temperatures and heart rates decreased similarly from day 1 to day 8 in both CF and control subjects. However, the sweat chloride concentrations of a control group decreased significantly from day 1 to day 8, whereas the sweat chloride concentrations of the CF patients remained high. The chloride loss in sweat was associated with a decreased serum chloride concentration in the CF patients. In spite of the daily ion loss during exercise, the serum electrolyte concentrations of the CF patients returned to normal levels by the start of the next day's exercise session. It should be noted that each exercise bout in the heat was relatively short, and the possible adverse effects of longer bouts of exercise in the heat have yet to be determined. With regard to the present findings, we encourage ample fluid intake and free use of the salt shaker.

SUGGESTED READING

American College of Sports Medicine. Guidelines for graded exercise testing and exercise prescription. 3rd ed. Philadelphia: Lea & Febiger, 1985: 13–15.

Benson LN, Newth CJD, de Souza M, et al. Radionuclide assessment of right and left ventricular function during bicycle exercise in young patients with cystic fibrosis. Am Rev Respir Dis 1984; 130:987–992.

Canny GJ, de Souza ME, Gilday DC, et al. Radionuclide assessment of cardiac performance in cystic fibrosis. Am Rev Respir Dis 1984; 130:822–826.

Cerny FJ, Pullano TP, Cropp GJA. Cardiorespiratory adaptations to exercise in cystic fibrosis. Am Rev Respir Dis 1982; 126:217–220.

Coates AL, Boyce P, Muller D, et al. The role of nutritional status, airway obstruction, hypoxia, and abnormalities in serum lipid composition in limiting exercise tolerance in children with cystic fibrosis. Acta Paediatr Scand 1980; 69:353–358.

Cropp GJ, Pullano TP, Cerny FJ, et al. Exercise tolerance and cardiorespiratory adjustments at peak work capacity in cystic fibrosis. Am Rev Respir Dis 1982; 126:211–216.

Cystic Fibrosis Foundation. Data Registry Report 1987. CFF. 6931 Arlington Road, Bethesda, MD 20814.

Dantzker DR, Patten GA, Bower JA. Gas exchange at rest and during exercise in adults with cystic fibrosis. Am Rev Respir Dis 1982; 125:400–405.

Gettman LR, Pollock ML, Durstine JL, et al. Physiological responses of men to 1, 3, and 5 day per week training programs. Res Q 1976; 47:638–646.

Godfrey S. Exercise testing in children. Philadelphia: WB Saunders, 1974:66–101.

Godfrey S, Mearns M. Pulmonary function and response to exercise in cystic fibrosis. Arch Dis Child 1971; 46:144–151.

Henke KG, Orenstein DM. Oxygen saturation during exercise in cystic fibrosis. Am Rev Respir Dis 1984; 129:708–711.

Hjeltnes N, Stanghelle JK, Skyberg D. Pulmonary function and oxygen uptake during exercise in 16 year old boys with cystic fibrosis. Acta Paediatr Scand 1984; 73:548–553.

Issekutz R Jr, Birkhead NC, Rodahl K. The use of respiratory quotients in assessment of aerobic work capacity. J Appl Physiol 1962; 17:47–50.
Keens TG, Krastins JRB, Wannamaker EM, et al. Ventilatory muscle endurance training in normal subjects and patients with cystic fibrosis. Am Rev Respir Dis 1977; 116:853–860.
Orenstein DM, Franklin BA, Doershuk CF, et al. Exercise conditioning and cardiopulmonary fitness in cystic fibrosis. Chest 1981; 80:392–398.
Orenstein DM, Henke KG, Costill DL, et al. Exercise and heat stress in cystic fibrosis patients. Pediatr Res 1983; 17:267–269.
Orenstein DM, Henke KG, Green CG. Heat acclimation in cystic fibrosis. J Appl Physiol 1984; 57:408–412.
Pollock ML, Gettman LR, Milesis CA, et al. Effect of frequency and duration of training on attrition and incidence of injury. Med Sci Sports 1977; 9:31–36.
Taussig LM, Landau LF, Marks MI. Respiratory system. In: Taussig LM, ed. Cystic fibrosis. New York: Thieme-Stratton, 1984:115.
Wood RE, Boat TF, Doershuk CF. State of the art: cystic fibrosis. Am Rev Respir Dis 1976; 113:833–878.
Zach M, Oberwaldner B, Hausler F. Cystic fibrosis: physical exercise versus chest physiotherapy. Arch Dis Child 1982; 57:587–589.
Zach MS, Purrer B, Oberwaldner B. Effect of swimming on forced expiration and sputum clearance in cystic fibrosis. Lancet 1981; 2:1201–1203.

EXERCISE IN CHRONIC AIRWAY OBSTRUCTION

NORMAN L. JONES, M.D.

Patients with chronic airflow limitation that is due to asthma, chronic bronchitis, or emphysema commonly present to the physician with a complaint that their activity is restricted. Usually they have found themselves progressively handicapped by the disability, imposed through an impairment of pulmonary function. The three terms *impairment, disability*, and *handicap* are now generally used in a specific sense, and an attempt to quantify each is clinically worthwhile. *Impairment* indicates a reduction of some physiologic function; in patients with chronic respiratory disorders, ventilatory capacity is impaired by airflow limitation, while pulmonary gas exchange function also is often impaired owing to an abnormal distribution of ventilation and perfusion and a reduced diffusing capacity in the lungs. *Disability* refers to a reduction in the capacity to exercise when the individual is compared with a healthy person of the same sex, age, and stature. *Handicap* indicates a reduction in the individual's own activities of everyday life. Since all three of these clinical indices vary widely, they require separate assessment. The aim of clinical management then becomes reversal of handicap, reduction in disability, and improvement of physiologic function.

CLINICAL SYNDROMES

Although the three clinical entities are frequently considered as expressions of one disease (chronic obstructive pulmonary disease), they have separate definitions and the clinical features of each should thus be assessed. Since it is quite possible for someone to have features consistent with asthma, chronic bronchitis, and emphysema, the aim of assessment is not to provide a single diagnosis, but rather to identify clinically relevant expressions of the three conditions.

Asthma refers to an airflow limitation that varies from time to time, either spontaneously or as the result of treatment, at least at some time in its clinical course. Thus, the severity of airflow limitation, its response to treatment with bronchodilators or steroids, and its variability, especially after exercise, is worth assessing in all patients.

Obstructive chronic bronchitis consists of airway narrowing, due to bronchial wall thickening and excess mucus production. Infective episodes are frequently experienced by such patients, and in many there is coexisting bronchiectasis. The affected individuals show airway limitation during both expiration and inspiration, but gas exchange function, as measured by the carbon monoxide transfer (or "diffusion") capacity, is relatively normal. However, when chronic airflow obstruction in such patients is severe, underventilation and carbon dioxide retention occur; these findings are accompanied by polycythemia and pulmonary heart failure. Such patients are commonly described as "type B" or "blue and bloated."

Emphysema indicates a destruction of alveolar walls and enlarged airspaces distal to the terminal bronchiole. Lung elastic recoil is lost and the lungs are large in volume. Expiratory airflow obstruction is severe, owing to lack of support in the small airways, and the expiratory difficulty often contrasts sharply with a relatively normal inspiratory flow. Gas exchange is impaired as a result of the loss of alveolar surface area, and the carbon monoxide transfer capacity is reduced. In spite of these abnormalities and even in the presence of severe dyspnea, resting arterial blood gases are often surprisingly well maintained. Right heart failure is also uncommon until late in the course of the condition. Such patients are often described as "type A" or "pink and puffing."

PHYSIOLOGIC ASSESSMENT OF IMPAIRED FUNCTION

Although the clinical features of airway obstruction are well known, they are notoriously misleading, and symptoms alone do not enable a quantitative estimate of severity to be made. For this reason, both the diagnosis of airflow limitation and an assessment of its severity are dependent on pulmonary function tests. The necessary techniques are widely available, and normal standards have been well established, thus enabling an individual patient's results to be expressed as a percentage of the expected values for a given sex, age, and stature.

All patients with clinical symptoms or other features suggestive of airflow obstruction should undergo spirometry, with the measurement of vital capacity and the volume expired in 1 second (FEV_1). This information is as essential as the measurement of blood pressure in the management of hypertension. Measurements may also be used to assess the efficacy of bronchodilators, acutely administered, or other therapeutic measures continued over a longer period. In patients with mild airflow obstruction, or those in whom the airflow obstruction is completely reversed by an inhaled bronchodilator, spirometry may be the only measurement required for assessment. However, in patients with more severe impairment, other techniques may be needed to assess specific respiratory functions.

The flow-volume loop allows flow to be measured throughout inspiration and expiration, and thus yields a more complete assessment of ventilatory capacity than that provided by spirometry alone.

Measurement of static lung volumes (residual volume, functional residual capacity, and total lung capacity) provides information regarding ventilatory capacity. It is also used to identify the presence of emphysema; in this condition, very large lung volumes are observed.

Carbon monoxide uptake yields an overall index of pulmonary gas exchange. It is characteristically impaired in severe emphysema.

Respiratory muscle strength may be simply assessed by the measurement of maximal inspiratory and expiratory pressures. Patients with chronic pulmonary disorders frequently exhibit respiratory muscle weakness, which may be difficult to detect.

When ventilatory capacity and gas exchange function are severely impaired, normal blood-gas status may not be maintained. Ventilatory failure is defined by an arterial CO_2 tension ($PaCO_2$) higher than the normal range (35 to 45 mm Hg), and it is recognized noninvasively by the finding of an elevated rebreathing P_{CO_2}, or invasively by analysis of arterial blood. Pulmonary gas exchange failure is defined in terms of the arterial O_2 tension (PaO_2), assessed noninvasively by oximetry or directly by the taking of an arterial blood sample.

ASSESSMENT OF DISABILITY

In patients with severe symptom limitation, particularly when treatment with simple bronchodilators and antibiotics has not led to improvement, further assessment is helped by noninvasive exercise testing. The essential features of this technique are that the patient exercises on a cycle ergometer, progressive small increases in exercise work rate are imposed every minute, and the test is continued to the point at which the patient is unable to continue, usually because of dyspnea, fatigue, or both. During the test, respiratory responses are measured in terms of ventilation, tidal volume, and frequency of breathing, and the arterial oxygen saturation may be monitored by an ear oximeter. Symptoms of dyspnea and leg effort are quantified, using a sensory rating scale. The maximal power output developed is compared with normal standards. This test allows exercise tolerance to be measured objectively and the factors contributing to a limitation of performance may be identified. In most patients with chronic airflow limitation, dyspnea is the symptom that causes them to stop exercising. The results of the study are then examined to identify specific factors contributing to dyspnea and disability.

Increased Ventilatory Demands. Ventilation may be high because of unfitness; this may lead to excess CO_2 production, inefficient gas exchange (high dead-space ventilation), or the presence of a hypoxic drive to breathing in patients in whom arterial O_2 saturation falls.

Increased Impedance to Breathing. Increases in resistance to airflow during inspiration and/or expiration may impose a severe load upon breathing, increasing the demands made on respiratory muscles and in this way contributing to dyspnea. Ventilation at maximal exercise is usually close to the ventilatory capacity, as assessed by spirometry and estimated either by multiplying the FEV_1 by an arbitrary factor of 35, or by a more complex analysis of the flow-volume loop.

Respiratory Muscle Weakness. Reduction in maximal inspiratory pressure, severe dyspnea during the exercise test, and a pattern of breathing with a restricted tidal volume and high frequency of breathing are clues that respiratory muscle weakness may play an important role in the limitation of exercise.

Skeletal Muscle Weakness. Many patients with chronic airflow obstruction indicate that in addition to dyspnea, leg muscle fatigue becomes intense and may actually be the dominant cause for stopping the cycle ergometer exercise. Skeletal muscle weakness is a common finding in patients with chronic pulmonary disorders, because of long-standing inactivity, steroid myopathy, electrolyte disturbances secondary to administration of diuretics, and poor nutrition. Such weakness may result in a lack of improvement in exercise tolerance in the face of improved pulmonary function.

ASSESSMENT OF HANDICAP

Handicap usually may be recognized as appropriate in terms of the patient's disability and the demands imposed by his or her activities of daily living. Thus, a patient may be very disabled, with impaired function and poor exercise tolerance, but the demands of living may be so small that little handicap is experienced. In contrast, a person employed in a heavy industrial occupation may be very handicapped, in spite of little disability in terms of exercise capacity. Handicap is assessed by a careful clinical interview; the distress experienced in everyday activities is identified and is related to the degree of pulmonary function impairment and the disability observed in terms of the objectively measured exercise capacity.

Exercise test results are helpful in the assessment of handicap; the rating of symptom severity obtained under standardized test conditions may be compared with the symptoms encountered at comparable levels of activity in daily life. In a large population of patients with chronic airflow limitation, there is a reasonable concordance between the severity of handicap, the extent of disability, and the degree of impairment (Table 1), but in a given individual, for the reasons already mentioned, large discrepancies may exist.

MANAGEMENT OF PATIENTS WITH CHRONIC AIRFLOW LIMITATION

A logical approach to management may be followed on the basis of the clinical assessment, pulmonary function measurements, and exercise test results.

Airway narrowing, as reflected in reductions of FEV_1, is managed mainly by the use of bronchodilator (beta-2 agonist) aerosols (salbutamol, terbutaline, or fenoterol) and by aminophylline products. If an adequate trial of these measures does not lead to a significant improvement in symptoms and spirometric scores, a short course of steroids is considered. This is carried out over 2 to 3 weeks; prednisone is used in high dosage and its effect is monitored by measurements of FEV_1. If a significant improvement in symptoms and FEV_1 is observed, the dosage of oral prednisone is tapered and inhaled steroid (beclomethasone) is introduced.

If sputum examination and culture reveal evidence of infection, a short course of antibiotics is given. The most common organism is *Haemophilus influenzae*, which usually responds to ampicillin, tetracycline, or trimethoprim.

Treatment may also be required for fluid retention and cardiac dysfunction.

Exercise rehabilitation programs may be considered if a significant handicap remains after optimal medical treatment. The program is carefully prescribed on an individual basis, and specific objectives need to be identified for each patient.

In patients with relatively mild airflow obstruction who complain of significant limitation in activity and who have a reduced exercise capacity, unfitness may play a large part in the symptoms. Such patients may enter a general fitness program, exercise being prescribed on the basis of heart rate, as in cardiac patients.

Patients with respiratory muscle weakness may be helped by a respiratory muscle training program in which they breathe through graded inspiratory resistances; this is usually accompanied by a prescription to increase regular walking activity on a gradual basis.

Very disabled patients may find it difficult to take part in endurance exercise training programs because of dyspnea. Such individuals may quickly become disheartened at a lack of progress; since poor function of skeletal muscles frequently accompanies disability in such patients, short-duration resistance training may be helpful.

In patients in whom arterial oxygen desaturation develops, oxygen supplements during exercise may make possible an increase in activity.

TABLE 1 Suggested Grading of Impairment, Disability, and Handicap

Grade	*Impairment*	*Disability*	*Handicap*
0	$FEV_1 > 3$ $D_{CO} > 25$	$\dot{W}max > 150$ $\dot{V}O_2max > 25$	Full-time work Walks briskly up hills
1	$FEV_1 < 3$ $D_{CO} < 25$	$\dot{W}max < 150$ $\dot{V}O_2max < 25$	Co-workers help Dyspnea on hills
2	$FEV_1 < 2$ $D_{CO} < 15$	$\dot{W}max < 100$ $\dot{V}O_2max < 15$	Part-time work Dyspnea on level
3	$FEV_1 < 1$ $D_{CO} < 15$	$\dot{W}max < 50$ $\dot{V}O_2max < 10$	Not working Dyspnea on slow walking
4	$FEV_1 < 0.75$ $D_{CO} < 10$ $PO_2\downarrow$ $PCO_2\uparrow$	$\dot{W}max < 25$ $\dot{V}O_2max < 7$	Limited to house Requires help in activities of daily living

Units are as follows: FEV_1 (liters); D_{CO} (ml/min/mm Hg); Wmax (watts); $\dot{V}O_2max$ (ml/kg/min). Values are approximate for a 50-year-old male, but relative changes apply for other patients.

In some very disabled patients, anxiety and depression may be prominent features. Such individuals may have adapted poorly to their limitations in terms of everyday activities. They may be helped by admission to a multidisciplinary rehabilitation program in which they are educated to conserve energy and are given advice and reassurance with the aim of increasing daily activities, both physical and social. Frequently, such patients have very limited social activity. They may thus respond well, and an increase in confidence and self-reliance may lead to less dependence on family members or colleagues at work.

SUGGESTED READING

Jones NL. Clinical exercise testing. 3rd ed. Philadelphia: WB Saunders, 1988.

Jones NL, Berman LB, Bartkiewicz PD, Oldvidge NB. Chronic obstructive respiratory disorders. In: Skinner JS, ed. Exercise testing and exercise prescription for special cases. Philadelphia: Lea & Febiger, 1987: 175.

EXERCISE TESTING IN PEDIATRIC CARDIOLOGY

ROLF MOCELLIN, M.D.

Exercise testing is one tool used by the pediatric cardiologist when assessing the functional status of the cardiovascular system before and after cardiac surgery. At present, corrective surgery of most hemodynamically relevant heart malformations is performed in infancy or before the child reaches school age. Accordingly, a preoperative ergometric assessment of the functional ability of the cardiovascular system is possible only in children with less severe malformations in whom surgery may not be indicated, or in children with complex cyanotic lesions in whom corrective surgery may not be possible. In the group of children with minor malformations that remain uncorrected at school age, discrimination from normal children is hampered, because the heart muscle has a strong tendency to compensate for the specific defect. Unlike the situation in adults who have developed coronary heart disease, the heart muscle generally remains healthy in children with congenital heart disease, and it may thus compensate for a mild to moderate pulmonary stenosis or an atrial septal defect by right ventricular hypertrophy or dilatation, reestablishing a fairly normal functional ability. If ergometry reveals a certain reduction of cardiovascular performance in an individual of this group, it can be supposed that this is not due to the cardiac malformation itself, but rather to a low level of habitual physical activity or to an inferior genetic endowment, just as in the healthy population.

In children whose cardiac malformation has been surgically corrected in infancy or early childhood, later exercise testing is one of the tools available to assess the success of surgery. The main question posed in such patients is whether normal or approximately normal functional capacity has been achieved by the operation. If function remains subnormal, it may also be asked whether a residual malformation is responsible. In patients with cyanotic congenital heart disease, considerable improvement of functional ability is the rule after corrective surgery. Nevertheless, distinct limitations of functional ability remain in most patients. This situation is especially likely when the "correction" must be considered as nothing more than a palliation, as in some modifications of the Fontan operation, where separation of the pulmonary and the systemic circuits can be established, but an absence or hypoplasia of one ventricular chamber cannot be overcome by the rather direct communication between the right atrium and the pulmonary artery without residual functional disturbances.

In assessing postoperative cardiovascular performance in this group of children, more detailed information about cardiac output, stroke volume, and pressure gradients during exercise may be required, especially if reoperation may be necessary. Some of this information may be supplied by echocardiography, but sometimes central venous catheterization and arterial cannulation are required, especially when it is necessary to determine the cardiac output and stroke volume during exercise. A careful decision is needed as to whether the information that is expected justifies the use of invasive methods.

Postoperative cardiac function may be impaired by dysrhythmias, especially if the sinus node region or the conducting tissue has been injured during the operation. Exercise may reveal rhythm disturbances not present at rest, and it may also exacerbate or attenuate abnormalities already observed at rest.

MAXIMAL VERSUS SUBMAXIMAL EXERCISE TESTS

Cardiovascular performance capacity is best reflected by maximal oxygen intake or aerobic power. The determination of maximal oxygen intake is performed with the child sitting and pedaling on a cycle ergometer or running on a treadmill. Both maximal heart rate and maximal oxygen intake are higher (the latter by about 10 percent) with a treadmill test than with a cycle ergometer test. We prefer the cycle ergometer test, however, because additional measurements such as electrocardiographic (ECG) and blood pressure recordings are less subject to motion artifacts than would be the case with treadmill exercise. The normal values presented below refer to cycle ergometry, with the child sitting in an upright position.

Because equipment for the measurement of oxygen intake is not always available, indirect methods have been suggested as useful for the determination of cardiovascular performance capacity. All indirect tests, however, are based on specific assumptions, which unfortunately apply to only a minority of children with cardiac diseases. Indirect tests are usually submaximal in type, and performance is gauged from the increase of heart rate in relation to mechanical power. This was originally thought to be justified because the heart rate shows a linear increase with augmentation of mechanical power output, the individual heart rate at a given absolute power output depends on sex, age, and constitution as well as training status, and the maximal heart rate is independent of sex, age, constitution, and level of training. However, despite the constancy of the mean maximal heart rate at a level of 195 to 200 beats per minute throughout adolescence, individual maxima vary between 180 and 210 beats per minute. The difference between group mean and individual maximal value can be even more pronounced in children with cardiac diseases. Accordingly, extrapolation to constant supposed maximal values, inherent in such indirect cycle ergometer tests as the PWC_{170} (the power output at a heart rate of 170 beats per minute) is a significant source of error, which increases the more the individual maximal heart rate differs from the group mean value.

Another assumption that is necessary to make submaximal indirect tests meaningful if oxygen intake is not determined, is that the physical power output bears a consistent relationship to oxygen intake. However, individual variations in mechanical efficiency may amount to more than 20 percent in children, so that this assumption is not valid. A certain power output, expressed in watts or in kilopond-meters per minute, may signify a very different oxygen intake for different individuals. However, oxygen intake is the variable that reflects the performance of the cardiovascular system at a given mechanical power output, while the mechanical power output itself also reflects skill and dexterity.

A further problem with indirect cycle ergometer tests is that measurements performed with different types of ergometer may not be strictly comparable despite careful calibration.

One way to overcome some of these difficulties might be to replace indirect submaximal cycle tests with indirect maximal effort tests. By use of a treadmill, calibration problems could also be reduced. However, in view of the multiple inaccuracies inherent in indirect determinations of cardiovascular performance, and the need for precise determinations (especially in children who have undergone surgical repair of cardiac malformations), we prefer to make direct measurements of aerobic power.

This can be done by application of a stepwise or continuously increasing load. When determined with a stepwise protocol, three stages are generally sufficient, particularly if the third stage is properly selected on the basis of the observed heart rate increase during the preceding stages. The third stage should correspond to a slightly "supermaximal" load. The first stage should be chosen according to body mass (a loading of 1 watt per kilogram of body mass in lean children and 1 watt per kilogram of the theoretical body mass expected for height in children who are overweight). The main criterion indicating that the maximal oxygen intake has been reached is a leveling off or "plateauing" of oxygen consumption (in other words, the increase of oxygen consumption at the third stage is less than would be expected from the mechanical power that is exerted). However, such a plateau is not always demonstrable in children. In such cases, a respiratory gas exchange ratio (CO_2 output divided by O_2 intake) that exceeds 1.0, and a blood lactate concentration of at least 6 mmol per liter in children up to 10 years of age or 8 mmol per liter in older children, are indicative of a true maximal effort. During the test, a rapid respiratory rate together with deep and noisy breathing and a heart rate that is close to or above 200 beats per minute are further indications that maximal oxygen intake has been achieved, especially when the child cannot continue in spite of adequate encouragement. To keep variations of mechanical efficiency as low as possible, a constant rate of pedal revolutions, 60 per minute, is mandatory at submaximal loads; this remains true even if an adjustment of power output at different pedaling rates is assured automatically (as is the case in some designs of electromagnetically braked ergometer). Standard values for maximal oxygen intake are presented in Table 1.

The anaerobic threshold has recently been proposed as a complementary measure of cardiovascular performance. The anaerobic threshold is here defined as a certain exercise intensity or percentage of maximal oxygen intake (differing interindividually) at which a steeper increase in blood lactate can be observed. In essence, it is the point at which the rate of lactate production exceeds its rate of elimination from the blood. Work intensities below the anaerobic threshold can be continued for long periods, whereas above the anaerobic threshold the possible duration of work is very limited. The higher

TABLE 1 Standard Values (Means) of Maximal Aerobic Power in Relation to Sex and Age

	Boys		*Girls*	
Age (yr)	*$\dot{V}O_2max$ (L/min)*	*$\dot{V}O_2max/BH^2$ (L/min/m²)*	*$\dot{V}O_2max$ (L/min)*	*$\dot{V}O_2max/BH^2$ (L/min/m²)*
6.5	1.04	0.71	0.93	0.66
7.5	1.17	0.72	1.03	0.66
8.5	1.29	0.74	1.14	0.67
9.5	1.41	0.75	1.24	0.67
10.5	1.53	0.76	1.35	0.67
11.5	1.65	0.77	1.47	0.67
12.5	1.81	0.79	1.62	0.68
13.5	2.05	0.81	1.73	0.69
14.5	2.32	0.84	1.80	0.70
15.5	2.55	0.88	1.86	0.71
16.5	2.71	0.91	1.87	0.71
17.5	2.81	0.93	1.87	0.71

$\dot{V}O_2max$ = maximal aerobic power; BH = body height.

the anaerobic threshold in relation to maximal oxygen intake, the higher is the percentage of the cardiovascular performance capacity that can be used without fatigue. For a precise determination of anaerobic threshold, an exercise protocol with a relatively continuous increase of work rate is preferable to a stepwise increase, and blood lactate determinations should be performed at frequent intervals. A small quantity of blood is collected from the hyperemized earlobe for each lactate determination. Note that equal absolute increments of work rate per minute correspond to a smaller relative increase per minute for larger children, and to a longer duration of the test procedure with older individuals. The time factor itself, however, may have an influence on the results. Therefore, the increments of power output should, as far as possible, be related to the body mass of the child who is being tested.

Whether or not the ventilatory anaerobic threshold can substitute for the anaerobic threshold (as measured by lactate concentrations) is still a matter of some controversy, especially as the mechanism triggering a disproportionate nonlinear increase of ventilation in relation to oxygen consumption is not yet fully understood. Whereas the transition to a steep increase of blood lactate with increasing work rate occurs at a blood lactate concentration of about 4 mmol per liter, the transition from a proportionate to a disproportionate increase of ventilation in relation to oxygen consumption occurs at a blood lactate concentration of about 2 mmol per liter. The ventilatory anaerobic threshold is easily determined by frequent measurements of ventilation and oxygen consumption as the patient exercises against a more or less continuously increasing workload. As maximal oxygen intake can be measured during the same test procedure, both the anaerobic and the ventilatory anaerobic threshold can be expressed as percentages of aerobic power. The percentage of maximal oxygen intake at which the anaerobic or the ventilatory anaerobic threshold is observed differs between individuals, depending on the velocity of release and removal of lactate from the blood. The thresholds are set higher in young than in older children, and modification of the threshold by training seems less possible than in adults. In a typical 11-year-old child, the anaerobic threshold is at about 84 percent of maximal oxygen intake, and in a 14-year-old child it is at about 74 percent of maximal oxygen intake. The corresponding ventilatory anaerobic thresholds for these ages are 65 and 60 percent of maximal oxygen intake, respectively. The anaerobic or ventilatory anaerobic threshold is now increasingly determined in addition to maximal oxygen intake. Determination of the work rate or the oxygen consumption at the anaerobic threshold is clinically useful because it enables the physician to offer advice concerning the optimal intensity of training. However, anaerobic threshold should not be regarded as an indirect measure of cardiovascular performance capacity or aerobic power.

STANDARDIZATION OF NORMAL VALUES

The appraisal of individual values requires a comparison with mean normal values, selected according to sex and age. Mere consideration of chronologic age, however, is insufficient. For instance, a healthy child who is small for his or her age generally shows a correspondingly reduced functional ability, because cardiovascular performance capacity is primarily related to biologic age, including such parameters of body development as height, total body mass, and lean body mass. The most appropriate single reference standard is height; if one relies on body mass, an undue significance is attributed to the fat component of the body. Therefore, the use of body mass as a reference standard for cardiovascular performance capacity becomes merely an attempt to estimate overweight indirectly. Similarly, body surface area does not appear to be a suitable reference standard, particularly since it cannot be measured directly.

TABLE 2 Standard Values (Means) of Maximal Cardiac Output and Stroke Volume During Exercise in Relation to Sex and Age

	Boys				Girls			
Age (yr)	*$\dot{Q}max$ (L/min)*	*$\dot{Q}max/BH^2$ (L/min/m²)*	*SV (ml)*	*SV/BH^3 (ml/m³)*	*$\dot{Q}max$ (L/min)*	*$\dot{Q}max/BH^2$ (L/min/m²)*	*SV (ml)*	*SV/BH^3 (ml/m³)*
6.5	7.7	5.3	39	21.9	6.9	4.9	35	20.4
7.5	8.7	5.4	43	21.1	7.6	4.9	38	19.5
8.5	9.6	5.4	48	20.4	8.4	5.0	42	19.0
9.5	10.4	5.5	52	19.9	9.2	5.0	46	18.4
10.5	11.3	5.6	57	19.7	10.2	5.0	50	17.6
11.5	12.2	5.7	61	19.3	10.9	5.0	55	16.8
12.5	13.4	5.8	67	19.0	12.0	5.0	60	16.3
13.5	15.2	6.0	76	18.9	12.8	5.1	64	16.1
14.5	17.2	6.3	86	19.0	13.3	5.2	67	16.2
15.5	18.9	6.6	94	19.3	13.8	5.3	69	16.3
16.5	20.1	6.7	100	19.5	13.9	5.3	69	16.2
17.5	20.8	6.9	104	19.7	13.9	5.2	69	16.2

$\dot{Q}max$ = maximal cardiac output; SV = stroke volume; BH = body height.

When using body height as the reference standard, it is essential to realize that older children are generally more fit than younger children who have attained the same height. This implies that height standardization of normal values is only meaningful if age is considered simultaneously; i.e., standardization in relation to height must be performed separately for each age group.

The standard deviation of the proposed standard values listed in Tables 1 and 2 cannot be evaluated precisely, because the means have been calculated from the data of different authors. However, a standard deviation of about 10 percent can be assumed for the relative values. The absolute, age-dependent values have higher standard deviations, especially during puberty, when interindividual developmental differences are pronounced. When considering results for an individual, it is not possible to distinguish among the error of the method, the influence of any residual heart malformation, the training status, and the effect of any genetic predisposition to an unusual level of performance.

CARDIAC OUTPUT AND STROKE VOLUME

The mean maximal cardiac output for boys and girls of any age can be calculated from the corresponding maximal oxygen intake if the mean maximal difference of oxygen content between arterial and venous blood (a-vDO_2) is known. Above 10 years of age, a mean maximal av-DO_2 of about 13.5 ml per 100 ml can be assumed. In younger children, the maximal av-DO_2 is somewhat lower, because of their lower hemoglobin concentration. However, this small discrepancy can be ignored for the purpose of calculating the mean maximal cardiac output, and a constant av-DO_2 of 13.5 ml per 100 ml may be used for the calculations, regardless of age. The resultant values are presented in Table 2, together with the corresponding values for cardiac stroke volume (SV), as calculated by applying a mean maximal heart rate of 200 beats per minute. The relative values in Table 2 were evaluated with regard to body height squared ($\dot{Q}max/BH^2$) and body height cubed (SV/BH^3), following a suggestion of B. Eriksson.

In order to ensure a meaningful interpretation of individual submaximal cardiac output values, sex- and age-specific regressions are needed relating oxygen consumption to cardiac output. Children typically have a smaller cardiac output than adults at a given oxygen consumption. The use of an adult regression line for the interpretation of exercise cardiac output is therefore misleading.

In Figure 1, two lines have been drawn linking all potential cardiac output readings with an av-DO_2 of 11 and 13.5 ml per 100 ml, respectively. The illustration also shows the regression line linking oxygen consumption ($\dot{V}O_2$) and cardiac output ($\dot{Q}$) in male adults as derived from the equation:

$$\dot{Q}\ (L/min) = 5.1 + 5.8\ \dot{V}O_2\ (L/min)$$

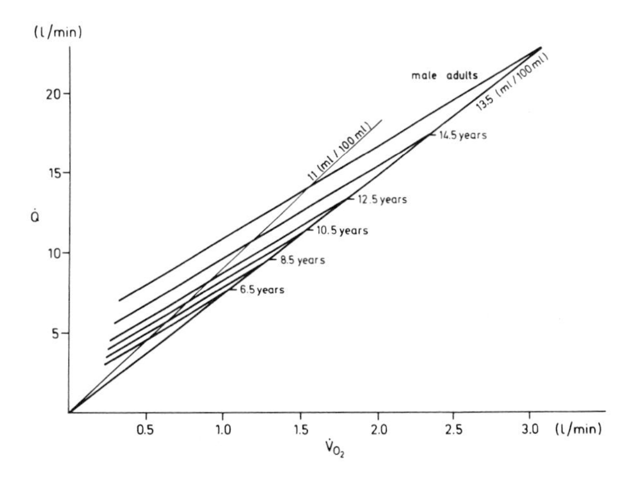

Figure 1 Standard regression lines relating oxygen consumption ($\dot{V}O_2$) and cardiac output ($\dot{Q}$) for boys in different age groups. For details see text.

Parallel to this regression line, and starting from the respective mean maximal values as taken from Tables 1 and 2, regression lines have been drawn for boys of five different age groups, on the basis that the av-DO_2 is always about 11 ml per 100 ml, at 50 percent of maximal oxygen intake. The intercept for each regression line has been calculated as summarized in Table 3. By subtracting the respective intercept from a measured individual value of cardiac output at rest and during exercise, the influence of age and sex on the measured values can be eliminated, and comparability of the individual values can be established. The standard regression equation, valid for boys and girls in all age groups, is then:

$$\dot{Q}corr\ (L/min) = 5.8\ \dot{V}o_2\ (L/min)$$

CARDIAC FUNCTION AFTER SURGERY

As the cardiac performance of many patients with congenital heart disease is not substantially impeded before surgery, an operation does not necessarily bring about any direct increase in functional ability. However, the prognosis for cardiovascular performance capacity will be better, the more completely a malformation of the heart or great vessels has been corrected. Complete anatomic correction is possible, for example, in patients with patent ductus, coarctation of the aorta (sometimes only after reoperation), atrial septal defect, total anomalous pulmonary venous connection, valvular pulmonary stenosis (including patients who have received balloon dilatation), and ventricular septal defect (especially when transatrial closure of the defect has been performed). However, postoperative function may be impaired by cardiac dysrhythmias attributable to intraoperative lesions of the sinus node region or of the conducting tissue. After valvotomy or balloon dilatation of an aortic stenosis, aortic insufficiency is generally present, especially if the valve was considerably malformed. It may indeed happen that functional disability is more pronounced after surgery than before treatment. Moreover, if valvotomy is performed for aortic stenosis during infancy and childhood, it is usually a palliative measure, to be followed by valve replacement when the patient is an adult.

TABLE 3 Intercepts (a) of Regression Lines Relating Cardiac Output and Oxygen Consumption in Boys and Girls of Different Ages

Age (yr)	*Boys (a, L/min)*	*Girls (a, L/min)*
6.5	1.7	1.5
7.5	1.9	1.7
8.5	2.1	1.8
9.5	2.3	2.0
10.5	2.5	2.2
11.5	2.7	2.4
12.5	2.9	2.6
13.5	3.3	2.8
14.5	3.7	2.9
15.5	4.1	3.0
16.5	4.4	3.0
17.5	4.6	3.0

In tetralogy of Fallot, the mean postoperative aerobic power is about 85 percent of normal. The extent of the residual limitation of performance in these patients depends in part on the degree of pulmonary insufficiency, which may be especially pronounced in patients who needed a transannular patch plastic of the right ventricular outflow tract. A reduced compliance of the right ventricle, especially in the presence of a moderate residual pulmonary stenosis, may be another factor leading to a persistent limitation of performance. A restriction of maximal heart rate, resulting from impaired electromechanical activity and associated with the right bundle branch block that is generally present postoperatively, may further inhibit cardiovascular performance.

In patients with transposition of the great arteries who have undergone a Senning or Mustard procedure, normal functional ability should not be anticipated if there is significant tricuspid regurgitation, caval or pulmonary vein obstruction, left ventricular outflow tract obstruction, or cardiac dysrhythmias. With improvement in surgical techniques, residual defects are now seen less frequently and a better functional result may be anticipated. However, the right ventricle remains the systemic ventricle, and hemodynamic studies in such patients have shown a postoperative right ventricular ejection fraction of about 50 to 55 percent, compared with the normal value of 65 percent. Thus, normal cardiovascular performance after a Senning or Mustard procedure is generally possible only if stroke volume can be maintained by a compensatory enlargement of the right ventricle, and as long as maximal heart rate is not reduced. Whether functional results will be better after anatomic correction of transposition of the great arteries by an "arterial switch" operation remains uncertain. The fact that both aortic insufficiency and pulmonary stenosis have been observed in many patients after completion of this procedure is less ground for optimism with regard to the likely functional result.

Impaired cardiovascular performance is to be expected especially after the Fontan procedure, which is applied more and more frequently not only in patients with tricuspid atresia, but also in those with a double-inlet ventricle or a univentricular atrioventricular connection. Even if the result of the operation is optimal, a normal increase of cardiac output during exercise cannot be expected in these patients, since flow through the pulmonary circuit depends mainly on the pressure gradient between the right and the left atrium. In some patients, the oxygen consumption does not correspond to mechanical power output even during submaximal exercise, so that anaerobic energy sources must be used.

SPORTS PARTICIPATION AND TRAINING RESPONSE

Cardiovascular performance is only one of the factors that determine physical fitness. Others include anaerobic capacity and neuromuscular performance, the latter subsuming a variety of skills including the velocity of movement, coordination, balance, and manual dexterity. Each of these components of fitness can be trained and each varies more or less independently. All are usually involved in sport activities, although to different extents and in different combinations, depending on the kind of activity that is undertaken. Cardiovascular performance does not generally play a dominant role in competitive athletics. In the technical disciplines and in activities for which short-term efforts are required, the prevailing factors lie outside the cardiovascular system. This implies that even if the cardiovascular performance is impaired, quite good results can often be achieved. Certainly, if aerobic power is found to be reduced, this does not imply that participation in sports is impossible. Rather, one should consider recommending types of physical activity that are less dependent on cardiovascular performance and are determined more by factors such as motor skills.

Given the residual functional and anatomic disorders of the cardiovascular system present in many children after open heart surgery, it is difficult to offer generalized advice concerning physical training. Some investigators have demonstrated a significant improvement in maximal work capacity when children have undertaken 6 to 9 weeks of training after the repair of various cardiac malformations. Interestingly, no significant increase of aerobic power has been observed after such training, and the tolerance of a higher workload must be attributed either to a significant improvement in mechanical efficiency or to an upward shift of the anaerobic threshold. If a higher mechanical efficiency is responsible for the increased maximal work rate after training, the coordination of movements must have improved. At all events, there is evidence that submaximal training has a positive influence on exercise capacity despite the lack of any increase of aerobic power. A more intensive training program might increase aerobic power, but it does not seem indicated when anatomic disorders are still present after "corrective" surgery.

EXERCISE THERAPY IN PEDIATRIC CARDIOLOGY

GORDON CUMMING, M.D.

For physicians caring for children with heart lesions, the overall therapeutic goal is to help their patients to become as close as possible to normal children in terms of cardiac function, exercise capacity, mental function, social function, and general well-being. This goal is generally achieved when function is deemed to be normal in the various spheres, when only infrequent special medical follow-up is needed, and when no special attention is required. Fortunately, for most children with heart abnormalities these goals are attainable without the need for special exercise classes and special supervision.

Table 1 lists the cardiac lesions that are considered mild. Patients with these lesions can be allowed unrestricted exercise and sport. Sport training and competition can also be allowed without special monitoring or advice. It is not unreasonable for these children to be given a maximal treadmill test in order to reassure both parents and children that intense exercise is possible and safe, and to exclude any unforeseen problems such as arrhythmia, exercise asthma, or occult impairments. For patients who choose intense sport training, a review every 2 to 3 years is in order.

TABLE 1 Lesions Compatible With Competitive All-Out Sports and Unrestricted Training

Lesion
Ventricular septal defect: small and trivial, normal pressures $\dot{Q}p/\dot{Q}s < 1.4$
Atrial septal defect: small, $\dot{Q}p/\dot{Q}s < 1.4$
Pulmonary stenosis: RV < 50 mm Hg
Aortic stenosis: peak gradient < 20 mm Hg
Bicuspid aortic valve: zero or mild insufficiency
Aortic insufficiency 1–2+, $< 25\%$ regurgitant fraction
Idiopathic dilatation of pulmonary artery
Mitral valve prolapse with zero or trivial mitral insufficiency, no arrhythmia
Mild mitral insufficiency
Patent ductus arteriosus within 3 months of surgery
Ventricular septal defect within 3–6 months of surgery
Atrial septal defect within 3 months of surgery
Pulmonary stenosis with mild residual stenosis and up to 2+ insufficiency
Coarctation of aorta within 4 months of surgery: very selective cases only
Tetralogy of Fallot 6–12 months after surgery: selected cases only
Total anomalous pulmonary venous return 6 months after surgery

$\dot{Q}p$ = pulmonary blood flow; $\dot{Q}s$ = systemic blood flow; RV = right ventricular.

Even moderate exercise is unsuitable and potentially dangerous in the situations listed in Table 2. Many of these children can still take part in light play activities, walking programs, calisthenics, or flexibility programs, in which exercise activities of 30 to 60 seconds are followed by pauses of 2 or 3 minutes. Assessment needs to be on an individual basis, and specific recommendations should be sought from a pediatric cardiologist. For some patients, activities of daily living are all that can be managed, and in extreme cases a wheelchair existence has to be enforced.

COMPARISON WITH ADULTS

Adults with coronary heart disease or who have undergone surgery for coronary vascular disease can benefit from structured supervised exercise programs that provide motivation, instruction, monitoring, and emergency care. Unrestricted competitive sport is never recommended for adults with coronary heart disease, because of the ever-present risk of infarction or arrhythmia.

For children with heart disease management is much simpler. In many the disease is mild, no restrictions are necessary, and there is no risk from vigorous competitive sports. Most young children want to be active, whereas many adults need to be led or even coerced out of a sedentary lifestyle. Children want to do what their friends are doing, and most of those with cardiac lesions can do just that. Children with structural heart defects seldom have life-threatening rhythm disturbances, and with a few exceptions sudden death precipitated by exercise is rare.

TABLE 2 Lesions Dictating Avoidance of any Significant Sports Competition or Serious Sports Training

Lesion
Aortic stenosis: peak gradient >40 mm Hg
Pulmonary stenosis: RV pressure >80
Pulmonary hypertension: mean PA pressure >30; pulmonary vascular resistance >5 units
Ventricular septal defect with $\dot{Q}p/\dot{Q}s > 2.5$
Ventricular septal defect with pulmonary stenosis: RV pressure >0.8 LV pressure
Tetralogy of Fallot unoperated
Transposition of great arteries: post-Mustard surgery
Hypertrophic cardiomyopathy
Congestive cardiomyopathy
Ebstein's malformation with significant tricuspid valve malfunction
Kawasaki's syndrome with coronary aneurysm or occlusion
Anomalous left coronary artery arising from pulmonary artery
Cyanotic heart disease uncorrected
Post-Fontan surgery
Myocarditis
Rheumatic pancarditis
Mitral regurgitation 3+ or worse
Marfan's syndrome with any aortic dilatation

$\dot{Q}p$ = pulmonary blood flow; $\dot{Q}s$ = systemic blood flow; RV = right ventricular; LV = left ventricular.

Because of the safety of exercise in this age group, children with major cardiac defects can be left to exercise on their own, with instructions to stop when they feel fatigued, short of breath, or light-headed. The supervision required in adult cardiology rehabilitation programs is not necessary.

SAFETY OF EXERCISE ACTIVITIES IN CHILDREN WITH HEART DISEASE

I have used maximal exercise to assess functional capacity in virtually every cardiac patient aged 4 years and over seen in a busy cardiology practice for 30 years. There has been no incident of ventricular fibrillation. About 20 patients with ventricular tachycardia of more than 30 seconds' duration have been encountered, but all reverted spontaneously to a normal rhythm, and none required cardioversion. A few patients changed from sinus rhythm and rates of 180 to 2:1 atrioventricular (AV) block and ventricular rates of about 90 with acute symptoms; again, there was spontaneous recovery within a few minutes. A few patients developed complete AV block during exercise, but there were no drastic consequences. Near-syncope during exercise occurred in one patient with moderately severe aortic stenosis. Postexercise syncope occurred in over a dozen normal patients, but in no child with significant heart disease. Nearly all patients were encouraged to exercise to the point of near-exhaustion, probably more intensely than in most exercise laboratories as judged by maximal heart rate values and postexercise lactate values. Only patients with cardiomyopathy, manifest cardiac failure, Marfan's syndrome, or severe aortic stenosis were excluded from performing near-maximal exercise.

In the same laboratory, serial exercise tests were carried out in a population of 510 "normal" men aged 40 to 64 years, with one case of ventricular fibrillation (successfully resuscitated) and several instances of ventricular tachycardia, atrial fibrillation, and flutter requiring medical intervention. Also in the same laboratory, adults with heart disease showed a 1 in 1,000 incidence of ventricular fibrillation (these also were successfully resuscitated). There is a definite difference between the vulnerability of the adult with or without manifest heart disease and that of children with various forms of heart disease.

Lambert and colleagues collected data from 20 pediatric centers on 254 cases of sudden unexpected death in patients 1 to 21 years of age with known heart disease. Ten percent of these occurred during or after sports participation. Over 50 percent had hypertrophic cardiomyopathy or aortic stenosis. No patient with rheumatic valvular disease died suddenly. It can be concluded that vigorous exercise activities are safe for children with mild and moderate heart anomalies (with the exception of those who have hypertrophic or dilated cardiomyopathy) and moderate aortic stenosis.

POTENTIAL DANGERS OF EXERCISE TRAINING IN CHILDREN WITH HEART LESIONS

Myocardial infarction occurs only rarely in patients under the age of 18 years. Occasionally, coronary atherosclerosis is severe enough to cause infarction at a young age in patients with homozygous familial hypercholesterolemia, or diabetes. Very rarely, myocardial bridges may cause ischemia, and anomalous origins of the left coronary artery have been implicated in exercise-induced infarction.

Sudden death during activity has occurred in some patients 1 to 10 years old after surgery for tetralogy of Fallot. Most of these children had poor right ventricular function, residual pulmonary stenosis, and resting ventricular ectopic activity; they are thus readily identified. Intense exercise programs are obviously contraindicated for such individuals.

Exercise-induced AV block can occur in patients with levotransposition of the great vessels, or in other patients with normal resting conduction. Patients who underwent surgery several years previously for ventricular septal defect or atrioventricular canal may have had a transient AV block in the postoperative period. These patients can develop exercise-related AV block of the second or third degree, and in such cases intense sport training is contraindicated. Maximal treadmill tests should be carried out periodically if these children are to engage in more than just recreational activities.

Patients with coarctation of the aorta, sometimes undiagnosed, can develop systolic blood pressures in excess of 275 mm Hg with exercise, and subarachnoid hemorrhage or other intracranial catastrophes have occurred.

After surgery for coarctation of the aorta, the resting blood pressure may be in the range of 130/70 mm Hg, but exercise can still lead to pressures in the 250/100 mm Hg range. Intense regular exercise training should not be allowed unless exercise pressures can be kept below 200 mm Hg systolic by medication, further surgery, or aortic ballooning. All patients with a history of coarctation of the aorta require treadmill or ergometer testing, with measurement of right arm blood pressure during exercise. Occasional late aortic rupture can occur at the anastomotic site in patients with coarctation. Yearly radiologic examination is required in patients of this group who are actively engaged in sports activities.

Patients with dilatation of the aorta secondary to congenital weakness, as in Marfan's or Ehlers-Danlos syndrome, should restrict exercise activities to the light recreational variety, because aortic rupture with strenuous activity has occurred even in 10-year-olds. Patients with significant aortic dilatation secondary to aortic stenosis, aortic injury, or other congenital anomalies should probably not take part in vigorous sport training.

There does not appear to be any danger of cardiac rupture when patients who have undergone ventriculotomy undertake vigorous exercise activities. Patients with right ventricular outflow tract patches, including those with moderate aneurysm formation, can exercise quite vigorously without obvious problems, but it would be foolhardy to recommend vigorous sports training for these individuals.

Exercise-induced syncope can occur in patients with pulmonary hypertension. Cardiac output fails to increase in a normal fashion, and with systemic vasodilatation systemic blood pressure falls, leading to cerebral anoxia. If postoperative heart catheterization studies are performed, exercise studies are also required to assess pulmonary hemodynamics. Occasional patients with resting pulmonary artery pressures in the range of 35/15 have pressures of 100/60 during intense exercise, since their pulmonary vasculature has lost the ability to dilate and accommodate an increase of blood flow without a large increase in pressure.

Exercise syncope also occurs in patients with aortic stenosis, who should not be exercising vigorously.

In patients with chronic hemodynamic overload due to mitral insufficiency, ill-advised daily exercise regimens can lead to manifestations of congestive heart failure that disappear with rest alone. Such individuals are not able to exercise vigorously, and even low-grade exercise programs can cause problems in patients who are just getting by without symptoms either at rest or with slow walking.

Cardiologists have different degrees of comfort or anxiety when an exercise test reveals arrhythmias in a child. Advice should not be based on adult experience of the potential danger of ventricular extrasystoles. In children who have had ventricular surgery, or in patients with lesions such as mitral valve prolapse, it is not unusual to precipitate bigeminy or over 10 extrasystoles per minute with exercise, most often in the first few minutes after stopping exercise.

These arrhythmias seem to be fairly benign. Regular exercise activities usually do not need to be restricted or monitored but intense sports training is probably unwise for such individuals. Occasionally, such patients demonstrate short runs of ventricular tachycardia or three to 10 beats, or multifocal ectopic beats that would be considered quite serious in an adult. These children, if asymptomatic, are generally given no treatment. Some physicians may wish to curtail these patients' activities, and others may prescribe ambulatory monitoring, but in general ordinary recreational activities are permissible. Some of these children engage in competitive sports at the intramural level, but serious sports training would be unwise.

When symptoms develop with arrhythmia, there is the danger that more serious arrhythmias may occur, and either exercise activities should be curtailed to intensities below which the arrhythmia is precipitated, or the arrhythmia should be controlled by medication. It is unlikely that intense sport training would ever be recommended for such patients.

ADVICE ON ALLOWABLE ACTIVITY

Physicians may wish to "play it safe" and advise any child with a heart lesion (or even with a normal murmur) to avoid strenuous exercise and competitive sports. Reasons for this approach may include genuine concern, lack of knowledge, or the fear of wrong diagnosis and litigation. Before the activity of any child is restricted, the advice of a pediatric cardiologist should be sought.

At each medical follow-up in children with heart defects (which may be as infrequent as once every 5 years for patients with trivial ventricular septal defect), the history should include exercise participation and exercise symptoms. Actual performance is easily assessed by a "level one" treadmill test. At the end of the medical review, child and parent should receive specific advice on the level of sports participation as listed in Table 3. Over 80 percent of patients fit into category 3 and above.

Under age 10 years, even children with significant residual defects can be allowed some competitive team sports, common sense being used to guide the level of participation. In this way, children usually decide on their own (along with 80 percent of their "normal" classmates) that their interest in athletics lies in the recreational and fun activities, not at levels that require training and intense competition. When a child over the age of 10 with a residual lesion wishes to pursue intense competition the extent of such competition and the type of sport require individual assessment and discussion. For many who want to follow this route, a suitable sport is available.

Immediately after surgery, children are advised to increase their activity gradually, building up walking from a few blocks to several kilometers over 2 weeks, bicycling by 14 days after most surgery, and resuming physical education in 2 months. Special rehabilitation measures are seldom required. I have encountered children who in error went into field-day competitions at school within 2 weeks after heart surgery with no adverse results. This is not advisable, but it does illustrate the adaptability of children.

Some special situations regarding exercise in children with cardiovascular disease are discussed below.

HYPERTENSION

Essential hypertension may have its onset during adolescence. Various population studies in children have found significant persistent hypertension in 2 percent of adolescents, and less severe and persistent blood pressure elevations in another 5 percent of "healthy" adolescents. The 95 percent confidence ceiling of blood pressure in adolescents is about 130/75 mm Hg.

Hagberg and colleagues reported the beneficial effects of endurance exercise in nine adolescents with essential hypertension. These authors also were able to obtain a 17/0 mm Hg reduction in blood pressure with weight training in adolescents.

TABLE 3 Levels of Physical Activity

Category	*Highest Activity Level*	*Example*
1	Intense sport training Interschool athletics: Tier 1 hockey	Trivial VSD Postoperative ASD
2	Moderate competitive sports participation in intramural athletics	Postoperative coarctation with good result
3	Regular physical education Avoidance of all-out competitive sport but able to go to the point of dyspnea, fatigue; recreation-level sports	Mild ASD: gradient 25 Postoperative tetralogy with good result
4	Regular physical education but letter to school giving medical permission to ease off when fatigued; recreation at own speed	Postoperative TGA with mild arrhythmia
5	Restricted physical education; limited running, no competitive games; recreation at own speed	ASD: gradient >40
6	Very limited physical education, observer, scorekeeper; walking or light bicycling only	Pulmonary atresia, inoperable
7	No activity other than attending class	Hypertrophic cardiomyopathy with arrhythmia
8	Wheelchair	Dilated cardiomyopathy with heart failure; considering transplant
9	Formal cardiac exercise class; appropriate to adult program as numbers do not justify a children's program	Rarely for child with exercise-induced arrhythmia

VSD = ventricular septal defect; ASD = atrial septal defect; TGA = transposition of great arteries.

One year after extra exercise lessons ceased, blood pressures were back to pretraining levels.

Weight training is often condemned as being unsuitable for patients with hypertension, coronary disease, or other structural diseases of the heart. However, there is no proof that mild or moderate work-outs with weights are in any way harmful.

Strong and associates studied the blood pressure response of black children to ergometer exercise and 50 percent of maximal hand grip sustained for 30 seconds or longer. At an age of 12 to 13 years, ergometer exercise increased systolic pressure an average of 34 mm Hg, and hand grip an average of 18 mm Hg. This suggests that there has been unwarranted concern about the dangers of isometric exercise in cardiac patients.

In adolescents with mild essential hypertension, systolic pressure during maximal ergometer exercise increases by about 55 mm Hg, the same as in normal patients. If it is assumed that exercise should cease when systolic pressure exceeds 230 mm Hg, adolescents with pressures over 175 mm Hg at rest should have their hypertension controlled before taking part in all-out sports.

Fixler and colleagues found that static exercise (a hand grip of 25 percent held for 4 minutes) increased systolic pressure by only 16 mm Hg in a group of hypertensive adolescents, much less than the value observed during cycle ergometer work; this suggests that isometric exercise or weight training is not particularly hazardous for children with mild hypertension.

The dramatic rise in blood pressure that occurs during exercise in some patients with coarctation of the aorta has already been mentioned.

THE FONTAN OPERATION

The right ventricle can be excluded from the circulation without greatly affecting overall resting cardiac performance. Fontan of France is given credit for showing that the right atrium can be connected directly to the pulmonary artery, with a consequent low mortality rate, excellent long-term results, and reasonable cardiac function. This operation opened the way for children with many complex congenital intracardiac lesions to have surgery that completely eliminated their cyanosis.

The common lesions suitable for this palliative therapy are those involving underdeveloped right ventricles (such as tricuspid atresia, pulmonary atresia, Uhl's anomaly, and lesions with single ventricles). In the last instance, the single ventricle is utilized to pump blood out of the aorta, and the pulmonary artery is blocked off from the single ventricle and is supplied by systemic venous blood directly from the right atrium. After the Fontan operation, resting cardiac index averaged 2.5 liters $\cdot min^{-1} \cdot m^{-2}$ (normal 4.1 liters$\cdot min^{-1} \cdot m^{-2}$), and in the same units the maximal exercise index averaged 6.2 (normal 11.1). The low cardiac output was partially compensated for by a lower mixed venous oxygen content and a resultant widening of the AV oxygen difference. Endurance times were below average in all patients, and below the tenth centile values for normal in 75 percent.

These patients cannot undergo serious sport training, but can take part in normal physical education and all recreational activities. Most can take part in recreational sports such as soccer to the best of their ability, with no concerns about safety; they simply slow down when they become tired.

TRANSPOSITION OF THE GREAT ARTERIES AFTER THE MUSTARD OPERATION

After undergoing the Mustard repair procedure, patients are acyanotic, are outwardly normal, and appear to lead normal lives. However, they have very abnormal cardiac anatomy; the right ventricle supports the systemic circulation, and interference with the sinus node and atrial conduction pathways may lead to problems of rhythm. Their exercise capacities in terms of endurance times are generally in the low-normal range, and seldom above the 50th centile. Ninety-three percent have a subnormal exercise heart rate, which likely is due to sinoatrial node dysfunction. The right ventricular ejection fraction fails to increase with supine exercise in 60 percent of such patients. Their exercise capacity correlates with the right ventricular ejection fraction. Such children are usually asymptomatic. They often claim to keep up with their friends in regular physical education, but on closer questioning admit to easier fatigability with running or other endurance activities. Except in those with significant rhythm problems or serious impairment of right ventricular function (RV ejection fraction less than 0.40), unrestricted recreational sport is permissible. There is no reason for these children not to take part in training programs to improve the strength and endurance of skeletal muscle, but regular treadmill tests are required to monitor for arrhythmias.

The arterial switch operation provides an anatomic correction for patients with transposition. There may be a narrowing at the pulmonary artery connection, there may be some aortic insufficiency, and there is a possibility that some coronary osteal stenosis may occur. Exercise performance in children without these complications should be normal, and regular physical education activities and recreational sport are possible. Theoretically, the child with a perfect anatomic result should be normal, with no contraindication to serious sports training.

SPONTANEOUS ACTIVITY

Most young children are active in their play, particularly when given the opportunity of outdoor freedom, away from the television set. In a group of 40 3- to 5-year-olds observed at a family summer camp, heart rates were above 150 percent of resting about 65 percent of the time. Average maximal free-time heart rates were 172 ± 9 for boys and 165 ± 10 for girls.

Spontaneous activity in this situation should have been sufficient for a training effect in children previously less active, e.g., those whose activity had been limited by a cardiac condition that was now corrected by surgery. For children aged 3 to 5 years with congenital heart disease, there is probably no better training than free-play activities with normal children.

Once children enter the controlled environment of school, and acquire the habit of watching television with less time devoted to free play, the heart rate of many is seldom above 130 beats·min^{-1}. Freedom to choose activities results in low fitness in many. It is all too easy for the child with a congenital heart anomaly to join the sedentary group; parents and teachers should see that these children have at least 1 hour each day of vigorous activity, provided that there is no medical contraindication.

AEROBIC TRAINING IN CHILDREN WITH HEART DISEASE

Training studies in normal children have not shown consistent increases of aerobic power. On the surface, it should be easy to enroll a group of children in a running program of at least one-half hour daily, which over 3 to 6 months produces definite gains in aerobic power. Numerous training studies have been carried out in normal children, as reviewed briefly by Bar-Or. As many reports show the absence of any significant improvement in aerobic power as show such improvements. Generally there has been improvement in running performance, and in ergometer studies improvement in work time or maximal workload. Gains in aerobic power were less consistent in 5- to 10-year-olds than in adolescents.

Training studies should follow a strict protocol. Both control and training groups should have three or four initial maximal exercise tests to allow familiarization with test methods, and appreciation of what is expected and what a maximal test is all about. Less than 50 percent of children develop a plateau of oxygen intake as the work rate is increased, so that there is no foolproof means of knowing whether a truly maximal effort and a maximal oxygen intake have been achieved. Average maximal heart rates should be about 205 in children aged 12 years and under, and 202 in children aged 13 to 16 years. Lactate should be at least 6.0 mmol per liter and preferably over 10 mmol per liter in children over the age of 12 years, and respiratory quotient should be 1.1 or greater, but in reported studies these ideals often have not been achieved. The maximal oxygen intake in normal boys in many studies is around 56 ml·kg^{-1}·min^{-1}. It is difficult to improve much beyond an average of 60 ml·kg^{-1}·min^{-1} unless the training is intense and is accompanied by a reduction in total body fat.

Given that consistent improvements in aerobic power have not been achieved in normal children (when there are large numbers of willing, almost captive, and motivated subjects), it is not surprising that consistent results have not been obtained in the few studies carried out in cardiac patients. These studies have all suffered from problems of small numbers, short training periods, lack of adequate practice sessions, failure to obtain true maximal efforts as judged by available indices, and lack of suitable controls. Miller and associates found no improvement in maximal oxygen intake in 12 children enrolled in ergometer training after heart surgery. This study is suspect because the maximal heart rates were low to begin with and even lower after the training, suggesting that the children could not be motivated to produce maximal efforts. Bradley and colleagues produced a 20 percent improvement in aerobic power in nine postoperative patients with tetralogy or transposition who were exercised twice weekly for 12 weeks. The mean maximal heart rate was 164 beats·min^{-1} for the first test and 181 beats·min^{-1} after training, suggesting that some patients did not make a true maximal effort in the initial assessment.

Goldberg and associates found an increase of maximal workload but not maximal oxygen intake with home ergometer training in 16 children after surgery for ventricular septal defect or tetralogy of Fallot, and Ruttenberg and associates obtained similar results. Galioto and colleagues produced a 23 percent increase in exercise cardiac output in eight postoperative patients who were given a hospital-based exercise program, but the degree of improvement that might have occurred by simply increasing activities at home and at school was not assessed.

One study with practical appeal was carried out at the Hospital for Sick Children in Toronto. Heart surgery children and parents were given instructions on a home program of progressive walking, calisthenics, and other exercises. Post-testing not unexpectedly showed improvement in most performance items in the group who were given specific instruction compared with those given none.

This type of specific advice costs little and may be preferable to general advice, although it has not been determined whether there is any difference 2 to 5 years later.

Our own studies on the treadmill endurance times in a general population of cardiac children showed that most children with cardiac lesions have fitness levels well within the normal range. Those who do not usually have serious heart lesions or are obese. The children with mild cardiac lesions and those with good results after cardiac surgery were encouraged to participate fully in school sports, and many took part in competitive activities such as hockey, soccer, skating, and track clubs. It would thus be expected that some of these children would have had treadmill endurance times above the 90th centile of a comparable normal group if high values of aerobic power (above 62 $ml \cdot kg^{-1} \cdot min^{-1}$ for males and 55 $ml \cdot kg^{-1} \cdot min^{-1}$ for females) were possible in these children. Overall, only 4 percent of the children with cardiac conditions were above the 90th centile, 40 percent of expected, and no children after surgery for pulmonary stenosis, aortic stenosis, coarctation of the aorta, patent ductus, tetralogy of Fallot, or other cyanotic lesions exceeded the 90th centile level for treadmill endurance.

This result suggests that such children have difficulty reaching superior levels of aerobic fitness. However, 43 percent of the entire group had treadmill endurance times in the 51st to 90th centile range, an indication that above-average fitness levels are certainly possible for a good many cardiac children in the absence of specific training programs.

There is no information available on strength or anaerobic training in cardiac children.

SUGGESTED READING

Bar-Or O. Pediatric sports medicine for the practitioner. New York: Springer-Verlag, 1983:46.

Benson LN, Bonet J, McLaughlen P, et al. Assessment of right ventricular function during supine bicycle exercise after Mustard's operation. Circulation 1982; 65:1052–1059.

Bradley LM, Galioto FM, Vaccaro P, et al. Effect of intense aerobic training on exercise performance in children after surgical repair of tetralogy of Fallot or complete transposition of great arteries. Am J Cardiol 1985; 56:816–818.

Cumming GR. Maximal exercise capacity of children with heart defects. Am J Cardiol 1979; 42:613–619.

Cumming GR. Maximal exercise hemodynamics after the Fontan procedure. In: Doyle EF, Engle MA, Gersony WM, et al, eds. Pediatric cardiology. New York: Springer-Verlag, 1985:257.

Cumming GR, Everatt D, Hastman L. Bruce treadmill test in children: normal values in a clinic population. Am J Cardiol 1978; 41:69–75.

Fixler DE, Laird P, Braune R, et al. Response of hypertensive adolescents to dynamic and isometric exercise stress. Pediatrics 1979; 64:579–583.

Fontan F, Baudet E. Surgical repair of tricuspid atresia. Thorax 1971; 26:240–248.

Galioto FM, Tomassoni MA, Vaccaro P, Vaccaro J. Effect on cardiac output of a cardiac rehabilitation program in children after repair of congenital heart disease. JACC 1988; II:250A (abstract).

Goldberg B, Fripp RR, Lake LG, et al. Effect of physical training on exercise performance of children following surgical repair of congenital heart disease. Pediatrics 1981; 68:691–699.

Hagberg JM, Ehsani AA, Godring D, et al. Effect of weight training on blood pressure and hemodynamics in hypertensive adolescents. J Pediatr 1984; 104:147–151.

Hagberg JM, Ehsani AA, Heath GW, et al. Beneficial effects of endurance exercise training in adolescent hypertension. Am J Cardiol 1980; 45:489.

Hesslein PS, Gutgesell HP, Gillett PC, McNamara DG. Exercise assessment of sinoatrial node function following the Mustard operation. Am Heart J 1982; 103:351–357.

Kucera M. Spontaneous physical activities in preschool children. In: Binkhorst RA, Kemper HCG, Saris WHM, eds. Children and exercise XI. Chicago: Human Kinetics, 1985:175.

Lambert EC, et al. Sudden unexpected death from cardiovascular disease in children. A cooperative international study. Am J Cardiol 1974; 34:89–97.

Longmuir P, et al. The benefits of a postoperative exercise program for children with congenital heart disease. Clin Invest Med 1983; 5(Suppl 1):45 (abstract).

Miller WW, Young DS, Bloomqvist CG. Physical training in children with congenital heart disease. In: Lavallee H, Shephard RJ, eds. Frontiers of activity and child health. Limites de la capacité physique obese l'enfant. Quebec: Pelican, 1977: 363.

Murphy JH, Barlai-Kovach MM, Mathews RA, et al. Rest and exercise right and left ventricular function late after the Mustard operation: assessment by Radionuclide ventriculography. Am J Cardiol 1983; 51:1520–1526.

Ruttenberg HD, Adams TD, Orsmond GS, et al. Effects of exercise training on aerobic fitness in children after open heart surgery. Pediatr Cardiol 1983; 4:19–24.

Strong WH, Miller MD, Striplen M, Salehbhai M. Blood pressure response to isometric and dynamic exercise in healthy black children. Am J Dis Child 1978; 132:587–591.

EXERCISE AND PREGNANCY

DAVID YOUNG, M.D., M.Sc., F.R.C.S.(C)

Together with the general increased interest and participation in exercise by our fitness-conscious society, there has been an increase in exercise among women who are pregnant. Special concerns in pregnancy relate to the effects of maternal exercise on the fetus and the mother, subsequent to the maternal physiologic adaptations that occur during pregnancy. There is no consistent evidence to support the popular notion that regular exercise improves the outcome of pregnancy. For the pregnant exerciser who experiences an injury, the proposed therapy must take into account the potential effects on the fetus.

Although there is a rapidly expanding research literature on exercise during pregnancy, the mother and her physician must continue to be conservative and prudent. The guidelines for exercise developed by the American College of Obstetrics and Gynecology remain appropriate for most of our patients.

MATERNAL PHYSIOLOGIC CHANGES DURING PREGNANCY

During normal pregnancy, the maternal blood volume increases by about 30 percent, and the resting cardiac output increases by 30 to 50 percent by midpregnancy. The increase of cardiac output is accomplished by an increase in stroke volume and a rise in resting maternal heart rate. These changes reduce the cardiac reserve that would otherwise be available during increased physical activity.

Another important physiologic adaptation is the increased capacitance of the venous system. This allows the maternal blood volume to increase without a significant growth in preloading of the heart. The supine hypotensive syndrome is a well-recognized phenomenon after the first trimester; the enlarged uterus obstructs venous return by compressing the inferior vena cava, and subsequently affecting cardiac output and potentially the uterine circulation. The pregnant exerciser should avoid the supine position.

Many women experience discomfort and an air hunger as the enlarging uterus displaces the diaphragm upward. However, lateral expansion of the rib cage compensates, so that pulmonary function is not impaired at rest. The hormones of pregnancy, in particular progesterone, lead centrally to an increase in tidal volume, so that the resting respiratory minute ventilation increases. There is no change in lung capacity, so that the functional residual capacity decreases. Blood gas measurements taken during a normal pregnancy, at rest, would show a mild compensated respiratory alkalosis.

An additional 1,200 kilojoules (300 kcal) per day are required to meet the metabolic needs of pregnancy; actively exercising women need even more. During pregnancy, fasting blood glucose levels are lower than in nonpregnant women, and carbohydrates form the primary substrate during exercise. Hypoglycemia and starvation ketosis may thus develop more readily during exercise in pregnancy. The pregnant exerciser should increase her fluid intake during exercise, and probably not exercise in the truly fasting state, i.e., before breakfast. The risk of exercise-induced dehydration is increased in pregnant women, and this in turn could lead to a dangerous increase of core temperature. There is a risk that an increased core temperature during the first trimester may give rise to congenital anomalies.

Under the hormonal influences of pregnancy, the connective tissues become softer and more easily stretched. Although this may be beneficial for pelvic compliance during delivery, it may lead to joint instability and increased susceptibility to injury during exercise. As the uterus enlarges, there is a change in the body's center of gravity and an increasing lumbar lordosis. Balance problems increase the risk of falls. Further stress on the sacroiliac and hip joints may create back strain and hip pain.

EFFECT ON THE FETUS

After the first trimester, the greatest danger that maternal exercise presents to the fetus stems from the potential redistribution of blood flow from the viscera (including the uterus) to the exercising muscles. In nonpregnant women, this redistribution is well established as being largely mediated by the sympathetic hormones, epinephrine and norepinephrine, leading to visceral vasoconstriction. Acute or chronic fetal deprivation of oxygen and nutrients could result. Animal research suggests that uterine blood flow must be reduced by more than 50 percent before fetal compromise occurs. There is also evidence that the action of catecholamines upon the blood vessels is blunted during pregnancy, although the mechanism is as yet undefined. Possible explanations include the generalized effect of increased steroid levels in pregnancy, or the local release of prostaglandins and their precursors. It has not been possible to study uterine blood flow in pregnant human females in the past. However, with the advancing technology of Doppler ultrasonography, a better appreciation of uterine blood flow and the response to maternal exercise may soon be forthcoming.

It is difficult to draw conclusions concerning the effects on the fetus of maternal exercise during pregnancy. The number of women studied in controlled circumstances is not substantial. With the overall low incidence of an abnormal fetal outcome in the 1980s, large sample sizes would be needed to determine with confidence that exercise has no harmful effect. In addition, existing studies have been of pregnant women at differing levels of general physical condition (some being involved in vigorous exercise before pregnancy, and others not); different types of exercise (weightbearing activity such as jogging or treadmill exercises versus nonweightbearing such as cycle ergometry); and differing duration, intensity, and frequency of exercise.

No consistent and clinically significant abnormalities have been found with regard to perinatal mortality, morbidity, birth weight, or Apgar scores in the fetuses of exercising mothers. A prospective study by Clapp suggested that women who continued endurance exercise at or near preconception levels during pregnancy on average gained 4.6 kg less body mass, delivered 8 days earlier, and had offspring that were 500 g lighter than those who stopped exercising before the 28th week of pregnancy. Another study by Kulpa revealed no difference in pregnancy outcomes. A third study from Hall proclaimed improved outcomes in the exercised group, particularly those exercising at high levels. Unfortunately, the numbers of women who continued to exercise regularly in the third trimester in these studies were only 29, 38, and 61, respectively.

The biophysical variables of fetal movement (by maternal perception or real-time ultrasound visualization) and fetal heart activity (electronic monitoring of fetal heart rate) are commonly used to assess fetal well-being. Nearly all existing evidence on these biophysical variables has been collected before and after exercise testing. Technical problems, related to movement of the maternal abdomen, have limited the collection of data during exercise. Maternal exercise of moderate intensity has generally produced a fetal tachycardia of 10 to 30 beats per minute (bpm) above the pre-exercise baseline, a change not clinically significant in most circumstances. Whether the fetal tachycardia is influenced by gestational age or the intensity of maternal exercise remains in doubt. Of concern are reports of fetal bradycardia in approximately 10 percent of fetuses during or after moderate to strenuous aerobic exercise (maternal heart rates of 130 to 150 bpm). In some cases, fetal heart rates reached levels that would normally reflect severely compromised fetal cardiac output. In all cases, the birth outcome of these pregnancies was favorable. Recent publications have questioned whether some of this may have been artifact. Our own research in 16 pregnant women, physically fit before pregnancy, whose fetuses were monitored electronically during exercise and observed by ultrasonography afterward, has not encountered significant fetal bradycardia. We observed fetal heart rate accelerations, generally accepted as ruling out significant fetal compromise, in four fetuses while their mothers were exercising on a cycle ergometer with maternal heart rates greater than 130 bpm.

Little has been reported on the effect of maternal exercise on fetal limb or breathing movements. One small study of 17 subjects observed by real-time ultrasonography before and after mild exercise found no change in the percentage of time that the fetus was involved in fetal breathing or in the number of fetal limb movements.

EXERCISE GUIDELINES

The following conditions are contraindications to vigorous exercise during pregnancy: ruptured membranes, preterm labor, multiple gestation, incompetent cervix, antepartum bleeding, intrauterine growth retardation, maternal cardiac disease, and hypertension or other medical problems leading to maternal or fetal compromise.

Any unusual signs and symptoms should alert the patient to stop exercise and seek medical attention. Particular attention should be paid to pain, bleeding, dizziness, shortness of breath, palpitations, faintness, and difficulty in walking.

In the light of current information, much common sense needs to be applied to the development of an appropriate exercise program for pregnant mothers. The program should be individualized, taking into consideration the mother's preferences, her level of fitness, the facilities available, her current health, and the progress of the pregnancy. Nonweightbearing exercises such as swimming and bicycle riding are to be encouraged. Exercise and sports involving jumping, twisting, or rapid turning should be avoided. A warm-up session is recommended for joints and muscles. The supine position should be avoided. A reasonably safe maximal intensity of exercise during pregnancy would be 60 to 70 percent of the age-adjusted maximal heart rate (220 minus the age in years). Environmental conditions must be watched more closely. In an exercise program that maintains fitness and yet is safe, the pregnant woman should exercise for no more than 30 minutes three times weekly, followed on each occasion by a cool-down session. Fortunately, even the most competitive athlete requires little persuasion to discontinue contact sports and to avoid striving for personal bests during pregnancy.

MANAGEMENT OF EXERCISE-INDUCED MATERNAL INJURY

External treatment of limb joints involving heat, cold, or physiotherapy can carry on as usual. When considering use of systemic analgesics and anti-inflammatory agents, the risk for the fetus must be weighed against the probable benefit to the mother. Indomethacin and the nonsteroidal anti-inflammatory agents should be avoided because of the potential intrauterine effects on closure of the fetal ductus arteriosus. The usual therapeutic doses of acetylsalicylic acid give rise to the same concerns, plus a prolonged effect upon maternal and fetal platelet function. Acetaminophen with or without codeine seems the safest choice at the present time. Steroids may be used if necessary, although one must remember the possible association of cleft lip with the chronic use of steroids during the first trimester. Prednisone is the steroid of choice when indicated for the mother, because it seems to have the poorest placental transport.

SUGGESTED READING

ACOG Home Exercise Programs. Exercise during pregnancy and the postnatal period. Washington, DC: American College of Obstetrics and Gynecology, 1985:1–6.

Artal R, Romem Y, Paul RH, Wiswell R. Foetal bradycardia induced by maternal exercise. Lancet 1984; 2:258–260.

Artal R, Rutherford S, Romem Y, et al. Fetal heart rate responses to maternal exercise. Am J Obstet Gynecol 1986; 155:729–733.

Artal R, Wiswell RA. Exercise in pregnancy. Baltimore: Williams & Wilkins, 1986.

Berkowitz RL, Coustan DR, Mochizuki TK. Handbook for prescribing medications during pregnancy. Boston: Little, Brown, 1986.

Carpenter MW, Sady SP, Hoegsberg B, et al. Fetal heart rate response to maternal exertion. JAMA 1988; 259:3006–3009.

Clapp JF, Dickstein S. Endurance exercise and pregnancy outcome. Med Sci Sports Exerc 1984; 16:556–562.

Dale E, Mullinax KM, Bryan DH. Exercise during pregnancy: effects on the fetus. Can J Appl Sport Sci 1982; 7:98–103.

Hall DC, Kaufmann DA. Effects of aerobic and strength condi-

tioning on pregnancy outcomes. Am J Obstet Gynecol 1987; 157:1199–1203.
Jovanovic L, Kessler A, Peterson CM. Human maternal and fetal responses to graded exercise. J Appl Physiol 1985; 58:1719–1722.
Kulpa PJ, White BM, Visscher R. Aerobic exercise in pregnancy. Am J Obstet Gynecol 1987; 156:1395–1403.
Morton MJ, Paul MS, Metcalfe J. Exercise in pregnancy. Med Clin North Am 1985; 69:97–108.
Paolone AM, Shangold M, Paul D, Minnitti J, Weiner S. Fetal heart rate measurement during maternal exercise—avoidance of artifact. Med Sci Sports Exerc 1987; 19:605–609.
Platt LD, Artal R, Semel J, Sipos L, Kammula RK. Exercise in pregnancy. II. Fetal responses. Am J Obstet Gynecol 1983; 147:487–491.

PHYSIOTHERAPY IN SPORTS MEDICINE

MAUREEN E. HUNT, B.Sc. (P.T.)

Although the first illustrated text on the relationship between medicine and sports and the role of exercise in gaining and preserving health was written in 1569 by Geronimo Mercuriale, we are still striving to improve upon this important union of disciplines. The liaison among physicians, physiotherapists, and trainers is invaluable.

The field of sports physiotherapy in recent years has become more specific, as therapists perform more basic research and conduct well-designed clinical trials.

The physiotherapeutic management of athletes should begin before any injury occurs. Physiotherapists should be part of any athlete's "coaching squad" to ensure that training, from basic to advanced levels, is well designed for the individual and the specific activity. Preventive training is the best form of management. Faults in movement patterns must be recognized and corrected before injuries occur.

When assessing the individual athlete, whether a recreational amateur or a highly competitive professional, the physiotherapist is alert to problems related to posture, muscle-strength imbalance, flexibility, and orthopaedic anomalies that may be the primary, underlying cause of injury. These factors must be dealt with, both to prevent injury and (if injury has already occurred) to render treatment more effective. Treating an injury that may be secondary to some unrecognized problem is frustrating for both the athlete and the therapist, because it will be less successful and more time consuming than necessary. For example, treating a shoulder lesion when there are muscle imbalances secondary to poor cervical posture may eventually be successful, but the success is likely to be only temporary, with recurrence of the problem when normal physical activity is resumed.

Athletic injuries, 80 percent of which affect soft tissues, fall into a few common categories: strains and sprains, overuse syndromes, direct trauma, and hematomas. Most frequently seen are injuries to the ankles, knees, shoulders, and spine.

There is a wide spectrum of physiotherapy modalities, from moist heat and ice to ultrasonography and lasers (Table 1). Each modality, if used with specific objectives, has value as an adjunct to enhance healing. However, the physiotherapeutic manage-

TABLE 1 Summary of Common Physiotherapeutic Modalities and Their Effects

Modality	*Healing Phase*	*Effect*
Ice/cold	Acute inflammatory phase	Reduction of local blood flow, swelling, and edema Local analgesic to reduce pain and spasm
Heat	Chronic maturation phase	Local rise in tissue temperature Increased metabolism and blood flow with increased oxygen supply to tissue Local analgesic
Ultrasonography	Subacute chronic maturation phase	As for heat Increased tissue permeability Increased collagen extensibility Local analgesic Assists in resolution of chronic inflammatory process
Electrical stimulation	Chronic maturation remodeling phase	To enhance muscle contraction
Transcutaneous-electrical nerve stimulation (TENS)	Subacute chronic maturation phase	To reduce pain and permit controlled mobilization

ment of any condition requires thorough assessment, not only initially but throughout the healing process, in order to ensure that the chosen modalities or techniques of treatment are having the desired effect. Unless there is regard for a total rehabilitation program, most modalities are of little, if any, value.

Treatment begins with first aid, to make sure that the effects of the injury are minimized. Elevation is a form of therapy that is always available and effective. Compression with wet, preferably cold, wraps should be applied and repeated for 20 to 30 minutes every 2 to 3 hours. Positioning of the injured tissue for rest or more active intervention must be optimized. Often, patients are simply advised to rest, and little emphasis is placed on the correct positioning, which may be vital to optimal tissue healing.

After the initial inflammatory stage, "early, controlled mobilization" of the tissue is important to minimize pain and maximize healing. Control of pain, with low-grade mobilization, allows gentle, directional stress to be applied to tissue earlier, so that strength is restored to tissue along the appropriate stress lines. Correct realignment of collagen fibrils during healing is important for the future strength of the tissue and success of the athlete.

Early mobilization with controlled, active movement also limits atrophy and loss of coordination. Movement permitted within a specified range, with appropriate external support such as taping or splinting, minimizes time lost and secondary complications.

Secondary complications, such as a diminished range of joint motion secondary to immobilization after an anterior cruciate repair, are often more difficult to treat and more time consuming than the original injury. Early intervention is therefore important, as long as it is appropriate and does not impede natural healing.

Early, controlled mobilization, be it passive or active, also benefits the athlete psychologically. There is less pain, and it is always encouraging when movement of the part is permitted. However, there must be adherence to a very specific regimen, so that the individual appreciates that there are limits and does not become too enthusiastic.

As reassessment is ongoing, the physiotherapist is able to increase the angular range through which the tissue can safely be moved, and the degree of resistance can also be increased without fear of further damage to the healing tissue.

Therapeutic exercise, which falls under the domain of rehabilitation, must be distinguished from exercise per se. A therapeutic exercise program must take into account many factors, the most important of which is the stage of healing of the tissue being considered. Once healing has reached the maturation phase, more appropriately patterned movements must be used. Uniplanar movements must be replaced with normal patterns of movement, so that each component of the normal physiologic action of the part may be assessed and restored where necessary. The use of normally patterned movements also restores correct muscle firing and coordination. Adaptive changes that take place are specific to the tissues and the manner in which they are used, so it is imperative that the physiotherapist appreciate the specific movements required by an athlete when performing in a particular discipline. If the therapist has not observed the athlete's performance before the injury, a videotape of someone performing the same skill may be helpful. Videotaping the athlete later in the rehabilitation period may also be useful, in order to point out postural or habitual movement errors that may lead to renewed injury.

Selection of specific exercises must be based on an analysis of the muscles and the joint angles to be trained. Specific goals must be set that are realistic, so that the athlete is not discouraged by a failure to satisfy excessive expectations.

As treatment progresses, it expands into the retraining phase. The greater the need for transfer of the effects of training to the specific skills required by the athlete, the more important it is that the exercises selected closely mimic the angles, speed, and type of muscle contraction used in the specific sport skills.

Perhaps the most important attribute of the physiotherapist is a knowledge of arthrokinematics and the mechanisms of joint lubrication. Ongoing analysis of movement patterns and the end-feel of tissue and its relationship to pain is our greatest tool. With this knowledge, the physiotherapist can determine just how much stress tissue can tolerate at any moment during healing. Diminished accessory joint motion can be restored, so that normal movement patterns are possible and the tissue heals with correct alignment of collagen fiber.

SPECIAL CONCERNS OF THE FEMALE ATHLETE

MONA M. SHANGOLD, M.D.

There has been a tremendous increase in the participation of women in regular exercise programs and a much greater awareness of the importance of exercise for the long-term health and well-being of women. The increased participation of women in both recreational and competitive exercise programs has increased our awareness of special problems that concern women athletes: menstrual disturbances, delayed puberty, fertility, pregnancy, contraception, dysmenorrhea, stress urinary incontinence, and breast support.

MENSTRUAL DISTURBANCES

The menstrual problems that are more common among athletes than among the general population are often multifactorial in etiology. Athletes who develop amenorrhea (cessation of menstruation) are more likely to experience stress, weight loss, thinness, and nutritional inadequacy than athletes who continue to menstruate regularly. Some disturbances are obvious; others are subtle.

The three major types of menstrual disturbances are luteal phase inadequacy, anovulatory oligomenorrhea, and hypoestrogenic amenorrhea. Luteal phase inadequacy is more common among athletes than among the general population. However, this abnormality can be detected only if the problem is sought. In women who experience luteal phase inadequacy, the second half of the menstrual cycle (following ovulation) may be of reduced duration or there may be decreased levels of progesterone in that portion of the cycle. This condition may be associated with infertility and warrants treatment only if pregnancy is desired.

Anovulatory oligomenorrhea is a condition in which women produce estrogen but do not ovulate. This leads to continuous stimulation of the endometrium (the inner lining of the uterus) and may lead to endometrial hyperplasia or adenocarcinoma, if untreated. Although there are no studies showing the prevalence of this condition among athletes and no case reports of endometrial carcinoma in athletes, athletes can develop hyperplasia and cancer and probably should be treated to prevent it. It is my impression that few athletic women experience anovulatory oligomenorrhea long enough to be endangered by it. However, the unpredictable and occasionally profuse bleeding that may occur in women who have this condition is certainly inconvenient. Therefore, I recommend treating women who have anovulatory oligomenorrhea, even if this condition lasts for only a short time.

The most serious condition that athletic women experience is hypoestrogenic amenorrhea, a disorder in which they do not menstruate and make very little estrogen. These women have an increased risk of developing osteoporosis because they lack the normal protective effect of estrogen on the bones. It is impossible to predict how long an athlete will have this condition. If it lasts for more than 3 years, she will probably have lost a significant amount of bone density that cannot subsequently be regained. For this reason, I recommend treating any woman who has had hypoestrogenic amenorrhea for longer than 6 months.

Before a woman with any of these conditions is treated, a thorough evaluation is necessary. Any woman who bleeds more often than every 25 days or less often than every 35 days warrants a thorough evaluation, including history-taking and physical examination. Laboratory tests should include thyroid function tests and measurement of serum prolactin, thyrotropin (TSH), follicle-stimulating hormone (FSH), luteinizing hormone (LH), dehydroepiandrosterone sulfate (DHEAS), testosterone, and beta-human chorionic gonadotropin (hCG). These tests will detect any serious causes of the menstrual disturbance (e.g., a pituitary tumor, hypothyroidism, hyperandrogenism, premature menopause, or pregnancy). Athletes are not immune to serious pathologic conditions, and such conditions can be detected only if they are sought. Once pregnancy has been ruled out, it is useful to perform a progestin challenge test to determine the endogenous estrogen level. Women who have sufficient endogenous estrogen to have withdrawal bleeding after progestin administration require monthly administration for endometrial protection. Women who do not have withdrawal bleeding after progestin administration do not have enough endogenous estrogen to protect their bones and require estrogen replacement therapy for skeletal protection. Any woman who has a uterus and who is treated with estrogen should also be given a progestin to protect the endometrium.

Athletes with anovulatory oligomenorrhea should be given monthly progestin therapy. I prescribe medroxyprogesterone acetate, 10 mg daily for 12 consecutive days of each calendar month. If the athlete desires pregnancy, ovulation should be induced with clomiphene citrate. An anovulatory athlete may be treated instead with oral contraceptives, which provide endometrial protection and contraception.

Women who have hypoestrogenic amenorrhea may also be treated with oral contraceptives. These agents provide both estrogen and progestin, thereby protecting bones and endometrium, as well as contraception. Oral contraceptive agents provide pharmacologic doses of estrogen and progestin, whereas skeletal and endometrial protection may be achieved with physiologic replacement therapy. I usually prescribe conjugated estrogens (0.625 to 1.25 mg daily on the first 25 days of each calendar month) and medroxyprogesterone acetate (10 mg daily on days 14 to 25 of every calendar month).

Although many athletes have an aversion to hormone ingestion, they should be informed about the risks of their condition and encouraged to undergo hormonal therapy.

Some athletes may choose to alter their training in an attempt to regain normal menstrual function. This plan is accepted best when it is the patient's suggestion, rather than the physician's. Any athlete who wishes to modify her training or weight in an attempt to regain normal menstrual function should be permitted to do so. However, hypoestrogenic amenorrhea should not be allowed to continue for more than 6 months without treatment.

DELAYED PUBERTY

Athletic girls tend to experience menarche (first menstruation) at a later age than the general population. Any girl who has not begun to menstruate by the age of 16 should be examined and further evaluated. Any girl who has not experienced thelarche (breast development) or adrenarche (appearance of pubic and axillary hair) by the age of 14 should be examined and evaluated also. No girl should avoid exercise for fear of delaying puberty. If puberty is delayed, the problem should be dealt with at that time. There are no medical hazards from delayed puberty, but psychological harm may result in an adolescent whose secondary sexual development lags behind that of her peers. Those who remain hypoestrogenic beyond the age of 18 should be treated with hormone replacement therapy for skeletal protection because they will otherwise be losing bone at a time when they should be adding it.

FERTILITY

Running and other endurance sports do not impair future fertility. However, the prevalence of menstrual disturbances among athletes would increase the likelihood of infertility if these women desired pregnancy at this time. Surveys of athletic women have revealed no greater an incidence of infertility than exists among the general population. This may be because many athletes do not desire pregnancy at the time of intensive training. The infertility experienced by athletes who have luteal phase inadequacy, anovulatory oligomenorrhea, or hypoestrogenic amenorrhea appears to be transient and reversible, resolving with medication, with reduced exercise, or spontaneously.

PREGNANCY

Prudent exercise may be continued throughout uncomplicated pregnancies by women who were accustomed to aerobic sports before becoming pregnant. It is probably reasonable for a trained athlete to continue exercising in the same aerobic sport she was accustomed to before pregnancy, although at a slower pace. The pregnant body is doing more work merely by virtue of being pregnant, and if the woman exercises with the added weight of pregnancy, she is doing even more work. Women who were not accustomed to any aerobic exercise before pregnancy should engage in no aerobic activity more vigorous than brisk walking. Sports should be avoided if they reduce oxygen availability to the fetus or cause hyperthermia. Thus, maximal exertion should be avoided because of the risk of decreased uterine blood flow and a decreased oxygen supply to the fetus. Although moderate exercise appears to be safe, the limits of safety have not been determined. For this reason, it is best for pregnant athletes to limit any aerobic exercise to 30 minutes at a moderate intensity. Axillary or rectal temperature should be assessed at the end of a customary exercise session, preferably early in pregnancy, in order to ensure that hyperthermia is avoided. Hyperthermia in early pregnancy is associated with an increased risk of neural tube defects in the fetus, while hyperthermia in later pregnancy may induce premature labor.

Direct abdominal trauma is undesirable during pregnancy, but the fetus is actually quite well protected during early pregnancy by the bones and muscles of the maternal pelvis and in later pregnancy by a cushion of amniotic fluid. The bouncing and shaking movements of running and aerobic dancing pose no dangers for the fetus.

Weight training and stretching exercises are safe for pregnant women, even if they never practiced them before pregnancy.

CONTRACEPTION

The choice of a contraceptive agent is rarely affected by the fact that a woman is an athlete. Oral contraceptives are acceptable for women provided there are no medical contraindications (e.g., a history of thromboembolic disease, hyperlipidemia, liver disease, breast cancer, or cigarette smoking), particularly if they have coitus at least twice a week. Oral contraceptive agents have not been shown to affect athletic performance. The major side effects associated with oral contraceptives are amenorrhea and breakthrough bleeding, both of which can be treated by manipulation of dose.

Intrauterine devices (IUDs) are acceptable for women who have completed childbearing, particularly if they are in monogamous sexual relationships. A slight risk of pelvic infections is associated with the use of such devices in those who have more than one sexual partner or whose partners have more than one sexual partner. This increased risk makes IUDs less desirable for women who want more children. Such devices may increase menstrual blood loss and pelvic pain in some women, who may experience impaired athletic performance as a result. IUDs remain in position during all types of exercise and are never dislodged by either endurance sports or contact sports.

Mechanical contraceptives are an excellent choice for motivated, disciplined couples practicing any coital frequency. The diaphragm must be left in place for at least 6 hours after each ejaculation. However, it is safe and not uncomfortable for a woman to exercise while her diaphragm remains in proper place in the vagina. Those who experience discomfort while wearing a diaphragm during exercise should be examined to check its proper placement and size. Some women may benefit from wearing a diaphragm that is one size smaller.

DYSMENORRHEA

Dysmenorrhea (menstrual cramps) results from myometrial contractions induced by prostaglandins, which are released by the endometrium at the time of menstruation. The most effective way of preventing menstrual cramps is to administer prostaglandin synthetase inhibitors, which are usually needed only for a day or two at the time of menstruation. Some athletes experience less dysmenorrhea during exercise, but exercise is rarely effective in providing total, lasting relief of pain.

STRESS URINARY INCONTINENCE

Stress urinary incontinence (involuntary leakage of urine during the Valsalva maneuver) is more common during exercise than during rest because intra-abdominal pressure rises during exercise. Women who have an anatomic defect that causes stress incontinence are more likely to be symptomatic when they exercise. However, exercise does not cause or worsen the underlying anatomic abnormality. The pelvic organs are very adequately protected by the bones and muscles surrounding them. Endurance sports pose no dangers to the function or support of the female pelvic organs.

BREAST SUPPORT

The breasts rarely present problems or dangers for female athletes. Composed mostly of fat, the breasts resist trauma well and heal quickly and completely when injury does occur. Most women who have large breasts find it physically and psychologically uncomfortable to exercise without wearing a supportive bra. However, such a garment is needed merely for comfort rather than for medical indications. The bouncing of the breasts that occurs during exercise is not harmful.

Many competitive athletes have very little body fat. Since the breast is composed mostly of fat tissue, breast size usually reflects body fat levels. Therefore, thin women usually have small breasts and may find it more comfortable to exercise without wearing a bra.

Exercise does not enlarge a woman's breasts, although exercises that strengthen the pectoral muscles may give the illusion of a fuller chest. Endurance exercise usually promotes an overall loss of body fat, which usually leads to a reduction in breast size.

Loss of breast support generally occurs with aging and is related to hereditary tendencies. There are no data suggesting that exercise hastens this loss of support.

SUGGESTED READING

Bullen BA, Skrinar GS, Beitins IZ, et al. Induction of menstrual disorders by strenuous exercise in untrained women. N Engl J Med 1985; 312:1349.

Cumming DC, Vickovic MM, Wall SR, Fluker MR, Belcastro AN. The effect of acute exercise on pulsatile release of luteinizing hormone in women runners. Am J Obstet Gynecol 1985; 153:482.

Drinkwater BL, Nilson K, Chesnut CH, et al. Bone mineral content of amenorrheic and eumenorrheic athletes. N Engl J Med 1984; 311:277.

Frisch R, Gotz-Welbergen A, McArthur J, et al. Delayed menarche and amenorrhea of college athletes in relation to age of onset of training. JAMA 1981; 246:1559.

Lotgering FK, Gilbert RD, Longo LD. The interactions of exercise and pregnancy: a review. Am J Obstet Gynecol 1984; 149:560.

Malina R, Spirduso W, Tate C, et al. Age at menarche and selected menstrual characteristics in athletes at different competitive levels and in different sports. Med Sci Sports 1978; 10:218.

Prior JC, Cameron K, Ho Yuen B, et al. Menstrual cycle changes with marathon training: anovulation and short luteal phase. Can J Appl Sport Sci 1982; 7:173.

Prior JC, Ho Yuen B, Clement P, Bowie L, Thomas J. Reversible luteal phase changes and infertility associated with marathon training. Lancet 1982; 2:269.

Schwartz B, Cumming DC, Riordan E, et al. Exercise-associated amenorrhea: a distinct entity? Am J Obstet Gynecol 1981; 141:662.

Shangold MM. The pain of dysmenorrhea. J Am Med Wom Assoc 1983; 38:12.

Shangold MM, Freeman R, Thysen B, et al. The relationship between long-distance running, plasma progesterone and luteal phase length. Fertil Steril 1979; 31:130.

Shangold MM, Levine HS. The effect of marathon training upon menstrual function. Am J Obstet Gynecol 1982; 143:862.

Warren MP. The effects of exercise on pubertal progression and reproductive function in girls. J Clin Endocrinol Metab 1980; 51:1150.

EXERCISE-INDUCED BRONCHIAL OBSTRUCTION

ALAN R. MORTON, M.Sc., Ed. D., F.A.C.S.M.
KENNETH D. FITCH, M.D., F.A.C.S.M.

Asthma, one of the most common respiratory disorders, is a major cause of morbidity in childhood and adolescence and carries a significant mortality rate throughout life. The incidence is greatest during primary school age; it is more common in boys than in girls (1.5:1 ratio), but is also higher in older women than in older men.

The airways may be narrowed by contraction of bronchial smooth muscle, swelling of the mucous membrane, or an increased mucous secretion from goblet cells. The result is an increase of airway resistance, and recruitment of accessory respiratory muscles may be necessary in order to maintain a now noisy or wheezing bronchial airflow. The bronchoconstriction and mucosal edema serve to increase the unfavorable transmural pressure gradient of the intrathoracic airways to such an extent that small airway closure may occur. This results in air trapping, which causes hyperinflation of the lungs, increases the residual volume, and decreases vital capacity.

Hyperinflation is a physiologic response of the lung to maintain airflow after early airway closure. However, this breathing at high lung volumes in order to maintain an adequate flow rate increases the work of breathing and can lead to respiratory muscle fatigue.

Infection, irritating dusts, air pollutants, exposure to allergens (such as pollens, house dust, animal danders, and specific foods), and nervous tension can all induce episodes of asthma in some people. Not all asthmatics respond to the same allergens. In fact, some patients (called "intrinsic asthmatics") do not respond to any. Bronchoconstriction is provoked by exercise in almost all asthmatics, but individuals vary greatly in the magnitude of the exercise response. A few rarely develop exertional asthma; others, in the absence of pharmacologic protection, become symptomatic almost every time they exercise. In some cases, exercise is apparently the only stimulus that provokes asthma.

The aggravation of asthmatic symptoms correlates well with the severity of the asthma. Historically, asthma sufferers have either avoided or been deliberately excluded from exercise, but recent studies of the pulmonary effects of various exercise regimens (including a demonstration of the long-term benefits of physical training), together with the development of certain drugs having a protective effect against exertional asthma, suggest that the avoidance of exercise is unwarranted and even detrimental to asthmatic patients.

ETIOLOGY

Despite extensive research efforts, the cause of exercise-induced bronchospasm (EIB) is still unknown. Metabolic acidosis, hypoxemia, hypocapnia from hyperventilation, abnormal catecholamine metabolism, and other autonomic nervous system abnormalities; release of bradykinin during sweating; fluid leaking from pulmonary capillaries; and exercise hyperpnea per se have all been considered and rejected as possible mechanisms. At present, the best hypothesis appears to be that EIB is caused by the release of some bronchoconstrictor substance, perhaps in response to changes in osmolarity of the periciliary fluid as a result of loss of fluid from the airways during the conditioning of cold, dry inspired air.

The bronchoactive mediators may include histamine, leukotrienes, and prostaglandins released from mast cells and epithelial cells lining the airways. These substances may act directly on smooth muscle or they may stimulate irritant receptors, which in turn causes bronchoconstriction via vagal influences or produces an inflammatory reaction via constituents such as the neutrophil chemotactic factor. Cooling of the airways may in itself enhance the response to water loss.

The extent of respiratory water loss may account for much of the variability in the exercise response as far as specificity, intensity, and duration of exercise are concerned, but it certainly does not appear to explain all aspects. It probably helps us to understand the lower asthmogenicity of swimming, in which one inhales highly saturated air from just above the surface of the water, but it does not seem to provide the whole answer. For instance, it has been shown that when asthmatics breathe dry air during swimming, they have smaller reductions of lung function than after running with a similar humidity of inspirate and an equivalent level of ventilation. Furthermore, breathing dry air during swimming at a given metabolic rate has been shown to induce lung function changes that do not differ significantly from those obtained while inhaling moist air under identical conditions. Thus, the cause of EIB has still to be clarified.

DIAGNOSIS

Susceptibility to EIB can be determined by comparing pulmonary function scores (FEV_1 or peak expiratory flow rate, PEFR) before and after 6 to 8 minutes of exercise at 65 to 75 percent of maximal oxygen intake (75 to 85 percent of maximal heart rate). If EIB occurs, the patient shows a decrease of at least 15 percent in FEV_1 or PEFR, usually within 3 to 10 minutes after cessation of the bout of activity. The FEV_1 or PEFR then gradually returns toward its pre-exercise level, generally recovering over about 60 minutes. Usually, there is some increase in FEV_1 or PEFR immediately after exercise; this is probably due to the bronchodilator effect of an exercise-induced increase in circulating catecholamines, an increase in mean alveolar volume causing a mechanical expansion of the airways, or an improvement in airway conductance due to reopening of collapsed airways. Nonasthmatic individuals may show a small subsequent postexercise decrease in FEV_1 or PEFR, but the magnitude of change is less than 10 percent.

Airway obstruction may develop during exercise, but more commonly occurs afterward. Some asthmatics develop a late reaction; this takes the form of a second increase in airway resistance, which may not develop until 3 to 4 hours after exercise and may take a further 3 to 9 hours to reach a peak. A significant number of asthmatics do not exhibit a spontaneous recovery, and such patients may require postexercise medication to reverse the EIB.

The severity of EIB increases with the intensity of exercise, at least up to 75 to 85 percent of maximal heart rate; severity is also augmented by an increase of exercise duration, although this effect appears to plateau at about 8 minutes. The severity can be decreased if the work is broken into short bursts of activity interspersed with short rest periods (interval training), if low asthmogenic activities such as swimming and walking are undertaken or if exercise is pursued in a warm and moist environment.

VALUE OF CHRONIC AEROBIC EXERCISE (TRAINING)

With few exceptions, everyone should undertake a daily period of physical activity. This recommendation is as important for asthmatics as for nonasthmatics, if not more important. Too often, the asthmatic patient manipulates unwary physicians, parents, and school administrators in order to obtain unnecessary exclusion from physical education classes and sports programs. This avoidance of physical activity leads to low fitness levels, a poor physique, chest deformity, and a profound lack of motor skills. There often are associated psychological problems, deriving from a poor self-image. Physically inactive asthmatics may also suffer socially and emotionally, since failure to participate in regular childhood or adolescent activities leads to poor peer group acceptance. Frequent absences from school may further result in poor academic achievement.

Regular and frequent aerobic exercise at a moderate to heavy intensity has proven physiologic benefits that apply to both asthmatic and nonasthmatic individuals. Research has indicated that enhanced aerobic fitness increases the tolerance and threshold levels of asthmatic patients so that a higher level of provocation is required in order to produce symptoms. In adults, it has been shown to decrease absenteeism attributable to the disease process and to decrease the amounts of medication required.

It is possible that the psychological and sociologic benefits of increased aerobic fitness, resulting improvements in self-image, and greater recognition and acceptance by peer groups and parents help to remove the "cripple" stigma from which many asthmatics suffer. It is thus of great importance that asthmatic patients practice and improve their skills in sports as a means of gaining greater status and recognition by others. Young asthmatic individuals should realize that with dedication and application they can usually compete quite well with nonasthmatic peers, given adequate training and medication before the event. Asthmatic individuals have demonstrated an ability to reach top international competition standards in almost all sports. Twenty-one members of the Australian team attending the Montreal Olympic Games in 1976 were asthmatics, and they competed in eight of the 18 events for which Australia was entered. Olympic gold medals were won by asthmatics on the Australian team in Melbourne (1956), Rome (1960), Tokyo (1964), Mexico City (1968), Moscow (1980), and Seoul (1988). Of the 597 US athletes who participated in the 1984 summer Olympic Games, 67 (11.2 percent) suffered from exercise-induced asthma and these same athletes won a total of 41 medals (15 gold, 20 silver, and six bronze).

Therefore, even though exercise can induce asthma, sports and regular physical activity are accepted components in the total management of this condition.

MANAGEMENT OF EXERCISE-INDUCED BRONCHOSPASM

To minimize the incidence and severity of exercise-induced bronchospasm, it is first necessary to maximize control of the asthmatic condition. This may necessitate a variety of measures, physical, immunologic, and pharmacologic.

Once the asthma is controlled and airway inflammation has been reduced, the adverse response to exercise will be minimized. The physician should regularly check that the patient is using the correct technique to administer the various aerosol medications that have been prescribed.

If asthmatics are expected to participate fully in physical education, recreational games, and competitive sports, it is necessary that they be provided with the means to maximize control over their labile bronchial system during activity sessions. The asthmatic patient should become aware of the preventive benefits of the various antispasmodic drugs, and of the most effective pharmacologic agents to reverse bronchoconstriction should a severe attack develop during exercise. If the asthmatic athlete reaches national or international standards of competition, he or she, together with the coach and team physician, must know which medications are permitted and which are illegal to use during competition (Table 1).

TABLE 1 Drugs Used for Treating Asthma: Effectiveness with EIB and Legal Status for Competition

Class of Drug	*Drug*	*Route of Administration*	*Usual Dosage (Adults and Adolescents)**	*Effectiveness in EIB*	*Legal or Banned*	*Prophylactic (P) or Bronchodilator (B)*	*Possible Side Effects or Adverse Reactions*
Kellin derivatives	Cromolyn sodium	Aerosol spray	1 mg 2 inhalations 4× per day	Good	Legal	P	
		Aerosol powder	20 mg spincap, 1 dose q 4–6 hr	Good	Legal	P	Virtually none—bitter taste. Transient irritation of the throat
	Nedocromil sodium	Aerosol	4 mg (2 mg per actuation) 4× daily	Good	Legal	P	
Sympathomimetic	Nonspecific β agonists						
	Epinephrine (α, β_1, and β_2 activity)	SC	Not recommended	Fair	Banned	B	Very short acting, tachyphylaxis
		IV	Not recommended	Fair	Banned	B	
	Ephedrine (α, β_1, and β_2 activity)	Oral	Not recommended	Fair	Banned	B	Large doses can cause headaches, sweating, thirst, tachycardia, palpitations, and tremor
	Isoproterenol (β_1 and β_2 activity)	Aerosol	Not recommended	Fair	Banned	B	Tachycardia, decreased diastolic pressure, skeletal muscle tremor, myocardial ischemia
	Specific β_2 agonists						
	Salbutamol β_2	Aerosol inhaler	100 μg per actuation, 1–2 actuations q 4 hr	Excellent	Legal	B	
		Rotocaps	200 μg per Rotocap, 1–2 inhalations 3–4× daily	Excellent	Legal	B	
		Respirator solution	5 mg per ml or 1 ml q 4–6 hr	Excellent	Legal	B	
		Oral	2–4 mg 3–4× daily	Good	Banned	B	
		SC & IM	1 ml (500 μg) q 3–4 hr	Good	Banned	B	
	Terbutaline β_2	Aerosol	1 puff = 0.25 mg, 1–2 puffs, repeated up to q 4 hr	Excellent	Legal	B	Administration of β_2 agonists by the aerosol route have minimal adverse reactions when given in recommended doses. Large doses, especially when administered orally or by injection, can cause tremor, nervousness, tachycardia, and palpitations.
		Oral	Tablet 2.5–5 mg 3× daily	Good	Banned	B	
		SC	0.25 mg (0.5 ml) up to 4× daily	Good	Banned	B	
	Metaproterenol β_2	Aerosol	1–2 actuations 3–4× per day (750 μg per puff)	Excellent	Legal	B	
	Rimiterol β_2	Aerosol	1–2 actuations up to 4× daily (200 μg per puff)	Excellent	Legal	B	
	Bitolterol β_2	Aerosol	1–2 actuations up to 4× daily (370 μg per puff)	Excellent	Legal	B	
	Fenoterol β_2	Aerosol	200 μg per actuation, 1–2 puffs 3–4× per day	Excellent	Banned	B	
		Oral	1–2 tablets 3× per day (2.5 mg tablets)	Good	Banned	B	

Table 1 continues on following page

TABLE 1 (continued) Drugs Used for Treating Asthma: Effectiveness with EIB and Legal Status for Competition

Class of Drug	*Drug*	*Route of Administration*	*Usual Dosage (Adults and Adolescents)**	*Effectiveness in EIB*	*Legal or Banned*	*Prophylactic (P) or Bronchodilator (B)*	*Possible Side Effects or Adverse Reactions*
Methylxanthines	Theophylline	Oral	125–200 mg q 6 hr	Good	Legal	B	Side effects less with controlled-release theophylline
		Oral	Controlled release 250–300 mg 2× per day	Good	Legal	B	Gastrointestinal—nausea, vomiting, epigastric pain; CNS—headaches, irritability, restlessness, insomnia
			To attain serum level of 10–20 mg· L^{-1} (50–100 µmol·L^{-1})				
	Aminophylline	IV for acute severe asthma	Not recommended		Legal	B	Cardiovascular—palpitations, tachycardia, extrasystole hypotension, tachypnea
Belladonna alkaloids	Ipratropium bromide	Aerosol	1 puff = 20 µg; adult 2 puffs (40 µg) 3–4× daily; Some may need up to 4 puffs (80 µg)	Fair	Legal	B	Some patients experience dryness of the mouth (xerostamia)
Glucocorticosteroids	Beclomethasone dipropionate	Aerosol	Inhaler—50 or 100 µg per actuation 1–2 inhalations (50–200 µg) 4× per day; Rotocap (100 µg per cap) or 1 cap 3–4× daily	Uncertain	Legal		Hoarseness, sore throat, oral and pharyngeal *Candida albicans* infection
	Systemic corticosteroid (for severe attacks of asthma and status asthmaticus)	Oral IV	Not recommended		Banned		Obesity, retardation of growth in children, hypertension, diabetes, and susceptibility to infections

NOTE: Where a drug is not recommended, the usual dosage is not provided.
* If recommended for EIB.

To inhibit EIB, the drugs of choice are the beta-2 agonists (Fig. 1 and Table 1). All of these have an approximately equal ability to inhibit exertional asthma. All except fenoterol are acceptable during international sporting competition, provided that the aerosol route of administration is used. Fenoterol is banned because it is metabolized to parahydroxyamphetamine.

The beta-2 agonists have a rapid action (onset within 60 seconds) and are effective over a relatively long time (3 to 4 hours). It is recommended that a medication of this class be administered by inhalation 5 or 10 minutes before exercise is begun. Irrespective of the question regarding the legality of these agents in sport, the aerosol route is preferred to the oral route, because their action has a more rapid onset, their efficacy is superior, the necessary dosage is greatly reduced, and side effects such as tremor and palpitations are lessened.

If administration of the beta-2 agonists does not block EIB, a combination of these drugs with cromolyn sodium, using single or even double doses of each, or a combination of beta-2 agonists with cromolyn sodium and theophylline should be tried, in that order (see Fig. 1). Theophylline is administered orally, and serum levels of 50 to 100 µmol·L^{-1} (10 to 20 µg·ml^{-1}) should be achieved to ensure a therapeutic effect. Cromolyn and theophylline are of approximately equal effectiveness in protecting against EIB, but they are inferior to beta-2 agonists. Research has shown that about 70 percent of asthmatics gain some protection from EIB after inhalation of cromolyn sodium, while 45 percent gain complete protection for about 1 hour. Effectiveness is minimal beyond 4 hours. Whereas cromolyn is virtually free of side effects, the usual preparations of theophylline can cause adverse reactions such as nausea, vomiting, and gastroesophageal reflux in some people; however, sustained release preparations of theophylline are better tolerated (see Table 1).

For individuals who continue to experience EIB, aerosol ipratropium bromide may be added to the medication regimen. Aerosol ipratropium bromide is a belladonna alkaloid that has proved a useful bronchodilator for patients who cannot tolerate or do not respond to beta-2 adrenoceptor stimulants.

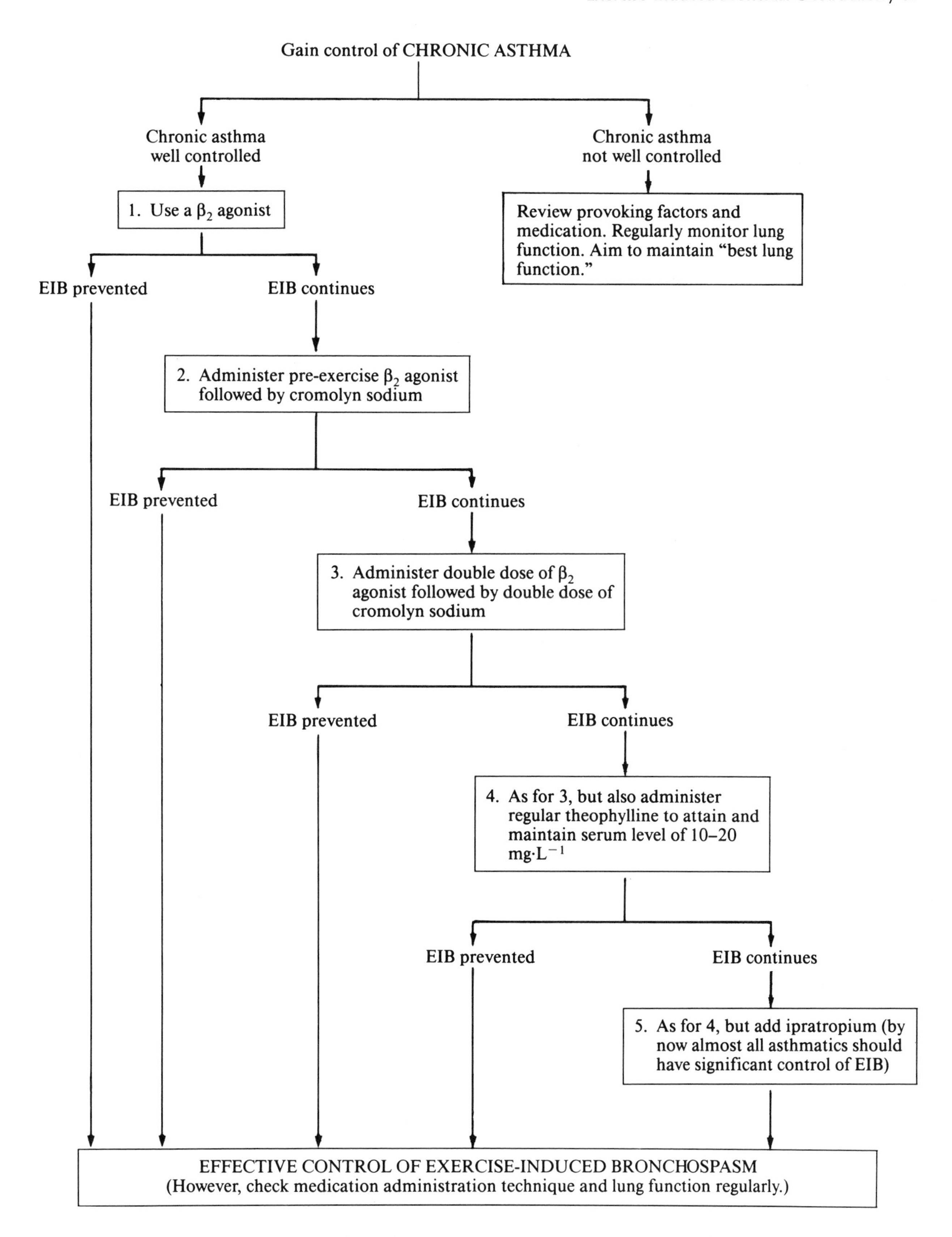

Figure 1 Flow diagram for prevention of exercise-induced bronchospasm. NOTE: Immediate pre-exercise administration of corticosteroids is relatively ineffective in preventing EIB. Corticosteroids may play an important role in controlling chronic asthma and thus allow effective control of EIB when used with the above medications. Use may also allow control of EIB with reduced amounts of other medication.

Glucocorticoids, both oral (e.g., prednisone) and aerosol (e.g., beclomethasone dipropionate), are excellent drugs to stabilize asthma, but they have little capacity to prevent EIB if administered just before exercise. The H_1 antagonists have no significant role in the management of asthma, but are often prescribed to control symptoms associated with other manifestations of atopy, including nasal and dermatologic reactions.

To allow a more complete participation in games and other physical activities, most asthmatic patients are thus advised to inhale either an aerosol preparation of a beta-2 adrenoceptor stimulant immediately before exercise, or a beta-2 agonist plus cromolyn 15 minutes before exercise (20 mg spincap or two to four puffs of an aerosol that delivers 1 mg per actuation). If both of these drugs are indicated, the beta-2 agonist should always be administered first, since the resultant bronchodilation permits a more effective distribution of cromolyn throughout the airways.

It is also recommended that the asthmatic patient take a beta-2 agonist aerosol spray to all exercise sessions, and ask the coach or referee to carry it during the game or training session, so that it is readily available if EIB supervenes.

TABLE 2 Fitness Training Program for Asthmatic Patients

When	Consider the climatic conditions
Intensity	75–90% of maximal heart rate (Stress the system, don't strain it)
Duration	15–60 minutes of continuous aerobic activity. Duration is dependent on intensity; a lower intensity activity should be performed over a longer period, and is the recommended approach for the nonathletic adult.
Mode of Activity	Any rhythmic aerobic activity that utilizes large muscle groups, including walking, jogging, running, swimming, cycling, rowing, rope skipping, and various endurance game activities
Frequency	3–5 sessions per week

Based on the recommendations of the American College of Sports Medicine.

PRESCRIBING EXERCISE FOR THE ASTHMATIC PATIENT

With the benefit of pre-exercise medication, most asthmatic patients can participate equally with nonasthmatics of similar size, skill, and fitness levels. As the training program for top level performers in a given sport is the same, regardless of whether they are asthmatic, only a general aerobic fitness program is outlined in Tables 2 and 3.

OTHER CONSIDERATIONS

1. Asthmatic patients who train either for general fitness or for a competitive sport may find it beneficial to wear a face mask during training. Such masks increase the temperature and humidity of the inspired air, thus reducing the likelihood of EIB; they are especially useful during cold weather, but in most instances are impractical for use during competition.
2. Immediately after completion of training, the asthmatic individual should take a warm shower and dress in a tracksuit or other suitable warm clothing. Many asthmatic patients are susceptible to sudden changes in body temperature.
3. If possible, asthmatics should select the time of training to coincide with the most favorable environmental conditions. For instance, they should not train early in the morning or in the evening if the weather is cold, and they should also refrain from training when pollens, dust, or air pollution levels are high. Under certain of these environmental conditions, it is unwise for asthmatic patients to exercise outside air-conditioned premises.
4. Asthmatics who are reluctant to take preventive medication before their exercise sessions would benefit by selecting swimming as their preferred mode of exercise. Alternatively, they could select games and activities that require intermittent periods of intense exercise, followed by brief rest periods (e.g., rugby, soccer, tennis, or squash).

TABLE 3 Suggested Exercise Session

	Segment	*Intensity*	*Duration*
1.	A warm-up period	Below 75% of max heart rate	5 min
2.	Set of exercises to maintain or increase flexibility		5 min
3.	Conditioning segment: program of activities to maintain or improve stamina (aerobic power). You may also add activities to increase strength and muscle endurance: e.g., weight training or calisthenics.	Below 75–90% of max heart rate	15–30 min
4.	Cool-down activities, including repeat of flexibility (stretching) exercises used in 2 above. Slow walking is an excellent cool-down activity.	Below 75%	5–10 min

SUGGESTED READING

Anderson SD. Current concepts of exercise-induced asthma. Allergy 1983; 38:389–402.

Anderson SD. Issues in exercise-induced asthma. J Allergy Clin Immunol 1985; 76:763–772.

Fitch KD. Use of anti-asthmatic drugs: do they affect sports performance? Sportsmedicine 1986; 3:136–150.

Fitch KD, Godfrey S. Asthma and athletic performance. JAMA 1976; 236:152–157.

Fitch KD, Morton AR. Specificity of exercise in exercise-induced asthma. Br Med J 1971; 4:577–581.

Fitch KD, Morton AR, Blanksby BA. Effects of swimming training on children with asthma. Arch Dis Child 1976; 51:190–194.

Hahn A, Anderson SD, Morton AR, Black JL, Fitch KD. A reinterpretation of the effect of temperature and water content of the inspired air in exercise-induced asthma. Am Rev Respir Dis 1984; 130:575–579.

Haynes RL, Ingram RH, McFadden ER. An assessment of the pulmonary response to exercise in asthma and an analysis of the factors influencing it. Am Rev Respir Dis 1976; 114:739–752.

Inbar O, Dotan R, Dlin RN, Nueman I, Bar-Or O. Breathing dry or humid air and exercise-induced asthma during swimming. Eur J Appl Physiol 1980; 44:43–50.

Jones RS, Buston MH, Wharton MJ. The effect of exercise on ventilatory function in the child with asthma. Br J Dis Chest 1962; 56:78–86.

Jones RS, Wharton MJ, Buston MH. The place of physical exercise and bronchodilator drugs. Arch Dis Child 1963; 38:539–545.

Mertens DJ, Shephard RJ, Kavanagh T. Long-term exercise therapy for chronic obstructive lung disease. Respiration 1978; 35:96–107.

Morton AR, Fitch KD, Hahn AG. Physical activity and the asthmatic. Physician Sportsmed 1981; 9:50–64.

Morton AR, Hahn AG, Fitch KD. Continuous and intermittent running in the provocation of asthma. Ann Allergy 1982; 48:123–129.

Silverman M, Anderson SD. Standardization of exercise tests in asthmatic children. Arch Dis Child 1972; 47:882–889.

Sly RM. Exercise-induced asthma. In: Weiss RB, Segal MS, eds. Bronchial asthma: mechanisms and therapeutics. Boston: Little, Brown, 1976; 537.

Voy R. The US Olympic Committee experience with exercise-induced bronchospasm 1984. Med Sci Sports Exerc 1986; 18:328–330.

Woolcock AJ. The difficult asthmatic: diagnosis and management. Patient Man 1987; 11:73–91.

BLOOD DOPING AND PERFORMANCE

NORMAN GLEDHILL, Ph.D.

Lasse Viren's brilliant double victories in the 5,000 and 10,000 meter races at the 1972 and 1976 Olympiads, with only erratic performances in the intervening years, parachuted the issue of "blood doping" into the public limelight. Viren's evasive nonanswers to reporters' questions about his suspected use of this performance-enhancing manipulation enabled him to sidestep the controversy at the time, but to this day his reputation is clouded by the alleged blood doping scandal. Since that time, the issue has received renewed attention in the news media with every Olympiad.

"Blood doping," "blood boosting," and "blood packing" are terms used to describe a medical intervention that produces an abnormally high concentration of red blood cells (induced erythrocythemia). The scientific basis for the effectiveness of blood doping is that an elevation in the red blood cell count augments the ability of the blood to carry oxygen, and hence increases the transport of oxygen by the circulatory system. With additional oxygen available to the working muscles, the expected result is an increase in aerobic power ($\dot{V}O_2max$) and thus endurance performance.

Blood doping can be accomplished by two approaches: (1) by transfusing matched blood from a donor into a recipient; or (2) by removing a volume of blood from an individual, separating and storing the red cells for a prescribed period, and then reinfusing the cells back into the donor. With the former approach (which was employed by some members of the US cycling team in the 1984 Olympiad), once the excess fluid has been excreted and the normal fluid volume of the cardiovascular system has been reestablished, there is an immediate increase in the red blood cell count. In the latter approach (the method generally employed in laboratory investigations of blood doping), the body manufactures red cells at an accelerated rate and returns the hematocrit to normal levels while the blood is in storage. Thus, when the stored cells are subsequently reinfused, the red cell count is increased above normal. Early investigations of the effects of blood doping were contradictory and inconclusive, and reviewers generally concluded that research did not support the theory that blood doping has a beneficial effect on endurance (aerobic) performance. However, subsequent studies that avoided a major flaw in early investigations (described later) have shown conclusively that blood doping increases aerobic power and improves endurance performance.

HEMOGLOBIN AND ATHLETIC PERFORMANCE

In males, approximately 45 percent of the volume of a normal blood specimen is made up of red blood cells, and the corresponding hemoglobin concentration is 15.5 g per 100 ml of blood. Muscle requires a great deal of oxygen during heavy exercise, and any change in the oxygen-carrying ability of blood induced by an altered hemoglobin concentration affects the amount of oxygen presented to the working muscles. Although it is not the only factor, the amount of oxygen presented to the muscles does, to a large degree, determine how much work the muscles can perform in a given time. In fact, an endurance athlete's capacity to utilize oxygen (the aerobic power, or $\dot{V}o_2max$) is widely accepted as the single most important factor in determining success or failure in aerobic events. Training programs are designed to maximize aerobic power, and any external manipulation that could likewise increase the $\dot{V}o_2max$ would be a distinct advantage for competition in endurance events.

First let us consider the donation of blood. The key consideration is not the reduction in blood volume, but the decrease in the red blood cell and hemoglobin concentrations. When 450 to 500 ml of blood is withdrawn from the circulation, the blood volume is restored to normal in a few hours. The regeneration of hemoglobin, however, is a much slower process, occurring over an average of 5 to 10 weeks. For example, athletes who are training heavily during a period in which they donate blood may require 8 to 10 weeks for their hemoglobin level to be restored to normal. The reduction in hemoglobin concentration after blood donation is not a factor that affects day-to-day living, but it can noticeably impair heavy training or performance in endurance competitions. This impairment of maximal effort was reported many years ago by Peter Karpovich at Springfield College. He conducted experiments with varsity athletes before and after blood donation and concluded that the withdrawal of 450 ml of blood unfavorably affected performance. This conclusion has since been confirmed in a number of studies. According to Karpovich, it took 10 to 20 days for the athletes' performance to return to normal.

Because of the relationship between a reduction in hemoglobin concentration and a deterioration in endurance performance, it is often recommended that blood (hemoglobin) analysis be included in the periodic fitness assessments of endurance athletes. Moreover, it follows from this relationship that an increased hemoglobin concentration should have a beneficial effect on endurance performance.

METHODOLOGY OF BLOOD DOPING

As mentioned previously, it is possible to increase the hemoglobin concentration by transfusing fresh blood from a matched donor. This procedure is employed when blood is transfused for therapeutic reasons. There is an acceptable risk-to-benefit ratio associated with this procedure that is justified in life-threatening situations. However, when dealing with healthy individuals, the potential for transmitting viral hepatitis, acquired immunodeficiency syndrome, and other infectious diseases such as malaria or syphilis, and the remote possibility of death from acute or delayed hemolytic reactions due to improper blood matching, far outweighs any potential benefits. Matched blood transfusions have been described as liquid organ transplants, with all the same possible complications. Therefore, investigations that involve healthy human participants should not be conducted using blood from matched donors.

The customary research approach to blood doping, and one that is considerably safer, involves removing blood from an individual, storing the cells for a prescribed time, and then reinfusing the cells into the donor. Unless there is an error in the labeling of the blood, and hence the possibility of a hemolytic reaction, the risks involved are minimal. When the blood is removed from the donor, it is centrifuged to separate the cells from the plasma. The cells are then stored, but the manner of storage is extremely important.

The most common method of storing blood is by refrigeration at 4°C. This procedure results in a considerable loss of red cells, owing to the normal aging process. In addition, health regulations in North America dictate that the maximal duration of storage for refrigerated blood is 3 weeks. Since it takes 5 to 10 weeks after blood donation for the body to restore the red cell level to normal, this storage technique does not allow sufficient time for red cell regeneration to be completed. It therefore is not possible to increase the hemoglobin concentration significantly when using refrigerator-stored cells.

An alternative process of blood storage is by means of a special freezing technique that is relatively inaccessible to the normal population and very expensive. This procedure is used by blood banks in order to maintain an adequate reserve of rare blood types. Unlike the usual refrigeration technique, when blood is stored as frozen cells the aging process is interrupted for an unlimited period, and the only cell loss occurs in handling. Thus, there is only a minimal loss of red blood cells during storage, and it is possible to wait as long as necessary for the donors' hemoglobin concentration to be restored to normal before reinfusing the additional cells.

In early studies of blood doping, the cells were stored by refrigeration. Thus, any resultant increase in the hemoglobin concentration was minimal, and it is not surprising that the findings of these early studies did not support the theory of an enhancement of aerobic performance by blood doping. However, if 900 to 1,000 ml of blood are removed and stored by the special freezing technique for the required time, it is possible to increase the hemoglobin concentration by approximately 10 percent.

RECENT EVIDENCE ON BLOOD DOPING

Once this major flaw in previous studies had been rectified, the topic of blood doping could be properly investigated. The first study in which the appropriate blood storage technique was employed was conducted at York University in Toronto. Eleven elite endurance runners took part in the study. In the initial phase of the investigation, control measurements of $\dot{V}o_2$max and endurance performance were conducted both before and 10 weeks after the removal of 900 ml of blood. It was thus possible to confirm that the athletes were at their initial hemoglobin and performance levels at the time of the blood reinfusion. The study was conducted using a double-blind design, so that neither the athletes nor the researchers knew on which occasion the blood had been reinfused. Six of the athletes initially received a sham reinfusion of a saline solution, and their actual blood reinfusion occurred later. The remaining five athletes received their actual reinfusion initially, with a sham reinfusion later. At the time of the reinfusion, the athletes wore blacked-out goggles and listened to music on headphones in order to remain unaware of the order of treatment. The effectiveness of this blind was confirmed by a questionnaire that was administered after the actual and sham reinfusions.

Twenty-four hours after the sham and actual reinfusions, the runners were retested. Following the reinfusion, there was a 10 percent increase in hemoglobin concentration, a 5 percent increase in $\dot{V}o_2$max, and a 35 percent increase in treadmill running time to exhaustion. These results established conclusively the physiologic and endurance performance benefits of blood doping.

However, concern was expressed over a potentially dangerous side effect of blood doping. When the red blood cell count is increased, there is also an increase in the viscosity of the blood. This increases the resistance to the flow of blood through the blood vessels, and could reduce the heart's maximal ability to pump blood to the muscles. Therefore, in a subsequent York University study, the potential health hazard of reinfusing up to 1,500 ml of freeze-preserved blood into elite endurance runners was examined. The primary aim of this study was to assess whether there was any evidence that the reinfusion of blood compromised the cardiovascular system during light to maximal exercise. For this reason, the athletes underwent very sophisticated instrumentation, allowing direct blood pressure and cardiac output measurements. As observed in the initial study, with the increase in hemoglobin concentration there was an increase in aerobic power. However, there was no evidence of any functional impairment or complication in the cardiovascular system. Nevertheless, it seems prudent to avoid the infusion of still greater volumes of blood.

Several subsequent studies in which the freeze-preservation technique was used have confirmed that blood doping has a beneficial effect on aerobic performance. For example, Williams and co-workers at Old Dominion University in Virginia observed that after reinfusion of 900 ml of blood, the performance time in an 8 km (5-mile) race was 49 seconds faster than in the control and sham conditions. Goforth and co-workers, in a study conducted at Georgia State University, reported that when the hematocrit was elevated by 10 percent, the $\dot{V}o_2$max was increased by 11 percent and 4.8 km (3-mile) run time was 23.7 seconds faster. It must be concluded, therefore, that blood doping improves performance in endurance events.

DOPING CONTROLS

The use of physiologic substances in abnormal amounts, by abnormal methods, and with the exclusive aim of obtaining an artificial or unfair increase in performance in competition is prohibited by doping control regulations. In 1985 the International Olympic Committee added blood doping to the list of banned substances and procedures. When doping controls are conducted at a competition, selected athletes must provide a urine sample in the presence of a doping control official, and in principle they could also be required to give a blood sample. In the studies of blood doping conducted at York University, the average hemoglobin concentration of the athletes increased from 15.1 to 16.7 g per 100 ml of blood after reinfusion. The average hemoglobin concentration in individual normal and athletic males varies from 14 to 18 g per 100 ml of blood. Thus, the problem facing doping control officials is that although a high hemoglobin concentration is relatively simple to detect, it currently is not possible to determine why it is high. For example, it may be elevated by either altitude acclimatization or genetic endowment.

Several investigations are currently under way to develop an effective technique for detecting blood doping, and a Swedish researcher recently announced preliminary evidence that it can be detected from a blood sample and an algorithm incorporating hemoglobin, erythropoietin, and serum iron or bilirubin. There is considerable optimism that a detection technique will be available for inclusion in the doping control procedures in the near future, but at present the only deterrents to the use of blood doping in athletic competitions are concern over the potential risks involved, accessibility to the appropriate blood storage technique, and the integrity of the athletes and coaches involved. We can only hope that these deterrents are sufficient!

SUGGESTED READING

American College of Sports Medicine. Position stand on blood doping as an ergogenic aid. Med Sci Sports Exerc 1987; 19:540–543.

Berglund B. Development of techniques for the detection of blood doping in sport. Sports Med 1988; 5:127–135.
Buick FJ, Gledhill N, Froese AB, Spriet L, Meyers EC. Effect of induced erythrocythemia on aerobic work capacity. J Appl Physiol 1980; 48:636–642.
Dugal R, Bertrand M. Doping. In: IOC Medical Commission booklet. Montreal: Comité Organisateur des Jeux Olympiques, 1976: 1.
Gledhill N. Blood doping and related issues: a brief review. Med Sci Sports Exerc 1982; 14:183–189.
Goforth HW, Campbell NL, Hodgdon JA, Sucec AA. Hematological parameters of trained distance runners following induced erythrocythemia. Med Sci Sports Exerc 1982; 14:174 (abstr).
Karpovich PV, Millman N. Athletes as blood donors. Res Q 1942; 13:166–168.
Spriet LL, Gledhill N, Froese AB, Wilkes DL. J Appl Physiol 1986; 61:1942–1948.
Spriet LL, Gledhill N, Froese AB, Wilkes DL, Meyers EC. The effect of induced erythrocythemia on central circulation and oxygen transport during maximal exercise. Med Sci Sports Exerc 1980; 12:122 (abstr).
Valeri CR. Blood banking and the use of frozen blood products. Cleveland: CRC Press, 1976:9–174.
Williams MH, Wesseldine S, Somma T, Schuster R. The effect of induced erythrocythemia upon 5-mile treadmill run time. Med Sci Sports Exerc 1981; 13:169–175.

AIR POLLUTION AND EXERCISE

SUSAN M. TARLO, M.B., B.S., M.R.C.P. (UK), F.R.C.P. (C)
ROBERT BRUCE URCH, M.Sc., C.A.C.P.T. (P)
FRANCES SILVERMAN, B.Sc., M.Sc., Ph.D.

The cardiorespiratory benefits of exercise are well documented. However, less attention has been directed toward the risk of adverse health effects from inhaled pollutants during exercise outdoors, particularly in urban environments.

Major pollutant sources in urban areas include both industry and vehicular exhaust, producing primary pollutants (such as sulfur dioxide, carbon monoxide, nitric oxide, and particulates) and secondary pollutants resulting from reactions between primary pollutants, ultraviolet light, and other ambient chemical compounds (such as ozone, nitrogen dioxide, peroxyacetyl nitrate, and aldehydes).

Although the concentration of pollutants is of primary concern when examining the health effects of exercise outdoors, other factors may exacerbate the response. The magnitude of the respiratory minute ventilation is roughly proportional to the intensity of exercise or work rate. Thus, at high work rates the pollutant dose (pollutant concentration × respiratory minute ventilation) is substantially increased over the resting condition. When estimating pollutant dose, a third factor must also be considered: exercise duration. Furthermore, at respiratory ventilations above 35 liters per minute, people tend to breathe oronasally, thus partially bypassing the normal filtration mechanisms of the nose. Other variables that can influence the response to pollutants include environmental factors such as temperature and humidity, physiologic factors such as age (children, adults, elderly), fitness level (a social exerciser versus a competitive athlete), the presence of underlying disease (particularly respiratory disease), and tobacco smoking.

Although many of the effects produced by normal ambient levels of pollutants are relatively small, they may have serious consequences for an elite competitive athlete, whose performance is timed to the millisecond. Therefore, in assessing the effects of air pollutants on exercising individuals, consideration must be given to (1) the ambient air conditions (type and concentration of pollutants), (2) the intensity and duration of exercise being undertaken, (3) environmental factors, and (4) the age of, level of fitness of, and presence of any underlying disease in the person exercising.

An excellent review of the biologic effects of ozone, sulfur dioxide, and carbon monoxide was given by Folinsbee in the first edition of this book. In this chapter we discuss the same pollutants in the light of subsequent research and briefly consider some additional pollutants. However, air pollution mixtures in indoor and outdoor air are very complex, varying in both constituents and concentrations. To date many contaminants have not been demonstrated to have significant effects on the exercising individual, or have not been systematically examined with respect to their impact.

OZONE

Ozone (O_3), a photochemical oxidant, is formed by an interaction of oxygen, nitrogen oxides, hydrocarbons, and sunlight. Concentrations are generally highest in warm, sunny climates and (in more northern climates) during the summer months.

Of ambient pollutants, ozone (a respiratory irritant) has probably been the most thoroughly investigated both in the laboratory and in the ambient environment. The United States National Ambient Air Quality standard for ozone is 0.12 part per million (ppm) for a 1-hour averaging time, although in high pollution areas, such as parts of the Los Angeles basin, levels of 0.12 to 0.2 ppm are common in the summer months for 1- to 3-hour periods. Longer but less marked elevations, often exceeding 5 or 6 hours, occur in other urban areas such as parts of New York and New Jersey.

Under resting conditions, ozone levels of less than 0.12 ppm produce no measurable change in the pulmonary function of either normal adults or asthmatics. However, with exercise, concentrations as low as 0.12 ppm can induce cough, discomfort on deep inspiration, and a reduction in forced inspiratory and expiratory flow rates and vital capacity. The extent of decrements in pulmonary function cannot be predicted on the basis of a diagnosis of asthma or preexisting airway hyperresponsiveness to agents such as methacholine. However, impairment increases with increasing concentrations of ozone, duration of exposure, increasing respiratory minute ventilation, and increasing ambient temperature. Thus, endurance athletes are likely to be more affected than those exercising for shorter periods or intermittently, or than the less fit recreationally exercising population. For example, endurance cyclists exercising at 31°C and 70 percent of their maximal oxygen uptake ($\dot{V}O_2max$) for 1 hour and then at maximal capacity until exhaustion show substantial decreases in 1-second forced expiratory volume (FEV_1) after maximal exercise (5.6 percent at 0.12 ppm ozone, 21.6 percent at 0.2 ppm relative to exercise in filtered air). An ozone concentration of 0.12 ppm does not limit the ride time, or reduce the work rate achieved, maximal oxygen intake ($\dot{V}O_2max$), or minute ventilation ($\dot{V}_E$), but 0.2 ppm reduces ride time by 30 percent, peak work rate by 8 percent, tidal volume by 22 percent, $\dot{V}_E$ by 18 percent, and $\dot{V}O_2max$ by 16 percent. In addition, about half of the cyclists develop an increased airway reactivity to histamine after the 0.2 ppm exposure.

Longer exposure to ozone has an increased effect on exercise tolerance. Levels as low as 0.12 ppm during an exposure of 6.5 hours with six 50-minute exercise periods have been compared with clean air exposure, as reported by Folinsbee. At a mean respiratory ventilation of about 40 liters per minute, normal individuals develop significant reductions in inspiratory and expiratory flow rates, associated with cough and pain on deep inspiration. These symptoms peak 3 to 5 hours after the onset of exposure. The mean decrement in FEV_1 and forced inspiratory vital capacity (FIVC) is about 13 percent under these conditions. As in shorter exposures to higher ozone concentrations, airway reactivity to methacholine is increased, although there is no relationship between individual changes in FEV_1 or forced vital capacity (FVC) and pollution-induced changes in airway reactivity, which suggests that different mechanisms are involved. However, there is an association between FVC, FEV_1, and subjective discomfort on deep inspiration, suggesting a primary limitation of inspired volume, either reflexly or from a voluntary inhibition of inspiration.

Healthy adolescents bicycling in Los Angeles for 1 hour at an ozone level of 0.144 ppm with a temperature of 32°C and relative humidity of 45 percent did not develop any symptoms, as compared with exercise in clean air, but they did develop a significant decrement in FEV_1, with only partial recovery after 1 hour.

Ozone might be expected to cause greater impairment in asthmatics than in normal individuals, but this has not been observed. Nevertheless, any factor that increases the effect of exercise alone on the airways may produce significant limitation in an asthmatic and should thus be considered in the choice of management. Men with coronary artery disease, similarly, have no increase in sensitivity to ozone. The factor limiting their exercise is often angina, so that the dose of ozone reaching the airways is probably insufficient to cause an effect.

Adaptation to ozone (a diminished response to the same level of exposure) may occur with three to four consecutive daily exposures to ozone at 0.4 to 0.5 ppm—levels that are rarely encountered in ambient air on consecutive days. However, the reduction in pulmonary function changes on successive days is less in those who are sensitive to ozone than in less responsive individuals. In addition, there is concern that the reduced response to ozone may result from damage to vagal sensory nerves or from changes in the protective mucus in the airways or lung tissue injury. Therefore, "acclimatization" to ozone cannot be recommended.

Management of the exercising individual exposed to ozone is mainly prophylactic. The chances of a person's developing symptoms, impairment in exercise performance, and postexercise pulmonary function changes can be assessed to some extent from knowledge of ambient ozone concentrations, the age and level of fitness of the individual, the duration and severity of exercise, and the presence of asthma. It currently appears that no special measures need be taken for athletes exposed to less than 0.12 ppm of ozone. Therefore, when possible, athletic events should be held in areas where the ozone level is less than 0.12 ppm. Long distance runners and cyclists are particularly advised to exercise when ozone levels are low. Less concern is needed for the recreational exerciser, who is less likely to inhale a significant local dose of ozone into the airways.

Use of charcoal-lined masks reduces ozone exposure, but these are impractical and uncomfortable during exercise. Medications have no clearly established preventive value. Inhaled beta-adrenergic agents reduce exercise-induced changes in asthmatics, but inhaled albuterol is ineffective in preventing ozone effects in nonasthmatics. However, postexposure airway narrowing may improve after the use of bronchodilators. Inhaled atropine, although not indicated clinically, blocks ozone-induced increases in airway resistance and airway reactivity to histamine, but does not prevent respiratory symptoms or the reduction in FVC after ozone exposure. Anti-inflammatory medications such as indomethacin inhibit ozone-induced airway hyperresponsiveness in dogs, but have not been assessed in humans. Results from large oral doses of vitamins C and E are inconclusive.

SULFUR DIOXIDE, SULFURIC ACID, AND SULFATES

Sulfur dioxide, sulfuric acid, and sulfates such as ammonium sulfate and ammonium bisulfate are combustion products of fossil fuels. The US Environmental Protection Agency's federal primary standard for sulfur dioxide is set at 0.14 ppm averaged over 24 hours, and 0.5 ppm averaged over one hour. In 1986 concentrations in New York City ranged from less than 0.1 ppm to occasional readings of 0.5 ppm; levels of 0.3 ppm were often present.

The concentrations of sulfur dioxide present in ambient air do not impair respiratory function in normal individuals, at rest or with exercise. However, strenuously exercising asthmatics develop significant exacerbation of symptoms and airflow limitation at values as low as 0.25 ppm. A minority of nonasthmatic but atopic individuals develop similar changes if exposed to 0.6 ppm of sulfur dioxide during exercise. Respondents show a dose-response effect with increasing concentrations of sulfur dioxide, but the extent of the response cannot be predicted from the severity of asthma. The impact is transient, with no measurable residual changes 1 day or 7 days after exposure. Effects usually clear in less than 1 hour after exercise, only occasionally persisting to 2 hours, even if sulfur dioxide exposure continues at rest. Subsequent exercise on the same day produces less reduction in pulmonary function.

Nose breathing reduces the effect of sulfur dioxide on asthmatics. The mouth breathing that develops during moderate exercise potentiates the effects on the airways, probably through vagal stimulation of the laryngopharynx and trachea. No synergism between sulfur dioxide and cold air has been found in asthmatics.

Management of sulfur dioxide effects is thus required by the exercising asthmatic individual. Prophylaxis is the key. Preferably, asthmatics should avoid areas of high sulfur dioxide concentration when exercising. Light exercise, in which nose breathing remains possible, is likely to minimize adverse responses. Premedication with cromolyn (disodium cromoglycate) 20 to 30 minutes before exercise also reduces the response, and albuterol or other inhaled beta-adrenergic medications can prevent the sulfur dioxide–induced bronchoconstriction if taken a few minutes before exercise. Optimal treatment of the asthmatic with limitation of relevant allergen exposure, use of appropriate bronchodilators, and (when indicated) inhaled steroids is necessary to control the independent response to exercise alone.

Sulfuric acid and sulfates are often present in the water of naturally occurring fogs, which can have a pH as low as 2, compared with the usual pH of atmospheric water and carbon dioxide, which is 5.6. The highest exposure to sulfuric acid occurs in industry, where the permissible exposure limit has been set at 1,000 μg per cubic meter based on an 8-hour averaging time and a 40-hour work week (US Occupational Safety and Health Administration); however, this standard is not recommended for assessing the health effects of ambient air pollution. Consideration has to be given to the size of the particles produced, because the mass mean aerodynamic diameter influences the site of airway deposition. In the upper airway, sulfuric acid may be neutralized by ammonia from the mouth. Individuals with high oral levels of ammonia are less affected by sulfuric acid inhalation than those with low oral ammonia levels, although other studies have suggested no difference in airway effects between the oral and nasal routes of breathing.

Normal persons have exercised in sulfuric acid levels of 100 μg per cubic meter or less without any measurable pulmonary function change or symptoms. Alternating 20-minute bouts of exercise and rest over 2 hours, with exposure to 950 μg per cubic meter of sulfuric acid at a mass mean aerodynamic diameter (MMAD) of 0.9 μm, lead to marginal but significant FEV_1 reductions (average 101 ml), as well as cough and throat irritation. An exposure to 450 μg per cubic meter, MMAD 0.8 μm sulfuric acid with moderate exercise (50 watts) for 4 hours resulted in mild throat irritation in half the subjects and a significant increase of bronchial reactivity to carbachol 24 hours later. Other reports have suggested changes in resting subjects at levels of 350 μg per cubic meter, although the MMAD was not specified.

Few studies of asthmatics have been reported. At rest, 450 μg per cubic meter sulfuric acid and 1,000 μg per cubic meter of ammonium bisulfate delivered by mouthpiece for 16 minutes resulted in a reduction of specific airway conductance, while levels as low as 100 μg per cubic meter resulted in increased bronchial reactivity to carbachol. Nevertheless, the levels producing changes are generally found only in industry, and ambient levels do not conclusively affect either normal or asthmatic exercising adults.

CARBON MONOXIDE

Outdoor ambient carbon monoxide results mainly from incomplete combustion of fuel from motor vehicles. Adverse effects in humans result from the formation of carboxyhemoglobin in the blood, as hemoglobin has 200 to 300 times more affinity for carbon monoxide than for oxygen. Carboxyhemoglobin causes a leftward shift of the oxyhemoglobin dissociation curve, resulting in less delivery of oxygen to the tissues. In addition, carbon monoxide has a strong affinity for myoglobin and cytochromes, and so may interfere with intracellular oxygen transport. A major source of carbon monoxide exposure, other than traffic exhaust, is tobacco smoking: even passive exposure to smoke can elevate carboxyhemoglobin levels by 1 to 2 percent.

The US Environmental Protection Agency has set ambient carbon monoxide levels with the intent of keeping blood carboxyhemoglobin levels below 2 percent. The maximal 1-hour ambient level is 35 ppm, and the 8-hour average is 9 ppm. Levels of 50 ppm correspond to a first-level alert in Los Angeles. Levels up to 90 ppm have been measured in hockey arenas after the use of resurfacing machines on the ice.

High levels of carboxyhemoglobin can be lethal, but even relatively low levels can significantly impair athletic performance. In addition, the rate of carbon monoxide uptake increases three- to fourfold with exercise, primarily because of an increased ventilation, thus delivering an increased dose of carbon monoxide to the blood. In Harvard hockey players exposed to 22.5 ppm carbon monoxide, carboxyhemoglobin levels increased from 1.1 to 3.2 percent after 90 minutes of exercise. Joggers in Denver showed elevated end-alveolar carbon monoxide levels when ambient concentrations were greater than 6.5 ppm, but lower levels resulted in a net loss of expired carbon monoxide.

Impaired dexterity and coordination have been found with carboxyhemoglobin levels around 5 percent, as have impaired choice responses in firefighters. Visual acuity is measurably reduced at levels around 10 percent, but lower levels may cause slight changes. Maximal oxygen intake is significantly reduced when carboxyhemoglobin levels are as low as 4 percent. However, no reduction of aerobic power was seen in normal men exercising maximally at 35°C when ambient carbon monoxide levels were 50 ppm, although the respiratory rate was increased and the duration of exercise was reduced. The effects of carbon monoxide on myocardial oxygenation are exacerbated in persons with underlying cardiac disease, who may experience angina, myocardial infarction, and sudden death. Similarly, ischemic events may be precipitated by increased carboxyhemoglobin levels in individuals with generalized atherosclerosis.

Management includes monitoring and control of ambient carbon monoxide levels, particularly in enclosed areas such as hockey arenas, with provision of adequate ventilation and exhaust systems. In addition, the exercising individual emphatically should not increase baseline carbon monoxide levels by smoking. Awareness and avoidance of potential sources of carbon monoxide exposure are the best safeguards and should be particularly emphasized to persons with atherosclerosis or heart disease.

OTHER POLLUTANTS

Lead is now becoming recognized as a potentially serious airborne pollutant, particularly in individuals exercising in urban areas. Urban road runners in South Africa showed average blood lead concentrations of 52 μg per deciliter, compared with 20 μg per deciliter in rural runners and 9.7 μg per deciliter in urban controls. Such individuals are potentially at risk of cumulative effects of lead absorption such as encephalopathy, peripheral neuropathy, anemia, and colic, although we have not found documented evidence of such effects in athletes. Nevertheless, awareness of local ambient lead levels and appropriate avoidance are suggested.

Peroxyacetyl nitrate (PAN) is an oxidant that coexists with ozone in photochemical smog. In ambient air it can cause significant eye irritation. Concentrations of 0.27 ppm have no significant effect on the maximal exercise response of normal men at 35°C. Near-ambient levels of nitrogen dioxide, likewise, do not affect normal individuals, but the bronchoconstriction of exercising asthmatics is increased at levels of 0.3 ppm for 30 minutes, and levels as low as 0.1 ppm can produce a subsequent increase in bronchial reactivity.

POLLUTANT COMBINATIONS

Coexisting factors can modify responses. High ozone levels often coexist with high temperatures, which may increase respiratory minute ventilation. Exercise in higher temperatures (e.g., 35°C versus 24°C) increases symptoms and causes greater impairments of FEV_1 and FVC. Particulate pollution in Los Angeles (295 μg per cubic meter) at mean ozone levels of 0.15 ppm gave similar responses to a laboratory exposure of 0.16 ppm ozone without particulate pollution, suggesting that in Los Angeles there was little added effect from particulates. Similarly, in normal exercising individuals, addition of sulfur dioxide at 1 ppm to ozone at 0.3 ppm produced no greater response than the ozone alone, and PAN, when added to ozone or to carbon monoxide (50 ppm), had no statistically significant additive effect.

Likewise, there are no significant additive effects when nitrogen dioxide is combined with ozone at ambient levels in normal individuals. However, studies of interactions, as well as the effects of many other gaseous and particulate pollutants, are still very limited; thus, specific therapeutic measures cannot be advised on the basis of the levels of these pollutants alone.

The effects of ambient concentrations of many air pollutants are currently unknown. Short-term effects of ozone, sulfur dioxide, and carbon monoxide have been described, but many laboratory studies have used higher concentrations than would be expected in the ambient air to which athletes are exposed. Even for ozone, sulfur dioxide, and carbon monoxide, the effects of months or years of exposure during exercise remain unknown. Therefore, management strategies must take account of these limitations in knowledge, and appropriate changes must be made as new information becomes available.

SUGGESTED READING

Adams WC. Effects of ozone exposure at ambient air pollution episode levels on exercise performance. Sports Med 1987; 4:395–424.

Folinsbee LJ. Air pollution and exercise. In Welsh RP, Shephard RJ, eds. Current therapy in sports medicine. 1st ed. Toronto: BC Decker, 1985:54.

Pierson WE, Covent DS, Koenig JQ, Nainekata T, Kim YS. Implications of air pollution effects on athletic performance. Med Sci Sports Exerc 1986; 18:322–327.

CONTROL OF DRUG ABUSE

M. T. LUCKING, M.D.

Table 1 provides the current list of drugs and related compounds that have been banned by the International Amateur Athletic Federation. Being specifically a list of prohibited drugs for track and field athletes, it does not necessarily follow that the contents are relevant to all other sports. The list has been drawn up and amended over decades in response to the use of drugs and other substances by athletes to enhance their training or competitive performance, or to mask a positive response to tests for active substances. Year by year the list grows, as sports contestants, or more probably their advisers, experiment with different drugs or groups of compounds in order to achieve some advantage.

The use of drugs to enhance the effect of sports performance is against the rules of all Olympic sports and many non-Olympic competitions. To use banned substances, either intentionally or otherwise, is just as much against the rules as to use an underweight throwing implement or to step over the throwing line, stop board, or jumping board. Such action renders the drug user, together with the coach or doctor aiding and abetting drug use, subject to the full penalties for breaking the rules.

HISTORY

Both the history of and information on the current use of drugs for nontherapeutic purposes in sport are based largely on hearsay. Since the rules of sport are against administration of drugs, whatever use has occurred has been clandestine and unpublished. It is probable that contestants have experimented with drugs from the very beginnings of organized sports, back even to the times of the ancient Greeks. In modern sports it is probable that stimulants have been used by humans and both stimulants and sedatives have been used in horse racing for a century or more. It was not until the later 1950s and early 1960s, when athletes took seriously to the use of sex hormones (and their derivatives), that drug taking became widespread. It may be that the rather crude use of virilizing compounds by women athletes was the origin of doubts about the gender of certain Eastern European athletes at about that time. Several "women" athletes declined to be subjected to appropriate tests, giving rise to even greater suspicions. Certainly, the use of anabolic steroids by university athletes in the United States was becoming an established practice by the early 1960s. Whether this practice derived from the knowledge that similar use was prevalent in Eastern Europe, or arose spontaneously in the United States, only those closely associated with the practice at that time knew in detail. It is certain that several athletes in the Tokyo Olympics in 1964 were using anabolic compounds, and it is probable that by 1968 most athletes in the "power" events were taking such substances.

The rules of sport at that time did not specifically legislate against the administration of sex hormones and their derivatives. In any case, it was not feasible to detect their use until 10 years later, when Professors Raymond Brooks and Arnold Becket, working in London, developed the techniques to identify even minute traces of such drugs in the urine. Anabolic agents were then added to the banned list, and the first Olympics to institute comprehensive testing were those celebrated in Mexico in 1968. The banning of synthetic anabolic steroids soon led to the increased use of the natural male hormone, testosterone. Initially, testosterone was frequently given to bridge the gap between ceasing administration of the detectable synthetic anabolic steroid and the event itself. The trend became to use anabolic steroids until just before a major tested event, and to switch over to testosterone dosage during the event itself. In the early 1980s a ratio of testosterone to epitestosterone was agreed that defined acceptable "normal" levels. The establishment of a limiting natural testosterone ratio immediately made use of the natural hormone more risky from the viewpoint of detection, and at about this time athletes started to experiment with the administration of pituitary hormones, including growth hormone, luteinizing hormone, and follicle-stimulating hormone, either singly or in various mixtures and cocktails. Some individuals seemed prepared to try anything in an attempt to achieve an increased anabolic status and a faster recovery.

Throughout the "anabolic period" the use of stimulants to "pep up" performance continued, mostly at events in which there was no drug testing. Additionally the use of anxiolytics in the form of alcohol, hypnotics, and latterly beta-blockers has become increasingly favored in skill events in which nervousness can hinder performance. These preparations have been especially useful in events such as shooting and archery. Participants in some endurance sports have also used morphine (or its derivatives) to numb the feeling of fatigue and actual pain induced by the effort.

SPOT TESTING

In recent years it has become increasingly evident that the only way to counteract the illegal administration of hormones is to test athletes during their training period. Before the introduction of randomly timed spot checks, it was necessary only for a treating physician to be cautious in prescribing such drugs when a major event was imminent. Practicing physicians now need to be aware of spot testing when treating any condition. Problems can arise when the condition requiring treatment is unrelated to the sport and the prescribing doctor is unaware of the patient's sporting prowess. In these cases, the onus must always be on the athlete to inform the treating doctor of his or her liability to spot testing. It is possible to envisage a scenario in which a doctor unwittingly prescribes a banned compound. The athlete subsequently has a positive spot test and is suspended, in some cases for life. In amateur sports this would be serious; in professional sports, it is disastrous. The legal implications are manifold.

The International Amateur Athletics Federation has urged all countries to establish spot testing programs. So far, only a handful of countries have managed to do so. Spot testing has now become an established procedure for most Olympic sports in the United Kingdom and also in the Scandinavian countries. The testing is based on a register. The principle is that any athlete who has ambitions to represent his or her country is asked to agree to spot testing at any venue, at any time, throughout the year. Similarly, an up-and-coming or improving athlete can be asked to be on the register. The act of signing an agreement to testing is voluntary, and it does not place the governing body of a sport in the position of infringing upon personal liberties by insisting on testing. However, an athlete will be considered for international competition only if entered on this register.

Spot testing is carried out in addition to random testing at major events. It could happen by chance that an athlete was spot tested one week and tested again at an actual event the following week. In the United Kingdom, spot testing is now in its third year. For the most part the procedure runs smoothly. The random selection has been criticized on the basis that it has picked out athletes in events in which the temptation to use drugs that influence training is low, whereas more suspect categories of contestants have not been tested. Such selection problems can be remedied. A more difficult problem is that of spot testing athletes who are training overseas, at high altitude, in warmer climates, or who are attending overseas universities. The cost of spot test collection in distant locations can be high. However, it has currently been recognized as a loophole in the spot testing system and is being used as such. Overseas collections have been made with positive results. Ideally, a worldwide international system of spot testing is required, with built-in provision for international cross-checking.

MORAL AND ETHICAL ISSUES

Until the advent of spot testing, the role of the physician in drug abuse in sport was largely that of the villain. As the rules of Olympic sports legislate against the use of drugs to enhance performance, any physician or pharmacist who promotes or monitors such action must be guilty of compounding a felony. It is well known that in some academic institutions, scientists, pharmacists, and doctors are striving to produce compounds or cocktails of compounds designed to enhance performance or evade testing, whereas in a laboratory "down the corridor" another group is striving to perfect analyzing and detecting techniques. Some physicians take the view that it is perfectly acceptable and ethical for athletes to use whatever chemical means they can to influence training or performance. It is maintained that a properly based scientific approach to nontherapeutic drug taking would in the long run be more informative and less hazardous than the current pattern of clandestine use, with very little surveillance or analysis and a greater chance of hazardous side effects. This school of thought campaigns to bring the rules of sport into line with such an open and free attitude.

It is possible to see a certain logic in this approach, but it flies in the face of most moral and scientific thinking with regard to the nontherapeutic use of drugs throughout the civilized world. This is true not just of drugs that influence sports performance, but also of hallucinatory and addictive narcotic drugs, the use of which for the purpose of mood changes has become so prevalent in the second half of the 20th century. There can be no doubt in anyone's mind that such drug taking is physically and emotionally very harmful to the participants. The underworld business of producing and distributing drugs is a source of much crime, undermining the very foundations of civilized societies. Likewise, the illicit use of drugs in sport has become an internationally based clandestine smuggling operation, attracting all the unpleasantness and crime associated with such activities when large amounts of money are involved. The hazardous effects of drug use in sport are poorly documented. Very few properly devised trials have tested either their efficacy or their effects upon the metabolism, physiology, and hemodynamics of the athlete. Any liberalization of the use of drugs in sport could soon become the thin end of the wedge, encouraging such activities as genetic engineering and Nazi-style selective breeding to produce super specimens. We have already heard horrific stories of the hormonal manipulation of adolescents to influence height and weight ratios. There are current rumors of the deliberate fertilization of women athletes to take advantage of the anabolic effects of the hormones of early pregnancy, with subsequent termination of the pregnancy. All these activities are directly contrary to the moral, ethical, and religious principles on which human relationships have evolved throughout the ages. The governing bodies of international sport are right to legislate against the use of drugs and other artificial means of enhancing performance. Their stand must be supported, and a means of enforcing that stand worldwide should be found wherever possible.

Where does this now place the physician responsible for the care of the athlete? If the normal standards of morality are accepted, the maverick doctor who wittingly prescribes a drug to place the patient at odds with the rules of a sport is manifestly out of order. Indeed, the International Amateur Athletic Federation rules on the subject specifically identify any person "assisting or inciting others to use doping substances" as being in contravention of the rules. In the case of a physician, the possible disciplinary measures open to the Administration of the Federation are few. It is not much of a penalty to prevent a physician from seeing an athlete at an event. The only significant sanction would be for that physician's responsible ethical council to bring pressure on the individual, as currently occurs when the General Medical Council of the United Kingdom takes action against the irresponsible prescribing of narcotic agents.

PRESCRIBING FOR REGISTERED ATHLETES

Undoubtedly, the list of banned drugs must influence the medical management of problems encountered by registered athletes. Even the simple prescription of a compound containing codeine can place both patient and physician in breach of the rules. There are numerous pharmaceutical alternatives making it possible to avoid the prescription of banned substances, but there will be circumstances when a physician feels that only a banned drug would be appropriate. What should the procedure then be?

There could be room for some compromise in the legislation, depending on the circumstances of the medical condition and the proximity in time to an event. Spot testing outside of the event has been introduced to prevent the use of drugs that influence training. Therefore, it seems appropriate that compounds that do not have anabolic effects and do not improve recovery rate could be permitted until 48 hours before an event. In principle, this would ban the administration of sex and pituitary hormones (and related compounds) permanently, but other substances would be banned only for 2 days before and during an event. This would free a physician to treat all but the most obscure conditions during the training period. There remain some anomalies, such as the athlete in need of beta-blocking agents for a cardiac or circulatory condition, the contestant needing a psychotropic drug for psychiatric purposes, or an injured individual requiring a strong analgesic. However, a line must be drawn somewhere, and if a banned list is to be effective, there is likely always to be someone on the "bad luck" side of the line. Thus, if an athlete should suffer from a condition requiring treatment with sex or pituitary hormones (other than contraceptives at normally accepted doses), he or she would be ineligible to compete within the rules during the period when such compounds were administered. Likewise, competitors using beta-blockers, banned psychotropic drugs, or analgesics would need to change their medication or lose competitive eligibility while using these preparations. The athlete ideally should be given a list of banned substances, together with a list of alternative drugs that can be legally used (see Tables 1 and 2).

Athletes and their physicians are advised to contact their governing bodies for advice when there is doubt. It is surely preferable to withdraw temporarily from a register or not take part in an event than to risk the possibility of prolonged banishment.

TABLE 1 Drugs and Related Substances Currently Banned by the International Amateur Athletic Federation

Stimulants, e.g.,

Amiphenazole	Etafedrine	Morazone
Amphetamine	Ethamivan	Nikethamide
Amphetaminil	Ethylamphetamine	Pemoline
Benzphetamine	Fencamfamin	Pentetrazol
Cathine	Fenethylline	Phendimetrazine
Chlorphentermine	Fenproporex	Phenmetrazine
Clobenzorex	Furfenorex	Phentermine
Cocaine	Meclofenoxate	Phenylpropanolamine
Cropropamide*	Mefenorex	Pipradrol
Crotethamide*	Methoxyphenamine	Prolintane
Diethylpropion	Methylamphetamine	Propylhexedrine
Dimethylamphetamine	Methylphedrine	Pyrovalerone
Ephedrine	Methylphenidate	Strychnine

and chemically or pharmacologically related compounds.

Narcotic Analgesics, e.g.,

Alphaprodine	Diamorphine	Morphine
Anileridine	Dihydrocodeine	Nalbuphine
Buprenorphine	Dipipanone	Pentazocine
Codeine†	Ethylmorphine	Pethidine
Dextromoramide	Levorphanol	Phenazocine
Dextropropoxyphene	Methadone	Trimeperidine

and chemically or pharmacologically related compounds.

Anabolic Steroids, e.g.,

Bolasterone	Methyltestosterone
Boldenone	Nandrolone
Chlordehydromethyltestosterone	Norethandrolone
Clostebol	Oxandrolone
Fluoxymesterone	Oxymesterone
Mesterolone	Oxymetholone
Methandienone	Stanozolol
Methenolone	Testosterone‡

and chemically and pharmacologically related compounds.

Miscellaneous—Diuretic compounds
—Probenecid

* Component of Micoren.
† Permitted for the treatment of a disorder.
‡ And any other substance that has the effect of increasing the testosterone to epitestosterone ratio.

TABLE 2 Proposed List of Medicines That May be Taken by Competing Athletes*

Antacids	
Actal	Alexitol sodium
Actonorm	Dried aluminum hydroxide gel, magnesium hydroxide, and activated dimethicone
Altacite Plus	Hydrotalcite and activated dimethicone
Alu-Cap	Dried aluminum hydroxide gel
Aludrox	Aluminum hydroxide gel
Andursil	Aluminum oxide, magnesium hydroxide, aluminum hydroxide/magnesium carbonate codried gel, and activated dimethicone
Antasil	Dried aluminum hydroxide gel, magnesium hydroxide, and activated dimethicone
Asilone	Activated dimethicone and dried aluminum hydroxide gel
Diloran	Magnesium oxide, aluminum hydroxide/magnesium carbonate codried gel, and activated dimethicone
Diovol	Aluminum hydroxide, magnesium hydroxide, and dimethicone
Droxalin	Alexitol sodium and magnesium trisilicate
Gastrils	Aluminum hydroxide/magnesium carbonate codried gel
Gastrocote	Alginic acid, dried aluminum hydroxide gel, magnesium trisilicate, and sodium bicarbonate
Gaviscon	Alginic acid, magnesium trisilicate, dried aluminum hydroxide gel, and sodium bicarbonate
Gelusil	Magnesium trisilicate and dried aluminum hydroxide gel
Maalox	Dried aluminum hydroxide gel and magnesium hydroxide

Table 2 continues on following page

TABLE 2 (continued)

Malinal	Almasilate
Mucaine	Oxethazaine, aluminum hydroxide gel, and magnesium hydroxide
Mucogel	Dried aluminum hydroxide gel and magnesium hydroxide
Nulacin	Whole milk solids combined with dextrins and maltose, magnesium trisilicate, heavy magnesium oxide, calcium carbonate, and heavy magnesium carbonate
Phazyme	Activated dimethicone and pancreatin
Polyalk	Dimethicone and dried aluminum hydroxide gel
Polycrol	Activated dimethicone, magnesium hydroxide, and aluminum hydroxide gel
Prodexin	Aluminum glycinate and magnesium carbonate
Siloxyl	Dried aluminum hydroxide gel and activated dimethicone
Sylopal	Dimethicone, light magnesium oxide, and aluminum hydroxide gel
Synergel	Aluminum phosphate gel and pectin and agar gel
Titralac	Calcium carbonate and glycine
Topal	Dried aluminum hydroxide gel, light magnesium carbonate, and alginic acid
Unigest	Dried aluminum hydroxide gel and dimethicone
Gastrointestinal sedatives, antacid-sedative combinations, and other ulcer-healing drugs	
Actonorm	Papaverine hydrochloride, atropine sulfate, thiamine hydrochloride, magnesium carbonate, diastase, pancreatin, dried aluminum hydroxide gel, calcium carbonate, light kaolin, and magnesium trisilicate
Actonorm-Sed	Belladonna tincture, dried aluminum hydroxide gel, magnesium hydroxide, and activated dimethicone
Aludrox SA	Ambutonium bromide, aluminum hydroxide gel, and magnesium hydroxide
Aluhyde	Aluminum hydroxide gel, magnesium trisilicate, and belladonna liquid extract
Antepsin	Sucralfate
APP	Papaverine hydrochloride, homatropine methylbromide, calcium carbonate, magnesium carbonate, magnesium trisilicate, bismuth carbonate, and aluminum hydroxide gel
Bellocarb	Belladonna dry extract, magnesium trisilicate, and magnesium carbonate
Biogastrone	Carbenoxolone sodium
Buscopan	Hyoscine butylbromide
Cantil	Mepenzolate bromide
Carbellon	Belladonna dry extract, magnesium hydroxide, charcoal, and peppermint oil
Caved-S	Deglycyrrhizinized licorice, aluminum hydroxide gel, magnesium carbonate, and sodium bicarbonate
Colofac	Mebeverine hydrochloride
Colpermin	Peppermint oil
De-Nol	Tri-potassium di-citrato bismuthate
De-Noltab	Tri-potassium di-citrato bismuthate
Duogastrone	Carbenoxolone sodium
Emetrol	Levulose, dextrose, and phosphoric acid
Gastrozepin	Pirenzepine hydrochloride
Kolanticon	Dried aluminum hydroxide gel, magnesium oxide, dicyclomine hydrochloride, and dimethicone
Kolantyl	Dried aluminum hydroxide gel, magnesium oxide, and dicyclomine hydrochloride
Libraxin	Chlordiazepoxide and clidinium bromide
Maxolon	Metoclopramide hydrochloride
Merbentyl	Dicyclomine hydrochloride
Metox	Metoclopramide
Monodral	Penthienate methobromide
Nacton forte	Poldine methylsulfate
Neutradonna	Hyoscyamine and aluminum sodium silicate
Ovol	Dicyclomine hydrochloride and dimethicone
Parmid	Metoclopramide hydrochloride
Peptard	Hyoscyamine sulfate
Piptal	Pipenzolate bromide
Piptalin	Pipenzolate bromide and activated dimethicone
Primperan	Metoclopramide hydrochloride
Pro-banthine	Propantheline bromide
Pyrogastrone	Carbenoxolone sodium, magnesium trisilicate, and aluminum hydroxide gel
Rabro	Deglycyrrhizinized licorice, magnesium oxide, calcium carbonate, and frangula
Robinul	Glycopyrronium bromide
Roter	Magnesium carbonate, bismuth subnitrate, sodium bicarbonate, and frangula
Spasmonal	Alverine citrate
Stelabid	Trifluoperazine hydrochloride and isopropamide iodide
Tagamet	Cimetidine
Zantac	Ranitidine hydrochloride

TABLE 2 (continued)

Antidiarrheals	
Arobon	Ceratonia and starch
Celevac	Methylcellulose
Dioralyte	Sodium chloride, potassium chloride, sodium bicarbonate, and dextrose
Enteromide	Calcium sulfaloxate
Guanimycin	Dihydrostreptomycin sulfate, sulfaguanidine, and light kaolin
Imodium	Loperamide hydrochloride
Kaopectate	Kaolin
Lomotil	Diphenoxylate hydrochloride and atropine sulfate
Rehidrat	Sodium chloride, potassium chloride, sodium bicarbonate, citric acid, glucose, sucrose, and levulose
Streptotriad	Streptomycin, sulfadimidine, sulfadiazine, and sulfathiazole
Analgesics and antipyretics	
Acupan	Nefopam hydrochloride
Benoral	Benorylate
Breoprin	Aspirin
Brufen	Ibuprofen
Cafadol	Paracetamol and caffeine
Calpol Six Plus	Paracetamol
Caprin	Aspirin
Claradin	Aspirin
Dolobid	Diflunisal
Equagesic	Ethoheptazine citrate, meprobamate, and aspirin
Fenopron	Fenoprofen
Ibu-Slo	Ibuprofen
Laboprin	Aspirin and lysine
Levius	Aspirin
Medised	Paracetamol and promethazine hydrochloride
Meptid	Meptazinol hydrochloride
Meralen	Flufenamic acid
Nu-Seals Aspirin	Aspirin
Panadol	Paracetamol
Panasorb	Paracetamol
Paynocil	Aspirin and glycine
Ponstan	Mefenamic acid
Progexic	Fenoprofen
Safapryn	Aspirin and paracetamol
Salzone	Paracetamol
Solprin	Aspirin
Suprol	Suprofen
Synflex	Naproxen
Tegretol	Carbamazepine
Unigesic	Paracetamol and caffeine
Zactirin	Ethoheptazine citrate, aspirin, and calcium carbonate
Hypnotics (See MPA warning)†	
Amytal	Amylobarbitone
Dalmane	Flurazepam
Dormonoct	Loprazolam
Euhypnos	Temazepam
Halcion	Triazolam
Heminevrin	Chlormethiazole edisylate
Loramet	Lormetazepam
Medomin	Heptabarbitone
Mogadon	Nitrazepam
Nembutal	Pentobarbitone sodium
Nitrados	Nitrazepam
Noctamid	Lormetazepam
Noctec	Chloral hydrate
Noludar	Methyprylone
Normison	Temazepam
Phanodorm	Cyclobarbitone calcium
Rohypnol	Flunitrazepam
Seconal	Quinalbarbitone sodium
Sodium amytal	Amylobarbitone sodium
Somnite	Nitrazepam
Soneryl	Butobarbitone
Surem	Nitrazepam
Trancopal	Chlormezanone
Tuinal	Quinalbarbitone sodium and amylobarbitone sodium
Unisomnia	Nitrazepam
Welldorm	Dichloralphenazone

Table 2 continues on following page

TABLE 2 (continued)

Sedatives and Tranquilizers (See MPA warning)†	
Almazine	Lorazepam
Alupram	Diazepam
Anquil	Benperidol
Anxon	Ketazolam
Atarax	Hydroxyzine hydrochloride
Atensine	Diazepam
Ativan	Lorazepam
Centrax	Prazepam
Clopixol	Clopenthixol hydrochloride
Clopixol injection	Clopenthixol decanoate
Dartalan	Thiopropazate hydrochloride
Depixol	Flupenthixol decanoate
Diazemuls	Diazepam
Dolmatil	Sulpiride
Droleptan	Droperidol
Equanil	Meprobamate
Evacalm	Diazepam
Fentazin	Perphenazine
Fortunan	Haloperidol
Frisium	Clobazam
Haldol	Haloperidol
Heminevrin	Chlormethiazole
Heminevrin syrup	Chlormethiazole edisylate
Integrin	Oxypertine
Largactil	Chlorpromazine hydrochloride
Largactil forte suspension	Chlorpromazine embonate
Lexotan	Bromazepam
Librium	Chlordiazepoxide
Limbitrol	Amitriptyline and chlordiazepoxide
Mellaril	Thioridazine hydrochloride
Milonorm	Meprobamate
Modecate	Fluphenazine decanoate
Moditen	Fluphenazine hydrochloride
Moditen enanthate	Fluphenazine enanthate
Motipress	Fluphenazine hydrochloride and nortriptyline
Motival	Fluphenazine hydrochloride and nortriptyline
Neulactil	Pericyazine
Nobrium	Medazepam
Orap	Pimozide
Paedo-Sed	Dichloralphenazone and paracetamol
Piportil depot	Pipothiazine palmitate
Redeptin	Fluspirilene
Serenace	Haloperidol
Serenid-D	Oxazepam
Solis	Diazepam
Sparine	Promazine hydrochloride
Stelazine	Trifluoperazine
Stemetil	Prochlorperazine maleate
Stemetil syrup	Prochlorperazine mesylate
Stesolid	Diazepam
Taractan	Chlorprothixene
Tenavoid	Bendrofluazide and meprobamate
Tranxene	Clorazepate potassium
Triperidol	Trifluperidol
Triptafen	Amitriptyline hydrochloride and perphenazine
Valium	Diazepam
Valrelease	Diazepam
Xanax	Alprazolam

TABLE 2 (continued)

Antidepressants (See MPA warning)[†]	
Allegron	Nortriptyline
Anafranil	Clomipramine hydrochloride
Aventyl	Nortriptyline
Bolvidon	Mianserin hydrochloride
Camcolit	Lithium carbonate
Concordin	Protriptyline hydrochloride
Domical	Amitriptyline hydrochloride
Elamol	Tofenacin hydrochloride
Evadyne	Butriptyline
Fluanxol	Flupenthixol
Gamanil	Lofepramine
Lentizol	Amitriptyline hydrochloride
Limbitrol 5	Amitriptyline and chlordiazepoxide
Liskonum	Lithium carbonate
Litarex	Lithium citrate
Ludiomil	Maprotiline hydrochloride
Marplan	Isocarboxazid
Marsilid	Iproniazid
Merital	Nomifensine hydrogen maleate
Molipaxin	Trazodone hydrochloride
Motipress	Fluphenazine hydrochloride and nortriptyline
Motival	Fluphenazine hydrochloride and nortriptyline
Nardil	Phenelzine
Norval	Mianserin hydrochloride
Optimax	L-tryptophan, pyridoxine hydrochloride, and ascorbic acid
Optimax WV	As Optimax but vitamin free
Pacitron	L-tryptophan
Parnate	Tranylcypromine
Parstelin	Tranylcypromine and trifluoperazine
Pertofran	Desipramine hydrochloride
Phasal	Lithium carbonate
Priadel	Lithium carbonate
Prondol	Iprindole
Prothiaden	Dothiepin hydrochloride
Saroten	Amitriptyline hydrochloride
Sinequan	Doxepin
Surmontil	Trimipramine
Tofranil	Imipramine hydrochloride
Triptafen	Amitriptyline hydrochloride and perphenazine
Tryptizol	Amitriptyline hydrochloride
Vivalan	Viloxazine
Antiemetics and antinauseants	
Ancoloxin	Meclozine hydrochloride and pyridoxine hydrochloride
Benadon	Pyridoxine hydrochloride
Dramamine	Dimenhydrinate
Equivert	Buclizine hydrochloride and nicotinic acid
Lipoflavonoid	Choline bitartrate, inositol, methionine, ascorbic acid, lemon bioflavonoid complex, thiamine hydrochloride, riboflavine, nicotinamide, pyridoxine hydrochloride, panthenol, and hydroxocobalamin
Maxolon	Metoclopramide hydrochloride
Metox	Metoclopramide
Motilium	Domperidone
Parmid	Metoclopramide hydrochloride
Primperan	Metoclopramide hydrochloride
Serc	Betahistine dihydrochloride
Stelazine	Trifluoperazine hydrochloride
Stemetil	Prochlorperazine maleate
Stugeron	Cinnarizine
Torecan	Thiethylperazine maleate
Valoid	Cyclizine hydrochloride
Vertigon spansule	Prochlorperazine maleate

Table 2 continues on following page

TABLE 2 (continued)

Nonsteroid anti-inflammatory drugs	
Alrheumat	Ketoprofen
Ananase	Bromelains (proteolytic enzymes)
Benoral	Benorylate
Breoprin	Aspirin
Brufen	Ibuprofen
Caprin	Aspirin
Chymar	Chymotrypsin
Chymoral	Trypsin
Claradin	Aspirin
Clinoril	Sulindac
Deanese D.C.	Delta-chymotrypsin
Disalcid	Salsalate
Distamine	Penicillamine base
Equagesic	Ethoheptazine citrate, meprobamate, and aspirin
Feldene	Piroxicam
Fenopron	Fenoprofen
Flenac	Fenclofenac
Froben	Flurbiprofen
Ibu-Slo	Ibuprofen
Imbrilon	Indomethacin
Indocid	Indomethacin
Indolar	Indomethacin
Laboprin	Aspirin and lysine
Lederfen	Fenbufen
Levius	Aspirin
Meralen	Flufenamic acid
Methrazone	Feprazone
Mobilan	Indomethacin
Myocrisin	Sodium aurothiomalate
Naprosyn	Naproxen
Nu-Seals	Aspirin
Orudis	Ketoprofen
Oruvail	Ketoprofen
Palaprin	Aloxiprin
Paynocil	Aspirin and glycine
Pendramine	Penicillamine
Plaquenil	Hydroxychloroquine sulfate
Ponstan	Mefenamic acid
Potaba	Potassium *p*-aminobenzoate
Progesic	Fenoprofen
Rheumox	Azapropazone dihydrate
Safapryn	Aspirin and paracetamol
Solprin	Aspirin
Surgam	Tiaprofenic acid
Synflex	Naproxen
Tolectin	Tolmetin
Trilisate	Choline magnesium trisalicylate
Voltarol	Diclofenac sodium
Zactirin	Ethoheptazine citrate
Bronchospasm relaxants	
Alupent	Orciprenaline sulfate
Atrovent	Ipratropium bromide (inhaler)
Becloforte	Beclomethasone‡ dipropionate (inhaler)
Becotide	Beclomethasone‡ dipropionate (inhaler)
Berotec	Fenoterol hydrobromide (inhaler)
Bextasol	Betamethasone‡ valerate (inhaler)
Bricanyl	Terbutaline sulfate
Bronchodil	Reproterol hydrochloride
Brontina	Deptropine citrate
Choledyl	Choline theophyllinate
Duovent	Fenoterol hydrobromide and ipratropium bromide (inhaler)
Etophylate	Acepifylline
Eumydrin	Atropine methonitrate (drops)
Exirel	Pirbuterol hydrochloride
Intal	Sodium cromoglycate (*N.B.* Intal compound also contains isoprenaline and hence is not allowed.)
Labophylline	Theophylline and lysine
Millophylline	Etamiphylline camsylate
Nuelin	Theophylline
Nuelin SA	Theophylline
Phyllocontin continus	Aminophylline

TABLE 2 (continued)

Pro-Vent	Theophylline
Pulmadil	Rimiterol hydrobromide (inhaler)
Pulmicort	Budesonide (inhaler)
Sabidal SR	Choline theophyllinate
Silbephylline	Diprophylline
Slo-Phyllin	Theophylline
Thean	Proxylline
Theodrox	Aminophylline and dried aluminum hydroxide gel
Theo-Dur	Theophylline
Theograd	Theophylline
Theosol	Theophylline
Uniphyllin Unicontin	Theophylline
Ventide	Salbutamol and beclomethasone‡ dipropionate (inhaler)
Ventolin	Salbutamol
Zaditen	Ketotifen
Expectorants, cough suppressants, mucolytics, and decongestants	
Airbron	Acetylcysteine
Alevaire	Tyloxapol
Alupent expectorant	Orciprenaline sulfate and bromhexine hydrochloride
Benylin expectorant	Diphenhydramine hydrochloride, ammonium chloride, sodium citrate, and menthol (*N.B.* Benylin Decongestant contains pseudoephedrine and that and Benylin with Codeine are not allowed.)
Bisolvomycin	Bromhexine hydrochloride and oxytetracycline hydrochloride
Bisolvon	Bromhexine hydrochloride
Bricanyl compound	Terbutaline sulfate and guaiphenesin
Copholco	Pholcodeine, menthol, cineole, and terpin hydrate
Copholcoids	Pholcodeine, menthol, cineole, and terpin hydrate
Cosylan	Dextromethorphan hydrobromide
Dia-Tuss	Pholcodine
Dimyril	Isoaminile citrate
Fabrol	Acetylcysteine
Guanor	Ammonium chloride, diphenhydramine hydrochloride, sodium citrate, and menthol
Histalix	Diphenhydramine hydrochloride, ammonium chloride, sodium citrate, and menthol
Mucodyne	Carbocisteine
Mucolex	Carbocisteine
Muflin	Dextromethorphan hydrobromide, sodium citrate, pheniramine maleate, and citric acid
Organidin	Iodinated glycerol
Pavacol-D	Papaverine hydrochloride and pholcodine
Phenergan compound	Promethazine hydrochloride, ipecacuanha, potassium guaiacolsulfonate, and citric acid
Pholcomed	Pholcodine and papaverine hydrochloride (*N.B.* Pholcomed Expectorant contains methylephedrine and is not allowed.)
Pholtex	Pholcodine and phenyltoloxamine
Robitussin	Guaiphenesin (*N.B.* Robitussin AC contains codeine phosphate.)
Sancos	Pholcodeine and glycerol (*N.B.* Sancos Co contains pseudoephedrine hydrochloride and is not allowed.)
Syrtussar	Dextromethorphan hydrobromide, pheniramine maleate, sodium citrate, and citric acid
Tussifans	Belladonna liquid extract, potassium citrate, tolu syrup, ipecacuanha liquid extract, and squill syrup
Visclair	Methylcysteine hydrochloride
Local reactants on the nose	
Afrazine	Oxymetazoline hydrochloride (spray and drops)
Antistine-Privine	Antazoline sulfate and naphazoline (spray and drops)
Beconase	Beclomethasone‡ dipropionate
Betnesol	Betamethasone‡ sodium phosphate
Dexa-Rhinaspray	Tramazoline hydrochloride, dexamethasone‡-21-isonicotinate, and neomycin sulfate
Iliadin-Mini	Oxymetazoline hydrochloride
Lomusol	Sodium cromoglycate
Naseptin	Chlorhexidine hydrochloride and neomycin sulfate
Otrivine	Xylometazoline hydrochloride
Otrivine-Antistin	Xylometazoline hydrochloride and antazoline hydrochloride
Pabracort	Hydrocortisone‡ acetate (insufflation)
Rynacrom	Sodium cromoglycate
Syntaris	Flunisolide
Vista-Methasone N	Betamethasone‡ sodium phosphate and neomycin sulfate

* This list is only a guide, is not intended to be comprehensive; and should not be taken as a recommendation of the efficacy of the various substances. Care should be taken when selecting proprietary preparations since formulations change from time to time. The list has been compiled by Dr. D. A. Cowan considering the known rules of British Sports Organizations. Care should be taken to ensure no contravention of the rules of overseas sports organizations nor the laws of overseas countries.

† MPA warning: The UIPMB bans the use of hypnotics and sedatives and includes under these categories preparations containing barbiturates, benzodiazepines, phenothiazines, tricyclic antidepressants, and anticonvulsants. They also ban the use of beta-adrenergic blocking drugs.

‡ Steroid warning: Listed preparations contain corticosteroids and may thus be considered as not allowed by the International Cycling Union.

NEUROMUSCULAR PHYSIOLOGY

GARY KAMEN, PH.D., F.A.C.S.M.

Compared with other exercise science subdisciplines, the areas of neuromuscular physiology and motor control are not usually as familiar to sports medicine professionals as are topics in exercise physiology, exercise biochemistry, and biomechanics. However, one need only recognize the fact that the nature of the neural stimulus largely determines such features as the kinematic movement pattern, muscle enzymatic profiles, and muscle fiber type composition to understand why neuromuscular physiology is as important as any other aspect of sports medicine discussed in this book. This chapter focuses on a few of the current concerns in neuromuscular physiology of particular interest to sports medicine clinicians.

SPECIFICITY OF TRAINING

It is now accepted that exercise training follows well-described laws of specificity. Previous authors have stated the theory of exercise specificity as follows: a specific exercise elicits a specific response in a specific individual at a specific time. Although the theoretical basis for the specificity of exercise is still the subject of research, some coaches have long practiced a form of specificity training. For example, wrestling coaches used to say that wrestling was an arrhythmic sport and that accordingly, wrestlers should not perform rhythmic activities such as swimming or bicycling.

The basic principle of exercise specificity can be used to predict alterations in the neuromuscular profile that occur with training. Early experimenters demonstrated that weight training was an appropriate stimulus for increasing strength, while long-term aerobic exercise was necessary for increasing endurance. More recent studies have served to refine fundamental rules of specificity. For example, high-resistance exercise results in increases in maximal strength, but only moderate improvements in the maximal rate of force production. On the other hand, an exercise program that is geared toward improving explosive strength improves the rate of force production, with only a limited increase in maximal strength.

These findings and other research observations suggest that some types of training can be detrimental to the athlete in a specific discipline. Simultaneous strength and endurance training seems to have a positive impact on endurance as measured by maximal oxygen uptake. Also, there may be some improvement in muscular strength, especially at low velocities (e.g., isometric or slow isotonic contraction). However, as shown schematically in Figure 1, this type of training has a negative impact on high-power activities during which the muscle is working at a high velocity and somewhat reduced forces. Thus, we may still have a lot to learn about how some athletes (such as basketball players) should train to optimize both muscular power and aerobic endurance.

ROLE OF THE NERVOUS SYSTEM IN SPORTS MEDICINE

Unfortunately, there seems to be a tendency among exercise scientists to ignore the nervous system. The emphasis appears to be on studying behavior in the circulation, in respiration, and in skeletal muscles, without regard to neural influences. A number of examples demonstrate that the human neuromuscular system does not always behave as predicted from isolated animal muscle experiments. Consider the muscle force–velocity relationship as an example. For decades we have recognized the inverse relationship between muscle force and velocity, as predicted by Hill's classical experiments. However, this relationship is disturbed in intact human muscle (Fig. 2). The reason for this difference is not entirely clear, but at least one plausible explanation is that at relatively high force levels the input from force-sensitive proprioceptors (Golgi tendon organs) prevents the production of an injury-causing force level. There is some indication that classical stretch reflexes may be altered in some athletes. Ballet dancers and endurance runners have notoriously poor tendon reflexes. However, it is not entirely clear whether these changes are due to dif-

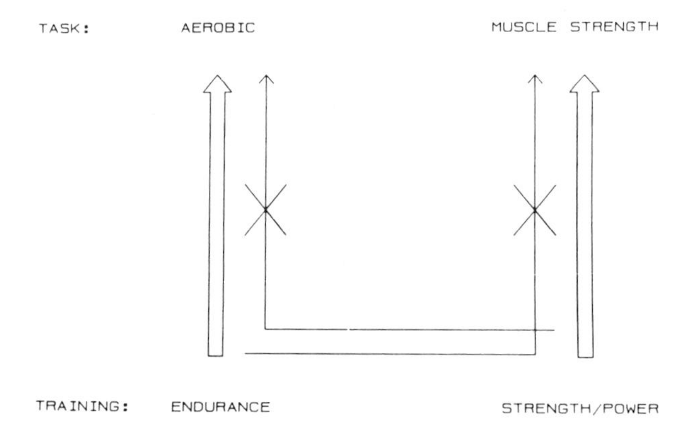

Figure 1 The specificity of exercise principle. Aerobic tasks require aerobic-endurance training, while muscular strength or power tasks require strength-power training. However, using only one type of training may have a detrimental effect on performance in another type of task. The most frequent observation has been that combined endurance and power training may attenuate gains in activities requiring muscular power.

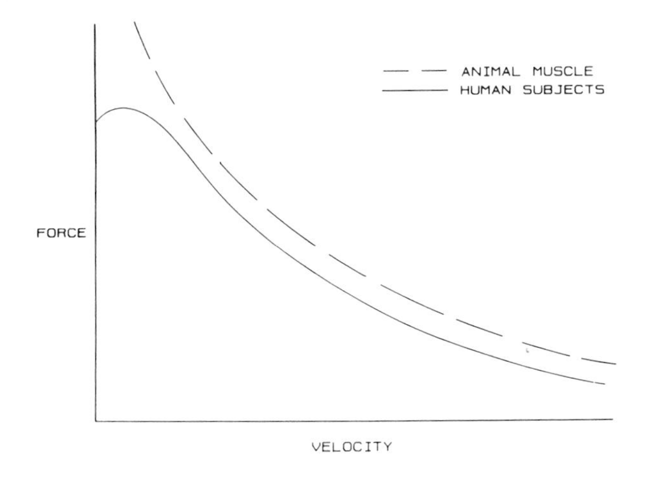

Figure 2 The inverse, curvilinear relationship between muscle force and velocity (dotted line) is well known in animal experiments. This relationship does not hold in human subjects, however, particularly in the high-force, low-velocity region.

ferences in synaptic excitability, or whether they should be attributed to changes in muscle-tendon compliance.

The role of classical reflex pathways in motor control can be demonstrated in a variety of ways. A muscle group that is forcibly stretched during the course of an active contraction produces a greater force than would be developed during an isometric contraction. It has been recognized for some time that a lengthening or eccentric contraction produces greater force than an isometric contraction. However, the effect from such an imposed stretch has a significant neural component. For example, let us assume an individual is producing a knee extension contraction simultaneously in both left and right legs. If the right leg is stretched while the individual maintains maximal effort in both legs, the observed strength of the left leg extensors declines. A likely neural mechanism, predicted from classical Sherringtonian neurophysiology, is the crossed extensor reflex. Contracting one muscle group inhibits the contralateral homonymous musculature. This reflex helps us to maintain an upright posture by increasing the extensor force in the quadriceps when balance in the contralateral leg has suddenly been disrupted (e.g., by one leg slipping on the ice or by stepping on a nail).

It may also be tempting to attribute this effect to divided attention. In other words, perhaps the individual is incapable of exerting maximal effort simultaneously in both limbs, and thus chooses to concentrate on producing as much strength as possible in the stretched leg. This divided attention concept can be dismissed by a second experiment. If the individual now performs a maximal knee flexion contraction in the left leg while the right leg is stretched, the strength of the left leg increases during the stretch, which is in perfect accord with a neural explanation.

Another example, consistent with the idea that neural reflex pathways are important in strength production, comes from the observation of bilateral contractions. A simultaneous bilateral contraction produces less force than the sum of the individual unilateral contractions. For example, exerting a simultaneous knee extensor contraction produces less force than if one were to measure left leg extensor strength and right leg extensor strength separately and sum the two scores. Some investigators have suggested that the pattern of motor unit recruitment may be different in these types of bilateral contractions. Of course, there are some activities (e.g., weight lifting) in which there is no choice but to perform the bilateral contraction. It may well be that some alternative training techniques would be more beneficial for individuals whose athletic activities involve simultaneous bilateral contractions.

NEUROMUSCULAR PRINCIPLES OF TRAINING

Until recently, strength training research has focused on the obvious question of how best to use high-resistance exercise in order to increase muscular strength. Regardless of whether the contraction is isometric, concentric, eccentric, or isokinetic, muscular strength gains occur in response to the overload principle developed by DeLorme. Of course, there are ways of optimizing the exercise training schedule. The number of repetitions, sets, and the like in isotonic exercise can be controlled, and unless isometric exercise is used appropriately, strength gains from this type of exercise tend to be joint-angle specific. The newer, computer-aided exercise machines utilize the idea that motivation can be enhanced by visual feedback, but the ultimate result still is generally guided by overload principles.

It is unfortunate that the role of the nervous system in strength training has generally been overlooked. A common misbelief, for example, is that when one begins a high-resistance exercise program, the most important goal is to increase muscle girth and thereby increase muscular strength. Although muscle cross-sectional area is reasonably well correlated to total muscle force in isolated animal muscle, initial gains in strength are usually unaccompanied by increases in muscle size. The greatest strength gains occur in the early stages of a strength training program, and during this period researchers have noted little change in muscle fiber size or type, anaerobic enzyme activity, or energy substrate levels. In other words, at a time when strength is increasing the most, there seems to be little change in muscle physiology. It is only after the first month or so that it is possible to detect muscle fiber hypertrophy.

So what does cause the initial improvement in muscular strength? Several researchers have suggested that some kind of "motor learning" occurs whereby the individual "learns" how to produce greater functional strength. In fact, we now know that during this early strength training interval there are changes in coordination patterns that involve agonist and antagonist muscles, and that we seem to learn to increase the pattern of activity of the motor units responsible for the contraction. So at least the gains seen in the early part of the training period appear to be mediated by neural mechanisms, while muscle hypertrophy plays a greater role later on. In some Eastern European countries, the importance of increasing muscle size has been de-emphasized. However, we still have much to learn about neural coordination and about how elite power athletes can optimize motor unit firing patterns.

NEW TECHNIQUES TO IMPROVE MUSCULAR STRENGTH

Functional Electrical Stimulation

Functional electrical stimulation (FES) is hardly a new modality of therapeutic treatment. During the 18th century the electric discharges from torpedo fish were used for a variety of therapeutic purposes. In the sports medicine arena, FES has found a number of applications. Orthopaedic surgeons often use stimulators to promote bone growth. Portable TENS (transcutaneous electrical nerve stimulation) units have long been used for pain control. Although the use of functional electrical stimulation to increase muscular strength has received added attention during the last few years, the idea that muscular strength can be increased with protocols other than the "no pain, no gain" approach is still novel.

The question of whether electrical stimulation can produce greater gains in functional strength than those achieved with high-resistance exercise training alone is still the subject of dispute. The earlier studies, in particular, often noted greater success from exercise than from electrical stimulation. It now appears that stimulation can be successfully applied, but we have yet to determine the optimal parameters (stimulation waveform, frequency, duration, and so on). Some researchers have also reported success in using FES to promote more coordinated muscular activity during rapid, complex movements. FES will probably enjoy increasing use for therapeutic purposes such as pain relief and the prevention of muscular atrophy. The growing use of stimulation to increase muscular strength awaits further progress from the basic research laboratory.

Imposed Stretch Training

Stretching a muscle group while it is actively contracting results in the development of more force than can normally be exerted during a maximal muscle contraction. Some exercise machines are now available that use this eccentric mode of muscle contraction. One of the problems of eccentric exercise is that it produces greater muscle soreness than either concentric or isometric contractions. It is possible that some use of eccentric exercise training may produce greater gains in muscular strength, partly owing to the greater use of the overload principle. However, one might also speculate that greater activation may be necessary to train the nervous system to produce higher motor unit firing rates. Such a suggestion is clearly speculative, and awaits testing by motor unit researchers.

Postcontraction

The phenomenon of post-tetanic potentiation has long been recognized in studies of animal muscle. A brief tetanic stimulus given to a muscle results in the development of a greater force during a subsequent twitch contraction. This phenomenon can be applied to human studies and is often called "post-contraction." The post-contraction effect can be elicited by standing in a doorway, closing your eyes, and pressing your arms against the side of the doorway. When you step out of the doorway, your arms feel as if they want to float upward.

Using an isokinetic dynamometer, postcontraction can be used to effect brief increases in muscle strength. If one performs a maximal isometric contraction followed by an isokinetic contraction, the peak force obtained during the isokinetic contraction is often higher than it would be without the preceding maximal isometric contraction. Strength coaches may be able to devise more effective ways of utilizing the post-contraction phenomenon during functional activity.

WHAT LIES AHEAD FOR NEUROMUSCULAR PHYSIOLOGY?

The neurosciences comprise one of the largest and fastest growing areas of scientific investigation. There are many examples of applications from the basic research laboratory that have found their way into the sports medicine arena. These include (1) the application of functional electrical stimulation to promote bone growth, (2) the increased use of imaging for injury diagnosis, (3) changes in training programs, and (4) the use of proprioceptive neuromuscular facilitation techniques to enhance flexibility.

There are many new and exciting developments in basic neuroscience research laboratories that will have significance for sports medicine in future years. Are there genetically defined limits on the extent to which physical training can alter neuromuscular characteristics? If so, can we (or should we) use this information to counsel young athletes to perform activities appropriate for their individual profile? Can we use FES, nerve growth factor, and other types of therapy to treat spinal injuries? What role does biofeedback have in the acquisition of motor skill? Can we model the motor unit activity pattern and develop ways to train individuals to replicate the optimal pattern? What features of spinal reflexes are alterable and trainable? The answers to these and other questions await further research from both the basic and applied research laboratories.

SUGGESTED READING

Edstrom L, Grimby L. Effect of exercise on the motor unit. Muscle Nerve 1986; 9: 104–126.

Henatsch, H-D, Langer HH. Basic neurophysiology of motor skills in sport: a review. Int J Sports Med 1985; 6: 2–14.

Kamen G. Serial isometric contractions under imposed myotatic stretch conditions in high-strength and low-strength men. Eur J Appl Physiol 1979; 41: 73–82.

Kamen G. Neuromuscular adaptations to exercise. In: Seefeldt V, ed. Contributions of physical activity to human well-being, Reston, VA: AAHPERD Publications, 1986.

Kamen G, Taylor P, Beehler PJ. Ulnar and posterior tibial nerve conduction velocity in athletes. Int J Sports Med 1984; 5: 26–30.

Koceja DM, Kamen G. Conditioned patellar tendon reflexes in sprint and endurance-trained athletes. Med Sci Sports Exerc 1988; 20: 172–177.

Moritani T, DeVries HA. Neural factors versus hypertrophy in the time course of muscle strength gain. Am J Phys Med 1979; 58: 115–130.

Sale DG, MacDougall JD, Upton ARM, McComas AJ. Effect of strength training upon motoneuron excitability in man. Med Sci Sports Exerc 1983; 15: 57–62.

EXERCISE IN THE PRIMARY PREVENTION OF ISCHEMIC HEART DISEASE

STEVEN N. BLAIR, P.E.D.
NEIL F. GORDON, M.B., B.Ch., Ph.D.
JESUS VILLEGAS, M.D.

ISCHEMIC HEART DISEASE

Death rates for ischemic heart disease (IHD) declined in many countries, including the United States and Canada, over the past 20 years, but heart disease remains the leading cause of death in the industrialized world. The burden of this disease on the population is considerable, accounting for significant medical care costs, lost productivity, and much suffering. Treatment of IHD is only marginally effective, and for many persons the first symptom is sudden death. Thus, prevention of IHD must have a high priority.

Pathology

The primary cause of IHD is atherosclerosis in the coronary arteries. Much has been learned about the atherosclerotic process from such diverse medical subdisciplines as epidemiology, nutrition, physiology, pathology, molecular biology, and genetics. A detailed discussion of the atherosclerotic process is beyond the scope of this chapter, but recent reviews are readily available. In brief, atherosclerosis is initiated by injury to the arterial endothelium by trauma, infection, or metabolic factors. Recurrent injury results in further damage to endothelial integrity and smooth muscle cell proliferation. This is followed by an accumulation of lipids and other material resulting in growth of the atherosclerotic plaque and protrusion into the arterial lumen. The mature lesion incorporates additional fibrous material and inorganic compounds. The end result is an encroachment into the arterial lumen that may significantly impede or block blood flow. The impact of the atherosclerotic plaque may be increased further by arterial spasm or by pieces of plaque that break free and lodge in a narrowed artery downstream. When blood flow in the coronary arteries is reduced to a critical level, myocardial ischemia occurs and the clinical signs and symptoms of disease may become evident. Thus, angina pectoris, ischemic changes on the electrocardiogram (ECG), myocardial infarction, or sudden death are the final product of decades-long atherosclerotic disease progression.

Risk Factor Theory

Epidemiologic studies provided clues to the factors that initiate and promote atherosclerosis before the process itself was very well understood and described. Research over the past 40 or 50 years has refined the risk factor theory of atherosclerosis and integrated this knowledge with pathophysiologic findings. One of the major features of the risk factor theory is that atherosclerosis has many causes and must be considered a multifactorial disease. The risk factors interact with one another and may impact at various points in the atherosclerotic process. For example, cigarette smoking may be one of the factors causing the initial injury to the arterial endothelium; thus, smoking may have a role in initiation of the disease. In addition, nicotine causes arterial constriction, and carbon monoxide reduces the oxygen-carrying capacity of the blood. These effects of smoking worsen the clinical manifestations in persons with advanced atherosclerosis.

Epidemiologic, clinical, and experimental studies clearly implicate several major risk factors for IHD. Elevated levels of blood cholesterol (particularly low-density lipoprotein–cholesterol), hypertension, and cigarette smoking are well established as risk factors, and their role in the pathogenesis of atherosclerosis is generally well understood. The presence of one of these factors increases the risk of developing IHD two- or threefold. The relationships between these characteristics and the risk of disease are continuous and graded, and have been documented in many studies in diverse populations. The evidence for the causal role of these risk factors in atherosclerosis is substantial. Studies also show that combinations of risk factors are especially disadvantageous, the risk increasing exponentially with the addition of factors.

Physical Activity and Ischemic Heart Disease

Sedentary living as a risk factor for IHD was first examined scientifically in the 1950s, and several dozen studies since then have further examined the issue. Scientists and clinicians typically have viewed lack of physical activity as one of the minor risk factors for IHD. A recent comprehensive review by Powell and colleagues challenges that position. The authors reviewed 43 prospective studies on physical activity and IHD. As in previous reviews, about two-thirds of the studies showed a significant inverse relationship between habitual physical activity and IHD. An important contribution of the paper of Powell and colleagues was that they critically evaluated methods in each of the studies, categorizing the studies as good, satisfactory, or unsatisfactory. When only the good studies were considered, more than 80 percent showed a strong inverse association between habitual physical activity and IHD. This important result strengthens the inference that a sedentary lifestyle is a causal risk factor for IHD. These authors reported that the risk of developing IHD was approximately twice as great in sedentary as in active persons. This relative risk is of the same order of magnitude as for high cholesterol, hypertension, and cigarette smoking. Thus, it seems appropriate to begin considering lack of physical activity as a major, rather than minor, risk factor for IHD.

Prevalence of Sedentary Habits

Consideration of the public health impact of a risk factor for disease requires attention to the prevalence of the disease and its impact, the strength of the association between the risk factor and the disease, and the distribution of the risk factor in the population. The impact of IHD in the industrialized world is abundantly clear. It is certainly one of the major health problems today, and its impact on society is enormous. As briefly reviewed above, sedentary living is an important risk factor for IHD.

Physical activity is difficult to assess accurately, but several survey questionnaires have been developed and validated. Large-scale surveys of representative samples of North Americans have been undertaken over the past decade. These surveys used different assessment techniques, and it is difficult to know exactly how to categorize respondents as sedentary or active. Survey limitations notwithstanding, there is a general consensus that a large percentage of North Americans are less than optimally physically active. A reasonable estimate of the prevalence of sedentary individuals in the United States and Canada is approximately 40 to 50 percent. In the United States, this totals approximately 80 million adults. Thus, the public health impact of sedentary living is considerable. If we consider the prevalence of sedentary persons in the United States to be 45 percent and set the relative risk of IHD mortality at 2.0, we can estimate the percentage of deaths from IHD attributable to sedentary habits. In this example, the estimate is that 32 percent of IHD deaths are due to sedentary habits. For comparison, if 25 percent of adults smoke cigarettes and if the risk of IHD mortality in smokers is 2.5 compared with non-smokers, 27 percent of all IHD deaths can be attributed to smoking. If 15 percent of a population are hypertensive and the relative risk of IHD mortality is 2.0 in hypertensives, 17 percent of IHD deaths are due to hypertension. These examples show that there is considerable potential for saving lives by getting patients to exercise regularly. In fact, a physician might prevent as many deaths by encouraging sedentary patients to become more active as if the time were spent on other interventions or treatments.

PHYSICIANS AND EXERCISE PROMOTION

One of the important interventions a physician can make to help prevent IHD is to encourage regular physical activity. Advice is given below on the specific actions physicians can take to promote more activity in their patients. These recommendations have been used successfully, but as with all medical interventions, exercise counseling is not effective for every patient. Physicians who persist and encourage activity in their patients will see progressively more of their patients adopt a physically active lifestyle.

Exercise History

One of the objectives proposed by the Surgeon General of the United States was that by the year 1990 more than 50 percent of primary care physicians should include a careful exercise history as part of their initial examination of new patients. A physician who does so is demonstrating to the patient the importance of exercise in disease prevention and health promotion. Furthermore, the history provides the physician with information that can be used in counseling patients about how to increase their activity levels. The exercise history can be a series of relatively simple questions asked by the physician, as illustrated in Table 1. A more detailed self-report of exercise habits (Table 2) can be completed by the patient, with review and follow-up questions by the physician in the counseling session.

Medical Evaluation

Exercise is a normal human function that can be undertaken with an extremely high level of safety by most adults. There are, however, certain conditions that constitute either an absolute or a relative

TABLE 1 Clinical Exercise History Questions

1. Do you think that exercise is an important health habit? Why?
2. How much exercise do you think you need?
3. For the past 3 months, have you regularly participated in an exercise program for the purpose of improving your health and physical fitness? If no, continue with question 4. If yes, skip to question 6.
4. When was the last time you exercised regularly?
5. What kind of exercise program would possibly interest you to increase your physical activity?
6. What has been the pattern of exercise throughout your life? How much did you do? What type of exercise did you do?
7. What type of activities do you do in your current exercise program?
8. How strenuous is your exercise work-out? (May get a subjective rating, heart rate data, distances, and times for walk/jog/run participants).
9. How long is your average exercise session?
10. How many days a week do you exercise?

(Republished with permission from Blair SN, Oberman A. Epidemiologic analysis of coronary heart disease and exercise. Cardiol Clin 1987; 5: 271–283.)

TABLE 2 Detailed Exercise Participation Questions for Medical History Questionnaire

1. Are you currently involved in a routine of regular exercise (moderate continuous exertion of at least 15–20 minutes' duration at least 3 days a week?) ____ Yes ____ No
2. How long have you been exercising regularly?
   ____ Years ____ Months ____ Weeks
3. For the last 3 months, which of the following activities have you performed regularly? (Please check YES for all that apply and NO if you do not perform the activity; provide an estimate of the amount of activity for all marked YES. Please be as complete as possible.)

Walking ____ Yes ____ No	How many work-outs per week? ____ How many kilometers (or fractions) per work-out? ____ Average duration of work-out? ____ (min) Average time per km? ____
Jogging or running (outdoors or on track) ____ Yes ____ No	How many work-outs per week? ____ How many kilometers per work-out? ____ Average duration of work-out? ____ (min) Average time per km? ____
Treadmill (walking or running) ____ Yes ____ No	How many work-outs per week? ____ Average duration of work-out? ____ (min) Speed? ____ Grade? ____ % Heart rate? ____
Bicycling (outdoors) ____ Yes ____ No	How many work-outs per week? ____ How many kilometers per work-out? ____ Average duration of work-out? ____ (min) Average time per km? ____
Stationary cycling ____ Yes ____ No	Type of stationary cycle? ____ How many work-outs per week? ____ Average duration of work-out? ____ (min) Heart rate during exercise? ____
Swimming laps ____ Yes ____ No	How many work-outs per week? ____ How many kilometers per work-out? ____ (880 yards = 0.5 miles = 0.8 km) Average duration of work-out? ____ (min) How many months per year? ____
Aerobics dance or floor exercises ____ Yes ____ No	How many work-outs per week? ____ Average duration of work-out? ____ (min) Heart rate during exercise? ____
Vigorous racquet sports (e.g., racquetball, singles tennis) ____ Yes ____ No	How many work-outs per week? ____ Average duration of work-out? ____ (min)

TABLE 2 (continued)

Other vigorous sports or exercise (e.g., basketball or soccer)
Please specify: How many work-outs per week? ____
____ Yes
____ No

4. How do you rate the physical activity that you are now getting compared with that of others of your same age and sex? Think about both your leisure and work activities. (Please check your response.)
____ A. Extremely inactive
____ B. Inactive
____ C. Somewhat inactive
____ D. About average
____ E. Somewhat active
____ F. Active
____ G. Extremely active

5. Compared with a year ago, how much regular exercise do you currently get?
____ A. Much less
____ B. Somewhat less
____ C. About the same
____ D. Somewhat more
____ E. Much more

6. Have you continuously followed your program?
____ Yes
____ No

Approximately how many times have you stopped for at least 6 months? ____

What is the longest period that you were continuously active? ____

What is the longest period that you were not on any program? ____

Since you started an exercise program, how many total years have you been regularly active? ____

7. What exercise equipment, if any, do you own? (Check those that apply.)
____ Running shoes
____ Stationary cycle
____ Bicycle
____ Rowing machine
____ Cross country ski simulator
____ Treadmill
____ Other (specify) ____________

8. To what exercise facilities do you have easy access? (Check those that apply.)
____ Fitness club
____ Bicycle path
____ Swimming lap pool
____ Jogging path
____ Aerobic exercise class
____ Suitable area for walking

9. If you are not exercising regularly, what exercise activities might be of most interest to you? (List in order of decreasing preference.)
A. ____________ C. ____________
B. ____________ D. ____________

10. Are you currently involved in a muscle-strengthening program? ____ Yes ____ No (go on to question 11)

If yes, what type? (Check those that apply.)
____ Calisthenics
____ Free weights
____ Weight training machines
____ Other: (Specify) ____________

How many days per week do you do these exercises? ____
Average duration of work-out? ____ (min)
How long have you been involved in this routine? ____

11. Are you currently involved in exercises to maintain or improve your joint flexibility? ____ Yes ____ No (go on to question 12)

If yes, what type?
____ Stretching
____ Calisthenics
____ Exercise class

How many days per week? ____
Average duration of exercise? ____
How long have you been involved in this routine? ____

12. Exercise Safety

Do you warm up before exercise?	____ Yes	____ No
Do you cool down slowly after exercise?	____ Yes	____ No
Do you know how to take your pulse?	____ Yes	____ No
Do you monitor your heart rate when exercising?	____ Yes	____ No
If you bicycle, do you wear a protective helmet?	____ Yes	____ No
If you exercise outdoors at night, do you use reflective gear or light?	____ Yes	____ No

contraindication to exercise, and others that require special consideration. Physicians who counsel patients on exercise should be familiar with these conditions and should attempt to identify them at the time of the medical evaluation. This can be adequately accomplished by means of an appropriate medical history (Table 3), physical examination (Table 4), blood lipid analysis, and, where indicated, a graded exercise test. Because advanced coronary atherosclerosis is the principal cause of sudden death during exercise, the medical evaluation should focus primarily on the cardiovascular system. In certain instances, additional laboratory tests may be required to clarify a patient's clinical status before permitting exercise training.

Maximal graded exercise testing with electrocardiographic (ECG) monitoring is now widely used for the purpose of exercise prescription. Baseline graded exercise testing is often of immense value, in that it may help to detect previously undiagnosed IHD or other diseases of the cardiovascular system; to establish safe levels of exertion for patients with known cardiovascular disease; to evaluate hemodynamic responses to exercise; to determine maximal exercise capacity; and to motivate patients to adopt a physically more active lifestyle. Follow-up graded exercise testing may be of equal importance. It serves to detect changes in clinical status, exercise capacity, and exercise hemodynamics. However, it must be realized that the indiscriminate use of graded exercise testing by physicians for the purpose of exercise prescription does have drawbacks. In particular, unacceptably high rates of false-positive tests are likely to be found in patient populations with low IHD rates. In view of this, and because the risk of exercise-induced cardiac complications is very small, we do not recommend that physicians perform exercise tests on all their adult patients before prescribing exercise for them.

At the Aerobics Center in Dallas, we perform graded exercise testing before exercise training in individuals aged 40 years or older, individuals aged 35 years or older with one or more major IHD risk factors, and (irrespective of their age) those with known or suspected cardiopulmonary or metabolic disease. Repeat exercise tests are conducted at least every 3 years in apparently healthy individuals who are 40 years or older, every 2 years in individuals who are 35 years or older with one or more major IHD risk factors, and in those with symptoms suggestive of cardiopulmonary or metabolic disease, and every year in individuals with known cardiopulmonary or metabolic disease or a previously positive exercise test. To reduce the incidence of false-positive exercise tests, we recommend that physicians consider multiple ECG and non-ECG responses to exercise testing rather than simply the presence or absence of ST-segment abnormalities when interpreting the results of such tests. Important exercise responses that should be taken into consideration include maximal exercise duration, systolic and diastolic blood pressure responses at

TABLE 3 Major Components of the Medical History*

Individuals should be questioned about a history of the following:
Heart attack, coronary bypass, or other cardiac surgery
Chest discomfort—especially with exertion
High blood pressure
Extra, skipped, or rapid heart beats or palpitations
Heart murmurs, clicks, or unusual cardiac findings
Rheumatic fever
Ankle swelling
Peripheral vascular disease
Phlebitis, emboli
Unusual shortness of breath
Lightheadedness or fainting
Pulmonary disease including asthma, emphysema, and bronchitis
Abnormal blood lipids
Diabetes
Stroke
Emotional disorders
Medications of all types
Recent illness, hospitalization, or surgical procedure
Drug allergies
Orthopaedic problems, arthritis
Family history should be explored for the following:
- Coronary disease—at what age
- Sudden death—at what age
- Congenital heart disease

Other habits
- Caffeine including cola drinks
- Alcohol
- Tobacco
- Other unusual habits or dieting
- Exercise history with information on habitual level of activity: type of exercise, frequency, duration, and intensity

* Republished with permission from American College of Sports Medicine. Guidelines for exercise testing and prescription. Philadelphia: Lea & Febiger, 1986.

TABLE 4 Major Components of the Physical Examination*

The physical examination should specifically assess:
1. Weight/body composition
2. Orthopaedic problems including arthritis
3. Presence of any acute illness
4. Most significant noncardiac problems that might influence exercise testing and prescription will be identified through the medical history. Areas of possible concern revealed by the history should be evaluated in the physical examination.
5. Cardiovascular evaluation:
   a. Pulse rate and regularity
   b. Blood pressure: supine, sitting, and standing
   c. Auscultation of the lungs with specific attention to:
      i. rales, wheezes, and rhonchi
      ii. uniformity of breath sounds in all areas
   d. Palpation for carotid, femoral, and pedal pulses and for cardiac impulse and thrills
   e. Auscultation of the heart with specific attention to murmurs, gallops, clicks, and rubs
   f. Carotid, abdominal, or femoral bruits
   g. Edema
   h. Xanthoma and xanthelasma

* Republished with permission from American College of Sports Medicine. Guidelines for exercise testing and prescription. Philadelphia: Lea & Febiger, 1986.

submaximal and maximal exercise, the peak heart rate achieved, the development and characterization of arrhythmias, the time of onset and duration of ST-segment changes, the magnitude and character of ST-segment changes, and the development and nature of clinical symptoms. When the probability of IHD is low (in healthy young athletes, for example), ST-segment changes are not likely to indicate disease. Thus, a false-positive test should be suspected. Additional recommendations for test interpretation are given by the American College of Sports Medicine.

Exercise Prescription

A great deal is now known about the physiologic adaptations that result from exercise conditioning. The exercise stimuli needed to evoke improvements in maximal oxygen uptake, the most widely accepted index of cardiorespiratory fitness, have been well documented. On the basis of existing research, the American College of Sports Medicine has formulated guidelines for the quality and quantity of exercise required to promote and maintain cardiorespiratory fitness. Briefly, they recommend that aerobic exercise be performed at an intensity corresponding to 65 to 90 percent of maximal heart rate, or 50 to 85 percent of maximal oxygen intake, for 15 to 60 minutes on 3 to 5 days each week. Because cardiorespiratory fitness and health are frequently considered synonymous, these guidelines are often extrapolated to the prescription of exercise for the purpose of disease prevention. In reality, changes in clinical health status do not necessarily parallel increases in maximal oxygen intake, and the precise exercise stimuli needed to produce health-related benefits currently are not well defined.

Recent epidemiologic studies strongly suggest that moderate levels of leisure time physical activity may be sufficient for reducing IHD mortality rates. These studies demonstrate that frequent participation in light to moderate intensity activities, which are unlikely to have a profound impact on maximal oxygen intake, is beneficial for IHD prevention and that more vigorous exercise in fact may not offer substantially greater protection. Unlike improvements in maximal oxygen intake (which are closely coupled to the intensity of exercise training), it appears that the effectiveness of exercise in the prevention of IHD may be primarily dependent on total energy expenditure. Thus, activities performed for an appropriate duration, but at an intensity below the threshold needed to elicit a significant cardiorespiratory training effect, may be beneficial for IHD prevention. Such activities are of particular relevance for counseling individuals who currently lead a totally sedentary lifestyle and may not be ready to make the major transition needed to comply with a formal exercise training program. Rather than encouraging them to participate in aggressive exercise conditioning, physicians should probably simply counsel these patients about activities, such as brisk walking, gardening, and yard work, which can be engineered into their lifestyle with relative ease. Once the sedentary individual has become accustomed to an active lifestyle, a more formal approach to exercise prescription may be adopted.

Although much research is still required to clarify the situation, it appears from the above mentioned epidemiologic studies that a threshold level of energy expenditure during leisure-time or job-related exercise must be exceeded to reduce IHD risk. Available data suggest that the reduction in risk commences at an energy expenditure of about 4,000 kilojoules (approximately 1,000 kcal) per week and the risk subsequently declines as energy expenditure increases up to about 12 MJ (3,000 kcal) per week. Therefore, when prescribing exercise for their patients, physicians should modulate the precise frequency, intensity, and duration of the activity in question to elicit a weekly energy expenditure of more than 4,000 kilojoules. Activities that can be performed for prolonged periods, use large muscle groups, and are rhythmical and aerobic in nature are recommended because they constitute the most effective means of attaining the desired level of energy expenditure. In healthy adults, such activities (which probably are best epitomized by a brisk walk) need to be performed on at least 3 to 4 days each week for a minimum of about 30 minutes. If the patient expresses a desire to increase habitual physical activity further, the exercise prescription should be gradually altered to conform more closely with the recommendations of the American College of Sports Medicine. Such an approach will enable the patient to derive many of the other benefits of exercise training, in addition to reducing the risk for IHD.

Finally, when counseling patients about exercise participation, physicians should educate them about the factors necessary for safe exercise. These include, but are not limited to, the warning symptoms and signs of cardiac complications; the importance of an adequate warm-up and cool-down; the dangers of adverse environmental conditions, inadequate fluid replacement, and exercising while suffering or recuperating from an acute viral illness; and the need to begin and proceed gradually with exercise training.

SUGGESTED READING

American College of Sports Medicine. Guidelines for exercise testing and prescription. Philadelphia: Lea & Febiger, 1986.

Caspersen CJ, Christenson GM, Pollard RA. Status of the 1990 physical fitness and exercise objectives—evidence from NHIS 1985. Pub Health Rep 1986; 101: 587–592.

Caspersen CJ, Heath GW. The risk factor concept of coronary heart disease. In: Blair SN, Painter P, Pate RR, Smith LK, Taylor CB, eds. Resource manual for guidelines for exercise

testing and prescription. Philadelphia: Lea & Febiger, 1988:111.
Department of Health and Human Services. Promoting health/ preventing disease: objectives for the nation. Washington, DC: US Government Printing Office, 1980.
Leon AS, Connett J, Jacobs DR Jr, Rauramaa R. Leisure-time physical activity levels and risk of coronary heart disease and death. JAMA 1987; 258:2388–2395.
Morris JA, Heady JA, Raffle PAB, et al. Coronary heart disease and physical activity of work. Lancet 1953; 2:1053–1057.
Paffenbarger RS Jr, Wing AL, Hyde RT. Physical activity as an index of heart attack risk in college alumni. Am J Epidemiol 1978; 108:161–175.
Powell KE, Thompson PD, Caspersen CJ, Kendrick JS. Physical activity and the incidence of coronary heart disease. Annu Rev Public Health 1987; 8:253–287.
Ross R. The pathogenesis of atherosclerosis—an update. N Engl J Med 1986; 314:488–500.
Stephens T. Secular trends in adult physical activity: fitness boom or bust? Res Q Exercise Sport 1987; 58:94–105.
Superko HR. The atherosclerotic process. In: Blair SN, Painter P, Pate RR, Smith LK, Taylor CB, eds. Resource manual for guidelines for exercise testing and prescription. Philadelphia: Lea & Febiger, 1988:101.
Thompson PD. The safety of exercise testing and participation. In: Blair SN, Painter P, Pate RR, Smith LK, Taylor CB, eds. Resource manual for exercise testing and prescription. Philadelphia: Lea & Febiger, 1988:273.

EXERCISE PRESCRIPTION FOR HEART DISEASE

ELIEZER KAMON, Ph.D.

The question whether exercise is "good for you" is no longer debated. The facts are that in people who exercise regularly the resting heart rate goes down, the glycogen level decreases, and the satiety problem takes care of itself, since they feel less hungry. According to Blackburn, selected patients who have had myocardial infarctions can attain improved work performance and greater endurance on the treadmill. This chapter does not deal with these aspects, but with people who need to exercise for the self-esteem it provides. Although some people must be encouraged to exercise, the final result is well worth the persuasive effort involved. Patients with heart problems form one such group. Of course, there are other patients with different problems and different situations who can also profitably follow the program for people with heart disease, including those who have diabetes or suffer from obesity. People with heart disease, however, serve as a model for appropriate procedures. It is a simple matter to adjust this program for other special populations.

CORONARY HEART DISEASE

This chapter focuses on the exercise prescription for patients recovering from myocardial infarction, cardiac arrest, angina pectoris, left ventricular dysfunction, and similar conditions. We must follow the patient from the time of entering a hospital bed until months later when she or he is ready to return to work. A patient may suddenly obey advice to exercise because of concern about hospitalization for an unhealthy heart. Now, at least, there is a willingness to hear what the physician has to say. The patient will listen to us and we can start the exercise program. This is a long process; many do not continue with the program. Initially, however, the patient usually complies and wants to exercise.

The paramedical exercise specialist does not take charge of the patient with myocardial infarction or a coronary artery bypass graft when the latter is in a hospital bed. Patients usually stay in the hospital 5 to 9 days and have a light daily exercise routine supervised by hospital staff. Only when they leave the hospital and start to exercise from their homes or a gym are the family physician and the exercise specialist responsible for them.

PRESCRIBED EXERCISE

The Wisconsin Heart Association Program is a convenient model program that is divided into three phases of exercise. Phase I is when the patient is in bed, usually a day after entering hospital, whether or not there has been a cardiac operation. The doctor and the patient both know there is a heart problem. The patient is usually confined to bed for 2 to 5 days. In general, the heart problem will be described as coronary artery disease (CAD), but treatment is varied according to the specific problem.

The program is detailed in Table 1. Particular parts need emphasis. First, the patient must pay attention to the exercise heart rate. The immediate task is to learn how to measure it, either by palpating the wrist or by palpating the neck. It is a very easy technique to learn. The beats are counted for 10 seconds and then multiplied by six to approximate the count per minute.

As a patient first starts to walk or to undertake some other prescribed exercise, the heart rate is palpated at some point during exercise. For someone in phase I who is walking 15 to 20 m (50 ft), the heart rate should be about 80 beats per minute (bpm). If there is no untoward response to a given level of effort, the intensity of exercise is progressively increased. The heart rate is monitored regularly. For example, if the patient is operating a cycle ergometer at a loading of 50 watts (300 kg per minute),

TABLE 1 Prescription of Exercise in Heart Disease

Event	*Phase*	*Calisthenics and Walk-Run*	*Frequency*	*Duration*
1–2 days after surgery or acute episode	I	Start walking 15–20 m (50 ft) from bed, increasing to 150–200 m (500 ft). Lie and move legs and hands.	3 times a day	10–20 min
Going home until 3 mo after hospitalization	II	Warm-up 5 min. Calisthenics: arms, trunk, abdomen. Sit and exercise, walk or jog, lift weights. Cool down.	3–5 times a wk at 60–70% of max*	Start with 20-min bouts, increase to 60-min bouts by end of 3 mo
3 mo and later	III	Bike, jog, or swim. Do calisthenics.	3–5 times a wk, starting at 80% max	60-min bouts with warm-up and cool-down

* Max = maximal consumption of oxygen. For the healthy 60-year-old male, max is about 2.0 L/min, but immediately after hospitalization it may be 1.5 L/min or less.

the heart rate should be about 100 bpm, 30 bpm above resting heart rate. This heart rate is appropriate for a patient who is at the end of phase II and is about to start phase III.

Second, the patient must perform calisthenics on a regular basis. These are done as a warm-up for 5 to 10 minutes prior to endurance exercise in phase II and phase III. The exercises to strengthen the back are very important.

EXAMPLES OF CALISTHENIC EXERCISES

The patient should raise the arms sideways while standing erect. The arms should then be moved backward and the patient should next bend forward and downward as much as possible. After the patient stands erect again, the cycle is repeated for a total of about five times.

Bending to the side is also important. The exercise begins while the patient stands erect, with hands on the waist; the patient bends from side to side and performs trunk rotations.

The patient should also sit down on the floor with the legs extended forward and bend slowly forward until the toes are touched.

In another possible exercise, the patient spreads the legs while sitting on the floor, and bends forward over the right leg; after straightening, the trunk is bent over the left leg. Each position is held for about 5 seconds, and the entire maneuver is repeated five to six times.

The patient can also lie on the back and raise the feet about six times. In this way, responsibility is taken for the abdominal muscles. Of course, the exercise may be repeated a greater number of times if desired.

These exercises provide a minimal calisthenic warm-up, but there are many more that can be performed. Several of the books listed as suggested reading are full of possible exercises.

MYOCARDIAL INFARCTION PROGRAM

Paramedical instructors at The Pennsylvania State University deal with only phases II and III following myocardial infarction. The patient should start with a little fast walking or running with others, maybe one or two laps around the gym or field as the initial part of the warm-up. The pulse rate, taken once during this activity and also afterward, should be between 120 and 150 bpm. Then, with the instructor and others, the patient should perform supervised group calisthenics. After the bout of calisthenics, the pulse rate should be around 100 bpm. Particular importance should be attached to developing muscle strength, from arms to abdomen, back, and legs. Next, the group of patients should play some active game such as kicking a ball along the gym, softball, or volleyball. This part of the program should take 30 to 40 minutes in addition to the 10 minutes of warm-up. The patient should then be allowed a 5-minute cool-down, slow walking in the gym or in the field.

As patients become more fit they should be encouraged to run more. They often desire to increase the exercise intensity somewhat anyway. In general, they start at a speed of about 1.6 km (1.0 mile) per hour and after a few months they can move at a speed of over 3.2 km (2.0 miles) per hour, depending on their condition. In order to perform calisthenics with the group, patients should begin running earlier. Eventually, they should learn to do everything by themselves or at most with one or two members of the group. This is very important, because our goal is to make them independent.

OTHER MEANS OF EXERCISE

Cycling Exercise

Some people may decide to select an alternative mode of exercise, such as cycling instead of fast walking or running. Cycling can take two forms: rolling or stationary. The stationary cycle ergometer uses a mechanical brake, a weighted belt running around the rim of the flywheel. In some designs, an electrical resistance is produced and is altered electronically to adjust for changes of pedaling speed. Many people in the United States now have some kind of stationary bicycle at home.

Schwinn Air-Dyne have designed a machine that exercises both the arms and the legs. It is air braked, the arm levers and foot pedals being connected to an air-resistant flywheel.

Usually as a warm-up, patients start to pedal without resistance for about 5 to 10 minutes. Next they move on to calisthenics, followed by cycling with resistance for 30 to 40 minutes. Finally, there is a cool-down of 5 minutes, the patient sitting on the ergometer and slowly turning the unloaded pedals.

At the beginning of resistance cycling, the work rate should be 25 to 50 watts (150 to 300 kg per minute), adjusted according to the heart rate. In fact it is best to start, at the most, 20 beats above the resting heart rate, corresponding to a work rate of around 25 watts.

When the patient begins phase III, the recommended setting is about one-third of maximal aerobic effort, around 50 watts or 300 kg per minute. After that, the patient progresses to 70 to 80 percent of max, corresponding to a heart rate of about 130 bpm for a 60-year-old person. Table 2 shows the recommended energy expenditure and heart rate for the various phases of the exercise program.

At any given oxygen consumption, cycling is a little harder than walking or running, but it is great in wintertime. So if the patient can do it, it should be encouraged.

Roller bicycling is a great deal of fun. Of course one must warm up on level ground. After 5 minutes of warm-up, one can start cycling up and down hill. However, after a heart attack it usually takes a lot of time before a patient is ready to start such a program.

Swimming Program

Another exercise that can be used in place of running is swimming. The water needs to be warm. For heart patients, a water temperature of 27° to 29°C (80° to 84°F) is recommended. The patient must also enter the water gradually. In our pool, we have a wooden incline that allows patients to walk down gradually into the water.

The best start is usually the breast stroke, although some patients suffer from back pain; in such instances, we suggest they warm up with the side stroke for about 5 minutes. The patient then checks the heart rate, and if it is no more than 90 bpm, swimming is begun for up to 20 minutes. Of course, in the early stages of the program, the patient often swims for less than 20 minutes, because it is difficult for an inexperienced person to swim for even 5 minutes continuously. But with time, this can be increased to 20 minutes. Finally, there is a cool-down phase in the water for about 5 minutes.

The literature contains some references to swimming programs for patients who have had myocardial infarction, angina, and coronary artery bypass graft surgery. Swimming demands less oxygen than the treadmill for equal heart rates, but this is not of concern to those prescribing exercise, because it is the heart rate that is important and must be checked. As long as cardiovascular fitness is being stimulated, the exercise is good and intense enough.

INTENSITY OF EXERCISE

When a patient is lying in a hospital bed he begins the exercise program with foot motion in order to restore self-confidence. After a day or so, walking is begun. From then on, the exercise is increased gradually, and again the patient is reassured that she or he will be all right. Development of confidence may take time, because we are trying to build some attitudes that may always have been lacking.

We should remember that exercise is a positive action. We are asking the patient to do something we think will be good for health. But the question remains, what happens in the long run? Does the patient continue the exercise program or become a drop-out? Unfortunately, as many as 50 percent of patients drop out within a year. The drop-out rate for females is supposedly larger than for males, although one study showed no sex difference.

DISCUSSION

It is interesting that exercise programs today are not reducing morbidity or improving mortality rates in cardiac patients, although there is possibly an increase in productivity. However, most patients feel much better after exercise. What creates this feeling of well-being in most, but not all, people?

TABLE 2 Apparatus, Recommended Work Rate, and Heart Rate for the Patient

*Treadmill (METs)**	*Cycling (w/kg/min)*	*Phase*	*Day in Hospital or at Home*	*Heart Rate (bpm)*
1.5–2	Not used	I	2 (or 6 in severe condition)	70 (rest) to 80
2 –3	25/150		Discharged from hospital	Up to 95–100
3 –4	50/300	II	At home	Up to 110
5 –6	100/600	II	With group	Up to 130
6 –?	>100/600	III	Advanced program	Up to 155 (seldom more)

* The MET is the ratio to resting energy consumption that is spent during this activity. One MET is equivalent to an oxygen consumption of 3.5 $ml \cdot kg \cdot min^{-1}$.

The exerciser feels better and wants to run at least every other day. Work capacity and the attitude to work also improve. The patient feels much better at work. Exercise improves cardiovascular efficiency, coronary blood flow, and myocardial oxygen consumption. Following a period of supervised training, postmyocardial infarction patients show an improved treadmill performance, in addition to a reduction in blood pressure–heart rate product at a fixed work rate.

One thing is noticeable: those people who persist with exercise programs are the self-employed and those who have freedom in what they produce. An assembly-line worker who does nothing more than turn a wheel does not generally want to exercise. Those who have no motivation to work equally have no motivation to exercise. This makes it important to motivate the whole group, so that they will at least discuss their exercising rather than just mention it in passing. Sometimes we can persuade them, for example, to describe their gym and be enthusiastic about their exercise program.

Patients are thus asked to report on the efficiency and effectiveness of their exercise program. Unfortunately, the problem remains that those who do not exercise do not report, and it is very difficult even to maintain contact with them. We do not have enough data on those who do not exercise, and more research and follow-up is needed for individuals who do not continue with their program.

How can we increase sports participation? One study found that it was helpful if the class leader was responsible to the program. Participants should also have social support from friends and family. Family encouragement and the attention of the leader may encourage more regular participation, increasing class numbers. Nonetheless, the only groups that show increased participation are those with a strong leader and family encouragement.

To summarize, I would like to quote the opinion of Karl Stoedefalke. He describes an appropriate exercise as enjoyable, individual, educational, relaxing and recreative, controlled, isotonic and innovative, safe, and energetic. The primary problem is that of motivation. Stoedefalke believes that the leader should be held responsible for the regularity of participation. Self-determination and freedom of choice are also important aspects of a program. A clean and aesthetically attractive area is also essential. The prescribed exercise must give pleasure without pain or discomfort, and most important must offer fun.

The drop-out rate in Dr. Stoedefalke's program at Penn State is almost zero, but of course Penn State is a university, and universities generally contain type A characters who are more persistent in achieving goals, whether at work or in an exercise program.

SUGGESTED READING

American Heart Association/Wisconsin Affiliate. Recommendations for insurance coverage of supervised cardiac exercise rehabilitation programs. Milwaukee: American Heart Association/Wisconsin Affiliate, 1980.

Blackburn H. Physical activity and coronary heart disease: a brief update and population view (Part I). J Cardiac Rehab 1983; 3:101–111.

Howley ET, Franks DB. Health/fitness instructor's handbook. Champaign, IL: Human Kinetics Publishers, 1986.

Oldridge NB. Efficacy and effectiveness: critical issues in exercise and compliance. J Cardiac Rehab 1984; 4:119.

Pollock ML, Wilmore JH, Fox SM. Exercise in health and disease. Evaluation and prescription for prevention and rehabilitation. Philadelphia: WB Saunders, 1984.

Skinner JS. Exercise testing and exercise prescription for special cases. Theoretical basis and clinical application. Philadelphia: Lea & Febiger, 1987.

Stoedefalke KG. Motivating and sustaining the older adult in an exercise program. TGR 1985; 1:78–83.

Thompson DL, Boone TW, Miller HS Jr. Comparison of treadmill exercise and tethered swimming to determine validity of exercise prescription. J Cardiac Rehab 1982; 2:363–372.

Wankel LM. Decision-making and social-support strategies for increasing exercise involvement. J Cardiac Rehab 1984; 4:124–135.

Ward A, Morgan WP. Adherence patterns of healthy men and women enrolled in an adult exercise program. J Cardiac Rehab 1984; 4:143–152.

EXERCISE AND MUSCLE SORENESS

PETER M. TIIDUS, M.Sc.

The sensation of delayed-onset muscle soreness (DOMS) that results from muscular overuse is an almost universal experience. Anyone involved in exercise, athletics, heavy manual labor, or other forms of occasional muscular overexertion has at times experienced the temporary stiffness and tenderness associated with DOMS. Despite the ubiquitous nature of this experience, the underlying causes of DOMS are not yet fully understood. In 1951 the noted muscle physiologist A. V. Hill wrote, "I know of nothing which prevents muscular soreness, except previous training, nor anything that quickens its disappearance; when others have asked me, I have often been forced with shame to confess ignorance."

Almost four decades have passed since Dr. Hill penned the above confession. However, despite significant advances in our understanding of exercise-induced muscle pain and damage, the fundamental causes and means of prevention of DOMS remain almost as elusive as they were then.

This article offers a review of our current understanding of the etiology of DOMS and a discussion of various therapeutic attempts at attenuating its severity, time course, and onset. Although DOMS usually is not sufficiently debilitating to warrant significant medical intervention, an appreciation of its physiology can assist the medical profession in understanding other forms of more chronic or severe muscle pain and their more debilitating effects.

SORENESS SENSATION

DOMS usually appears after unaccustomed or severe exercise, particularly if it involves eccentric muscular contractions such as downhill running. Armstrong described the following typical time course for DOMS sensation. A postexercise pain-free period of 5 to 8 hours is followed by a gradual increase in discomfort sensation, reaching maximal intensity 1 to 3 days after exercise (usually 2 days). The pain then gradually subsides until it disappears completely within 5 to 6 days after exercise.

The DOMS sensation has generally been characterized as one of "stiff" or "tender" muscles. These sensations, although they cause considerable discomfort, are usually not severe enough to be considered debilitating (nonetheless, in some cases further exercise can be difficult). As noted above, the sensations usually disappear within several days of onset and do not appear to be accompanied by any lasting damage.

Unmyelinated group IV afferent neurons (those nerve fibers associated with diffuse muscle pain) are the most probable transmitters of the DOMS sensation. While the exact muscular location of the DOMS sensation varies, depending on the muscle involved and the type of exercise performed, many DOMS sufferers report that the greatest pain sensations occur near myotendinous junctions. Some researchers have attributed this localization of DOMS sensation to associated tendon trauma. However, the concentration of unmyelinated group IV afferents near myotendinous junctions suggests that the location of the DOMS sensations may be due as much to afferent localization as to any particular area of trauma.

EFFECT OF DOMS ON MUSCLE FUNCTION

During the DOMS time course, the range of movement about the joint that is flexed or extended by the affected muscles is usually noticeably reduced. Temporary losses in muscle strength and power also coincide with DOMS sensation. Strength loss may persist for several weeks, even after the sensation of pain has disappeared.

Neither of the limitations of muscular function are necessarily caused directly by the DOMS sensation itself; they may be attributable to other physiologic changes associated with exercise-induced muscle trauma, such as edema or disruption of the sarcomere. This issue is discussed in greater detail in the section dealing with causes of DOMS.

CLINICAL MEASURES

Elevations in a number of clinical indices have been reported to occur coincident with DOMS, although not necessarily following a similar time course. These indices include serum enzyme activities of creatine kinase (CK) and lactate dehydrogenase (LDH), as well as their more muscle-specific isozymes. Serum and urinary hydroxyproline concentrations may also be elevated. Hemoglobinuria and myoglobinuria have also been reported coincident with DOMS.

Changes in other less traditional indices that occur coincidentally with DOMS have been recently described. Using 31P nuclear magnetic resonance measures (NMR), McCully and associates reported elevated inorganic phosphate-to-phosphocreatine ratios that persisted for up to 7 days in the muscles of patients experiencing exercise-induced DOMS.

Newham and colleagues demonstrated an enhanced 99m-technetium pyrophosphate (Tc-PYP) uptake by some muscles in patients experiencing exercise-induced DOMS. In addition, Friden and associates noted microscopic evidence of sarcomere and Z-line disruptions in biopsies obtained from sore muscles.

Since all the above changes can occur in muscular conditions that do not induce DOMS sensation, their value in the clinical confirmation of DOMS is questionable. Their relationship to the causes of DOMS is discussed later in this article.

Extreme forms of DOMS that result from very severe unaccustomed exercise have been clinically characterized as an exertional rhabdomyolysis. In addition to the normal characteristics of DOMS (tender and stiff muscles, elevated serum CK levels, and so on), patients exhibit several more severe symptoms. These include nausea, hypocalcemia, and hypoalbuminemia, as well as a hemoglobinuria and a myoglobinuria that may sometimes progress to renal failure.

Another form of exercise-induced muscle pain is known as the compartment syndrome. Unlike DOMS, its onset occurs during exercise and it may be severe enough to force the patient to stop exercising. It is generally believed to be caused by abnormally elevated intramuscular pressures, exacerbated by a lack of distensibility of the surrounding fascia. Since the formation of edema and elevated intramuscular pressures have also been associated with the development of DOMS, the compartment syndrome is likely an extreme version of DOMS that occurs in certain susceptible individuals.

ETIOLOGY

In 1902 Hough suggested that muscle soreness was caused by some form of microtearing or structural damage to the tissue that had occurred as a result of unaccustomed physical activity. Most subsequent research has continued to link DOMS to some form of contraction-induced muscular and/or connective tissue damage and to the subsequent necrosis-repair process. However, the exact nature of the damage–pain sensation link has proved elusive.

Two other causes of DOMS have had some degree of popularity (particularly among the lay exercise community) over the years. These theories can be classified as the metabolic waste accumulation theory and the muscle spasm theory.

The metabolic waste (or lactic acid) premise for DOMS was first proposed by Scandinavian researchers as early as the 1930s. The most convincing evidence against this theory involved observations on the eccentric muscle contractions developed during activities such as downhill running. Eccentric muscle contractions generate a relatively greater force than concentric contractions, but require a lesser expenditure of energy and thus result in a much smaller accumulation of lactic acid. Despite the lesser lactic acid accumulation, eccentric contractions have been repeatedly reported to induce significantly greater DOMS sensation than concentric contractions.

DeVries proposed that exercise-induced muscle pain caused a feedback cycle, leading to muscle spasm. This in turn induced yet more pain due to local ischemia and metabolic waste accumulation. However, subsequent research did not find increases in EMG (which would have been anticipated if there was increased electrical activity associated with muscle spasm in the sore muscles). Nor has there been any evidence of an accumulation of metabolites such as lactic acid in sore muscles.

Exercise-induced morphologic muscle damage has commonly been reported to occur in association with DOMS sensation. Such damage is usually seen immediately after exercise as small areas of focal damage. These become more extensive over the next several days. The main signs are Z-line and myofibrillar disruption. Severe damage is readily evident in transverse sections, using a light microscope, and there may be a reversible atrophy of some affected fibers.

In animal studies, exercise-induced muscle damage is accompanied by activation of lysosomal enzymes and invasion of macrophages. Fiber necrosis is evident for several days and is accompanied by inflammation and edema. Regenerative processes are evident after 3 days. Most of the degeneration and damage is delayed and thus cannot be seen until some hours after exercise. Macrophage invasion of exercise-damaged rat muscle does not peak until several days after exercise. Free radical–linked indices of lipid peroxidation are also seen some hours after exercise. Thus, the animal model suggests that most of the exercise-induced muscle damage is not produced directly by the exercise, but rather results from necrotic processes associated with the postexercise period and/or the resultant regeneration. How these necrotic-regenerative developments relate to the DOMS sensation in humans is uncertain.

In most patients, complete recovery from exercise-induced muscle damage requires less than 10 days, although in severe cases a complete regeneration of atrophied fibers may take 20 days or longer. As previously mentioned, the time course of DOMS sensation is usually much shorter than this. Thus, although muscle damage and DOMS can occur concurrently, they do not necessarily occur simultaneously. Some damage is evident immediately after exercise, while DOMS may not be felt until 8 to 24 hours after exercise. Similar muscular damage may occur in trained athletes without accompanying DOMS sensation. Moreover, patients with muscular dystrophy commonly exhibit muscular damage, although they do not usually develop any accompanying DOMS sensation.

Indices of muscle membrane disruption such as the efflux of soluble enzymes, or radiolabeled isotope uptake can occur in association with DOMS sensation. However, the time course of these disturbances does not usually coincide with that of the DOMS sensation. Marked enzyme efflux can occur in trained athletes without any DOMS sensation. Increased isotope uptake is also common in the muscles of patients suffering from such diseases as muscular dystrophy, polymyositis and McArdle's syndrome, none of which is usually accompanied by DOMS sensation. Finally, not all muscles that exhibit DOMS sensation take up radioisotopes.

DOMS-associated muscle damage is usually accompanied by inflammation and edema. While evidence from animal studies has been interpreted to suggest an association between DOMS sensation, inflammation, and edema, studies involving humans appear to make this link more tenuous.

Inhibition of prostaglandin-mediated vasodilatation in mice appears to protect their muscles partially from exercise-induced damage. However, prostaglandin inhibition does not appear to have any effect on the degree of exercise-induced DOMS sensation in humans.

Friden and colleagues reported that eccentrically exercised muscles that exhibited marked muscle soreness also had elevated tissue fluid pressures as measured by the slit-catheter technique. Thus, edema may be a factor in DOMS sensation. However, intramuscular fluid pressure was elevated immediately after exercise and did not increase further at the time when DOMS sensation peaked (some 24 hours after exercise), thus bringing into question a direct association between these two events.

Armstrong and Edwards both suggested that abnormally elevated calcium ion concentrations in the muscle cytoplasm may be a factor in the cascade of events that lead to postexercise muscle damage and regeneration, as well as the DOMS sensation. Structural damage to the muscle sarcolemma could lead to abnormally high intracellular calcium concentrations that could inhibit mitochondrial respiration. Recent evidence of an elevated inorganic phosphate-to-phosphocreatine ratio that persists for up to 10 days in muscles experiencing exercise-induced DOMS lends support to this hypothesis.

The elevated calcium concentrations could also activate certain protease and phospholipase enzymes, which could ultimately create an intracellular environment that would activate lysosomal enzymes and attract monocytes. The resultant accumulation of histamine and kinins that inevitably accompany lysosomal enzyme activity and monocyte invasion may then be factors in stimulating the type IV afferent nerves that transmit the DOMS sensation.

Armstrong discussed some evidence for the attenuation of muscle pain by drugs that lower calcium concentrations, but this has been reported only for patients with chronic muscular pain. The possible link to the short-term exercise-induced DOMS sensation of normal individuals remains unconfirmed.

Although there appears to be a strong link between exercise-induced muscle damage and DOMS sensation, the factor or factors directly responsible for the sensation have yet to be clearly identified.

SIMILARITIES BETWEEN DOMS AND MUSCULAR DEGENERATIVE DISEASES

The etiology of the exercise-induced muscle damage associated with DOMS is in many ways similar to the more extensive damage seen in a number of degenerative muscular diseases, particularly the muscular dystrophies. Elevated cytosolic calcium ion concentrations have been linked to the muscular degenerative process in such conditions as polymyositis, various muscular dystrophies, general muscle atrophy, and reperfusion injury. Evidence of free radical–induced lipid peroxidation is also a characteristic common to numerous degenerative conditions and exercise-induced muscular damage.

Recently Round and associates proposed that exercise-damaged muscle may be a suitable model for studying some of the factors involved in inflammatory muscular diseases. They noted that macrophage invasion is common to both exercise-induced muscle damage and polymyositis. However, macrophage invasion does not occur until some hours or days after the cessation of exercise. Thus, it is unlikely to be the direct cause of the exercise-induced damage, although it may be a reaction to it. By analogy, Round and associates proposed that the macrophage invasion associated with polymyositis and dystrophic muscle was again not the cause of the damage (as has usually been proposed) but rather a similar reaction to it.

PREVENTION AND TREATMENT

Since the exact causes of DOMS are as yet undefined, it is not surprising that the various interventions that have been attempted in order to prevent and treat the DOMS sensation have met with only limited success.

In his pioneering work on muscle soreness, Hough noted that exercising sore muscles appeared to relieve the soreness temporarily. Personal observation supports this conclusion. Armstrong suggested that the most likely explanation for this seemingly paradoxical observation could be exercise-induced increases in afferent discharge from low-threshold sensory fibers of groups Ia, Ib, and II. These fibers could partially block the pain sensation carried by the small, DOMS-sensing, group IV fibers through interneurons located in the spinal cord. Another possible explanation could involve the elevated endorphin levels that accompany exercise. Nevertheless, exercise offers only temporary relief, and the DOMS sensation returns shortly after exercise is stopped.

A common treatment, popular among the exercising public, is the application of creams containing methylsalicylate, menthol, or camphor. While the local sensation of cutaneous heat generated by the creams may temporarily attenuate the DOMS sensation (possibly owing to the blocking mechanism discussed above), it is unlikely to have any effect on the underlying causes of DOMS.

Attempts have been made to relieve or prevent DOMS by reducing inflammation and the resultant edema formation. Experiments using ice massage, antihistamines, and prostaglandin-blocking drugs have not reduced DOMS sensation. Since inflammation or edema may not be primary or singular causes of DOMS, this result is not surprising.

The use of saunas, whirlpool baths, and massage has become popular among competitive athletes and their coaches. It is alleged that their regular use assists in quicker "rejuvenation" between workouts (personal communication, Canadian Coaching Association). What effects these interventions may have on DOMS or exercise-induced muscle damage are unknown.

A belief common to the exercising public is that "warm-up" and "cool-down" exercises combined with stretching prevent exercise-induced DOMS. Shephard noted that while there are other benefits of this practice, there is little experimental evidence to suggest that it has any effect on the development of DOMS.

The only effective method for preventing DOMS is previous exercise training. Surprisingly, only one or two training sessions are necessary to prevent the recurrence of DOMS. It has been suggested that unaccustomed exercise damages a pool of susceptible muscle fibers. The subsequent degeneration-regeneration of these fibers decreases their susceptibility to further exercise-induced damage.

Although very limited amounts of training are needed to prevent DOMS, such conditioning is usually insufficient to prevent other aspects of muscle damage such as temporary strength reductions. Therefore, while small amounts of training can prevent DOMS, only well-trained individuals are likely to avoid the other adverse consequences of exercise-induced muscle damage.

SUGGESTED READING

Abraham W. Factors in delayed muscle soreness. Med Sci Sports 1977; 9:11–20.

Armstrong R. Mechanisms of exercise-induced delayed onset muscular soreness: a brief review. Med Sci Sports Exerc 1984; 16:529–538.

Armstrong R, Ogilvie R, Schwane J. Eccentric exercise-induced injury to rat skeletal muscle. J Appl Physiol 1983; 54:80–93.

Asmussen E. Observations on experimental muscle soreness. Acta Rheum Scand 1956; 2:109–116.

Byrnes W, Clarkson P, White S, et al. Delayed onset muscle soreness following repeated bouts of downhill running. J Appl Physiol 1985; 59:710–715.

DeVries H. Quantitative electromyographic investigation of the spasm theory of muscle pain. Am J Phys Med 1966; 47:175–181.

Edwards R. Hypotheses of peripheral and central mechanisms underlying occupational muscle pain and injury. Eur J Appl Physiol 1988; 57:275–281.

Friden J. Muscle soreness after exercise: implications of morphological changes. Int J Sports Med 1984; 5:57–66.

Friden J, Seger J, Ekblom B. Sublethal muscle fiber injuries after high-tension anaerobic exercise. Eur J Appl Physiol 1988; 57:360–368.

Friden J, Sfakianos P, Hargens A. Muscle soreness and intramuscular fluid pressure: comparison between eccentric and concentric load. J Appl Physiol 1986; 61:2175–2179.

Friden J, Sjöstrom M, Ekblom B. A morphological study of delayed muscle soreness. Experimentia 1981; 37:506–507.

Hill A. The mechanics of voluntary muscle. Lancet 1951; 261:947–954.

Hough T. Ergographic studies in muscular soreness. Am J Physiol 1902; 7:76–92.

Howell J, Chila A, Ford G, David D, Gates T. An electromyographic study of elbow motion during postexercise muscle soreness. J Appl Physiol 1985; 58:1713–1718.

Jenkins R. Free radical chemistry: relationship to exercise. Sports Med 1988; 5:156–170.

Kelly D. The role of endorphins in stress-induced analgesia. Ann NY Acad Sci 1982; 398:260–270.

Kuipers H, Keizer H, Verstappen F, Costill D. Influence of a prostaglandin-inhibiting drug on muscle soreness after eccentric work. Int J Sports Med 1985; 6:336–339.

McCully K, Argov Z, Boden B, et al. Detection of muscle injury in humans with 31-P magnetic resonance spectroscopy. Muscle Nerve 1988; 11:212–216.

McGlynn G, Laughlin N, Rowe V. Effect of electromyographic feedback and static stretching on artificially induced muscle soreness. Am J Phys Med 1979; 58:139–148.

Newham D. The consequences of eccentric contractions and their relationship to delayed onset muscle pain. Eur J Appl Physiol 1988; 57:353–359.

Newham D, Jones D, Clarkson P. Repeated high-force eccentric exercise: effects on muscle pain and damage. J Appl Physiol 1987; 63:1381–1386.

Newham E, Jones D, Tolfree S, Edwards R. Skeletal muscle damage: a study of isotope uptake, enzyme efflux and pain after stepping. Eur J Appl Physiol 1986; 55:106–112.

Noakes T. Effect of exercise on serum enzyme activities in humans. Sports Med 1987; 4:245–267.

Pierrynowski M, Tiidus P, Plyley M. Effects of downhill or uphill training prior to a downhill run. Eur J Appl Physiol 1987; 56:668–672.

Round J, Jones D, Cambridge G. Cellular infiltrates in human skeletal muscle: exercise-induced damage as a model for inflammatory muscle disease. J Neurol Sci 1987; 82:1–11.

Salminen A, Kihlstrom M. Protective effect of indomethacin against exercise-induced injuries in mouse skeletal muscle fibers. Int J Sports Med 1987; 8:46–49.

Schwane J, Watrous B, Johnson S, Armstrong R. Is lactic acid related to delayed-onset muscle soreness? Phys Sportsmed 1983; 11:124–131.

Shephard R. Physiology and biochemistry of exercise. New York: Praeger, 1982:92.

Tiidus P, Ianuzzo D. Effects of intensity and duration of muscular exercise on delayed soreness and serum enzyme activities. Med Sci Sports Exerc 1983; 15:461–465.

Vihko V, Salminen A. Propagation and repair of exercise-induced skeletal fiber injury. In: Biochemical aspects of physical exercise. Elsevier Science, 1986:337.

Wallensten R, Eriksson E. Intramuscular pressures in exercise-induced lower leg pain. Int J Sports Med 1984; 5:31–35.

Yackzan L, Adams C, Francis K. The effects of ice massage on delayed muscle soreness. Am J Sports Med 1984; 12:159–165.

EXERCISE IN THE SECONDARY PREVENTION OF ISCHEMIC HEART DISEASE

DAVID L. ANDERS, M.D.
JOHN D. CANTWELL, M.D.

The health benefits of exercise were recognized long before the development of the scientific methods currently used to demonstrate them. Cicero (108–46 BC) instructed his pupils "to resist old age . . . practice moderate exercise," and yet not until the last half of the 20th century were adequate epidemiologic studies designed to demonstrate the health-related advantages of exercise. Recent studies indicate that individuals who exercise regularly show reductions in both cardiovascular disease–related deaths and nonfatal myocardial infarction (MI). Research will certainly continue to refine our understanding of the protective role of exercise and activity in reducing the incidence of primary cardiovascular morbidity and mortality. Equally significant are studies that address the benefits and risks of exercise in patients with established coronary artery disease.

Despite a recent decrease in the incidence of cardiovascular deaths in the United States, the natural history of atherosclerotic coronary vascular disease and the health practices of many North Americans indicate that thousands of patients will continue to develop cardiovascular disease every year. Those who survive the initial manifestations of their disease (i.e., those who do not die of sudden ventricular fibrillation with or without acute MI as the first indication of their coronary artery disease) will require continued medical management. These patients may have a variety of cardiac conditions, including recent acute MI, stable angina, silent myocardial ischemia, and previous percutaneous transluminal coronary angioplasty or coronary artery bypass grafting surgery. Exercise for rehabilitation and secondary prevention has become a well-accepted component of the total therapeutic plan of cardiac rehabilitation designed for these patients.

To appreciate adequately the current role of exercise in the treatment of heart disease, one should first know the history of cardiac rehabilitation. Such a review is beyond the scope of this chapter, but excellent sources are available. In the 1950s the standard management of the post-MI patient included 6 weeks of strict bed rest. Over the past four decades, cardiac rehabilitation has developed into a multifaceted discipline designed to address the physical, social, emotional, psychological, and vocational-economic needs of the individual patient. Current methods are vastly different from those of the 1950s and will certainly continue to be modified into the twenty-first century.

THE BENEFITS OF EXERCISE IN ISCHEMIC HEART DISEASE

The physiologic benefits of exercise training are well documented. One objective parameter used to evaluate exercise performance is oxygen uptake ($\dot{V}O_2$), expressed in milliliters of oxygen uptake per kilogram of body weight per minute. The maximal oxygen uptake or aerobic power ($\dot{V}O_2max$) that can be achieved during endurance exercise is an indicator of work capacity; it depends on both general physical condition and cardiac status. Exercise training leading to an enhanced work capacity (as measured by increased $\dot{V}O_2max$) is a proved effect of cardiac rehabilitation programs. The primary cause of an increase of $\dot{V}O_2max$ is likely a peripheral adaptation of conditioned skeletal muscle, with a resultant reduction of vascular resistance in the exercising muscles, rather than a central or direct enhancement of myocardial contractility. The augmentation of $\dot{V}O_2max$ increases the probability of a successful resumption of work and leisure activities, even in patients with significant left ventricular dysfunction.

More recent information indicates that a central improvement in myocardial function is possible, in addition to the peripheral adaptations noted above. The "double product" (product of heart rate and systolic blood pressure) reflects myocardial oxygen consumption. In a given patient with stable angina, the double product defines a fairly constant threshold for the onset of angina. In cardiac rehabilitation programs, exercise training lowers the double product for a given submaximal workload in individual patients, while raising the maximal double product (and thus the anginal threshold) in some patients; the latter change suggests a direct rather than a peripheral improvement in myocardial function or myocardial oxygen supply. Further research is needed to determine the possible limits of improvement in $\dot{V}O_2max$ from either peripheral or central cardiovascular changes after exercise training.

Other studies have shown that participation in exercise programs may lead to improved left ventricular function, cardiac thallium image scores, increased blood fibrinolytic activity, decreased platelet aggregation, and an improved plasma lipid profile. Reports on changes in exercise-induced ST-segment depression have been conflicting, and researchers have not shown any increase in resting left ventricular ejection fraction after exercise training.

The protective role of exercise following infarction is not yet clearly defined. The first of several prospective randomized controlled trials to study the impact of exercise training on death and nonfatal reinfarction in the postinfarction patient was reported by Wilhelmsen and colleagues in 1975 (Table 1). Over a 4-year period in a training group of 158 patients, there were 21 percent fewer deaths and 11 percent fewer nonfatal MIs, but neither differ-

TABLE 1 Randomized Controlled Clinical Trials Evaluating Cardiac Rehabilitation After Myocardial Infarction

			Overall Mortality			*Nonfatal MI*		
Study	*Number of Patients*	*Duration of Study*	*Exercise Group*	*Control Group*	*p*	*Exercise Group*	*Control Group*	*p*
Wilhelmsen	315	4 yr	17.7%*	22.3%	0.40	15.8%	17.8%	N.S.
Kallio	375	3 yr	18.6%†	29.4%	0.02	18.1%	11.2%	0.10
Shaw	651	3 yr	4.6%*	7.3%	0.22	4.6%	3.4%	N.S.
Rechnitzer	733	4 yr	4.0%‡	3.7%	N.S.	10.3%	9.3%	N.S.

* Total deaths.
† Coronary deaths.
‡ Infarction deaths.
N.S. = not significant.

ence was statistically significant. Kallio and associates reported a significant (36.7 percent) decrease of cumulative cardiac mortality in 183 patients who participated in a 3-year physical exercise program, compared with a control group of 187 patients who did not. Exercise patients also had an increase in nonfatal MI, but this was not statistically significant. These changes cannot be attributed solely to exercise, however, because the exercised group participated in an associated multifactorial intervention program. Reductions in mortality may have been due to intergroup differences with respect to the number of physician visits, the amounts of medications prescribed, or the degree of blood pressure control. Mortality rates in the National Exercise and Heart Disease Project (reported by Shaw) did not differ significantly between exercised and control groups, although again there was a lower incidence of death in the 323 patients who exercised over 3 years as compared with the 328 controls. In 1983 Rechnitzer and colleagues reported a 4-year trial that failed to show any difference in either infarction deaths or nonfatal MI during a study in which 733 males were allocated randomly to vigorous and light exercise programs after infarction. When reviewing the above and other trials, Shephard concluded that "no single team of investigators has accumulated a sample of sufficient size to allow adequate statistical evaluation of the exercise hypothesis for a 30% or even a 50% therapeutic effect." He predicted that a trial to do so would cost at least $10 to $15 million. By making several assumptions, Shephard was able to show a significant reduction in mortality for the post-MI group, using combined data from the several published studies. No similar random studies have evaluated exercise training in patients with coronary artery disease after cardiovascular surgery or percutaneous transluminal coronary angioplasty.

EXERCISE AND CARDIAC REHABILITATION

The role of exercise in the management of a patient with ischemic heart disease is best put into perspective by an initial evaluation of current methods of cardiac rehabilitation. Several different protocols exist, but the overall goals are similar (Table 2). The process described below is applied to the patient who has had a recent acute MI, but with certain modifications it can be applied to most patients with coronary artery disease.

Phase I

Cardiac rehabilitation has been divided functionally into four phases. Phase I covers the period of hospitalization that begins as soon as the physician decides that the patient has been stabilized hemodynamically. Working with a nurse, a physical therapist, or another member of the cardiac rehabilitation team, the patient begins range-of-motion exercises and gradually progresses to a level of activity that allows him or her to function as an outpatient, e.g., walking 100 m. These sessions allow a close monitoring of the patient's reactions to exercise; any significant hemodynamic changes or other signs or symptoms of cardiac dysfunction may indicate the need to reevaluate the management regimen or diagnosis. During phase I, it is equally important to provide counseling and patient education covering

TABLE 2 Goals of Cardiac Rehabilitation

To return the individual to optimal physiologic and psychological function.
To reverse the adverse effects of physiologic deconditioning, resulting from a sedentary lifestyle and accelerated by bed rest.
To prepare the individual and his or her family for a lifestyle that may reduce the risk of future coronary heart disease and hypertensive cardiovascular disease. This will involve activities to control smoking, high blood pressure, diabetes mellitus, lipid disorders, and emotional stress. It will also involve discussion and clarification of the cardiac disease process, vocational guidance, and the importance of regular participation in a physical activity program.
To assist the individual with heart disease to return to activities that were important to the quality of life before the onset of the cardiac illness.
To reduce the emotional disorders frequently accompanying serious disorders of health.
To reduce the cost of health care through a shortening of treatment time and a reduced use of drugs.
To prevent premature disability and lessen the need for institutional care of elderly patients.

Modified from Parmley WW. President's page: position report on cardiac rehabilitation. J Am Coll Cardiol 1986; 7:451–453.

a broad area of related subjects, including modification of cardiac risk factors, basic aspects of cardiovascular disease, and instruction in newly prescribed drugs. Family members may be included in these sessions. In addition to such an educational program, specific reassurance should be given to both the patient and the spouse concerning the safe resumption of sexual activity at the time when other usual prehospital activities are resumed. Patients who have undergone coronary artery bypass grafting surgery are also candidates for phase I rehabilitation, with appropriate modifications of the program to allow for postoperative wound healing.

Shortly before or after hospital discharge, submaximal stress testing may be performed safely to assure both the patient and the physician that there is now an adequate cardiac reserve. Several different protocols have been designed to screen for significant residual ischemia and arrhythmias and to document safe levels of physical activity. The test results reassure the patient and allow the physician to prescribe a level of outpatient activity to keep the heart rate below the level achieved during submaximal testing. The target heart rate during the submaximal test is adjusted to take account of several factors, including the patient's age and current therapy with beta-adrenergic receptor blocking agents. Failure to reach the target heart rate because of angina or early ST-segment depression may indicate that the patient has a higher risk of subsequent cardiac morbidity, and further evaluation may then be appropriate.

Phase II

Phase II of rehabilitation begins upon discharge from the hospital and continues for 2 to 4 months. During this time the patient participates in prescribed individual and group activities such as walking, jogging, swimming, cycling, or other aerobic activities at an outpatient rehabilitation center. Because some patients show unstable angina, dangerous dysrhythmias, or other contraindications to cardiac rehabilitation (Table 3), not all participants in phase I will be candidates for progression to phase II. Others, for example, patients with stable angina who are being managed medically, or individuals who have undergone recent percutaneous transluminal coronary angioplasty, may begin exercise in a phase II program without first participating in phase I (although the counseling and patient education otherwise provided in phase I should be available). Those who progress to phase II exercise are carefully monitored, initially with continuous electrocardiographic (ECG) monitoring, and they are taught not to exceed their prescribed target heart rates (usually established at 70 to 85 percent of the rate safely attained during submaximal testing). The level of activity is gradually intensified during each week of phase II. Selected low-risk patients who cannot or will not participate in a supervised program may be instructed in a home walking program (Table 4). Such individuals are taught to count their pulse rate and are warned not to exceed preestablished limits.

TABLE 3 Contraindications to Cardiac Rehabilitation

- Unstable angina pectoris
- Severe ventricular dysfunction manifested by a drop in systolic blood pressure or limited cardiac output in response to exercise, or severe dyspnea at low workloads
- Active cardiomyopathy or myocarditis during the previous year
- Uncontrolled hypertension
- Complex dysrhythmias
- Second- and third-degree atrioventricular block
- Uncontrolled atrial fibrillation
- Substantial cardiomegaly
- Hemodynamically relevant valvular or congenital heart disease, as well as important noncardiac illnesses: orthopaedic, pulmonary, gastrointestinal, and other systemic diseases, particularly the following: recent pulmonary embolism; anemia; uncontrolled metabolic diseases (e.g., diabetes mellitus, uremia, thyrotoxicosis); transient febrile illnesses

Republished with permission from Council on Scientific Affairs, American Medical Association. Physician-supervised exercise programs in rehabilitation of patients with coronary heart disease. JAMA 1981; 245:1463–1466. (Copyright 1981, American Medical Association.)

Phases III and IV

After several weeks of monitored exercise, most patients can progress to phase III, an unmonitored

TABLE 4 Standard Home Walk Program for Cardiac Rehabilitation at Georgia Baptist Medical Center

Week After Discharge	*Distance*	*Allotted Time*
Week 1	Walk 400 m (¼ mile) daily	Leisurely pace, 5 min
Weeks 2–3	Walk 400 m (¼ mile) twice daily	Leisurely pace, 5 min
Week 4	Walk 800 m (½ mile) daily or twice a day if the above is tolerated	Leisurely pace, 10 min
Week 5	Walk 1,200 m (¾ mile) daily	Leisurely pace, 15 min
Weeks 6–7	Walk 1.6 km (1 mile) daily	Leisurely pace, 20 min
Week 8	Walk 2.4 km (1½ miles) daily	Leisurely pace, 30 min
Week 9	Walk 3.2 km (2 miles) daily	Leisurely pace, 40 min
Week 10	Walk 3.2 km (2 miles) daily	Moderate pace, 30 min
Weeks 11–12	Walk 4.8 km (3 miles) daily	Leisurely pace, 60 min
Week 13	Walk 4.8 km (3 miles) daily	Moderate pace, 50 min
Week 14	Walk 6.4 km (4 miles) daily	Moderate pace, 60 min

but supervised program at a center where cardiac monitoring and resuscitative equipment is available if needed. Not all phase II patients should be advanced to unmonitored exercise, however; restriction is usually imposed when there is more serious underlying cardiac disease (Table 5). Those patients who successfully accomplish several months of a phase III program are then encouraged to graduate to phase IV, a lifelong fitness maintenance program without further direct medical supervision. The patient may elect to continue to exercise at the cardiac rehabilitation center, to join a fitness center or health club, or to exercise at home. Throughout phases II, III, and IV, continued check-ups by the primary care physician or cardiac rehabilitation team are an important aspect of continued surveillance and patient education.

THE SAFETY OF EXERCISE IN ISCHEMIC HEART DISEASE

Two large studies have evaluated the safety of prescribed exercise in patients with ischemic heart disease (Table 6). Haskell's study, started in 1960, showed a decreased mortality rate during the latter years, probably a result of program modifications introduced by the reporting centers. Haskell concluded that post-MI patients who participated in an exercise program did not place themselves at greater risk of death than patients who chose to remain inactive. A subsequent study by Van Camp showed an even lower risk of cardiac arrest during exercise in a cardiac rehabilitation program, perhaps a reflection of better patient selection and program application. When Van Camp compared his results with the anticipated morbidity and mortality rates in joggers without known cardiovascular disease, he concluded that patients attending a cardiac rehabilitation center were more likely to develop an acute cardiac event, but were less likely to die, possibly because of the ready availability of trained personnel and equipment for cardiac resuscitation. Additional evidence of the safety of appropriately prescribed exercise is provided by Shephard and colleagues, who carefully supervised a select group of 50 cardiac patients; these individuals trained for and ran in over 300 marathons, with no exercise-related deaths.

To further minimize risks, investigators have attempted to identify features of patients who, despite preexercise evaluation and testing, experience a cardiac arrest or infarction during an exercise training program. High-grade coronary artery stenosis, failure to follow the prescribed limitations of maximal heart rate, male gender, and ECG ST-segment depression during exercise testing are all common conditions in patients experiencing ventricular fibrillation or cardiac arrest during supervised exercise.

TABLE 5 Definite Indications for ECG Monitoring During a Cardiac Rehabilitation Exercise Program

Severely depressed left ventricular function (ejection fraction < 30%)
Resting complex ventricular arrhythmia (Lown type 4 or 5)
Ventricular arrhythmia appearing or increasing with exercise
Decrease in systolic blood pressure with exercise
Survivor of sudden cardiac death
Myocardial infarction complicated by congestive heart failure, cardiogenic shock, and/or serious ventricular arrhythmia
Severe coronary artery disease with marked exercise-induced ischemia
Inability to self-monitor heart rate because of physical or intellectual impairment

Modified from Parmley WW. President's page: position report on cardiac rehabilitation. J Am Coll Cardiol 1986; 7:451–453.

FUTURE TRENDS IN EXERCISE PROGRAMS FOR ISCHEMIC HEART DISEASE

Undoubtedly, future studies will continue to refine our present understanding of the categories of patients who are most likely to benefit from exercise training. One select group whose numbers will probably grow consists of those who have undergone cardiac transplantation. Kavanagh and associates demonstrated the utility of exercise in this group, and additional information should be most interesting. Patients in whom revascularization has been successfully achieved by thrombolytic therapy, percutaneous transluminal coronary angioplasty, coro-

TABLE 6 Complications Encountered in Outpatient Cardiac Rehabilitation

	Study	
	Haskell	*Van Camp*
Years covered	1960–77	1980–84
Number of patients	13,570	51,303
Number of patient-hours observed	1,629,634	2,351,916
Cardiac arrest rate: patient-hours of exercise		
Nonfatal	1:38,801 (n = 42)	1:130,662 (n = 18)
Fatal	1:203,704 (n = 8)	1:783,972 (n = 3)
Myocardial infarction: patient-hours of exercise		
Nonfatal	1:325,927 (n = 5)	1:293,990 (n = 8)
Fatal	1:814,816 (n = 2)	n = 0
Overall mortality rate: patient-hours of exercise	1:116,402	1:783,972

nary artery bypass surgery, or a combination of these techniques make up a larger group that also merits in-depth study.

Further investigation is needed to determine the optimal level of exercise for maximal therapeutic benefit. One 3-month trial showed no significant difference between the effects of high-intensity (65 to 75 percent of maximal oxygen consumption rate) and low-intensity (less than 45 percent of maximal oxygen consumption rate) exercise in a group of patients who had recently sustained an acute MI. However, 3 months may not be sufficient time for a significant difference in results to develop.

Research currently under way will assess the effect of moderate-intensity versus high-intensity exercise programs over a prolonged time. In a 5-year trial supported by the National Institutes of Health, patients with cardiovascular disease will be compared after training at either 50 or 85 percent of maximal heart rate. The results of this study should influence future exercise guidelines for the cardiac patient.

Specific types of exercise will continue to be compared to determine the relative advantages of each. Cardiac rehabilitation has traditionally been built around a program of aerobic activity such as jogging or cycling, but a controlled study by Kelemen and colleagues demonstrated an additional increase in both aerobic endurance and musculoskeletal strength when a small group of patients added circuit weight training to their walk-jog exercise program.

Changes are likely to occur in the structuring of exercise programs. According to recent US estimates, only 15 percent of eligible patients enter a monitored phase II program. Reasons for this low percentage are multiple, but certainly include financial, logistical, and emotional obstacles encountered by patients. To increase the number of patients involved in phase II activity, several authors have suggested that home training is possible and safe for selected individuals. Further study is needed to show just how much electrocardiographically monitored exercise the patient should perform in phase II before progressing to unmonitored activity. Guidelines are not yet established on if, how, or when patients training at home should be monitored electrocardiographically to detect exercise-induced cardiac ischemia or dysrhythmias. For patients training at home who require intermittent monitoring, transtelephonic transmission of ECG signals is now playing an increasing role, allowing patients to pass to the physician postexercise ECG data for rhythm analysis and ST-segment evaluation. Improved continuous ambulatory ECG monitoring may also allow more sensitive analysis of exercise-induced ST-segment changes, in addition to traditional evaluation for dysrhythmias. Exercise videotapes for home use are currently marketed by professional and commercial organizations, and may become yet another widely used way to encourage continued outpatient participation.

Such developments will allow for broader application of the outpatient phases of cardiac rehabilitation. Continued clinical research and economic pressures have diminished the duration of the inpatient component of cardiac rehabilitation. The median length of hospitalization for an uncomplicated MI in 1970 was 21 days; by 1979 that period had decreased to 14 days, and it has certainly decreased further during the 1980s. Recent investigators have shown that carefully selected patients with uncomplicated MI can be discharged from the hospital after 3 days without increased risk. Thus, the challenge of defining and prescribing safe, effective, and cost-efficient outpatient exercise programs will carry researchers well into the next century.

SUGGESTED READING

Blumenthal JA, Rejeski WJ, Walsh-Riddle M, et al. Comparison of high- and low-intensity exercise training early after acute myocardial infarction. Am J Cardiol 1988; 61:26–30.

Clausen JP. Circulatory adjustments to dynamic exercise and effect of physical training in exercise and effect of physical training in normal subjects and in patients with coronary artery disease. Prog Cardiovasc Dis 1976; 18:459–495.

Cole HM, ed. Diagnostic and Therapeutic Technology Assessment (DATTA)—coronary rehabilitation services. JAMA 1987; 258:1959–1962.

Conn EH, Williams RS, Wallace AG. Exercise responses before and after physical conditioning in patients with severely depressed left ventricular function. Am J Cardiol 1982; 49:296–300.

Council on Scientific Affairs, American Medical Association. Physician-supervised exercise programs in rehabilitation of patients with coronary heart disease. JAMA 1981; 245:1463–1466.

DeBusk RF, Blomqvist CG, Kouchoukous NT, et al. Identification and treatment of low-risk patients after acute myocardial infarction and coronary artery bypass graft surgery. N Engl J Med 1986; 314:161–166.

DeBusk RF, Haskell W. Symptom-limited vs heart-rate limited exercise testing soon after myocardial infarction. Circulation 1980; 61:738–743.

Dressendorfer RH, Amsterdam EA, Mason DT. Therapeutic effects of exercise training in angina patients. In: Physical conditioning and cardiovascular rehabilitation. John Wiley, 1981:122.

Ehsani AA, Biello DR, Schultz J, Sobel BE, Holloszy JO. Improvement of left ventricular contractile function by exercise training in patients with coronary artery disease. Circulation 1986; 74:350–358.

Ehsani AA, Heath GW, Hagberg JM, Sobel BE, Holloszy JO. Effects of 12 months of intense exercise training on ischemic ST-segment depression in patients with coronary artery disease. Circulation 1981; 64:1116–1124.

Fardy PS. Home-based cardiac rehabilitation. Phys Sports Med 1987; 15:89–94.

Fletcher GF, Cantwell JD. Ventricular fibrillation in a medically supervised cardiac exercise program. JAMA 1977; 238:2627–2629.

Froelicher V, Jensen D, Genter F, et al. A randomized trial of exercise training in patients with coronary heart disease. JAMA 1984; 252:1291–1297.

Hartung GH, Squires WG, Gotto AM. Effect of exercise training on plasma–high density lipoprotein cholesterol in coronary disease patients. Am Heart J 1981; 101:181–184.

Haskell WL. Cardiovascular complications during exercise training of cardiac patients. Circulation 1978; 57:920–924.

Hellerstein HK. Cardiac rehabilitation: a retrospective view. In: Pollock ML, Schmidt DH, eds. Heart disease and rehabilitation. New York: John Wiley, 1986:701.

Hellerstein HK, Friedman EH. Sexual activity in the postcoronary patient. Arch Intern Med 1970; 125:987–999.

Hertanu JS, Davis L, Focseneamu M, Lahaman L. Cardiac rehabilitation exercise program: outcome assessment. Arch Phys Med Rehabil 1986; 67:431–435.

Hossak KF, Hartwig R. Cardiac arrest associated with supervised cardiac rehabilitation. J Cardiac Rehabil 1982; 2:402–408.

Hung J, Gordon EP, Houston N, et al. Changes in rest and exercise myocardial perfusion and left ventricular function 3 to 26 weeks after clinically uncomplicated myocardial infarction: effects of exercise training. Am J Cardiol 1984; 54:943–950.

Kallio V, Hamalainen H, Hakkila J, Luurila OJ. Reduction in sudden death by a multifactorial intervention programme after acute myocardial infarction. Lancet 1979; 2:1091–1094.

Kavanagh T, Yacoub MH, Mertens DJ, et al. Cardiorespiratory responses to exercise training after orthotopic cardiac transplantation. Circulation 1988; 77:162–171.

Kelemen MH, Stewart KJ, Gillilan RE, et al. Circuit weight training in cardiac patients. J Am Coll Cardiol 1986; 7:38–42.

Kitamura K, Jorgensen CR, Gobel FL, Talor HL, Wang Y. Hemodynamic correlates of myocardial oxygen consumption during upright exercise. J Appl Physiol 1972; 32:516–522.

Laslette LJ, Paumer L, Amsterdam EA. Increase in myocardial oxygen consumption indexes by exercise training at onset of ischemia in patients with coronary artery disease. Circulation 1985; 71:958–962.

Leon AS, Connett J, Jacobs DR Jr, Ravramaa R. Leisure-time physical activity levels and risk of coronary heart disease and death. The multiple risk factor intervention trial. JAMA 1987; 258:2388–2395.

Levine FA, Lown B. The "chair" treatment of acute coronary thrombosis. Trans Assoc Am Physicians 1951; 64:316–326.

Martin WH III, Ehsani AA. Reversal of exertional hypotension by prolonged exercise training in selected patients with ischemic heart disease. Circulation 1987; 76:548–555.

Mead WF, Pyfer HR, Tronbole JC, Frederick RJ. Successful resuscitation of two near simultaneous cases of cardiac arrest with a review of 15 cases occurring during supervised exercise. Circulation 1976; 53:187–189.

Miller NH, Haskell WL, Berra K, DeBusk RF. Home versus group exercise training for increased functional capacity after myocardial infarction. Circulation 1984; 70:645–649.

Myers J, Ahnve S, Froelicher V, et al. A randomized trial of the effects of 1 year of exercise training on computer-measured ST segment displacement in patients with coronary artery disease. J Am Coll Cardiol 1984; 4:1094–1102.

National Exercise and Heart Disease Project. Effects of a prescribed supervised exercise program on mortality and cardiovascular morbidity in patients after a myocardial infarction. Am J Cardiol 1981; 48:39–46.

Naughton J, Haider R. Methods of exercise testing. In: Naughton J, Hellerstein HK, eds. Exercise testing and exercise training in coronary heart disease. New York: Academic Press, 1973:79.

Oberman A. Rehabilitation of patients with coronary artery disease. In: Braunwald E, ed. Heart disease. Philadelphia: WB Saunders, 1987:1384.

Paffenbarger RS Jr, Hyde RT, Wing AL, Hsieh C. Physical activity, all-cause mortality, and longevity of college alumni. N Engl J Med 1986; 314:605–613.

Parmley WW. President's page: position report on cardiac rehabilitation. J Am Coll Cardiol 1986; 7:451–453.

Rechnitzer PA, Cunningham DA, Andrew GM, et al. Relation of exercise to the recurrence rate of myocardial infarction in men. Am J Cardiol 1983; 51:65–69.

Rowell LB. Human cardiovascular adjustments to exercise and thermal stress. Physiol Rev 1974; 54:75–159.

Sami M, Kraemer H, DeBusk RF. The prognostic significance of serial exercise testing after myocardial infarction. Circulation 1979; 60:1238–1246.

Sebrechts CP, Klein JL, Ahnve S, Froelicher VF, Ashburn WL. Myocardial perfusion changes following one year of exercise training assessed by thallium-201 circumferential count profiles. Am Heart J 1986; 112:1217–1226.

Shephard RJ. The value of exercise in ischemic heart disease: a cumulative analysis. J Cardiac Rehabil 1983; 3:294–298.

Shephard RJ, Kavanaugh T, Tuck J, Kennedy J. Marathon jogging in post-myocardial infarction patients. J Cardiac Rehabil 1983; 3:321–329.

Squires RW, Gau GT. Cardiac rehabilitation and cardiovascular health enhancement. In: Brandenburg RO, Fuster V, Giuliani ER, McGoon DC, eds. Cardiology: fundamentals and practice. Chicago: Year Book, 1987:1944.

Starling MR, Crawford MH, Kennedy GT, O'Rourke RA. Exercise testing after myocardial infarction: predictive value for subsequent unstable angina and death. Am J Cardiol 1980; 46:909–914.

Stern MJ, Cleary P. National Exercise and Heart Disease Project. Psychosocial changes observed during a low-level exercise program. Arch Intern Med 1981; 141:1463–1467.

Strauss MD. Familiar medical quotations. Boston: Little, Brown, 1968:164.

Theroux P, Waters DD, Halphen C, Debaisieux JC, Mizgala HF. Prognostic value of exercise testing soon after myocardial infarction. N Engl J Med 1979; 301:341–345.

Thompson PD, Funk EJ, Carlton RA, Sturner WQ. Incidence of death during jogging in Rhode Island from 1975 through 1980. JAMA 1982; 247:2535–2538.

Topol EJ, Burek K, O'Nell WW, et al. A randomized controlled trial of hospital discharge 3 days after myocardial infarction in the era of reperfusion. N Engl J Med 1988; 318:1083–1088.

Van Camp SP, Peterson RA. Cardiovascular complications of outpatient cardiac rehabilitation programs. JAMA 1986; 256:1160–1163.

Waters DD, Bosch X, Bouchard A, et al. Comparison of clinical variables and variables derived from a limited predischarge exercise test as predictors of early and late mortality after myocardial infarction. J Am Coll Cardiol 1985; 5:1–8.

Wenger NK. Rehabilitation after myocardial infarction. JAMA 1979; 242:2879–2881.

Wenger NK, Fletcher GF. Rehabilitation of the patient with atherosclerotic coronary heart disease. In: Hurst JW. The heart. New York: McGraw-Hill, 1986:1025.

Wenger NK, Hellerstein HK, Blackburn H, Castranova FJ. Uncomplicated myocardial infarction—current physician practice in patient management. JAMA 1973; 224:511–514.

Wenger NK, Hellerstein HK, Blackburn H, Castranova SJ. Physician practice in the management of uncomplicated myocardial infarction: changes in the past decade. Circulation 1982; 65:421–427.

Wilhelmsen L, Sanne H, Elmfeldt D, et al. A controlled trial of physical training after myocardial infarction—effects on risk factors, non-fatal reinfarction and death. Prev Med 1975; 4:491–508.

Williams RS, McKinnis RA, Cobb FR, et al. Effects of physical conditioning on left ventricular ejection fraction in patients with coronary artery disease. Circulation 1984; 70:69–75.

Williams RS, Miller H, Koisch FP, Ribisl P, Graden H. Guidelines for unsupervised exercise in patients with ischemic heart disease. J Cardiac Rehabil 1981; 1:213–219.

Wolthuis RA, Froelicher VF Jr, Fischer R, et al. New practical treadmill protocol for clinical use. Am J Cardiol 1977; 39:697–700.

DIETARY PROTEIN REQUIREMENTS FOR THE ATHLETE

PETER M. TIIDUS, M.Sc.

The ingestion of protein in the form of red meat has been associated with strength and power development since antiquity. Many ancient cultures encouraged their young hunters and warriors to eat the flesh of large animals so as to gain something of their power. Even relatively recent history has seen training meals for athletes consisting primarily of steak.

More recently, health care professionals have encouraged athletes to focus on a balanced diet. Recommended daily allowances (RDA) of protein for the general North American population are usually around 0.8 mg per kilogram of body mass per day. In fact, many normal individuals can maintain nitrogen balance on as little as 0.57 mg per kilogram per day. These levels of protein ingestion can easily be exceeded by consuming no more than 15 percent of one's energy intake as protein.

For example, a moderately active 70-kg male consuming a diet of 12 to 13 megajoules (3,000 kcal) per day, of which 15 percent was protein, would be eating approximately 112 g of protein (assuming 4 calories per gram of protein). This would ensure a consumption of 1.6 g of protein per kilogram of body mass, double the recommended daily allowance for sedentary subjects. Such levels of protein consumption are common in typical North American diets. Also, most nutrition textbooks suggest that supplementing protein intake for athletes is unnecessary.

Despite these assurances, many athletes, particularly those concerned with muscle bulk or power, believe that supplementation of their protein intake is necessary in order to achieve optimal training results (Lemon, 1987). It is commonly held among these individuals that by enhancing their intake of protein, particularly the essential amino acids, they can enhance the synthesis of muscle proteins in response to a training bout. This enhanced protein synthesis would exceed that which could be obtained by the RDA of protein and is believed to be necessary for the maximal bulk and strength gains sought by these individuals. Normal diets, although usually maintaining nitrogen balance, are not believed by some athletes to promote optimal results.

Capitalizing on these beliefs, the marketing of amino acid supplements has helped create a significant subpopulation of consumers who are concerned about boosting their protein intake primarily by ingesting specific amino acid tablets. In addition, athletes using anabolic steroids believe that very high intakes of proteins along with a heavy training schedule are necessary for maximal anabolic steroid effects on muscle hypertrophy.

Research findings related to these beliefs are still equivocal. Dragan and colleagues suggested that consuming 500 percent of the RDA of proteins may enhance strength and muscle bulk gains in weight lifters. However, more controlled and objective studies are needed to confirm the validity of these results.

Some review papers have also recommended that active individuals ingest up to 3.0 g of protein per kilogram of body mass to maintain a positive nitrogen balance. These recommendations are based on observations of elevated amino acid catabolism, protein turnover, and total nitrogen excretion following physical activity.

Lemon reviewed several nitrogen balance studies performed on athletes in training, and concluded that during training it is possible for certain individuals to be in negative nitrogen balance, even though they maintain protein intakes significantly higher than the RDA. However, many of these studies were not totally objective or well controlled. Lemon suggested that a number of variables should be taken into account when assessing the protein requirements of athletes. These include the intensity and duration of the exercise performed, the energy balance of the athlete, the training status, and the time after initiation of training program that the measurements were taken.

For example, some studies suggested that exercise intensity or duration may affect protein turnover and utilization, and hence dietary protein requirements. Lemon and colleagues reported increased branched chain amino acid oxidation with increased work intensity in rats.

Low liver and muscle glycogen levels (which may develop during exercise of long duration) can enhance amino acid oxidation. As well as acting as a potential source of adenosine triphosphate (ATP), amino acids can be used as gluconeogenic precursors during times of glucose and glycogen depletion. Goldstein and Newsholme described a metabolic pathway by which de novo alanine synthesis can occur entirely from amino acid sources in exercising muscle (Fig. 1). The alanine would be deaminated in the liver and the resultant pyruvate used for gluconeogenesis.

Lemon and Nagel equated the metabolic state toward the end of a long-term bout of exercise with that seen in short-term (several days) starvation. In both cases, gluconeogenesis is heavily dependent on protein sources.

Several studies have estimated that the protein contribution to total energy liberation during exercise exceeds 5 percent in certain conditions. It has been suggested that exercise alone can induce acti-

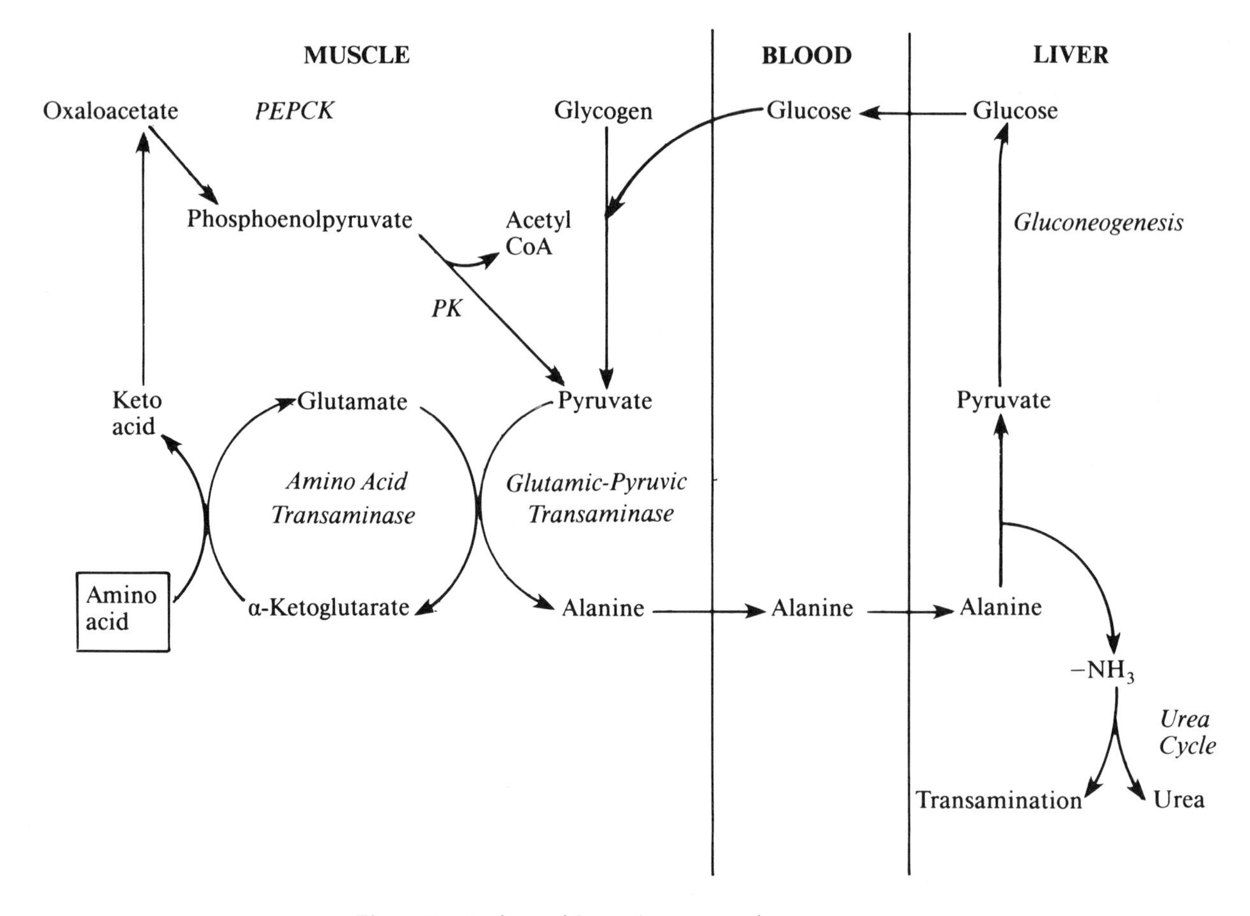

Figure 1 Amino acids as gluconeogenic precursors.

vation of muscular branched-chain keto-acid dehydrogenase enzymes, thereby facilitating amino acid breakdown and metabolism.

Dohm and associates reported that training increases the ability of rats to oxidize amino acids during exercise, by enhancing the concentration of enzymes peculiar to protein breakdown. Thus, increased protein turnover and utilization as a result of exercise and training is a distinct possibility.

These findings tend to suggest that physically active individuals may require greater dietary protein intakes than a normal population in order to remain in protein balance.

Another factor to be considered when assessing protein turnover is the potential for exercise-induced muscle damage. Numerous studies with animals and humans have demonstrated that various degrees of muscle damage can result from intense or long-duration exercise. This can include sarcomere disruption, Z-disc damage, edema, inflammation, and increased lysosomal enzyme activity.

Increasing intensity or duration of muscular activity also results in indirect evidence of muscle and muscle sarcolemma disruption in the form of increased intracellular enzyme leakage (particularly creatine kinase). Eccentric contractions seem to be the cause of most of this type of muscular disruption.

If this exercise-induced muscle damage results in greater protein turnover (which is by no means certain), athletes experiencing it may require increased dietary protein to maintain nitrogen balance.

Despite the preceding speculations, many researchers continue to downplay the need for protein consumption beyond RDA levels in order to achieve optimal gains in training-induced strength and muscle bulk.

In a critical interpretation of the literature, Butterfield suggested that the amount of nitrogen retention by active individuals is related to energy balance. She noted that when protein requirements are examined in the context of total energy balance, the vast majority of experimental evidence indicates the following:

1. When energy intake exceeds expenditure, nitrogen retention even with marginal protein intakes will improve with exercise.
2. When energy balance is negative, protein requirements during exercise may exceed intake even when intake is well above RDA levels.
3. When energy expenditure and intake are balanced, increases in protein intake beyond 0.8 g per kilogram of body mass per day do not result in improved nitrogen retention.

Thus, athletes who are in negative energy balance may be in negative nitrogen balance despite protein intakes exceeding the RDA, whereas athletes who are in positive energy balance may not improve their nitrogen retention by increasing protein intake beyond the RDA.

Butterfield and Calloway reported results indicating that moderate-intensity exercise itself stimulates nitrogen retention in humans. When untrained subjects increased their exercise time at 50 percent $\dot{V}O_2max$. from 1 hour to 2 hours, their rate of nitrogen retention also increased.

The duration of the training program may also affect nitrogen retention. Gontzea and colleagues reported that immediately after initiation of an exercise program nitrogen balance begins to decline toward the negative. However, after approximately 4 days this trend stops and within 2 weeks the nitrogen balance is restored to pretraining levels without any dietary manipulation. Therefore, the results of nitrogen balance studies may depend on how long after the initiation of training the studies are carried out. Also, evidence indicates differential effects of exercise on the rates of degradation of contractile and noncontractile proteins in muscle. Whether this may affect dietary protein requirements is uncertain.

Although numerous studies have demonstrated increased branched-chain amino acid oxidation as a result of increasing intensity of exercise, this fact alone does not necessarily imply nitrogen loss. Wolfe reported tracer study results indicating that much of the nitrogen that leaves the muscle as a result of amino acid oxidation does so as alanine. In the liver, much of this nitrogen may be involved in the formation of new amino acids via transamination. The remainder would be lost as urea (see Fig. 1). Thus, even though amino acid carbon skeletons may contribute significantly to ATP generation during certain types of exercise, nitrogen conservation by the liver may limit any increase in overall protein loss.

In summary, some experimental evidence indicates that there may be a small added requirement of dietary protein above the RDA of 0.8 g per kilogram of body mass per day in athletes. Other evidence indicates that as long as energy balance is maintained, the increased requirement is minimal and well within the RDA. This conclusion still needs to be rigorously examined over long periods, with a variety of exercise modes, intensities, and durations. Also, controlled experiments examining the effects of protein supplementation on the magnitude of training-induced muscle hypertrophy need to continue.

Despite these disclaimers, there currently is not enough evidence to warrant prescribing large increases in protein intake to any athletic population. Normal individuals who continue to consume approximately 15 percent of their total energy intake

TABLE 1 Diet of 12 to 13 Megajoules (3,000 Kcal), 18 Percent of Calories as Protein

		Protein	
Food Description	*Kcal*	*(g)*	*(kcal)*
Breakfast			
Milk (500 ml)	320	18	72
Cornflakes (33 g)	133	3	12
1 orange (180 g)	65	1	4
2 slices whole wheat toast (50 g)	120	6	24
Butter (14 g)	100	–	–
3 slices bacon (45 g)	90	8	32
Total Breakfast:	828	36	144
Lunch			
Brussel sprouts (78 g)	28	4	16
2 slices whole wheat bread (50 g)	120	6	24
Butter (14 g)	100	–	–
Corned beef (85 g)	185	22	88
3 chocolate chip cookies	180	3	12
Lemonade (250 ml)	110	–	–
Total Lunch:	723	35	140
Dinner			
Hamburger (170 g)	245	21	84
Hamburger bun	140	2	8
Ketchup (15 g)	15	1	4
Mashed potatoes (200 g)	190	2	8
Milk (500 ml)	320	18	72
Tomato salad (120 g)	50	5	20
Total Dinner:	960	49	196
Snacks			
Peanuts (72 g)	420	18	72
Grapefruit juice (250 ml)	100	2	8
Apple (200 g)	90	–	–
Total Snacks:	610	20	80
TOTAL:	3,121	140	560

as protein will far exceed the protein RDA, and if they include meat and dairy products in their diet, all the essential amino acids will be adequately consumed.

Increasing energy expenditure with training, if it results in an adequate increase of food intake with no change in the distribution of nutrients, should ensure an increase in protein consumption that exceeds any increase in requirements. For example, assume an athlete's energy expenditure and consumption were to increase by 4 megajoules (1,000 kcal.). If the diet continued to contain 15 percent of the energy as protein, this would already add a total of 37 g of protein to the diet.

Protein and amino acid supplements are expensive and totally unnecessary. Even individuals who continue to believe that they require dietary protein far in excess of the RDA can easily consume over 250 percent of the RDA on a relatively inexpensive, well-balanced, and normal diet. Table 1 illustrates 1 day of a 12- to 13-megajoules (3,000-kcal) diet that would supply almost 140 g of protein. If consumed by a 70-kg individual, this diet would supply 250 percent of the RDA of high-quality protein.

Thus, the best dietary advice to give competitive athletes is to continue to consume a normal, well-balanced diet.

SUGGESTED READING

Armstrong RB. Mechanisms of exercise-induced delayed-onset muscular soreness. Med Sci Sports Exerc 1984; 16:529–538.
Briggs GM, Calloway DH. Nutrition and physical fitness. New York: CBS College Publishing, 1984.
Brooks GA, Fahey TD. Exercise physiology: human bioenergetics and its applications. New York: John Wiley, 1984.
Butterfield GE. Whole-body protein utilization in humans. Med Sci Sports Exerc 1987; 19:S157–S165.
Butterfield GE, Calloway DH. Physical activity improves protein utilization in young men. Br J Nutr 1984; 51:171–184.
Dohm GL, Hecker AL, Brown WE, et al. Adaptation of protein metabolism to endurance training. Increased amino acid oxidation in response to training. Biochem J 1977; 164:705–708.
Dohm GL, Tabscott EB, Kasperek GJ. Protein degradation during endurance exercise and recovery. Med Sci Sports Exerc 1987; 19:S166–S171.
Dragan GI, Vasiliu A, Georgescu E. Effect of increased supply of protein on elite weight-lifters. In Galesloot T, Tinbergen B, eds. Milk proteins. Wageningen, Netherlands: Pudoc, 1985.
Friden J. Muscle soreness after exercise; implications of morphological change. Int J Sports Med 1984; 5:57–66.
Goldstein L, Newsholme EA. The formation of alanine from amino acids in diaphragm muscle of the rat. Biochem J 1976; 154:555–558.
Gontzea I, Sutzescu P, Dumitrache S. The influence of adaptation to physical effort on nitrogen balance in man. Nutr Rep Intern 1975; 11:131–136.
Katch FI, McArdle WD. Nutrition, weight control and exercise. Boston: Houghton Mifflin, 1977.
Lemon PW. Protein and exercise. Med Sci Sports Exerc 1987; 19:S179–S190.
Lemon PW, Nagel FJ. Effects of exercise on protein and amino acid metabolism. Med Sci Sports Exerc 1981; 13:141–149.
Lemon PW, Nagel FJ, Mullen JP, Benevenga NJ. In vivo leucine oxidation at rest and during two intensities of exercise. J Appl Physiol 1982; 53:947–954.
Tiidus PM, Ianuzzo CD. Effects of intensity and duration of muscular exercise on delayed soreness and serum enzyme activities. Med Sci Sports Exerc 1983; 15:461–465.
Williams MH. Nutrition for fitness and sport. Dubuque, IA: WC Brown, 1983.
Wolfe RR. Does exercise stimulate protein breakdown in humans? Isotope approaches to the problem. Med Sci Sports Exerc 1987; 19:S172–S178.
Worthington-Roberts BS. Proteins and amino acids. In Worthington-Roberts BS, ed. Contemporary developments in nutrition. Toronto: CV Mosby, 1981.

ANABOLIC STEROIDS AND INJURY TREATMENT

MAURO G. DI PASQUALE, B.Sc., M.D.

The anabolic influence of androgenic-anabolic steroids, and in particular their effect on the musculoskeletal system, makes this class of compound therapeutically useful for the treatment of sports injuries.

When an athlete is injured, performance deteriorates in proportion to the severity of the injury and its effect on training. In most injuries the competitor is forced to protect the injured part; that part then does less work than usual and therefore begins to undergo a catabolic response (a normal phenomenon in well-nourished athletes between seasons). The degree of the catabolic response is usually proportional to the mass of the structures involved and the severity of the injury. The result is a decrease in the strength (and in the size and density) of the involved muscles, tendons, ligament, joints, and bones in the injured area.

The catabolic response that follows most injuries may also be due to a hypogonadotropic hypogonadic state, in which there is a decrease in the production of luteinizing hormone (LH) and subsequently in testosterone. This is commonly seen in persons who have sustained major medical insults, especially in brain injuries, in which the magnitude of the hormonal dysfunction is dependent on the severity of neurologic damage.

Since the dominant action of testosterone is a stimulation of protein anabolism in most tissues, it is reasonable to assume that testosterone (and its synthetic analogues) may counteract the catabolic response that occurs in injured tissues (as a result of the relative inactivity of the injured area, and a possible reduction in testosterone secretion).

It may be questioned whether the catabolic response to injury can be modified significantly by androgens, and if so whether a clinical advantage can be gained by administration of such substances. It may also be asked whether androgenic-anabolic steroids can counteract the catabolic influence of the glucocorticosteroid injections often used in the treatment of athletic injuries. Certainly, use of glucocorticosteroids results in a catabolic response in skeletal muscles, bone, and skin and quickly leads to protein depletion. Moreover, in animal experiments, Beyler and colleagues showed that anabolic steroids reversed the catabolic effects of cortisone acetate.

For many athletes, conservative treatment for chronic injuries is often insufficient. Moreover, some athletes find the alternative of surgery (for conditions that lend themselves to effective surgical treatment) less palatable than a curtailment of their athletic careers.

Because of the gap between conservative treatment and surgery, I began using localized injections of androgenic-anabolic steroids to treat some chronic athletic injuries. These injections were used only after the potential of other therapeutic modalities, including physiotherapy, anti-inflammatory drugs, and graduated exercises had been exhausted.

After experimenting with various compounds, used alone and in combination with one another, I discovered what worked best for my patients. I found that anabolic steroids increased tissue anabolism during the period of recovery from injuries. In most patients whom I have treated with injectable anabolic steroids (and in some in whom I have used therapeutic levels of oral anabolic steroids), the overall effect has been sufficient improvement in the injury to allow the athlete to resume normal training after an appropriate period of rehabilitation and graduated exercises.

It would appear from these results that the repair that takes place under the influence of the anabolic steroid goes beyond the anticipated initial effects of the anabolic steroid itself, provided of course that the athlete's training program is modified so as to avoid reproducing the injury. It seems that once the injured tissue has been strengthened and "reinforced," it becomes better able to handle an increased workload, and the increased workload in turn has an anabolic effect on the injured tissues. Also, the rebound increase in the production of endogenous testosterone that occurs several weeks after the injection may have a further anabolic effect on the injured tissues.

INJURIES TREATED BY INJECTIONS

The two most common types of injuries that I treat with injections of anabolic steroids are chronic strains (muscle and tendon injuries) and sprains (injuries to the joint capsule and ligaments). These injuries often are a result of overuse and they involve relatively avascular tissue (tendons, ligaments, and the joint capsule).

At the time I see most of these injuries, they have become refractory to conservative treatment and have already received extensive first-line therapy (including ice, heat, rest, massage, ultrasonography, and anti-inflammatory drugs). The tissues involved in the injury have usually undergone an extended catabolic response as a result of relative inactivity, chronic inflammation, and (usually) one or more glucocorticoid injections.

The sites I most commonly use for injection are the tendons (tendinitis), the tendinous insertions, the linings of the tendons (tenosynovitis), the joints (arthritis and synovitis), and the various bursae (bursitis).

Chronic injuries that often respond to injections of anabolic steroids include the following:

1. *Injuries in and around the shoulder joint.* Rotator cuff tendinitis involving the infraspinatus, supraspinatus, and teres minor including the impingement syndrome—inflammation of the supraspinatus tendon, and possibly of the biceps tendon deep to the supraspinatus insertion); acromioclavicular inflammation and arthritis (the injections are less effective if there is radiologic evidence of arthritic changes); deltoid tendinitis, most commonly near its insertion on the shaft of the humerus; coracobrachialis tendinitis at its insertion at the coracoid process; and tendinitis involving the other rotator muscles such as the latissimus dorsi, subscapularis, teres major, and pectoralis major.

2. *Injuries in and around the scapula* (inferiorly, the latissimus dorsi; superiorly, the levator scapulae and rhomboideus minor; medially, the rhomboideus major; and laterally the teres minor and triceps).

3. *Biceps tendinitis.* The biceps tendon can be strained at the glenoid attachment, or more commonly in the bicipital groove, producing a tenosynovitis.

4. *Tennis elbow.* This group of conditions includes radiohumeral bursitis, radioulnar bursitis, and strain of the extensor-supinator aponeurosis, either at its attachment to the lateral epicondyle or directly over the radial head.

5. *Medial epicondylitis* (golfer's or Little League elbow). This condition is similar to tennis elbow except that the medial flexor-pronator muscle group is involved.

6. *Injuries to the sternoclavicular ligaments.* Anterior sprains are much more common than poste-

rior ones. Extensive disruption of these ligaments should not be treated with anabolic steroid injections; it requires surgical treatment as soon as possible.

7. *The trapezius insertion* at the base of the skull.

8. *The various musculotendinous units of the forearm.*

9. *Quadriceps tendon insertion,* with pain just above and on top of the kneecap.

In certain cases of tendinitis (especially those involving the Achilles and quadriceps-patellar tendons) the injection should not be given into the tendon proper, because the injection itself can be disruptive and can weaken the tendon's tensile strength. There is an increased incidence of rupture after injection into these particular sites.

In treating such tendons (and others that may be liable to unusual amounts of stress, such as the biceps brachii tendon in power lifters), the injection is made into the tendon sheath and the surrounding tissues, rather than the tendon substance.

Anabolic steroid injections should not be used for the treatment of acute injuries.

SIDE EFFECTS

In men, all the studies completed so far show a reversal of any side effects with a return of normal testicular function and sperm count 4 to 8 weeks after one to three therapeutic injections of an anabolic steroid. The esters of testosterone, in normal therapeutic doses, are quite safe and do not result in hepatotoxicity or any of the other severe side effects sometimes seen in athletes who chronically use high doses of oral anabolic steroids.

ANABOLIC STEROID PREPARATIONS

The compounds I now use almost exclusively are the long-acting testosterone esters. In the past I used other compounds, including nandrolone and methenolone esters, methandrostenolone tablets and suspension, and stanozolol tablets and suspension. Only the testosterone and nandrolone esters and the methandrostenolone and stanozolol tablets are available in North America. In the occasional athlete, because the type of injury did not lend itself to localized injections of anabolic steroids, I have used oral anabolic steroids. However, the results were usually not as favorable as with the injections, and the side effects were potentially more serious.

The esters of testosterone, when de-esterified or hydrolyzed by esterase enzymes, produce active testosterone, which then enters the systemic circulation. The tissues around the site of injection thus contain higher concentrations of active testosterone for a longer period than those found elsewhere in the body.

Nandrolone decanoate (Deca-Durabolin), can be detected several months after injection, it should thus be avoided in athletes who may be tested for performance-enhancing drugs.

The two compounds that I normally use are testosterone enanthate (a commercial preparation is Delatestryl) and testosterone cypionate (Depo-Testosterone). These two compounds, the longest-acting testosterone esters currently available, have proved most effective. A new testosterone ester may ultimately prove to be even more effective than the cypionate and the enanthate esters. In a 1986 study the new ester, testosterone-trans-4-N-butylcyclohexylcarboxylate (or 20-Aet-1) in an aqueous suspension, was compared with testosterone enanthate in sesame seed oil. The new ester sustained physiologically active concentrations of testosterone eight times longer than the enanthate form of testosterone. Because of its extremely long duration of action, this new ester should not be used by injured athletes who may be drug tested within 6 months of treatment.

DRUGS USED

At present I use a cocktail containing testosterone enanthate or cypionate, triamcinolone acetonide or methylprednisolone acetate, and lidocaine with epinephrine. I put the measured amounts of each compound in a vial and shake the vial vigorously to get as good a mix of water and oil as possible. For example, in treating a chronic anterior deltoid injury, I use 2 to 3 ml of testosterone enanthate (depending on the extent of the injury), 1 ml of triamcinolone acetonide, and 1 ml of 2 percent lidocaine with epinephrine.

The anesthetic agent relieves initial pain from the injection itself, but more importantly serves as a marker of the injection site.

The corticosteroid preparation reduces the acute or chronic inflammatory process, and because of the presence of the anabolic steroid, the usual catabolic response is avoided. I use the longer-acting preparations to give extended effects, thus complementing the prolonged effects of the depot testosterones.

Technique of Injection

After the usual preparation of the injection site (cleansing, draping, and so forth), I usually inject a small amount of anesthetic subcutaneously to decrease the pain of the subsequent injection with the larger-gauge needle.

Using a 5-ml syringe with a 4-cm, 21-gauge needle, I inject the solution that I have previously prepared into and around the injured area. Many of the injuries can be treated by infiltrating the preparation into the area of greatest tenderness (see earlier discussion), taking into account the local anatomy. The injection is performed carefully and slowly, periodically pulling the plunger outward to ensure that a blood vessel has not been penetrated.

During injection, the area can be palpated to make sure that the solution is reaching the desired location (as indicated by the disappearance of pain). By withdrawing the needle partly, other areas can be injected without having to repuncture the skin.

After injection, the patient is reexamined and the injured area is taken through a complete range of motion to make sure that the injected area is pain free. When a significant amount of pain or discomfort remains, the injured area can be immediately reinjected with up to one-half the initial amount of all three compounds (anabolic steroid, corticosteroid, and anesthetic agent). Treatment failures most often reflect failure to inject the appropriate space or trigger area.

RECOVERY

Within a few hours after injection, the injected site usually becomes painful, swollen, and warm, although a few athletes whom I have successfully injected have reported very little discomfort at any time. For the next 24 to 48 hours, the site is typically very tender to both palpation and movement. This tenderness is normal and lessens considerably over the ensuing 24 to 48 hours. Ice is often effective in alleviating acute discomfort. Once the tenderness and pain subside, the athlete is ready to begin rehabilitating the injured area.

The secret of a successful comeback after the anabolic steroid injection is essentially the same as when the athlete is rehabilitated by means of other, nonsurgical therapies. Function must be encouraged as quickly as possible by putting the injured area through a graduated series of exercises, each one a little more demanding than the last, until the athlete is close to the preinjury level, usually over a 6- to 8-week period.

It is important while the injured part is healing that there be no significant pain during exercise. At the first sign of pain, the exercise or movement that is causing the pain must be stopped. The movement concerned is reassessed and the style modified as needed, to spare the injured part. The athlete must also gain some insight into how the injury occurred in the first place, and training should be modified if the initial injury was thought to be secondary to faulty style or overuse.

Since no two injuries are alike, the rate of recovery varies from athlete to athlete. Most athletes are able to get the injured area into reasonable (but not top) shape within 4 to 6 weeks. Attempts to get ready for competition too soon (especially if a competitor is encouraged to work through the pain) is the most frequent cause of relapse.

SUGGESTED READING

Beyler AL, Arnold A, Potts GO. Methods for evaluating anabolic and catabolic agents in laboratory animals. J Am Med Wom Assoc 1968; 23:708–721.

Danyo JJ, Kruper JS. The illustrated handbook of injection techniques. Rahway, NJ: Merck, 1975.

Di Pasquale MG. Drug use and detection in amateur sports. Warkworth, Ontario: MGD Press, 1984.

Di Pasquale MG. Drug use and detection in amateur sports. Updates 1 to 5. Warkworth, Ontario: MGD Press, 1985–1988.

Kochakian CD, ed. Anabolic androgenic steroids. Berlin: Springer-Verlag, 1976.

Woolf PD, Hamill RW, McDonald JV, et al. Transient hypogonadotrophic hypogonadism after head trauma: effects on steroid precursors and correlation with sympathetic nervous system activity. Clin Endocrinol (Oxf) 1986; 25: 265–274.

Weinbauer GF, Marshall GR, Nieschlag E. New injectable testosterone ester maintains serum testosterone of castrated monkeys in the normal range for four months. Acta Endocrinol (Copenh) 1986; 113: 128–132.

ANABOLIC STEROIDS TO ENHANCE PERFORMANCE

MAURO G. DI PASQUALE, B.Sc., M.D.

For almost a century androgens, or at least substances produced by the testes, have been known to exert an anabolic effect on the musculoskeletal system. In 1895 Sacchi described a 9-year-old boy who at the age of 5 started growing rapidly, both in height and physical development. In 1929 Rowlands and Nicholson reported another case of a virilized 9-year-old boy. The advanced physical development in both cases was due to hormone-secreting testicular tumors. These two case reports (and many others since published) constitute the early evidence of the anabolic influence of testicular androgens and specifically of testosterone.

A comprehensive examination of the metabolic effects of testosterone in man was carried out by Kenyon in studies extending from 1938 to 1944. Kenyon described the potential of the male hormone to affect muscular growth and development, and was one of the first authors to outline possible clinical uses for testosterone.

It did not take the athletic community very long to put some of the principles outlined by Kenyon and others into practice. Since the early 1950s, the use of testosterone and testosterone analogues by athletes has escalated dramatically. Today, most world-caliber athletes use these compounds at some time during their training.

There are valid clinical reasons for using androgenic-anabolic steroids: for replacement therapy in cases of deficiency; to treat some malnourished states, osteoporosis, carcinoma of the breast, and aplastic anemias; and more recently for bleeding disorders. Unfortunately, by far the largest users of anabolic steroids (obtained by prescription or through the black market) are athletes.

DO THEY WORK?

Athletes use anabolic steroids or exogenous testosterone in an attempt to increase their muscular size and strength. Although there is some controversy in the literature about the effectiveness of anabolic steroids in enhancing performance, there is no doubt in most athletes' minds that they do work.

The predominant attitude of the scientific community has been that anabolic steroids do not enhance performance. The 1985 edition of *Goodman and Gilman's The Pharmacological Basis of Therapeutics* states that "the use of these agents does not cause an increase in muscle bulk, strength, or athletic performance—even when phenomenally large doses are used. The commonly observed increase in body weight (seen secondary to steroid use) is due to the retention of salt and water." The authors base this conclusion on the results of 25 papers that have addressed the effects of androgenic-anabolic steroids on physical strength and athletic performance in men.

Despite this, there has been some acceptance of the ergogenic effects of anabolic steroids. In a review of the literature, Haupt and Rovere concluded that if certain criteria are met (e.g., intensive training, a high protein diet, and specific measurement techniques), anabolic steroids do appear to enhance athletic performance.

The studies done so far are not comprehensive enough to provide the information needed to assess the efficacy of anabolic steroids conclusively. More work needs to be done to determine the effect of the long-term use of high dosages of anabolic steroids on athletic performance.

The efficacy of anabolic steroids as an ergogenic aid will undoubtedly be found to be dependent on many variables, including individual genetic characteristics such as receptor response and affinity, the dosage and duration of treatment, the physiologic and psychological state of the individual before and during their use, and other factors such as diet, training intensity, and the concomitant use of other hormones, drugs, and nutritional aids. It must also be remembered that the primary reason for the banning of anabolic steroid use in amateur sports by such bodies as the International Olympic Committee (IOC) is that it is suspected that they may enhance athletic performance—not their potential side effects.

DOPING CONTROL

In 1967 the IOC established a medical commission that banned the practice of doping, which it defined as the use of substances or techniques in any form or quantity alien or unnatural to the body, with the exclusive aim of obtaining an artificial and unfair increase of performance in competition. Having specified an initial list of banned substances, the IOC carried out limited doping tests at the 1968 Olympics. By 1972, new scientific and technologic knowledge enabled the IOC to increase the scope and rapidity of its testing. At the 1976 Olympics, anabolic steroids were included in the testing program, and in 1984 at Los Angeles testosterone was added. In 1987 the IOC Medical Commission changed their definition of testosterone abuse, which now reads: "For testosterone, the definition of a positive depends on the following: the administration of testosterone or the use of any other manipulation having the result of increasing the ratio in the urine of testosterone/epitestosterone to above 6."

COLLECTION AND TESTING OF SAMPLES

The procedures for selecting the athletes to be tested, and for collecting and transporting samples of urine to the testing laboratories, have been standardized for each particular athletic activity. At the laboratory, a urine sample is subjected to sophisticated, precise tests to determine whether a banned substance is present in the urine, and if so, in what concentration.

The testing of urine samples involves three basic steps: extraction, screening, and confirmation. The first step, extraction, prepares the urine for analysis. Multiple extractions are usually necessary, because many drugs are excreted not only in their original form, but also as by-products resulting from the metabolic breakdown of the original compound.

The second step, screening, is a systematic search for traces of banned substances within the extracted solutions. The screening is carried out by gas chromatography, a procedure used to distinguish individual drugs present in the urine, based on their relative volatility and solubility. The individual drugs are transported through the chromatographic column (a long, thin glass tube coated on the inside with a polymeric substance) by an inert carrier gas (such as helium). The carrier gas transports any drugs in the gaseous phase, but has no other part in the chromatographic process.

Different drugs emerge from the column at different times (depending on their special characteristics). The time when a drug appears is known as its retention time. If the retention time of the drug being analyzed is the same as the retention time for a known sample drug, the two drugs are likely to be the same, but this is not necessarily so, since many compounds can be crowded together in the same 0.1 second of retention time.

Thus, the initial screening, which serves to indicate the possible presence of a banned substance, is not specific enough to constitute definitive proof of a positive doping test.

The final identification of a substance, and confirmation of its presence, requires further testing, using a computerized gas chromatography–mass spectrometry system (GC/MS). The GC serves as a purification technique (distinguishing the banned component from all the rest), whereas MS identifies the substance by ion bombardment. In the mass spectrometer, an electron beam bombards the compound with electrons, imparting a charge to the molecules of the isolated substance, causing some of the molecules to fragment into charged particles or ions. These charged particles (which also include the charged parent compound or molecular ion) are sorted magnetically according to size and charge. An ion detector then records the presence and amount of these ions, producing a mass spectrum for the sample compound. The pattern of fragments and their proportional abundance (the mass spectrum consists of a plot of fragment mass versus relative abundance) is characteristic enough to allow a positive identification of the unknown molecule.

A computer compares the resulting mass spectrum with the many thousands of mass spectra contained in its memory banks; an exact match identifies the unknown compound. If an exact match is not made, the compound cannot be identified for the purposes of a positive doping test, even though the laboratory may suspect that the compound present in a urine sample is an anabolic steroid.

Mass spectrometry is extremely accurate in identifying substances in the urine, but it is not overly sensitive (even when selected ion monitoring is used), and if the concentration of a drug isolated by the screening process is too low, mass spectrometry will not be able to detect it and confirm its identity (hence the rationale for athletes drinking large amounts of water to produce a diluted urine sample, and for using drugs such as probenecid, which may decrease the amount of drug excreted).

In the event of a positive test, the athlete is notified of this finding and is asked to come to the laboratory (or send a representative) to observe the identical testing of a second urine sample. If the banned substance is again found in the athlete's urine, the contestant is disqualified from immediate competition, and possibly from future competitions (for whatever period the governing sports federation decides).

The IOC has imposed severe penalties on athletes found positive for certain substances. For anabolic steroids (including testosterone), amphetamine-related and other stimulants, caffeine, diuretics, beta-blockers, narcotic analgesics, and designer drugs, the penalty is a 2-year ban for a first offense and a life ban for a second offense.

ANABOLIC STEROID PREPARATIONS

The phenotypic effects produced by testosterone can be subdivided into two somewhat arbitrary categories: androgenic (producing secondary male sexual characteristics) and anabolic (mainly increasing muscle size and strength).

Most of the synthetic derivatives of testosterone have been designed to try to dissociate these two effects, and to increase the bioavailability of the steroid when it is taken orally. There is, however, no purely anabolic steroid; all have some androgenic effects. In early experimental work with animals, the dissociation was significant, but in humans it is less so. The lack of complete dissociation has led to much confusion of terminology. The terms "anabolic steroid," "androgenic steroid," "anabolic-androgenic steroid," and "androgenic-anabolic steroid" are often used interchangeably. Testosterone itself can be described as an anabolic steroid, although in practice the term usually refers to its synthetic derivatives.

Modifications of structure at any of the 19 carbon groups of testosterone are made for many reasons, including an alteration of the anabolic-androgenic ratio or the therapeutic index (ideally, anabolic effects will be increased and androgenic effects decreased); increasing the bioavailability of the drug when it is taken orally; decreasing its absorption time when it is given parenterally; and increasing the potency of the drug so that a smaller dose produces for similar results.

Current preparations of testosterone and testosterone derivatives that are used by athletes despite their official banning by the IOC include: bolasterone, boldenone, chloroxomesterone (dehydrochlormethyltestosterone), clostebol, fluoxymesterone, mesterolone, methandienone (methandrostenolone), methenolone, methyltestosterone, nandrolone, norethandrolone, oxandrolone, oxymesterone, oxymetholone, stanozolol, and testosterone in its many forms (oral and injectable).

Administration and Metabolism

Testosterone, when taken orally, is partially destroyed by the chemical and enzymatic processes of the gastrointestinal tract. The remaining testosterone crosses the gastrointestinal mucosa, whence it is conveyed to the liver by the portal system. It is promptly metabolized by the liver, so that only very small amounts (at most 5 to 10 percent of the absorbed dose) reach the systemic circulation and, therefore, the target tissues.

The 17α-alkylated compounds (methyl or ethyl groups are added at the C17α position in the steroid nucleus) are more effective when administered orally, because they largely escape degradation by the liver during their initial passage from the gut.

When given parenterally, crystalline testosterone is rapidly absorbed into the systemic circulation; the result is a relatively short burst of androgen exposure to the peripheral tissues. Several injections per day would be needed to sustain effective serum levels.

Reaction of the 17-hydroxy group with an acidic compound results in the formation of an ester; this is less soluble in water and more soluble in lipids than is crystalline testosterone. The larger the carbon chain of the acid reactant, the more insoluble is the salt formed, and the more prolonged the action of the preparation. For example, testosterone propionate (short carbon chain) is short-acting in comparison to testosterone enanthate (longer carbon chain). The esters of testosterone, when deesterified or hydrolyzed by esterase enzymes, produce active testosterone, which enters the systemic circulation.

Detection

Certain changes to the steroid molecule alter the normal process of metabolic inactivation, resulting in differences in the rate of excretion of both 17-keto steroids and the anabolic compound itself. Thus, some anabolic steroids are largely excreted unchanged, while others are highly metabolized, resulting in a large urinary output of excretory steroids. Detection of a synthetic anabolic steroid (but not testosterone) is thus possible by urinary identification of either the free form of the compound or one or more of its metabolites (depending on the metabolic and excretory profile of the specific anabolic steroid).

For example, 17-alkylation, changing the position of the double bond in ring A, methyl substitution on atoms C-1, C-2, and C-6, and 4-chloro substitution all influence the pattern of metabolism and the excretory end products of a synthetic compound as compared with testosterone. Thus, while 17α-methyl steroids (such as methandrostenolone) are mostly excreted in the free form and are not significantly metabolized to 17-ketosteroids, the 17α-ethyl and the 19-nortestosterone analogues are rapidly metabolized. The resulting metabolites, which are subsequently conjugated in the liver and excreted in the urine, can be used to identify the latter group of compounds.

Detection of testosterone is difficult, since it is endogenously produced in both males and females, and is therefore naturally present in the urine. The exogenous administration of testosterone can nevertheless be detected. It alters the endogenous hormonal profile, and it is thus a matter of comparing the relative amounts of certain hormones found in the urine.

The test now being used by IOC-accredited laboratories compares the ratio of testosterone to epitestosterone, which is normally around 1 in both males and females. Administration of exogenous testosterone increases the urinary output of testosterone, but has little effect on urinary epitestosterone. The accepted upper limit of the testosterone-epitestosterone (T-E) ratio is 6, with no units.

The upper limit for the T-E ratio is deliberately set high, so that the vast majority of drug-free steroid profiles fall well below the prescribed limit. However, it is both theoretically and clinically possible to increase the T-E ratio without administering exogenous testosterone. The question is whether the ratio under any of these conditions would exceed 6. More studies are still needed before the T-E ratio can be universally accepted as an unequivocal sign of exogenous testosterone administration.

Analytical testing for anabolic steroids and testosterone is not welcomed by everyone. Laboratory evaluation is especially unpopular with athletes who constantly seek a competitive edge by abusing drugs. Since the advent of analytical doping control, athletes have tried various ruses to make the testing procedures ineffective. They have sent impersonators to the drug-testing station; diluted the urine by using diuretics to reduce the concentration of banned substances; introduced "clean" urine into the bladder through a catheter; simulated the passage of "clean" urine from an external source; ingested such chemicals as sodium bicarbonate, phenylbutazone, probenecid, antiprostaglandins, and other compounds to mask or reduce the rate of elimination of banned substances; introduced exogenous chemicals or bacteria into the urine specimen at the time of voiding; used compounds that are obscure, such as veterinary anabolic steroids; and used compounds not yet on the banned list, such as growth hormone and human chorionic gonadotropin.

Some sophisticated and pharmacologically minded athletes are now attempting to avoid detection of their use of exogenous testosterone by taking injections of one or more of epitestosterone, dehydroepiandrosterone, and androstenedione before and/or during competitions, or by adding small amounts of crystalline, and have even conjugated glucuronide and/or sulfate forms of epitestosterone directly to the urine samples.

The list of techniques for invalidating the tests can never be complete. The inventive mind of the athlete is always searching for new methods to beat the system and the system in turn is always refining its techniques in an attempt to keep up.

SUGGESTED READING

Haupt HA, Rovere GD. Anabolic steroids: a review of the literature. Am J Sports Med 1984; 12:469–484.
Kenyon AT. The effect of testosterone propionate on the genitalia, prostate, secondary sex characters, and body weight in eunuchoidism. Endocrinology 1938; 23:121–134.
Kenyon AT. The first Josiah Macy Jr Conference on bone and wound healing. September, 1942.
Kenyon AT, Knowlton K, Lotwin G, Sandford I. Metabolic response of aged men to testosterone propionate. J Clin Endocrinol 1942; 2:690–695.
Kenyon AT, Knowlton K, Sandford I. The anabolic effects of the androgens and somatic growth in man. Ann Intern Med 1944; 20:632–654.
Rowlands RP, Nicholson GW. Growth of left testicle with precocious sexual and bodily development (macro-genitosomia). Guy's Hosp Rep 1929; 79:401–408.
Sacchi E. A case of infantile gigantism (pedomacrosomia) with a tumor of the testicle. Riv Sper Freniat 1895; 21:149–161.

EXERCISE IN DIABETIC PATIENTS

FRIEDRICH W. KEMMER, M.D.

Active participation in various kinds of physical exercise and training has become very popular both for recreational and social reasons and for its beneficial effects on general health. Thus, for almost half a century exercise was strongly recommended as a cornerstone in the treatment of diabetes because of its ability to lower blood glucose. However, during the last two decades it was realized that physical exercise should not be used indiscriminately to treat diabetes mellitus for several reasons. First, the particular effects of physical exertion differ fundamentally between type 1 and type 2 diabetes. Second, defined physical activity prescribed as a means to improve metabolic control in type 1 diabetic patients should nowadays be regarded as obsolete. Third, the overall end results from a large number of elaborate investigations are disappointing as far as the beneficial effect of physical activity on improvement of glucose tolerance in the group of non–insulin-treated type 2 diabetic patients as a whole are concerned. Nevertheless, diabetic patients should be encouraged to exercise for the same reasons as the nondiabetic population rather than for therapeutic reasons. In this context, modern diabetes therapy should preferably aim at teaching diabetic patients to reduce or prevent exercise-associated complications such as hypoglycemia or hyperglycemia and coronary events. Since many physiologic and pathophysiologic mechanisms operative during exercise in diabetes have already been reviewed in detail, we will briefly summarize the pathophysiologic background and focus mainly on reviewing the practical aspects of exercise in the management of diabetes.

GLUCOREGULATION DURING EXERCISE IN NORMAL INDIVIDUALS AND INSULIN-TREATED DIABETIC PATIENTS

In normal humans the major energy-yielding substrates for resting and working muscles are glucose and free fatty acids (FFA). Glucose and FFA are derived from the circulation and depots in the liver, in adipose tissue, and in the muscle itself. Their relative contribution to the energy needs of the muscle depends on the state of nutrition and training as well as the duration and intensity of exercise. In the postabsorptive state, the resting muscle oxidizes mainly FFA stemming from adipose tissue. With the onset of exercise the muscle increases the use of glucose, which during the initial exercise period is mainly derived from glycogen stores in the working muscle. As exercise continues, plasma glucose serves as the major source for the increased glucose needs of the working muscle.

The increased glucose uptake during exercise in normal humans is precisely matched by glucose originating from the liver, from intestinal absorption, or both. This mechanism makes it possible to maintain normoglycemia and to supply sufficient energy for all vital organs during the performance of exercise. Although the precise nature of the coordination of glucose production and glucose utilization during exercise is not yet completely understood, the principal role of insulin in regulating hepatic glucose production during exercise is fairly well established. With the onset of exercise, insulin secretion decreases almost instantaneously. As a result, hypoinsulinemia and relative hyperglucagonemia can be found in portal blood, facilitating an increased hepatic glucose output that exactly matches the increased peripheral uptake of glucose (Fig. 1). Catecholamines released from the adrenal medulla or from nerve endings in the liver and the pancreas appear to play an important role in the immediate suppression of insulin and in stimulating hepatic glucose production rapidly, while cortisol and

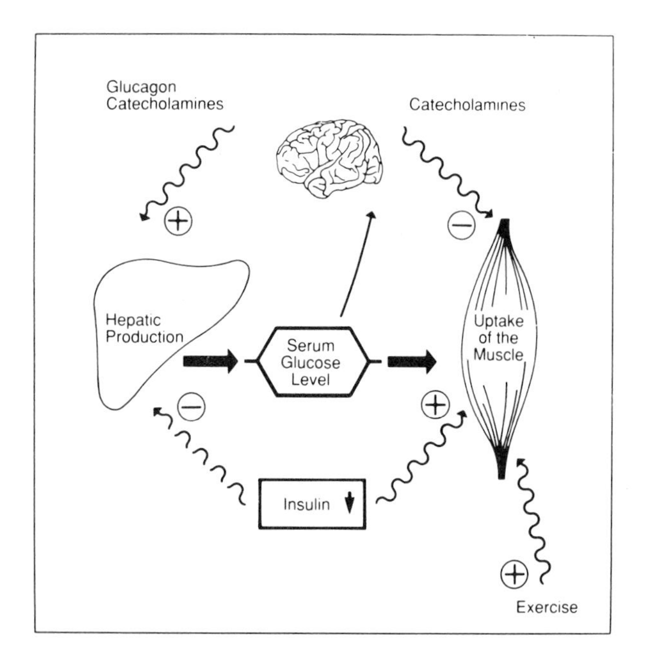

Figure 1 Schema of glucose homeostasis during exercise under physiologic conditions. Straight arrows indicate fuel fluxes. Curved arrows indicate stimulatory and inhibitory effects. (Republished with permission from Kemmer FW, Berger M. Exercise. In: Alberti KGMM, DeFronzo RA, Keen H, Zimmet P, eds. The international textbook of diabetes mellitus. New York: John Wiley, 1988.)

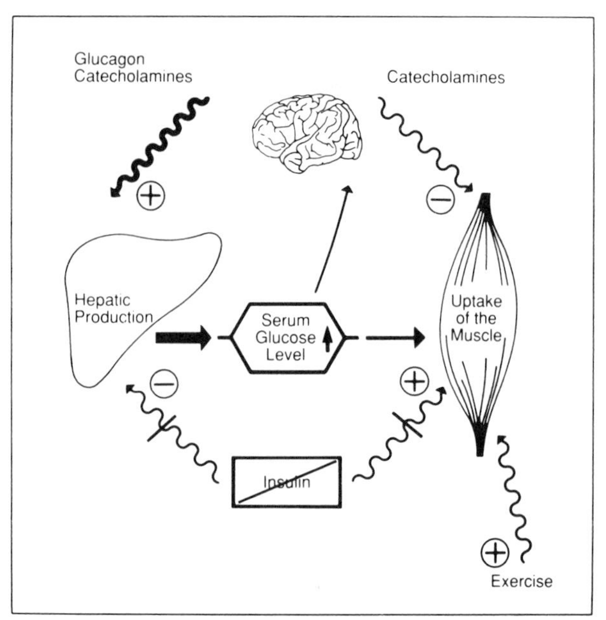

Figure 2 Schema of glucose homeostasis during exercise in the presence of insulin lack. Straight arrows indicate fuel fluxes. Curved arrows indicate stimulatory and inhibitory effects. (Republished with permission from Kemmer FW, Berger M. Exercise. In: Alberti KGMM, DeFronzo RA, Keen H, Zimmet P, eds. The international textbook of diabetes mellitus. New York: John Wiley, 1988.)

growth hormone are apparently less important in increasing hepatic glucose production at the onset of muscular activity. The decrease in plasma insulin levels has no bearing on glucose uptake during exercise, because the working muscle needs only minute concentrations of insulin to increase glucose uptake.

In type 1 diabetic patients, the basic mechanism of glucoregulation during exercise is impaired because various states of insulin deficiency or excess may be present in peripheral and portal blood. Depending on the circulating insulin levels, physical activity in insulin-treated diabetic patients may therefore lead to a deterioration in or improvement of metabolic control, i.e., a rise or fall in glycemia, ketone bodies, and FFA. If usual insulin injections are withheld for any reason, severe insulin deficiency occurs. Under this condition, during performance of physical exercise, hepatic glucose production will rise without restraint and exceed peripheral glucose uptake, which is impaired owing to insulin lack. As a consequence, blood glucose levels increase progressively (Fig. 2). Under usual circumstances, subcutaneous insulin administration is associated with hyperinsulinemia. In this situation, glucose utilization is not restrained, but the excess insulin prevents an adequate rise in hepatic glucose production. As a result, glycemia falls gradually and hypoglycemia is likely to develop (Fig. 3). These

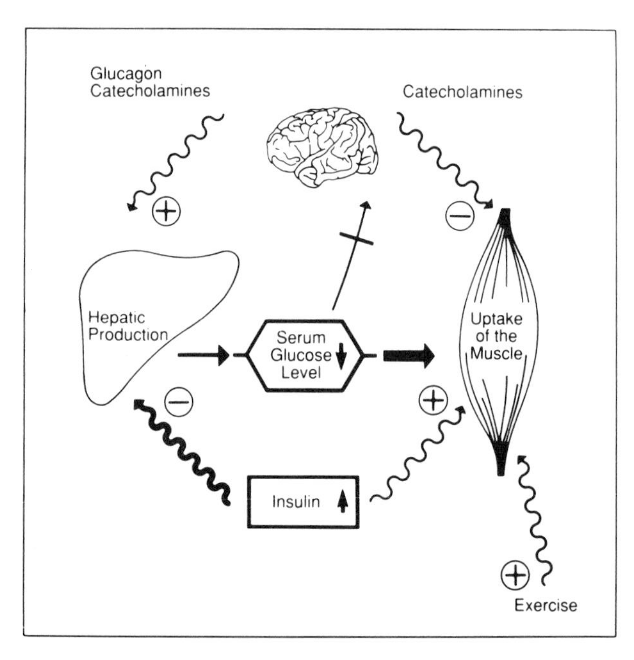

Figure 3 Schema of glucose homeostasis during exercise in the presence of hyperinsulinemia. Straight arrows indicate fuel fluxes. Curved arrows indicate stimulatory and inhibitory effects. (Republished with permission from Kemmer FW, Berger M. Exercise. In: Alberti KGMM, DeFronzo RA, Keen H, Zimmet P, eds. The international textbook of diabetes mellitus. New York: John Wiley, 1988.)

mechanisms represent the principal impairments of glucoregulation during exercise in diabetes, and serve to explain two serious but preventable metabolic complications: hyperglycemia and hypoglycemia.

PHYSICAL EXERCISE IN PATIENTS WITH TYPE 1 DIABETES MELLITUS

The principal problem in using exercise for treatment of type 1 diabetic patients is that the amount by which exercise lowers glycemia is hardly predictable. Factors that influence the glycemic response to exercise include the blood glucose level and the state of nutrition before exercise, the time of day exercise is begun, the duration and intensity of exercise, the state of physical training of the patient, and the type and dose of insulin injected. Thus, in order to take systematic advantage from physical exercise on a long-term basis, the patient would need to exercise every day, preferably postprandially for a defined period and at a defined workload. Unfortunately, this kind of treatment would add even more restrictions on the daily schedule, which already is largely determined by insulin injections at mealtimes. In addition, several studies have clearly demonstrated that no improvement of metabolic control can be achieved by regular performance of physical exercise. Since good metabolic control can be achieved and maintained by much simpler means, such as adaption of the insulin dose on the basis of regular glucose self-monitoring, only a minority of type 1 diabetic patients may agree to such a rigid exercise regimen.

Nevertheless, like most healthy people, type 1 diabetic patients like to exercise to promote general health and for recreational or competitive purposes. Because most patients exercise mainly on weekends, in the evenings, and during holidays, physical activity is largely spontaneous, and the time, duration, and intensity of exercise vary. Consequently, type 1 diabetic patients must be able to prevent the development of hyper- and hypoglycemia during their physical activity.

GUIDELINES TO PREVENT METABOLIC COMPLICATIONS DURING EXERCISE IN TYPE 1 DIABETES

The guidelines for preventing severe ketoacidoses during exercise can be laid down very briefly. Blood glucose levels above 300 or 350 mg per deciliter associated with marked acetonuria indicate severe insulin deficiency. Exercise performed in this state is likely to deteriorate metabolic control even further. Therefore, patients who detect these indices of insulin deficiency should not exercise, but instead should first administer adequate amounts of insulin to restore satisfactory metabolic control. Only after glycemia has been normalized may these patients start to exercise.

Patients usually are faced with the problem of how to prevent hypoglycemia during exercise. Considering that in normal individuals circulating insulin levels decrease during exercise, the most logical approach would be to mimic this situation in diabetic patients by reducing the insulin dose before the onset of exercise. However, this approach is useless if the patient has already injected the insulin. In this case, supplementation of hepatic glucose production by increasing carbohydrate ingestion before, during, and after the physical activity remains the only way to prevent exercise-induced hypoglycemia.

The injection of insulin in a nonmoving part of the body has been shown to be ineffective as a safeguard against hypoglycemia during exercise. Thus, only a reduction of insulin dosage or the intake of additional amounts of carbohydrate can be used to minimize the risk of hypoglycemia during or after exercise. This recommendation sounds simple, but in clinical practice it meets with a number of difficulties with regard to how much the insulin dosage should be reduced and how much additional carbohydrate should be consumed. When adapting the insulin dose or carbohydrate intake to prevent hypoglycemia during exercise, the patient has to take into consideration the time, duration, and intensity of exercise; the level of glycemia and the state of nutrition at the onset of exercise; and last but not least his or her physical fitness. Consequently, a specific recommendation to fit every diabetic patient and every conceivable condition can hardly be given. Nevertheless, a few general rules of thumb can be laid down.

Short and relatively mild physical exercise, such as a sprint, walking, ½ hour of light swimming, and so forth, does not require changes of insulin dosage. Additional carbohydrates taken before or after such mild physical activity will be sufficient to cover the increased energy needs of the working muscle and to prevent hypoglycemia. In such situations a reduction of the insulin dosage may result in hyperglycemia a few hours after the physical activity.

If the patient expects to exercise for a longer time, e.g., taking part in a hiking tour, long distance running, jogging, or cross-country skiing, he or she should preferably reduce the insulin dose. When the patient has a normal blood sugar level and starts to exercise in the morning 30 to 60 minutes after breakfast, a drastic reduction of the morning insulin dose by more than 50 percent appears to be necessary to sustain exercise for 3 or more hours. At blood sugar levels above normal, e.g., between 200 and 300 mg per deciliter, a less substantial reduction of the insulin dosage will be sufficient. In any case, a dosage reduction of only a few units of insulin would be entirely sufficient to prevent exercise-induced hypoglycemia.

The dosage reduction, however, is practicable only when the patient can foresee the time and duration of physical activity. When exercise is spontaneous, only ingestion of extra carbohydrates can prevent hypoglycemia. No doubts exist about the efficacy of this measure, because glucose stemming from intestinal absorption is oxidized almost completely by the working muscle if sufficient amounts of insulin are available. The additional carbohydrates should be ingested in small amounts before, during, and/or after the physical activity to avoid exercising on a full stomach. In addition to the usual carbohydrate-containing food, other rapidly absorbable carbohydrates, in the form of liquids or chocolate bars, may be used to supplement the increased glucose needs of the working muscle.

Since many patients exercise during the late afternoon or early evening, prevention of exercise-induced nocturnal hypoglycemia needs particular attention from both patient and physician. Nocturnal postexercise hypoglycemia is likely to occur because the muscle continues to take up more glucose after cessation of exercise in order to replenish its glycogen stores. In order to prevent hypoglycemia, patients should be advised to reduce the insulin dosage in the evening, and also after they have performed physical exercise. If both regular and intermediate-acting insulin are usually injected in the evening, the dosage reduction should focus mainly on the regular insulin and less on the intermediate-acting insulin. In addition to the dosage reduction of insulin, supplementary amounts of carbohydrates may be taken after physical activity of more than half an hour in the afternoon or evening, in order to facilitate replenishment of muscular glycogen stores.

Continuous subcutaneous insulin infusion (CSII) is now an established form of insulin therapy that many patients use as their preferential form of treatment. For such patients, in principle the same rules apply to prevent metabolic complications during exercise as for people on conventional insulin treatment. If, for example, a patient wants to exercise at a mild workload for 30 to 40 minutes and starts the exercise 60 minutes after the previous meal, it is sufficient to reduce the "basal rate" by 50 percent during the exercise period. When moderate exercise of longer duration is performed, e.g., jogging or swimming, the patient should be advised to take off the pump altogether as long as he or she exercises and to reduce the "basal rate" afterward by 25 percent for up to several hours, depending on the blood sugar level. In addition to this measure, the last premeal bolus before the exercise period may be reduced by 50 percent if the physical activity is more exhausting and of very long duration, e.g., mountain climbing or a long hiking tour.

These general guidelines can serve only as a starting point for individual patients to discover how they personally react to the physical exercise of their choice under varying conditions. Thus, diabetic patients who want to exercise must be offered an intensive and comprehensive teaching program for self-management of metabolic control. In applying frequent blood glucose measurements, they will know the actual blood glucose level before they start to exercise, and may discover how they personally react to the physical exercise of their choice under various conditions. On the basis of their own observations and measurements, patients must decide which preventive measure is the most appropriate for the actual situation. Large variations among patients are likely to occur, underlining the absolute necessity for individual experience. As the personal experience of patients grows and their success in preventing hypoglycemia and other exercise-related complications increases, exercise can be performed safely and with optimal physical performance. The success of diabetic athletes and the activities of the International Diabetic Athletes Association have impressively documented that this is wholly possible.

Other Exercise-Related Complications in Type 1 Diabetic Patients

Previous restrictions for diabetic patients on participation in certain sports disciplines have largely been abandoned by many leading diabetes centers around the world. As for nondiabetic individuals, safe participation in more dangerous sports activities, such as alpine mountaineering or diving, requires thorough counseling and, in particular, adequate information for the teammates. Any sport or game is suitable as long as it increases the quality of life.

Last, and perhaps most important, there are a number of exercise-related contraindications of which both the physician and diabetic patient must be aware. Autonomic neuropathy may interfere with the cardiovascular reflexes necessary to maintain cardiac output and blood pressure during physical exertion. Such patients may be at risk of developing hypotensive episodes during or after exercise. Loss of sensory function due to peripheral polyneuropathy may create a serious risk of traumatic injury to the feet. Finally, an exercise-induced increase in blood pressure may cause acute complications in diabetic patients with (pre-) proliferative retinopathy. For these last, the advice of an ophthalmologist should be sought and laser treatment carried out before participation in physical activities may be recommended.

PHYSICAL ACTIVITY IN THE TREATMENT OF TYPE 2 DIABETES MELLITUS

In patients with type 2 diabetes mellitus a complex syndrome of hyperglycemia, insulin resistance, and often a variety of interrelated cardiovascular risk factors such as hypertension and hyperlipoproteinemia can be found. As a consequence, longevity in these patients is primarily influenced by the development of macroangiopathy rather than by diabetic microvascular complications. Whereas in type 1 diabetic patients deficiency of endogenous insulin is the primary defect, the metabolic disorder in type 2 diabetic patients is linked to insulin resistance due to a receptor or postreceptor defect. Therefore, any treatment of this metabolic syndrome should aim at increasing insulin sensitivity. From a pathophysiologic point of view, such a therapeutic approach would be fundamental, as opposed to any treatment involving beta-cytotropic drugs. Along with weight reduction, physical exercise and training must a priori be regarded as a rational approach to the treatment of type 2 diabetes mellitus.

Although the beneficial effects of physical training in reducing cardiovascular risk factors are fairly well established, the ability of increased physical activity to improve glucose tolerance together with insulin sensitivity in patients with type 2 diabetes mellitus is less well documented. The evidence in support of such an association between increased physical activity and glucose metabolism has been largely derived from experiments in nondiabetic animals. Prospective studies in Zucker rats, genetically hyperglycemic obese rodents, have documented that physical activity may be instrumental in preventing the development of insulin resistance.

In humans only epidemiologic studies in Pacific populations are suggestive of a possible role of physical inactivity in increasing the incidence of type 2 diabetes in this region of the world. In contrast, in glucose-intolerant or type 2 diabetic men, a multitude of studies have been carried out aiming to demonstrate improved glucose tolerance or glycemic control.

In most of these studies exercise training improved insulin sensitivity, decreased fasting blood glucose levels, and improved Hemoglobin A_{IC}, but the studies have not shown the anticipated beneficial effects of physical training on glucose tolerance. Only in a few selected subgroups of type 2 diabetic patients, i.e., in relatively healthy, fairly young, and hyperinsulinemic patients, have clear-cut positive effects of physical activity and training on glucose tolerance been documented. Nevertheless, even in such favorable circumstances the duration of the beneficial training effects remains to be elucidated. The critical evaluation of these overall disappointing results from a large number of elaborate investigations at a recent National Institutes of Health Consensus Development Conference gave rise to skepticism as to the general beneficial effects of physical training programs as part of the treatment of type 2 diabetes mellitus.

Against these potential and as yet not fully explored benefits of physical training programs, one has to balance the possible risks and disadvantages associated with physical training programs. First, many of these patients manifest atherosclerosis and coronary heart disease that may precipitate acute cardiovascular complications. Thus, type 2 diabetic patients need to be specifically screened for cardiovascular risks and diseases before participation in any such training program. Second, training programs should be designed and carried out under professional and medical supervision, taking into account that most elderly type 2 diabetic patients have not been physically active for some time and thus are particularly vulnerable to all kinds of injuries. Third, patients treated with insulin, oral sulfonylureas, or both are likely to develop exercise-induced hypoglycemia. Such patients must be advised to adapt their insulin dosage and reduce the sulfonylurea dosage, respectively, before exercise. Finally, the age-related multimorbidity, physical disability, and apparent lack of motivation for prolonged cooperation have been shown to interfere heavily with the feasibility of physical training programs in elderly type 2 diabetic patients.

Thus, physical training programs may be of benefit only for certain subgroups of type 2 diabetics, mainly those below the age of 60 who have not yet developed cardiovascular complications, and those who are at risk of developing diabetes or have just manifested the disease.

SUGGESTED READING

Assal JP, Mühlhauser I, Pernet A, et al. Patient education as the basis for diabetes care in clinical practice and research. Diabetologia 1985; 28:602–613.

Becker-Zimmerman K, Berger M, Berchtold P, et al. Treadmill training improves intravenous glucose tolerance and insulin sensitivity in fatty Zucker rats. Diabetologia 1982; 22:468–474.

Berger M, Berchtold P, Cüppers HJ, et al. Metabolic and hormonal effects of muscular exercise in juvenile type diabetics. Diabetologia 1977; 13:355–365.

Kemmer FW. Diabetes und Sport ohne Probleme: Praktische Hinweise für diabetische Kinder und Jugendliche sowie deren Eltern. Mainz: Kirchheim Verlag, 1986.

Kemmer FW, Berchtold P, Berger M, et al. Exercise-induced fall of blood glucose in insulin treated diabetics unrelated to alteration in insulin mobilization. Diabetes 1979; 28:1131–1137.

Kemmer FW, Berger M. Exercise and diabetes mellitus: physical activity as a part of daily life and its role in the treatment of diabetic patients. Int J Sports Med 1983; 4:77–88.

Kemmer FW, Berger M. Therapy and better quality of life: the dichotomous role of exercise in diabetes mellitus. Diabetes/Metabolism Rev 1986; 2:53–68.

Kemmer FW, Berger M. Exercise. In: Alberti KGMM, DeFronzo RA, Keen H, Zimmet P, eds. The international textbook of diabetes mellitus. New York, John Wiley, (in press).

Kemmer FW, Tacken M, Berger M. On the mechanism of exercise induced hypoglycemia during sulfonylurea treatment. Diabetes 1987; 36:1178–1187.

Kemmer FW, Vranic M. The role of glucagon and its relationship to other glucoregulatory hormones in exercise. In: Orci L, Unger RH, eds. Glucagon. Contemporary endocrinology series. New York: Elsevier North Holland, 1981:297–331.

Krzentkowski G, Pirnay F, Pallikarakis N, et al. Glucose utilization during exercise in normal and diabetic subjects: the role of insulin. Diabetes 1981; 30:983–989.

National Institutes of Health. Consensus Development Conference on diet and exercise in non–insulin-dependent diabetes mellitus. Diabetes Care 1987; 10:639–644.

Skarfors ET, Wegener TA, Lithell H, Selinus I. Physical training as treatment for type 2 (non–insulin-dependent) diabetes in elderly men. A feasibility study over 2 years. Diabetologia 1987; 30:930–933.

Vranic M, Berger M. Exercise and diabetes mellitus. Diabetes 1979; 28:147–167.

Wallberg-Henriksson H, Gunnarson R, Henricksson J, et al. Increased peripheral insulin sensitivity and muscle mitochondrial enzymes but unchanged blood glucose control in type I diabetics after physical training. Diabetes 1982; 31:1044–1050.

Wasserman D, Vranic M. Exercise, fitness and diabetes. In: Bouchard C, ed. The scientific proceedings of the International Conference on Exercise Fitness and Health. Champaign, IL: Human Kinetics, in press, 1989.

Yki-Järvinen H, De Fronzo RA, Koivisto VA. Normalization of insulin sensitivity in type 1 diabetic subjects by physical training during insulin pump therapy. Diabetes Care 1984; 7:520–527.

Zimmet P, Faaiuso S, Ainuu J, et al. The prevalence of diabetes in the rural and urban Polynesian population of Western Samoa. Diabetes 1981; 30:45–51.

EMERGENCY TREATMENT OF DIVING INJURIES

R. SUKE, M.D., B.Eng., C.C.F.P.
G.D. HARPUR, M.D., C.C.F.P.

In order to approach the management of diving injuries logically, some understanding of the way in which the diver is affected by the environment is essential. The aquatic environment exposes the diver to the usual risks of drowning and near-drowning shared with other swimmers. By virtue of the descents and ascents divers make, they are also subject to the effects of pressure changes, which can result in a series of problems unique to divers. Failure to understand these problems has resulted in unnecessary delays in treatment, aggravation of injuries, and death. Unfortunately, diving deaths usually involve fit, young people nearing their full potential.

DIVING PHYSICS

To understand the pressure changes, we must briefly review some principles of physics. Boyle's law states that if the absolute pressure acting on a given volume of gas is varied, that volume will vary in inverse proportion to the change of pressure. Therefore, taking 1 liter of air from the water surface (1 atmosphere absolute pressure or 1 ATA) to 10 m (33 feet) under water (2 ATA) doubles the pressure and reduces the volume to 500 ml. Conversely, bringing a volume of 1 liter from a depth of 30 m (99 feet) or 4 ATA to 10 m or 2 ATA will cause its expansion to 2 liters, and if ascent is continued to the surface it will yield 4 liters.

This effect has significant implications for all air-containing spaces, in or exposed to the body. Middle ears, sinuses, mask space, lungs, and gut must all be able to permit equalization of the gas that they contain, or injury may follow with either reduction or expansion of this gas. This type of injury is called barotrauma.

Henry's law deals with the effect that pressure has on the amounts of gas dissolved in body fluids. In simple terms, it states that reducing or increasing the pressure of a gas to which fluids are exposed will proportionately vary the amount of that gas held in solution (e.g., if 5 ml of nitrogen can be dissolved in 1 liter of blood at 1 ATA, 10 ml would dissolve at 2 ATA, 20 ml at 4 ATA, and so on). Conversely, blood saturated with nitrogen (N^2) at 4 ATA would seek to eliminate 15 ml of N_2 when the diver returned to a pressure of 1 ATA at the water surface. This effect has implications for all body fluids, but since exposure of tissues remote from the lungs is dependent on secondary transport of gas via the circulation, significant time elements become involved. Exceeding the limits imposed by this situation can result in supersaturation of body fluids, bubble formation within the tissues, and a series of effects together described as "decompression sickness."

The direct and immediate physiologic effects of gases are proportional to the absolute pressure (or partial pressure) of those gases in breathing mixtures. Therefore, carbon monoxide (CO) uptake from a gas mixture and the narcotic effect of nitrogen in breathing mixtures are both proportional to depth. For the same reason a gas mixture that contains some CO may be non-toxic at 1 ATA, but may become deadly at 4 ATA. Conversely, a diver who runs out of air at 30 m may be alert and conscious when he leaves the bottom of a lake, but may become critically hypoxic and unconscious during ascent, owing to the falling absolute pressure of the remaining oxygen(O_2).

SPECIFIC INJURIES

Squeeze and Reverse Squeeze

Those problems arising as a result of failure to equalize the air content of spaces during descent are called "squeezes."

Middle Ear

The most common space to be affected is the middle ear. The extent of injury depends on the overpressure encountered and on the specific strength of the tissues.

Mild stress (failure to equalize pressures for a water depth of 1.5 to 2 m) causes some pain in the ears and minimal injury to the eardrum. More severe pressure differentials increase the intensity of pain and can result in hemorrhage or rupture. If hemorrhage occurs into the middle ear at depth, it may equalize the space quite nicely, but on return to the surface the trapped gas will remain at the pressure of depth unless the blood can exit via the eustachian tube. If this is not possible, the tympanic membrane (TM) is stretched outward, with consequent pain and occasionally rupture and bloody discharge.

Similar problems may involve the sinuses, but owing to the absence of a tympanic membrane there may be much less awareness of the condition. Squeeze results if there is an obstruction to the ostium of a sinus due to allergy, polyp, infection, or upper respiratory infection. The pressure differential may cause mild pain during descent, and if the maxillary sinus is involved, it may also present as a toothache. On return to the surface, there may be slight epistaxis, or blood may be coughed up from the posterior pharynx, and there is also likely to be a residual ache in the region of the affected sinus. If the ache is severe and increases after surfacing, it is suggestive of a reverse squeeze, which occurs in the same manner as described for the ears.

Treatment. Although often painful, these conditions are not life threatening in themselves. Treatment is twofold. First, institute measures to reassure the diver and relieve pain. Mild analgesics are usually sufficient, but measures to reduce nasal congestion may also be helpful. Topical agents such as xylometazoline hydrochloride (Otrivin), phenylephrine hydrochloride (Neo-Synephrine), saline, or systemic pseudoephedrine hydrochloride (Sudafed) may prove effective. In severe reverse ear squeeze, myringotomy may be appropriate. The inferior anterior quadrant should be approached, and a minimal radial incision or prick with the point of a long No. 20 needle will suffice. If a chamber is available, a shallow (max 6 m) dive after decongestion may relieve the block in both reverse sinus and ear squeeze.

In the event of perforation of the eardrum, observation is generally all that is required. The defects are usually tiny, close with serum within hours, and are well healed in a week. Antibiotics are used only if unusual risk exists (e.g., after diving in contaminated water, or if a later indication arises such as fever, discharge, or pain). In all cases, the problems observed resolve with time, and the diver can return to underwater sport once any perforations are well healed and ear pressures can be equalized easily on the surface. There is no simple test for patency of the sinuses, but in all cases of continued difficulty correctable causes should be sought. This requires direct examination of the nose and nasopharynx for evidence of allergy, polyps, or infections. X-ray examination of the sinuses may also be necessary.

The second phase of treatment involves educating divers about the necessity to heed any discomfort in the ears and sinus regions, and making them aware of the importance of learning proper pressure equalization procedures.

Mask

Mask squeeze is frightening, but is not a serious injury. It results from a failure to equalize pressure in the space between the diver's face and the mask, and it causes a variable degree of edema and hemorrhage into the tissues of the face and eyes thus exposed. Signs can vary from just a few petechial hemorrhages in the skin and conjunctivae to a mask-shaped bruise and swelling of the face so severe as to close the eyes. Subconjunctival hemorrhage may be extensive enough to obscure the whole of the sclera.

Treatment. A mask squeeze requires only reassurance and education of the diver regarding equalization of the pressure within the mask space.

Gut

If a diver swallows much gas at depth, or drinks carbonated beverages just before a dive, the expansion of this gas can lead to severe abdominal pain during ascent and a crowding of the diaphragm. Similar consequences can result from evolution of bowel gas after some meals.

The principal hazard of this occurrence lies in the fact that the pain may induce panic and lead to other injury. Divers may present with concern about this sort of pain, which is typically terminated by a large expulsion of gas from either or both ends of the gastrointestinal tract. Persistent pain must be investigated, to rule out more serious causes, but the distended hyperresonant gut, the history, and the absence of other clinical findings usually make the cause obvious.

Treatment. Antacids with antifoaming agents may help the stomach. Breathing 100 percent 0_2 by mask speeds absorption of swallowed gas from the gut, and as time passes, so does the gas. Severe pain may require analgesics, and rarely a nasogastric tube may also be indicated. Education regarding dietary practices is important.

Lungs

A direct lung squeeze during descent is possible, but the conditions required to produce it are not likely to be encountered in normal sports diving.

In contrast, a reversed lung squeeze or burst lung syndrome can give rise to arterial gas embolism (AGE), the second most common cause of death in scuba divers after drowning and a frequent precipitant of drowning.

Burst lung can occur in one of two ways. If a diver panics or for some other reason holds the breath while ascending, the lungs expand to their full capacity as the gas within them obeys the dictates of Boyle's law. Once full capacity has been reached, further expansion will be resisted for a short distance until the overpressure caused by continued ascent reaches 75 to 100 cm of water pressure. The lung tissue then tears, and gas escapes. This degree of overpressure can be achieved in any body of water deeper than 1.5 m (including backyard pools), if the diver takes a full breath at the bottom and then holds the breath on ascent. The amount of gas released into tissues is usually large, and further expansion in volume will take place if the rupture has occurred at significant depth. The other manner in which this injury can occur is by obstruction of the airway to a small segment of the lung. This can arise as result of lung scars, mucous plugging, bronchospasm, congenital cysts or blebs, and in some circumstances dynamic airway closure with continuous exhalation during ascent. The last becomes more likely if the exhalation is especially forceful and continued to low lung volumes. Injury due to regional trapping of gas in the lungs will result in the release of smaller volumes of gas, perhaps only a few milliliters.

However the gas is released, the significance of the event depends on where the gas tracks. If it tracks into the pleural space, a pneumothorax results. If this occurs at depth, even a small amount of air can become a deadly tension pneumothorax as the diver surfaces. Gas can also migrate along the airways to the mediastinum, and result in a pneumomediastinum of a degree sufficient to compromise the circulation by exerting pressure on the heart and great vessels. Further migration along the trachea can give rise to dysphonia and emphysema of the neck structures.

Arterial Gas Embolism

The most devastating effects are caused by gas entering the circulation. Gas emboli may then be distributed by the arterial circulation as AGE. With massive volumes of gas, every tissue in the body becomes embolized. This situation rapidly results in death of the diver despite attempts at resuscitation.

Owing to the normal anatomy of vascular structures, the cerebral circulation is the most likely to be embolized in the upright diver. The consequences may range from minor dysfunction, for very small bubbles, to the equivalent of a massive cerebrovascular accident, with convulsion and coma. With minor degrees of embolization, the findings may be subtle, requiring meticulous neurologic evaluation, including the assessment of personality and complex functions. In more serious cases, emboli can be seen in the fundi and there may be a blotchy pattern on the tongue. Hemoptysis is frequently present. The burst lung syndrome often presents with a combination of the problems described (AGE and pneumothorax). Unconsciousness under water usually leads to drowning, and therefore minimal cerebral AGE should be suspected in all drownings or near-drownings in divers.

Despite the extent of injury that can result, victims who receive proper treatment and support can survive lesser degrees of injury and make a total recovery. Treatment guidelines are outlined in the section on management of serious injuries, and in Figure 1.

Dissolved Gas

Carbon Monoxide

The next group of injuries are those resulting from dissolved gas. First, because of the effects of increased pressure, toxic material in air supplies rapidly becomes more toxic at depth. CO is the commonest toxic agent encountered. A bad air supply must be suspected if a diver becomes confused at depth and unconscious when returned to the surface; suspicion is particularly great if several divers are afflicted. Treatment is the same as for any other cause of CO intoxication, but care must be taken to exclude other disorders.

Narcosis

Confusion at depths greater than 30 m may be caused by nitrogen narcosis, but this vanishes with return to the surface and thereafter requires no treatment. Narcosis may affect judgment and thus lead to other injuries.

Decompression Sickness

While under water a diver's body absorbs nitrogen in accordance with Henry's law. Owing to variations in circulation and diffusion rates, more time is required for some tissues to take on and eliminate gas. On ascent, an excess of gas accumulates in parts of the body. This gas must be eliminated, or significant numbers of tiny bubbles will develop. Such bubbles have various effects, depending on their location.

Chokes. Blood equilibrates rapidly as it passes through the lungs, but if a very rapid ascent from a long, deep dive is made, enough bubbling can occur to affect the lung. This will cause the "chokes,"

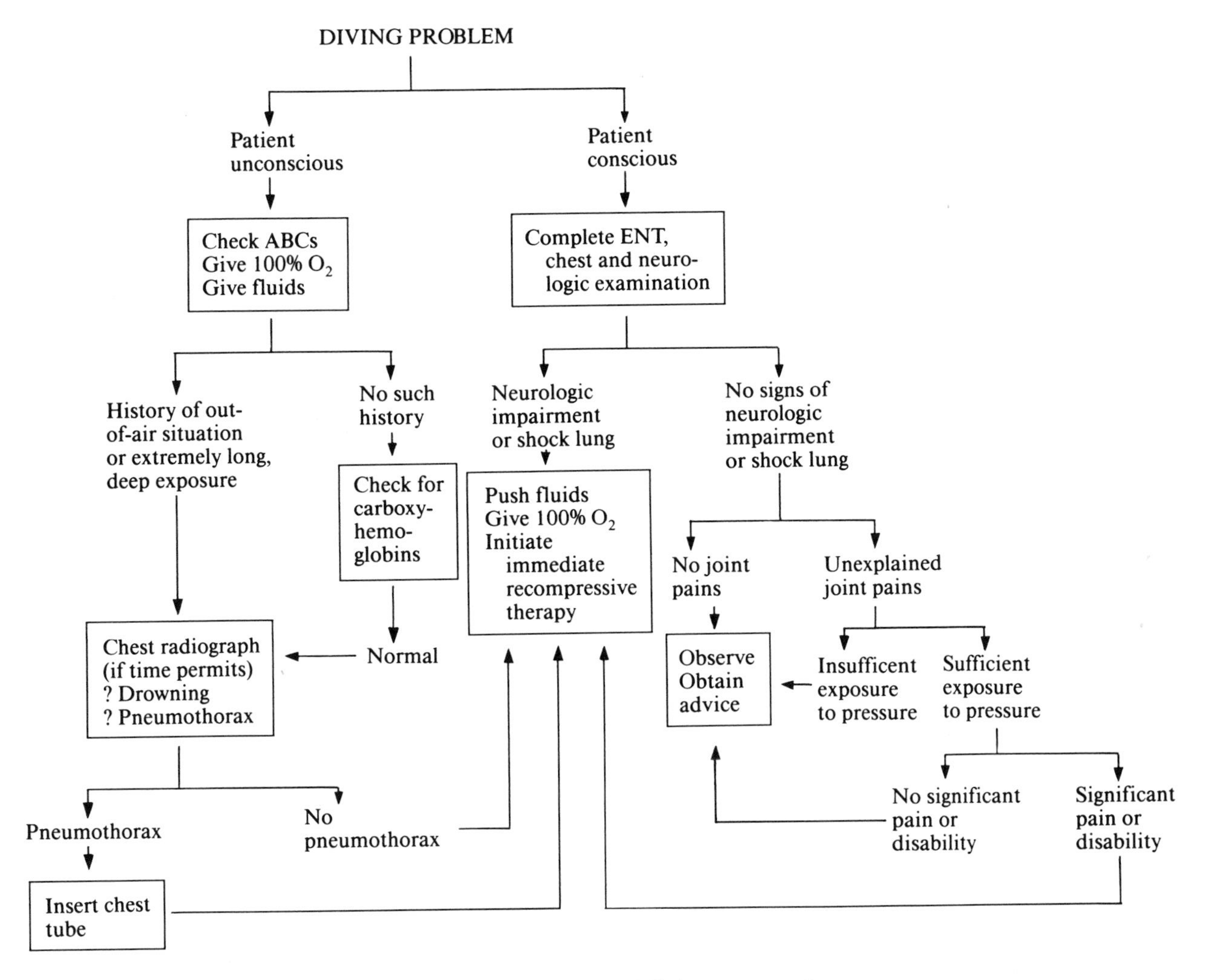

Figure 1 Management of diving emergencies.

a tight cough, tachycardia, tachypnea, and retrosternal chest pain. Without prompt recompression, severe cases usually lead rapidly to cardiovascular collapse, shock, and death.

Neurologic Conditions. Although less life threatening, the sequelae of neurologic decompression sickness are significant.

The problems can range from an alteration in cerebral function that can mimic AGE or a cerebrovascular accident to spinal cord dysfunction affecting only the lower limbs, or on occasion just bladder function. Spinal cord lesions are more common with decompression sickness than with AGE, and often start with a girdle-like pain and paresthesia in the lower limbs.

Owing to the many small bubbles involved, the neurologic picture is often one of multiple small defects; it may involve disturbances of vision, coordination, and balance. Distinction from AGE is difficult, and makes little difference to treatment.

Pain. The most common problem arising with decompression sickness (70 to 80 percent of cases) is pain in the extremities. The shoulder is the most frequent site, followed by the knee and then other joints of the upper limb or hip. It is usually described as a deep pain, difficult to localize, and aggravated by movement. There frequently are associated paresthesia in the region, and multiple joints may be affected, occasionally in a migratory fashion. Encircling the affected part with a sphygmomanometer cuff inflated to above arterial pressure may temporarily abolish the pain. The severity varies from minor "niggles" to severe and boring sensations, like a toothache. Such pain may precede the onset of more serious symptoms in 30 percent of cases. Whether late sequelae will arise in cases of decompression sickness causing only pain is not clear, but because of the risk of progression, most patients should be moved to a facility capable of recompression therapy with support as outlined.

Skin Conditions. Simple skin itching after dives is probably not a true manifestation of decompression sickness, and it requires no treatment. More significant itching or burning with wheals, the appearance of ecchymoses, or erythematous blotches is probably significant, but still requires only observation for 6 to 12 hours to ensure early detection of any progression to other more serious forms. Patches of edema may occur; while slightly more ominous, they are managed in the same way.

Fluid Loss. Hemoconcentration is common in decompression sickness and to a lesser extent in AGE owing to fluid leakage into tissues. This causes sludging, and aggravates the problems present. Consequently, close attention to circulatory parameters and hematocrit values is essential.

Onset. There is usually a latent period between surfacing and the onset of decompression sickness. In most cases, this is 30 minutes to 2 hours, but it may extend to 24 hours or beyond. More serious forms can arise during ascent, but are exceedingly rare after 2 to 3 hours. Onset during ascent usually signifies a very serious insult. The risk of decompression sickness is low when dives are kept within the limits prescribed by the various tables in use, but can occur without a violation of these tables. At 18 m (60 feet), the diver can ascend directly, unless bottom time exceeds 60 minutes, but by 30 m (100 feet) this is down to 10 minutes. Time, depth, age, and obesity are just a few of the factors that increase risk. More than one dive in a 12-hour period has an additive effect on the quantities of N_2 in the tissues, and this accumulation is frequently overlooked by sports divers.

Treatment. The first step is a rapid assessment to separate the serious injuries, such as AGE, neurologic decompression sickness, and shock lung, from the minor ear, sinus, and skin problems.

The serious cases must be separated into life-threatening and less serious categories. In dealing with unconscious victims, the usual ABC approach should be followed and standard therapeutic measures applied. An F_IO_2 100 percent should be used whenever possible to speed inert gas elimination and ensure maximal O_2 delivery. Close attention to hematocrit and urine output, with copious fluid replacement using crystalloids, is essential for the same reasons.

Neurologic decompression sickness can be difficult to distinguish from AGE, but in its serious forms it makes no difference to management. All unconscious divers should be managed as AGE until the diagnosis is disproved. Complications such as pneumothorax should be sought and relieved. The 30-degree head-low position is appropriate for the first 15 to 20 minutes after the victim surfaces, but it will also impair respiration and hinder care, with little proven benefit, beyond this period. Definitive care for all these injuries consists of recompression and administration of hyperbaric O_2, so contact should be made early with the nearest facility for advice on management and transport. Details of the dive leading to the accident may be important to diagnosis of the injury and should always be sought.

Chest x-ray examination can be useful, but delay in achieving recompression is to be avoided except for essential procedures. Details of recompression therapy are not described here, but are included in the list of suggested reading.

Transport

1. All victims of serious accidents should be given 100 percent oxygen via an anesthetic circuit or some form of demand mask.
2. Adequate hydration with crystalloids adjusted by hematocrit, urine output and hemodynamic signs is essential.
3. There should be continued observation of ABCs and support as required.
4. High altitude is to be avoided, as it causes gas expansion and aggravates injuries. If aircraft are used, it must be possible to pressurize the cabin to sea level.
5. Do not forget the bladder, especially in *conscious* victims with spinal cord injury.
6. Establish and maintain contact with the receiving unit for advice.
7. In conscious, less threatened victims, oral rehydration may be appropriate and important, while oxygen is still indicated.
8. Remember that significant injuries may still respond to recompression therapy after 48 hours, but the response is less likely to be effective and complete with the passage of time.
9. Young people have died because the emergency physician did not realize that divers *may present with injury due to pressure exposure that mimics other illness (e.g., heart attack, stroke, sprains, and strains) but requires different and specific therapy.*

Dizzy Divers

Dizziness can be a presenting complaint in divers, but usually is not significant unless it is persistent. It may be caused by difficulty with clearing the ears, especially if excessive force has been used. In this case a tear of the round or oval window may have occurred, with a subsequent fistula and hearing loss. An ear, nose, and throat consultation and audiogram may be required.

Decompression sickness as a cause of dizziness in sports divers is rare, but it must be considered if other causes have been eliminated.

Perforation of the tympanic membrane and pressure changes on ascent can both cause dizziness, but such dizziness is transient and easily recognized.

PREVENTION OF DIVING INJURIES

Prevention is still the most effective treatment for all diving disorders. It is best achieved by encouraging divers to obtain good instruction and to keep up-to-date and fit as divers in the broadest sense. Physicians should take advantage of any opportunity to supply current advice on effective first aid to diving groups.

ADVICE AND INFORMATION

The Diver Accident Network (DAN) can supply immediate advice regarding case management and access to the nearest hyperbaric chamber. It can be called from any place, at any time: (919) 684-8111. The Undersea and Hyperbaric Medical Society, Inc., has lecturers, a huge library, and numerous publications. Further information and a list of topics can be obtained from The Undersea and Hyperbaric Medical Society, 9650 Rockville Pike, Bethesda, MD 20814.

SUGGESTED READING

Davis JC. Hyperbaric and undersea medicine. San Pedro: Best Publishing Co., 1981.

Edmonds C, Lowry C, Pennefather J. Diving and subaquatic medicine. Mosman, Australia: Diving Medical Center, 1976.

Shilling C.W. The physician's guide to diving medicine. New York: Plenum Press, 1984.

Strauss RH. Diving medicine. New York: Grune & Stratton, Inc., 1976.

U.S. Navy Diving Manual Revision I. Washington DC: Navy Department; 1985.

EXERCISE REHABILITATION FOR CORONARY ARTERY BYPASS GRAFT PATIENTS

JACK GOODMAN, Ph.D.

CORONARY BYPASS SURGERY: DEVELOPMENTS AND POSTSURGICAL RESULTS

Coronary artery bypass grafting (CABG) has proved remarkably effective in reducing symptoms of angina pectoris and has been instrumental in prolonging life in high-risk patients with coronary artery disease (CAD). Surpassing simple endarterectomy procedures common in the late 1960s, since its inception 20 years ago CABG has become a common treatment of CAD, the most common indication for surgery being chronic stable angina. Surgical data indicate that CABG relieves anginal pain in 75 to 90 percent of patients. Relief of pain correlates well with the degree of revascularization and graft patency. Patency rates are quite high within 1 month after surgery (>85 percent), but decline to below 65 percent after 10 years. Recurrence of angina is approximately 5 percent per year and may be further reduced with platelet inhibition. Progression of atherosclerosis in graft bypasses is the most common long-term reason for graft attrition. More recently, however, internal mammary artery grafts have demonstrated higher patency rates and have become a more popular grafting technique when surgically feasible.

Bypass grafting may have little positive effect on resting left ventricular (LV) function; however, exercise LV function improves dramatically after CABG (typically through an increase in ejection fraction and improved wall motion). Exercise testing following CABG has been attempted as early as 24 hours after surgery, most patients demonstrating an improved exercise time and maximal oxygen intake ($\dot{V}O_2max$).

Although clinical exercise testing is a popular method to assess functional capacity after CABG, there is a paucity of data describing the effects of chronic exercise training during rehabilitation in CABG patients. Increased exercise time and $\dot{V}O_2max$ have been reported in a few studies, but fewer than 600 CABG patients have been investigated. Work by our group suggests that both young and old patients (those over 60 years of age) can benefit from training, and that like post-myocardial infarction (MI) patients, much of the improvement in cardiovascular function seen in CABG patients during rehabilitation is likely due to changes in the periphery, rather than in cardiac function per se. The CABG patient stands to gain as much from exercise rehabilitation as the MI patient. If MI or LV aneurysm is absent, improvements in $\dot{V}O_2max$ are more rapid at the onset of training, and potentially more substantial. A $\dot{V}O_2max$ of less than 20 ml per kilogram per minute is not uncommon for CABG patients at the onset of training, but within 1 year after beginning intensive exercise rehabilitation, values can exceed 30 ml per kilogram per minute. Because of the high number of bypass procedures now performed, rehabilitation programs originally designed for post-MI patients have expanded to accommodate the CABG patient. Since both types of patients often have similar initial $\dot{V}O_2max$ and convalescent time courses, the general principles of rehabilitation for the CABG patient are similar to those used after MI.

GENERAL PRINCIPLES OF EXERCISE PRESCRIPTION FOR CABG PATIENTS

Exercise training for CABG patients follows the general principles used for healthy adults. The initial fitness level and the rate of progression during training are the critical differences between CABG patients and healthy adults. The initial prescription is based on the initial level of fitness and general health; the primary objectives of the exercise prescription are the attainment of sufficient intensity, duration, and frequency, using dynamic, rhythmic aerobic exercise involving large muscle groups. Intensity and duration are closely linked in the training stimulus (in a general sense, intensity plus duration equals "volume"), but in order to maximize adherence and minimize musculoskeletal injuries, both must be advanced in a graduated manner over a period of more than 6 months.

Progression should initially be slow (before discharge), with a low energy expenditure (200 to 400 kJ, 50 to 100 kcal per session). However, within 24 weeks 1,200 to 1,600 kJ (300 to 400 kcal) per session should be attained, with an ultimate goal of reaching 6,000 to 8,000 kJ (1,500 to 2,000 kcal) of energy expenditure per week, similar to that recommended for healthy individuals. Many patients who are highly motivated and adapt well to exercise training can reach the final level within 18 to 24 weeks of training. CABG patients are likely to show more rapid improvements in the early stage of a rehabilitation program than post-MI patients; therefore, a less conservative approach to exercise prescription may be warranted during the first 3 months of rehabilitation.

The exercise session should incorporate a warm-up period, mild strength exercises, aerobic exercise (reaching a predetermined target heart rate), and a cool-down phase. The warm-up session should last approximately 15 minutes during phase 1 rehabilitation and can taper to 10 minutes during phase 2. This is a critical portion of the exercise session, facilitating an increased muscular blood flow, joint readiness, and mobility. A period of 5 minutes involving muscular strength exercises (toe standing, partial leg squats, arm rotation) should precede the aerobic exercise session. The aerobic exercise is followed by a cool-down period (5 to 10 minutes), essential for preventing orthostatic hypotension, augmenting blood lactate clearance, and reducing muscle stiffness. Cool-down activities should include light walking (30 to 40 percent of the target heart rate) followed by stretching.

There are three phases of the rehabilitation process: phase 1, for pre-discharge patients recuperating from surgery; phase 2, for outpatients attending a hospital or community service program; and phase 3, for fully independent, unsupervised exercise.

Phase 1 Rehabilitation

Inpatient rehabilitation is a critical component of postoperative care. In uncomplicated cases, earlier rehabilitation optimizes the surgical results. Increased range of motion (ROM), particularly in the upper body, helps to reduce adhesions and muscle stiffness typical of the postsurgical state, and will probably contribute to an expeditious return to a proper upright walking posture, flexibility, and muscle strength. Postsurgical discomfort typically arises from sternal wound pain and drainage, coughing (facilitating drainage), and saphenous vein graft sites. Despite these sources of discomfort, in most cases phase 1 rehabilitation can begin within 12 hours of surgery. Such strategy minimizes stiffness, postoperative atelectasis, and venous thrombosis and improves psychological status. The physiologic basis for early ambulation is based on the documented effects of prolonged bed rest, including hypovolemia, tachycardia, orthostatic hypotension, a reduced muscle mass, and $\dot{V}O_2max$. Absolute and relative contraindications precluding entrance into exercise programs, or suggesting caution during participation, are presented in Table 1.

TABLE 1 Contraindications to Exercise Training of CABG Patients

Absolute Contraindications
Unstable angina
Severe sitting or standing orthostatic hypotension
Severe conduction abnormalities
Severe aortic regurgitation (>50% gradient)
Thrombophlebitis
Perioperative myocardial infarction
Uncompensated heart failure
Dissecting aneurysm
Second- or third-degree heart block
Active myocarditis
Systemic illness or fever >39°C
Severe hypertension: diastolic, >120; systolic, >200
Relative Contraindications
Excessive sternal movement and/or incisional drainage
Surgically induced pericarditis
Hypertension: diastolic, >110, <120; systolic, >160, <200
Resting ST-segment depression >3 mm
Sinus tachycardia >120 at rest
Uncontrolled diabetes
Musculoskeletal disorders preventing physical activity
Compensated heart failure
Mild orthostatic hypotension
Conditions Requiring Special Considerations
Fixed-rate pacemakers
Intermittent claudication
Obesity (>20–25% above ideal weight)
Conduction disturbances (e.g., left bundle branch and biphasicular block, Wolff-Parkinson-White syndrome)
Peripheral edema and/or incisional complications

Modified from Pollock M, Pels A, Foster C, Ward A. Exercise prescription for rehabilitation of the cardiac patient. In: Pollock M, Schmidt D, eds. Heart disease and rehabilitation. Toronto: John Wiley, 1986:477.

Phase 1 exercises may begin while patients are in bed, with daily progression. Passive ROM exercises of the upper and lower limbs, in addition to breathing exercises (coughing) should be included, gradually progressing to active ROM exercises, reaching an energy expenditure of approximately 2 MET (1 MET = basal energy expenditure). Within 24 hours, many patients can walk to a limited extent in the ward; activity should increase to an intensity of 3 MET (during ambulatory activity) two times per day (as tolerated) within 3 to 4 days after surgery, in addition to bedside therapy (ROM and breathing exercises). Exercises performed in the ward should be primarily walking, progressing to stair climbing. A fixed upper heart rate is not recommended, but rather 20 to 25 beats per minute above the resting heart rate should be used as a peak exercise intensity. If tolerated, the duration of walking should be extended 5 minutes per day, reaching 25 to 35 minutes upon discharge. Ongoing education is a crucial aspect of the exercise program; it should include information regarding exercise physiology, nutrition, stress management, risk-factor modification, and medication effects. Patients should be taught to measure their pulse rate immediately after exercise (within 10 seconds). Upon discharge, patients should be given detailed instructions for home training. Although pre-discharge low-level exercise tests are advocated by some and help to establish objective criteria for home training, a target heart rate not exceeding 25 beats above rest is a safe and practical guideline for home training, if such a test is not available. An initial comprehensive exercise test is a critical component of phase 2 rehabilitation.

Phases 2 and 3 Exercise Rehabilitation

Outpatient exercise training typically begins 6 to 8 weeks after surgery; however, there is growing support for an earlier onset of phase 2 exercise programs (4 weeks). Ideally, if recuperation and home exercise has progressed without complications, a symptom-limited maximal exercise test should be scheduled 4 to 6 weeks after surgery, with phase 2 exercise training beginning at that time. If patients have remained on beta-blocking medication, testing should be performed while they are on medication. Sophisticated centers offer comprehensive metabolic testing, including direct measurement of ventilation and expired gases using rapid response O_2 and CO_2 analyzers for the determination of $\dot{V}O_2max$ and anaerobic threshold. Use of objective criteria such as these allow a more precise determination of the exercise prescription, and typically the centers offering such testing have equally sophisticated programs. It is emphasized that the entire basis of exercise prescription, particularly the initial portion during phase 2 training, is dependent on the determination of $\dot{V}O_2max$, and that accurate and reproducible methods should be used in its determination.

The objective of phase 2 rehabilitation is to achieve 1,200 to 1,600 kJ (300 to 400 kcal) of energy expenditure per session within 18 to 24 weeks. Patients should exercise five times per week, the intensity and duration of activity increasing gradually, and with rest days spread evenly throughout the week. The initial intensity should correspond to 55 to 60 percent of estimated or measured $\dot{V}O_2max$, or 60 percent of maximal heart rate reserve (HRR) as determined during exercise testing (Training heart rate = $[HR_{max} - HR_{rest}] \times \%$ intensity + $[HR_{rest}]$). Since maximal heart rate decreases with age, and endurance training elicits bradycardia, a range of training intensity is advised (Table 2). Use of the Borg scale of perceived exertion as a method to establish intensity is advocated by some. However, others have found a poor relationship between symptoms or warning signs (particularly ST-segment depression) and perception of effort. Consequently, the use of age-dependent target heart rates is advised.

A walk-jog routine is recommended, since it requires no special facility or significant cost. Swimming is not advised until after 8 weeks of phase 2 exercise, and only if sternal healing shows no complications or delay.

Initially, the duration of the aerobic component should be 30 minutes, but it can be gradually extended to 45 to 60 minutes, the intensity reaching 80 percent of HRR after 24 weeks. The rate of progression should be based on the initial level of fitness of the patient. The combination of a moderate intensity and frequent exercise sessions will yield favorable cardiovascular adaptations, body composition changes (decreased body fat mass), and improved blood lipid profile (reduction in triglycerides and low-density lipoprotein cholesterol, increased high-density lipoprotein cholesterol).

Progression throughout the program is based on training volume (duration plus intensity) and the rate of improvement (heart rate response during exercise). After 8 weeks of training during phase 2, an exercise test determining the $\dot{V}O_2max$ should be performed to monitor progression and to detect potential advancement of the disease process and/or the adequacy of revascularization. It is theoretically appropriate if an exercise prescription is based on a fixed time requirement at a target heart rate, or a distance covered in a required time period, provided that a threshold intensity of effort is reached

TABLE 2 Recommended Training Intensity During Rehabilitation*

Age	*35–39 yr*	*40–44 yr*	*45–49 yr*	*50–54 yr*	*55–59 yr*	*60–64 yr*
THR_1	140	137	133	131	128	125
THR_2	151	147	143	140	136	133
THR_3	161	157	153	149	146	141

*Assuming a resting heart rate of 75 beats per minute.
THR_1 = Training heart rate at 60% maximal heart rate reserve.
THR_2 = Training heart rate at 70% maximal heart rate reserve.
THR_3 = Training heart rate at 80% maximal heart rate reserve.

(more than 60 percent of $\dot{V}O_2$max or of the maximal HRR). However, the latter technique is preferred, since energy expenditure is more readily monitored (walking and running speeds can easily be transformed into metabolic equivalents or O_2 cost), and the speed technique also allows a "progressing heart rate" method of increasing intensity. When the exercising heart rate is consistently below the training heart rate (using a percentage of the maximal HRR), the time to complete the distance is reduced, thereby maintaining a desired intensity of effort. This method requires patients to complete exercise diaries describing distance covered, symptoms, and exercise heart rate routinely. Such a process facilitates comprehensive monitoring on a weekly basis, thereby allowing rapid adjustments to the exercise prescription.

A critical feature of phase 2 rehabilitation is encouragement by both spouse and physician. A practical concern is the number of supervised sessions. Some patients may prefer to engage in supervised exercise three to four times per week, but for many this is both impractical and undesirable. A minimum of one supervised class per week is essential. Patients who experience frequent arrhythmias should be monitored (by electrocardiographic telemetry) during supervised exercise. Supervised pulse checks are also encouraged (palpation, or using devices such as "Exersentry" monitors), since many patients are inaccurate at recording postexercise pulse measurements.

The phase 3 rehabilitation program (unsupervised) is both a continuation and an expansion of the phase 2 prescription (Table 3). After 1 year of supervised exercise, patients should begin a maintenance program of prescribed but largely unsupervised exercise. Aerobic exercise should be performed for 45 to 60 minutes, five sessions per week, at an intensity of approximately 80 percent HRR. Since most post-CABG patients can attain a $\dot{V}O_2$max similar to that of healthy age-matched individuals, little supervision is required, and provided that the disease process has not progressed, patients showing no complications should be encouraged to participate in all activities. It is advised that a comprehensive exercise test be performed once a year after discharge from phase 2, facilitating patient motivation, feedback, and monitoring of the disease process.

TABLE 3 Exercise Prescription During Phases 2 and 3 Rehabilitation

	Phase 2	*Phase 3*
Frequency	5 times/wk	5 times/wk
Intensity		
% Max HRR	60–70%	80%
Duration	30–45 min	45–60 min
Kcal expenditure	300–400 kcal/session	400+ kcal/session

Exercise rehabilitation for the CABG patient is a critical extension of surgical therapy and may help to maximize the benefits of surgical intervention. Although current data suggest that only 60 to 75 percent of postsurgical patients return to work, exercise training indeed contributes to an enhanced physical work capacity and quality of life.

SUGGESTED READING

Bourassa M, Enjalbert M, Campeau L, Lesperance J. Progression of atherosclerosis in coronary arteries and bypass grafts: ten years later. Am J Cardiol 1984; 53:102C–107C.

Goodman J, Dornan J, Brown K, Plyley M. Exercise training following coronary artery bypass surgery in older patients. J. Clin Gerontol 1987; 9:19–29.

Goodman J, Plyley M, Rosenblatt D, et al. Central and peripheral adaptations to exercise training in cardiac patients. Med Sci Sports Exerc 1987; 19:23.

Kavanagh T. The healthy heart program. Toronto: Key Porter Books, 1985.

Manley J. Quantitative assessment of coronary artery bypass surgery results. In: Pollock M, Schmidt D, eds. Heart disease and rehabilitation. Toronto: John Wiley, 1986:247.

Pollock M, Pels A, Foster C, Ward A. Exercise prescription for rehabilitation of the cardiac patient. In: Pollock M, Schmidt D, eds. Heart disease and rehabilitation. Toronto: John Wiley, 1986:477.

PHYSICAL ACTIVITY IN MEDICAL CARE

ROD K. DISHMAN, Ph.D.

The prevalence of sedentary leisure time (exercise fewer than 3 days a week or less than 20 minutes per session) has remained at 30 to 60 percent in North America during the past 15 years, while the typical drop-out rate from supervised exercise programs has remained at roughly 50 percent. Only 10 percent of American and 25 percent of Canadian adults appear to be active at the minimal intensity (60 percent of maximal oxygen intake), duration (3 days a week and 20 minutes per session), and energy level (12 kilojoules or 3 kcal per kilogram of body mass per session) believed necessary to ensure fitness and optimize most health benefits.

The US participation rate objective for 1990 of 90 percent for children aged 10 to 17 years, 60 percent for ages 18 to 65, and 50 percent for persons over 65 will not be met. This is largely due to an incomplete understanding of the factors that determine free-living physical activity and adherence to supervised exercise programs. This chapter focuses on the important role that physicians and medical care professionals can play in promoting and increasing physical activity among their patients.

BELIEFS AND PRACTICES OF PHYSICIANS

In their review of physical activity promotion programs in the United States, Iverson and colleagues discussed evidence of the effectiveness of the physician's office as a method of promoting physical activity. They concluded:

> Health practitioners in medical care settings are in an excellent position to encourage and assist patients to become physically active. A majority of patients have a regular source of health care and most see a physician at least once per year.
>
> Physicians do not regularly ask about the physical activity patterns of their patients. Although most physicians believe that being physically active is important, most do not counsel their patients about physical activity....
>
> It appears that physicians can be effective in altering patient behavior.

It is important to address these conclusions in light of current evidence of the promotion of physical activity by physicians, and of tested techniques and principles of behavioral change that can be applied through the medical office to increase physical activity in patients.

It was estimated that in 1984 slightly less than 50 percent of US physicians routinely asked their patients about exercise. Although this rate approximates the 1990 US Department of Health and Human Services national objective that more than 50 percent of primary care physicians should include a careful exercise history in their initial examination of new patients, guidelines for taking an exercise history are neither established nor widely available, and it appears that many physicians do not fully believe in the health benefits of exercise. In recognition of these concerns, the US Department of Health and Human Services' midcourse review of the 1990 objectives for physical fitness and exercise has recommended a modified objective for the year 2000: "By 2000, 65 percent or more of primary medical care providers will inquire about the frequency, duration, type, and intensity of most new patients' exercise habits." Some evidence suggests that this recommended objective may already be met. A nationally representative random sample of 2,000 pediatrician members of the 22,000-member American Academy of Pediatricians indicated that more than 70 percent of primary care pediatricians encouraged exercise for well children 6 years or older, even if they were not at high risk for illness (Fig. 1). Among primary care physicians, 50 to 65 percent believed that exercise was very important for patients in these age groups: more so than for diet, but less so than for cigarette smoking.

The more striking result from the national survey of pediatricians, however, was that only 25 percent believed they could be effective in changing patient behavior. Other studies agree in their estimates that only 10 to 40 percent of physicians consider themselves successful in helping patients change behavior. Population estimates are not available to evaluate the true success rates for increasing patient exercise, but a lack of confidence in behavioral change approaches could hinder physicians' attempts and their effectiveness. Only 17 percent of primary care physicians in Massachusetts believed that training in behavior modification would be valuable.

Despite these beliefs, several lines of research suggest that behavior modification may facilitate the promotion of physical activity through medical care settings. Available evidence indicates that advice and counseling that relies solely on educational approaches, including health risk appraisal and fitness testing, has only modest effects on exercise behavior. Behavior modification, together with the teaching of self-regulation, may hold more promise.

HEALTH RISK APPRAISAL AND FITNESS TESTING

Early studies suggested that health risk appraisal might increase physical activity. Lauzon reported that health risk appraisal had no effect on smoking, blood pressure, or seat-belt use, but that it increased physical activity, particularly in high-risk males. Leppink and DeGrassi reported that 6 months after health risk appraisal of 144 patients, 37 percent had increased, 4 percent had decreased, and 59 percent showed no change in their exercise habits. After 18 months, 34 percent reported increased exercise, 11 percent decreased exercise, and 55 percent no change. These studies were uncon-

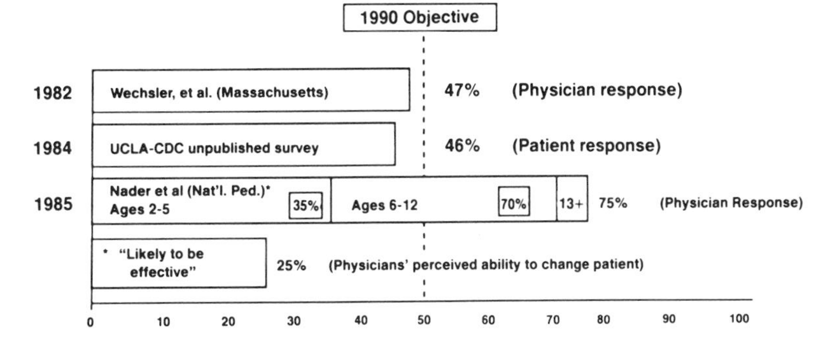

Figure 1 Percentage of physicians who counsel patients about exercise. Adapted from (1) US Department of Health and Human Services. Midcourse review 1990 objectives for physical fitness and exercise. Washington, DC: US Government Printing Office, 1986; and (2) Nader PR, et al. Adult heart disease prevention in childhood: a national survey of pediatricians' practices and attitudes. Pediatrics 1987; 79:843–850.

trolled, however, and the accuracy and validity of the self-reports of activity were not demonstrated. It was thus unclear how many patients might have begun exercising without a health risk appraisal. Establishing an objective baseline for expected improvement is particularly important in studies like these, because patients can be motivated to inflate their reports of physically active behavior in order to give the appearance of complying with their physician's advice.

Similar results have been observed for physical fitness testing. Bruce and colleagues examined the impact of a physician-supervised graded treadmill test on exercise habits 1 year later. Of 2,892 men sampled, 2,001 responded to a mail questionnaire; results indicated that 50 percent of the 1,384 initially sedentary men reported that "the exercise test motivated them to increase daily exercise." No objective measure of actual physical activity was obtained, however. Surprisingly, patients who showed functional aerobic impairment during the first treadmill test were no more active 1 year later than were functionally normal patients. A better controlled study by Driggers and associates subsequently demonstrated that exercise stress testing had no influence on health behavior, attitudes, objective health measures, or self-reported exercise. Likewise, Ewart and associates examined the effects of exercise testing on physical activity patterns 3 weeks after uncomplicated myocardial infarction. The patients' confidence was increased when performing activities similar to the treadmill exercise (e.g., walking, stair climbing, and running), but an increased confidence in performing other activities such as lifting and sexual intercourse required an explanation of the test results by a physician or nurse. Importantly, self-reported activity was verified in this study both by daily heart rate monitoring and by demonstration of a decreased heart rate response to standard exercise after training. Increased confidence for leg activity was correlated with an increase in self-reported activity, but there was only a weak association between fitness gains and increased physical activity.

ASSESSMENT AND EDUCATIONAL APPROACHES

Because of the modest influence of health and fitness appraisals, other studies examined the combined effects upon habitual activity of health risk appraisal, fitness assessment, and educational interventions. Reid and Morgan randomly assigned 124 firefighters to three groups: a control group that received a submaximal fitness test, an exercise prescription, and consultation with a physician; a group that also received a 1-hour media and verbal presentation; and a third group that was also taught to monitor exercise habits by pulse palpation and the use of Cooper's aerobic point system. After 3 months, compliance (as determined by self-report of two or more weekly exercise sessions of at least 15 minutes duration and a decreased heart rate during standard exercise testing) was 29 percent in the control group and 55 percent in pooled data from the two experimental groups. After 6 months, however, only about 33 percent of each group was participating in regular physical activity. Similar findings came from the Stanford Community study, which represents one of the few population-based attempts to modify health habits through intensive health education, media campaigns, and individual patient counseling. Although significant reductions in overall risk were observed in experimental subjects, exercise habits were not changed at 1 or 2 years.

Daltroy reported on the effectiveness of randomized educational intervention designed to increase compliance in cardiac patients during the initial 3 months of a prescribed exercise program. Telephone counseling for both patient and spouse, with mailing of an information brochure, increased program attendance by 12 percent when the groups were statistically equated in terms of entry characteristics, including coronary risk. However, without this adjustment, attendance rates were equivalent between the intervention (64%) and control (62%) gropus. Much of the increased attendance occurred in patients with a high school education or less. Although three-fourths of the patients reported that they continued to be active after dropping out of the formal program, only one-third remained active at an intensity that would maintain cardiorespiratory fitness.

Home-Based Approaches

Because limited access to facilities and inconvenience have been repeatedly cited as reasons for dropping out of supervised cardiac rehabilitation exercise programs, several studies have implemented home-based interventions. Acquista and colleagues combined health-risk appraisal with intensive educational and counseling sessions conducted by nurses in the home. Health behavior plans were tailored to individual risk profiles. On telephone and interview follow-up 1 year later, 61 (48 percent) of 126 persons who had reported no regular physical activity at the outset of the study indicated that they had increased their habitual activity. However, this study had no control group, and the self-selected participants (476 volunteered from a population of 3,800) could have been motivated to increase their activity patterns regardless of the intervention. Also, the validity of the interview assessment of physical activity is unclear, and the increase of activity was not quantified.

Controlled studies combining health risk appraisal with education or physical fitness assessment have not been successful in increasing physical activity on follow-up. Godin and associates examined the effect of the Canadian Home Fitness Test and the Health Hazard Appraisal on intentions to exercise and exercise behavior over a 3-month period. Importantly, mere administration of the tests was contrasted with personalized knowledge of the test results. Subjects were assigned to one of four groups: (1) control, (2) fitness appraisal only, (3) health-age appraisal only, or (4) appraisal of both fitness and health-age. Knowledge of results was given to half of the subjects in each group. The Health Hazard Appraisal had no impact on either intended or actual leisure time exercise. Although the fitness test and knowledge of results initially increased intentions to exercise, neither intentions to be active nor actual exercise behavior were changed after 3 months. Similarly, Desharnais and colleagues examined the Canadian Home Fitness Test and EvaluLife (a Canadian version of health risk appraisal) as possible tactics for increasing leisure exercise. As predicted, only subjects with a high health risk maintained an increased intention to exercise over a 3-month period. Exercise behavior was not assessed, however, and prospective studies have shown quite small relationships between intentions to exercise and subsequent behavior.

BEHAVIOR MANAGEMENT TECHNIQUES

Although exercise prescriptions tailored to health risk and fitness level deserve continued study, a feasible adjunct is to apply techniques of behavior modification. Reviews of the available technology for behavior management in exercising populations can be found in Knapp and in Martin and Dubbert. Techniques generally involve reinforcement and stimulus control. Self-regulation approaches such as relapse prevention appear particularly promising, because they address behavioral skills for planning, monitoring, and reinforcing exercise habits in the context of a person's existing lifestyle.

Behavior Modification

Behavior may be regarded as a function of the observable response to objective events in the environment. The emphasis of behavior modification is on reproducible changes in behavior or neuroendocrine symptoms that result from associations between an external stimulus and an action. Responses can be classically conditioned (pavlovian) to a single experience (e.g., some phobic and somatic disturbances) or operantly conditioned (to achieve a specific goal) through repeated pairing with a consequent event (a reinforcer) or an extraneous event (a secondary reinforcer) that increases (reinforcement) or decreases (punishment) the likelihood of the same response in the future. Removal of unpleasant (aversive) events associated with the absence of the desired response can also increase the desired behavior (negative reinforcement).

Desired behaviors can often be altered quickly by continuous reinforcement, or modified in a more long-lasting way by an intermittent schedule. Common behavior modification procedures include the following:

1. *Shaping.* Existing behaviors similar to the desired behavior or subparts of a desired complex behavior are progressively reinforced, or a behavior exhibited in many undesired settings is reinforced in only a few desired settings.
2. *Generalizing.* A behavior exhibited in a single setting is gradually reinforced when it is shown elsewhere, or additional desired behaviors related to an existing one are reinforced in the initial setting.
3. *Fading.* Reinforcement or punishment of a desired behavior by a professional is gradually made less frequent or less intense, so that self-reinforcement or punishment by the patient is increased.

These methods of behavior modification are typically implemented by such techniques as reinforcement or punishment control (e.g., social evaluation, feedback, prize lotteries, contingency contracts or tokens, awards, written agreements, withholding of rewards, or pain) or stimulus control (whereby naturally occurring secondary reinforcers are structured to cue or prompt the desired behavior).

A key to the effectiveness of behavior modification lies in the identification of critical behaviors. This can be relatively straightforward for simple overt behaviors such as exercise, but is more difficult for covert behaviors such as decision-making or planning to begin an exercise program. The finding of effective reinforcers for different individuals can also be difficult, and individual differences in the strength of various reinforcers is a serious limitation to any standardized application of behavior modification to physical activity.

Behavior modification techniques minimize the role of thoughts, emotions, and perceptions as determinants of behavior. The emphasis is on objective situations and overt responses. Clinical experience reveals, however, that people do not respond in identical ways to the same situations. Not only can humans learn without being reinforced (e.g., by observation), but people are motivated for future efforts by both a knowledge of behavioral outcomes and future expectations.

This has led some psychologists to modify the techniques developed by behaviorists for overt behaviors so that they can be used with covert behaviors such as emotions, self-confidence, and motivation. The underlying assumption is that a wide range of dysfunctional or maladaptive behaviors stem from irrational, unproductive thoughts and incompletely formed cognitions. By the application of learning principles, or sometimes by providing the patient with insight, faulty thoughts can be restructured, augmented, or replaced by beliefs and cognitive skills that are behaviorally more effective.

Cognitive Behavior Modification

In the initial stage of cognitive behavior modification, the health professional probes the thoughts and beliefs of the patient and determines the behavioral habits that result. This is followed by an educational stage that fosters an expectation of change and evaluates possible plans to promote change. Next the actual treatment plan is designed. Finally, an attempt is made to implement and maintain the plan in daily life. Relapse is common, so there is frequently a return to earlier stages among those who have difficulty in changing their behavior, but retain the desire to do so. Several procedures rely almost exclusively on eliminating or restructuring existing thoughts. It is assumed that the desired changes in behavior or emotion will follow, but neither are direct targets. This is a radically different approach from simple behavior modification, where the emphasis excludes conscious mediation of behavioral or somatic responses.

Cognitive behavioral procedures also emphasize the acquisition of coping skills. The construction of an active plan of behavior (an adaptive alternative) separates these techniques from classic behavior modification, which focuses primarily on eliminating maladaptive responses. An instructional focus makes cognitive behavioral procedures attractive for medical care settings, because self-regulation permits the patient to develop behavioral skills for responding to the demands of daily living.

Relapse Prevention

A popular example of self-regulation is relapse prevention, as developed by Marlatt & Gordon, and applied to exercise by Knapp. The principal components include (1) identifying situations with a high risk of relapse; (2) revising plans to avoid or cope with high-risk situations (e.g., time management, relaxation training, confidence building, reducing barriers to activity); (3) correcting expectations of a positive outcome so that the consequences of not exercising are placed in a proper perspective (e.g., people who are tired at the end of the working day may expect to feel refreshed if they rest rather than exercise; however, they may actually feel guilty while resting, whereas activity would likely have been invigorating); (4) expecting and planning for lapses, such as scheduling alternative activities while on vacation or after injury; (5) minimizing the tendency to interpret a temporary lapse as a total failure, with loss of confidence and complete cessation of activity; and (6) correcting a lifestyle imbalance in which "shoulds" outweigh "wants." The focus here is on optimizing the pleasure derived from physical activity, rather than viewing exercise as another obligation, avoiding urges to relapse by blocking self-dialogues and images of the benefits of not exercising.

Knapp correctly noted that relapse prevention is designed to reduce high-frequency addictive behaviors such as smoking and substance abuse, whereas exercise is generally a desired but low-frequency behavior. Thus, the relapse prevention model may require modification in the context of exercise. Nevertheless, several studies have reported increased activity rates when certain components of the model (identifying high-risk situations, planning for relapse, reducing barriers, and minimizing the effects of a lapse) were combined with broader approaches to cognitive behavior modification.

EXERCISE STUDIES

Behavior Modification

Written agreements, behavioral contracts, contingency schedules, and lotteries all increase exercise participation. In such approaches, a person signs an agreement to remain active for a certain period, and the consequences of keeping or breaking the contract may be specified. The amount of exercise required can be determined by a random drawing. Other examples involve the depositing of money or some valuable possession that will be returned when the exercise program has been successfully completed, or a behavioral contingency in which a valued goal or activity is attained when the person has undertaken a predetermined amount of exercise.

Cognitive Behavior Modification

Various goal-setting and reinforcement techniques have been used, including self-monitoring, stimulus control, and self-reinforcement. With self-monitoring, patients record completion of specific types of exercise; stimulus control involves the use of objects, ideas, or other behaviors associated with exercise to create an environment that promotes exercise. While these approaches capitalize on associational learning, they also make it more difficult for a patient to ignore either a previous decision to be active or a discrepancy between intention and actual behavior. Stimulus-control techniques may restructure the environment (e.g., taking a homeward route past an exercise facility or keeping exercise clothes in the car or at the office), and they may remove or diminish real (e.g., inconvenience) or imagined (e.g., excuses) barriers to activity. Perhaps the best tested and most easily implemented technique is the decision balance sheet. This involves a careful evaluation by the patient of the expected or experienced benefits and costs of activity; the medical professional can actively reinforce positive outcomes and diminish negative expectations. The consequences of activity are considered not only for the patient, but also for a spouse, friends, or other family members. Importantly, reinforcement of the decision to begin or resume activity is accompanied by planned strategies for overcoming perceived or real barriers to exercise. In this way, the decision balance sheet shares common aspects with the relapse prevention model of Marlatt and Gordon. The decision balance sheet has been effectively implemented by direct patient counseling, and also by telephone.

Methodology Problems

It is not known how effective behavior management is compared with other possible program changes (such as altering the type of activity or the intensity in order to fit a patient's existing preferences); however, behavior modification and cognitive behavior modification techniques typically achieve a 60 to 80 percent exercise adherence or attendance rate, compared with control rates of 40 to 60 percent.

However, research designs have not discounted generalized treatment effects, therapist effects, or participant expectations as explanations of effectiveness. Moreover, some of the most impressive results have been based on a "treatment package" that encompasses various principles of behavior management, including shaping, reinforcement control, stimulus control, behavioral contracting, cognitive strategies, generalization, reinforcement fading, and relapse prevention. Although these are all sound principles, and attempts have been made to ensure compatibility with other program factors believed to influence adherence (e.g., convenience and social support), the complexity of treatment does not allow specific evaluation, or indeed a decision as to whether any intervention is better than none.

The use of placebo groups has been infrequent, yet when more than one intervention has been used, changes of exercise behavior effects have often been similar for each treatment. Some 50 percent of those who opt for behavior management exercise programs claim to have previously attempted exercise unsuccessfully on their own; it is thus unclear to what degree self-referred patients may be responsive to program packages that strongly emphasize social support. In one study, over 50 percent of individuals who had previously failed to maintain a program stated that they had attempted exercise alone, even though more than 80 percent said they would have preferred to exercise with someone else. Some factor common to the interaction between the patient and treatment, such as social reinforcement, may thus account for most of the increased activity apparently induced by behavior modification.

Many interventions have lasted for only 3 to 10 weeks, while exercise involvement of 3 to 12 months or longer is needed in preventive exercise programs. Thus, even if short-term studies suggest an increase of physical activity, a longer follow-up is needed. About one-half of the studies included follow-ups after the intervention, but few showed long-term (3 to 12 months) maintenance of any initial behavioral change. A period of 10 to 20 weeks is necessary for the training adaptations that may provide reinforcing feedback, and adherence through an initial 3 to 6 months appears to increase the odds of a long-term increase of physical activity. Behavior management may provide important support in the early months of treatment, with later reinforcement from other factors, including the personal changes induced by training. This concept is consistent with studies showing that behavioral change is effective for a 3 or 6-month period.

The value of behavior modification as a means of increasing exercise taken outside supervised programs is unclear. Several studies demonstrated behavioral success using the Cooper aerobic point system as the dependent variable. However, the volume of activity needed for either a decreased risk of coronary disease or an increase of physical fitness would require an aerobic point total two or more times greater than those achieved following behavior modification. The probable explanation is that behavior modification does not impart skills for self-regulation. Thus, continued supervision by a health professional is needed. However, a further source of uncertainty is a lack of consensus over a standardized method to assess a patient's leisure-time physical activity accurately and validly.

Extensive reviews note the difficulty of measuring unsupervised exercise. A self-report can be an accurate means of identifying highly active and sedentary patients, but the accuracy of a self-report for individuals who sporadically pursue various types and intensities of activity is unclear, and such individuals make up a large segment of the population. Electronic movement counters appear to estimate the energy cost of walking and running accurately, while moderate to vigorous intensity activity can be estimated from heart rate monitoring. Neither of these last approaches assesses the type of activity performed, but with medical advice both offer the advantage of patient self-monitoring and in this way can be an adjunct to behavior modification.

In conclusion, an unvalidated self-report is unlikely to provide a true measure of a patient's physical activity. Likewise, it is unlikely that health risk appraisal, fitness testing, medical advice, or education about why exercise is a healthy habit will lead to sustained increases of physical activity in most patients. As illustrated in Table 1, each of these procedures contributes to the promotion of physical activity, but they alone do not induce sufficient increase of physical activity to improve health.

TABLE 1 Recommendations for Promoting Physical Activity

1. Promote specific exercises (jogging, swimming, walking):
   a. Emphasize the positive personal consequences that will result from performing the exercise
   b. Explain how negative personal consequences that can result from the exercise are avoidable
2. Communicate the negative personal consequences of not exercising ("fear appeals"), but also include information about how to avoid those consequences (i.e., how to begin exercising)
3. Create perceived social pressure for exercising:
   a. Communicate that "important others" want the target person to perform specific exercises
   b. Involve "opinion leaders" from the community in the campaign
4. Increase perceived control over exercising:
   a. Explain that exercising regularly is compatible with any lifestyle
   b. Explain that everyone can engage in some form of activity
5. Provide basic detailed information about how to perform the exercise (or specify where such information can be obtained)

Reproduced with permission from Olson JM, Zanna MP. Understanding and promoting exercise: a social psychological perspective. Can J Public Health 1987; 78:S1–S14.

Roughly 70 percent of American adults already know how often and how long they should exercise for health outcomes or for fitness, yet 60 percent of Americans do not reach this level of activity. Medical care offers many opportunities to educate patients about health problems that may be prevented or diminished by prudent exercise. The effectiveness of medically based exercise deserves particular study among racial and ethnic minorities, women, children, the elderly, and patients undergoing rehabilitation.

Patient advice and education should move beyond the health outcome message, teaching about effective plans that remove barriers and move patients safely toward their own rather than solely medical goals. Equally important are the teaching of behavioral skills, including self-monitoring, correcting and rewarding progress, and social support; such measures make possible and reinforce exercise programs that often disrupt an existing lifestyle. Examples of educational materials for physicians can be found elsewhere. The September/October 1987 issue of *Rx Being Well*, a waiting room magazine published by Biomedical Information Corporation and McGraw-Hill, includes a good example of patient education material; this informs the patient not only how to begin and stay with an exercise program but also why this is a good idea. Medical care offers unique opportunities for promoting physical activity that should not be missed

SUGGESTED READING

Acquista VW, Watchtel TJ, Gomes CI, Salzillo M, Stockman M. Home-based health risk appraisal and screening program. J Commun Health, 1988; 13:43–52.

American College of Sports Medicine. Guidelines for exercise testing and prescription. 3rd ed. Philadelphia: Lea & Febiger, 1986.

Belilse M, Roskies E, Levesque J. Improving adherence to physical activity. Health Psychol 1987; 6:159–172.

Bruce RA, DeRoven TA, Hossack KF. Pilot study examining the motivational effects of maximal exercise testing to modify risk factors and health habits. Cardiology, 1980; 11: 1119.

Caspersen CJ, Christenson GM, Pollard RA. Status of the 1990 physical fitness and exercise objectives—Evidence from NHIS 1985. Pub Health Rep 1986; 101:587–592.

Daltroy LH. Improving cardiac patient adherence to exercise regimens: a clinical trial of health education. J Cardiac Rehabil 1985; 5.

Desharnais R, Godin G, Jobin J. Motivational characteristics of EvaluLife and the Canadian Home Fitness Test. Can J Public Health 1987; 78:161–164.

Dishman RK. Determinants of physical activity and exercise for persons aged 65 years or older. Am Acad Phys Ed Papers 1989; 22:146–162.

Dishman RK. Determinants of participation in physical activity. In: Bouchard C, ed. Physical activity, fitness, and health. Champaign, IL: Human Kinetics, 1989.

Dishman RK, Sallis JF, Orenstein DR. The determinants of physical activity and exercise. Public Health Rep 1985; 100:158–171.

Driggers DA, Swedberg J, Johnson R, et al. The maximum exercise stress test: is it a behavior modification tool? J Fam Pract 1984; 18:715–718.

Epstein LH, Koeske R, Wing RR. Adherence to exercise in obese children. J Cardiac Rehab 1984; 4:185–195.

Ewart CK, Taylor B, Reese LB, DeBusk RF. Effects of early post-myocardial infarction exercise testing on self-perception and subsequent physical activity. Am J Cardiol 1983; 51:1076–1080.

Godin G, Desharnais R, Jobin J, Cook J. The impact of physical fitness and health-age appraisal upon exercise intentions and behavior. J Behav Med 1987; 10:241–250.

Godin G, Shephard RJ. Physical fitness promotion programmes: effectiveness in modifying exercise behavior. Can J Appl Sports Sci 1983; 8:104–113.

Iverson DC, Fielding JE, Crow RS, Christenson GM. The promotion of physical activity in the United States population: the status of programs in medical, worksite, community, and school settings. Public Health Rep 1985; 100:212–224.

King AL, Frederiksen LW. Low-cost strategies for increasing exercise behavior: relapse preparation training and social support. Behav Mod 1984; 8:3–21.

Knapp DN. Behavioral management techniques and exercise promotion. In: Dishman RK, ed. Exercise adherence: its impact on public health. Champaign, IL: Human Kinetics, 1988: 203.

Lauzon RRJ. A randomized controlled trial of the ability of health hazard appraisal to stimulate appropriate risk reduction behavior. In: Proceedings of the 13th Annual Meeting of the Society of Prospective Medicine, Health Education Resources. 1977: 102–103.

Leppink HB, DeGrassi A. Changes in risk behavior: a two-year follow-up study. In: Proceedings of the 13th Annual Meeting of the Society of Prospective Medicine, Health Education Resources. 1977: 104–107.

Logsdon DN, Rosen MA, Demak, MM. The Insure project on lifestyle preventive health services. Public Health Rep 1982; 97:308–317.

Marlatt GA, Gordon JR. Determinants of relapse: implications for the maintenance of behavior change. In: Davidson P, Davidson S, eds. Behavioral medicine: changing health lifestyles. New York: Brunner-Mazel, 1980:410.

Martin JE, Dubbert PM. Behavioral management strategies for improving health and fitness. J Cardiac Rehabil 1984; 4:200–208.

Meyer A, Nash J, McAlister A, et al. Skills training in a cardiovascular health education campaign. J Consult Clin Psychol 1980; 48:129–142.

Montoye HJ, Taylor HL. Measurement of physical activity in population studies: a review. Hum Biol 1984; 56:195–216.
Mulder JA. Prescription home exercise therapy for cardiovascular fitness. J Fam Pract 1981; 13:345–348.
Oldridge NB, Jones NL. Improving patient compliance in cardiac rehabilitation: effects of written agreement and self-monitoring. J Cardiac Rehabil 1983; 3:257–262.
Reid EL, Morgan RW. Exercise prescription: a clinical trial. Am J Public Health 1979; 69:591–595.
Rogers F, Juneau M, Taylor CB, et al. Assessment by a microprocessor of adherence to home-based moderate-intensity exercise training in healthy sedentary middle-aged men and women. Am J Cardiol 1987; 60:71–75.
Stephens T. Secular trends in adult physical activity: exercise boom or bust? Res Q Ex Sport 1987; 58:94–105.
Wankel LM. Decision-making and social-support strategies for increasing exercise involvement. J Cardiac Rehabil 1984; 4:124–135.
Washburn RA, Montoye HJ. The assessment of physical activity by questionnaire. Am J Epidemiol 1986; 123:563–576.
Wells KB, Ware JE, Lewis CE. Physicians' practices in counseling patients about health habits. Med Care 1984; 22:240–246.
White CC, Powell KE, Hogelin GC, Gentry EM, Forman MR. The behavioral risk factor surveys. IV. The descriptive epidemiology of exercise. Am J Prev Med 19XX; 3:304–310.

BIOMECHANICS IN SPORTS MEDICINE

DAVID J. SANDERSON, B.Sc., M.Sc., Ph.D.

Over the past few years there has grown the perception that biomechanics, as a discipline, holds the potential to help the human machine perform sports with better speed, power, and economy. This may indeed be the case, but biomechanics as a discipline also offers something to other fields of human endeavor. Evidence of its potential for cross-disciplinary interaction can be seen in published articles dealing with ergonomics, tissue mechanics, and sports medicine, to name just three related areas. The aim of this presentation is to focus on the role of biomechanics in sports medicine. Is there a role for biomechanics in sports medicine, and if so, what is it?

The biomechanist studies how the mechanical environment impinges on human movement in general, while the sports biomechanist is the one who focuses primarily on sport. The focus may be on the achievement of the best possible performance or on an understanding of how athletic performance is achieved under the constraints of a given mechanical environment. The sports medicine specialist, on the other hand, is the one who examines the damage that sometimes results from impingement of the environment on the athlete, and identifies ways and means to return the athlete to the field.

By the biomechanical aspects of sports injuries, we are referring to the mechanical factors that may have resulted in or contributed to the injury. Pierrynowski argued in 1985 that forces of excessive magnitude (e.g., impact injuries such as being struck on the head by a rapidly moving cricket ball) are a major cause of sports injuries. Forces have also been implicated in the chronic injuries that occur as a result of, or in conjunction with, repeated loading. The classic example is an injury to a joint of the lower limb because of accumulated running distance. However, not all impulsive or frequently applied forces result in injuries, either chronic or acute, in all individuals. The relationship between biomechanical force and injury is complex. The question is not simply how much force causes an injury, but whether the force acts alone or in conjunction with some other factors to cause injury. The biomechanist and the sports medicine practitioner must strive to answer this question as a team. The development of successful diagnostic and treatment strategies depends in part on the interaction of these professionals.

Early sports medicine practitioners were concerned primarily with surgical intervention, but many other specialists are now involved with the surgeons, including physiotherapists, podiatrists, physicians, and other rehabilitation personnel who have specialized in treating sports-related injuries. This development has occurred along with, or as a result of, the increased involvement of the general population in sporting activities, which has set the stage for a considerable expansion of sports medicine.

Two major factors have resulted in increased interest in biomechanics and recognition of the possible contributions it can make to sports medicine. First, the increased ease with which biomechanical information can be obtained has brought the discipline of biomechanics into everyday discussions. The modern biomechanics laboratory bristles with cine and video recording systems, force platforms, and multisensor pressure mats, all controlled by one or more computer systems. Second, the development of equipment to make possible real-time recording and processing has enabled biomechanics to expand beyond the research laboratory. As Taunton and colleagues pointed out, the increased sophistication of biomechanical analysis has contributed to a much better understanding of the etiology and management of sports-related injuries.

However, in spite of this "high-tech" approach to the study of human movement, there remain many problems in assuming that biomechanics has all the answers, or indeed can provide a means to obtain all the answers. For example, while the external forces applied to the foot during walking can be measured accurately, the biomechanist relies on theoretical constructs or models to compute the magnitudes and direction of forces within the body. Such models require a number of assumptions regarding segment anthropometry, muscle orientation and activation, joint structure, and so on before they can be used. The assumptions themselves limit the confidence with which the results can be applied to any given real-life situation.

It is clear that biomechanics has made a contribution to the development of healthy athletic performance and to the information useful to the sports medicine practitioner. Running shoes of 20 years ago had little to recommend them for any athletic activity; they were inadequate for their task. With the development of a large public interest in running as a recreational pursuit, magazines for runners responded with running shoe tests. Reports were at first based on subjective impressions by runners. The implementation of objective tests by the Runner's World magazine in 1977 resulted in a major shift in shoe design. This testing was conceived, developed, and implemented in a university based biomechanics laboratory. The objectivity of the tests gave them added credence. Manufacturers responded to negative test results by increasing their commitment to the design of more effective footwear. They also recruited biomechanists to assist in the development of a more effective product. Today, experts in biomechanics and sports medicine work with the designers of footwear to ensure a safe product.

This development has helped to foster interest in the achievement of good health through athletic participation. The medical community responded by examining the traditional means of dealing with sports-related injuries. Practitioners developed areas of specialty in sports injuries, and began to examine whether surgical intervention was the best or the only solution. The end result of these developments was a population that demanded more information from the manufacturers and a better product. They also expected medical personnel to have available other methods for rehabilitation of injuries.

Arising from the running shoe tests and the enormous interest in the design of running shoes was a recognition that the biomechanics of the foot under dynamic loading might contribute to chronic foot, knee, or other lower limb injuries. In response to such questions, a number of studies examined how much pronation occurred during the support phase of running, how fast it occurred, and whether the amount and/or rate of pronation were factors in running-related injuries. As a consequence of these studies, more information was obtained on how in-shoe orthoses affected motion of the foot. These data have made a significant contribution to the health of runners through increasing our understanding of the etiology and management of such injuries.

There is a caveat, however, to this apparent success. Biomechanics provides only a partial picture of factors contributing to sports-related injuries. Often the questions posed are superficially simple. To illustrate my point, I would like to discuss two problems that have been presented to the University of British Columbia biomechanics laboratory from local sports medical personnel, and to comment on how the expertise of the laboratory is being geared to address these specific problems. One issue concerns chronic knee pain during cycling. The second concerns the influence of leg-length differences on locomotion mechanics, and in turn how possible compensation may result in chronic lower leg injuries.

KNEE PAIN DURING CYCLING

Increased use of the bicycle for transportation, recreation, and sport has led to a concomitant increase in knee injuries. This is not surprising, because the knee joint bears most of the load during cycling. It has been hypothesized that healthy function of the knee joint is closely related to a pattern of motion of the legs that minimizes joint loading. It has further been hypothesized that orthotics and/or pedal adjustments can be introduced that will compensate for movement pattern problems, reducing both knee loading and knee injuries.

There is an abundance of literature on how orthoses affect pronation during the support phase of running. However, cycling differs from running in that the foot is fixed firmly to the pedal. The knee joint is the primary limiting link between the bicycle and the cyclist. Injuries may arise because of the restricted degrees of freedom of movement in association with joint loading. Solutions to chronic knee pain have included adjusting the position of the foot on the pedal, or using orthotics to alter the foot position in the hope of reducing joint loading. The hypothesis is that, either alone or together, the pattern of motion of the knee joint and joint forces have resulted in a loading pattern that causes injury. From the sports medicine perspective, the request is quite clear: how can orthotics be used to reduce loading and the associated injury? From the biomechanical perspective, a few more issues must be resolved before the question can be addressed.

Subjective observation and subject reporting support these hypotheses. The specialist must devise a way to test these hypotheses objectively. A literature search revealed little hard data on coronal plane knee motion in cycling. We therefore filmed the pattern of knee motion in the coronal plane as cyclists rode a stationary ergometer. The coordinates of markers placed on the tibial tuberosity of the left and right legs and on the pedals were digitized from the film and were used to compute the trajectory over successive pedaling cycles. The medial-lateral motion of these markers with respect to the pedals could then be quantified.

We observed a wide variation in the medial-lateral motion of the knee between individuals, as well as differences between the left and right legs. Such asymmetries explain why some individuals complain of pain in only one knee, although the sore knee may occur because the rider compensates for a problem in the contralateral knee.

The next step was to examine how movement patterns would be affected by canting the foot on the pedal. This time, the foot position was adjusted using aluminum wedges bolted to the back rail of the pedal. While canting appeared to cause some changes in knee motion, those changes were much smaller than anticipated. The riders apparently accommodated to the canting, so that the knee motion remained as in the control condition. This suggests that a more careful examination of the rider-bicycle system is required. For example, we have not yet addressed the issue of lower limb alignment and its effect on knee motion, nor have we correlated the incidence of injury with specific patterns of coronal-plane knee motion. Finally, the pattern of motion may not necessarily reflect the forces developed within the knee joint itself. We need to devise a method of directly measuring the forces within the joint under various riding conditions.

LEG LENGTH AND RUNNING MECHANICS

In most reports on locomotion, film and force platform data are collected from one side of the body. Assumptions of symmetry are made to simplify data collection and analysis. However, the issue of asymmetry must be clarified when diagnosing factors contributing to an injury.

The question posed to our biomechanics laboratory was whether middle distance runners with a measurable leg-length difference presented different biomechanical characteristics of running style that would correlate with their injury history. Could the runner accommodate a shorter leg (structural asymmetry) by adjusting some biomechanical variable (functional asymmetry) to achieve smooth locomotion? This information may contribute to both the design of shoes and corrective orthotics, and the diagnosis and rehabilitation of running-related injuries, while providing insight into the mechanics of compensation for existing injuries.

In order to assess asymmetries, it is necessary to collect data from both legs during a typical running stride. To limit variability, an extensive training period is required. What constitutes a typical running stride? If these data are to be recorded in a laboratory, will they reflect outdoor running patterns? Can one force platform be used, or will two platforms be needed to record successive left-right footfalls? Finally, we must define the method by which leg lengths are measured.

When these decisions have been made, cine and ground reaction force data will be used with link-segment models to summarize the estimated joint reaction forces that, when examined with respect to the external limb kinematics and the ground reaction forces, should provide some clues regarding the influence of difference in leg lengths.

The two studies described above illustrate how biomechanics and the sports medicine specialist can interact to deal with problems arising from sporting activities.

As Taunton and colleagues concluded, there is an obvious relationship between biomechanics and sports injuries. Large forces can exceed tissue tolerances. There are other cases, however, in which the relationship is less clear. Do differences in leg length really affect running mechanics? If so, to what extent does the runner have to compensate? Can altering foot position on the pedals really alter the pattern of forces within the knee joint? It seems that whenever one question is posed, many more arise.

There will be a continued refinement of and spread of equipment employed in biomechanics and sports medicine. However, what is needed is not more sophisticated equipment, but rather a careful examination of movement characteristics with the aim of identifying and quantifying underlying principles. These principles will help to enhance diagnosis, prognosis, and the quality of rehabilitation. The biomechanist and the sports medicine specialist must work closely together to identify these factors before appropriate treatment strategies can be developed.

SUGGESTED READING

Pierrynowski M. The role of biomechanics in sports medicine. In: Shephard RJ, Welsh RP. Current therapy in sports medicine. Toronto: BC Decker, 1985.

Taunton J, McKenzie D, Clement D. The role of biomechanics in the epidemiology of injuries. Sports Med 1988; 6:107–120.

CARDIOPULMONARY PHYSIOLOGY

WALTER P. VANHELDER, M.D., M. Eng., Ph.D.

The cardiopulmonary system has a number of important functions. The primary goal of this system is to deliver oxygen to target tissues of the human body to meet their ever-changing needs. The logistics of this delivery are quite dynamic, especially in exercising athletes in whom various organs have different oxygen requirements depending on the type, intensity, and duration of the activity. Further important functions of the cardiopulmonary system are the removal of carbon dioxide (CO_2), body temperature regulation, immunologic support, transport of metabolites, and many others.

A functional approach to the oxygen delivery system can lead to the following classification of its components:

1. Prepulmonary factors.
2. Pulmonary ventilation and exchange of gases.
3. Pulmonary circulation.
4. Heart function.
5. Coronary circulation.
6. Systemic circulation and vascular resistance.
7. Oxygen transport in blood and gas exchange in target tissues.

It is necessary that all these components function properly in a person striving for excellence in athletic achievements. On the other hand, physical training can influence the function or structure of these several subsystems. Examples of such changes include an increased capacity of the blood to carry oxygen, a decreased resting heart rate, and cardiac hypertrophy (athlete's heart).

The above-mentioned changes occur in response to the training of a healthy athlete, but there are also implications for people who exercise with a preexisting illness. First, it is important to understand the limitations imposed by the existing disease. Second, the illness can sometimes be alleviated by the proper physical training.

PREPULMONARY FACTORS

Inspired gas has a certain oxygen content. As the gas is inspired, it is warmed to body temperature and is humidified. This process is normally completed before the gas reaches the bronchi. When the gas is saturated by water vapor, the partial pressure of this water vapor amounts to 47 mm Hg at the body temperature of 37°C, irrespective of the barometric pressure. Barometric pressure (P_B) and the fraction of oxygen in the inspired gas (F_IO_2), however, determine the partial pressure of oxygen (PiO_2) delivered to the lungs.

$$PiO_2 = F_IO_2 \, (P_B - 47)$$

Dramatic changes in P_B and/or F_IO_2 can occur with increases of altitude or in scuba divers (in hypobaric and hyperbaric conditions, respectively).

PULMONARY VENTILATION

Pulmonary ventilation ($\dot{V}_E$) is a function of respiratory rate (RR) and tidal volume ($\dot{V}_T$).

$$\dot{V}_E = RR \times \dot{V}_T$$

The partial pressure of oxygen at the alveolar level can be calculated, knowing the partial pressure of inspired oxygen (PiO_2), the partial pressure of CO_2 at the alveolar level (P_ACO_2) and a respiratory quotient (RQ).

$$RQ = CO_2 \text{ generated}/O_2 \text{ consumed}$$

In a normal adult at rest, RQ $\doteq$ 200 ml CO_2/250 ml O2, or RQ $\doteq$ 0.8. The actual ratio of gases exchanged with the atmosphere sometimes differs a little from the RQ, and is designated as R, the respiratory gas exchange ratio. P_ACO_2 (alveolar) can be approximated by $PaCO_2$, which is the arterial partial pressure of CO_2. Alveolar O_2 can be calculated as follows:

$$P_AO_2 = PiO_2 - (P_ACO_2)/R$$

This is called the alveolar gas equation.

Hyperventilation (occurring, for example, in exercise, fever, and asthma) or a period of breath holding can temporarily change these approximations. Thus, the ratio of gases actually exchanged with the atmosphere (R) can temporarily differ from the tissue RQ. For example, exercise above the anaerobic threshold leads to an additional CO_2 liberation, owing to anaerobic effort. In such cases, R may exceed 1.0. However, over a longer period, R = RQ.

The difference between alveolar and arterial oxygen tension ($P_AO_2 - PaO_2$) is also called an "A-a gradient." It reflects the efficiency of oxygen exchange at the interface between alveoli and pulmonary blood. This gradient is not affected by changes in ventilation. It equals about 10 mm Hg in a normal young person breathing at sea level. In comparison with this, P_ACO_2 is very nearly equivalent to $PaCO_2$ even in disease. This is due to the fact that CO_2 diffuses across the blood-alveolar gas interface many times more easily than does O_2.

PULMONARY CIRCULATION

The pulmonary vessels are much more compliant than the systemic ones, and they can accommodate an increased blood flow with a minimal increase of pulmonary blood pressure. The normal resting mean pulmonary artery pressure is about 15 mm Hg. Usually, at least a three- to fivefold increase in cardiac output is needed to increase pulmonary pressure. This can occur, for example, during exercise or in patients with left-to-right cardiac shunting (as in various types of septal defect).

Normally, ventilation ($\dot{V}$) and perfusion ($\dot{Q}$) are relatively well matched in healthy lungs. $\dot{V}/\dot{Q}$ mismatch occurs when parts of the lungs are well ventilated but not well perfused, as in emphysema. Conversely, parts of the lungs may be unventilated and the blood passing through these regions does not gain any oxygen on its way to target tissues. This is called a pulmonary shunt. The shunted blood with a low oxygen content mixes later with oxygenated blood coming from normal parts of the lungs, thus lowering the total oxygen content of arterial blood.

HEART FUNCTION

Cardiac output (CO) is the product of stroke volume (SV) and heart rate (HR).

$$CO = SV \times HR$$

A normal CO is approximately 2.5 to 3.5 liters per minute per square meter of body surface, or about 5 to 6 liters per minute in a 70-kg man with a SV of 60 to 90 ml per beat and an HR of 80 beats per minute. Exercise-evoked increases in CO entail early increases in SV and HR at the beginning of physical activity, but an increase of HR is mainly responsible for further increases of CO as exercise progresses. In moderate exercise, HR, SV, and CO can reach 130 beats per minute, 130 ml per beat, and 17 liters per minute, respectively. In maximal exercise, these indices can reach 200 beats per minute, 150 ml per beat, and 30 liters per minute in healthy young athletes.

In healthy resting individuals SV can also increase when the heart rate decreases; the left ventricular filling time is increased, and thus the CO is maintained. This can be seen, for example, in long distance runners with a resting bradycardia. The healthy heart empties between 60 and 80 percent of the end-diastolic volume (EDV). The ejection fraction is the ratio of SV to EDV.

$$SV/EDV = 0.6 - 0.8$$

The magnitude of the SV is determined by preload (EDV), afterload (the pressure against which the heart must contract), inotropy (myocardial contractility), and proper synchronization of ventricular contraction.

CORONARY CIRCULATION

The resting coronary blood flow in a 70-kg man is approximately 225 ml per minute, or about 5 percent of the total CO. The coronary arteries supply the myocardium with oxygen according to its varying needs. When a normal person exercises, there is a proportional increase in both CO and coronary blood flow. Increased blood flow through the coronaries is by far the most important factor in meeting the increasing myocardial oxygen needs during physical exertion. The myocardium cannot generate energy by anaerobic glycolysis, and oxygen extraction from the coronary vessels (their arteriovenous oxygen difference) can increase only negligibly (normally, the heart extracts about 65 percent of the oxygen carried by arterial blood). Thus, the narrowing of a coronary artery by 50 percent or more can impair oxygen delivery during exercise, leading to myocardial ischemia, with consequences that may or may not be reversible.

SYSTEMIC CIRCULATION AND VASCULAR RESISTANCE

Systemic blood pressure (BP) is determined by CO and total peripheral resistance (TPR).

$$BP = CO \times TPR$$

TPR is affected by a large number of factors, including neural and hormonal regulation of the cardiovascular system, as well as the structural composition of the blood vessels. The systolic pressure increases readily with dynamic exercise, while the diastolic pressure increases much more slowly, with a resultant increase in pulse pressure. During isometric exercise, both systolic and diastolic pressures increase considerably.

OXYGEN TRANSPORT IN BLOOD AND GAS EXCHANGE IN TARGET TISSUES

The oxygen-carrying capacity of the blood depends on its hemoglobin content (Hgb; g per 100 ml blood), the percentage of O_2 saturation of the hemoglobin (So_2) and the partial pressure of O_2 in arterial blood (PaO_2).

$$O_2 \text{ capacity} = 0.0139\,(Hgb)\,(So_2) + 0.003(PaO_2)$$

Only a negligible part of the total O_2-carrying capacity represents oxygen physically dissolved in plasma ($0.003 \times PaO_2$) at normal barometric pressure. However, this component could be augmented by increasing the barometric pressure, e.g., in a hyperbaric chamber, thus increasing the oxygen-carrying capacity; this type of emergency treatment can have value in a person with acute loss of hemoglobin and no suitable replacement available.

The oxyhemoglobin dissociation curve is curvilinear, with the bend of the curve occurring at an oxygen partial pressure of 60 mm Hg, corresponding to approximately 90 percent O_2 saturation of hemoglobin. Events associated with exercise, such as increased temperature or Pco_2 and acidosis, shift the oxygen dissociation curve to the right, facilitating desaturation and thus the delivery of oxygen to target tissues. The opposite is true for a decreased temperature or Pco_2 and alkalosis. Oxygen delivery can be monitored by the difference between arterial and venous oxygen content, multiplied by the CO.

Blood flow redistribution in exercise favors the exercising muscle by an increase that can reach 25 to 50 times the resting flow. In addition, there is a threefold increase in patency of capillaries in the exercising muscle.

The complexity of the oxygen delivery system implies that this delivery can be impaired on its way from the inspired gas to the target tissues by a defect in any one or more of the interplaying factors. People at risk are primarily those with a preexisting illness, whether or not it has been diagnosed. However, exercise can frequently be used to alleviate such a condition, or at least to diagnose it correctly.

Two of the most prevalent diseases in our society are ischemic heart disease and hypertension. High blood pressure is the most significant risk factor for cardiovascular disease.

EXERCISE IN HYPERTENSION

It has generally been accepted that regular dynamic exercise may lower blood pressure in patients with mild hypertension, while isometric (static) exercise can cause temporary increases in both systolic and diastolic pressure. The decrease of blood pressure in mildly hypertensive people is often accompanied by decreases in plasma norepinephrine (sympathetic activity) and cholesterol and an improvement in glucose utilization. There is some evidence that in more severe hypertension, exercise may be beneficial after some control of blood pressure has been achieved by means of drug therapy.

Even a single training session seems to have a beneficial effect. A reduction in systolic and diastolic blood pressure lasting for several hours has been reported after a single bout of submaximal exercise. Furthermore, exercise has predictive value in patients who are presently borderline hypertensive. Many of those who have hypertension during exercise develop established hypertension later in life. Conversely, if the blood pressure response to a dynamic exercise in borderline hypertensive individuals is normal, it seems possible to dismiss the diagnosis of hypertension. For example, the Canadian Aerobic Fitness Test (CAFT) has been used for this purpose. Thus, exercise can offer multiple benefits, including prevention of premature death from cardiac-related causes, as suggested by earlier more recent reports. (See also subsequent chapters.)

EXERCISE TESTING

An exercise stress test conducted before embarking upon an exercise program is a very useful clinical tool. It can be used both in screening asymptomatic individuals who wish to start an exercise program and in those with diagnosed cardiac disease, myocardial infarction, or coronary artery disease. Patients are usually exercised on a treadmill, and the 12-lead electrocardiogram (ECG) is analyzed continuously for ST depression or elevation, T-wave changes, rhythm disorders, and atrioventricular block. Symptoms and physical signs are carefully monitored, including chest pain, shortness of breath, blood pressure changes, exhaustion, pallor, and confusion. Whenever the result of the test is doubtful, thallium scintigraphy can follow. This considerably increases the sensitivity of the test, as the heart image can be screened for uneven thallium uptake. An exercise ECG alone has a sensitivity of about 65 percent, while a exercise ECG combined with an exercise thallium test has a sensitivity of 90 percent in terms of detecting myocardial ischemia and infarcted areas.

Thallium-201 concentrates in myocardial cells, where it is transported by the Na-K-ATPase system through the cell membrane. The emission of the thallium taken up by the myocardial cells is recorded by a gamma camera. An irreversible defect in such activity (an image defect) represents dead myocardium—an area of infarction. Defects that appear during exercise, but reperfuse later, signify areas of transient myocardial ischemia.

SUGGESTED READING

Balady GJ, Weiner DA. Exercise testing for sports and the exercise prescription. Cardiol Clin 1987; 5:183–196.

Franz IW. Exercise hypertension: its measurement and evaluation. Herz 1987; 12:99–109.

Kannel WB. Some lessons in cardiovascular epidemiology from Framingham. Am J Cardiol 1976; 37:269–282.

Massie BM, Botvinick EH, Bristow JD. Myocardial perfusion scintigraphy with thallium-201: current status and further prospects. In: Yu PN, Goodwin JF, eds. Progress in cardiology Number 11. Philadelphia: Lea & Febiger, 1982:19.

Pekkanen J, Marti B, Nissinen A, Tuomilehto J, Punsar S, Karvonen MJ. Reduction of premature mortality by high physical activity: a 20-year follow-up of middle-aged Finnish men. Lancet 1987; 1:1473–1477.

Pickering TG. Exercise and hypertension. Cardiol Clin 1987; 5:311–318.

TIME ZONE SHIFT AND SLEEP DEPRIVATION PROBLEMS

THOMAS REILLY, B.A., Dip. P.E., M.Sc., Ph.D., M.I.Biol., F.Erg.S.

CIRCADIAN RHYTHMS

It is obvious that humans have become habituated to the alternations of light and darkness by fitting activity to daylight hours and sleep to nighttime. There was probably a strong teleologic drive to do so in the course of evolution, as well as sound practical reasons. The practical consequence for the athlete of today is that the level of arousal varies throughout the solar cycle, sleep and wakefulness being associated with night and day, respectively. The arousal level is not constant during wakefulness, rising in the morning and falling in the evening before the individual retires to sleep. A cycle of about 24 hours' duration is known as *circadian* and that of arousal is recognized as a basic biologic rhythm.

A myriad of circadian rhythms has been documented, but body temperature is regarded as the fundamental physiologic variable. The body's core temperature tends to peak at 1800 to 1900 hours, the amplitude or mean to peak variation in temperature amounting to 0.3° to 0.4°C. Many performance rhythms, including important components of sports performance, vary with the time of day, in phase with the curve of body temperature variations.

Circadian rhythms connote the existence of internal biologic clocks. There is extensive evidence favoring the cells of the suprachiasmatic nucleus of the hypothalamus as the site of a master clock. Similarly, the pineal gland has important time-keeping functions associated with circadian rhythmicity. There are also local timekeepers, such as those in heart, muscle, and liver cells, that are partly independent of these master clocks. Endogenous rhythms are not easily dislodged by a change in environmental conditions such as exposure to 24 hours of darkness (or light), nocturnal shiftwork, or the time zone transitions involved in transcontinental and intercontinental travel.

Exogenous rhythms, on the other hand, are easily influenced by environmental factors such as light, temperature, physical activity, feeding, and social patterns. They are easily manipulated by changes in the environment and adapt quickly to a new environmental profile.

Normally, circadian rhythms pass unrecognized until normality is so disturbed as to disrupt them. In contemporary society, this occurs most often with nocturnal shiftwork, employees rotating in shifts around the solar day to avoid the costs of having expensive factory machinery idle at night. It is estimated that 20 percent of employees in developed countries have now experienced some form of shift system; the possible impacts of operating nocturnal shift systems upon the physical performance and health of the work force that is implicated are still a matter of concern. The ease of modern air flight allows large numbers of people to travel internationally each year, passing through time zones and disturbing their body rhythms in the process. Many of those involved are athletes traveling to participate in international competitions. The disorientation that ensues is commonly called "jet lag." Either of these factors—shift work or time zone transitions—can impair sleep, which may also be affected by worry (including precompetitive anxiety), environmental noise (e.g., noisy hotel rooms), children in the household, unsettled diurnal routines, and other factors.

The remainder of this chapter concentrates on two major situations in which the circadian rhythms of an athlete are commonly disturbed. The first is time zone shifts: consideration is given to the ways in which effects of jet lag may be minimized. The second is sleep deprivation, when the individual either partially or completely loses the normal daily ration of sleep. Ways in which a person may cope with such deprivation, either short-term or long-term, will be described.

TIME ZONE SHIFTS

When a competitor travels through a series of time zones, the activity of the biologic clocks becomes at odds with signals from the environment that normally lock the body's rhythms into a 24-hour period. The major endogenous rhythms show a resistance to change in response to the new environmental cues, different rhythms varying in their rate of adaptation to the new local time. Thus the body's rhythms become desynchronized for a while after entering the new time zone. The cluster of symptoms known as jet lag may include fatigue, loss of drive, poor concentration, inability to sleep at the proper time, headaches, indigestion, loss of appetite, diarrhea, and so on.

Travel northward or southward does not entail crossing any time zones and simply results in so-called "travel fatigue." Generally the traveler is refreshed after a wash or shower or perhaps a short rest. Long eastward or westward journeys necessarily involve time zone shifts. The duration and severity of the resultant jet lag depend largely on the number of time zones that have been crossed. Other factors affecting the extent of jet lag symptoms include the direction of travel, the times of take-off and arrival, and individual differences in susceptibility.

Physiologic rhythms affected by time zone shifts include body temperature, the sleep-wake cycle, heart rate, ventilation, blood pressure, and renal function. The important external signals that determine the rate of adaptation to the new local time are the patterns of sleep and inactivity imposed by the new community, the timing and type of meals, the exposure to social influences, and the alternation of natural daylight with nocturnal darkness. In general, the body temperature rhythm adapts to the time zone shift at a rate of 1 day for each time zone that has been crossed. The sleep-wake cycle may adapt more rapidly than this, while the excretion of electrolytes adapts more slowly. The rate of adaptation can be accelerated by complying with the time-giving external signals.

Jet lag symptoms are more severe and more prolonged when travel is in an easterly rather than a westerly direction. The traveler gains time when going westward, and the body's rhythms adjust more readily to a lengthening rather than a shortening of the day. In "free-wheeling" conditions, such as exposure to periods of continuous light or continuous darkness (a situation encountered in northerly communities and in cave exploration), the body temperature rhythm slows down to a 25- to 27-hour cycle. In near-maximal time zone shifts, for example, during travel between Britain and Australia (Fig. 1), there does not appear to be any difference in symptoms between the outward and return legs of the journey.

Individuals seem to differ in the severity of jet lag symptoms they encounter. Young and generally fit individuals tend to suffer less than their older or more sedentary counterparts. Nevertheless, individual susceptibility is not consistent from one visit to the next, and one symptom-free journey provides no guarantee of subsequent immunity against jet lag. Owing to this variability, it is unlikely that key characteristics of "good" or "poor" adapters could be identified and used in team selection for international travel.

MINIMIZING JET LAG

Individuals who are crossing time zones for a short stay (1 to 2 days at their destination) may be able to organize the timing of their daily activities to conform with the time of day in their city of origin. This is achieved by the discipline of altering mealtimes, time of arising from bed, timing of training sessions, and time of retiring for sleep. It would generally be possible when traveling between the East and West Coasts of North America, for example, to accommodate such changes. In the case of longer journeys, there would be little possibility of avoiding the influence of the strong environmental cues upon the body's circadian timekeepers. The strategy of anchoring circadian rhythms to the time zone of departure has been employed successfully by some airline personnel on quick-return flights, but it would be a risky tactic to suggest for athletes engaged in strenuous competitive activity.

In the main, it is to the advantage of the individual to adjust to the new environment as quickly as possible. The strategies available to the physician and coach in aiding this forced adjustment can be classified according to behavioral, dietary, and pharmacologic methods.

BEHAVIORAL METHODS

Preparation can sometimes be made for a time zone shift by altering the athlete's bedtime for a few days before the date of departure. The individual can retire to bed 1 to 2 hours earlier or later than usual and get up 1 to 2 hours earlier or later, depending on the intended direction of travel. For many people, even this maneuver may be impractical, and any greater change before departure is likely to interrupt the normal habitual activity unduly.

Once on the plane, watches should be reset according to the time zone of destination. It is important to tune mentally into the time of day at the city of arrival. It is a good idea to try to sleep on the plane when it is nighttime at the destination. At other times, it is advisable to stay awake; a regimen of mental work, reading, or similar activity can be helpful. Sometimes muscle contractions can be performed while sitting, and stretching (flexibility) exercises can be conducted in the aisle or at the rear of the plane; either should help to maintain alertness and avoid stiffness.

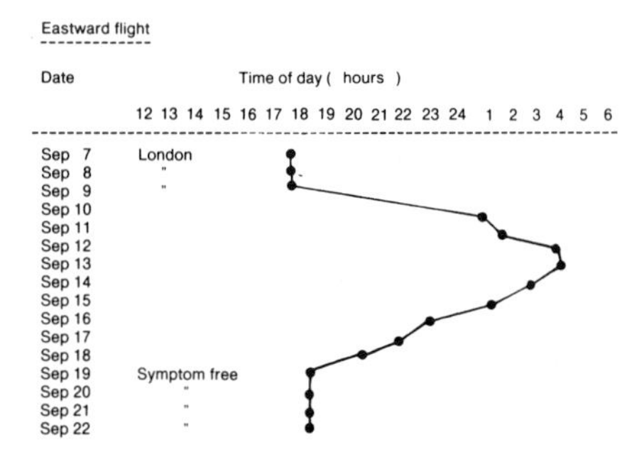

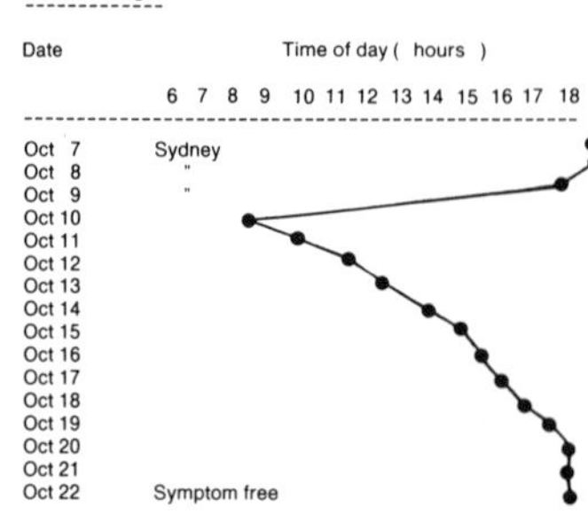

Figure 1 The time of day at which the oral temperature attained a peak is plotted according to local time on outward (eastward) and return (westward) journeys between England and Australia. There was a stop-over of 1 night in Singapore on both journeys. The points were determined using cosinor analysis of data collected throughout each day. Data are for a single individual.

After the flight has been completed, it is important to fit into the local pattern of activity as quickly as possible. However, a 1- to 2-hour adjustment of rising and retiring time can be allowed. Early rising for a day or two after a westward flight is advocated. There may be a temptation to take a nap if the athlete feels tired during the day; this should be avoided if possible, because a prolonged nap would keep circadian rhythms anchored to their former phases and would resist the replacement of the obsolete rhythms.

It is likely that exercise helps adaptation to a new time zone. It is nevertheless recommended that such exercise be light in intensity for a few days, until the worst of the jet lag symptoms have passed. Athletes may need to alter the time of day at which they train, so that this coincides with the time of day when they are now likely to be most alert. For athletes who have traveled westward, this should be in the morning, whereas those who have traveled eastward should train in the evening. For some days after a near-maximal time zone shift, training is best conducted in the morning, after the athlete has benefited from a night of sleep.

Athletic teams are advised to plan friendly or trial matches first, to ease themselves into the new time zone. Important engagements may follow, once all members of the squad have overcome the effects of jet lag.

DIETARY APPROACHES

A problem may be presented by dryness of the air in a pressurized aircraft; this promotes dehydration. The diuretic effects of caffeine and alcohol make them unsuitable as in-flight drinks. It is preferable to drink fruit juices, mineral drinks, or even water, and these can be taken more copiously than normal.

The meals provided on a plane tend to be scheduled on the basis of the local time of departure. The traveler with an eye toward the time zone at the final destination can prudently miss those meals that do not fit into the projected schedule.

It is prudent also to avoid alcohol in the days immediately after arrival at the destination. Caffeine (in coffee) and theophylline (in tea) help to maintain arousal levels during the course of the day, but should be avoided as the local bedtime approaches.

Scheduling of mealtimes is an important factor in helping to adapt to the new time zone. It can be complemented by the daily schedule of social activity. The proportions of macronutrients in the meal may also be relevant. A breakfast biased toward protein stimulates epinephrine and promotes arousal. A light carbohydrate snack in the evening stimulates the synthesis of serotonin in the brain; this neurotransmitter has an important function in the regulation of sleep, and thus carbohydrate foods increase drowsiness. These principles can be applied to the choice of diet by athletes until their symptoms of jet lag have abated.

PHARMACOLOGIC MEASURES

The use of methylxanthines (caffeine, theophylline, aminophylline) in the early part of the day, especially after an eastward flight, and in the afternoon, particularly after traveling westward, can help to establish circadian rhythms in their new phases. It has already been mentioned that alcohol is not advisable because of its diuretic effect; taken late in the evening, it can have the adverse effect of disrupting badly needed sleep.

The family of drugs known as hypnotics have been touted as promoting adjustment to a new time zone. Such agents may be effective in getting the individual to sleep, but offer no guarantee of preventing an early awakening. They may have a role in promoting the onset of sleep on the nights immediately after a long flight in the minority of individuals who have extreme difficulty in getting to sleep.

A similar caveat applies to the use of benzodiazepines. Even short-acting benzodiazepines are known to cause hangovers, which simply aggravate the symptoms of jet lag. The subsequent effects on exercise performance have not been thoroughly researched.

Athletes should be particularly cautious about using chronobiotic drugs. Apart from producing unwanted side effects, the substances may be on the list of those barred to competitors (see the chapter entitled *Control of Drug Abuse*).

Orally ingested melatonin, a hormone produced by the pineal gland, has been suggested as an effective counter to the symptoms of jet lag. Synthetic versions of this hormone are not yet commercially available, and apart from an encouraging pilot study, there is no conclusive evidence that administration of melatonin eliminates jet lag symptoms.

SLEEP DEPRIVATION

Sleep is an enigma in the sense that it has never been conclusively explained why we need it. One school of thought relates sleep to the restitution of the body's tissues; an alternative view is that the need for sleep is specific to nerve cells—the so-called "brain restitution theory." Nevertheless, sleep is essential, and this need becomes most apparent when we look at how human functioning deteriorates after a severe loss of sleep.

Sleep loss interacts with circadian rhythms, in that the adverse effects of sleep deprivation are most keenly noted at nighttime. In self-paced work sustained for 3 to 4 days, the activity level peaks at about 1800 hours, coinciding with the peak of body temperature. This peak persists on as many days as the individual can be kept awake. The effects of 3 to

4 days of complete sleep loss can be seen as a trend to deteriorating performance on which a circadian rhythm is superimposed. The trend is not evident in all functions; gross motor functions such as muscle strength are highly resistant to the effects of sleep loss, while cognitive functions are easily affected. Complex and challenging mental tasks are less affected than monotonous or boring ones. Strong motivation can often override the effects of sleep loss. Sleep loss and environmental factors interact, but not in a predictable or additive manner: heat, for example, compounds the effects of loss of sleep, while noise tends to partly offset them. Individual expectations and previous experience of sleep deprivation may also be relevant, so that it is not easy to ascertain the interplay of the various factors affecting performance after sleep loss.

Complete Sleep Loss

Many individuals who have suffered a complete loss of sleep for two consecutive nights experience temporary visual hallucinations. Most people have such an experience by the third night without sleep. At this time, behavior becomes bizarre, and psychotic-like symptoms are displayed. Phenylethylamine, a naturally occurring amine in the brain, may play a role in such cycles of behavior and mood. By the third night of complete sleep deprivation, the levels of this substance that are being excreted in the urine approach the values normally observed in psychiatric patients. Individuals experiencing such trances may be abruptly snapped out of them if their companions provide strong verbal encouragement to keep awake.

Such extreme losses of sleep are rarely met in normal clinical practice. They may be experienced by sports medical personnel on hospital duty. They may also be encountered for a single night by those participating in 24-hour sports events or charity sports activities that attempt to set unofficial endurance records. Exercise itself has a powerful arousing effect, and is a good antidote to sleepiness.

Frequently we hear people say that they require a "sleeping pill" as they were unable to sleep at all during the previous night. Such accounts may be untrue and need independent corroboration. Short periods of sleep, snatched unwittingly during the night, serve a significant restorative function. Individuals who go without sleep for some time derive considerable benefit from such naps, and those deprived of sleep for 2 to 4 days usually recover from their ordeal after one complete night of uninterrupted sleep.

Partial Sleep Loss

For the traveling sports competitor, partial sleep loss is a more common problem than total sleep deprivation. Although there is a large variability in the amount of sleep normally taken by adults, most athletes are convinced that they need a good night's sleep if they are to perform well. This is commonly interpreted to mean 8 hours of uninterrupted sleep. Sports competitors accept uncritically the need for good sleeping habits, despite many examples of colleagues who cope well with athletic engagements after a poor night's sleep.

Disrupted sleep can promote anxiety in those who believe that good-quality sleep is essential. Coordination tasks seem to be more easily affected than gross motor tasks such as running, cycling, or exerting maximal muscle tension. This assumes that the individuals concerned are strongly motivated to perform at their maximum.

There appears to be no difference between the sexes in terms of responses to partial sleep loss. In both men and women, adverse effects are most pronounced in tasks demanding muscle coordination; effects are less marked in gross motor tasks. Indeed, the variation in performance of tasks such as a maximal hand grip is much greater with the time of day than with partial sleep loss.

Individuals forced to reduce their normal sleep ration may adapt to their new regimen without any obvious consequences for performance, provided the reduction does not exceed 2 hours. Otherwise, they may need to reorganize their daily routine to accommodate an afternoon nap. The practicality of such a nap depends on personal and occupational circumstances.

Sleeplessness

Although true insomnia is rare, a large number of people, perhaps 10 to 15 percent of the population, have difficulty in sleeping. Causes include anxiety, depression, bereavement, stress, overwork, and environmental noise such as that from motor vehicle traffic. Some of these problems are transient and self-limiting; others may persist and become chronic.

It is generally thought that exercise promotes sleep, and so regular bouts of physical activity are recommended as therapy for individuals who are having difficulty in sleeping. The effect of exercise is likely to be indirect, sleep being promoted by an alleviation of the anxieties that prevented it. Athletes exhibit different sleep patterns from those of their sedentary peers according to electroencephalographic (EEG) observations. However, EEG characteristics are only marginally altered by a regimen of physical training. Strenuous exercise shortly before retiring to sleep is likely to cause arousal rather than induce drowsiness, owing to an increase in circulating catecholamine levels. Thus, if exercise therapy is prescribed for sleeping problems, it should not be strenuous and it should be performed early rather than late in the evening.

A more usual prescription for insomnia is some type of sleeping pill. People taking sedatives or hypnotics for a prolonged period develop a dependence upon them, and the drugs progressively lose their effectiveness. The minor tranquilizers, the benzodiazepines, are probably now being overprescribed, both in Europe and in North America. Habitual users also become dependent on benzodiazepines and suffer severe withdrawal symptoms when the drug is withdrawn. Even normal doses impair reaction time and reduce mental concentration the morning after the medication is taken. Consequently, such a prescription should be considered for athletes only in cases of dire necessity.

Effective nonpharmacologic methods of treating sleeplessness include hypnotherapy. Biofeedback of skin resistance and EEG may also be employed to induce relaxation, thus training individuals to overcome the emotional tension that keeps them awake. Psychological techniques such as visualization of tranquil scenes, concentration on relaxing muscle activity, and deep breathing provide alternative methods of treatment. Stimulus control therapy refers to a mental strategy whereby bed and sleeplessness are dissociated; the individual goes to bed only when sleepy, avoids eating, reading, or watching television in the bedroom, and does not "sleep in" during the morning. Sensible eating and drinking habits (such as avoiding large meals, heavy alcoholic beverages, or caffeine late at night) also promote sleep, and so help "knit up the ravelled sleave of care."

SUGGESTED READING

de Looy A, Minors D, Waterhouse J, et al. The coach's guide to competing abroad. Leeds: National Coaching Foundation, 1988.

Horne J. Why we sleep: the function of sleep in humans and other mammals. Oxford: Oxford University Press, 1988.

Minors DS, Waterhouse J. Circadian rhythms and the human. Bristol: John Wright, 1981.

Reilly T. Circadian rhythms and exercise. In: Macleod D, Maughan R, Nimmo M, et al, eds. Exercise: benefits, limits and adaptations. London: E. and F.N. Spon, 1987: 346.

PHYSIOLOGIC PRINCIPLES OF EXERCISE TESTING

MICHAEL J. PLYLEY, Ph.D.

Exercise is a natural stressor for the human body, and one which is routinely encountered to various degrees during daily living. Exercise testing provides a reproducible means by which the body's capacity for physical effort can be assessed. To be effective, the exercise test must stress all components of the system in order to evaluate any limitation(s) that exist. The risk of complications during exercise testing has been reported to be 0.04 percent, making exercise testing, especially submaximal testing, relatively safe for evaluating the integrity of the cardiorespiratory system. This chapter examines the types of equipment and some of the protocols commonly used in conducting an exercise test.

DESIGNING AN EXERCISE TEST

The general requirements for the design of an exercise test include the following:

1. The work should involve large muscle groups.
2. The nature of the work should be familiar to the test population, to ensure a consistent mechanical efficiency.
3. The protocol and test conditions should be reproducible, to allow comparisons between tests.
4. The test conditions and protocol should maximize yield, but minimize time and expense.
5. The test must be safe and acceptable to a majority of the population.

CHOOSING AN ERGOMETER

The choice of ergometer is based on a number of factors. When evaluating athletes, the primary factor to consider is specificity; the ergometer should utilize the same movement patterns as those used in training and competition. For assessing the general population, the most frequently chosen ergometers are the cycle ergometer and the stepping bench (Table 1). Other types of ergometers include treadmill, arm-crank, SwimBench, and those used for rowing, kayaking, cross-country skiing, wheelchair, tethered swimming, and stair climbing.

Stepping Bench

The stepping bench provides the simplest means of assessing the cardiorespiratory response to an increasing work rate. It represents an activity commonly carried out by most individuals and therefore requires little habituation. The apparatus requires little maintenance, and once built to specifications it requires no further calibration. The major disadvantage of the stepping bench is that it is nearly impossible to conduct a graded exercise test to exhaustion because the subject either fails to

TABLE 1 Choosing an Ergometer: Comparison of the Advantages and Disadvantages of Various Ergometers.

Cycle Ergometer	*Treadmill*	*Stepping Bench Ergometer*
Advantages:		
Seated subject facilitates ancillary physiologic assessment	Effort limited by "central" cardiovascular function, i.e., yields a plateau in oxygen uptake	Simple design
Reproducible workloads	Effort paced by ergometer	Little maintenance
High mechanical efficiency	Familiar exercise	No regular calibration required
Easily calibrated		Portable
Takes up little space		Familiar exercise
Mobility		No electrical requirements
		Inexpensive
		Easily stored
Disadvantages:		
Loading varies with pedaling frequency	Costly	Restricted to only submaximal testing
Often limited by muscle strength	Noisy	Ancillary physiologic assessment is difficult
Regular calibration is necessary	Requires considerable space	Hazardous at high rates of stepping
Electrically braked models are expensive	Requires special electrical wiring	Different sizes are necessary for testing all segments of population
	Requires considerable habituation	
	Hazardous	
	Anxiety provoking	
	Ancillary physiologic assessments are difficult	
	Emergency treatment is difficult	

Modified from Shephard RJ. Exercise physiology. (1987). Toronto: BC Decker, 1987; and Andersen KL, Shephard RJ, Denolin H, et al., eds. Geneva: World Health Organization, 1971.

maintain the proper cadence or trips. The apparatus consists of either a single step (Balke step test), a double step (Master two step, Canada Home Fitness test), or a multistep (e.g., Stair Master). The subject alternately ascends and descends the step(s) at a rate established by a metronome; the usual frequencies of stepping range from 24 to 36 cycles per minute (cpm) on the single step, 11 to 28 cpm on the double step, and 20 to 40 cpm on the multistep; the setting on the metronome is based not on the number of cpm, but on the number of footplants per minute (i.e., 96 to 144 on the single step, which has four footplants per cycle; 66 to 168 on the double step, which has six footplants per cycle; and 40 to 80 on the continuous stair, which has two footplants per cycle). Stepping rates above 150 footplants $\cdot$ min^{-1} are not advised, because there is an increased danger of tripping at such high rates. The "resistance" to the effort of stepping is provided by the subject's body mass, which represents a force against which the individual must work; it can be expressed in newtons (= mass $\times$ 9.81 m $\cdot$ sec^{-2}) (Appendix 1). The resistance can be increased for testing at a fixed step height and cadence by using a weight belt or pack for loading additional mass, although this means of loading can lead to difficulties in performance by altering the center of gravity of the individual. The work done while stepping (in joules) is determined as the product of (force, in newtons) (step height, in meters) (Appendix 2). The rate of doing work (power output, in watts) is given by the product of (work, in joules) (step frequency, in c $\cdot$ s^{-1}). The work done in stepping down (approximately 33 percent), and that due to stepping forward and backward (fre-

Appendix 1 Standard International (SI) Units of Scientific Measurement and Conversion Factors From Previously Used Units

Variable	*Dimensions*	*SI Units*	*Previous Units*
Mass	kg	kilogram	pound (= 0.454 kg)
Distance	m	meter	foot (= 0.305 m) yard (= 0.914 m) mile (= 1.609 km)
Time	s	second	
Frequency	s^{-1}	hertz	
Speed	$m \cdot s^{-1}$	$m \cdot s^{-1}$	$foot \cdot min^{-1}$ (= 0.508 $cm \cdot s^{-1}$) $mile \cdot hour^{-1}$ (= 0.446 $m \cdot s^{-1}$) (= 1.606 $km \cdot h^{-1}$)
Force	$kg \cdot m \cdot s^{-2}$	newton	kg-force (= 9.81 N) kilopond (= 9.81 N) lb-force (= 4.448 N)
Work	$kg \cdot m^2 \cdot s^{-2}$	joule	calorie (= 4.186 J) ft·lb-force (= 1.356 J)
Power	$kg \cdot m^2 \cdot s^{-3}$	watt	$kg \cdot m \cdot min^{-1}$ (= 0.164 W) horsepower (= 745.7 W)

Appendix 2 Examples of Work, Power, and Oxygen Consumption Calculation on Stepping Bench, Cycle ergometer, and Treadmill

1. *Stepping Bench*

Body mass	70 kg
Step height	40 cm
Stepping frequency	30 steps·min^{-1} (= 0.5 steps·s^{-1})
Body surface area	2 m^2

a. Force = mass × acceleration
= 70 kg × 9.81 m·s^{-2}
= 686.7 kg·m·s^{-2}
= 686.7 N

b. Work = force × displacement
= 686.7 N × 0.40 m
= 274.7 N.m
= 274.7 J (per step)

c. Power = work / time
= 274.7 J / 2.0 s
= 137.4 J·s^{-1}
= 137.4 W (per step) *or*
$= \frac{\text{force} \times \text{displacement}}{\text{time}}$
$= \frac{686.7 \text{ N} \times 0.4 \text{ m}}{2.0 \text{ s}}$
= 137.4 N·m·s^{-1}
= 137.4 W (per step) *or*
= force × velocity
= 686.7 N × 0.2 m·s^{-1}
= 137.4 W (per step)

d. $\dot{V}O_2$ = [(0.0179 power) + (0.134 BSA)]
= [(0.0179 L·min^{-1}·W^{-1}) (137.4 W) + (0.134 L·min^{-1}·m^{-2}) (2.0 m^2)]
= 2.73 L·min^{-1}

2. *Cycle Ergometer*

Mass (load)	5.0 kp (= 5.0 kg)
Frequency	50 rev·min^{-1} (= 0.83 rev·s^{-1})
Circumference (2 πr)	2.0 m
Gear ratio (ie. pedal: flywheel)	1:3
Body surface area	2.0 m^2

a. Force = mass × acceleration
= 5.0 kg × 9.81 m·s^{-2}
= 49.1 kg·m·s^{-2}
= 49.1 N

b. Work = force × displacement
= force × circumference × pedal:flywheel
= 49.1 N × 2.0 m × 3
= 294.6 N·m
= 294.6 J (per revolution)

c. Power = work / time
= 294.6 J / 1.2 s
= 245.5 J·s^{-1}
= 245.5 W (per revolution) *or*
$= \frac{\text{force} \times \text{displacement}}{\text{time}}$
$= \frac{\text{force} \times \text{circumference} \times \text{pedal : flywheel}}{\text{time}}$
$= \frac{49.1 \text{ N} \times 2.0 \text{ m} \times 3}{1.2\text{s}}$
= 245.5 N·m·s^{-1}
= 245.5 W (per revolution) *or*
= force × velocity
= 49.1 N × 5.0 m·s^{-1}
= 245.5 W

d. $\dot{V}O_2$ = [(0.0125 power) + (0.134 BSA)]
= [(0.0125 L·min^{-1}·W^{-1}) (245.5 W) + (0.134 L·min^{-1}·m^2) (2.0 m^2)]
= 3.34 L·min^{-1}

3. *Treadmill*

Mass	70 kg
Speed	10 km·h^{-1} (= 2.78 m·s^{-1})
Incline	10.5% (= 6, i.e., 1 degree = 1.75%)

a. Force = mass × acceleration
= 70 kg × 9.81 m·s^{-2}
= 686.7 kg·m·s^{-2}
= 686.7 N

b. work = force × vertical displacement
= 686.7 N × (2.78 m × sine 6 degrees)
= 686.7 N × 0.29 m
= 199.4 N·m
= 199.4 J

c. Power = work / time
= 199.4 J / 1.0 s
= 199.4 J·s^{-1}
= 199.4 W

d. $\dot{V}O_2$ = 61.6 ml·min^{-1}·kg^{-1} (from Fig. 1)

quency dependent), also contribute to oxygen consumption; in most calculations, these other sources of work are incorporated into the mechanical efficiency value assumed for this type of work (approximately 16 to 19 percent). Since oxygen intake and work rate are linearly related (until near-maximal effort), the calculated power output can be converted into an oxygen consumption by the equation:

$$\dot{V}O_2 (\text{L·min}^{-1}) = [(0.0179 (F) (f) (H) + (0.134 \text{ BSA})]$$

where F, f, H, and BSA are force, stepping frequency, step height, and body surface area, respectively. Because oxygen intake and heart rate are also linearly related during exercise, exercise can be prescribed on the basis of heart rate (or alternatively by work rate, power output, or oxygen intake). Because stepping is a weightbearing activity, the oxygen intake is properly expressed as ml·min^{-1}·kg^{-1}.

Cycle Ergometer

The cycle ergometer is the most commonly used form of ergometer; there are two types, the mechanically braked and the electrically braked. The advantage of the cycle ergometer is that the subject is in a relatively stable, upright body position, which allows easy assessment of ancillary physiologic variables such as blood pressure, heart rate and rhythm, and blood sampling via indwelling catheters, and also facilitates conversing with the individual about perceived exertion or other symptoms. A second advantage of the cycle ergometer is that it can be used for arm-crank ergometry by placing the ergometer on a table or bench. (Specially designed arm-crank ergometers with smaller flywheels are also available.) The major disadvantage of the cycle ergometer is that the exercise is often limited by leg strength and local muscular endurance rather than by the cardiovascular transport system. In addition, for proper use, the cycle ergometer requires daily calibration and minor but regular maintenance of the belt and flywheel. Resistance to pedaling on the mechanically braked cycle ergometer is provided by a belt that passes around a flywheel; by increasing the tension (measured in kiloponds; 1 kp = 9.81 newtons) on the belt, it can be made increasingly difficult to pedal. Pedaling frequency is again indicated by a metronome, and is recorded as the number of complete revolutions (rev) of one foot per minute (usually 50 or 60 rev $\cdot$ min^{-1}). The frequency setting for the metronome during cycle ergometry is based on the number of revolutions of both feet per minute (100 to 120). Note that this is not necessarily the number of flywheel revolutions per minute, because the cycle ergometer may have a specific gearing that provides more, or less, than one revolution of the flywheel per single revolution of the pedals. Therefore, the pedal:flywheel revolution ratio (or gear ratio, p:f) must be taken into account in the calculation of the work rate. The work done while cycling (in joules) is determined as the product of (resistance setting, in newtons) (circumference [= $2\pi r$ 2 r] of the flywheel, in m) (pedal: flywheel ratio) (see Appendix 2). Power output (work/time, in watts) is determined as the product of (work, in joules) (frequency of pedaling, in rev $\cdot$ s^{-1}). Again, assuming a standard mechanical efficiency (usually 21 to 23 percent), oxygen intake can be calculated from the power output by the equation:

$$\dot{V}o_2\ (L \cdot min^{-1}) = [(0.0125)(R)(C)(f)(p{:}f) + (0.134\ BSA)]$$

where R, C, f, p:f, and BSA are resistance, circumference, pedaling frequency, gear ratio, and body surface area, respectively. Unlike stepping, cycling is a weight supported activity, and $\dot{V}o_2$ is best expressed as L $\cdot$ min^{-1}.

Treadmill Ergometer

The treadmill, in many ways, represents the best choice in ergometers. The activities of walking and running utilize large muscle groups and are natural forms of exercise for everyone. However, considerable habituation is often required for treadmill exercise, because the kinesthetic feedback during this form of exercise is different from that received during normal physical activity. The problem is one in which the frame of reference has been changed from running through a "stationary world" to one in which the individual is stationary and the "world" moves beneath the individual. A second major advantage of treadmill ergometry is that the machine, not the person, paces the exercise; therefore, tests of oxygen intake measured from treadmill exercise are viewed as the "gold standard" against which values from the other ergometers can be compared (Table 2). The disadvantages of the treadmill include cost, a need for special electrical wiring, its bulk and noise, and the apprehension caused because it seems intimidating and somewhat disorienting. It would be safer for those using a high-speed treadmill for exercise testing if the treadmill were placed in a "pit," so that the bed of the treadmill is level with the floor of the laboratory or office. The calculation of power output on the treadmill ergometer is complicated by two factors (see Appendix 2). First, because the center of gravity of the body is not lifted to any great extent during level walking or running, there is no accumulation of potential energy, and little or no physical work is done. In essence, the mechanical efficiency for this type of activity is zero. Once the subject begins walking or running on an incline, work can be calculated as the product of (body mass, in newtons) (vertical distance climbed, in meters); the vertical distance is computed as the product of (treadmill speed, in m $\cdot$ min^{-1}) (slope of the incline, in percent, but expressed as a decimal fraction). The efficiency of climbing the incline is quite variable, and is dependent on both the slope of the incline and the skill of the subject. Calculation of oxygen consumption for exercise on the treadmill ergometer is not as straightforward as with the stepping bench or cycle ergometer because of the complications in calculating the work performed; however, several equations have been developed for use with specific treadmill protocols or for specific exercise levels on the treadmill. A nomogram for determining the oxygen cost of treadmill running was developed by Shephard (Fig. 1).

TABLE 2 Comparison of Maximal Oxygen Intake Measurements from Various Ergometers

Ergometer	*Relative $\dot{V}o_2max$ Value**
Treadmill	100%
Cycle : upright exercise	93–96%
: supine exercise	82–85%
Steptest	88–92%
Arm crank	65–70%

*Relative to the treadmill value.

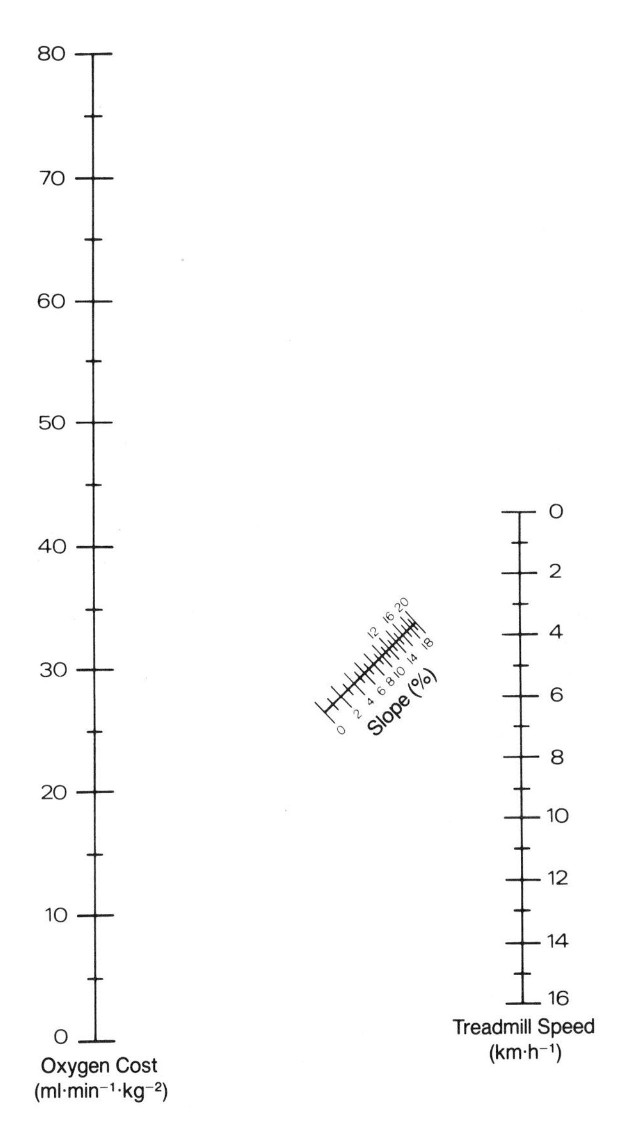

Figure 1 Nomogram for the determination of the oxygen cost (ml·min^{-1}·kg^{-1}) of treadmill running from the speed (km·h^{-1}) and grade (%). (Modified from Shephard RJ. A nomogram to calculate the oxygen cost of running at slow speeds. J Sports Med 1969; 9:10.)

CHOOSING A PROTOCOL

The choice of protocol is often dictated by the particular test situation and by the overall goals of the test. Decisions to be made include the following: (1) Will the test be a maximal one, a submaximal one with prediction of maximal aerobic power via extrapolation to maximal heart rate, or a submaximal one with no prediction? (2) Will the test be conducted using continuous or discontinuous progressive loading? (3) Will the test examine submaximal, steady-state, or maximal responses? For the healthy general public, it is more effective to use one or more steady-state loads with no prediction of aerobic power. Testing in this way does not necessitate extrapolation of data, and improvement of the individual's condition is easily documented as the ability to perform the same test with a lower heart rate at a subsequent testing. The major difficulty with this procedure is that exercise prescription is usually based on a percentage of maximal aerobic power. With elite athletes (especially those with an endurance component), it is usually of interest and important for performance that both the steady-state and the maximal responses be evaluated. In developing a testing protocol, the following principles should be applied:*

1. The exercise should begin at an intensity level that can easily be handled by the individual.
2. The increases in intensity should be gradual, and observations should be made at each stage.
3. Heart rate, blood pressure, the appearance of the subject, rating of perceived exertion, and any other symptoms (either observed or verbally reported) should be monitored regularly.
4. Contraindications to further testing and the reasons for stopping a test should be closely monitored.
5. Recovery of the individual should be followed for 7 to 10 minutes after the test is stopped. Any abnormal responses during recovery require additional monitoring or follow-up.
6. The room temperature should be 22°C or less, with a relative humidity of 60 percent or less.

The most popular types of testing protocols (Fig. 2) include (1) discontinuous step incremental, (2) continuous step incremental, and (3) continuous ramp incremental. With the discontinuous step incremental test, the load is assigned for 4 to 6 minutes and then the subject is allowed to rest for 2 to 3 minutes before undertaking the next load; this type of protocol is used when evaluating cardiac output by the CO_2 rebreathe technique. With the continuous step incremental test, the load is increased every 1 to 2 minutes and the subject is not given a period of rest between increases; this type of protocol is most often used for measurement of maximal oxygen intake. The continuous ramp incremental test is similar to the step incremental, but the increases in load (steps) are so small as to give the impression of being continuously increasing throughout the time interval rather than being increased at the end of a time interval as in the step incremental; this type of protocol is used with the computer-driven, electronically braked cycle ergometers that have recently come onto the market.

The criteria for the acceptance of a valid test of maximal oxygen intake include (1) a "plateau" in oxygen intake of 2 ml · (min · kg)$^{-1}$ or less with increasing workload; (2) reaching a heart rate that would be expected for the age of the individual (at

---

*Guidelines for Exercise Testing and Prescription, American College of Sports Medicine, 1986.

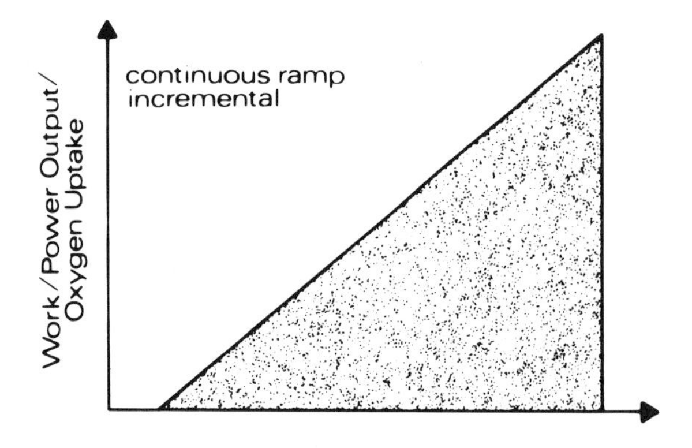

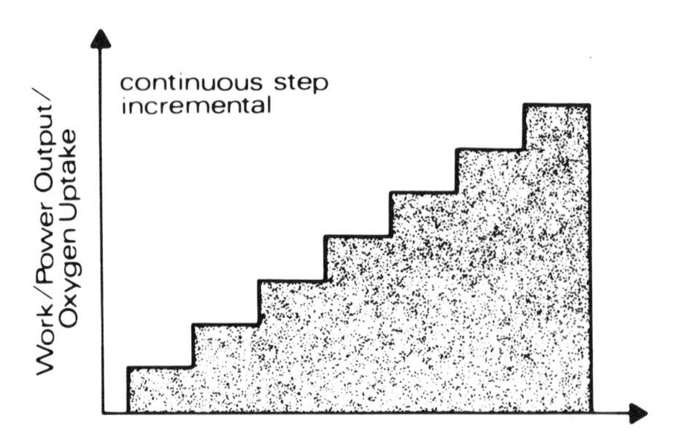

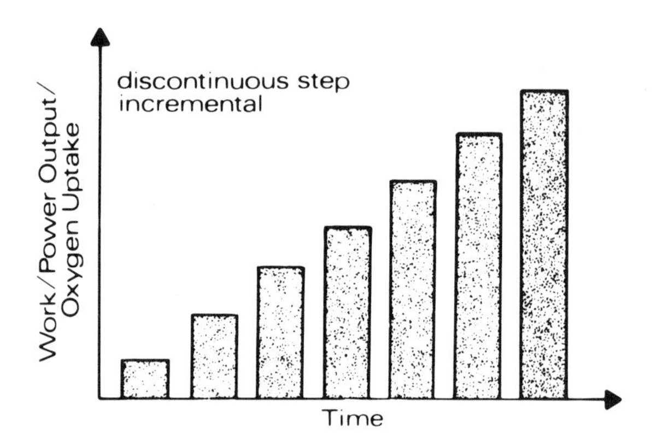

Figure 2 Loading schedules for protocols of exercise testing.

least 220 – age in years); (3) development of a respiratory exchange ratio (= $\dot{V}CO_2/\dot{V}O_2$) of 1.05 or higher; and (4) a post-test blood lactic acid level of greater than 10 mM · L^{-1} (children and older individuals may exhibit lower values, even at maximal effort). The best of these criteria is the observation of a "plateau" in oxygen consumption with increasing levels of power output; however, many individuals who have not experienced a maximal effort voluntarily stop the exercise before reaching this plateau stage. In this case, the other three criteria are used to establish the validity of the test as a maximal effort, and the oxygen intake value is referred to as $\dot{V}O_2$ peak.

Oxygen intake can be expressed in several formats; the two most commonly used are gross oxygen intake (in L · min^{-1}) and relative oxygen intake (in ml · $[min \cdot kg]^{-1}$). Maximal oxygen intake when expressed in L · min^{-1} is used for activities in which the body mass is supported (e.g., cycling, rowing, and swimming). The expression of $\dot{V}O_2$max as ml · $(min \cdot kg)^{-1}$ is determined by dividing the gross oxygen consumption (in ml · min^{-1}) by the body mass (in kilograms), and is used when the activity under examination is one in which the individual must carry that mass. Thus, in activities such as cycling, rowing, and swimming, the individual does not pay as great a price for being bigger and heavier as those engaged in walking- or running-based activities.

SUGGESTED READING

Andersen KL, Shephard RJ, Denolin H, et al. Fundamentals of exercise testing. Geneva: World Health Organization, 1971.

Blair SN, Gibbons LW, Painter P, et al. Guidelines for exercise testing and prescription. 3rd ed. Philadelphia : Lea & Febiger, 1986.

Rochmis P, Blackburn H. A survey of procedures, safety and litigation experience in approximately 170,000 tests. JAMA 1971; 217:1061.

Shephard RJ. A nomogram to calculate the oxygen cost of running at slow speeds. J Sports Med 1969; 9:10–16.

Shephard RJ. Exercise Physiology. Toronto : BC Decker, 1987.

FLUID AND MINERAL NEEDS

TIMOTHY DAVID NOAKES, M.B., Ch.B., M.D., F.A.C.S.M.

The relatively recent increase in the popularity of endurance sporting events such as ultradistance running and triathlon races has had one less than desirable effect: a large increase in the number of participants who are sufficiently incapacitated at the finish of these events to require medical attention. This has focused attention on the role that fluid and electrolyte balance plays in the etiology of the exercise-related collapse that occurs in these otherwise healthy athletes, and how the condition should be managed and prevented.

FLUID REQUIREMENTS DURING EXERCISE

The traditional belief is that fluid must be ingested during exercise in order to prevent the serious consequences of dehydration. Dehydration is believed to impair both thermoregulatory function and physical performance during exercise, leading to postexercise collapse, often with heat stroke, acute renal failure, or both.

There is no doubt that all these possibilities continued to be a real concern in competitive sport until as recently as the mid-1970s. One of the greatest marathon runners of all time, former world record holder Jim Peters, wrote in 1957 that "... (in the marathon race) there is no need to take any solid food at all and every effort should be made to do without liquid, as the moment food or drink is taken, the body has to start dealing with its digestion and in so doing some discomfort will almost invariably be felt." The fact that Peters retired from athletics after developing near-fatal heat stroke during the 1954 Empire Games Marathon in Vancouver is frequently quoted as anecdotal proof that an inadequate fluid intake causes heat stroke, particularly during marathon running.

However, partly because of further tragedies like that which befell Peters, but more especially as a result of the publicity given to the studies of Wyndham and Wyndham and Strydom and the work of organizations such as the American College of Sports Medicine, the past decade has witnessed a profound change in the manner in which endurance athletic events are now managed.

Thus, with the notable exception of the 226-km Hawaiian Ironman Triathlon, these demanding events are no longer held in the heat of the day during heatwaves, as was the 1954 Empire Games Marathon. In addition, the organizers of all the world's major endurance events now ensure that adequate fluid is readily available for all participants at regular intervals during these races. For example, more than 150,000 liters of fluid (approximately 15 liters per participant) is provided at 57 refreshment stations in the 90-km Comrades Marathon run annually between Durban and Pietermaritzburg, South Africa.

The question that needs to be asked is whether the relatively high frequency of postexercise collapse in athletes competing in these events can really be ascribed to "dehydration" and heat injury, given the change in race organization that has occurred in the past decade and the high degree of competitor awareness of the need to drink adequately during these events. Is the condition that we see in these collapsed athletes really the same as that which struck Jim Peters? Or is another explanation more likely? For example, the increased popularity of these ultradistance events has resulted in a major change in the personal characteristics of the participants from the exclusively highly talented and highly trained to a situation in which the less well trained and less athletic are in the majority. It would be extremely surprising if the risk of postexercise collapse was not influenced by the physical abilities and levels of training of most of the participants in any particular race.

It is appropriate to review the scientific basis for the belief that a failure to drink fluid in the appropriate amounts is the major factor causing the syndrome of postexercise collapse.

The landmark scientific study that is most frequently quoted as proof of the twin dangers of dehydration and heat stroke developing during prolonged exercise was performed by Wyndham and Strydom. They showed that runners who became dehydrated by more than 3 percent during races of 32 km had elevated body temperatures. They concluded that dehydration was the most important determinant of the rectal temperature during prolonged exercise. Interestingly, this conclusion failed to take account of their own and others' findings, which showed that metabolic rate is a significant determinant of body temperature during exercise.

On the basis of their findings, Wyndham and Strydom and, later, Wyndham suggested that runners need to drink at least 900 ml of fluid per hour during competition in order not to collapse from heat stroke. Remarkably, this belief has persisted for nearly two decades, despite a wealth of clinical and experimental evidence to the contrary.

First, as reviewed in detail elsewhere, the overwhelming majority of athletes competing in marathon and ultramarathon running events are only mildly hyperthermic at the finish of these races. The range of average postexercise rectal temperatures in

The work on which this article is based is supported by the Staff Research Fund of the University of Cape Town, the Medical Research Council of South Africa, the South African Association for Sport Science, Physical Education and Recreation, and G. W. Leppin (Pty) (Lta).

all studies of runners reported in the literature is between 38.0° and 40.0°C, most runners having postexercise rectal temperatures below 38.9°C. The same has been found in those collapsed marathon and ultramarathon runners in whom rectal temperatures have been measured. Paradoxically, some are even hypothermic.

The reason why these athletes do not become hyperthermic during prolonged exercise is almost certainly because the running speed, and therefore the rate of energy production, falls with the distance run. Metabolic rate (which is determined principally by the athlete's mass and running speed), rather than the level of dehydration (as proposed by Wyndham and Strydom), is the more likely determinant of thermoregulatory strain during exercise. Thus, it follows that rectal temperatures, sweat rates, and the risk of development of heat stroke will actually be lowest in runners competing the longest distances. Only those running very fast for short distances in severe environmental conditions are at high risk of developing environmentally and exercise-induced heat stroke (Fig. 1.).

Second, clinically significant levels of dehydration have never been recorded in large numbers of individuals competing in any modern ultradistance event, including some that were run in very severe environmental conditions. The average mass loss during long distance races is seldom more than 3 kg, of which at least 2 kg represents the obligatory losses of oxidized metabolic fuel (200 to 400g) and the water stored with glycogen (1.8 kg) that is released as the glycogen is mobilized during exercise. Thus, a mass loss of even 3 kg after very prolonged exercise would represent a real fluid loss of less than 1 kg, or about 2 percent of total body water. It seems unlikely that such a small reduction in body water could have a serious impact on an athlete's performance capacity.

There seems to be a need for more modern studies on the effect of such small degrees of dehydration on exercise performance. Those studies that are most frequently quoted as evidence that dehydration impairs physical performance do not, in my opinion, address the question satisfactorily. If the degree to which body water is reduced during prolonged exercise is really quite small, it should not be surprising that plasma volume and renal function are relatively well preserved during very prolonged exercise, even in athletes who lose up to 3 kg of body mass during exercise and who drink considerably less than the volumes suggested by Wyndham and Strydom. In women, there may even be an expansion of plasma volume during prolonged exercise, suggesting that these women may actually have been overhydrated.

Third, the fluid volumes ingested by runners during competition are considerably less than those advocated by Wyndham and Strydom, and seldom

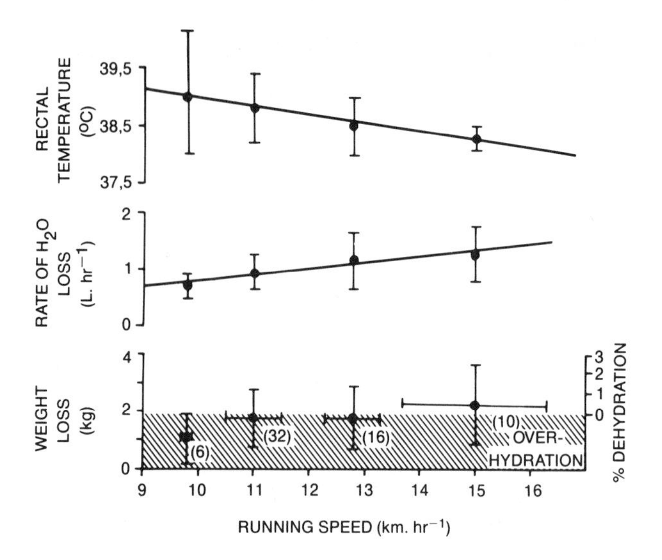

Figure 1 Postrace rectal temperature, rate of water loss, weight loss, and percentage of dehydration in runners of 70 to 80 kg completing different 42.2-km marathon races at different running speeds. Note that (1) the mean rectal temperatures are below 39.5°C in all groups, (2) the rate of water loss increases with running speed, and (3) only the fastest runners are dehydrated (mass losses greater than 1.8 kg). Slower runners finished the marathon races marginally overhydrated. (Based on data from Noakes TD, et al. The danger of an inadequate water intake during prolonged exercise. A novel concept re-visited. Eur J Appl Physiol 1988; 57:210–219.)

exceed 500 ml per hour. I have never encountered an athlete who was able to drink 1 liter of fluid per hour for any length of time *while continuing to run at a competitive pace.* Such high rates of fluid intake are possible only in participants who become exhausted and start to walk near the end of ultradistance running events. Paradoxically, their fluid requirements are greatly reduced when they start walking.

For reasons that are not clear but are probably related to the absence of weight bearing during cycling, cyclists are able to ingest considerably more fluid during prolonged exercise both in the laboratory and during competition. Rates of fluid intake of up to 2 liters per hour have been estimated in competitors in the Tour de France who were cycling in very hot conditions (more than 35°C). However, in the laboratory more modest intakes of 750 ml per hour have been recorded in professional cyclists.

The fact that athletes do not become seriously dehydrated during prolonged exercise, even when they ingest about half the fluid volume recommended by Wyndham and Strydom, can be explained on the basis that (1) these authors overestimated the sweat rates, particularly of the heavier runners who tend to run more slowly than lighter runners; and (2) the authors failed to adjust their data for the weight loss attributable to fuel oxidation and the obligatory exercise-induced release of the water stored with glycogen. As neither of these contributes to the level of the athlete's dehydration, both must be subtracted from the weight loss if the true water deficit at the end of exercise is to be calculated correctly.

When these corrections are applied, the data of Wyndham and Strydom predict that fluid intakes of 400 ml per hour should be adequate to prevent significant dehydration during prolonged running in moderate environmental conditions in most athletes. The finding that most runners ingest about 500 ml per hour during exercise is therefore in accord with that prediction.

In summary, it appears that the fluid requirements of runners during prolonged exercise in moderate environmental conditions can, in most instances, be adequately covered by an intake of 500 ml per hour. Higher rates of intake are usually associated with nausea and gastric distention in runners, but may be better tolerated by cyclists. Given the thermoregulatory advantages of cycling, in particular the greater capacity for convective heat loss, it is unlikely that the fluid requirements of cyclists are much different from those of runners. Indeed, they may even be less.

Participants in events of high intensity that last less than 1 hour are at much lesser risk of becoming seriously dehydrated, even if they drink sparingly. This is because the rate of glycogen breakdown is rapid during high-intensity exercise, with an obligatory release of the large volume of fluid stored with that glycogen. Paradoxically, for reasons given above, heat stroke is more likely to develop in athletes participating in high-intensity exercise, even when they do *not* become severely dehydrated. The prevention of heat stroke during high-intensity exercise of short duration hinges on factors other than the exclusive prevention of dehydration.

MINERAL AND ELECTROLYTE REQUIREMENTS DURING EXERCISE

Sweat is a hypotonic solution whose major constituent is sodium chloride. Thus, the loss of water from the body during prolonged exercise exceeds the loss of electrolytes (especially sodium), producing hypertonic hypernatremia in the vast majority of athletes. For this reason, the traditional teaching has been that water is the most important constituent that must be replaced during and after exercise. The addition of sodium chloride delays the gastric emptying of an ingested solution, at least at rest, thereby potentially exacerbating dehydration. This finding has been evoked as another important reason why only water should be drunk during exercise. However, three new findings suggest that this belief is due for revision.

First, the presence of sodium chloride has been shown to stimulate glucose transport across the intestinal villi, at least at low glucose concentrations. At high glucose concentrations, similar to those found in the 5 to 10 percent glucose solutions commonly ingested during exercise, the effect would likely be very small. Nevertheless, the presence of sodium chloride in an ingested fluid could potentially increase the rate of carbohydrate delivery from that solution, if the magnitude of the positive effect of sodium chloride on intestinal absorption was greater than the negative effect of these ions on gastric emptying.

Second, it appears that at least during prolonged running or cycling exercise, the rate of gastric emptying is less dependent on the osmolality of the ingested fluid than was believed on the basis of studies performed at rest. During exercise, electrolyte- and carbohydrate-containing solutions of quite widely differing osmolalities empty from the stomach at the same rate as does water. Thus, there appears to be no particular advantage to ingesting water alone during exercise; electrolytes and carbohydrates can be added, at least in relatively modest concentrations.

Third, there is the finding that a few competitors develop profound, life-threatening hyponatremia during very prolonged exercise (usually bouts lasting more than 8 hours). The exact cause of this condition is still in doubt, but during prolonged exercise sodium chloride ingestion may be of some value and is unlikely to be harmful, at least for the small group of athletes at risk of developing hyponatremia.

Furthermore, if, as has been proposed, depletion of the extracellular volume is the method whereby the body prevents the development of hyponatremia when there is a reduction of body sodium stores, maintenance of optimal hydration demands that these sodium chloride losses be replaced as they develop during prolonged exercise. This would require that athletes ingest solutions with a sodium chloride content of at least 40 to 60 mmol $\cdot$ liters $^{-1}$, equivalent to the sodium chloride content of sweat. However, it is likely that such solutions would be unpalatable.

For all these reasons, it seems logical that sodium chloride should be added to the solution ingested during exercise. The optimal concentration that should be added remains unknown. Most current research has been with sodium chloride concentrations of up to 20 mmol (1.2 g) $\cdot$ liters $^{-1}$. These concentrations have been shown to increase the rate of both water and carbohydrate absorption during exercise.

With regard to other electrolytes and minerals, there is no good scientific evidence to suggest that athletes eating a typical Western diet can develop significant electrolyte deficiencies, even during heavy training; nor does supplementation with the common minerals enhance performance.

ENERGY REQUIREMENTS DURING EXERCISE

Hypoglycemia is a factor that explains exhaustion in some athletes during prolonged exercise. Ingestion of high-carbohydrate solutions can thus enhance performance during prolonged exercise of moderately high intensity, by preventing hypoglycemia and maintaining a high rate of carbohydrate combustion. In the conclusive study of Coyle and colleagues, exercising athletes who did not ingest carbohydrate became exhausted when their blood glucose levels fell below 3.0 mmol · liters $^{-1}$, and the rate of carbohydrate oxidation fell below 1.4 g per minute. Carbohydrate ingestion during exercise prevented the development of hypoglycemia and maintained the rate of carbohydrate oxidation at more than 1.8 g per minute. Muscle glycogen depletion did not explain exhaustion, because when ingesting carbohydrate the athletes were able to continue exercising for 60 minutes, even though their muscle glycogen levels were very low and did not decrease further during the additional hour of exercise. This suggests that carbohydrate ingested during exercise may not decrease the rate of muscle glycogen utilization in cycling or in running.

A carbohydrate intake of between 20 and 50 g per hour optimizes performance. It is not clear whether any particular carbohydrate source is superior. Solutions of glucose polymers (which are the products of the partial digestion of starch, in which the glucose molecules remain bound to each other in chains comprising up to 10 or more glucose units) should provide a more rapid rate of carbohydrate delivery than solutions of mono- or disaccharides such as glucose, maltose, fructose, or sucrose. For the same total carbohydrate content, solutions of glucose polymers have lower osmolalities and should therefore empty more rapidly from the stomach. However, this possibility either has not been realized or has been found only with solutions of high carbohydrate content.

The optimal carbohydrate concentration is about 10 percent, which at a rate of ingestion of 500 ml per hour provides 50 g of carbohydrate per hour.

MANAGEMENT OF COLLAPSED ATHLETES AFTER PROLONGED EXERCISE

If most participants can complete ultradistance athletic events without becoming either severely hyperthermic or dehydrated, why do so many collapse, how should they be treated, and how can the condition best be prevented?

Clearly, some runners collapse because they fail to drink adequately and to ingest sufficient carbohydrate either before ("carbohydrate loading") or during marathon and ultramarathon races, thereby becoming hypoglycemic. A small percentage may also become hyponatremic, possibly because they fail to prevent an expansion of extracellular volume when a sodium chloride deficit is induced by sweating. Some may even develop heat stroke, but it is likely that such runners have a hereditary predisposition; they may in fact be suffering from stress-induced malignant hyperthermia, particularly if they collapse when running in relatively mild environmental conditions. Still others may suffer acute myocardial infarction or ventricular fibrillation.

It is important to recognize that these specific medical conditions may be present in some runners, but the vast majority of collapsed runners do not fit into any of these diagnostic categories. The common assumption is that they are dehydrated and must therefore be in hypovolemic shock. Against this, there is no firm evidence for clinically significant dehydration. Also, such athletes do not recover sufficiently fast when given intravenous fluid therapy to suggest that fluid depletion was an important cause for the collapse.

In addition, there is no satisfactory evidence that these athletes are severely shocked. The supine blood pressures of the collapsed ultramarathon runners that were studied were 115 ± 14 (mean ± standard deviation) mm Hg systolic over 77 ± 9 mm Hg diastolic; their heart rates were 72 ± 18 beats per minute and their 24-hour postrace rates of creatine clearance were normal. Such values are no different from findings in noncollapsed athletes studied immediately after they had completed the Hawaiian Iron Man Triathlon. Postrace creatinine clearance in eight collapsed hyponatremic runners studied after the 1988 90-km Comrades Marathon was considerably elevated (174.8 ± 28.2 ml per minute). These findings are incompatible with a diagnosis of significant shock.

The principal physical sign common to all collapsed runners is postural hypotension, shown by an inability to stand without support. The cardiovascular adaptations necessary for upright posture include sympathetically mediated vasoconstriction in the splanchnic, renal, skin, and skeletal muscle vasculature to compensate for a redistribution of blood volume. The athlete who stops running immediately after completing a long distance race develops postural hypotension if these sympathetically mediated reflexes are not activated immediately to vasoconstrict arterioles in the previously active skeletal muscles. This vasoconstriction helps to maintain blood pressure in the face of the precipitous fall in cardiac output that develops on cessation of exercise.

It is therefore proposed that the collapse seen after prolonged exercise is generally due to a persistence of vasodilation in the active muscles after exercise. This may be compounded by a redistribution of blood volume to the dilated capacitance vessels of the arms and legs, and the end of the assistance to venous return provided by contracting leg muscles.

This mechanism would explain why most athletes collapse almost immediately after they stop running. Furthermore, if this theory is correct, thc rationale of treatment of these patients is not to infuse intravenous fluids, but to induce vasoconstriction in the persistently dilated areterioles of the previously active skeletal muscles.

Whether or not this proves to be correct, it serves as a reminder that each collapsed runner deserves a firm clinical diagnosis made on the basis of a carefully taken medical history and clinical examination. The history should determine whether the athlete has specific symptoms; whether too much or too little fluid was drunk during exercise; whether sufficient carbohydrate was ingested before and during exercise; and whether there is progressive clouding of consciousness, suggesting hyponatremia, hypoglycemia, or even hypo- or hyperthermia. The presence of muscle twitching, muscle fasiculation, or an epileptic fit suggests hyponatremia. The clinical diagnosis should be confirmed by at least some basic tests, including measurement of rectal temperature and blood glucose level. If both are normal and the runner reports an adequate fluid intake (500 ml or more of fluid per hour of exercise), the temptation to give intravenous fluids should be resisted, at least until a high serum sodium level has been demonstrated. It is no longer acceptable simply to conclude that all collapsed runners are "dehydrated" and require intravenous fluids, particularly when such treatment may exacerbate life-threatening hyponatremia. This condition not only carries a high mortality rate, but also may result in permanent brain damage.

Until the results of controlled clinical trials are available, conservative management, including oral rather than intravenous fluids, seems the most appropriate treatment for most athletes who develop postural hypotension after prolonged exercise, particularly if they lack evidence of hypoglycemia, hypo- or hyperthermia, or hyponatremia, and have drunk appropriate amounts of fluid during exercise.

The natural history of most patients is to recover spontaneously 1 to 5 hours after stopping exercise. This suggests that the cardiovascular disturbance causing the postural hypotension is self-righting, given sufficient time. A controlled study to determine whether vasoconstrictor medication would expedite recovery appears worthy of consideration.

SUGGESTED READING

American College of Sports Medicine. The prevention of thermal injuries during distance running. Med Sci Sports Exerc 1987; 19:529–533.

Costill DL, Kammer WF, Fisher A. Fluid ingestion during distance running. Arch Environ Health 1970; 21:520–525.

Coyle EF, Coggan AR, Hemmert MK, Ivy JL. Muscle glycogen utilization during prolonged strenuous exercise when fed carbohydrate. J Appl Physiol 1986; 61:165–172.

Davidson RJL, Robertson JD, Galea G, Maughan RJ. Hematological changes associated with marathon running. Int J Sports Med 1987; 8:19–25.

Douglas PS, O'Toole ML, Hiller WDB, Hackney K, Reichek N. Cardiac fatigue after prolonged exercise. Circulation 1987; 76:1206–1213.

Irving RA, Noakes TD, Irving GA, Van Zyl-Smit R. The immediate and delayed effects of marathon running on renal function. J Urol 1986; 136:1176–1180.

Jardon OM. Physiologic stress, heat stroke, malignant hyperthermia—a perspective. Milit Med 1982; 147:8–14.

Maughan RJ, Leiper JB, Thompson J. Rectal temperature after marathon running. Br J Sports Med 1985; 19:192–196.

Noakes TD. Editorial: why marathon runners collapse. S Afr Med J 1988; 73:569–571.

Noakes TD, Adams BA, Myburgh KH, et al. The danger of an inadequate water intake during prolonged exercise. A novel concept re-visited. Eur J Appl Physiol 1988; 57:210–219.

Noakes TD, Goodwin N, Rayner BL, Branken T, Taylor RKN. Water intoxication: a possible complication during endurance exercise. Med Sci Sports Exerc 1985; 17:370–375.

Rowell LB. Adjustments to upright posture and blood loss. In: Human circulation. Regulation during physical stress. New York: Oxford University Press, 1986:137.

Sandell RC, Pascoe MD, Noakes TD. Factors associated with collapse following ultramarathon foot races: a preliminary study. Phys Sports Med, 1988; 16 (Sept): 86–94.

Sawka MN, Francesconi RP, Young AJ, Pandolf KB. Influence of hydration level and body fluids on exercise performance in the heat. JAMA 1984; 252:1165–1169.

Wyndham CH. Heatstroke and hyperthermia in marathon runners. Ann NY Acad Sci 1977; 301:128–138.

Wyndham CH, Strydom NB. The danger of an inadequate water intake during marathon running. S Afr Med J 1969; 43:893–896.

Wyndham CH, Strydom NB, van Rensburg AJ, Benade AJS, Heyns AJ. Relation between Vo_2 max and body temperature in hot humid air conditions. J Appl Physiol 1970; 1:45–50.

HAZARDS OF COLD WATER

THOMAS J. DOUBT, Ph.D.
T.J.R. FRANCIS, Surgeon Commander, Royal Navy

The principal hazards of exposure to cold water are related to the cooling of tissues. Initially, this cooling is limited to the peripheral tissues. However, if exposure persists, a further loss of body heat may result in hypothermia, which is defined as a core temperature one standard deviation (SD) below the mean value (about 37 ± 1°C) under normal resting conditions.

Thermal balance (S) is the algebraic difference between heat production and loss as given in the equation below. Metabolic heat production (M) is always positive in life. Losses are governed by evaporative heat loss (E), which is always negative and radiation (R), convection (C), and conduction (D), each of which may have either a positive or a negative sign, depending on the environmental conditions. During cold water immersion E is negligible; R, C, and D are negative, with D being the principal avenue of loss.

$$S = M + (E + R + C + D)$$

Table 1 lists some of the factors that determine whole body heat balance under immersed and nonimmersed conditions. Water temperature and duration of exposure have the most direct bearing on the rate of heat loss. The external passive thermal insulation provided by protective clothing modifies the rate of heat loss. Personal variables include the importance of the subcutaneous fat layer as a source of insulation. Large body surface area to volume ratios, typically found in infants, dramatically increase the rate of cooling. Another source of individual variability is the response to hypothermia. One person with a core temperature of 32°C may be conversant, while another with a core temperature of 35°C may be somnolent. As discussed later, physical activity generates additional metabolic heat, but this is often inadequate to counterbalance an associated increase in the rate of heat loss.

This chapter focuses mainly on the hazards of cold water immersion and discusses preventive measures, physiologic effects, and general principles of treatment. Special sections are devoted to the effects of nonimmersion cold water exposure and nonfreezing cold injury. Emphasis is placed on aspects that pertain to what might be encountered in the field, distant from a hospital setting. The material presented addresses the hazards of cold water encountered in athletic endeavors; for more comprehensive reviews of hypothermia and its treatment, consult the list of suggested reading.

COLD WATER IMMERSION

Preventive Measures

Sporting events which are often associated with prolonged cold water immersion include long distance open-water swimming, surfing, triathlons, spear fishing, and scuba diving. These activities involve intentional immersion; therefore, preventive measures can be taken to minimize the hazards involved. In selecting appropriate protective clothing, consideration should be given to the temperature of the water, the level of activity, and the likely duration of the exposure. Data such as those presented in Figure 1 can be used to help select the amount of thermal protection required to maintain the core temperature within the normal range.

In other recreational activities conducted on or around cold water, accidental immersion may occur. Typical examples include fishing, boating, or events taking place on a frozen pond. By definition, immersions under these conditions are unplanned and

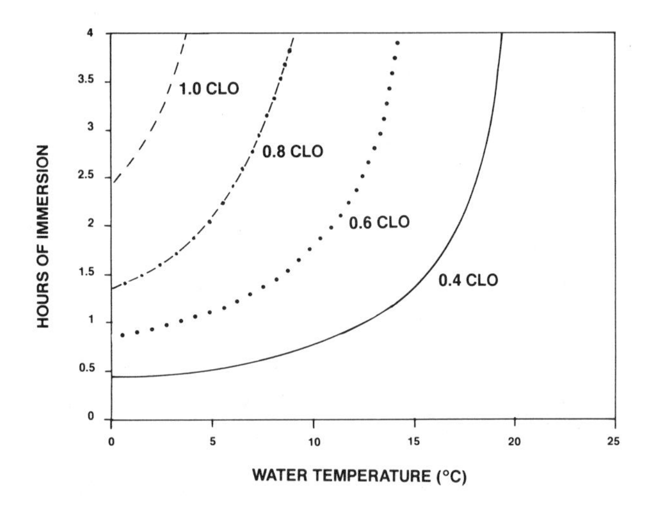

Figure 1 Curves are plotted for levels of passive insulation (0.4–1.0 CLO) that describe the maximal allowable duration of immersion. The maximal allowable duration is defined as maintenance of core temperature between 36° and 37°C, and heat loss not to exceed 3 kcal per kilogram. The curves were constructed for an individual performing light exercise ($\dot{V}O_2$ = 0.85 liters per minute). Similar curves can be constructed for other levels of activity and insulation. For reference, a ¼-inch neoprene wet suit has a CLO value of 0.8. (Data courtesy of Dr. R.P. Weinberg, NMRI.)

Acknowledgments. This study was funded by the Naval Medical Research and Development Command Work Unit No. M0099.01A-1003. The opinions and assertions contained herein are the private ones of the authors and are not to be construed as official or reflecting the view of the United States Navy, the Royal Navy, or the naval service at large.

are often complicated by the absence of protective equipment (such as adequate thermal insulation or flotation devices).

THE PHYSIOLOGIC EFFECTS OF COLD IMMERSION

Acute Effects

The most immediate physiologic response to cold water immersion is a dramatic, involuntary hyperventilation, which may last for several minutes. This hyperventilation reduces breath-holding time and, coupled with the potential for panic (particularly during an unintentional immersion), increases the risk of drowning, especially in rough water. Hyperventilation may also interfere with the normal coordination of breathing and swimming motions. It has been postulated that this is why good swimmers have drowned while attempting to rescue themselves or others from cold water, although development of sudden cardiac arrhythmias may also be a factor.

We have observed that the immediate hyperventilation subsequently gives way to a relative hyperventilation, compared with a euthermic immersion. The relative hyperventilation may persist until the respiratory drive is depressed by severe hypothermia. Hyperventilation, by provoking a reduction in arterial P_{CO_2} and cerebral blood flow, may of itself be hazardous, since it can result in an alteration of mental function that may compromise any attempt to survive.

Cold water immersions, particularly those that are rapid or unplanned, often result in an apparent failure of the victim to execute any effort to swim or stay afloat. These "nonstruggling" experiences have been described by survivors as involving a sense of complete helplessness or weakness. In such instances, rescue becomes an immediate concern, particularly if the victim has no means of passive flotation.

An immediate, profound peripheral vasoconstriction occurs upon exposure to cold water; this can provoke a transient elevation of systolic blood pressure to values exceeding 200 mm Hg. Baroreceptor reflexes, coupled with facial immersion (the "dive reflex"), should theoretically result in a slowing of the heart rate. However, this reflex is weak in humans. More commonly, an exercise-independent tachycardia occurs, owing to the stressful nature of the exposure. Cardiac arrhythmias are common and can range from multifocal premature ventricular contractions (PVCs) early in immersion to sinus dysrhythmias with prolonged exposure. Sudden cardiac arrest has been implicated as the cause of death in many cold water immersions.

The rapid loss of heat that occurs immediately upon immersion in cold water induces peripheral vasoconstriction and shivering thermogenesis. However, these mechanisms may fail to reverse the negative thermal balance. Thus, survival time becomes a function of water temperature. There are equations to predict survival time versus water temperature on the basis of declines in core temperature, but other factors such as hyperventilation, impaired neuromuscular function, and the lack of a flotation device may lead to drowning before the core temperature is reduced to lethal levels.

Chronic Effects

There are effects of cold water immersion that may compromise athletic performance. As muscles cool, their strength, coordination, and flexibility are all decreased. Cold exposure has also been associated with increased lactate production and a more rapid depletion of muscle glycogen stores. These factors have a strong association with reduced performance, and the poor performance of the cooled muscles in turn increases the risk of musculoskeletal injury. Furthermore, cold exposure may result in acute or chronic injuries being exacerbated. This is because the pain and numbness of the extremities that commonly accompany cold water exposure may confound the awareness of any traumatic injury until the affected area is rewarmed.

Exercise performed during cold immersion (e.g., competitive swimming) has two effects that may contribute to greater rates of body heat loss, even though heat production is increased. First, the increase in arterial blood flow to the working muscles delivers warm blood to the periphery, where heat loss is greatest. Second, movement through the water disturbs the boundary layer of warmer water that develops next to the body during static immersion, thus increasing rates of convective and conductive heat loss. The exercise intensity that produces enough metabolic heat to offset losses thus depends on complex interactions with the other factors listed in Table 1 (including clothing and the thickness of subcutaneous fat).

It is well recognized that immersion results in a diuresis that is secondary to a central shift of blood volume. In general, this diuresis reaches a peak in 1 to 3 hours, although the timing depends on environmental circumstances, the level of physical activity, and the degree of preimmersion hydration. In the absence of fluid intake, a marked dehydration results; this further degrades athletic performance and thermogenic responses.

Finally, with the development of hypothermia, there is a gradual loss of mental function that can impair performance and judgment. For example, we have measured decrements in several neuropsychological functions that were inversely related to core temperature. Ultimately, progression of hypothermia can result in loss of consciousness.

TABLE 1 Factors Related to Heat Loss

Factor	*Term in Heat Balance Equation*	*Comments*
Water temperature	C, D	Any temperature less than ∼25°C
Exposure time		Loss proportional to time
Protective clothing	E, R, C, D	See also Fig. 1
Personal variability	M, D	Subcutaneous fat layer Shivering response Body surface-to-volume ratio Diet Hydration status
Activity level	M, C, D	Increased heat production with increased activity. Movement may disrupt boundary layer and increase rate of loss
Wind-chill factor	E, D	Relevant to nonimmersed conditions

RESCUE AND TREATMENT

The basic concept behind the rescue of victims of cold immersion is to remove them safely from the water, prevent injury, and minimize further loss of body heat. Rescuers need to remember that the victim of a prolonged cold immersion, even if apparently conscious, may be unable to render any self-help or even to comprehend verbal instructions. The victim should be handled gently, because the usual sense of pain and the associated protective reflexes may be blunted by the cold and because careless blows to the chest may induce ventricular fibrillation.

Sudden cardiovascular collapse may occur during or shortly after rescue from prolonged immersions. This is the consequence of a number of factors. During exposure, both immersion-induced diuresis and the redistribution of body fluid result in a reduction of circulating blood volume. Extended exposure to water at temperatures below 15°C directly reduces peripheral vascular tone, and eventually cooling of the hypothalamus also leads to a depressed neurogenic control of blood pressure. While immersed, the central circulation is supported by the external hydrostatic pressure of the water. Upon removal from the water, the sudden loss of hydrostatic support results in a peripheral pooling of blood and a potentially life-threatening reduction of cardiac output. This last effect is most dramatic if the immersion victim is removed from the water in a vertical position. It is therefore advantageous, if possible, to remove the victim horizontally.

There is considerable individual variability in the response to hypothermia. Most persons with mild hypothermia (core temperature 34° to 36°C) are fully awake but distressed, and shivering may be violent. With moderate hypothermia (core temperature 30° to 34°C), there is generally some loss of mental acumen. At the lower limit, the victim may not be easily roused but is generally still shivering. When core temperature falls below 30°C, patients are usually unconscious, and shivering may have ceased. With increasing depth of hypothermia, particularly if combined with submersion, it may be difficult to detect either pulse or respiratory movements. The pupils may react very sluggishly to light and appear fixed and dilated. Furthermore, the extremities may be rigid, giving the appearance of rigor mortis. The absence of detectable vital signs in the field shortly after rescue is not a reason for abandoning care; the principles of basic life support should be applied. Under the circumstances surrounding most sporting events, these principles include airway management and effective ventilation, preferably with 100 percent oxygen. Further reduction of heat loss is achieved by removing wet clothing and providing dry, passive insulation. It is important to insulate the head as well as other body parts, because of the head's propensity to lose large amounts of heat. Transportation to a hospital in a vehicle equipped with life support apparatus should be carried out expeditiously.

Cardiac resuscitation by first responders is a controversial issue in the absence of an electrocardiographic (ECG) recording. Some experts consider that effective cardiac resuscitation of the victims of cold water submersion is a vital part of first aid treatment. Others believe that the victims of cold, dry exposures should be transported without cardiac compressions until rewarming has begun. There are reports of successful field CPR in severely hypothermic patients, but external chest compressions may induce ventricular fibrillation in a hypothermic heart. This is of particular importance, because the hypothermic myocardium has a reduced response to drugs and defibrillation, making cardioversion difficult until the myocardium is rewarmed. Bretylium tosylate seems to be the only drug in the ACLS arsenal that is an effective treatment of ventricular tachycardia or fibrillation in a cold heart.

Near-drowning must be suspected in any case of immersion, even if the patient is asymptomatic upon initial examination, because hypoxemia and pulmonary insufficiency can develop 12 to 24 hours after the aspiration of water.

Fluid replacement is required after prolonged cold exposure. Opinions differ somewhat on

TABLE 2 Selected Methods of Rewarming

Method	*Comments*
Spontaneous passive rewarming	Self-production of body heat; may be ineffective in severe cases. Most effective in warm air with increased insulation garments.
Active Methods:	
External methods	
Warm shower, bath,	Water temperature 38° to 40°C. If too hot, can cause burns.
heating pads/blankets	
Internal methods	
Respiratory heating	Humidified gas at 40° to 42°C. Ineffective unless used with other methods.
Peritoneal dialysis	Lactated Ringer's or saline at 42°C
Lavage	Colonic or gastric, with Ringer's or saline at 42°C
Extracorporeal circulation	Warm blood delivered directly to core. Preferred to immersion when ACLS needed.
Diathermy	Microwave rewarming method

whether oral fluids should contain glucose and electrolytes, but hyperosmotic solutions should be avoided because of their propensity for provoking gastrointestinal disturbances. Warm, nonalcoholic beverages provide some psychological comfort, but deliver only neglible heat. In contrast, cool beverages (about 10°C) empty more quickly from the stomach than warm beverages, and also transiently raise metabolic heat production in mild cases of cold water exposure. Comatose victims should be rehydrated with warm intravenous fluids (lactated Ringer's or saline). The infusion rate should initially be kept low until the victim's cardiopulmonary and renal function status can be assessed.

It is likely that most patients with cold water exposure associated with sporting events will have a rectal temperature above 34.4°C (the lowest reading on many clinical thermometers). Such mild cases of hypothermia can be effectively managed by spontaneous, passive rewarming (Table 2). The basis of this treatment is that metabolic heat production gradually increases the core temperature once the negative elements of the heat balance equation have been minimized by the provision of adequate insulation. Our approach for rewarming cold divers is presented here as a general paradigm. After removal from the cold water, dry clothing and an insulating garment are provided. We have found that it normally takes 2 to 3 hours to restore a 1° to 2°C decrease in rectal temperature if the diver is reclining and inactive. Light activity, such as walking or jogging, speeds the rewarming process considerably. Warm showers or baths are psychologically and physiologically beneficial, but when the initial rectal temperature is 35°C or lower, the person is kept in the insulating garments until a definitive increase in temperature is observed.

Skin exposed to cold water is usually pale and numb. Hands and feet may ache. For mild to moderate hypothermia, rapid rewarming by immersion in 38° to 40°C water is usually effective and has no adverse consequences. Chilled hands and feet may be rewarmed in the same manner, although this is often somewhat painful. With any attempt at active external rewarming, the temperature of the rewarming fluid is important. Burns may be caused by water temperatures above 40°C, because the cold, vasoconstricted skin is unable to dissipate heat rapidly. Since the skin is initially numb, a burn may be ignored until well into the rewarming period.

Rectal temperature should be monitored throughout rewarming. The subjective opinion of the patient is often unreliable, because either passive insulation or active rewarming raise the skin temperature faster than the core. This imparts a sensation of warmth that may be deceptive. The well-publicized afterdrop phenomenon (a further decrease in core temperature following rescue from cold immersion) is of little clinical importance in these cases.

The active rewarming methods listed in Table 2 are best applied in a hospital setting (see suggested reading list for details). In general, the methods of choice for conscious patients are those using external devices, while unconscious patients may be treated with internal active rewarming at those facilities with expertise in such techniques.

NONIMMERSION HAZARDS OF COLD WATER

Cold water may present a nonimmersion hazard in activities such as windsurfing, water skiing, cycling, long distance running or walking, hiking, and mountaineering. The rate of heat loss is less than with immersion, but the cold, wet, and windy conditions can nonetheless pose a threat of hypothermia to participants. Sweating can reduce the effective insulation of protective garments and lead to increased rates of heat loss, most noticeable during periods of rest. Events such as hiking are best undertaken in groups, so that the development of hypothermia can be recognized and treated by colleagues. Competitive events should be well marshaled so that hypothermic participants can be identified and treated. Individual athletes should give serious consideration to not competing in an event if preventive or management issues relating to hypothermia are not sufficiently addressed.

Approaches to reducing the cold water risk in such sports are generally the same as outlined for the immersed condition, with emphasis on preplanned strategies. Preventive measures can often be quite simple yet effective. For races when cold rain is forecast, marathon runners may carry plastic bags, with holes cut for the arms and head. Donning the bag during the storm lessens the rate of heat loss, and the covering can easily be removed at other times to allow the dissipation of excess heat. For events such as water skiing and windsurfing, a wide array of sophisticated protective equipment is available.

It is difficult for an exercising athlete to notice the relative hyperventilation that occurs with cold exposure. Nonetheless, trained athletes can generally sense when they are breathing harder than they should be for a given intensity of physical activity. This "body sense," developed in the course of training, can be a valuable clue to thermal status in the cold.

Hypothermia is a particular risk at times of reduced activity in a sporting event (e.g., during a transition phase in a triathlon, if a runner slows or stops, or during a break in the action of a soccer game). Once the person is stationary, the rate of heat loss may be slightly reduced, but the rate of metabolic heat production is greatly decreased. When pronounced shivering occurs, it should serve as a warning sign of a negative heat balance. Resuming exercise will again increase metabolic heat production, but it may not be adequate to restore the body heat lost while the athlete was stationary. Any shivering that persists after resumption of competition is a probable reason to suspect a core temperature below normal, and the athlete should seek additional thermal protection or withdraw from the race.

NONFREEZING COLD INJURY

When most people think about localized injury caused by cold, they think of frostbite. This condition, in which tissues undergo freezing, is usually restricted in the sporting community to skiers and mountaineers. Although skin freezes at approximately −0.5°C, even a brief exposure to a very cold (below −15°C) environment or contact with cold objects can produce frostbite. It is not, however, a common hazard of cold water.

The fact that cold water is capable of inducing nonfreezing cold injury (NFCI) has been known for many years. Most commonly, the NFCI involves the feet or the hands. It is a consequence of prolonged cooling in a moist environment. Historically, such injuries have occurred in foot soldiers engaged in combat in cold, wet climates. Factors that increase the risk of NFCI include the duration of exposure (normally more than 24 hours), dehydration, hypothermia, fatigue, stress, and a history of cold injury. Knowing this, it is possible to identify sports in which NFCI poses a threat, either through accidental or deliberate exposure to cold water. These include yachting, long distance swimming, backpacking, and cave exploration. The condition has also been diagnosed in scuba divers who have undertaken repetitive dives in very cold water.

During exposure to cold, the limb is numb, and although intricate manual dexterity is not possible in the case of the hand, a person developing NFCI of the foot is quite capable of swimming or walking. The problems begin when the cold limb is rewarmed. At this stage, the cold, pale, soggy, numb periphery is transformed into a swollen, dry, red, tender, or exquisitely painful limb that, in the case of the foot, can no longer support weight or permit walking. Depending on its severity, this acute phase of NFCI may last from a few days to a month or more. In severe cases gangrene may develop requiring surgical intervention. With the passing of the acute phase, normal function may return to the limb. Unfortunately, it is common for the limb to develop a more chronic condition, characterized by extreme cold sensitivity and excessive sweating. Studies of veterans of World War II and the Korean war show that this chronic phase may last indefinitely.

Fortunately, the vast majority of athletes are rarely exposed to sufficiently prolonged cold, wet conditions to develop NFCI. However, awareness and prevention of the problem is important. There is currently no satisfactory treatment, and even the mechanism of the disease is unclear. Where exposure to the appropriate conditions exists (e.g., during hill walking and backpacking), preventive measures should include regular inspection, massage and drying of the feet or hands (at least three times a day), and, when possible, a change of socks or gloves. Adequate fluid intake and the prevention of hypothermia reduce the risk of factors that promote NFCI. Footwear must fit well and not restrict circulation. If, during a routine foot check, the feet remain numb and cold, the early stages of NFCI may be present. In such situations, especially in remote locations, it is probably best to avoid active rewarming of the feet. Instead, while the feet are still usable, the footwear should be replaced and a warm, dry shelter should be sought. If the acute phase of NFCI occurs, mobility is reduced and the risk of developing hypothermia is significant while rescue is awaited. In this situation, concern about NFCI becomes secondary to the avoidance of life-threatening hypothermia.

SUGGESTED READING

Deuster PA, Smith DJ, Smoak BL, Doubt TJ. Fluid and electrolyte changes during cold water immersion. Undersea Biomed Res 1987; 14:11–12.

Doubt TJ, Deuster PA, Haberman K, et al. Fluid replacement during cold water immersion: hydration and thermal status. In: Ilmarinen R, Pasche A, eds. Proceedings of 3rd Int. Conf. Environ. Ergonomics. Helsinki, 1988.

Doubt TJ, Mayers DL, Flynn ET. Transient cardiac sinus dysrhythmia occurring after cold water immersion. Am J Cardiol 1987; 59:1421–1422.

Epstein M. Renal effects of head out water immersion in man: implications for understanding volume homeostasis. Physiol Rev 1978; 58:529–581.

Francis TJR. Non-freezing cold injury: a historical review. J R Nav Med Serv 1984; 70:134–139.

Francis TJR, Golden F. Non-freezing cold injury: the pathogenesis. J R Nav Med Serv 1985; 71:3–8.

Harnett RM, Pruitt JR, Slas FR. A review of the literature concerning resuscitation from hypothermia. Part I: The problem and general approaches. Aviat Space Environ Med 1983; 54:425–434.

Harnett RM, Pruitt JR, Slas FR. A review of the literature concerning resuscitation from hypothermia. Part II: Selected rewarming protocols. Aviat Space Environ Med 1983; 54:487–495.

Hayward JS, Eckerson JD, Collis ML. Thermal balance and survival time predictions of man in cold water. Can J Physiol Pharmacol 1975; 53:21–32.

Hsieh S, Bilanin J, Haberman K, Doubt T. Effects of caffeine and cold on exercise metabolism. Med Sci Sports Exerc 1988; 20:S84.

Jacobs T, Romet TT, Brown D. Muscle glycogen depletion at 9°C and 21°C. Eur J Appl Physiol 1985; 54:35–39.

Keatinge WR. London University: personal communication, 1988.

Mekjavic JB, Banister EW, Morrison JB, eds. Environmental ergonomics. New York: Taylor & Francis, 1988.

Nemiroff MJ. U.S. Coast Guard: personal communication, 1988.

Okada M. The cardiac rhythm in accidental hypothermia. J. Electrocardiol 1984; 17:123–128.

Pozos RS, Wittmers LE, eds. The nature and treatment of hypothermia. Minneapolis: University of Minnesota Press, 1983.

Riddell DI. A practical guide to cold injuries. J R Nav Med Serv 1986; 72:20–25.

Schechter DC, Sarot IA. Historical accounts of injuries to cold. Surgery 1968; 63:527–535.

Segarra F, Redding RA. Modern concepts about drowning. Can Med Assoc J 1974; 110:1057–1059.

EXERCISE AT HIGH ALTITUDES

JOHN R. SUTTON, M.D.

At a recent Continuing Medical Education conference in Breckenridge, Colorado (altitude: 2,770 m, 9,100 ft), I was giving an opening address on high-altitude medical illness. After briefly going through the list of symptoms that might be attributed to altitude, I surveyed the audience. Of all those who were attending the symposium for the first time, 100 percent had at least some symptoms of mild altitude illness. Those who had attended my session the previous year or were already aware of the potential problems of altitude had taken steps to reduce the likelihood of symptoms and were less affected. During the course of the week at Breckenridge, I saw no fewer than 30 of the 150 conference registrants whose symptoms of altitude illness were sufficient to warrant a medical consultation. Four of these people found it necessary to descend to a lower altitude.

What is altitude illness and how might we recognize it? Although we have known about altitude illness for several centuries, by and large it has been considered as a matter in the domain of the explorer and mountaineer. In more recent years, as society has become more affluent and many have begun to choose exotic holidays in locations such as the Rockies, the Andes, or the Himalayan ranges, the frequency of altitude problems affecting the general populace has increased dramatically. Family physicians and sports medicine practitioners should now be aware of such potential problems and advise their patients accordingly.

Under most circumstances, altitude illness is no more than an inconvenience, which lasts a few days at the most. However, there are several forms of altitude illness that are not benign and may end in death unless recognized and treated promptly.

PATHOPHYSIOLOGY

The crucial physiologic change induced by ascent to altitude is that of hypoxemia. The effect of a lower barometric pressure is to decrease the inspired oxygen pressure and, therefore, the arterial oxygen pressure; this change is responsible for all the altitude difficulties (Fig. 1). However, the pathophysiology is rather more complex; it is important to separate the effects of acute hypoxia per se from those of mountain sickness, which usually develops several hours or even days after ascent. The time relationship suggests that secondary events stimulated by hypoxemia result in the symptoms we know as mountain sickness (Fig. 2).

The major types of mountain sickness are (1) acute mountain sickness—a benign, usually self-limiting problem; (2) high-altitude pulmonary edema—a much more serious and potentially fatal condition; (3) high-altitude cerebral edema—again, less frequent but potentially deadly; and (4) high-

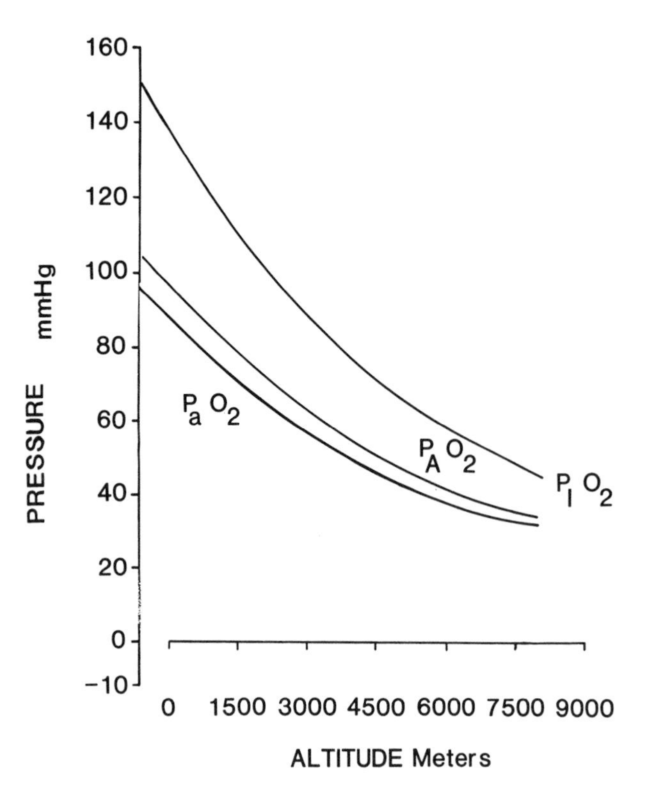

Figure 1 Changes of inspired, alveolar, and arterial oxygen pressures (P_IO_2, P_AO_2, and PaO_2) with altitude.

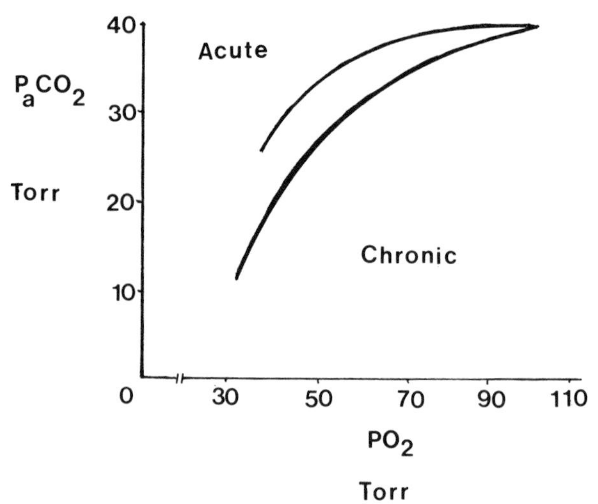

Figure 2 The relationship of alveolar CO_2 and oxygen pressures (the O_2-CO_2 diagram). On the "summit" of Mount Everest, $Po_2 = 30.3 \pm 2.1$ mm Hg and $Pco_2 = 11.2 \pm 1.7$ mm Hg (mean ± SD). (Data from the "Operation Everest II" study.)

altitude retinal hemorrhage. In addition, a variety of other medical conditions such as coronary artery disease, chronic obstructive pulmonary disease, and sickle cell disease are aggravated by high altitudes; the physician should thus be capable of appropriately counseling patients with these disorders. Chronic mountain sickness (Monge's disease), as its name implies, takes a substantial time to develop and is not seen in the short-term sojourner.

ACUTE MOUNTAIN SICKNESS

Acute mountain sickness (AMS) (Fig. 3) was first described by Jose de Acosta, a Jesuit with the conquistadores invading Peru. In 1569 he published a description of the symptoms. Today, one of the best descriptions we have is still that of Dr. Ravenhill, who was a physician with a mining company in the Andes during the early part of the present century. In 1913 he wrote:

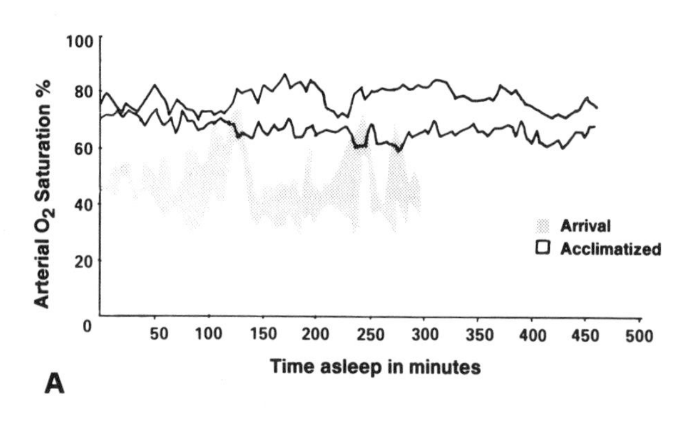

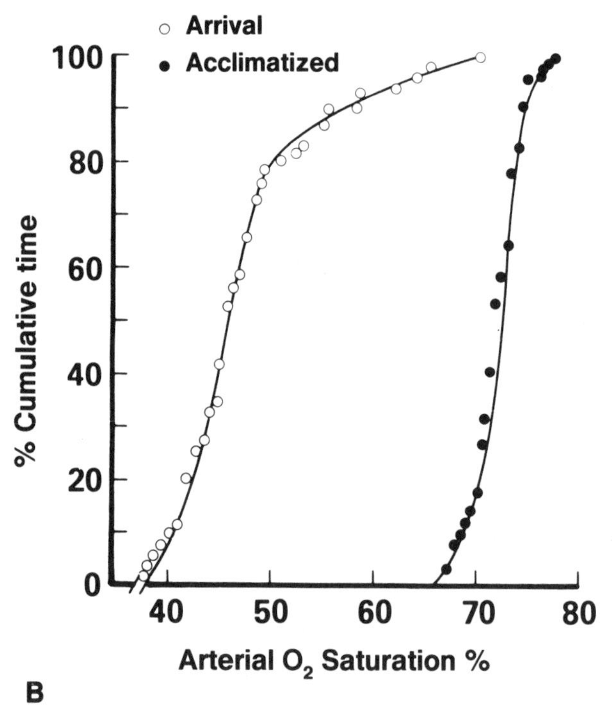

Figure 3 Effect of acclimatization on sleep hypoxemia. (From Sutton JR, ed. Man at altitude. Sem Respir Med 1983; 5:177.)

It is a curious fact that the symptoms of puna [AMS] do not usually evince themselves at once. The majority of newcomers have expressed themselves as being quite well on first arrival. As a rule, towards evening, the patient begins to feel rather slack and disinclined to exertion. He goes to bed, but has a restless and troubled night and wakes up the next morning with a severe frontal headache. There may be vomiting; frequently there is a sense of oppression in the chest, but there is rarely any respiratory distress or alteration in the normal rate of breathing so long as the patient is at rest. The patient may feel slightly giddy on rising from the bed, and any attempt at exertion increases the headache, which is nearly always confined to the frontal region. . . . The headache increases towards evening, so also does the pulse rate; all appetite is lost and the patient wishes to be alone—to sleep if possible. Generally, during the second night he is able to do so, and as a rule, wakes the third morning feeling much better. . . . By the fourth day, he is probably much better and at the end of a week is fit again.

Treatment

Usually, the symptoms of AMS are self-limiting and will pass. Nothing more than rest, hydration, and analgesia with aspirin is generally necessary. If symptoms prove more persistent, stronger analgesics may be required, and acetazolamide, 250 mg every 8 hours, has been found to be helpful.

HIGH-ALTITUDE PULMONARY EDEMA

The classical symptoms of high-altitude pulmonary edema (HAPE) are cough, excessive shortness of breath even at rest, cyanosis, and rapid, noisy breathing (Fig. 4). On physical examination, one sees the features of pulmonary edema, including loud rales and elevated jugular venous pressure. There may be no evidence of a third heart sound or peripheral edema. The patient is usually very distressed and cyanosed.

Treatment

HAPE is a medical emergency; if oxygen is available, it should be administered immediately. Furosemide (Lasix), 40 mg intravenously, should also be given both immediately and every 6 hours, with acetazolamide, 250 mg immediately and every 8 hours. Evacuation to a lower altitude should take place as soon as possible. In climbing circles, people with incipient pulmonary edema have often been traveling between camps; there is always a temptation to go higher rather than to descend what may be a further distance to an alternative camp. However, there is no question that descent is of the utmost importance; even a descent of 300 m may bring immediate relief. Evacuation with the patient sitting as in a "Sherpa chair" is ideal, as gravity will then aid redistribution of the edema fluid to the lung bases.

HIGH-ALTITUDE CEREBRAL EDEMA

The symptoms of high-altitude cerebral edema (HACE) are usually an exacerbation of those of AMS (Fig. 5); in addition, the headache becomes much more severe. The patient may be hallucinating, incoherent, weak, and ataxic. The state of consciousness may deteriorate until the patient becomes completely unconscious and unresponsive.

Treatment

HACE is also a medical emergency and evacuation should occur immediately if at all possible. Treatment should begin with betamethasone, 4 mg intravenously immediately and every 4 hours, and acetazolamide, 250 mg immediately and every 8 hours. Care of the airway and general management should be as is usual for an unconscious patient.

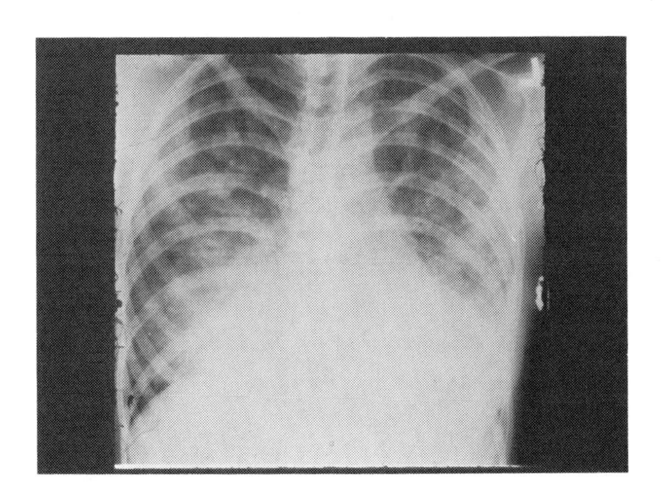

Figure 4 High-altitude pulmonary edema.

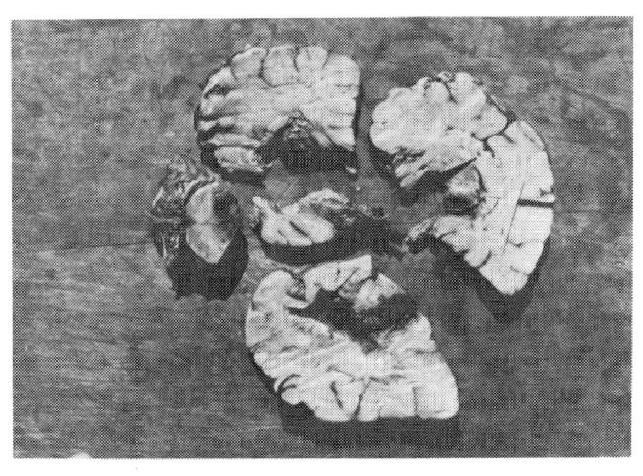

Figure 5 High-altitude cerebral edema, thrombosis, infarction, and hemorrhage.

HIGH-ALTITUDE RETINAL HEMORRHAGE

High-altitude retinal hemorrhage (HARH) was described only recently, but may occur in as many as 56 percent of people going to an altitude above 5,000 m (Fig. 6). Usually, it is asymptomatic, and visual symptoms appear only if a macular hemorrhage has occurred. On most occasions, a physician with an ophthalmoscope is not at hand. Visitors to high altitude are therefore usually unaware that HARH has occurred. Furthermore, many of these hemorrhages resolve while the patient is still at altitude. Thus, as a practical point, the retinal hemorrhage will not be recognized unless there are visual symptoms, and it is only under these circumstances that we would recommend descent to a lower altitude. No other treatment appears to be of value.

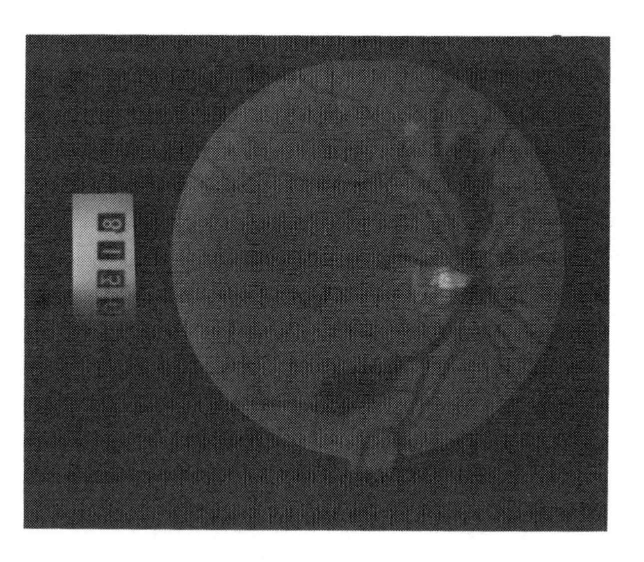

Figure 6 High-altitude retinal hemorrhage at 5,300 m on Mount Logan in the Yukon.

COLD AND ALTITUDE

Frequently, in the mountain world, the stress of hypoxia is combined with that of cold. The effects appear to be additive, both in the production of conditions such as HACE and HAPE and also in the development of cold-related injuries such as hypothermia and frostbite.

PREVENTION

High-altitude exposure carries with it potentially fatal medical situations, all of which are preventable. The most important means of prevention is a process of slow acclimatization. There is tremendous interindividual variation in susceptibility to high-altitude problems. Occasionally, a person may ascend as high as 3,000 to 4,000 m and suffer no ill effects; this is very rare. Most people experience at least mild symptoms of anorexia, headache, and insomnia at altitudes above 2,000 m. The following is a series of recommendations for those going to altitude:

1. Begin exposure at an altitude below 2,500 to 3,000 m if arriving by automobile or aircraft.
2. Exert yourself little for the first 24 hours.
3. Avoid or minimize alcohol consumption for the first 48 hours.
4. Keep the daily rate of ascent below 300 m.
5. If you climb high, sleep low (i.e., descend at night).
6. Keep yourself well hydrated and avoid using sedatives.

It is important that the physician recognize that these are only guidelines. Many people do not experience problems at this rate of ascent, but the occasional person will, showing that even this relatively conservative acclimatization regimen is too fast for that person. It is also important to appreciate that although acetazolamide may minimize the symptoms of AMS, there is no evidence that it will prevent HAPE or HACE. Furthermore, it is easy to be lulled into a false sense of security, in the expectation that by taking what appears a simple and effective panacea, there is no need to be concerned. Both physician and patient should play it safe so that altitude illness does not spoil a unique holiday experience.

ANXIETY AND DEPRESSION: EXERCISE FOR MOOD ENHANCEMENT

KENNETH H. SIDNEY, Ph.D.
WENDY C. JEROME, Ph.D.

Anxiety and depression are mood disorders that involve disturbances in self-awareness, self-perception, affect, and social interaction. These disorders, along with schizophrenia, are the most frequent causes of psychiatric hospitalization.

Anxiety may be defined as an unpleasant emotional experience varying in degree from mild unease to intense dread. Chronic anxiety is usually secondary to depression, schizophrenia, substance abuse, and an assortment of other medical problems; however, anxiety can also represent a primary mental disorder. Anxiety disorders include panic and generalized anxiety disorders (in which the eliciting stimuli are obscure, complex, and quite pervasive), obsessive-compulsive disorders (in which anxiety seems to be represented in intrusive thoughts and behaviors), and the phobias (which are irrational fears of objects or events). Generalized anxiety is characterized by excessive worry, muscle tension, restlessness, irritability, rapid heart rate, labored breathing, dizziness, sweating, and trembling. Compulsive disorders are associated with repetitive thoughts or actions. Phobias are characterized by both panic attacks and avoidance behaviors. In all anxiety disorders, traits characteristic of overarousal occur.

A variety of therapies and medications are used in the treatment of anxiety, but first it is important to restore a satisfactory cycle of sleep as soon as possible. Attention to diet and adequate exercise are helpful in assisting patients' general state of health and thereby increasing their resistance to stress.

In the major affective disorders, the primary symptoms are extremes of mood. These may alternate from mania to depression in the bipolar disorders, or may remain at the depressed end in major depression. Virtually everyone undergoes periods of depression in response to environmental stress. About 5 to 10 percent of men and 10 to 20 percent of women are diagnosed as clinically depressive at least once in their lives. Depressive illness ranks close behind coronary heart disease and hypertension as a major cause of morbidity. Its major complication, suicide, ranks high as a cause of death. Depressive psychoses account for 35 to 40 percent of all mental hospital admissions.

The word depression is used in at least three senses, to describe (1) a mood, (2) a syndrome, and (3) an illness. As a mood, depression is part of a universal human experience, usually developing in response to the frustrations and disappointments of life, but sometimes occurring for no apparent reason. The syndrome of depression consists of a depressive mood together with a combination of other symptoms, such as insomnia, weight loss, inability to concentrate, and suicidal ideas. As an illness, depression involves the presence of the syndrome. The condition is not transitory and is associated with significant functional impairment. The patient is unable to work, or does so with reduced efficiency, and has lost the capacity for enjoyment. In all depressed states, there are feelings of helplessness, guilt, and unworthiness. Depressed people characteristically blame themselves for whatever setbacks they encounter.

The clinical features of depressive disorders suggest a defect in hypothalamic function, possibly as a result of deficiency in a brain biogenic amine neurotransmitter (serotonin or norepinephrine). There is a strong genetic predisposition for the major depressions. There are also a variety of psychological theories of depression which revolve around the concept of loss (for instance, death of a loved one, or breakup of a friendship). Recurring depression is often seen in individuals with a long history of emotional deprivation.

The terms depression and anxiety do not necessarily refer to psychopathologic states. Rather, they can describe the subjective distress caused by the unpleasant emotions of sadness and fear that occur in both normal individuals and the mentally ill. This emotional dysphoria is associated with various behavioral patterns and physiologic signs and symptoms. The intensity and duration of subjective distress are frequently disproportionate to the importance of any cause that might be identified. Indeed, often no specific cause is identified by the sufferer.

This article summarizes the postulated benefits and risks of exercise as a means of alleviating the symptoms of depression and anxiety. It supports the proposition that regular aerobic physical activity contributes to improvements in mood states, and emphasizes that specific characteristics of the exercise program need to be carefully considered on an individual basis to better ensure a positive impact upon the participant's psychological state.

POSTULATED BENEFITS OF EXERCISE AND EXERCISE TRAINING

The beneficial effects of habitual exercise on physical health, fitness, and performance are fairly well documented (Table 1). The physiologic benefits include cardiovascular, metabolic, and hormonal adjustments that are observed at rest, and during and following both submaximal and maximal effort. In addition, there are favorable alterations of body size, structure, and composition. The type and

TABLE 1 Possible Physiologic Effects of Regular Exercise

Increases:	*Decreases:*
Blood volume	Appetite
Bone (calcium) mineral	Blood coagulability
Capillary: muscle fiber ratio	Body fat
Daily energy expenditure	Cardiac work
Diffusion of respiratory gases in lungs	Electromyographic activity
Efficiency of blood distribution and return	Heart rate at rest and during exercise
Enzymatic function in muscle cells	Lactate levels at submaximal effort
Fibrinolytic capability induced by vascular occlusion	Neurohormonal overreaction
Flexibility (range of motion)	Peripheral vascular resistance
Functional (work) capacity, aerobic power	Plasma catecholamines
Glucose tolerance	Plasma insulin level
Growth hormone production	Platelet stickiness
Heat tolerance (sweating rate)	Serum lipids (cholesterol, triglycerides)
HDL:LDL ratio	Systolic blood pressure at rest and during exercise
Immune function	Ventilatory minute volume at submaximal effort
Motor coordination	Vulnerability to cardiac dysrhythmias
Muscle mass	
Muscle strength and endurance	
Myocardial efficiency	
Number and size of blood vessels	
Orthostatic tolerance	
Rate of recovery from effort (heart rate, ventilation, lactic acid)	
Red blood cell mass	
Sensitivity to insulin	
Stroke volume	

HDL = high density lipoproteins; LDL = low density lipoproteins.

magnitude of training responses are dependent on two factors: (1) the characteristics of the exercise program employed (type of training; mode of exercise; intensity, frequency, and duration of effort) and (2) the physiologic and psychological characteristics of the participants (current health, initial fitness, age, and motivation).

Vigorous activity has also been claimed to affect the psychological characteristics of both normal individuals and those with clinical problems. Many health professionals argue that physical well-being is associated with positive mental health. It is widely believed that acute exercise reduces anxiety and depression and helps in venting tensions. When appropriate exercise is performed on a regular basis, the chronic mood and well-being of participants are favorably affected. In addition, one of the major effects of regular activity may be its ability to improve mood on a daily basis, thereby preventing the onset of chronic anxiety and depression. Thus, both acute and chronic psychological benefits are associated with exercise. Higher tolerance levels are developed, so that physically fit individuals are better able to cope with stress than those who are less fit and are sedentary.

A wide variety of psychological benefits have been associated with exercise (Table 2). These include increased arousal; optimization of intellectual development; improved self-confidence and body image; positive effects on attitudes to physical activity, mood, and well-being; relief of anxiety, depression, tension, and fatigue; and reduction of the stress response.

What Is Currently Known

In the United States, the National Institute of Mental Health consensus panel developed statements concerning the influence of exercise on mental health, as follows:

1. Physical fitness is positively associated with mental health and well-being.
2. Exercise is associated with the reduction of stress emotions such as state anxiety.
3. Anxiety and depression are common symptoms of failure to cope with mental stress, and exercise has been associated with a decreased level of mild to moderate depression and anxiety.
4. Long-term exercise is usually associated with reductions in traits such as neuroticism and anxiety.
5. Severe depression usually requires professional treatment, which may include medication, electroconvulsive therapy, and/or psychotherapy, with exercise as an adjunct.
6. Appropriate exercise programs result in reductions of various stress indices such as neuromuscular tension, resting heart rate, and blood levels of some stress hormones.
7. Current clinical opinion holds that exercise has beneficial emotional effects in all age groups and in both sexes.
8. Physically healthy people who require psychotropic medication may safely exercise, provided that exercise and medications are titrated under close medical supervision.

TABLE 2 Possible Psychological Benefits of Exercise

Increases:	*Decreases:*
Academic performance	Absenteeism at work
Arousal	Aggression
Assertiveness	Alcohol abuse
Attitudes toward job and work environments	Anger
Attitudes toward physical activity	Anxiety
Catharsis	Confusion
Confidence	Depression
Coping abilities	Destructive habits (cigarette smoking, substance abuse)
Emotional stability	Dysmenorrhea
Energy	Fatigue
Independence	Headache
Information processing	Hostility
Intellectual functioning	Loneliness
Internal locus of control	On-the-job fatigue
Joie de vivre	Perception of exertion
Memory	Phobias
Mood	Psychotic behaviors
Optimism	Reaction time
Pain tolerance	Stress response
Perception	Tension
Popularity	Type A behavior
Positive body image	Work errors
Prudent living habits	
Psychomotor development	
Self-control	
Self-esteem (concept)	
Self-perception	
Self-satisfaction and acceptance	
Sexual satisfaction	
Social interactions, contacts, and skills	
Tolerance to stress	
Well-being	
Work efficiency	

More recently, at the 1988 International Conference on Exercise, Health, and Fitness held in Toronto, a consensus panel of world experts with extensive research and clinical experience in exercise science and mental health attempted to identify what is known about the influence of exercise on mental health. Although their final report has not yet been published, the following statements were drafted and presented to conference delegates for discussion:

1. High levels of activity and/or high levels of physical fitness are associated with (a) reduced levels of autonomic arousal before, during, and after exposure to stressors, (b) quicker autonomic recovery following exposure to a stressor, and (c) attenuated emotional reactions in response to some stressors.

2. High levels of muscle tension are known to produce serious pain symptoms (headache, neck and back pain). Aerobic exercise of moderate to high intensity causes a rebound reduction in muscle tension for 2 to 5 hours after a bout of activity. Rest or relaxation training is as effective as exercise in reducing muscle tension. For some individuals, the acute experience of exercise may be noxious and uncomfortable, but for others it may reduce pain symptoms. The quality and quantity of sleep is influenced positively by exercise training and negatively by exercise deprivation.

3. Acute physical activity of low intensity and short duration is not associated with reductions in state anxiety, even though it is associated with reduced muscle tension. Acute vigorous physical activity of moderate duration is associated with reductions in state anxiety or muscle tension in male, female, young, middle-aged, elderly, physically impaired and nonimpaired, and high-, moderate-, and low-anxious individuals. Acute vigorous activity does not induce anxiety symptoms of a clinical magnitude or panic disorders. Chronic physical activity is often associated with lower levels of anxiety.

4. Chronic physical activity or high levels of fitness are associated with reductions in depression for (a) individuals from the general population who are initially mildly or moderately depressed and (b) noninstitutionalized outpatients suffering from clinical depression. Properly prescribed and monitored exercise appears safe to use for individuals who are taking a psychotropic medication. It is not uncommon for active and fit people to have lower levels of depression than the inactive or unfit, but the efficacy of intervention programs in improving the mood state of the masses has not yet been demonstrated.

5. High levels of activity or high fitness are associated with reduced levels of sympathetically mediated elevations in heart rate before, during, and after exposure to stress. However, oxygen consumption

values during psychological stress are not significantly related to the level of fitness. Regarding type of exercise training, it is clear that anaerobic (strength and sprint) training is not as effective as aerobic training in reducing cardiovascular reactivity.

Both consensus panels emphasized that the positive relationship among physical activity, fitness, and mental health were associative rather than causal. It is not known whether improvements of fitness induced by regular exercise actually cause improvements in affect.

THE BASIS OF MOOD ENHANCEMENT

Morgan and, later, Morgan and O'Connor reviewed various hypotheses that they believed could explain the effects of vigorous physical activity on well-being. One hypothesis was that exercise-induced affective changes are a result of diversion, distraction, or "time out" from stressful stimuli. A second hypothesis suggested that alterations in mood are due to alterations in brain neurotransmitters such as norepinephrine and serotonin. A third hypothesis was that endorphins or lipotropins that mediate the affective changes are produced during muscular effort. A fourth (thermogenic) hypothesis indicated that the effects of exercise on mood state are mediated via the elevations of body temperature that occur with vigorous physical activity.

Additional mechanisms by which physical activity programs might influence mood state are summarized in Table 3. For example, physical activity may provide a specific challenge that, when dealt with or removed, moderates both the intensity and the duration of anxiety and depressive states, enabling participants to return to a relaxed state and giving them a sense of accomplishment for having confronted and overcome a difficult physical or psychological challenge. In addition, physical activity may provide social support from others with similar goals, interests, and values.

TABLE 3 Possible Agents for Psychological Change in Exercise Programs

Acute physiologic responses to exercise
Alterations in brain neurotransmitters—serotonin, catecholamines
Production of endogenous opioids
Elevated body temperature
Increase in physical fitness
Increased aerobic (endurance) fitness
Increased muscle strength and endurance
Decreased response to (or quicker recovery from) various stressors
Increase in physical work capacity or performance
Increased total work done or rate of working
Change in physical appearance
Loss of body fat
Increased muscle tone, definition, or size
Goal achievement and sense of accomplishment
Feelings of somatic well-being
Sense of competence, mastery, or control of the events in one's life
Adoption of associated (prudent) health behaviors
Adoption of physically active lifestyle
Increased physical activity outside the exercise program during leisure or work—(walk more, take stairs, work in the garden or around the house)
Social experiences
Increased social competence
Identification with a group or individual
Increased social contacts
Reinforcement of significant others
Development of esprit de corps
Promotion of sound sleep

USE OF EXERCISE TO ACHIEVE PSYCHOLOGICAL BENEFITS

Individuals with affective disorders, and indeed even most persons judged to be normal, engage in insufficient physical activity to maintain desirable levels of cardiorespiratory fitness, body fat, muscular strength, muscular endurance, and flexibility. For such persons, an exercise program that improves general stamina and increases energy expenditure, perhaps supplemented by strength and flexibility activities, should be a major component of any prescribed treatment. Nevertheless, gains in mood state may be of more practical importance than physiologic gains in terms of the individual's well-being and overall performance. Furthermore, it does not appear that physiologic adaptations must develop in order for the participant to experience psychological benefits.

In comparison with other possible regimens, physical training is an active, aggressive approach. This may be effective in people whose personality type predisposes them to want to be involved in the resolution of their problems, i.e., the internalizers. Most patients are accustomed to being passive recipients of medical treatment and would benefit if they took a more active role in their "rehabilitation."

Physical inactivity leads to a loss of fitness and effort intolerance, which in turn can lead to diminished physical performance, reduced or impaired activities of daily living, or decreased independence. The decline in physical abilities and possible disengagement from social interactions, in turn, promotes poor self-confidence and self-concept, which contribute to such mood states as depression, anxiety, frustration, and unhappiness. These may further reduce participation in physical activity. By increasing personal activity levels, such persons may be able to break the vicious cycle, and in so doing achieve a more desirable mood state.

The development of an effective exercise program requires clinical judgment, which comes from experience and knowledge of exercise physiology, of psychological reactions to stress, and of various behavior modification techniques. The patient's physical work capacity, current and past health status, health habits, and psychological state must be considered. Too often, the physiologist neglects the psychological characteristics of the patient when prescribing exercise, just as the psychologist neglects physiologic aspects.

Health professionals have frequently argued that exercise must be carried out at a certain frequency, intensity, and duration for it to have any benefit. This is true for the augmentation of aerobic power, but the same attitude can be counterproductive during the early phases of an exercise program. This is particularly so for patients with an emotional disorder who have a myriad of real and perceived barriers to overcome in order to initiate, adopt, and sustain the exercise habit (Table 4). We do not know the minimal amount of exercise needed to bring about optimal psychological benefits, or how the characteristics of an activity regimen should be adapted to the physiologic and psychological profile of the participant.

The nature of a mood disorder probably determines the optimal exercise mode. Patients who are only mildly depressed are generally underaroused and will therefore be helped by the kinesthetic stimulation arising from vigorous movement. Activities performed in a group, with arousing, lively music under the guidance of an enthusiastic exercise leader, should further facilitate a beneficial response. For more severely depressed patients, their symptoms make exercising difficult. Exercise in a highly structured program with normal, happy people is recommended for such individuals.

Patients who suffer from an anxiety disorder are, in contrast, overaroused. Initially, these people need plenty of reassurance and close supervision by medical personnel in order to become accustomed to the feeling of muscular exertion and to attenuate the unpleasant symptoms often reported with exercise. Furthermore, anxiety patients with excessive muscular tension should engage in a preliminary extensive stretching routine, accompanied by easy aerobic warm-up activities. As the excessive muscle tension is alleviated, they may then proceed to a more vigorous exercise program. Individuals with less disabling anxiety should benefit most from relaxing physical activities that are rhythmical, repetitive, and prolonged (walking, hiking, cycling, swimming, or cross-country skiing). The activities should be performed at a leisurely pace, either alone or with an understanding and reassuring companion, in a pleasing and soothing environment (for instance, in a park or along the seashore). Anxious individuals who are chronically stressed should not participate in competitive programs in which their performance can be compared with that of others.

A training (treatment) program will be counterproductive if a person is required to perform an activity that either is not liked or produces excessive discomfort. The program will also be ineffective if the patient does not have the opportunity to carry it out, or must perform it in an intimidating environment. Exercising under such conditions, or skipping the prescribed activities, induces additional anxiety and feelings of guilt, fear, frustration, or monotony.

TABLE 4 Barriers to the Initiation and Maintenance of a Physical Activity Program

Barrier
Medical (Health) Status
Current minor illness (cold, flu)
Presence (or suspected presence) of cardiovascular, respiratory, neurologic, or metabolic disease
Physical
Orthopaedic or locomotor limitations
Restricted flexibility
Excess body fat
Physiologic
Poor cardiovascular fitness
Muscle weakness or imbalance
Poor skill development, balance, or coordination
Hearing or visual impairment
Psychological
Negative attitudes to physical activity
Fear of injury
Exercise-induced (or exercise-related) feelings of discomfort—muscle, joint, chest pain; shortness of breath; nausea; dizziness; awkwardness; self-consciousness; embarrassment
Lack of self-confidence, poor body image/self-esteem
Unsuccessful (or negative) previous experiences
Lack of motivation
Disabling mental illness—severe anxiety, depression
Social
Discouragement, lack of interest or negative attitudes of spouse, family members, friends, coworkers
Lack of exercise partner
No appropriate role model for emulation
Inadequate social contacts or support from exercise group
Insufficient encouragement from exercise personnel
Poor family or office social relationships
Educational
Inability to set realistic, achievable goals
Lack of knowledge (how to exercise, relationship among activity, health, and fitness); misconceptions about benefits and hazards of activity
Minimal or no perceived benefits from participating in exercise
Lack of specific advice from personal physician or other health professionals
Lack of (or inappropriate) feedback and counsel from exercise leader or supervisor
Environmental
Adverse weather
Absence of convenient and appropriate facility or exercise program in the community
Personal
Cost of joining program, testing, equipment and clothing, transportation
Lack of time—conflict with work, school, or social commitments, holidays
Incompatible or stressful personal lifestyle (health habits)—inadequate sleep, cigarette smoking, substance abuse, poor nutrition

Even though an improvement of fitness has not been proved to enhance mood state, we feel strongly that the key to an effective exercise program is the selection of activities that the patient enjoys and will perform long enough, often enough, and at sufficient intensity to elicit a training effect. Improvement of fitness has been found in many studies to be associated with physical and psychological well-being, which we feel will have a favorable effect on mood states.

Exercise programs should not be imposed. Program adherence is much better when the patient is involved in the decision making and design of the program. Particularly important for depressed and anxious clients is the fact that if a self-designed program is neglected, there are less likely to be attacks of conscience. Indeed, if a group leader or therapist sets goals or contracts that are excessively difficult for the patient to attain or that the patient has difficulty in internalizing, anxiety and depression may be exacerbated.

Both physiologic and psychological reactions of patients to the exercise sessions should be recorded in an exercise and mood diary closely monitored by experienced personnel. Careful and direct observation of the patient is recommended during the early phases of physical training, when the exercise prescription has not been fully evaluated; this precaution is particularly necessary in persons unaccustomed to exercise and in those considered to be at high risk. Moreover, in individuals with a type A personality, denial of symptoms should be anticipated. In such persons, symptom denial during exercise could lead to a hazardous situation in which the exercise prescription is exceeded.

POSSIBLE HAZARDS OF EXERCISE

Participation in an exercise program is associated with certain risks and discomforts, especially for individuals with specific cardiovascular, respiratory, or metabolic disorders and for those with significant emotional distress. In dealing with such individuals, the anticipated benefits must be carefully evaluated in relation to the risks of physical activity. Abnormalities of heart rate and blood pressure, fainting, and (in rare instances) myocardial infarction and death are acknowledged hazards of muscular exertion.

The therapist-clinician should also be aware of the possibility of overtraining. The signs and symptoms of chronic overexertion include diminished physical performance, excessive fatigue during and after effort, heaviness of limb movement, labored breathing during submaximal effort, loss of appetite, decreased body mass, anemia, and sore muscles and joints. In addition, when individuals augment the volume or intensity of effort or when they become progressively fatigued throughout an exercise session, there is a possibility of joint and musculoskeletal injury, dehydration, hypo- and hyperthermia, and (in women) dysmenorrhea.

A number of adverse psychological effects have been attributed to exercise (Table 5). Some runners have been described as addicted, compulsive, or obligatory, since their commitment and dedication to running exceed their commitments to personal relationshps, family relationships, occupation, or medical advice. In addition, the anxious type A person may experience frustration and tension as a result of overcompetitiveness in a zeal to "be the best."

When dealing with individuals considered to be at increased physical or psychological risk, it is important to evaluate carefully the anticipated benefits in relation to the possible hazards of augmented activity, and to take appropriate action to minimize the possibility of complications when exercise is to form a part of treatment. It is therefore appropriate to give careful, specific advice to individuals judged to be at increased risk. Their exercise response and progress should be monitored regularly through periodic testing and evaluation of mood and activity diaries. Patients should be taught to expect, recognize, and handle the various unpleasant symptoms of unaccustomed physical exertion and to distinguish the signs and symptoms of vigorous effort from those of overexertion.

Exercise performed at excessive intensity, duration, or frequency or activities of an inappropriate type not only increase the chance of physical injury or illness, but also make patient noncompliance more likely. Another negative result could involve a worsening of mood state (e.g., increased anxiety or depression) and a lowering of self-esteem when the patient fails to perceive meaningful improvements

TABLE 5 Possible Negative Psychological Effects of Exercise

Aggression
Anxiety
Compulsiveness
Decreased involvement in job and personal relationships
Depression
Distortion of normal sense of values
Escape from, or avoidance of problems
Exacerbation of anorexia nervosa
Exercise deprivation effects
Exposure to excessive total stress
Fatigue and tiredness
Fear of failure
Feelings of inadequacy, clumsiness, ridicule
Frustration
Irritability
Mood fluctuations
Nervousness, worry
Overarousal
Overcompetitiveness
Poor eating habits
Preoccupation with fitness, diet, and body image
Self-centeredness
Sleep disorders (difficulty in falling asleep, early morning awakening)
Tension

in fitness or performance. Furthermore, each patient should be counseled individually to ensure that the proposed program does not make excessive or unrealistic demands on time and financial resources, and that unrealistic expectations are not harbored by the patient or the family. The program should be designed and implemented so that its organization and administration does not become an additional source of stress to the participant, thereby negating any benefits that result from the exercise regimen itself.

The following strategies are recommended for the development of effective training programs:

1. Always have the patient warm up well before engaging in vigorous physical exertion, and always conclude each exercise session with a cool-down period that includes gentle stretching of major joints.

2. Monitor the intensity of effort frequently, especially in the early stages of an exercise program. Intensity can be monitored by palpating the pulse rate, or by exercising at a level that permits conversation to be carried on. The intensity of exercise should be held below a level that elicits adverse signs and symptoms, with periodic upward revision, according to the patient's responses to exercise as judged from direct observation, testing, and scrutiny of training and mood diaries.

3. Instruct the patient to exercise at a reduced intensity or for a shorter time when unusual fatigue or pressure is sensed. Exercise should not be performed when a fever is present or when the patient is feeling unwell.

4. Excessively anxious or fearful patients should exercise in a calm, relaxing environment under supervision until they become accustomed to both exercise and the exercise setting. Plenty of verbal reassurance and personal attention should be offered. Training should be performed at a comfortable low intensity, continuing for only a short period, so that recovery is rapid. The wearing of a heart rate monitor may provide both the patient and the exercise supervisor with immediate and accurate feedback. Instructions and practice of various relaxation or coping techniques (e.g., slowing down, stretching, and use of association-disassociation techniques) to monitor, control, and reduce any anxiety responses may be appropriate. Avoid including exercises that cause discomfort or are disliked; these activities, if judged to be necessary, should be introduced into the program in a gradual and controlled manner. As the patient overcomes the initial fear or anxiety, exercise in a less closely supervised situation in the company of a supporting friend or group should be attempted.

5. Patient compliance with any exercise program can be optimized by providing opportunities for them to engage in activities that interest them and at an intensity safe and vigorous enough to accomplish their specific objectives (weight loss, increase of muscle tone or size, venting of aggression and tensions). Patient progress should be monitored in terms of the minutes of activity completed or the number of exercise sessions attended, as well as the results of repeated physiologic, psychological, and performance testing. The activity routine and location of exercise sessions should be varied to avoid monotony and sustain interest. The program should provide opportunities for the participation and education of family members or significant others, and also provide plenty of opportunities for social interaction between patients, normal individuals, exercise staff and therapists.

SUGGESTED READING

Fasting K. Leisure time, physical activity and some indices of mental health. Scand J Soc Med 1982; Suppl 29:113–119.

Folkins CH, Amsterdam EA. Control and modification of stress emotions through chronic exercise. In: Amsterdam EA, Wilmore JH, DeMaria AN, eds. Exercise in cardiovascular health and disease. New York: Yorke Medical Books, 1977:280.

Folkins CH, Sime WE. Physical fitness training and mental health. Am Psychol 1981; 36:373–389.

Hughes JR. Psychological effects of habitual aerobic exercise: a critical review. Prev Med 1984; 13:66–78.

Leigh D, Pare C, Marks J, eds. Encyclopaedia of psychiatry for general practitioners. Great Britain: Lund Humphries, 1972.

Mihevic PM. Anxiety, depression and exercise. Quest 1981; 33:140–153.

Morgan WP. Affective beneficence of vigorous physical activity. Med Sci Sports Exerc 1985; 17:94–100.

Morgan WP, Goldston SE, eds. Exercise and mental health. Washington, DC: Hemisphere Publishing, 1987.

Morgan WP, O'Connor PJ. Exercise and mental health. In: Dishman RK, ed. Exercise adherence: its impact on public health. Champaign, IL: Human Kinetics, 1988:91.

Shephard RJ. Physical activity and the healthy mind. Can Med Assoc J 1983; 128:525–530.

Taylor CB, Sallis JF, Needle R. The relation of physical activity and exercise to mental health. Public Health Rep 1985; 100:195–202.

SPINAL CORD INJURIES AND NEUROMUSCULAR STIMULATION EXERCISE

ROGER M. GLASER, Ph.D.

Spinal cord injury (SCI) usually causes skeletal muscle paralysis and limited ability to exercise voluntarily. This situation frequently leads to a sedentary lifestyle and a marked loss of physical fitness, as well as an increased occurrence of secondary health complications (e.g., cardiovascular diseases, muscle atrophy, osteoporosis and decubitus ulcers). A major goal of our research effort is to develop and evaluate the effectiveness of specialized exercise techniques by which individuals with SCI can improve their physical fitness. This chapter presents current research data related to using functional neuromuscular stimulation (FNS) of paralyzed leg muscles for improving the physical fitness of individuals with SCI.

Patients with paralyzed legs typically use their functional arms for manual wheelchair locomotion, exercise training, and sports activities. However, because the relatively small muscle mass available limits arm exercise capability, paraplegics cannot develop the high levels of physical fitness (cardiopulmonary, aerobic) that can be achieved by able-bodied individuals through leg exercise. In this situation, upper body muscles tend to fatigue (because of peripheral factors) before the cardiopulmonary system is driven to sufficiently high output levels for long enough to enable substantial central training effects to occur. Quadriplegics have even lower exercise and fitness development capabilities.

Recently, the use of FNS-induced contractions to exercise paralyzed lower limb muscles of patients with SCI has received much attention. This technique has the potential for improving physical fitness to higher levels than can be accomplished through voluntary arm exercise alone. Apparent advantages of this technique include the activation of muscles that are usually dormant, the greater muscle mass that can be utilized, and improved circulation of blood. Quadriplegics will most likely find this involuntary exercise mode to be especially advantageous. However, FNS exercise does not "cure" SCI, and indeed any health and physical fitness benefits derived from participating in FNS exercise programs will most likely be lost several weeks after exercise is discontinued. Therefore, FNS exercise needs to become part of one's lifestyle if it is found to be beneficial.

Although some of the FNS exercise techniques to be presented are experimental and require specially constructed instrumentation, commercial electrical neuromuscular stimulator systems are now available to permit FNS exercise in a clinical or home setting.

CONSIDERATIONS FOR USE OF FNS

A major requirement for FNS use is that the damage to the spinal cord is upper motor neuron in nature (i.e., the motor units of the paralyzed muscles are intact and functional). Individuals who respond best to FNS typically exhibit reflex contractions and spasms in the affected muscles. Evaluation for FNS response may be accomplished by using a portable neuromuscular stimulator and skin surface electrodes placed over motor points (where motor nerves enter the muscle). Motor point location may be determined by placing a stationary electrode over the muscle and moving a small "probe" electrode around the muscle while stimulating in a pulsatile manner (e.g., 0.25-second pulses) at an intensity that causes weak contractions. At motor points, the threshold level will be lower and a greater contraction force will be obtained for a given stimulation level. When individuals respond well to FNS, gradual increases in stimulation intensity result in more motor unit recruitment and a greater contraction force. However, if the patient with SCI has some degree of intact sensory function, the FNS may be uncomfortable or painful, and higher levels of stimulation may not be tolerated.

For patient safety, a medical examination is necessary before FNS is used for exercise training. This should include an electrocardiogram, radiographs of the paralyzed limbs, range-of-motion testing, and a neurologic examination. FNS-induced contractions should be smooth and limited with respect to maximal force development, to prevent injuries to the deteriorated muscles, bones, and joints. Since FNS may trigger spasms and reflex contractions in the stimulated and other muscles, it is important to observe the activity closely to make certain that it is not hazardous. It is also advisable to monitor the heart rate and blood pressure, especially during initial FNS exercise sessions with quadriplegics. As with any mode of exercise, activity should be discontinued immediately if abnormal responses occur that place the user at risk.

DEVELOPING MUSCLE STRENGTH AND ENDURANCE WITH FNS

FNS-Induced Weightlifting Exercise

Training with FNS-induced contractions can result in greater strength and endurance of the paralyzed muscles (for this mode of exercise). However, early FNS exercise training techniques achieved only limited success. This may have been due to inadequate loading of the muscles, and the use of stimulation patterns and training protocols that were not highly effective. In contrast, recent studies that have followed well-established weight-training principles (progressive overload, exercise sets of relatively low number of repetitions at relatively high resistance), in conjunction with FNS of gradually ramped intensity levels, have resulted in substantially greater performance gains.

This FNS technique is readily applied to the paralyzed quadriceps muscles to make possible knee extension weightlifting. Protocols can be designed that use three to five lifts per minute for each leg (in a reciprocal pattern if two channels of stimulation are used), 10 to 30 repetitions per set, two to three sets per session, and two to four sessions per week. As performance improves, increments of 0.5 kg appear to be suitable for the load weight progression. Although most research studies have used specially designed and constructed stimulators and weightlifting devices such as illustrated in Figure 1, battery-powered commercial stimulators (which provide gradually ramped output intensity) and ankle weights may also be effective. It has been reported that by progressively increasing load resistance on the muscles as well as the number of repetitions per set, quadriceps strength and resistance to fatigue can be markedly increased over a period of several weeks. In addition, muscle hypertrophy can improve limb cosmesis. Similar protocols can be devised for use with other paralyzed muscles.

Although this quadriceps weightlifting exercise can result in peripheral adaptations to increase muscle strength and endurance, the aerobic metabolic and cardiopulmonary responses are not of sufficient magnitudes and durations to stimulate cardiopulmonary (central circulatory) training effects. In addition, there is no convincing evidence that this or any other form of FNS exercise can reverse osteoporosis. Therefore, it is conceivable that FNS weight training can eventually make the muscles capable of generating greater contraction force than the bones can withstand. Since standard radiographs are not sensitive enough to quantify osteoporosis precisely (e.g., a 30 to 50 percent change in bone mass can occur before it is observed), it is prudent to set practical limits to the maximal resistance used for training (for instance, 10 to 15 kg for knee extension exercise). When this maximal loading is achieved, the number of repetitions per set may be increased to enhance endurance rather than strength.

DEVELOPING CARDIOPULMONARY FITNESS WITH FNS

FNS Cycle Ergometer Exercise

In an effort to increase the capability of individuals with SCI to develop higher levels of cardiopulmonary fitness, a Monark cycle ergometer was modified to permit paraplegics and quadriplegics to pedal via computer-controlled FNS-induced contractions of the quadriceps, hamstring, and gluteus maximus muscles. Recently, highly sophisticated versions of this device became commercially available for clinical and home use (Fig. 2). When the patient pedals at the target rate of 50 rpm, these cycle ergometers induce 50 contractions of the contralateral muscle groups each minute. Therefore, FNS cycle ergometer exercise incorporates more muscle mass than the above-described FNS weightlifting exercise, and the muscles are stimulated to contract at a considerably higher rate. This exercise seems well suited for endurance (rather than strength) training, and many individuals with SCI can pedal continuously for 30-minute periods.

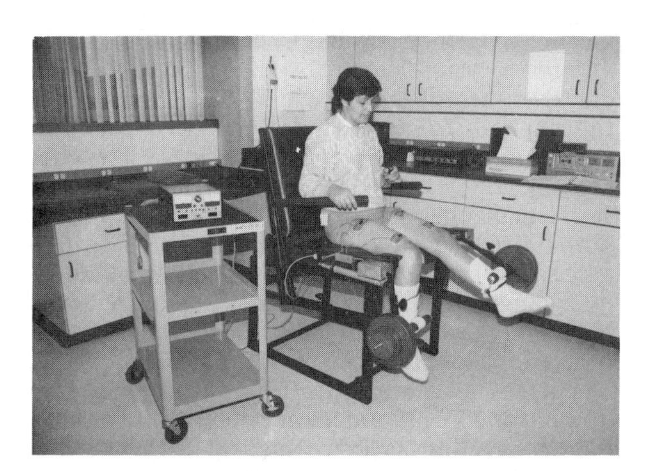

Figure 1 FNS-induced knee extension weightlifting exercise being performed by a person with SCI. The instrumentation illustrated was specially designed and constructed for this purpose.

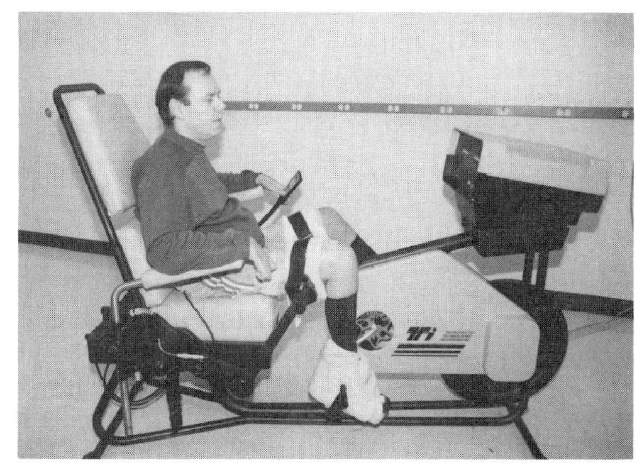

Figure 2 FNS cycle ergometer exercise being performed by a person with SCI on ERGYS (Therapeutic Technologies, Inc.).

In the typical protocol, individuals initially pedal this FNS cycle ergometer with no load resistance (0 watts). When 30 minutes of continuous pedaling can be accomplished, subsequent exercise sessions use greater load resistance to increase power output (PO) to 6.1 watts. When 30 minutes of continuous pedaling can be achieved at this higher PO, the PO is increased by a further 6.1 watts. This progressive intensity protocol is repeated, with gains in performance capability up to a maximum PO of 42.7 watts. Exercise is usually performed three times a week.

It appears that for some individuals with SCI (especially quadriplegics), FNS cycle ergometer exercise may provide more effective cardiopulmonary fitness training than voluntary arm exercise. In part, this is due to the high magnitudes of metabolic and cardiopulmonary responses that are elicited. Figure 3 provides data from 12 patients with SCI during steady-state FNS cycle ergometer exercise, and illustrates the near-linear relationship between PO and oxygen uptake ($\dot{V}O_2$), pulmonary ventilation ($\dot{V}_E$), and heart rate (HR). PO capability ranged from 0 to 30 watts for this group of individuals. The one patient who pedaled at 30 watts achieved a peak $\dot{V}O_2$ of 1.77 liters per minute, $\dot{V}_E$ of 45 liters per minute, and HR of 135 beats per minute. Since 42.7 watts is the maximal PO capability of this cycle ergometer, it appears that well-trained SCI individuals who can pedal at this PO may reach a $\dot{V}O_2$ of about 2 liters per minute (with concomitant $\dot{V}_E$ and HR responses). Considering that able-bodied individuals typically perform cardiopulmonary training at about 50 to 60 percent of their maximal $\dot{V}O_2$ (maximal $\dot{V}O_2$ may be about 3 to 4 liters per minute for leg exercise), FNS cycling offers a potential means for individuals with SCI to achieve a similar training metabolic rate. Indeed, able-bodied persons commonly jog at $\dot{V}O_2$ levels of 1.5 to 2.0 liters per minute. It is unlikely that such high $\dot{V}O_2$ levels can be elicited by arm exercise for a sufficient duration (e.g., 30 minutes) to stimulate substantial cardiopulmonary training.

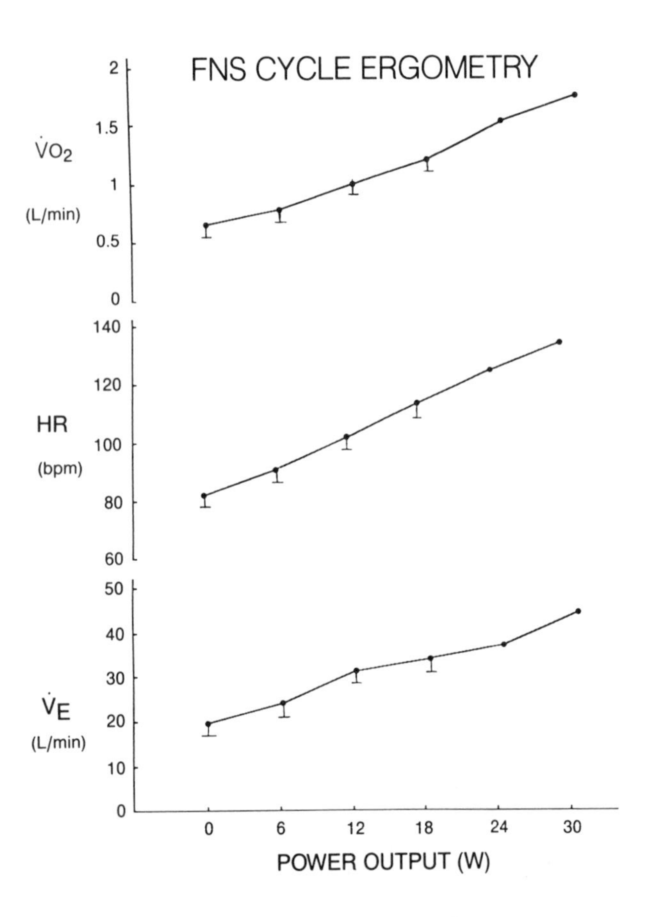

Figure 3 Steady-state oxygen uptake ($\dot{V}O_2$), pulmonary ventilation ($\dot{V}_E$), and heart rate (HR) responses of patients with spinal cord injury in relationship to power output for FNS cycle ergometry. (n = 12 at 0 W, 10 at 6.1 W, 9 at 12.2 W, 4 at 18.3 W, and 1 at 24.4 W and 30.5 W) (Modified from Glaser RM, Figoni SF, Collins SR, et al. Physiologic responses of SCI subjects to electrically induced leg cycle ergometry. Proceedings of the Annual International Conference of the IEEE Engineering in Medicine and Biology Society, Piscataway, NJ: IEEE 1988: 1638–1640.)

Mechanical efficiency for FNS-induced exercise is extremely low. This may be due to nonphysiologic activation of the muscles, histochemical changes in deteriorated muscles, and imprecise joint biomechanics. However, this is advantageous for the training of individuals with SCI. Such patients performing FNS cycling at 42.7 watts may have a $\dot{V}O_2$ of about 2.0 liters per minute, whereas able-bodied individuals cycling voluntarily at this same PO would have a $\dot{V}O_2$ of less than 0.9 liters per minute (which would not be very effective for aerobic training).

Another potential advantage of FNS cycling over arm-cranking is the superior central hemodynamic responses. In another study, six SCI quadriplegic men performed maximal FNS cycle ergometer exercise at a mean PO of 11 watts, and on another occasion maximal voluntary arm-crank ergometer exercise at a mean PO of 38 watts. Although both exercise modes produced peak $\dot{V}O_2$ levels of about 1.0 liters per minute, FNS cycling elicited a 59 percent greater stroke volume (92 versus 58 ml per beat), and a 20 percent greater cardiac output (8.01 versus 6.66 liters per minute). These response patterns may be due to activation of the venous muscle pump and facilitated venous return of blood to the heart during the FNS-induced contractions of the lower limb musculature. In addition, a 25 percent lower heart rate (87 versus 116 beats per minute) and 19 percent lower rate-pressure product for FNS cycling suggested that the higher cardiac volume load was accomplished with lower myocardial O_2 demands. Therefore, FNS cycling may be more effective and have a lower cardiovascular risk than arm-cranking as a means for the aerobic conditioning of quadriplegics.

Hybrid FNS Cycling and Voluntary Arm-Cranking Exercise

To further improve cardiopulmonary fitness training capability for individuals with SCI, a hybrid form of exercise was developed in which FNS cycling is performed simultaneously with voluntary arm cranking (Figure 4). This combined mode of exercise may provide a more superior training capability than either mode of exercise performed individually. This is due to the greater muscle mass used, the higher levels of metabolic and cardiopulmonary responses that can be elicited, and possibly the improved circulation of blood to both the upper and lower body muscles.

To demonstrate the additive effect of this hybrid exercise, Figure 5 illustrates the $\dot{V}O_2$ of a T8 male paraplegic subject at rest and during FNS cycling at 6.1 watts, voluntary arm-cranking at 25 watts, and hybrid exercise at a total of 31.1 watts. Individually, both modes of exercise increased $\dot{V}O_2$ above the rest level (0.25 liters per minute) by about 0.5 liters per minute for a total of about 0.75 liters per minute. When the two modes of exercise were performed simultaneously, however, the $\dot{V}O_2$ increased to 1.25 liters per minute. This hybrid exercise technique has been used to elicit $\dot{V}O_2$ levels of over 1.5 and 2.0 liters per minute for nonathletic quadriplegic and paraplegic persons, respectively. Considering that most data on maximal effort arm exercise for trained wheelchair athletes (paraplegics) have indicated peak $\dot{V}O_2$ values of slightly above 2.0 liters per minute, the hybrid exercise mode appears to be quite advantageous, since this same high $\dot{V}O_2$ level can be elicited from individuals with SCI from the general population. The combination exercise permits training at a higher $\dot{V}O_2$ level (as well as higher heart rate, stroke volume, and cardiac output), giving more effective aerobic conditioning, while providing training benefits for both the upper and lower body musculature. Because of the large muscle mass activated with this hybrid exercise, it appears likely that central circulatory factors, rather than peripheral factors, limit exercise performance capability.

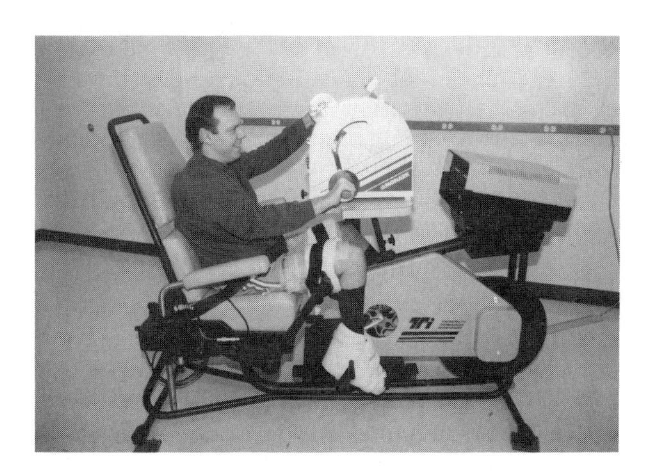

Figure 4 Hybrid (simultaneous FNS-induced cycle ergometer and voluntary arm-crank ergometer) exercise being performed by a person with SCI. The stand supporting the arm-crank ergometer was specially designed and constructed.

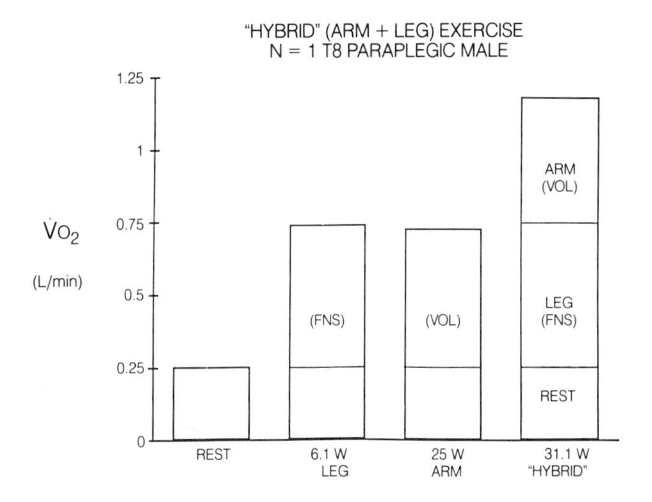

Figure 5 Oxygen uptake ($\dot{V}O_2$) of a T8 paraplegic male subject at rest, during FNS cycle ergometry at 6.1 watts, during voluntary arm-cranking at 25 watts, and during hybrid exercise at a total power output of 31.1 watts. Note the additive effect upon $\dot{V}O_2$. (From Glaser RM. Functional neuromuscular stimulation for physical fitness training of the disabled. Symposium, Osaka, 1988, in press.)

Acknowledgment. Most of the research projects described in this paper were supported by the Rehabilitation Research and Development Service of the Veterans Administration.

SUGGESTED READING

Åstrand PO, Saltin B. Maximal oxygen uptake and heart rate in various types of muscular activity. J Appl Physiol 1961; 16:977–981.

Bar-Or O, Zwiren LD. Maximal oxygen consumption test during arm exercise—reliability and validity. J Appl Physiol 1975; 38:424–426.

Clausen JP, Klausen K, Rasmussen B, Trap-Jensen J. Central and peripheral circulatory changes after training of the arms and legs. Am J Physiol 1973; 225:675–682.

Collins SR, Glaser RM. Comparison of aerobic metabolism and cardiopulmonary responses for electrically induced and voluntary exercise. Proceedings of the Eighth Annual Conference on Rehabilitation Technology, Washington, DC: RESNA, 1985:391–393.

Figoni SF, Davis GM, Glaser RM, et al. FNS-assisted venous return in exercising SCI men. Proceedings of the International Conference of the Association for the Advancement of Rehabilitation Technology, Washington, DC: RESNA, 1988:328–329.

Figoni SF, Glaser RM, Hendershot DM, et al. Hemodynamic responses of quadriplegics to maximal arm-cranking and FNS leg cycling exercise. Proceedings of the Annual International

Conference of the IEEE Engineering in Medicine and Biology Society, Piscataway, NJ: IEEE, 1988: 1636–1637.
Glaser RM. Exercise and locomotion for the spinal cord injured. In: Terjung RL, ed. Exercise and sport sciences reviews. Vol 13. New York: Macmillan, 1985:263.
Glaser RM. Physiologic aspects of spinal cord injury and functional neuromuscular stimulation. Cent Nerv Syst Trauma 1986; 3:49–61.
Glaser RM. Functional neuromuscular stimulation for physical fitness training of the disabled. Proceedings of the International Council for Physical Fitness Research: Symposium, Osaka, 1988, in press.
Glaser RM, Collins SR, Horgan HR. An electrical stimulator for exercising paralyzed muscles. Proceedings of the Tenth Annual Conference on Rehabilitation Technology, Washington, DC: RESNA, 1987:597–599.
Glaser RM, Collins SR, Strayer JR, Glaser M. A closed-loop stimulator for exercising paralyzed muscles. Proceedings of the Eighth Annual Conference on Rehabilitation Technology, Washington, DC: RESNA, 1985:388–390.
Glaser RM, Davis GM. Wheelchair-dependent individuals. In: Franklin BA, Gordon S, Timmis GC, eds. Exercise in modern medicine: testing and prescription in health and disease. Baltimore: Williams & Wilkins, 1988:237.
Glaser RM, Figoni SF, Collins SR, et al. Physiologic responses of SCI subjects to electrically induced leg cycle ergometry. Proceedings of the Annual International Conference of the IEEE Engineering in Medicine and Biology Society, Piscataway, NJ: IEEE 1988: 1638–1640.
Glaser RM, Rattan SN, Davis GM, et al. Central hemodynamic responses to lower-limb FNS. Proceedings of the IEEE Ninth Annual Conference of the Engineering in Medicine and Biology Society, Piscataway, NJ: IEEE, 1987: 615–617.
Gruner JA, Glaser RM, Feinberg SD, et al. A system for evaluation and exercise-conditioning of paralyzed leg muscles. J Rehabil Res Dev 1983; 20:21–30.
Petrofsky JS, Phillips CA. Active physical therapy: a modern approach to rehabilitation therapy. J Neurol Orthop Med Surg 1983; 4:165–173.
Petrofsky JS, Phillips CA, Heaton HH III, Glaser RM. Bicycle ergometer for paralyzed muscles. J Clin Eng 1984; 9:13–19.
Zwiren LD, Bar-Or O. Responses to exercise of paraplegics who differ in conditioning level. Med Sci Sports 1975; 7:94–98.

SPINAL DEFORMITY AND SPORTS

DAVID C. MANN, M.D.

Many spinal disorders become evident during late childhood and early adolescence, when young athletes begin to show interest in and aptitude for particular sports. Pain or deformity may threaten athletic participation and exclude special opportunities, such as a university athletic scholarship, if untreated or treated improperly.

SCOLIOSIS (ADOLESCENT IDIOPATHIC)

The prevalence of measurable scoliosis in competitive athletes has been reported to be 1.6 to 2.0 percent. The prevalence of spinal curves greater than 25 degrees is not known in athletes, but does occur (with a 10:1 female predominance) in 0.2 to 0.3 percent of the general population.

Diagnosis

After a spinal curve is detected, the patient should undergo a thorough examination to exclude nonidiopathic possibilities. A spinal curve and associated pain can result from an osseous tumor, such as an osteoid ostoma. Scoliosis and bilaterally tight hamstrings can indicate spondylolysis, and a unilaterally tight hamstring may be the only clue to a spinal cord tumor. The observed scoliosis may be a congenital curve (secondary to a failure of segmentation or formation) and is managed entirely different from an idiopathic lesion. Additionally, there can be a nonmusculoskeletal cause, such as a genitourinary or gynecologic condition.

If idiopathic scoliosis is diagnosed, the next task is to determine the patient's maturity and the size and type of spinal curve; these are important factors for estimating the probability of progression of the condition. The risk of progression is greatest during the adolescent growth spurt, corresponding with the appearance of breast development and pubic hair in girls and pubic hair in boys. About 66 percent of growth is completed in girls by the time they experience first menstruation, and in boys by the time they experience voice change and the growth of facial hair. In both sexes, radiographic evidence of absent or incomplete iliac apophyseal capping (Risser's sign) indicates skeletal immaturity; capping and fusion indicate skeletal maturity.

The patient is asked to make a forward-bend and is viewed from the back, front, and side; if a significant spinal curve is seen, the physician should obtain (on one long film) standing posteroanterior radiographs that include the thoracic and lumbar spines. The first radiograph should also include a sufficient amount of the pelvis to allow an estimate of Risser's sign. Follow-up posteroanterior radiographs should be filtered to limit the radiation of soft tissues (e.g., the breasts). The posteroanterior and lateral films should be measured, using the Cobb technique, to locate the curve(s) and apex(es).

Natural History

Published, long-term follow-up studies of untreated scoliosis give the physician some indication of the type and size of spinal curves that ultimately could be undesirable for patients. Pain, increased deformity, and disability are of particular concern here.

The incidence of back pain in untreated scoliotic adults is the same as in the general population. The percentage of severe pain, however, appears to be greater and is more a function of age. The relationship between pain and the degree of spinal curvature is less clear; some authors find no relationship, while others report more pain in those with a greater amount of curvature. Often the pain is caudal to the level of the original structural curve; apparently, it originates from the concavity of the curve and is characterized as discogenic, facet, or radicular. Pain is particularly related to lumbar and thoracolumbar curves. Untreated spinal curves of 50 to 60 degrees may be associated with back pain in patients during their fourth decade, and in their fifth decade these individuals may need surgery to control the pain if conservative management is unsuccessful. Additional factors related to pain include the presence of a translatory shift, an oblique takeoff from the sacrum, or decompensation. Curves less than 45 degrees often are not painful. Scoliosis that is treated, particularly with instrumentation in the lower lumbar region, is associated with more severe back pain 10 or more years after the operation.

Future cardiopulmonary dysfunction is often the stated justification for prophylactic fusion. In fact, only very large thoracic curves are associated with cardiopulmonary problems. Lordotic thoracic curves greater than 60 degrees are associated with decreased vital capacity. Curves greater than 80 degrees may be associated with pulmonary hypertension. Only curves greater than 100 degrees are associated with cor pulmonale, significantly lower vital capacity and forced expiratory volumes, and higher mortality rates than in the general population.

Curves greater than 30 degrees at skeletal maturity undergo some progression after maturation. The greatest average progression, 0.35 to 1.0 degrees per year, occurs in curves in the 50- to 75-degree range.

Curves that occur before skeletal maturity pose an increased risk for progression if they are sufficiently large to be discovered before or early during the growth spurt. The probability of spinal curve progression is easy to calculate. However, it is currently impossible to determine which individual patients will experience progression. Risk factors for progression include curve magnitude and pattern, Risser's sign, patient age and sex, and menarche. Double curves progress more than single curves, and lumbar or thoracolumbar curves of a double major usually progress more than thoracic curves.

Using the records of 727 patients with initial curves of 5 to 29 degrees, Lonstein developed the following expression:

$$\text{Progression factor} = \frac{\text{Cobb angle} - (3 \times \text{Risser's sign})}{\text{Chronologic age}}$$

He cautions that this relationship does not take into account the patient's sex, a female's menarchal status, or the location of the curve. Moreover, the formula should be used "to advise the family as to the chance of progression, not to help to decide whether treatment is indicated or not."

Management

Options for managing idiopathic scoliosis include observation, bracing, and surgery. The magnitude of the curve is not the sole factor in selecting an option. It must be kept in mind that during the growth spurt not all curves progress, not all curves progress after skeletal maturity, and not all large curves cause pain and disability in later adulthood. The patient and family must be made aware of risks and options, so that they may make informed decisions and be involved in all decisions about treatment from the first visit.

Nonsurgical Options

Observation should be the initial approach for any spinal curve. It is impossible to continue most competitive sports if the athlete must wear a brace. If a spinal curve is allowed to progress by 5 degrees, irreversible damage does not usually result, but if immediate bracing or surgery is used, it might.

Observation is especially indicated for any spinal curve of less than 25 degrees, regardless of the patient's age. Given that curves of less than 30 degrees do not usually progress after skeletal maturity and are not associated with an increased severity or incidence of back pain, it is reasonable to allow these curves to progress by 5 degrees before considering the use of a brace. All other factors, such as menarche and Risser's sign, should be considered before resorting to a brace. Curves of 20 to 29 degrees have a 70 percent risk of progression if accompanied by a Risser's sign of 0 or 1, but only a 25 percent risk if Risser's sign is 2 to 4. Bracing every Risser's 3 child with a 25-degree curve would be unnecessary in 75 percent of patients!

Lonstein's formula is particularly useful for determining the frequency of follow-up visits. Patients with high-risk curves should return every 2 or 3 months, but those with low-risk curves need return less often. Not every visit necessitates radiography; a clinical examination may be sufficient to monitor progression. A scoliometer is useful for measuring the amount of rotation. Radiography is indicated when the clinician suspects that or is unsure whether the rotation has increased, or when an extended period has elapsed since the last visit.

If the curve currently approaches 30 degrees and has been seen to progress by 5 degrees or more, *and* if the patient is skeletally and clinically immature, it is appropriate to consider a brace.

Nonsurgical, nonobservational options for scoliosis management should be limited to the use of a brace. Dramatic successes have been claimed for various other options. A careful review of these reports, however, generally reveals a mix of patients, many with no risk of progression when the particular treatment was initiated. Exercises, manipulation, and electrical stimulation have not affected the natural history of scoliosis in patients at risk for progression. Electrical stimulation has included both implanted and surface electrodes. Patients at the highest risk for progression have had the lowest likelihood of success with these treatments. The results were worse than observed in patients at similar risk who had been treated with a Milwaukee brace.

The purpose of a brace is to prevent progression of the curvature. A significant reduction of curvature occurs at the time of brace application. However, despite discontinuance of the brace at an appropriate time, the curve eventually collapses to its original magnitude. The brace should be a thoraco lumbosacral orthosis (TLSO) type; a Milwaukee-type brace with a neck ring is necessary only if the apex of the thoracic curve is cephalad to T7.

The most frequent questions to be asked about a brace are (1) how long must it be worn each day? and (2) when is it no longer needed? Most studies reporting success recommend wearing it for 23 hours a day. However, Green found that wearing the brace for 16 hours a day (most patients preferred not to wear it to school) produced results equal to full-time wear. Such findings have tremendous implications for adolescent athletes. A child who requires a brace can start by wearing it for 16 hours a day, and participate in sports without restriction. If the curve progresses, full-time wear should be considered.

The time to begin weaning from the brace, or ceasing to wear it, is best predicted by the same factors initially used to evaluate progression. Clinical (menarche, breast development) and radiographic (Risser's, bone age) signs of maturity serve as objective indicators, although not every patient needs to adhere to the same timetable. The use of a brace should not stop until the clinician considers the patient is at low risk for progression. The correct weaning sequence has yet to be established. It is probably safe to wean the patient rapidly from the brace once the risk of progression is low. The physician, patient, and family should not be surprised by the collapse of the curve to its original magnitude. Nighttime wear of the brace is well tolerated and is a reasonable step in the weaning process.

Currently there is interest in a nighttime brace that is molded while the patient is laterally bent in a direction opposite to the deformity. Preliminary results with this reverse brace are similar to those in earlier reports for the TLSO brace. This option should be considered experimental, however, until more patients have been followed for longer periods.

Surgical Options

Indications for surgery include a failure to control the curve to less than 50 degrees and an expected continuation of skeletal growth. All reports of any implant system describe at least a 50 percent correction of the instrumented curve; a 50-degree curve is routinely reduced to 25 degrees after the operation. If a 25-degree residual curve is acceptable (we do not start bracing until 25 degrees), and if curves of less than 50 degrees at skeletal maturity create a low risk of progression in adulthood, it is logical to use 50 degrees of curvature as one indication for surgery. Other indications include the presence of a large curve and associated thoracic lordosis. A brace should not be used when this combination occurs, because the lordosis may continue to develop and thoracic lordosis is associated with compromised pulmonary function. Surgery is also indicated if the patient has a large spinal curve and refuses to wear a brace, or if a curve becomes significantly larger while the patient is wearing a brace.

The physician should not be confused by the variety of instrumentation available and should remember that the purpose of the surgery is to create a solid fusion of the spine. Solid fusion is achieved by complete subperiosteal stripping, facetectomy, facet fusion, and sufficient bone grafting. Properly placed instrumentation is essential, and is ensured by preoperatively locating the end vertebra (both in the coronal and sagittal planes) and the stable vertebrae. Preoperative radiography is needed to determine the flexibility of structural and compensatory curves. This information is crucial to the making of decisions about the surgery.

Instrumentation to L4 and L5 should be avoided; there is a much higher incidence of severe, early postoperative back pain associated with fusion to these levels than to higher levels. If fusion to these low lumbar levels is indicated, anterior fusion and instrumentation, in addition to posterior fusion and instrumentation, should be considered to preserve mobile segments.

Before surgery, patients are encouraged to deposit their own blood, usually through the services of the local Red Cross. Average blood loss during surgery for adolescent scoliosis is about 750 ml. Three units of deposited blood and the use of the cell saver during surgery eliminate any need for donor blood in most cases.

Details that require perioperative attention include positioning of the patient, monitoring of the spinal cord, and maintenance of hypotensive anesthesia. When the patient is placed on the frame, particular attention must be given to eliminating pressure points, especially in the axilla and breast. Spinal cord monitoring allows the early detection, but not the prevention, of cord injury. Hypotensive anesthesia helps to decrease blood loss and should be maintained throughout the operation.

Instrument options include single or double Harrington rods alone, Luque rods, sublaminar or spinous process wires, and the Cotrel-Dubousset system. The latter system provides correction without distraction and allows some reduction of vertebral rotation. Currently, I use a sagittally contoured, square-end Harrington rod in the concavity, and a Luque rod on the convexity, segmentally secured with spinous process wires that have Drummond buttons. A brace is optional after the operation. The patient is unable to resume athletics for 1 year or until the fusion mass matures. General conditioning activities may start early (at 4 to 6 weeks) and progressively become more vigorous. Return to competitive sports is dependent on the patient, the level of fusion, and the type of sport.

KYPHOSIS (SCHEUERMANN'S)

Patients with kyphosis have increased roundback, pain, or both. Before reaching a diagnosis of Scheuermann's disease, the clinician should rule out other causes of roundback. Postural roundback is defined as kyphosis that is greater than 45 degrees, and that is supple without associated radiographic changes. The condition is treated by extension exercises. Congenital kyphosis secondary to anterior body fusion (failure of segmentation) may appear as a fixed kyphosis. Kyphosis may also be secondary to infection.

True Scheuermann's disease involves a rigid, hyperkyphosis and associated changes in vertebral structure. During adolescence, thoracic Scheuermann's disease may or may not be painful, whereas thoracolumbar Scheuermann's disease frequently is painful. On standing the patient exhibits kyphosis and an associated increase in lumbar lordosis or an anterior protrusion of the head relative to the trunk. The forward-bent patient, viewed from the side, usually shows a sharp bend at the apex of the spine. Posteroanterior and lateral radiographs of the standing patient should be obtained, plus a supine radiograph with a wedge or bolster at the apex of the spine, in order to determine the magnitude of the curve and associated scoliosis and rigidity. Radiographs reveal wedged vertebrae, irregular end plates, and often thinned disc spaces.

Indications for treatment include the elimination of pain and the prevention of further deformity. Pain at the level of the deformity or in the compensatory lumbar lordosis may occur in older adults, but it is rarely disabling for adolescents. The severity of pain does not seem to be related to the extent of curvature. Painful thoracic disease often is resolved with or without treatment, whereas thoracolumbar disease necessitates more aggressive conservative management. For athletes, pain may be managed with a short period of rest, anti-inflammatory medications, and possibly the use of a brace when the patient is not engaged in athletic activities. Thoracic disease cephalad to T7 necessitates use of a Milwaukee brace, whereas thoracolumbar Scheuermann's disease can be managed with a TLSO.

Cosmetic factors remain the primary indication for the extended management of Scheuermann's kyphosis; treatment is therefore primarily a decision to be made by the patient and family. Pulmonary compromise is not associated with kyphosis, and neurologic compromise secondary to kyphosis is rare unless the condition is severe and progressing rapidly. Brace treatment dramatically reduces kyphosis, but long-term follow-up studies reveal that most curves collapse to their prebrace level of deformity during the decade after the brace has been removed. For these reasons, it is reasonable to use short-term conservative treatment for athletes with painful Scheuermann's disease. Such an approach allows them to remain competitive during adolescence and young adulthood. If, after their skeleton has matured, patients have a personally objectionable kyphosis, they may want to undergo surgical reduction and fusion. If a clinically and skeletally immature athlete does not want to risk a progression of the deformity, but does want to avoid later surgery, a brace should be used. The part-time use of a brace (16 hours a day) for Scheuermann's disease has been reported and appears as effective as full-time use. The current bracing regimen involves the full- or part-time use of a brace for 1 year, followed by 1 year of weaning and 1 year of nighttime use only. The weaning and nighttime-only periods may be modified, depending on clinical and radiographic evidence of maturity. It may be possible to eliminate progression with other regimens, but to date there have been no reports to this effect.

Surgery is rarely indicated for adolescents. The potential need for anterior fusion, possible postoperative loss of correction, and instrumentation failure should temper one's enthusiasm for surgery. If the fixed deformity is greater than 50 degrees, anterior disc excision and fusion, in addition to posterior instrumentation and fusion, is necessary. Postoperatively, the fusion does not progress, but Bradford and colleagues noted that five of 24 patients who were fused both anteriorly and posteriorly later developed a significant loss of correction caudal to the fusion.

To treat a patient best, the physician needs to understand the natural history of the disorder. Unfortunately, much of our knowledge of the natural history of disease is derived from a relatively small number of cases, and many of our recommendations are based on the premise that the most disabling course is the one most likely to occur. In reality, sequelae are less than 100 percent certain. When this uncertainty is made known to patients and their families, they are better able to make decisions. A patient may decide to "play against the odds" and make an apparently wrong decision. This choice may be unsettling to the physician, but it is the very trait we admire in a competitive athlete.

SUGGESTED READING

Ascani E, Bartolozzi P, Logroscino CA, et al. Natural history of untreated idiopathic scoliosis after skeletal maturity. Spine 1986; 11:784–789.

Bradford DS, Khalid BA, Moe JH, et al. The surgical management of patients with Scheuermann's disease. J Bone Joint Surg 1980; 62A:705–712.

Bjerkreim E, Hassan I. Progression in untreated idiopathic scoliosis after end of growth. Acta Orthop Scand 1982; 53:897–900.

Bjure J, Nachemson A. Non-treated scoliosis. Clin Orthop 1973; 93:44–52.

Carman D, Roach JW, Speck G, et al. Role of exercises in the Milwaukee brace treatment of scoliosis. J Pediatr Orthop 1985; 5:65–68.

Carr WA, Moe JH, Winter RB, et al. Treatment of idiopathic scoliosis in the Milwaukee brace. Long-term results. J Bone Joint Surg 1980; 62A:599–612.

Goldberg C, Dowling FE, Fogarty EE, et al. Electro-spinal stimulation in children with adolescent and juvenile scoliosis. Spine 1988; 13:482–484.

Green NE. Part-time bracing of adolescent idiopathic scoliosis. J Bone Joint Surg 1986; 68A:738–742.

Gutowski WT, Renshaw TS. Orthotic results in adolescent kyphosis. Spine 1988; 13:485–489.

Jackson RP, Simmons EH, Stripinis D. Incidence and severity of back pain in adult idiopathic scoliosis. Spine 1983; 8:749–756.

King HA, Moe JH, Bradford DS, Winter RG. The selection of fusion levels in thoracic idiopathic scoliosis. J Bone Joint Surg 1983; 65A:1302–1312.

Kostuik JP, Bentivoglio J. The incidence of low back pain in adult scoliosis. Spine 1981; 6:268–273.

Krahl H, Steinbruck K. Sportsachaden und Sportverletzungen an der Wirbelsaule. Dtsch Arztebl 1978; 19.

Kuprian W. Physical therapy for sports. Philadelphia: WB Saunders, 1982.

Lonstein JE. Risk of progression of idiopathic scoliosis in skeletally immature patients. Spine: State of the Art Reviews 1987; 1:181–193.

Lonstein JE, Carlson JM. The prediction of curve progression in untreated idiopathic scoliosis during growth. J Bone Joint Surg 1984; 66A:1061–1071.

Montgomery F, Willner S. The natural history of idiopathic scoliosis. Spine 1988; 13:401–404.

Nachemson A. Adult scoliosis and back pain. Spine 1979; 4:512–517.

O'Donnell CS, Bunnell WP, Betz RR, et al. Electrical stimulation in the treatment of idiopathic scoliosis. Presented at the Scoliosis Research Society Meeting, Vancouver, BC, 1987.

Simmons EH, Jackson RP. The management of nerve root entrapment syndromes associated with the collapsing scoliosis of idiopathic lumbar and thoracolumbar curves. Spine 1979; 4:533–541.

Weinstein SL. The natural history of scoliosis in the skeletally mature patient. Spine: State of the Art Reviews 1987; 1:195–211.

Weinstein SL, Ponsetti IV. Curve progression in idiopathic scoliosis. J Bone Joint Surg 1983; 65A:447–455.

HYPNOSIS

DAVID R. BROWN, Ph.D.

> From hypnosis I have learnt that so great can be the power of suggestion that indeed, I now use simple suggestions extensively as a therapeutic weapon in my general practice.
>
> David Ryde

The purpose of this chapter is *not* to provide the reader with a thorough review of the literature in which hypnosis has been used in research or clinical practice in sports medicine. Indeed, if such a review were written, it would of necessity be brief, as "reference to the use of hypnosis, either as a research tool or clinical application, is almost completely absent in the sports medicine literature" (Morgan, 1980). This is surprising, since hypnosis has been used extensively as a research and clinical tool in several medical subspecialties, in subdisciplines within psychology (e.g., clinical and counseling), and in dentistry. Several members of these professions have affiliated with professional organizations representing sports medicine (e.g., the American College of Sports Medicine) and/or hypnosis (e.g., the American Society of Clinical Hypnosis [ASCH] and the Society for Clinical and Experimental Hypnosis [SCEH]). Of course, interest in and affiliation with one field, such as sports medicine, does not imply interest in or affiliation with the other field of hypnosis, or vice versa. Nevertheless, it seems unusual that empirical or clinical reports regarding the use of hypnosis in sports medicine are so sparse. This chapter explores possible reasons why hypnosis has not been used more extensively in sports medicine, challenges the barriers that have impeded the use of hypnosis in sports medicine, and (it is hoped) will encourage professionals in sports medicine to use hypnosis in research or clinical practice.

POSSIBLE REASONS WHY HYPNOSIS HAS NOT BEEN USED IN SPORTS MEDICINE

There are several possible reasons why workers in sports medicine have been reluctant to employ hypnosis in research or clinical practice. These may include (1) a misunderstanding of what hypnosis is, (2) a lack of training or experience in using hypnosis, (3) a belief that hypnosis requires a hypnotist to "control" an athlete, (4) a view that athletes are not good hypnotic subjects, or (5) the feeling that hypnosis provides an athlete with an unfair, unnatural advantage over a competitor, and therefore should be banned as an illegal or unethical ergogenic aid. These potential barriers to the use of hypnosis in sports medicine will be examined in greater detail, in an effort to separate fact from fallacy.

What Is Hypnosis?

The domain of hypnosis has been described by Hilgard (1987) as including posthypnotic amnesia, hallucinations, analgesia, and dissociation. In other words, forgetting, vivid perceptual images, reduction in pain, and focusing concentration on the dimensions of a relevant stimulus as opposed to many stimuli can all be promoted through suggestion during hypnosis. Ryde defined hypnosis as "a state of suggested relaxation in which the subject becomes amenable to the suggestions of the hypnotist." However, some hypnosis theorists do not view hypnosis as a unique domain or "state" position. Barber (1966), for example, reviewed research comparing the effects of hypnosis per se and motivational suggestions per se on muscular performance, and concluded that hypnosis that did not include suggestions for improved performance did not enhance muscular strength or endurance. In addition, Barber noted that motivational suggestions of improved muscular performance provided to individuals in the hypnotic state *and* motivated waking state were equally effective in enhancing performance. These findings indicate that *suggestions* of improved performance, rather than hypnosis, are what led to the increases in muscle strength and endurance observed by Barber.

Whether hypnosis is viewed as a "state" or "nonstate," a heightened susceptibility to suggestion is a part of the domain of hypnosis, and some individuals have more hypnotic talent than others. For persons exceptionally high on hypnotic talent, posthypnotic amnesia, hallucinations, and analgesia seem to be within the realm of the hypnotic experience. For individuals with less hypnotic talent, the hypnotic experience may be more appropriately defined as dissociation, rather than as a hypnotic state or trance. A distinction has been made between hypnotic talent or hypnotizability, and being hypnotized. Hypnotizability has been conceptualized as a *trait* characteristic, reflecting stable individual differences. Some individuals are high on hypnotizability while others are low, and the *state* experience to hypnotic instructions during hypnosis theoretically differs between those who are readily hypnotizable and those who are not.

The trait-state issue is important, but the hypnotic experience potentially contains several elements that should be attractive to workers in sports medicine. The induction procedure can be relaxing or alerting, suggestions and images can be heightened, and concentration on relevant stimuli can be promoted when necessary. Equally important for workers in sports medicine is the fact that some of the more successful uses of hypnosis have been in the areas of anxiety and pain reduction. Hypnosis has also been employed successfully to treat asthma, migraine, and burns. There is also some evidence that hypnosis may be effective in treating skin diseases and nausea and vomiting, and in improving recovery from surgery. More than two decades ago Ryde discussed the medical treatment of 35 cases of injury, several of which were sustained as a result of athletic competition. Hypnosis was successfully employed to treat "tennis elbow, shin soreness, chronic Achilles tendon sprain, bruised heels, arch sprains and other common ailments of uncertain minor pathology." Ryde states: "To the question 'Is hypnosis ethical in sport?' I reply . . . There is no clear margin between suggestion and hypnosis and if a pep talk is ethical to an athlete in training or under stress, likewise hypnosis is ethical. But I repeat it should be used only by a responsible person."

What Professional Training Is Required to Use Hypnosis?

Since hypnosis is normally used as an adjunct to other medical or psychological interventions, a primary requisite for the use of hypnosis is professional training in a helping profession such as medicine, psychology, or dentistry. In addition, training in hypnosis can be obtained through reading the hypnosis literature, taking formal university course work in hypnosis, or attending workshops such as those offered by ASCH or SCEH. Such workshops are normally approved for continuing education credit hours in medicine and psychology.

In terms of using hypnosis, Hilgard (April, 1979) pointed out that "lack of advanced degrees does not necessarily mean incompetence, and society memberships do not guarantee competence either." However, the well-trained professional "will know much more what is relevant about personality and individual differences than is implied by hypnosis," or than occurs as a result of training only in hypnosis. Morgan and Brown proposed that "hypnosis does not qualify a hypnotist to perform activities that he or she is not competent to perform without hypnosis."

Very little training is required to equip professionals with the ability to *induce* hypnosis in a willing, suggestible subject. In fact, it is not uncommon for people to teach themselves self-hypnotic techniques, avoiding the hetero-hypnosis relationship completely. *Training* in the use of hypnosis is required, however, in order to know when to employ hypnosis, with whom, and under what circumstances. This knowledge, as well as clinical intuition, becomes the "art" of hypnosis.

Training is needed because not all individuals are equally hypnotizable or susceptible to suggestions, and of those who are hypnotizable, some may need the proper structure and guidance offered by a supportive, well-trained professional during a hetero-hypnotic session. The unstructured freedom associated with self-hypnosis or an improperly structured experience during hetero-hypnosis can result in adverse consequences for an athlete. Hypnosis may have either positive or negative outcomes. For example, laboratory efforts to decrease muscular performance through hypnotic suggestion are almost always successful.

It seems much more difficult to increase the performance of well-trained athletes than that of untrained individuals. In addition, the use of a "relaxing" hypnotic induction procedure as opposed to an "alerting" induction procedure can theoretically affect an athlete's performance differently. For example, Sheehan and Perry noted that there is "the possibility that suggestions to be sleepy, drowsy, or relaxed may be antagonistic to suggestions of enhanced performance." Evans and Orne reported that the performance of subjects in a hypnosis experiment was adversely affected by suggestions of drowsiness and relaxation used during induction. This is interesting in light of the current Zeitgeist in sport psychology to relax entire athletic teams. The tasks employed in the Evans and Orne investigation (grip strength, weight-holding endurance, hand tremor, and rote learning) do not relate directly to athletic performance, but this study suggests that relaxation may have a negative effect on performance in some individuals. Whether such adverse effects generalize to athletic performance needs to be investigated.

Finally, the suggestions given an athlete during hypnosis may require involvement or relative uninvolvement in tasks that theoretically might influence performance. Morgan and Brown stated that "hypnotic suggestions of enhanced physical ability are effective if subjects scoring high on hypnotizability and low on physical performance are administered 'involving' instructions following an 'alerting' induction." Training in hypnosis is required if the nuances between hypnotist, subject, and setting are to be understood, and if hypnosis is to generate positive rather than negative outcomes.

With some effort, sports medicine professionals can avail themselves of training opportunities in hypnosis. Contacting ASCH* or SCEH† for information on training is an initial step.

Does the Hypnotist Control the Athlete?

The impression that a hypnotist controls the behavior of the person being hypnotized remains, perhaps, the biggest fallacy surrounding hypnosis. This inaccurate perception has been fueled by visions of theatrical stage hypnotists, who seemingly control behavior against the will of some member of the audience. In reality, the audience member is a "willing" participant, the demand characteristics of the situation are high, and the feats performed under hypnosis can also be performed in the motivated waking state. Traditional induction procedures used by clinicians have also at times seemed to border on the mysterious. This is changing, however. In an article entitled "The State of the Art of Clinical Hypnosis," Baker says, "Authoritarian and mystical inductions popular 50 years ago have fallen from vogue. In most instances, clinicians have increasingly come to employ permissive induction strategies that emphasize the patient's or subject's own capacities to alter consciousness and produce trance."

Whereas the hetero-hypnotic relationship has, in the past, tended to focus primarily on direct suggestions given by the hypnotist, and on the response to suggestions provided by the patient or subject, contemporary hypnosis places a greater reliance on self-hypnotic techniques, and also on "adaptation, problem solving, enhanced coping capacities, and mastery" (Baker) of skills on the part of a hypnotic subject. In addition, hypnosis has been used to support "self-actualization in a variety of arenas" including sports medicine. Indeed, Baker indicates that the use of hypnosis to maximize potential and improve creativity has only recently begun to be explored. An increasing use of hypnosis to promote psychological or physical self-improvement, to discover untapped potential, and to assist in optimizing performance should increase both interest in and use of hypnosis in sports medicine.

Are Athletes Good or Poor Hypnotic Subjects?

Hilgard (1979) reported that many athletes are unsusceptible and generally are not good hypnotic subjects. By nature of their athleticism, athletes are activity oriented, whereas the hypnosis process often stresses quiescence or a relaxed state. Athletes

---

* The American Society of Clinical Hypnosis, 2250 East Devon Avenue, Suite 336, Des Plaines, IL 60018. Phone (312) 297-3317.

† The Society for Clinical and Experimental Hypnosis, Inc., 128-A Kings Park Drive, Liverpool, NY 13090. Phone (315) 652-7299.

have also been conditioned to be sensitive to information obtained from the environment, to be actively involved in decision making, and to be in control of a situation. Traditionally, these behaviors would be counterproductive in relation to entering hypnosis. Whether this remains true in light of Baker's contention that there has been a shift in hypnosis from direct suggestion and behavioral manipulation to self-actualization, self-enhancement, and the inner experiences of a subject undergoing hypnosis remains to be seen. Perhaps athletes will perceive such a shift in hypnosis as less threatening and less controlling, and ultimately they will be more receptive to the hypnotic experience. More likely, there will remain a wide variability in the degree to which athletes are susceptible and hypnotizable. Hilgard (1979), for example, found that athletes who have a wide variety of experiences and interests other than athletics are more receptive, or may have more pathways leading to hypnosis than athletes who focus primarily on athletic competition. Also, athletes competing in sports emphasizing personal enjoyment or "individual" performances (e.g., skiing, swimming, tennis, and track events) seem to be significantly more hypnotizable than athletes competing in "team" sports (e.g., basketball, hockey, and volleyball).

Should Hypnosis Be Banned as Dangerous or as an Ergogenic Aid?

In 1976 Rosen stated that "athletes frequently apply for hypnosis to increase physical performance . . . This is inadvisable and can be dangerous." Rosen did not elaborate on why it is inadvisable to use hypnosis to improve performance, nor was any empirical evidence provided to substantiate the claim that doing so can be dangerous.

Certainly, hypnosis has a potential for negative as well as positive outcomes. However, when properly used, hypnosis has had many positive effects. In addition, arguing against the use of hypnosis with athletes implies also that suggestions, encouragement, and pep talks are dangerous or unethical interventions to employ with this population. Taken to the extreme, Rosen's recommendation would preclude the use of relaxation, visual imagery, concentration, attention, and cognitive strategies such as association and dissociation by athletes. In other words, the profile of the athlete would be one without a head.

It also makes little sense to be opposed to hypnosis on the basis of its effectiveness as an "unnatural" ergogenic aid. First, hypnosis may be used to tap the "natural" potential of the athlete and promote self-enhancement. Second, hypnosis does not appear to be consistently effective as an ergogenic aid. Earlier reviews in which hypnosis was used to enhance muscle strength or endurance led to equivocal findings, summarized by Morgan (1980) and Morgan and Brown: "Some studies have shown that hypnosis *per se* has no influence on muscular performance, whereas other studies have found performance increments or decrements. The literature is clearly equivocal regarding this area." The effects of hypnosis on hallucinated exercise, motor learning and performance, and clinical application in sport have been briefly described. There is reason to be optimistic regarding the use of hypnosis in exercise, sports sciences, and sports medicine. However, so little is known about the hypnotic experience in relationship to sports medicine that research and application possibilities seem limitless.

Application must be approached carefully, however. There have been case studies and reports in the lay press suggesting that hypnosis has enhanced athletic performance, but such reports have lacked the scientific controls necessary to attribute improvements in performance to hypnosis. Unlike their counterparts who treat patients, hypnotists who have used hypnosis to increase athletic performance have not been held accountable by the public or scientific community to document the efficacy of hypnosis as an intervention. The hypnotic experience has been obfuscated by such factors as suggestion, relaxation, and visual imagery, and the reasons for clinical improvement cannot be identified. In fact, the use of similar strategies in the waking state may be equally efficacious, and this has been documented in the case of suggestion. Other problems may be encountered when researchers evaluate the effects of hypnosis on performance, because issues related to subject, task, and research design interaction can confound the results obtained from such investigations. It is recommended that individuals using hypnosis to improve athletic performance be held to the same standards of accountability as medical doctors, dentists, and clinical psychologists who are treating patients for health rather than strictly performance-related problems. In short, it is critical that scientists and clinicians work together to advance the stature and credibility of hypnosis within the field of sports medicine.

HYPNOSIS AS AN EXPERIMENTAL AND CLINICAL TOOL IN SPORTS MEDICINE

The third purpose of this chapter is to generate interest in using hypnosis as a research or clinical tool within the sports medicine community. It is suggested that hypnosis by its very nature complements the nature of sports medicine. First, hypnosis is a psychophysiologic phenomenon. Second, the field of sports medicine is concerned with the maintenance or improvement of an athlete's physical or psychological health, and the prevention or reduction of an athlete's physical or psychological health problems, so that athletic performance can be maintained or enhanced. Thus, both somatic and psychic therapies should be appropriate options for use by sports medicine personnel in some circumstances. While individual disciplines within the field of sports medicine may not traditionally approach the athlete as a mind-body interactive entity, the field of sports medicine as a whole implicitly embraces a holistic concept of the athlete, thereby contributing to the multidisciplinary nature of sports medicine.

Hypnosis, when properly employed, has the potential to impact positively on clinical problems of either a psychological or a physical nature, and to provide insight into many questions of sports medicine research. In the future, hypnosis should be used more frequently in sports medicine, to generate greater knowledge and to elucidate the potential benefits derived from clinical use of hypnosis with athletes. It is hoped that the clinicians who are currently using hypnosis with athletes will embark upon more intensive efforts to document whether any claims of improved performance are really due to hypnosis, rather than to some artifact of the hypnotic experience, or to a hetero-hypnosis relationship. Only then will the efficacy of the "science" and "art" of hypnosis in sports medicine become known.

SUGGESTED READING

Baker EL. The state of the art of clinical hypnosis. Int J Clin Exp Hypn 1987; 35:203–204.

Barber TX. The effects of hypnosis and suggestions on strength and endurance: a critical review of research studies. Br J Soc Clin Psychol 1966; 5:42–50.

Barber TX. Hypnosis: a scientific approach. New York: Van Nostrand Reinhold, 1969.

Evans FJ, Orne MT. Motivation, performance, and hypnosis. Int J Clin Exp Hypn 1965; 13:103–116.

Frankel FH. Significant developments in medical hypnosis during the past 25 years. Int J Clin Exp Hypn 1987; 35:231–247.

Fromm E. Significant developments in clinical hypnosis during the past 25 years. Int J Clin Exp Hypn 1987; 37:215–230.

Gorton BE. Physiologic aspects of hypnosis. In: Schneck JM, ed. Hypnosis in modern medicine. Springfield, IL: Charles C Thomas, 1959.

Hilgard ER. More about forensic hypnosis. Am Psychol Assoc Division 30 Newsletter, April, 1979.

Hilgard ER. Research advances in hypnosis: issues and methods. Int J Clin Exp Hypn 1987; 35:248–263.

Hilgard ER, Hilgard JR. Hypnosis in the relief of pain. 2nd ed. Los Altos, CA: William Kaufmann, 1983.

Hilgard JR. Personality and hypnosis: a study of imaginative involvement. 2nd ed. Chicago: University of Chicago Press, 1979.

Hull CL. Hypnosis and suggestibility: an experimental approach. New York: Appleton-Century-Crofts, 1933.

Johnson WR. Hypnosis and muscular performance. J Sports Med Phys Fitness 1961; 1:71–79.

Morgan WP. Hypnosis and muscular performance. In: Morgan WP, ed. Ergogenic aids and muscular performance. New York: Academic Press, 1972.

Morgan WP. Hypnosis and sports medicine. In: Burrows G, Dennerstein LD, eds. Handbook of hypnosis and psychosomatic medicine. Amsterdam: Elsevier Biomedical Press, 1980.

Morgan WP, Brown DR. Hypnosis. In: Williams MH, ed. Ergogenic aids in sport. Champaign, IL: Human Kinetics, 1983.

Orne MT. On the social psychology of the psychological experiment: with particular reference to demand characteristics and their implications. Am Psychol 1962; 17:776–783.

Rosen H. Hypnosis and drug abuse in sports. In: Craig TT, ed. The humanistic and mental health aspects of sports, exercise and research. Chicago: American Medical Association, 1976.

Ryan AJ, Allman FL Jr, eds. Sports medicine. New York: Academic Press, 1974.

Ryde D. A personal study of some uses of hypnosis in sport and sports injuries. J Sports Med Phys Fitness 1964; 4:241–246.

Sarbin TR, Coe WC. Hypnosis: a social psychological analysis of influence communication. New York: Holt, Rinehart, & Winston, 1972.

Sheehan PW, Perry CW. Methodologies of hypnosis: a critical appraisal of contemporary paradigms of hypnosis. Chap 7. Hillsdale, NJ: Lawrence Erlbaum Associates, 1976: 225.

Spanos NP. Hypnotic behavior: a social psychological interpretation of amnesia, analgesia, and "trance logic." Behav Brain Sci 1986; 9:449–502.

Weitzenhoffer AM. Hypnotism: an objective study in suggestibility. New York: John Wiley, 1963.

ATHLETIC INJURIES AND THE USE OF MEDICATION

NETA A. HODGE, PHARM D

ANALGESIA IN SPORTS-RELATED INJURIES

Sports injuries vary widely from mild to severe, but a common ingredient of most is pain. Pain acts as an integral component of the body's defense system to alert an athlete that an injury or trauma has occurred so that the affected area can be protected from further injury. Regardless of the type of injury causing it, pain can be classified as mild, moderate, or severe; it is a universal symptom, but a highly personal experience.

Several classes of analgesic drugs are available to treat pain. The choice of agent depends on the severity of the pain and the individual patient variables, such as drug allergies or concomitant disease states. The spectrum of analgesics ranges from nonprescription drugs to opiates; proper characterization of the pain by means of patient interview can guide the clinician in the choice of appropriate analgesic therapy.

Cryotherapy

Immediately after an acute sports injury, the affected area should be immobilized and elevated, and ice should be applied. Ice may be applied in many forms (e.g., an ice bath, ice massage, or an ice pack), but speed is important. Ski patrols commonly use snow in a plastic bag, applied before the injured skier is transported from the slopes. When ice is applied to the traumatized area and tissue cooling occurs, several physiologic responses ensue locally: vasoconstriction, decreased inflammation, edema, and blood leakage. Impulses via cooled nerve fibers are slowed and pain is decreased. Local tissue metabolism is slowed, so that oxygen needs and histamine release are decreased. Monosynaptic stretch reflexes are suppressed and muscle spasm is retarded.

Ice should be applied to the affected area for 20 to 30 minutes several times a day. Although a feeling of cold and aching or burning may occur for the first 1 to 7 minutes after the application of ice, a local anesthetic action may be expected within 5 to 12 minutes. Some studies have demonstrated a reflex vasodilation after the local anesthetic effect occurs, but others have not corroborated this and it remains an area of controversy. Hocutt and colleagues demonstrated that immobilization, compression by taping, elevation, and ice (e.g., cryotherapy), when administered within 36 hours of the occurrence of grades 3 or 4 ankle sprains, were more effective than either cryotherapy initiated more than 36 hours after the injury, or of heat therapy begun within 36 hours of the injury. Patients receiving cryotherapy within 36 hours after the injury regained full activity in 13.2 days, whereas those who received heat therapy required 33.3 days. When cryotherapy was instituted after 36 hours, patients required 30.4 days to regain full activity.

There are dangers associated with the use of ice. Local frostbite should be avoided by limiting direct application of ice to the skin to periods of less than 30 minutes. Also, ice should not be used for any patient who has cold allergy, rheumatoid arthritis, peripheral vascular disease, or other vasoactive disorders such as Raynaud's phenomenon.

Nonopiate Analgesics

Although cryotherapy is commonly the initial therapy for most acute sports injuries, additional pharmacologic analgesia may be necessary. Several nonprescription analgesics are available to treat mild to moderate pain, including acetaminophen, the salicylates, and ibuprofen.

Acetaminophen

On a milligram-to-milligram basis, acetaminophen is equal to aspirin as an analgesic and antipyretic. The mechanism of action of acetaminophen is unknown. It is a very weak anti-inflammatory agent, and because of this is considered a weaker choice than aspirin for treating the post-traumatic pain and inflammation of sports injuries. It is not toxic to the gastrointestinal (GI) tract and does not affect platelet aggregation, so that it may have increased merit in patients with a history of peptic ulcer disease or in those with platelet disorders, closed head injuries, or hematomas incurred as a result of injury. The maximal recommended nonprescription adult daily dose of acetaminophen is 4 g in divided doses. An increase of individual dosages of aspirin or acetaminophen from 650 to 1,000 mg per dose does not increase the analgesic effect of these drugs; a ceiling analgesic effect occurs at 650 mg. Intentional or inadvertent overdosage of acetaminophen can be potentially lethal, if the antidote (*N*-acetylcysteine) is not administered in time and hepatic necrosis results. Hepatotoxic effects are more likely to develop in actively drinking alcoholic patients after an overdose than in patients who are not drinking at the time of the overdose. Children under the age of 10 to 12 years are generally the least likely to develop hepatotoxicity after an overdose.

Aspirin

Although several salicylate products are available, aspirin is discussed here as the prototype salicylate. Aspirin is an analgesic, antipyretic, and anti-inflammatory agent. Its mechanism of action, while not completely understood, is thought to be due to the blockade of the enzyme cyclo-oxygenase, which oxygenates arachidonic acid to produce prostaglandins. Prostaglandins are produced on a homeostatic basis in most cells of the body, and are necessary for the normal physiologic functioning of most major organs. When trauma occurs, as in acute sports injuries, prostaglandin production increases on demand at the site of injury and is thought to help mediate inflammation. Aspirin and the nonsteroidal anti-inflammatory drugs help to decrease edema, pain, and other signs of inflammation by blocking prostaglandin production. Low-dose aspirin (less than 3 g per day) is analgesic, but higher doses are anti-inflammatory. Great individual variation can occur in patients' responses to aspirin because elimination is nonlinear and accumulation of blood salicylate levels can occur. Because of this, it is difficult to specify a daily dose of aspirin for everyone; generally, anti-inflammatory doses are considered to range from 3 to 8 g per day in divided doses. Aspirin is available readily without a prescription, so many patients may be resistant to taking it and may ask for a "real" pain killer. Aspirin combined with cryotherapy provides excellent analgesia for mild to moderate pain with inflammation, as may occur with mild sprains or strains; patients should be told of its anti-inflammatory capabilities.

The side effect profile of aspirin can be extensive, and side effects or certain individual patient variables may preclude its use. GI effects such as gastritis, ulceration, or hemorrhage can occur, especially at high dosages, and aspirin should be avoided in patients with a history of peptic ulcer disease or GI tract hemorrhage. Aspirin, by blocking cyclooxygenase, inhibits platelet aggregation irreversibly for the life of the platelet. This effect may be of little consequence in most healthy athletes, but those with platelet disorders or bleeding diatheses should not use it. The antiplatelet effect of aspirin may be particularly dangerous in athletes who may have sustained an intra-articular hemorrhage or muscular hematoma, or a closed head injury. The use of aspirin after these types of injuries is contraindicated because of the danger of further bleeding.

Allergy to aspirin, termed "aspirin intolerance," may appear within hours of ingestion of the drug, and may take one of two forms: bronchospasm or urticaria-angioedema. Aspirin intolerance, not to be confused with GI upset due to aspirin, is more likely to occur in patients with a history of chronic urticaria, asthma, or chronic rhinitis. It may have a familial pattern, and many aspirin-intolerant patients are also allergic to tartrazine dye. Antibodies against aspirin have not been demonstrated, but prostaglandin inhibition has been implicated in the mechanism of the bronchospastic form of aspirin intolerance.

The use of aspirin, and of related drugs such as the nonsteroidal anti-inflammatory drugs, is strictly contraindicated in patients with a history of aspirin intolerance. It is exceedingly important to question patients about this before prescribing these drugs, because aspirin intolerance can be life-threatening.

Aspirin intoxication can occur during short courses of aspirin and at doses considered to be "therapeutic." Because of the nonlinear elimination of aspirin, small increases in dosage may result in disproportionate rises in serum salicylate levels. Therapeutic salicylate levels are considered to range from 20 to 30 mg per deciliter, but some patients may exhibit symptoms of intoxication, such as tinnitus or nausea at dosage and blood levels considered to be therapeutic. Individualization of dosage by the proper use of serum salicylate levels may alleviate these problems and allow anti-inflammatory therapy to continue. When given chronically, in anti-inflammatory doses, aspirin every 8 or 12 hours is sufficient to maintain therapeutic salicylate levels.

Acetaminophen or Aspirin in Combination With Opiate Drugs

A combination of aspirin or acetaminophen with opiate analgesics causes an additive increase in the amount of analgesia available with each dose. Depending on the opiate used, a combination of these drugs extends the spectrum of pain treatment to that of moderate to severe pain. The increase in analgesia may be offset, however, by the side effects of the opiates. Such combinations are indicated for the management of pain on a short-term basis only, because of the potential of drug dependency with long-term use.

Nonsteroidal Anti-inflammatory Drugs

The nonsteroidal anti-inflammatory drugs are as effective antipyretic and anti-inflammatory agents as aspirin. Several of these drugs have been shown to be more effective analgesics than aspirin alone, acetaminophen alone, or either aspirin or acetaminophen in combination with codeine in several pain models. Some nonsteroidal anti-inflammatory drugs have been shown to be equally effective as oral and injectable opiates for dental, postoperative, post-episiotomy, and cancer pain. Only some of the nonsteroidal anti-inflammatory drugs currently available in the United States are approved by the FDA to treat pain. Table 1 lists these agents and their recommended doses. Although many health care professionals believe that the nonsteroidal anti-inflammatory drugs are weak analgesics, these agents have been shown to control moderate to severe pain in many situations. They have the advantage over acetaminophen in that they are anti-inflammatory,

TABLE 1 FDA-Approved Nonsteroidal Anti-inflammatory Drugs for the Treatment of Pain

Generic Name	*Trade Name*	*Starting Adult Dose*	*Maximal Recommended Dose**
Ibuprofen	Motrin, Rufen	400 mg q 4–6 hr	2,400 mg
Nonprescription ibuprofen	Nuprin, Advil	200 mg q 4–6 hr	1,200 mg
Naproxen	Naprosyn	500 mg initially; 250 mg q 6–8 hr	1,250 mg
Naproxen sodium	Anaprox	550 mg initially; 275 mg q 6–8 hr	1,375 mg
Diflunisal	Dolobid	1,000 mg initially; 500 mg q 8–12 hr	1,500 mg
Fenoprofen calcium	Nalfon	200 mg q 4–6 hr	3,200 mg
Mefenamic acid	Ponstel	500 mg initially; 250 mg q 6 hr	250 mg q 6 hr
Ketoprofen	Orudis	25–50 mg q 6–8 hr	200 mg
Meclofenamate sodium	Meclomen	50–100 mg q 4–6 hr	400 mg

*Maximal analgesic dose per day.

over aspirin in that they are stronger analgesics, and over the opiates because they do not cause physical dependence in chronic dosages.

Although their exact mechanism of action is unknown, the nonsteroidal anti-inflammatory drugs, like aspirin, are believed to work by means of inhibition of prostaglandin production, thereby blocking the attendant effects of prostaglandins on inflammation. The use of nonsteroidal anti-inflammatory drugs in treating sports-related injuries is increasing, although studies of the use of these drugs in acute sports-related injuries have reported varying results and have been plagued with flaws in study design: very few studies have been double-blind or placebo controlled, and some drugs have been studied at suboptimal dosages. Despite this, the nonsteroidal anti-inflammatory drugs are a rational choice for analgesic and anti-inflammatory effects in acute and chronic sports-related injuries and have been reported to permit a faster recovery. However, these drugs have side effects that must be borne in mind during selection of patients for this therapy. The nonsteroidal anti-inflammatory drugs can cause GI toxicity (ulceration and/or hemorrhage), and although this occurs less frequently than with aspirin, the use of these drugs in patients with a history of peptic ulcer disease or GI bleeding is contraindicated. Platelet aggregation can be affected by nonsteroidal anti-inflammatory drugs, but this effect is reversible upon their discontinuation. Nevertheless, extreme caution should be exercised in using these drugs in patients with pre-existent platelet disorders, bleeding diatheses, or hematomas or closed head injuries. Patients with aspirin intolerance may have a more than 90 percent probability of cross-reactions when given nonsteroidal anti-inflammatory drugs; this constitutes a strict contraindication to their use in this patient group. All nonsteroidal anti-inflammatory drugs are more expensive than aspirin, and this may limit their use in some patients. It has been shown that nonsteroidal anti-inflammatory agents are more economical to use in hospitalized patients with moderate pain than the aspirin or acetaminophen combinations with opiates. DEA-controlled substances must be handled more, and require increased paperwork; as a result, hidden labor costs increase the cost of these drugs significantly. Nonsteroidal anti-inflammatory drugs have been reported to produce acute renal failure and concomitant electrolyte disturbances in patients with chronic renal insufficiency, congestive heart failure, systemic lupus erythematosus, cirrhosis with ascites, and various states of fluid depletion. This is thought to be a result of renal prostaglandin inhibition and may be of concern in athletes with fluid depletion or renal disease. Other side effects of nonsteroidal anti-inflammatory agents include central nervous system effects (headache, sedation) and skin rashes.

Opiate Analgesics

Opiate analgesics are indicated for severe pain such as may occur with a fracture, with a severe sprain, or after surgery. The term "narcotic" has been supplanted, since the discovery of the opiate receptor, with the more specific term "opiate agonist" to specify the action of this group of drugs at the receptor site. These drugs produce analgesia by competitively binding opiate receptors. Although the main pharmacologic action of the opiate agonists is analgesia, these drugs have many other effects throughout the body. Actions in the central nervous system include sedation, mental clouding, mood variations, nausea, vomiting, euphoria, and respiratory depression. The use of opiate agonists in patients with closed head injuries should be avoided so that changes in mental status are not masked by the drugs. Release of pituitary hormones such as thyrotropin and luteinizing hormone may be suppressed, while the release of prolactin and growth hormone may be enhanced by opiates. The opiate agonists can cause miosis and also can depress the cough reflex. Since a large number of opiate receptors are found in the GI tract as well as the central nervous system, it is not surprising that opiate agonists cause constipation; effects in the biliary tract include increased pressure. The clinical effects of the opiate agonists on the smooth muscles of the ureter and the sphincter of the urinary bladder can be especially troublesome and somewhat frightening to the recumbent postoperative patient who has difficulty urinating. Hypotension may occur in the nonrecumbent patient due to the release of histamine and the alpha-adrenergic effects of the opiate agonists. Many opiate agonists are available in oral and parenteral form. The route of administration of opiate agonists affects the dose: oral administration requires higher dosages than parenteral administration because significant first-pass metabolism occurs in the liver with oral dosing. The duration of action of these drugs is also affected by the route of administration, so that oral dosing generally increases the duration of action by at least 1 hour. Opiate agonists can cause tolerance, physical and psychological dependence, and a withdrawal syndrome; these side effects may limit long-term use of opiates in patients who do not have cancer. The effects of opiate agonists are blocked by opiate antagonists. Mixed opiate agonist-antagonist drugs are also effective in treating pain, but they can cause psychomimetic effects such as hallucinations, and may precipitate a withdrawal syndrome in patients who are physically dependent on opiate agonist drugs.

The long-term use of opiates to manage pain in the recovering and rehabilitating athlete is not routinely recommended, except in special circumstances, because of the potential for addiction.

Anti-inflammatory doses of aspirin or the nonsteroidal anti-inflammatory drugs should suffice for such patients.

SUGGESTED READING

Dunn MJ, Patroro C. Renal effects of nonsteroidal anti-inflammatory drugs. Am J Med 1986; 81:1–132.

Goodman, Gilman. The pharmacological basis of therapeutics. 7th ed. New York: MacMillan Publishing Company, 1985: 491, 674.

Hess EV. Nonsteroidal anti-inflammatory drugs: new perspectives in the inflammatory process and immunologic function. Am J Med 1984; 77:1–31.

Kastrup EK, ed. Drug facts and comparisons. 1989 ed. St. Louis: Facts and Comparisons Division, JB Lippincott, 1989:889–970.

Lasagna L, Prescott LF. Non-narcotic analgesics today: benefits and risks seminar-in-print. Drugs 1986; 32 (suppl):1–208.

Van Tyle WK. Handbook of nonprescription drugs. 8th ed. Washington DC: American Pharmaceutical Association—The National Professional Society of Pharmacists, 1986:191.

VITAMINS AND EXERCISE

RENA A. MENDELSON, M.S., D.Sc.

The purpose of this chapter is to discuss the usefulness of vitamins in improving performance during exercise. In general, professionals in the areas of nutrition and medicine advise that healthy adult men and healthy adult nonpregnant and nonlactating women who consume an adequate and varied diet do not need vitamin supplements. This recommendation would apply to individuals who are involved in normal everyday activities, as well as those who are participating in a variety of athletic endeavors. However, it is important to recognize that many people involved in athletic activities may have restricted both their total food and their energy intake for the purpose of weight reduction or the maintenance of a lower than optimal weight. This is especially true for athletes involved in body building, boxing, gymnastics, weight lifting, and other activities that involve a specific weight requirement. In general, individuals who have restricted their diets to less than 6 to 8 megajoules (1,500 to 2,000 kcal) per day may be consuming less than optimal amounts of specific vitamins and nutrients. Therefore, it may be appropriate to consider multivitamin supplements for those whose total energy intake has been restricted over an extended period (e.g., more than 6 months). In working with athletes, it is important to recognize the possibility not only of a restricted food intake, but of associated bulimia or anorexia; the latter type of eating disorders may lead to very severe restriction of food intake or (in the case of bulimia) the consumption of huge amounts of foods followed by self-induced vomiting.

The recommended intakes of vitamins have been established by a scientific advisory committee in order to meet the needs of most healthy adults; levels have been set at 2 standard deviations above what is considered the mean level required to maintain health. At these intakes, the probability of developing any nutrient deficiency is practically zero. So far, we have no evidence to suggest that exercise increases the need for specific nutrients. The one exception to this generalization is an increased need for the cofactors of energy metabolism: thiamine, niacin, and riboflavin. Requirements for these nutrients are established on the basis of energy intake. An increase of energy intake from a mixed diet of wholesome foods automatically increases the consumption of these vitamins; therefore, supplementation is not necessary. Table 1 lists recommended nutrient intakes for readers who wish to compare these values with supplements on the market.

Athletes are more likely than nonathletes to use nutritional supplements, but their knowledge of nutrition and their consumption of food nutrients are often less than desirable. In a survey of college athletes, 76 percent of the sample indicated that they used nutritional supplements, primarily multivitamins and vitamin C; 31 percent of the athletes and only 11 percent of nonathletic students used iron supplementation. In another study of intercollegiate athletes, males consumed almost twice as much energy as females. The average energy intake for the men was about 14 megajoules per day (3,500 kcal), whereas women consumed an average of about 7 megajoules (1,730 kcal). Of the 10 female basketball players evaluated, only two consumed a diet that met the definition of adequacy. Therefore, it is appropriate for women athletes who are restricting their total energy intake to consider the quality of their diet and to use nutrient supplements to provide an adequate vitamin intake.

Each vitamin has a specific function in intermediary metabolism or growth and development; however, some common characteristics can be identified.

In general, the water-soluble vitamins are found in the water-soluble portion of food and are stored within cells such as muscle and liver. Because of the body's limited water storage capacity, these vitamins are required on a more regular basis than the fat-soluble variety. Water-soluble vitamins include the B vitamins and vitamin C. Fat-soluble vi-

TABLE 1 Recommended Intakes of Vitamins for Adult Males and Females Aged 25 to 51 Years*

Vitamin	*Male*	*Female*
Fat-Soluble Vitamins		
Vitamin A (Retinol equivalents, µg/day)	1,000	800
Vitamin D (mg/day)	2.5	2.5
Vitamin E (mg/day)	9	6
Vitamin K	No recommended intake	
Water-Soluble Vitamins		
Vitamin C (mg/day)	60	45
Folic acid (mg/day)	220	175
Vitamin B_{12} (mg/day)	2.0	2.0
Thiamine	0.4 mg/1,000 kcal	
Riboflavin	0.5 mg/1,000 kcal	
Niacin	7.2 Nicotinic acid equivalents, mg/1,000 kcal	
Vitamin B_6	15 µg/g protein	

*From Bureau of Nutritional Sciences. Recommended nutrient intakes for Canadians. Ottawa, Canada: Health and Welfare, 1983.

tamins are stored in fat and liver, and may be consumed on a somewhat less regular basis. A well-nourished individual is unlikely to develop a deficiency of fat-soluble vitamins for a significant period, unlike a person placed on a diet inadequate in water-soluble vitamins.

The B vitamins (thiamine, niacin, and riboflavin) are involved in energy metabolism as cofactors of the tricarboxylic acid cycle. As such, they are critical to the synthesis of cellular energy (ATP) from glucose, fatty acids, and amino acids. An individual suffering from a deficiency of thiamine or niacin (riboflavin deficiency is exceedingly rare) suffers from a variety of symptoms, including a build-up of intermediary by-products. Advertising for the B vitamins suggests that they are a source of energy, or that they somehow unlock extra energy that can be available to the body. With an inadequate intake of B vitamins, it is true that energy metabolism is hampered; however, adding an excess of B vitamins to an already adequate diet does not enhance ATP production.

Two other major B vitamins, folic acid and vitamin B_{12} (cyanocobalamin), are required for the synthesis of DNA and RNA; they are thus particularly important during periods of growth. Deficiencies of either folic acid or vitamin B_{12} can lead to a macrocytic anemia, which can be treated by a therapeutic dose of B_{12} or folic acid, depending on the primary cause. It is essential that the characteristics of the macrocytic anemia be differentiated, in order to use the appropriate nutrient in treatment.

Vitamin B_6 (pyridoxine) is another of the so-called B-complex vitamins. It is also a cofactor in intermediary metabolism, and is especially important in amino acid synthesis and degradation. The dietary requirement for B_6 is thus determined by protein intake. The currently recommended level is 2.0 mg a day. This vitamin has been used therapeutically to treat a range of medical problems, including carpal tunnel syndrome, premenstrual syndrome, and nausea during pregnancy. Clinical trials have had mixed results. Some positive responses to B_6 may be related to its role in the synthesis of serotonin from the amino acid tryptophan. Unfortunately, self-administration of very large doses (1.2 to 6.0 g per day) has had adverse effects, including neuropathic conditions. Athletes do not appear to be susceptible to deficiencies of any of these B vitamins, in part because cereals and wheat flour in Canada and the United States arc fortified with thiamine, niacin, and riboflavin. Under specific circumstances, however, these vitamins may be needed to treat inherited metabolic disorders or, in the case of folic acid, to treat the side effects of some cancer treatments. Vitamin B_6 has also been used to treat the side effects of some prescription drugs such as oral contraceptives. Niacin, in the form of nicotinic acid, has also been used to treat hyperlipidemia. Thiamine provides a standard treatment for Wernicke's encephalopathy, a disorder resulting from thiamine deficiency induced by prolonged alcoholism. Thiamine may also be used for a form of heart disease that results from thiamine deficiency: beriberi.

The other important water-soluble vitamin is ascorbic acid, or vitamin C. This important nutrient is a cofactor in the synthesis of hydroxyproline, a basic building block of collagen, the protein necessary for connective tissue synthesis. Vitamin C (100 to 200 mg) has been used to help wound repair after surgery. Some periodontists and other oral surgeons recommend a moderate dose of vitamin C before oral surgery to saturate the tissues and facilitate tissue repair. Vitamin C has also been used to treat urinary tract infections, because it modifies the pH of urine and inhibits bacterial growth.

The use of water-soluble vitamins as supplements within an intake range compatible with dietary intake does not appear to have any special advantage or disadvantage for either athletes or nonathletes. However, it is important to recognize that very high doses of water-soluble vitamins such as vitamin B_6 can lead to neurologic complications. The use of large doses of folic acid may also mask a pernicious anemia in individuals who have vitamin

B_{12} deficiency. Although injections of B_{12} are popularly used, there is no clinical evidence to suggest that they are effective in improving athletic performance. Aldaheff and Gualtieri give a useful review of the toxic effects of water-soluble vitamins.

The four fat-soluble vitamins (A, D, E, and K) are of special concern with regard to supplementation, because they are stored in body tissues for a long time and are not excreted as readily as water-soluble vitamins. Vitamin A is essential for growth and development. Recently, it has been used in its analogue form to treat disfiguring cystic acne. However, it is especially dangerous for women who may become pregnant. A significant number of birth defects have been reported among children of women using a vitamin A analogue during various stages of pregnancy. Vitamin A deficiency is exceptionally rare in North America, and it is very unlikely that athletes will present with a Vitamin A deficiency unless they have a gastrointestinal disorder such as cystic fibrosis that inhibits fat absorption. This would present a problem for the absorption of all fat-soluble vitamins.

Vitamin D is a nutrient that is added to our milk supply, but it is also a hormone, because it is available through the body's own synthesis when the skin is exposed to ultraviolet rays. It is essential for the absorption and maintenance of calcium stores. Vitamin D deficiency in adults is extremely rare in North America. For athletes who train outdoors, exposure to sunshine provides adequate vitamin D. The only individuals thought to require a supplementation of vitamin D are newborns who are exclusively breast-fed and born early in the winter, without opportunity for exposure to sunshine for several months.

Vitamin K is synthesized in the gastrointestinal system by microorganisms, and it is a key cofactor in blood coagulation. Those who require a vitamin K supplement include newborn infants who have a sterile gut and lack the microorganisms to synthesize vitamin K, and individuals who have been treated by anticoagulants that are vitamin K antagonists. Long-term antibiotic use can diminish vitamin K production by the intestinal microflora and warrants supplementation. Healthy adults have no need of extra vitamin K.

Vitamin E is a nutrient found in the oils of vegetables and grains, and it has received a great deal of attention. The best-documented function of vitamin E is to work as an antioxidant, to protect vulnerable fatty acids from destruction. The protected substances include vitamin A, as well as the fatty acids that make up the cell membranes found in the red blood cell. A deficiency of vitamin E can lead to hemolytic anemia in which the red blood cell membrane breaks down in the presence of oxidative products. Vitamin E prevents retrolental fibroplasia in premature infants, and it has also been used to prevent postoperative thromboembolism. Vitamin E supplementation substantially increases the levels of this vitamin in plasma and in red blood cells. However, it does not affect platelet aggregation, nor does it alter the production of metabolites that would lower the risk of thrombosis and coronary disease. Vitamin E has been recommended for climbers at very high altitudes, where it appears to enhance oxygen uptake by red blood cells. Vitamin E also appears to protect red blood cells from hemostasis, and for athletes who are mountain climbers there may be some advantage to vitamin E supplementation.

Nevertheless, vitamin supplementation does not generally appear to provide athletes with any objective advantages. In a study of long distance runners, half of the group were given a multivitamin supplement for 3 months, and half received a placebo. After a 3-month wash-out period, the treatments were reversed. The multivitamin supplement contained levels in significant excess of those that might be consumed in a normal diet: anywhere from 100 to 1,000 times the recommended nutrient intake. There was no significant change in blood mineral concentrations during any stage of the study. The blood levels of all nutrients except vitamin C and pyridoxine (B_6) remained within the normal range. There thus appears little likelihood that toxic side effects will develop from the intermittent use of such supplements. However, there was also no effect on maximal oxygen consumption, blood lactate, peak treadmill running speed, or 15-km running time.

SUGGESTED READING

Aldaheff L, Gualtieri CT. Toxic effects of water-soluble vitamins. Nutr Rev 1984; 42:33–80.

Barr S. Nutrition knowledge of female varsity athletes and university students. J Am Diet Assoc 1981; 87:1664–1669.

Bureau of Nutritional Sciences. Recommended nutrient intakes for Canadians. Ottawa, Canada: Health and Welfare, 1983.

Nowack RK, Knudsen KS, Schulz LO. Body composition and nutrient intakes of college men and women basketball players. J Am Diet Assoc 1988; 88:575–578.

Schaumburg H, Kaplan J, Windebank A, et al. Sensory neuropathy from pyridoxine abuse: a megavitamin syndrome. N Engl J Med 1983; 309:445–448.

Stampfer MJ, Jakubowski JA, Faigel D, et al. Vitamin E supplementation effect on human platelet function. Am J Clin Nutr 1988; 47:700–706.

Weight LM, Noakes TO, Labadarios D, et al. Vitamin and mineral status of trained athletes including the effects of supplementation. Am J Clin Nutr 1988; 47:186–191.

MUSCULOSKELETAL INJURIES | FOOT

METATARSALGIA AND OTHER COMMON PROBLEMS

R. PETER WELSH, M.B., Ch.B, F.R.C.S.(C), F.A.C.S.

"When the foot aches, the whole body aches!" To the athlete with pain in the forefoot, the whole athletic performance is indeed compromised, and there are few injuries more frustrating to cope with than these ill-defined and often unresponsive maladies.

CLINICAL ENTITIES

Common foot problems include:

Intermetatarsal ligament strains and intermetatarsal bursitis
Morton's metatarsalgia
Stress fractures
Freiberg's infraction
Metatarsal prolapse and plantar callosities
Sesamoiditis
Bunions and bunionettes
Hallux rigidus
Hammer and claw toes

Intermetatarsal Ligament Strains and Intermetatarsal Bursitis

The running sports impose tremendous loads on the forefoot with impact forces of up to three times body weight at foot-plant and push-off. The intermetatarsal ligament complex is subject to tremendous strain, particularly with the demands of hard surface running, and with aging there is also a gradual splaying of the forefoot, imposing undue stress on this structure. Furthermore, inflammation of the intermetatarsal bursae occurs in response to the jostling motion with running activity, and this results in an ill-defined forefoot pain in the region between adjacent metatarsal heads and necks. Tender to touch, sensitive to loads, this condition may completely preclude running activity.

Morton's Neuroma

Morton's neuroma is a more distinctive entity; symptoms are quite specific, often with a lancinating jab of pain on footfall and an associated neuritis in the form of parasthetic sensations spreading down the adjacent borders of the affected toes in the digital nerve distribution. This condition is defined pathologically as a neuroma, but in reality is due to the bursitic involvement of the neurovascular complex at its intermetatarsal digital bifurcation.

Stress Fractures

Repetitive cycling of any structural element may lead to the development of fatigue fractures. Bone shows such a breach in the rigid cortex of the metatarsal neck area and occasionally near the base of the metatarsal.

In runners and dancers, other sites of these fractures are of course the distal fibular 2 inches above the tip of the lateral malleolus, the tibia about the junction of the proximal and mid one-third, and occasionally the tibial plateau and the femoral condyle. Very rarely a stress fracture may be seen in the neck of the femur.

The breach in the cortex sets up an intense subperiosteal reaction, which is very painful and does not settle until there is new bone formation sufficient to consolidate the fracture focus. Radiographs may not be positive in the initial stages, and changes may not be observed until periosteal new bone is noted 3 to 4 weeks after injury. A technetium bone scan is often helpful in the early stages in differentiating a stress fracture from a simple intermetatarsal foot strain. The scan is positive only if there is actual bone involvement.

Freiberg's Infraction

A rare avascular necrosis of the metatarsal head, most commonly the second, is occasionally seen as a cause of metatarsalgia. The condition is known as one of the osteochondroses and is in fact akin to Perthes' disease of the hip. The metatarsal head is rendered dysvascular, and then, with regeneration, new bone is laid down on the old scaffold, but not before a fracture or partial collapse of the head distorts the shape of the metatarsal and deranges the metatarsal phalangeal articulation, leading in late stages to degenerative arthritis of the joint.

Metatarsal Prolapse and Plantar Callosities

Abnormal weightbearing pressures beneath the metatarsal head result in the development of painful callosities. The collapse of the transverse arch of the foot sees the weight borne preferentially on the middle metatarsals instead of the first and fifth. Similarly, the development of an arthritic tendency at the base of the metatarsal may result in loss of flexibility in the foot and abnormal weight distribution across the forefoot without the normal resilience being shown at this level.

With prolapse of the metatarsal head, the prominence of the bone causes abnormal loading on the weightbearing bursal pad with secondary thickening of the overlying skin, producing a hard callus.

Sesamoiditis

If the abnormal pressures are maldistributed beneath the first metatarsal head, it is often the metatarsal sesamoids that bear the brunt of the load. Associated sesamoiditis and bursal inflammation may result. Furthermore, the sesamoids, which are bones in the tendon of the short flexor of the great toe, are also subject to fracture and developmental abnormalities (they are often bipartite), and in the older individual they are subject to arthritic change in their articulation with the metatarsal head.

Bunions and Bunionettes

A bunion is a painful bursitis overlying the medial prominence of the first metatarsal head. A bunionette is a similar condition on the lateral aspect of the foot in relation to the fifth metatarsal head. In the great toe a bunion may be associated with hallux valgus or hallux rigidus, whereas a bunionette may also be associated with abnormal weight bearing on the plantar aspect of the foot.

Hallux Rigidus

A disabling arthritis of the first metatarsophalangeal (MTP) joint results in gross limitation of first metatarsal joint movement, particularly in extension. This markedly limits participation in any of the running or jumping sports, for without adequate dorsiflexion, push-off is severely inhibited. Often there is a strong familial tendency in the development of this condition, although it may also arise as a consequence of trauma involving the first MTP joint.

Hammer and Claw Toes

A flexion deformity of the interphalangeal joints of the toes may result in abnormal pressure areas with callus or corn formation overlying the prominence of the angulated joint. A hammer toe is associated with flexion at the distal interphalangeal (DIP) joint and extension at the MTP joint. A claw toe maintains a normal articulation at the MTP joint that involves a clawing or flexion deformity at either the proximal interphalangeal (PIP) or DIP joints.

CLINICAL ASSESSMENT

The clinical diagnosis of the above conditions is obvious in most instances. In others, such as hallux rigidus, review of radiographs is required to confirm the extent of the condition, and if doubt exists in defining whether or not a metatarsal neck pain is related to a stress fracture, a technetium bone scan may be required.

In completing the assessment, particular care should be taken on examining the hindfoot, noting the mobility of associated ankle subtalar and midtarsal joints as well as the characteristics of the foot and the heel plant, and whether there is a varus or valgus disposition of the heel that will misdirect the forefoot placement. In all instances the neurovascular status of the extremities should be carefully evaluated. The foot itself should never be examined in isolation from the rest of the patient. Particular importance is placed in the overall examination, noting the total limb alignment and whether there is a varus or valgus deformity or rotational anomaly of the limb more proximally. Any limb length inequalities should be noted and any rotational abnormality in the hip, femur, or tibia documented. The knee joint function, particularly patellar mechanics, is of vital concern with regard to the functioning of the foot. A tendency to genu valgum with a subluxating patella due to an increased "Q" angle leads invariably to a displacement of the forefoot with a valgus tendency of the heel at foot-plant, resulting in abnormal hyperpronation of the forefoot.

Finally, in the clinical assessment, any abnormalities of the spine and its development should be noted; for example, scoliosis may affect foot mechanics.

MANAGEMENT OF METATARSALGIA AND FOOT DISORDERS

Management of these conditions may require (1) modification of sports activity, (2) footwear adaptation, (3) use of orthotics and other podiatric appliances, (4) physical therapies, (5) medications, and (6) surgery.

Modification of Sports Activity

Participation in many of the running and jumping sports have to be modified. Acute strains of the forefoot require rest from provocative loading; stress fractures cannot be subjected to more than normal daily walking and must heal completely before running can be resumed. Hallux rigidus may put an end completely to the career of a dancer or jumper because of the inability to dorsiflex the great toe joint.

Footwear Adaptation

Footwear must be both protective and supportive, comfortably conforming to the foot. An arch support system should be adequate, but not bulky; of particular importance is the adequacy of heel control, which directs forefoot plant and push-off. Pressure points should be eliminated by stretching at sites of local irritation, or areas of pressure should be bridged so that the sensitive area fits into a relative recess.

Different conditions dictate particular footwear requirements. With hallux rigidus, a stiff shank or even a rocker bottom sole may be of great assistance, whereas in many sports a stiff shank may result in excessive loading of the heel at the bone-tendon junction and a predisposition to Achilles tendinitis. Obviously, footwear requirements must be tailored to the needs and condition of the patient.

Use of Orthotics and Other Podiatric Appliances

The role of orthotic supports has unfortunately been grossly overplayed. Nonetheless, customized adaptation of footwear has played a major part in the management of foot disorders.

Orthotics should in most instances be regarded as a temporary aid, just as a back brace aids an acutely injured spine. Most foot disorders suffered acutely are self-limiting, and a soft orthotic may assist by allowing continuance of the sports activity while the healing process occurs. However, once the injury has healed, the device should be discarded. Therefore, it makes no sense for athletes who have run successfully for perhaps 5 or 10 years to feel that, because of a single foot injury, they must forever persist with an orthotic support in the shoe. Only if an injury proves recurrent and major structural abnormality is seen to benefit from the use of an orthotic should a more permanent device be prescribed.

It should be remembered that an orthotic device occupies space in a shoe and adds weight to the foot, and that by the employment of these aids, even a subtle alteration of foot-plant and push-off must call for compensatory adjustment in the gait pattern elsewhere, at the level of the knee, hip, or spine.

The type of orthotic employed varies according to the condition from which the patient suffers. Orthotics may be of great value in acute long arch strains, in which case an arch support and scaphoid cookie greatly reduce load on the arch structure. A more rigid device is required for the patient with hallux rigidus to restrict pressures on the great toe joint, but such rigidity may throw loads at the heel and cause Achilles tendinitis.

In managing metatarsal problems, there is no need for the major building-in of a long arch system into the orthotic; all that is required is a metatarsal pad support beneath the metatarsal neck to elevate and separate the metatarsal heads and reduce their compressive tendency on weight bearing. This device also may be very effective in the management of Morton's neuroma.

There has been a great tendency to overprescribe orthotics for what is termed the hyperpronated or flat foot. There is such a wide range of what may be considered the normal arch height that to offer orthotics arbitrarily to the flatter-appearing foot totally disregards how that individual may function with that particular foot form. The arbitrary prescription of orthotics in these instances can be more harmful than beneficial, but if injury does prove resistant to other forms of treatment, and proven benefit is obtained by a soft orthotic device, prescription of more permanent orthotics should be considered. Otherwise, most orthotics should be used on a temporary basis to assist the athlete through the healing of an injury. It is probably better to further customize the footwear itself than to add redundancy in the form of orthotic devices to the athlete's shoes.

In most instances, soft, resilient orthotics are preferred to the more rigid materials often prescribed. Even though these more rigid materials may prove more durable in regard to the life of the device itself, it is better to have a system that conforms more to the texture of both the shoe and the foot structures than to have a rigid interface between the foot and the shoe.

Other appliances that may be useful are doughnut protective devices over pressure points to prevent friction between the foot and the shoe, e.g., over a bunion or hammer toe prominence. Care must be paid in general to the skin of the foot, with careful attention to any cracks or ulcer areas. A tendency to interdigital fungal infection usually can be handled adequately with topical antifungal agents.

Physical Therapies

As a species, man has lost much of his capacity to individual control of the intrinsic musculature of the foot. Physical therapy aimed at assisting intrinsic function can be of extreme benefit. In this regard, faradic foot baths may be employed to initiate intrinsic response, and teaching of intrinsic exercises may be of considerable benefit.

Passive stretching of deforming digits and stiffening toes is a worthwhile endeavor.

Local measures, such as icing and ultrasound, may have empiric value; if no benefit is obviously arising from their employment, treatment should be discontinued.

Medications

Systemic medication has little place in the management of most of these conditions, but local steroid injections between the metatarsal heads may settle acute bursitis and benefit a Morton's neuroma. Sesamoiditis may also respond to local infiltration. As a general rule in most treatments, if one injection does not help, there seems little justification for continuing treatments of that type, and if one injection works, there is no cause for further treatment.

Surgery

Foot problems of some athletes prove to be both refractory to treatment and sufficiently disabling to preclude any sports participation. These require definitive surgical treatment.

Morton's Neuroma. Local interdigital exploration allows the resection of the involved bursal scar tissue enveloping the bifurcation of the digital nerve and interdigital space. Tourniquet control of circulation greatly aids the dissection in these instances, and a web space incision is favored: this gives a clear view of the whole intermetatarsal space both dorsally and on the plantar aspect.

Freiberg's Infraction. Metatarsal neck osteotomy decompresses the involved metatarsophalangeal joint in addition to easing the weightbearing load on the affected metatarsal head.

Metatarsal Prolapse and Plantar Callosities. Elevation of the affected metatarsal head by metatarsal neck osteotomy decompresses the lesser and overlying calloused skin. An oblique osteotomy just proximal to the head allows the head to slide up and shorten slightly. Weight bearing is allowed immediately, but the fracture requires 4 to 6 weeks to unite. The return to sport may be delayed 2 to 3 months by swelling and tenderness.

The patient should be closely observed postoperatively for transfer of weight from one metatarsal to the adjacent metatarsal head, which may necessitate another decompressive osteotomy.

Sesamoiditis. Excision of the sesamoids for nonunion, avascular necrosis, or osteoarthritis can be extremely rewarding. Care must be taken to avoid injury to the digital nerves or flexor tendon.

Bunions. If the bunion is associated with hallux valgus, the local excision of the bunion must always be carried out in conjunction with correction of the hallux valgus. In addition, any degree of metatarsus varus should be corrected by metatarsal osteotomy, preferably at the base of the first metatarsal.

Preservation of the intact joint should be practiced whenever possible, and procedures such as the McBride procedure are preferred to excisional remedies such as a Keller procedure.

Bunionettes. The fifth metatarsal head should never be excised in the athlete, or a tendency to rolling over and a sense of weakness will always prevail. Instead, in addition to a local bunionette excision, an oblique medializing osteotomy of the neck of the fifth metatarsal allows both correction of the lateral deviating metatarsal head and upward correction of any abnormal weightbearing pressure point.

Hallux Rigidus. In the athlete, excisional arthroplasty may be necessary, with excision of the base of the proximal phalanx removing sufficient bone to permit adequate dorsiflexion of the joint. Careful capsular reconstruction is essential, but tension on the great toe joint must be minimal at the conclusion of the procedure. The use of interposition material, as with Silastic arthroplasty, has little place in the athlete; these materials cannot prove durable to the repetitive load demands of active athletic endeavor.

Metatarsophalangeal fusion has a definite place in certain individuals. It provides a totally pain-free, strong push-off, but limits the type of footwear that can be used, and its success relies on complete mobility of the associated joints at the DIP and the base of the first metatarsal.

Greater morbidity of this procedure, the risk of nonunion, and the necessity for careful technical considerations in obtaining the correct angle of the MTP joint make this a demanding technique. In general, the excisional procedure is favored in dancers and jumpers.

Hammer and Claw Toes. For hammer toes with PIP hyperextension, if the joint remains mobile and the MTP joint is not subluxated, a flexor to extensor tendon transfer is recommended.

If the PIP deformity is fixed, an interphalangeal fusion is preferred; if the MTP joint is concurrently subluxated, a partial excision of the base of the proximal phalanx is added.

For claw toes at the DIP joint, a Jones repair, excising a transverse dorsal elipse of skin, tendon, and a bone wedge at the DIP joint, provides a completely durable correction.

SUGGESTED READING

Bossley CJ, Cairney PC. The intermetatarsophalangeal bursa: its significance in Morton's metatarsalgia. J Bone Joint Surg 1980; 62B:184.

Mann RA. DuVries's Surgery of the Foot. 4th ed. St. Louis: CV Mosby, 1978.
Mann RA, Clanton TO. Hallus rigidus: treatment by cheilectomy. J Bone Joint Surg 1988; 70A:400.
Myerson MS, Shereff MJ. The pathological anatomy of claw and hammer toes. J Bone Joint Surg 1989; 71A:45.
Richardson E. The foot in adolescents and adults in Campbell's operative orthopaedics. 7th ed., St. Louis: CV Mosby, 1987: 829.

SOFT TISSUE INJURIES

G. JAMES SAMMARCO, M.D., F.A.C.S.

Soft tissue in the foot serves to support, nourish, and provide sensation, in addition to controlling the position of the bone structures. At the same time, it acts as a shock-absorbing mechanism for high loads created during weight bearing.

The foot may be divided into the forefoot, midfoot, and hindfoot; special conditions occur in each of these areas. Two types of problems occur in soft tissue: the acute injury arising from a single traumatic event or several and the chronic tissue problems associated more commonly with overuse. Certain principles should be followed when treating injuries to soft tissue.

An acute injury is often the result of a single traumatic episode. This presents with swelling, tenderness, significant pain, and decreased joint motion, all of which interrupt sports activity. Restriction of motion and application of ice and a compression dressing while the leg is elevated above the level of the waist (acronym, RICE) are recommended as principles of acute care. Restriction of motion is achieved with a cast, splint, or brace. The principle of elevation is simply that "water flows downhill." Although it does not reduce edema, ice does provide a certain anesthetic effect to the skin, thereby reducing the pain. Restriction of motion relates to the particular part injured. The player is encouraged to move the remaining part of the foot: e.g., if the subtalar joint is injured and placed in a splint, the player is encouraged to elevate the leg and move the toes. This creates a "milking" action that helps reduce edema. The injury is reassessed in a few days and a rehabilitation program is started. This includes stretching, range-of-motion exercises, and power building to develop proprioception. The use of the foot and ankle exerciser board or "wobble board" is helpful (Fig. 1). If surgery is indicated, there should be a specific diagnosis; early return to the field should be expected if surgery is not required. During surgery a bloodless field is to be preferred in order to delineate tissue structures, avoid cutaneous nerves, and visualize vessels. For surgery on the toes and small joints, loupe magnification is helpful. When the athlete returns to sports activities, taping or bracing may be required with a modification of the shoe.

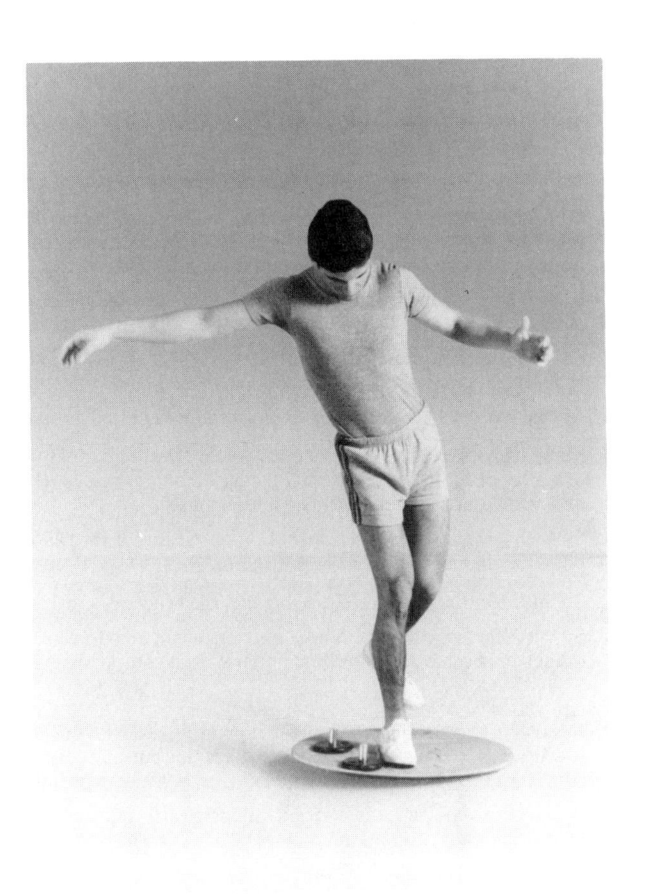

Figure 1 Athlete using the foot and ankle exercises board (BAPS BOARD). The foot is placed in the center and rotated. Proprioception, range of motion, and strength are developed after injury.

For chronic injuries due to overuse syndromes, a treatment regimen should include a warm-up program to deal specifically with the injured foot (Table 1). Warming up the foot before exercise is as important as stretching. Functional bracing and strapping, in addition to nonsteroidal anti-inflammatory drugs (NSAID) are important adjuncts to treatment.

NAIL INJURIES

Acute problems of the nails can occur from trauma such as a crush creating an acute *subungual*

TABLE 1 Flexibility Program for the Foot and Ankle

Non-Weightbearing Exercises

Do each exercise 10 times a day. Increase repetitions of each exercise by 5 each day up to a total of 30 repetitions.
Do the program 3 times daily.
Exercise slowly and to the maximal stretch.

1. Sit on floor with legs straight in front. Place towel around ball of foot. Grasp both ends of towel with hands, and pull foot toward knee. Stretch to a count of 5. Release.

   Repeat the above, except pull more with right hand to bring foot to the right, then pull with left hand to bring foot to the left.

   Repeat with knee bent about 30 degrees.

2. Sit on floor with legs straight out. Flex foot upward toward face and curl toes under at the same time. Now point foot downward and bring toes up at the same time. The sequence is: Foot up, toes down, foot down, toes up.

   Sit on floor with legs straight out in front, putting foot flat against wall. With heel and ball of foot flat against wall, pull toes toward face. Hold to a count of 5. Relax.

   Do the same exercise with knee bent 30 degrees.

3. Sit in chair with knee bent and foot flat on floor under knee. Keep heel and ball of foot on floor, and raise toes. Keeping toes up, slide foot back a few inches, and relax toes. Raise toes again and slide foot back a few more inches. Keep raising toes and sliding foot back until you can no longer keep heel on floor while raising toes. Bring foot back out to starting position.

   Repeat from starting position. Raise heel, keeping toes flat on floor, then press down again. Lean upper body forward for increased stretch.

   Same position as above. Slide foot forward as far as you can, keeping both toes and heels in contact with floor. At this point, keep heel in place and knee straight. Flex foot up toward knee, then point foot and press toes onto floor. Keep stretching and pointing foot.

   Repeat from starting position, except keep toes curled as you stretch and point foot.

4. Sit with knees parallel, foot flat on floor. Pull inside edge of foot toward you (supinate), keeping outside edge on floor. Hold to a count of 5. Flatten foot, then bring outside edge of foot toward you (pronate), keeping inside edge on floor, including big toe. Hold to a count of 5. Don't let knee move during this exercise.

   Sit with feet flat on floor. Claw toes and inch foot forward as toes claw, then release. Separate toes between clawing. Inch out as far as possible, then slide back and start again.

5. Sit with feet flat on floor. Raise big toe, then second, progressing to little toe. Reverse and go from little toe to big toe.

   Sit with feet flat. Slightly lift heel, putting weight on lateral borders of feet. Roll from little toe to big toe, then back through heel without letting heel touch floor. You are making a complete circle around ball of foot. Repeat and reverse.

Progressive Weightbearing Exercises

1. Between two chairs, using them for support: Stand with one foot 12 inches in front of the other, feet flat on floor. Rock forward onto front foot, so that weight is on this foot, leaving back foot in contact with floor, toes on floor, heel lifted. Rock all the way back so that front foot is on heel and toes are pulled back. Change position of feet and repeat.

   Between two chairs, stand on good leg. Swing affected leg all the way back, knee flexed, foot pointed, then swing leg forward to an extended leg, foot and toes pulled toward you (dorsiflexed). Keep repeating.

2. Stand with back to wall, feet directly under shoulders, weight evenly distributed. Slowly bend knees and do not raise heels. Go to point of maximal stretch and hold 5 counts, then rise up and repeat.

   Standing as above, at the bottom of knee bend, roll onto balls of the feet to maximal arch, then roll down, then straighten legs. Repeat.

3. Stand on a step with feet parallel, heels hanging off edge so that calves are maximally stretched. Pull all the way up onto toes, slowly, then lower all the way down to maximal stretch. Repeat up to 10 times. Repeat with feet turned out, then turned in. Progress to using 5 to 10 pound ankle weights.

4. Stand with all the weight on one leg. Keep knee straight and raise to a fully arched foot, slowly, then lower down. Repeat up to 20 times.

   Stand with all the weight on one leg. Bend knee and keep heel down, then straighten knee and pull up to a full arch. Slowly lower heel, keeping knee straight. Repeat.

5. Stand, rock back on heels, claw toes. Walk on heels and then walk with toes clawed around pencils.

   Walk on heels with 1 to 3 pound ankle weights wrapped around forefoot.

6. Standing, raise and lower inner sides of feet with toes clawed.

   Stand with feet parallel, on balls of feet, weight on outer borders of feet, knees about 4 inches apart. Roll the weight from fifth metatarsal to big toe in a circular motion. Heels stay off floor. Do this exercise with feet turned in, then with feet turned out.

hematoma. Repeated minitrauma of the toe may produce a chronic subungual hematoma, "black toe," and is usually asymptomatic. The acute subungual hematoma is drained by means of a small drill held through the nail into the hematoma, allowing the blood under pressure to escape. A second, more traditional method is to heat the end of a paper clip under an alcohol lamp until red hot (Fig. 2). The hot tip is pressed directly over the nail, creating a hole into the hematoma and allowing the blood under pressure to escape. The nail is not removed but is taped in place to protect the nail bed; it may be lost at a later date, but meanwhile the nail bed begins to heal. Removal of the nail exposes the tender matrix to repeated painful trauma, and it may take 1 year for the hallux toenail to regrow.

Onycholysis, delaminating of the nail on its end, occurs as a result of weight bearing on the tip of the toe or repeatedly striking a hard object with the end of the nail. Partial avulsion can occur, but if the condition is chronic, as in toe dancers, no treatment is needed since the condition is asymptomatic. This should not be confused with paronychia, ingrown toenail, or onychomycosis.

SKIN INJURIES

The skin of the sole may be 7 mm thick. It is well fixed through fibrous septa to deep tissue and lacks sebaceous glands. Beneath lies a compartmentalized subcutaneous fat layer that acts as a shock-absorbing cushion. This is in contrast to the skin of the dorsum of the foot, which may be less than 1 mm thick and overlies several fascial layers that permit excellent mobility.

A *tear of the plantar skin* is caused by overstretching of the flexion creases of the proximal hallux or small toes. Tension on the foot is caused by running, stopping, or turning either barefoot or in a light shoe. This is treated by gentle cleansing and prophylactic antibiotic ointment until healing occurs. This condition does not prevent participation in sport.

Ill-fitting shoes force the toes into a hammer toe position, causing ulceration and *corns* on the dorsal aspect of proximal interphalangeal joints and on the toe tufts and adjacent toes. The condition is corrected by changing shoes and padding the toes. In athletes with flexible hammer toe and chronic corns, a doughnut-shaped foam rubber pad is taped to the top of each corn. Such pads can also be placed between the toes to prevent soft corn formation. A neglected soft corn can become infected and develop a *web space abscess.* Diagnosis of an abscess is made by clinical examination that reveals tenderness and redness in the web space. A sinogram can help confirm the diagnosis. Treatment consists of incision and drainage of the abscess with administration of appropriate antibiotics. The player may resume activities in 10 days when healing has occurred. Recurrent or persistent soft corn formation is treated by excision of the underlying cartilaginous osteophyte through a longitudinal incision above the flexion crease line on the side of the toe (Fig. 3). The edges of the corn are not excised, because they will resolve when the underlying protuberance is removed. Sports activity is restricted until the wound heals.

Blisters result from two concomitant forces, normal force and shear force, applied to feet that are

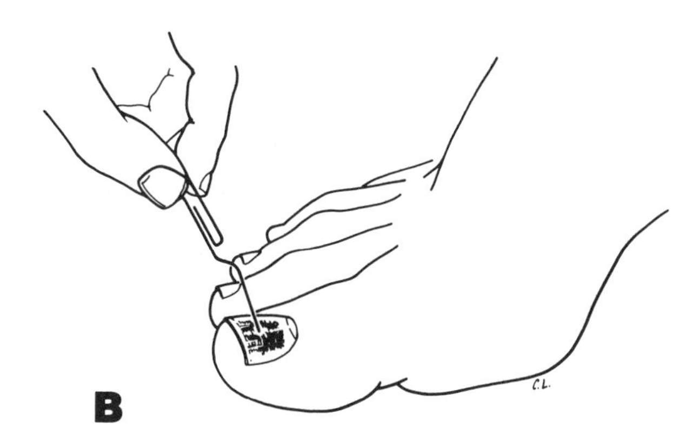

Figure 2 ***A, B,*** Acute hallux subungual hematoma causes pain from pressure beneath the nail. A paper clip is heated in the flame of an alcohol lamp and pressed through the nail, creating a hole into the blood and relieving pressure.

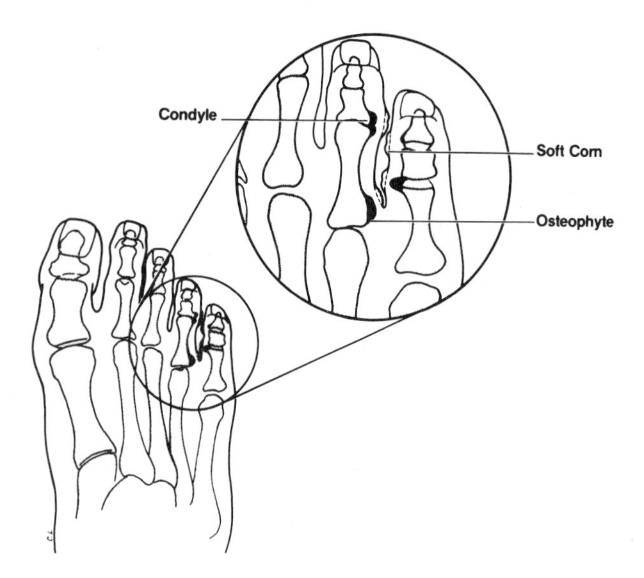

Figure 3 Diagram of the region of soft corn formation between the toes. As the toes are pressed together in the shoe, pressure against a condyle or osteophyte and sweat cause skin maceration, and chronic pressure necrosis develops.

not properly conditioned. The skin breaks down at the junction of the cornified and maturing cell layers. Fluid forms, creating a bleb. This occurs in the areas of high pressure.

Treatment is symptomatic, relieving the load-bearing surface by taping a closed cell foam rubber doughnut pad (¼-inch thick) to the bottom of the foot. The doughnut hole should be large enough to include the entire blister. An alternative method is to apply benzoin circumferentially about the blister, followed by a moleskin patch with a hole cut out for the blister. A small amount of Vaseline should be applied to the center area. To prevent recurrent blisters, recommended prophylaxis includes applying a single layer of Microcore paper tape over the area at risk, and wearing double-thickness socks and properly fitted shoes. A graduated fitness program increases skin tolerance. A thick sock or a special double-layered sock (Runique) also helps reduce normal and shear forces on the skin.

PUNCTURE WOUNDS

The puncture wound is the most underrated injury to soft tissues of the foot. Penetrating objects must pass through the shoe and sock before entering the skin, carrying both normal flora and pathogens. The most serious error is to underestimate the nature of the wound in light of a history of a penetrating injury and foot x-ray films revealing no evidence of radiopaque objects. In fact, most puncture wounds in which foreign bodies are found are caused by nonradiopaque objects such as ordinary glass, splinters, thorns, and plastic. Close follow-up is an important principle of treatment. X-ray examination using soft tissue technique, with special views such as metatarsal head views or lateral and oblique views of the heel with thick emulsion film, may be necessary. The history is important, since the patient may relate that only part of the object was recovered. Gentle cleansing and prophylactic antibiotics are recommended. The author prefers to use cephalexin (Keflex), 500 mg every 6 hours. The wound is examined after 48 hours for the presence of swelling, redness, increasing tenderness, and signs of early abscess formation. It may be necessary to perform incision and drainage. Magnetic resonance imaging (MRI) is helpful to determine whether there is a nonradiopaque foreign body within the foot. The incision should be positioned in the region of the puncture wound, avoiding a site directly beneath the metatarsal head or other bony weight-bearing prominence. Meticulous care is taken to explore the area of abscess thoroughly without violating the unaffected, compartmentalized fat pad on the sole. At the time of surgery, both aerobic and nonaerobic cultures are obtained. Polymicrobial infections are common (Fig. 4). Thorough examination of the wound is necessary to ensure that a foreign body is not present, since migration can occur quickly (Fig. 5). Postoperatively, a splint is applied. Cephalosporin antibiotic coverage is continued postoperatively until the operative culture and sensitivities are returned. The patient is then placed on appropriate specific antibiotics.

Rehabilitation is begun without weight bearing after 5 days. A weight-bearing program is added when the wound has healed.

LESSER TOE INJURIES

Soft tissue injuries of the lesser toes can have two causes: (1) external trauma related to jamming, crushing, and ill-fitting shoes; and (2) internal trauma due to lesser toe deformity or laxity of joint ligaments. Crushing injuries to the toes can occur either from player contact or from off-the-field injuries. Acute treatment includes elevation of and compression dressing to the forefoot. After edema begins to subside, active motion of the toes with elevation is started. If blebs have developed, the toe is protected with a soft dressing. The player is allowed to return to sports when symptoms permit. Uncommonly, dislocation of the proximal interphalangeal (PIP) or distal interphalangeal (DIP) joint can occur, usually associated with fracture. After closed reduction, the toe is "buddy" taped to the adjacent toes for 3 weeks.

If flexible hammer toes are repeatedly traumatized and become symptomatic, a flexor-to-extensor tendon transfer of the modified Girdlestone type or one of its variants is recommended. Such surgery should be timed for the off-season, since 1 month is necessary for healing. For players with toes prone to

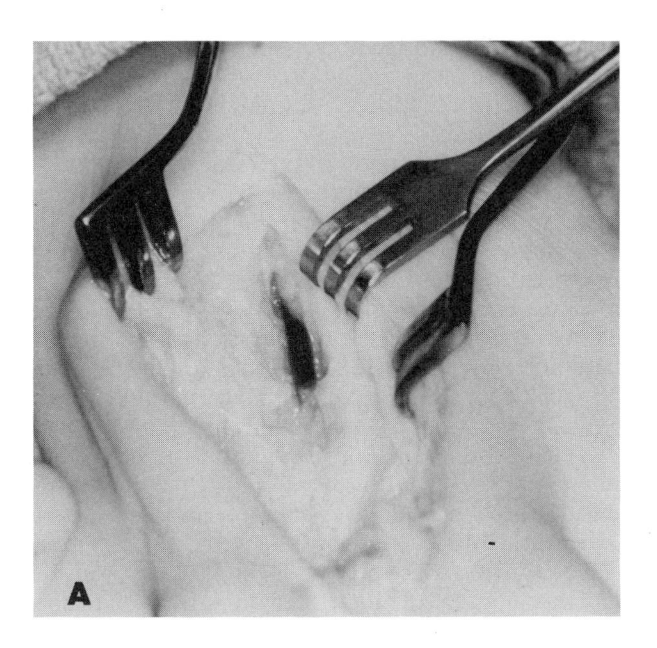

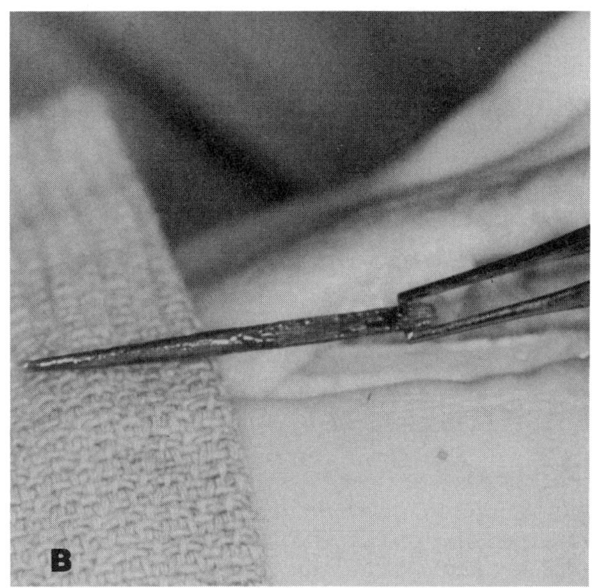

Figure 4 ***A, B,*** Operative photographs of a foot abscess with a toothpick 1 year after injury. The patient's report of recovering only a small amount of toothpick from the ball of the foot went unheeded. Two subsequent plantar incisions for the abscess failed to reveal the other half of the toothpick, which had migrated to the base of the metatarsal. A third dorsal incision revealed the source of the bimicrobial infection.

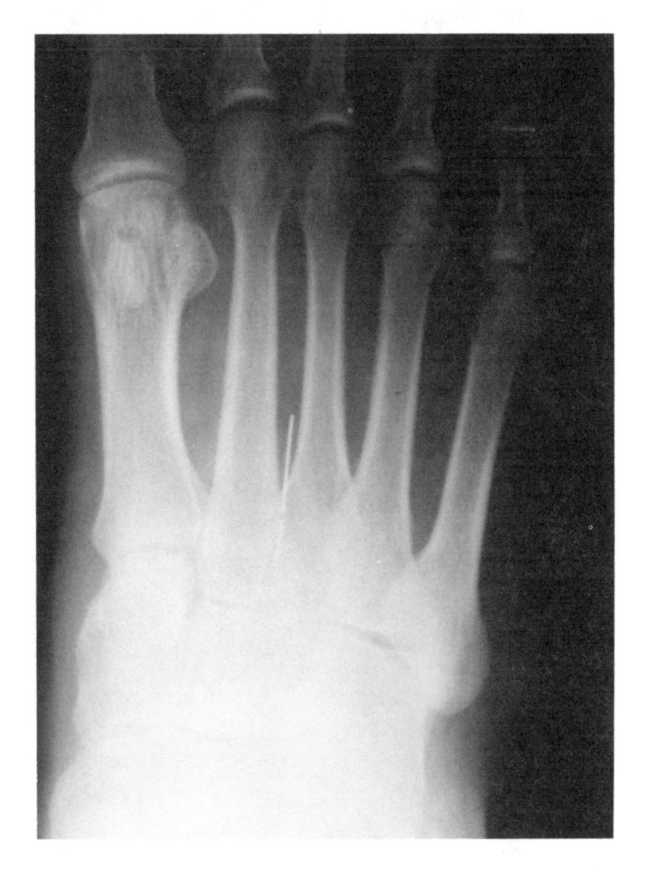

Figure 5 X-ray photograph of a foot 20 years after a puncture wound. No object was originally found at the entrance wound near the ball of the foot, no x-ray films were taken, and the pain and swelling eventually subsided. The needle has migrated to the midfoot.

repeated injury, a semirigid full-insole orthosis provides rigidity beneath the forefoot.

A player with cock-up fifth toe deformity is likely to injure the toe. Taping and padding between the fourth and fifth toes, as well as laterally, prevents corn and blister formation. Persistent symptoms warrant surgical correction and can be timed for a period of laying off. The author recommends a partial proximal phalangectomy with Z-plasty to release the contracted dorsal skin as necessary. Recovery takes 6 weeks.

HALLUX INJURIES

The great toe is subject to the most injuries. *Interphalangeal (IP) injuries* are usually caused by acute flexion either in a soft shoe or when barefoot. Repeated injury about the IP joint can cause arthritis and osteophyte formation, which predisposes the hallux to additional trauma. "Buddy" taping the hallux to the second toe helps prevent recurrence of the injury.

With the advent of artificial turf, the incidence of hyperextension injuries has increased. *Turf toe* is caused by jamming the forefoot, forcing the hallux into hyperextension at the metatarsophalangeal joint causing strain and avulsion of the plantar plate. To this is added a valgus stress, and the medial collateral ligaments may be partially avulsed. Although most such injuries are initiated on artificial turf, recurrent injuries occur on both artificial and natural turf. Symptoms include severe pain beneath the first metatarsal head medially, with swelling of the hallux and decreased range of motion. An antalgic gait is noted. X-ray examination may reveal avulsion fractures from the proximal phalanx or metatarsal head at the attachment of collateral ligaments. Rarely, a fractured sesamoid is noted. Treatment includes rest, ice application, elevation, and a compression dressing. The player is seen after 48 hours and, depending on the severity of the symptoms, a rehabilitation and stretching program is begun. Recurrence is prevented by restricting hyperextension of the hallux at the metatarsophalangeal joint. To achieve this, 1-inch tape is looped over the dorsum of the proximal phalanx, crisscrossing on the sole (Fig. 6*A*). Tight circumferential tape is not recommended, because it may cause circulatory compromise. Additional protection with a foot orthosis stiffened beneath the forefoot and hallux helps to prevent hyperextension. Counseling for acceptance of the orthosis may be required, since players often consider this to be a minor problem. Long-term sequelae of turf toe include hallux rigidus and hallux valgus. Surgical treatment of the acute injury is limited to the unreducible dislocation of the metatarsophalangeal joint.

Football players are prone to hyperextension injuries, *tripping injuries*, at the metatarsophalangeal joint, as well as ballet dancers and runners who also incur hyperflexion injuries at the metatarsophalangeal joint. The mechanism in noncontact activities such as running or dancing is simply that of tripping. In contact sports, blocking or tackling from behind, and landing on the hallux with the added force of a tackler, contribute to the force of the injury. Compression dressing, elevation, and ice are indicated, followed after 48 hours by a rehabilitation program as dictated by the subsidence of symptoms. A subsequent decrease in range of motion may occur. Long-term sequelae are similar to those for turf toe.

Acute bursitis of the metatarsophalangeal joint is caused by poorly fitted shoes or repeated medial trauma. Symptoms of pain and swelling may follow acute injuries, such as turf toe or tripping injuries, and may reflect an associated collateral ligament injury. The condition may also develop from chronic pressure and irritation at the medial metatarsal head. Treatment includes a doughnut-shaped closed foam pad taped over the medial first metatarsal head. The doughnut hole should be large enough to permit the tender area to settle within the opening. The pad should be thick enough (at least 5 mm) to prevent contact of the tender bursa with the shoe. NSAIDs are also prescribed.

PLANTAR FASCIITIS AND PLANTAR HEEL PAIN

Acute conditions of the plantar fascia include acute fasciitis in its proximal, middle, or distal parts. Complete rupture can occur at or near the calcaneal insertion. More commonly, *acute plantar fasciitis* is caused by strain with microrupture of the fascia following increased exercise after a period of laying off. The origin of the flexor digitorum brevis muscle is closely associated with the middle section of the plantar aponeurosis. The abductor hallucis and abductor digiti quinti muscles also take origin

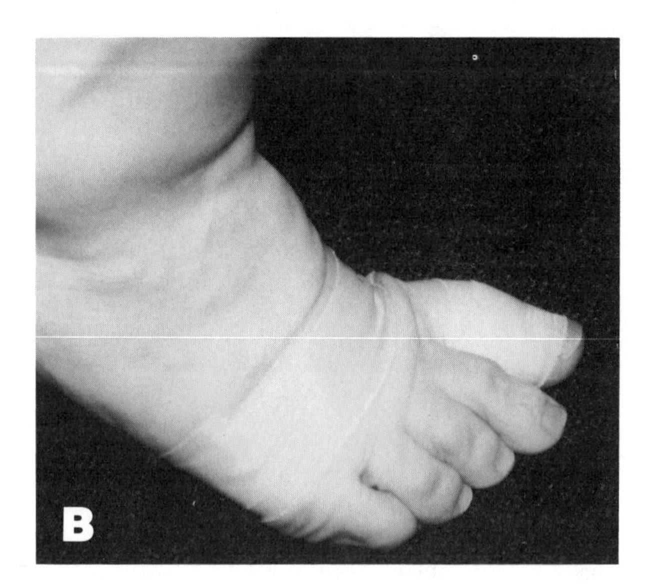

Figure 6 Recurrent turf toe prevention. *A*, The plantar aspect of the foot with dorsally looped 1-inch tape crisscrossed on the sole. *B*, Hyperextension of the hallux metatarsophalangeal joint is restricted. This may be combined with a stiff hallux extension in a foot orthosis to prevent reinjury.

in part from the medial and lateral portions of the plantar aponeurosis, respectively. Acute fasciitis in this region may be associated with acute intrinsic muscle strain. Diagnosis is made by palpation in the tender region. Dorsiflexion of the hallux and lesser toes tightens the plantar fascia, permitting localization to a specific point. The principle of treatment is to maintain flexibility while decreasing inflammation and protecting the foot from additional injury. Active motion with elevation and ice packs accompanied by NSAIDs is prescribed. A foot and ankle flexibility program is started (see Table 1). Shoes should be changed if needed and double-thickness socks worn. Taping the arch is helpful during the acute stages, but if symptoms persist a semirigid foot orthosis is recommended. These should be custom molded to the foot to provide an even distribution of load. *Acute rupture of plantar fascia* in the posterior medial portion requires time away from play until symptoms subside (Fig. 7). The diagnosis may be difficult to differentiate from a stress fracture since the tender area is near the calcaneal tuberosity.

Heel pain (calcaneodynia) can be caused by avulsion of the fascia from its insertion on the calcaneus, entrapment of the medial calcaneal nerve, or stress fracture of the calcaneal tuberosity. A thin or atrophic heel fat pad contributes to the symptoms. Diagnosis may be difficult since more than one condition may exist at the same time. The athlete complains of heel pain of acute onset, but not generally associated with a traumatic episode. Tenderness is present directly beneath the calcaneal tuberosity or slightly distal to it. Symptoms are present in the morning upon rising; they tend to subside during the day, only to increase at the beginning of practice. During strenuous activity the pain may decrease again, but recur after a work-out. Runners find that they are unable to sustain their usual distance.

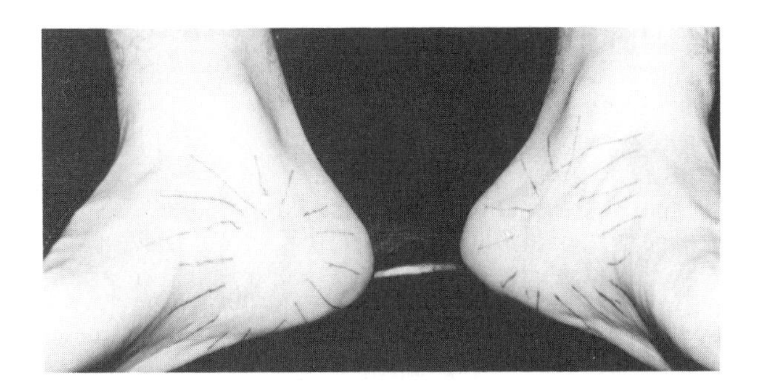

Figure 7 The foot of a 15-year-old male soccer player with acute bilateral plantar fascia rupture. The most symptomatic areas are plantar and plantar medial, as outlined on the skin. Conservative treatment failed, necessitating bilateral partial plantar fasciectomies. The player returned to practice 2 months postoperatively.

Radiography of the heel may reveal a heel spur, which is found in 50 percent of patients with calcaneodynia. However, it is difficult to implicate such a common finding as the sole cause of the pain. Bone scans may indicate periostitis or stress fracture in the tuberosity. A computed tomographic (CT) scan may confirm a stress fracture, but nerve conduction velocities are ineffective in revealing a nerve entrapment.

Treatment of calcaneodynia includes a heel lift fashioned from ½-inch-thick felt or closed foam rubber with a central cut-out in the tender area. The diameter of the aperture should be 4 cm so that the entire tender area is relieved of pressure. The hole may be eccentrically placed if the tender region extends into the distal medial aspect of the heel. This can be taped to the heel or glued into the shoe. A foot and ankle flexibility program is begun. If shoes are worn or cleats protrude against the soft tissue, new, properly fitted shoes are ordered. When symptoms persist, a foot orthosis with a similar cut-out in the heel is prescribed. NSAIDs are helpful.

Chronic pain in the heel may be related to repeated tearing and healing of the plantar fascia. An olive-sized mass may be palpable distal to the fascial insertion. Occasionally, injection of 1 ml of betamethasone (Celestone) mixed with 1 ml of 1 percent lidocaine (Xylocaine) is given. I do not recommend more than three injections at 1-month intervals. A 3-cm (1½-inch) 25-gauge needle is used and injection is made into the area of discrete tenderness. Relief of pain during injection indicates that the corticosteroid has been placed in the symptomatic region. Severe and disabling symptoms that last longer than 6 months and significantly alter performance may require surgical intervention. However, these patients represent a small percentage of symptomatic cases.

Surgical technique includes a plantar medial incision 5 cm in length above the heel pad, curving upward proximally at the heel and curving plantarward distally to the anteromedial border of the weight-bearing heel pad. Meticulous dissection is made with loupe magnification to avoid small branches of cutaneous nerves that may be present. The medial calcaneal nerve is identified posteriorly, and the nerve to the abductor digiti quinti is located at the posterior margin of the wound passing beneath the origin of the abductor hallucis muscle. Constricting bands of fascia are divided. The plantar fascia is then located deep to the heel fat pad and cleaned on its superficial and deep surfaces. An area of scarred aponeurosis may be visible, usually the size of a small olive; it may be more than 1 cm in length. The entire fibrotic region in the central part of the aponeurosis is excised. The specimen measures 2 cm. Palpation laterally in the wound ensures that the aponeurosis has been divided. Care is taken to protect neurocirculatory structures passing between the plantar aponeurosis and the inferior calcaneus. If a heel spur is present and palpable from beneath the heel, it is excised (Fig. 8). A compression dressing is applied postoperatively, and restricted weight bearing with crutches is prescribed until the wound heals. A foot orthosis is recommended early in rehabilitation. Competitive play is permitted when symptoms subside.

DISORDERS OF POSTERIOR HEEL

The differential diagnosis of disorders of posterior heel pad includes insertional tendinitis of the Achilles tendon, retrocalcaneal bursitis, and heel pain secondary to symptomatic posterolateral calcaneal process, "pump bumps," or calcaneal apophysitis (Sever's disease).

Insertional tendinitis of the Achilles tendon occurs at its insertion onto the posterior calcaneus; it encompasses the lower two-thirds of the surface of the latter. Diagnosis is made simply by palpating the posterior calcaneus at the insertion of the tendon. Tenderness is noted medially, posteriorly, and laterally. Radiographs are not helpful, although fragmentation of the posterior calcaneal apophysitis (Sever's disease) may be seen in athletes who have not completed their growth. A ½-inch elevation of the heel and NSAIDs are recommended for both conditions. A combined heel cord stretching and foot and ankle flexibility program is begun. Symptoms may continue for 6 months.

Retrocalcaneal bursitis (Haglund's disease) is caused by inflammation of the bursa that lies between the superior calcaneus and the anterior border of the Achilles tendon. The cause of retrocalcaneal bursitis is pressure and irritation on the bursa between the posterior superior calcaneal tuberosity and the Achilles tendon. Pain is elicited by medial and lateral palpation of the bursa anteriorly just above the tendon insertion. Symptoms are increased by passive dorsiflexion of the ankle. This can be confirmed by injecting 1 ml of 1 percent lidocaine into the bursa through a 25-gauge needle, with consequent relief of pain. X-ray films may reveal a prominent posterior superior tuberosity. Treatment includes a ½-inch heel lift, NSAIDs for 3 weeks, and a flexibility program for the foot and ankle. If symptoms do not subside over several months, excision of the bursa is recommended. The author prefers a medial longitudinal incision 3 cm long; the bursa is excised along with the portion of the posterior superior calcaneal tuberosity.

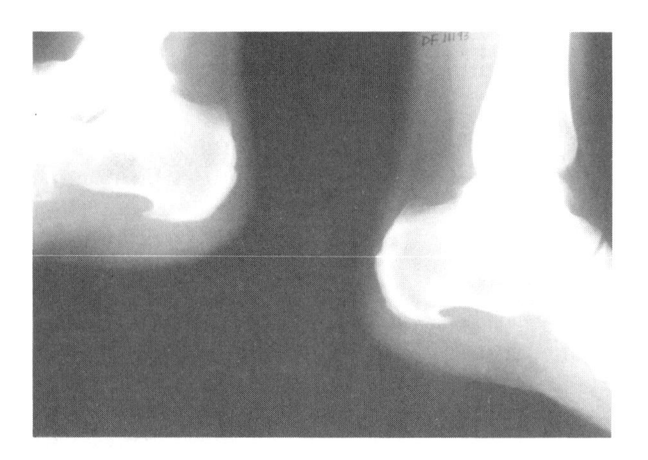

Figure 8 X-ray photograph of heels showing bilateral heel spurs. These lie beneath the plantar fascia and superficial to the nerve to the abductor digiti quinti. These may be removed during plantar fasciectomy to relieve pressure on the nerve if necessary.

A tight shoe with a stiff counter can irritate the posterior lateral calcaneus and cause a painful callus and periostitis ("pump bump"). A prominent lateral heel border emerges as a response to irritation from the shoe counter. Treatment includes changing the shoe type so that a padded heel counter comes into contact with the tender region. The shoe may be modified by cutting the counter to accommodate the tender area. A horseshoe-shaped pad made of ⅜-inch felt or closed cell foam rubber may be used to pad around the tender area. The aperture within the U should be large enough so that all the tender area is included in the opening. When the pad is placed in the shoe or taped to the heel, the entire area should remain nontender when pressure is exerted against the posterior lateral heel.

If these forms of conservative management fail to relieve symptoms, excision of the tuberosity is recommended. I prefer a medial longitudinal incision 4 cm in length. The posterior superior tuberosity of the calcaneus is removed along with the prominent "pump bump" on the lateral border with a high-speed oscillating micro-saw. A medial incision avoids a hypertrophic tender scar laterally. Palpation over the lateral area of prominence ensures that no bone protrusion remains. The attachment of the calcaneus is long and broad, and a portion of the tendon insertion is elevated to ensure that enough bone has been removed. If more than 50 percent of the Achilles tendon is detached, sutures are placed through the calcaneus to reattach that portion back to the bone. The patient is placed in a short leg cast. Failure of this procedure usually results from too little bone being removed. A cast will considerably decrease the amount of immediate postoperative pain. After 2 weeks the cast is removed and a foot ankle orthosis with a variable hinge is applied. Motion is increased gradually and the patient is permitted full weight bearing. The orthosis is removed 3 weeks later.

NERVE INJURIES

Traumatic neuritis can occur in any of the peripheral nerve branches to the foot. The *cutaneous branch of the superficial peroneal nerve* is irritated by pressure from a shoe at the tarsometatarsal or talonavicular joints more often than from a direct blow. Symptoms may be caused by osteophytes pressing upward from articular joint margins and entrapping the nerve against outer footwear. Symptoms are caused by stretching the irritated nerve. Irritation of the *lateral cutaneous branch of the superficial peroneal nerve* causes pain on the dorsum of the foot. A positive Tinel's sign may be elicited not only on the dorsum of the foot but also at the exit of the nerve from the deep fascia of the leg in the anterior compartment, 15 cm above the lateral malleolus. A fasciotomy may be necessary to relieve symptoms.

Trauma from both standing and walking may cause irritation of the *interdigital nerve* between the third and fourth metatarsal head (Morton's neuroma). The nerve in this area often receives branches from both the medial and lateral plantar nerves. It is less common for neuroma to occur in other interdigital nerves. Symptoms may be elicited by pressing the web space dorsally and plantarly between the finger and thumb while compressing the foot medially and laterally. The patient experiences paresthesia in the third and fourth toes. If symptoms are not relieved with a metatarsal pad or foot orthosis including a metatarsal pad, along with anti-inflammatory medication, surgical excision is indicated. A dorsal incision is recommended and loupe magnification is used to avoid injuring the artery that accompanies the nerve proximal to the neuroma. A flexibility program is started as soon as the wound heals, and return to play is permitted as symptoms subside.

Injury to the *proper digital nerve* is uncommon. Symptoms include metatarsalgia associated with paresthesia along the medial hallux. A Tinel's sign is elicited medially and proximally to the tibial sesamoid as the nerve passes through dense connective tissue before passing medially to the tibial sesamoid. If NSAIDs and appropriate padding do not relieve persistent symptoms that significantly alter performance, excision of the neuroma is recommended. The author's experience indicates that neurolysis on the weight-bearing aspect of the forefoot carries a poor prognosis. Neurectomy is the treatment of choice. The patient should be advised that the neuroma may recur proximally and require additional resection.

TARSAL TUNNEL SYNDROME

The tarsal tunnel syndrome is rarely caused by direct trauma to the tibial nerve at the posterior medial ankle. Post-traumatic causes are often associated with calcaneal or ankle fractures or dislocation at the subtalar or ankle joints. Unlike the carpal tunnel syndrome, the tarsal tunnel syndrome has many causes and occurs more often in middle-aged athletes. Symptoms begin insidiously, the only consistent symptoms being pain daily and occasionally at night, and burning on the sole with prolonged standing, walking, and running. Other symptoms are so variable and inconsistent that patients have often been diagnosed as having interdigital neuroma and undergo surgery, only for symptoms to persist postoperatively. Electromyography and nerve conduction velocity studies may give objective evidence of entrapment or injury to the posterior tibial nerve or its branches as it divides into the medial and plantar nerves.

Treatment of this condition is difficult. Anti-inflammatory medication together with a foot orthosis helps. A flexibility program performed twice daily is prescribed. Surgery is reserved for patients with symptoms that are significantly disabling and have caused modification of lifestyle. Neurolysis of the posterior tibial nerve and its branches is performed with loupe magnification under turniquet control.

The author has found that the most common causes of the tarsal tunnel syndrome are an abnormally low division of the posterior tibial nerve into the plantar nerves, a small vascular loop passing through the nerve at its terminus, giving a "vascular leash" effect, and varicosities encompassing the nerve. The most consistent operative finding is a thickened fibrotic region of the posterior tibial nerve within 1 cm of its division. Other anatomic variants of the nerve have been found in addition to those described. The ankle is splinted for 2 weeks postoperatively, after which a supervised physical therapy program is begun. The athlete should be advised that the recovery period may take 11 months.

ACUTE LIGAMENT SPRAINS

The mechanism of foot strain occurs most commonly through plantar flexion and inversion. Less commonly, forced dorsiflexion may occur. Strain is noted at the lateral tarsometatarsal joints, Chopart's joint, or subtalar joint. In addition to symptoms of lateral ankle ligament injuries, such as pain with giving way, tarsometatarsal strain produces pain with weight bearing at the fourth and fifth tarsometatarsal joints. Radiography may show only chip fractures dorsally. Treatment of the acute injury includes an Ace bandage, NSAIDs, and limited weight bearing with crutches. If symptoms are severe and pain persists, cast immobilization for 2 weeks may be necessary. A physical therapy program of whirlpool, power building, and use of a foot and ankle exerciser board follows. When the athlete returns to the field, a canvas ankle support may be necessary to help prevent plantar inversion. If symptoms persist, bone and CT scans help rule out stress fracture and arthritis. Subtalar strain is characterized by tenderness in the region of the sinus tarsi. This is treated in a similar manner. If symptoms persist, however, arthrography of the subtalar joint may reveal the formation of a cyst, a ligament tear, or outpouching of the posterior facet joint into the sinus tarsi. Symptoms may persist for several months. Surgical exploration is reserved only for the most severe cases unrelieved by conservative measures.

TRAUMATIC CYSTS

Traumatic cysts are uncommon in the foot but do occur at the metatarsophalangeal joints. They develop over a short time, giving symptoms of an expanding soft tissue mass in the web space, most commonly at the second metatarsophalangeal joint (Fig. 9). The forefoot appears broadened and the involved toe may become angulated, giving the appearance of a cross-over toe. The use of thick emulsion x-ray film and soft tissue technique may reveal the presence of a mass. CT scanning and MRI may confirm the presence of a mass, often shaped like a dumbbell, that is expanded superiorly and inferiorly. The cyst, filled with synovial fluid, is distinct from a ganglion cyst, which is chronic in nature and filled with gelatinous material. Treatment consists of simple excision through a dorsal incision, and the athlete is permitted to return to sports when the wound is healed.

TENDINITIS

Inflammation of tendons in the foot occurs primarily in those of the extrinsic muscles. The intrinsic muscles have short tendons with short excursions pulling generally in a straight line. Although cramping can occur, this is usually of short duration in the plantar aspect of the foot. Tendinitis occurs below the ankle. The most commonly affected tendon is the *tibialis posterior.* Tendinitis is present from the tendon insertion at the navicular tuberosity, extending beneath the medial malleolus into the posterior calf. Redness and swelling may accompany the symptoms. Painful active inversion against resistance aids in the diagnosis. Treatment of the mild condition includes NSAIDs, strapping, or an ankle orthosis as well as a foot and ankle flexibility program.

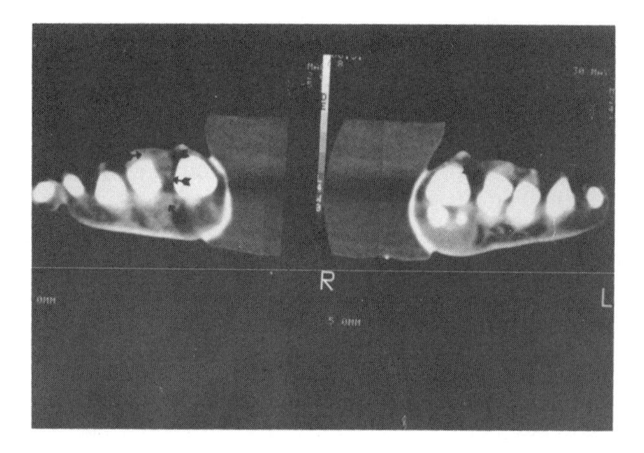

Figure 9 Axial CT scan of the right and left forefoot through the region of the metatarsal heads. Soft tissue view reveals "dumbbell"-shaped cystic mass between the right first and second metatarsal heads *(arrows)*. Simple excision allowed this dancer to return to the barre in 2 weeks.

Although uncommon, acute avulsion of the tendon from its insertion requires open repair. Through a 6-cm medial incision over the tendon, the ligamentous canal is opened and a tenosynovectomy performed if indicated. The tear may be transverse, in which case the tendon is advanced and attached through drill holes in the navicular tuberosity with 2–0 braided polyester sutures. A cast is applied for 6 weeks postoperatively. If a longitudinal disruption of the fibers is found, indicating a more chronic condition, this is repaired with 5–0 polyester sutures in a recurring manner. The tendon sheath is not closed. (The treatment of a chronic tear of the tibialis posterior tendon is not within the scope of this chapter.) Postoperatively, a cast is applied for 2 weeks followed by an ankle orthosis with a variable hinge. Therapy is then started. The brace is discontinued 6 weeks postoperatively.

Tendinitis or a partial tear of the *flexor hallucis longus*, seen primarily in dancers, is treated conservatively as above. The tear is longitudinal. If "trigger toe" occurs it is necessary to release the tendon in the tarsal tunnel through a posteromedial incision at the ankle. The tendon is repaired with a running 5–0 polyester suture and limited motion is begun after the wound heals.

Acute avulsion of the *peroneus brevis tendon* from its insertion into the fifth metatarsal styloid is caused by a lengthening contraction of the muscle with plantar inversion of the foot. Treatment includes ice, elevation, a compression dressing, and a limited weight-bearing (RICE) regimen until symptoms subside, usually in 3 weeks. A foot and ankle flexibility program is begun along with use of the foot and ankle exercise board as soon as symptoms permit. Longitudinal tears of the tendon are uncommon and often accompany disease of the ankle, including chronic lateral instability and dislocated peroneal tendons. Treatment includes repair at the time of correction of the underlying problem.

Acute tears of the *peroneus longus* are rare, occurring in middle-aged individuals. If chronic, the tear is resected and the proximal tendon is sutured to the peroneus brevis tendon.

SUGGESTED READING

Arrowsmith SR, Fleming LL, Allman FL. Traumatic dislocations of the peroneal tendons. Am J Sports Med 1983; 11:142–146.

Baxter DE, Thigpen CM. Heel pain—operative results. Foot Ankle 1984; 5:16–25.

Clanton TO, Butler JE, Eggert A. Injuries to the metatarsophalangeal joints in athletes. Foot Ankle 1986; 7:162–176.
DiRaimondo CV, Sammarco GJ. Tears of the peroneus brevis tendon. In: Proceedings of the Third Annual Summer Meeting of the American Orthopedic Foot and Ankle Society, Sante Fe, NM. Foot Ankle 1987; 8:113.
Jones DC. Bucket handle tears of the peroneus brevis. In: Proceedings of the Third Annual Summer Meeting of the American Orthopedic Foot and Ankle Society, Sante Fe, NM. Foot Ankle 1987; 8:113.
Miller CD. Personal communication. Cincinnati, OH, Blister Treatment Program, U.S. Naval Academy, 1987.
Sammarco GJ, Miller EH. Partial rupture of the flexor hallucis longus tendon in ballet dancers. J Bone Joint Surg 1979; 61A: 149–150.
Thompson F, Patterson AH. Rupture of the peroneus longus tendon. In: Proceedings of the Third Annual Summer Meeting of the American Orthopedic Foot and Ankle Society, Sante Fe, NM. Foot Ankle 1987; 8:114.

PLANTAR FASCIITIS

JOSEPH S. TORG, M.D.

Plantar fasciitis is characterized by low-grade pain, insidious in onset, located along the medial plantar fascia just distal to the calcaneus. Pain is often felt directly beneath the calcaneus at the insertion of the plantar fascia, and at times on the medial aspect of the calcaneus. It can be felt while walking, while running, and in mild cases only after running. The pain and inflammation is a result of repeated traction on the plantar fascia at its insertion into the calcaneus. Microtears and inflammation of the plantar fascia at the calcaneus can result from limited ankle dorsiflexion due to a tight gastrocnemius soleus complex. Swelling is not a predominant symptom and yet there is likely to be tenderness. A common roentgenographic finding is a heel spur on the lateral view.

An ice massage or a slush bath for 20 minutes several times a day can help alleviate discomfort temporarily, although it may not be successful for long periods.

Rest is often an effective early treatment for overuse injuries. For the treatment of plantar fasciitis, Clancy stated that rest is to be continued until there is pain-free palpation, at which point a gradual training program can be followed. Newell also prescribed the reduction of activity. Stretching and support are used in combination with rest to provide permanent relief.

Anti-inflammatory drugs are recommended for the treatment of plantar fasciitis. The injection of steroidal medication into the calcaneal attachment can help control inflammation, but care is necessary in cases in which symptoms persist, in order to avoid local iatrogenic complications. Oral medications include naproxen (Naprosyn), Feldene, indomethacin (Indocin), and ibuprofen (Motrin).

Furey presented a study of the treatment of 116 patients with plantar fasciitis. The characteristic physical findings were pain and tenderness in the area of the calcaneal tuberosity. Patients were treated with phenylbutazone, 100 mg four times a day for 1 week, then three times a day for 1 week. Heel pads and arch supports were also used. In 71 percent of the patients initially treated, there were excellent or good results after an average follow-up of 5.2 years. Aspirin and other anti-inflammatory agents can be used, but none of these should be administered without close supervision.

The pain that persists in plantar fasciitis can be alleviated with an adhesive strapping known as the low dye technique. Biomechanical problems, specifically abnormal pronation of the foot, have been identified as possible causal factors for plantar fasciitis. Whitesell stated that it stabilizes the head of the first metatarsal through plantar flexion, and decreases foot pronation. Newell reported that a positive response to this strapping is indicative of mechanical problems and can be used as a guide for orthotics. The use of moleskin instead of tape is suggested because it is stronger, provides more support, and wears better during exercise.

LOW DYE STRAPPING TECHNIQUE

Low dye strapping is recommended for treating conditions involving inflammation of plantar fascia, and traumatic or static sprains of the inner or outer longitudinal arches. It is also recommended for shin splints if the diagnosis is consistent with a musculotendinous inflammation along the medial border of the tibia.

Positioning. The foot is placed in a neutral position with plantar flexion of the first metatarsal ray (Fig. 1*A*).

Materials. The materials required are 1-inch adhesive tape and 3-inch moleskin. The moleskin is cut to approximate the plantar surface of the foot from just under the metatarsal heads to the calcaneus (Fig. 1*B*).

Instructions

Step 1. The moleskin is applied to the metatarsal head, pulled with slight tension downward through its midsection, and secured to the calcaneus (Fig. 1*C*).

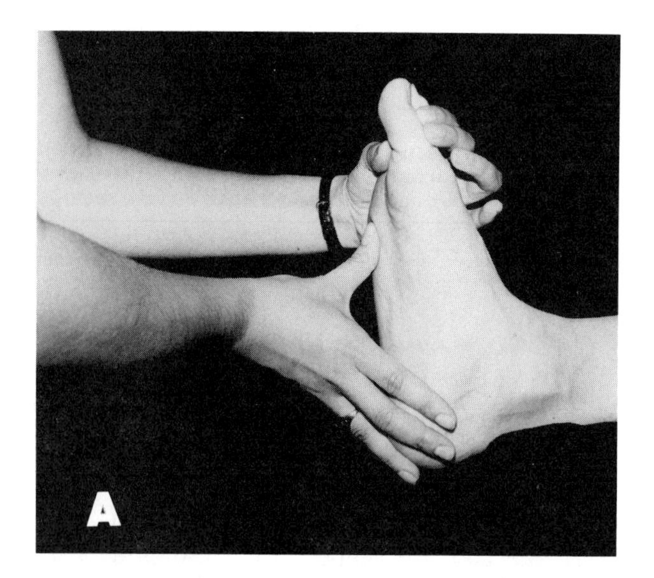

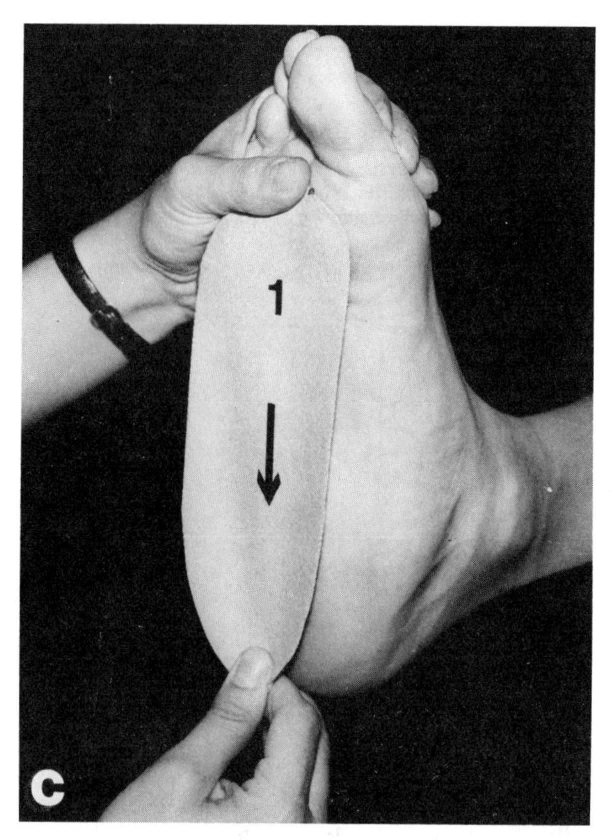

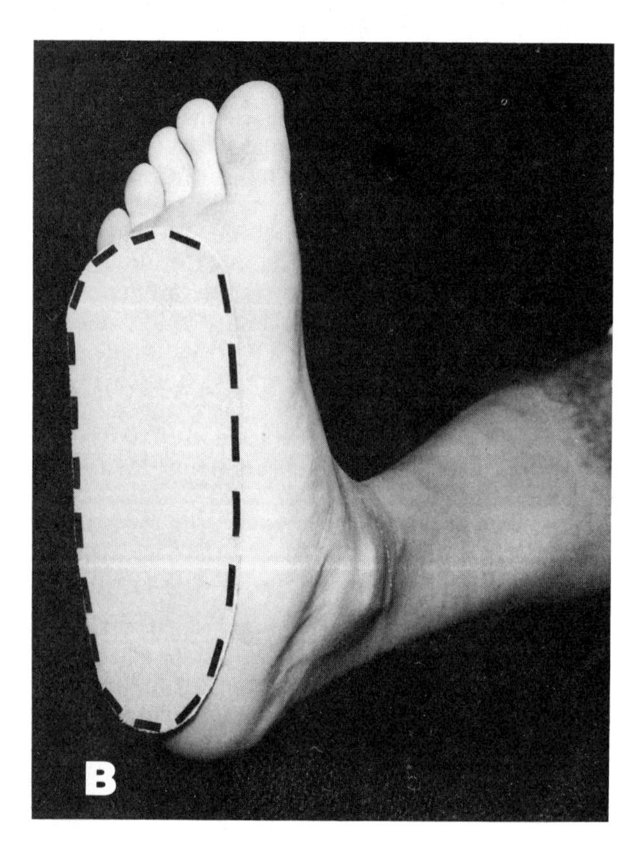

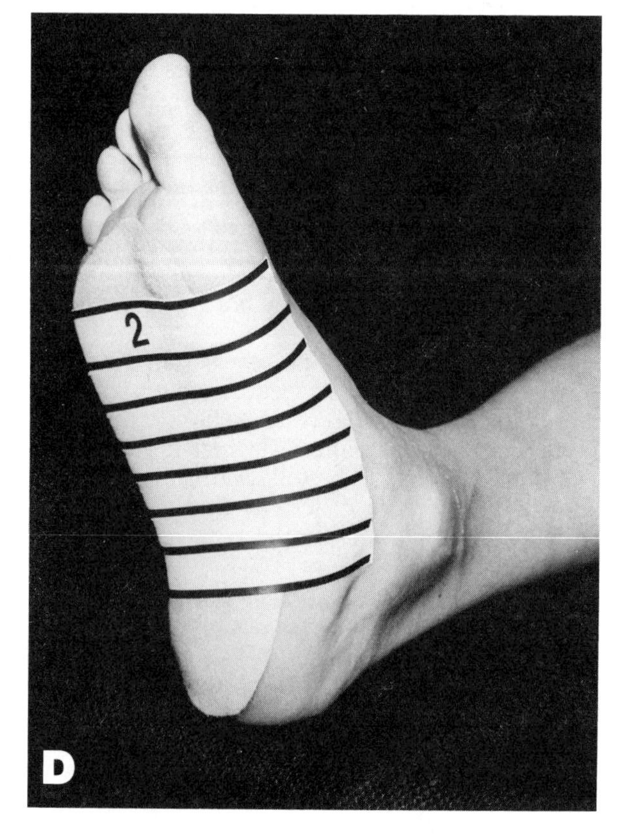

Figure 1 *A*, The foot is placed in the neutral position, with plantar flexion of the first metatarsal ray. *B*, A 3-inch moleskin is cut to fit the foot. *C*, The moleskin is applied to the plantar side of the foot, extending from just under the metatarsal heads to the calcaneus. *D*, The first piece of a 1-inch tape is applied, running upward underneath the plantar surface with equal pressure medially and laterally. Anchor strips are placed over the dorsal lateral aspect of the foot to secure the strapping. An additional anchor is placed around the posterior aspect of the calcaneus just beneath the malleoli.

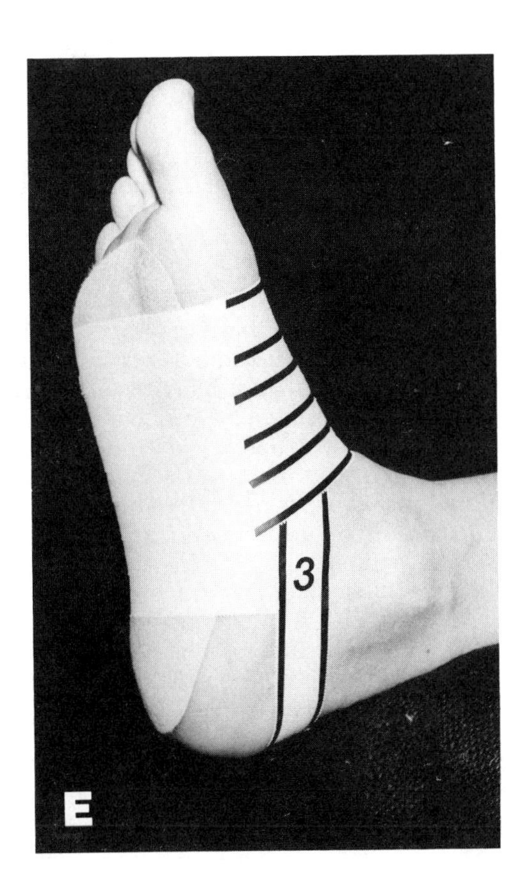

Step 2. Additional support is achieved by applying 1-inch strips of adhesive tape upward from underneath the plantar surface with equal pressure medially and laterally (Fig. 1*E*). The length of the tape should not exceed the height of an imaginary line running just beneath the malleoli to the outer borders of the first and fifth metatarsal heads.

Step 3. To secure the strapping, the anchor strips are placed over the dorsal aspect of the foot. An additional anchor is placed around the posterior aspect of the calcaneus just beneath the malleoli (Fig. 1*E*).

Orthotic correction is another effective method for treating plantar fasciitis. Similar in function to low dye strapping, orthotics correct the biomechanical problems responsible for the development of the injury. Refer to the chapter on orthotics.

There are several other methods for treating plantar fasciitis. Heel supports (which can be either soft or rigid: rigid when pain persists), arch supports, heel wedges, heel cups, donuts, and good running shoes are additional methods used to correct biomechanical problems.

Surgical treatment is advocated when conservative therapy fails. Clancy reported 15 patients in whom the results of surgical release of the plantar fascia were all excellent, and who returned to running in 8 to 10 weeks.

SUGGESTED READING

Bonci CM. Adhesive strapping techniques. Clin Sports Med 1982; 1:99–116.

Clancy WG. Runner's injuries. Part two: evaluation and treatment of specific injuries. Am J Sports Med 1980; 8:287–297.

Furey JG. Plantar fasciitis: the painful heel syndrome. J Bone Joint Surg 1975; 57-A:672–673.

Newell SG, Miller SJ. Conservative treatment of plantar fascial strain. Phys Sports Med 1977; 68–73.

Roy S. How I manage plantar fasciitis. Phys Sports Med 1986; 11: 127–131.

Whitesell J, Newell SG. Modified low dye strapping. Phys Sports Med 1980; 8:129–130.

STRESS FRACTURE OF THE TARSAL NAVICULAR

JOSEPH S. TORG, M.D.

Tarsal navicular stress fractures are an underdiagnosed source of prolonged disabling foot pain in young athletes. Eichenholtz and Levine, referring to all fractures of the tarsal navicular, stated that "the diagnosis is being missed with and without radiographs because this fracture is not being suspected." Towne and associates recognized the limitations of routine radiographs and, in a report of two stress fractures of this bone, suggested the need of "special roentgen views and laminography for detection," but without further elaboration. Goergen et al reported two stress fractures in runners and emphasized the importance of and difficulty involved in radiographic diagnosis. In the orthopaedic literature, Torg et al described the diagnosis, fracture patterns, complications, and possible etiology of 21 tarsal navicular stress fractures in 19 patients. They emphasized the orthopaedic management and stated that "the interval between the onset of symptoms and the diagnosis ranged from less than one month to thirty-eight months (mean interval 7.2 months)" because the fracture was not evident or because it was overlooked on the routine foot radiographs.

The tarsal navicular stress fracture is notoriously misdiagnosed. Because of the ill-defined nature of the pain and the difficulty of identifying the fracture in routine radiographs, there is often a sizable delay between the onset of symptoms and correct diagnosis.

Symptoms of the tarsal navicular stress fracture include the insidious onset of vague pain over the dorsum of the medial midfoot or over the medial aspect of the longitudinal arch. The pain is an ill-defined soreness or cramping, which is aggravated by activity and relieved by rest. Usually there is a well-localized tenderness over the tarsal navicular or along the medial longitudinal arch. There is little if any swelling and no discoloration or lumps. There may be an associated decrease in dorsiflexion or subtalar motion.

Stress fractures occur commonly in the weight-bearing bones of military recruits, distance runners, and others who participate in prolonged and vigorous activity. However, the occurrence of these lesions in the tarsal navicular appears to be either rare or infrequently recognized.

The circumstances surrounding the occurrence of navicular stress fractures suggest certain features that may contribute to the development of the lesion. The patients are all very active physically. Foot abnormalities, including a short first metatarsal and metatarsus adductus, as well as limited dorsiflexion of the ankle or limited subtalar motion, or both, are present in some patients and may concentrate stress on the tarsal navicular. The findings of sclerosis of the proximal articular border of the navicular narrowing of the talonavicular joint, talar breaking, accessory ossicles, and malalignment at the dorsal margins of the talonavicular and navicular-cuneiform joints in some patients may indicate the presence of some type of mechanical abnormality in the involved feet.

Microangiographic studies of the blood supply to the tarsal navicular demonstrate relative avascularity of the middle third of the bone. All these findings suggest the hypothesis that repetitive cyclic loading, associated with some as yet unidentified variations in foot structure, may result in fatigue failure through the relatively avascular central portion of the tarsal navicular.

Prompt diagnosis of tarsal navicular stress fractures requires appropriate radiographic studies. Routine standing anteroposterior, lateral, and oblique radiographs of the foot should be made when a tarsal navicular stress fracture is suspected. The tarsal navicular is frequently underpenetrated on these radiographs, and a coned-down anteroposterior radiograph centered on the tarsal navicular may be required for visualization. The continuity of the cortical bone of the navicular, especially on the anteroposterior radiograph, must be carefully examined, because when there is a fracture the lateral fragment resembles a separate tarsal bone and can easily be overlooked.

If the routine radiographic examination is normal or equivocal, a radionuclide bone scan of both feet should be obtained, using technetium-99m methylene diphosphonate. Localized augmented isotopic uptake is interpreted as abnormal (Fig. 1).

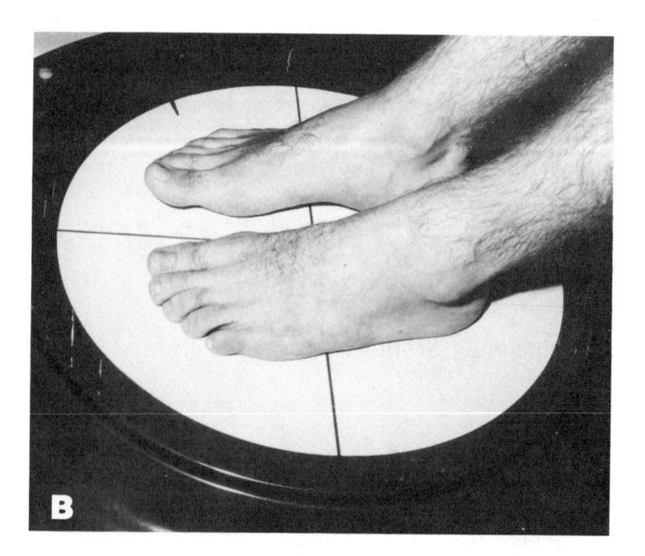

Figure 1 *A*, Radionuclide bone scanning was performed (starting in the upper left quadrant and moving clockwise) in the frontal, medial (right), plantar, and medial (left) positions. There is augmented isotope uptake in the left navicular and fourth metatarsal. In the frontal view the tarsal area is overlapped by that of the hindfoot, and it is difficult to localize the isotope uptake. On the medial (left) view the uptake is intensified in the region of the tarsal navicular; however, it is poorly localized because of other areas of augmented uptake. On the plantar view the areas of increased isotope uptake are best demonstrated and conform to the configuration of the navicular and the fourth metatarsal, respectively; stress fractures in both areas were documented. *B*, Plantar views are obtained with the soles of the patient's feet positioned on the face of the gamma camera. The patient leans posteriorly so that the isotope uptake from the body pool does not contribute to the uptake from the feet.

When the radionuclide bone scan indicates a lesion of the tarsal navicular but the routine radiographic examination is normal, tomograms of the tarsal navicular are required. The position of the foot for the tomographic examination is critical and should be established accurately under fluoroscopic guidance. Tomograms must be made with the tarsal navicular in the true anteroposterior position. To do this, the foot should be slightly inverted until the entire medial-lateral width of the tarsal navicular is demonstrated fluoroscopically (Fig. 2). Exact positioning for the anteroposterior tomogram is important because the typical stress fracture is in the sagittal plane through the center of the bone and is obscured by even slight obliquity with respect to the x-ray beam. Also, the dorsal surface of the tarsal navicular must be parallel to the plane of the tomographic cut, because in most cases an incomplete stress fracture is confined to the dorsal aspect of the bone and can be obscured if the tomographic plane is oblique (Fig. 3).

All the fractures in the series of Torg et al were in the sagittal plane and were located in the central third of the bone. Ten of the fractures were partial, involving only the dorsal cortex, and 11 were complete. Of the partial fractures, nine involved the proximal articular border (Fig. 4) and one the distal articular border (Fig. 5). Eleven of the fractures were complete (Fig. 6); 10 were nondisplaced and one was displaced. A transverse dorsal fracture fragment was associated with one partial fracture of the proximal articular border and with two complete fractures.

The 21 tarsal navicular stress fractures in this series could be divided into three separate groups: (1) uncomplicated fractures that went on to complete healing with treatment; (2) those in which there was a complication when they were first seen and in which treatment resulted in successful healing; and (3) those in which delayed union or nonunion developed despite treatment, or in which there was a recurrence of the fracture following treatment.

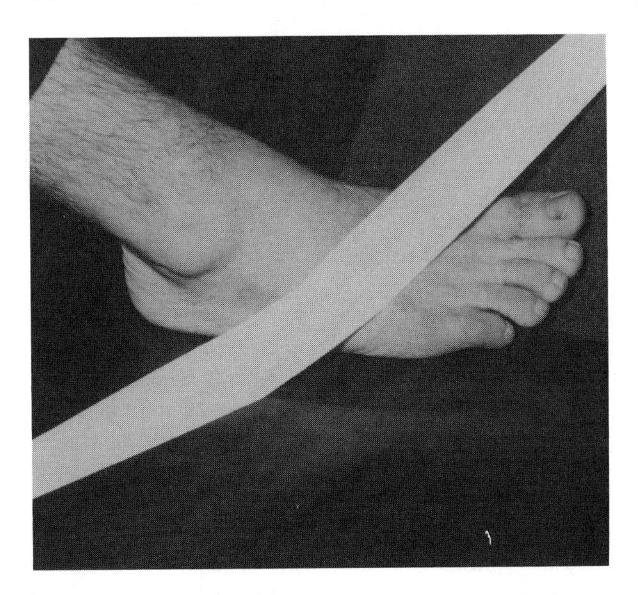

Figure 2 A foot is placed on a foam wedge and taped to the cassette in the correct position to make a so-called anatomic anteroposterior radiograph. The medial side of the forepart of the foot is elevated so that the entire foot is inverted. Fluoroscopy should be used to ensure proper positioning of the foot.

Of the 12 uncomplicated fractures that went on to successful healing, 10 were treated by immobilization in a plaster cast and non–weight bearing for 6 to 8 weeks, and two healed with only limitation of activity and continued weight bearing.

Two complicated fractures, one with acute displacement of the fragments and the other with an established nonunion and aseptic necrosis of the lateral fragment, were treated surgically at the outset, the first by open reduction and internal fixation and the second by medullary curettage and autogenous bone grafting (Fig. 7). Both fractures were immobilized in a non-weightbearing cast for 6 weeks postoperatively, and both healed (Fig. 8).

In seven patients the result of treatment was either a delayed union, a nonunion, or a refracture after healing. All seven had been permitted to continue weight bearing during the initial treatment. In two of these seven fractures, union was delayed, but healing occurred after immobilization in a non-weightbearing cast for 8 weeks in one and 18 weeks in the other. A third fracture, initially treated in a weightbearing cast for 8 weeks, went on to nonunion, which was successfully treated by an inlay bone graft and internal fixation, followed by immobilization in a non-weightbearing cast for 8 weeks. The other four patients were disabled and unable to participate in sports activity as a result of the fractures. One patient was a professional basketball player with a complete, nondisplaced fracture associated with a dorsal transverse fragment. Initially he attempted to continue playing on the injured foot, but eventually the fracture was immobilized in a series of partial-weightbearing casts. The fracture healed, but marked osteoporosis accompanied by pain developed. Subsequent attempts to return to playing basketball resulted in recurrence of the fracture and continued disability 42 months after the initial injury.

The other three fractures that resulted in disability were partial, proximal, undisplaced fractures, one having an associated dorsal transverse fragment. One was treated with a weightbearing plaster cast, and the other two with limitation of activity and weightbearing. Of these three patients, the first, a professional basketball player whose treatment consisted of limitation of activity and continued weight bearing, had a refracture at 12 months and was still disabled at 24 months. The second, a recreational distance runner who was similarly treated, had delayed union and was still disabled at 16 months. The third, a recreational tennis player who was treated with a weightbearing cast, had a nonunion and was still disabled at 30 months.

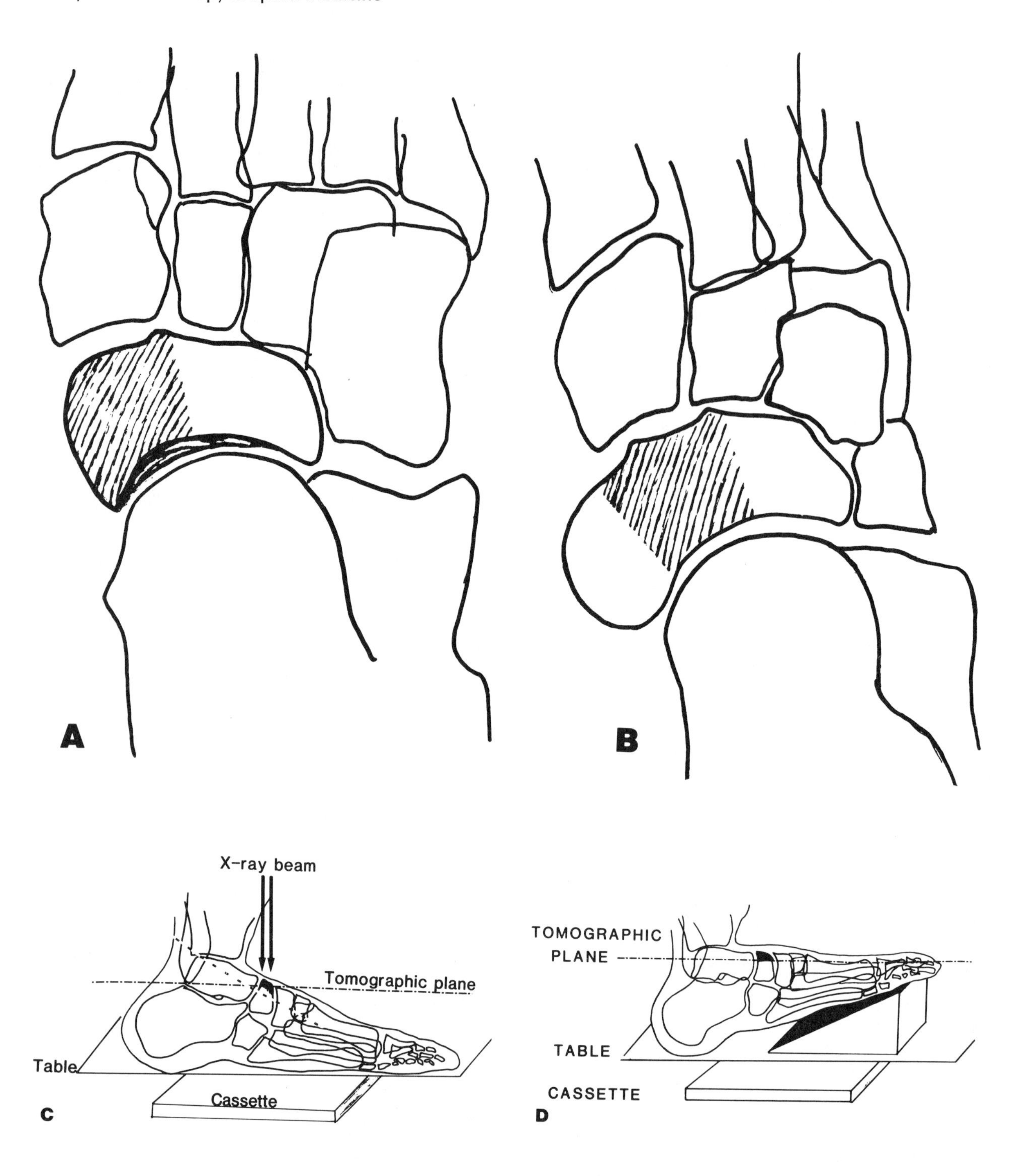

Figure 3 *A*, Standard anteroposterior tomogram position. The foot is flat on the table. The dorsal surface of the navicular (*shaded area*) and the long axis of the talus and the navicular are oblique to the tomographic plane. *B*, Anatomic anteroposterior tomogram position. The forefoot is lifted off the table with a wedge so that the dorsal surface of the navicular (*shaded area*) and the long axis of the talus and the navicular are parallel to the tomographic plane. *C*, Standard anteroposterior tomogram position. On this view the central third of the navicular (*shaded area*) is seen obliquely. Also, the undersurface of the navicular is usually seen because the x-ray beam is not tangential to the talonavicular joint. *D*, Anatomic anteroposterior tomogram position. On this view the central third of the navicular (*shaded area*) is seen en face and the x-ray beam is tangential to the talonavicular joint.

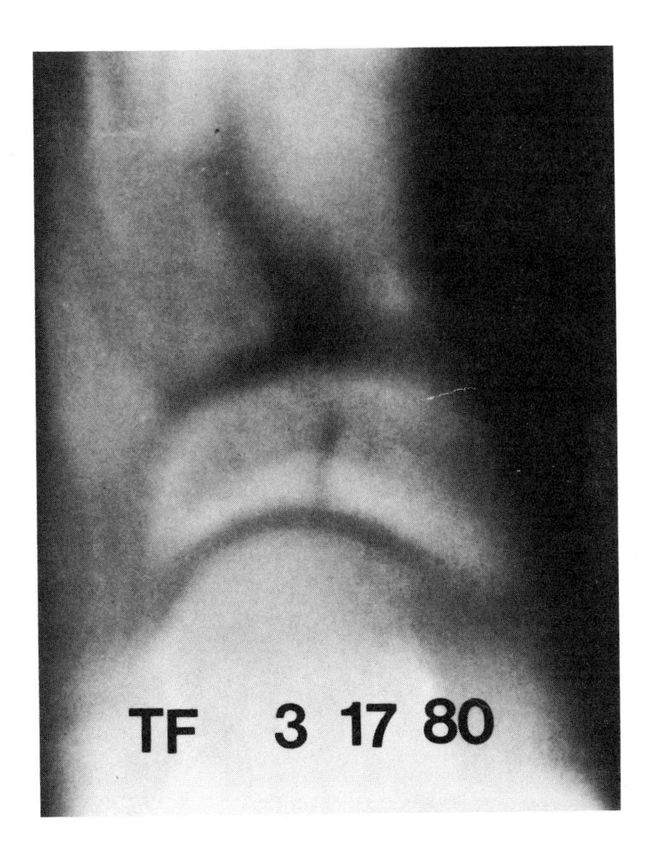

Figure 4 Anteroposterior tomogram of the right foot of a 17-year-old high-school player with a partial proximal stress fracture of the tarsal navicular. The tomogram was made 3 months after the onset of the symptoms and shows a partial stress fracture involving the proximal articular border of the tarsal navicular, but the distal articular border as seen here and on comparison cuts showed no evidence of fracture. Deeper sections also showed that the fracture was limited owing to the dorsal aspect of the bone.

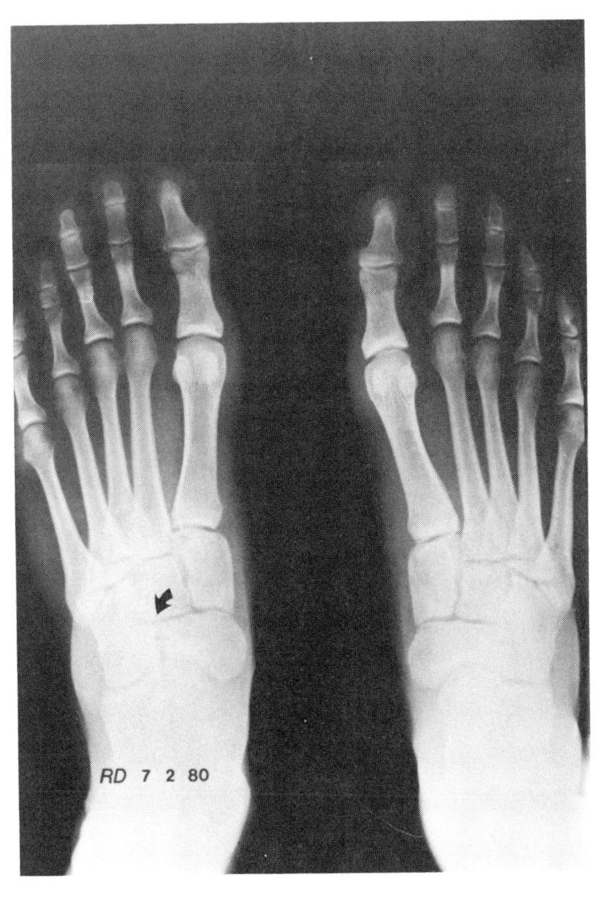

Figure 6 Complete stress fracture involving the left tarsal navicular in a 15-year-old high-school basketball player is visualized on routine anteroposterior roentgenographic views.

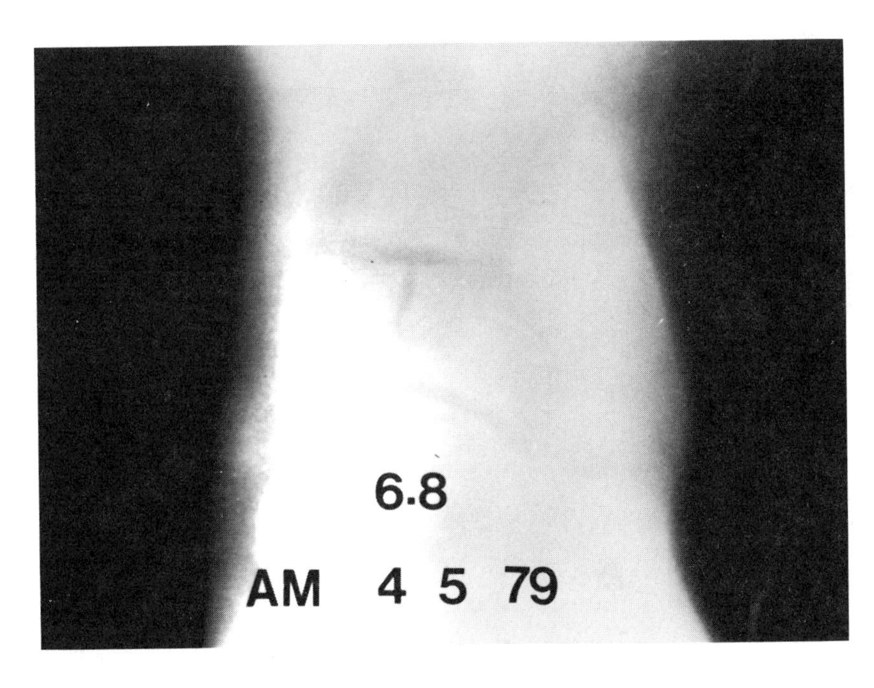

Figure 5 Tomogram of a 17-year-old middle-distance runner made 1 month after the onset of symptoms shows a partial stress fracture involving the distal articular border of the tarsal navicular. This tomogram and companion sections revealed that the proximal articular border was intact. A deeper selection did not show the fracture, which indicates that it was limited to the dorsal aspect of the bone.

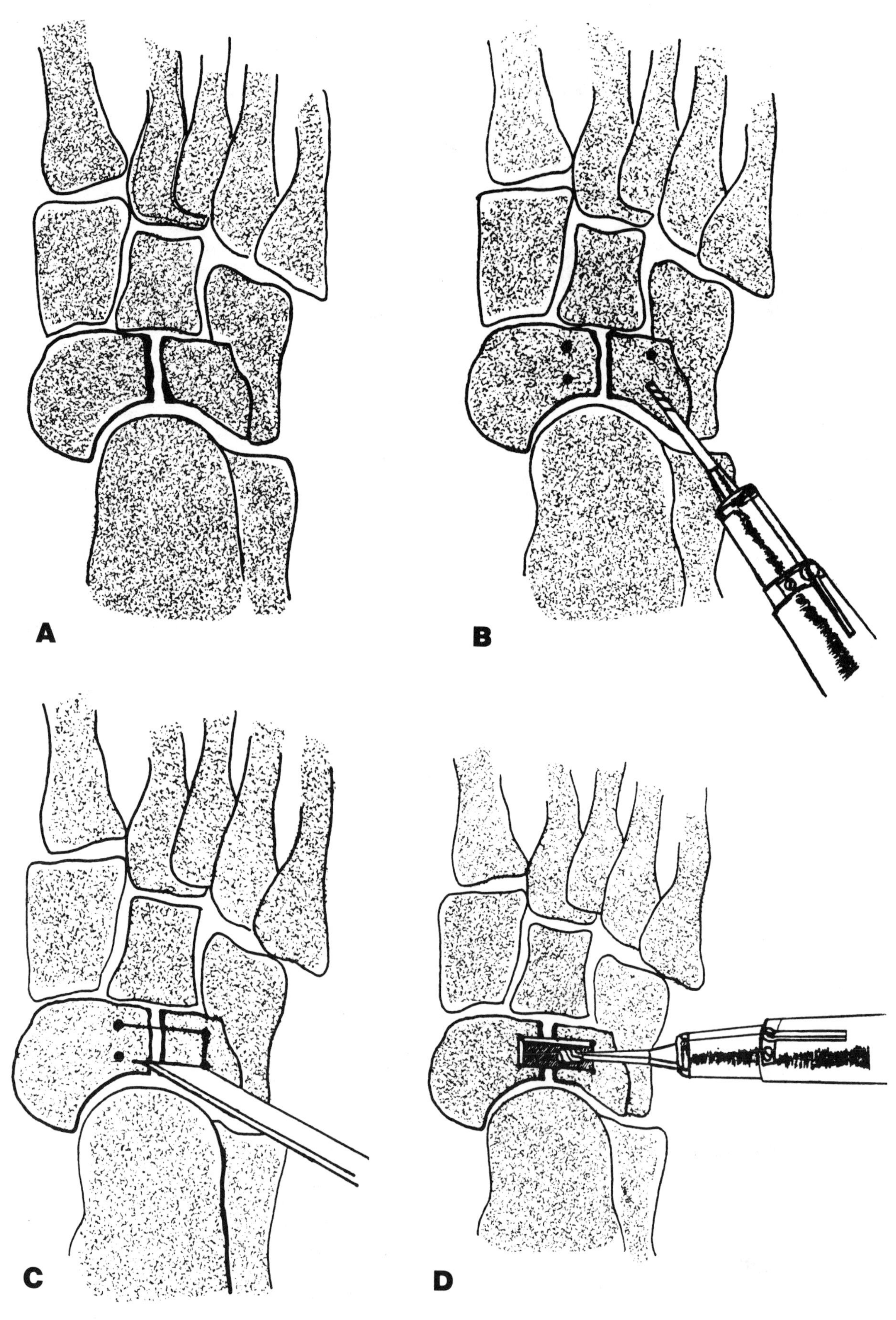

Figure 7 *See legend on opposite page.*

Figure 7 *A*, In instances of established nonunion of a tarsal navicular stress fracture, with or without aseptic necrosis of one of the fragments, medullary curettage and inlaid bone grafting is indicated. If a fibrous union exists, do not attempt to reduce the fracture. Do not excise sclerotic fragments. If there is motion, internal screw fixation is indicated. *B*, A rectangular piece of bone measuring approximately 0.7 by 2.0 cm, centered over the fracture, is outlined with four drill holes. *C*, The outlined cortical fragment is then excised with an osteome. *D*, The sclerotic bone in the medullary canal is removed with a drill. *E*, An autogenous cortical graft, obtained from the anteromedial aspect of the distal part of the tibia, is carefully contoured with a high-speed burr and placed in the previously created defect. The periosteum, subcutaneous tissues, and skin are then closed in layers, and immobilization in a non-weightbearing toe-to-knee cast is continued for 6 weeks.

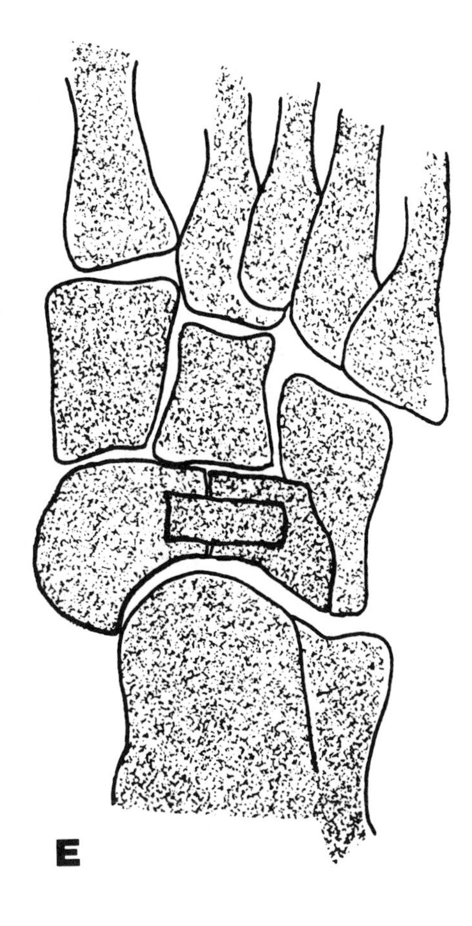

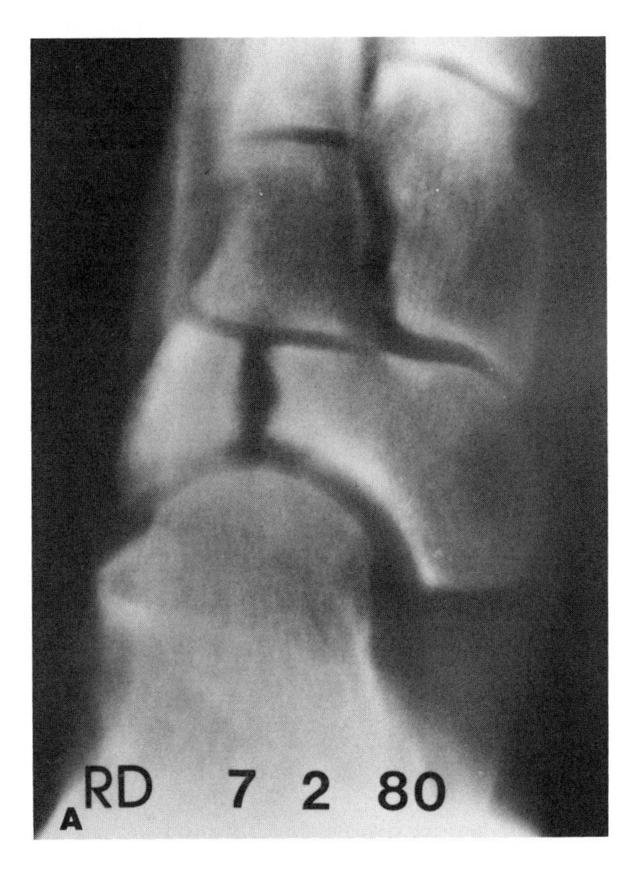

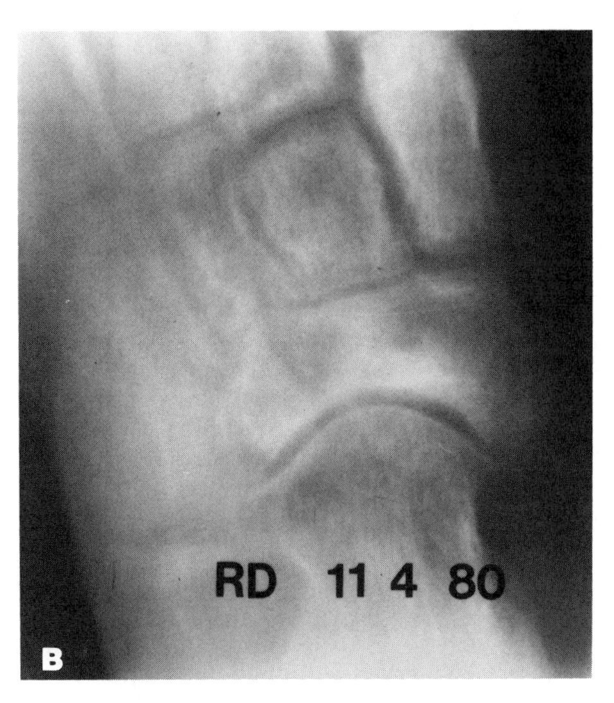

Figure 8 *A*, Nonunion of a stress fracture of the tarsal navicular with aseptic necrosis of the lateral fragment. *B*, Roentgenograms following medullary curettage and inlaid bone graft without attempt at reduction of fracture demonstrate complete healing.

TREATMENT GUIDELINES

On the basis of the above experience, the author recommends the following guidelines for management of tarsal navicular stress fractures:

1. Uncomplicated partial fractures and nondisplaced complete fractures of the tarsal navicular should be treated by immobilization in a plaster cast with non–weight bearing for 6 to 8 weeks. The decision to allow a return to weight bearing and activity should be guided by the patient's clinical picture as well as roentgenographic evidence of the union.

2. Complete displaced fractures can be treated with either immobilization in a plaster cast with non–weight bearing for 6 to 8 weeks or open reduction and internal fixation, followed by immobilization and non–weight bearing for 6 weeks.

3. Fractures complicated by delayed union or nonunion should be treated with medullary curettage and inlaid bone grafting. In these situations, a fibrous union may exist and no attempt should be made to reduce the fragments. If the fragments are mobile, internal fixation should be effected using a malleolar screw. After medullary curettage and inlaid bone grafting, with or without internal fixation, the patient should be placed in a non-weightbearing short-leg cast for 6 to 8 weeks. Again, mobilization and return to activity should depend on clinical and roentgenographic evidence of healing. It should be noted that in fractures treated by bone grafting, the healing course may be protracted and firm bony union may not occur for 3 to 6 months.

4. Partial fractures complicated with a small dorsal transverse fracture may require excision of the dorsal fragment.

5. Complete fractures complicated by a large dorsal transverse fracture will go on to union with immobilization and do not require excision of the fragment.

6. Associated dorsal talar beaks should be excised. Apart from these and the small dorsal transverse fragments, sclerotic fragments associated with delayed union and nonunion should not be excised, but treated with medullary curettage and inlaid bone graft as indicated.

SUGGESTED READING

Bateman JK. Broken hock in the greyhound: repair methods and the plastic scaphoid. Vet Rec 1958; 70:621–623.

Eichenholtz SN, Levine DB. Fractures of the tarsal navicular bone. Clin Orthop 1964; 34:142–157.

Goergen TG, Venn-Watson EA, Rossman DJ, et al. Tarsal navicular stress fractures in runners. Am J Roetgenol 1981; 136:201–203.

Pavlov H, Torg JS, Freiberger RH. Tarsal navicular stress fractures: radiographic evaluation. Radiology 1983; 148:641–645.

Torg JS, Pavlov H, Cooley LH, et al. Stress fractures of the tarsal navicular. J Bone Joint Surg 1982; 63-A:700–712.

Towne LC, Blazina ME, Cozen LN. Fatigue fracture of the tarsal navicular. J Bone Joint Surg 1970; 52-A:376–378.

FRACTURES OF THE BASE OF THE FIFTH METATARSAL DISTAL TO THE TUBEROSITY: THE JONES FRACTURE

JOSEPH S. TORG, M.D.

Proximal fifth metatarsal fractures can be separated into two distinct types: (1) a fracture of the tuberosity and (2) a fracture of the metatarsal shaft within 1.5 cm of the tuberosity.

The latter fracture distal to the tuberosity has recently been described as a troublesome fracture to manage. It requires a prolonged immobilization, has a high propensity for nonunion, and refracture after union is common after conservative treatment.

Fractures of the base of the fifth metatarsal distal to the tuberosity were first described by Jones in 1902. He reported four such fractures, including his own, which he sustained while dancing; all four healed with conservative treatment. In 1927 Carp reported 21 fractures, five of which went on to delayed union. He stated that these fractures tended to heal poorly and that a poor blood supply was the cause. In 1975 Dameron reported 20 patients, five of whom needed a surgical procedure to obtain union. He also reported prolonged healing times for 15 patients treated conservatively, but concluded that the initial treatment did not influence the final results. Dameron's surgical approach, a sliding bone graft procedure, was suggested early in the clinical course for professional athletes.

In 1978 Kavanaugh et al reported on 23 fractures of the base of the fifth metatarsal distal to the tuberosity. The average age of their patients was 20.3 years. The athletes sustaining this fracture most often were football and basketball players. Kavanaugh advised intramedullary screw fixation for young competitive athletes, selected recreational athletes, and nonathletes with nonunions. Delayed union occurred in 12 of 18 fractures treated conservatively. The fractures united in all of the 13 surgically treated patients, but in six of these patients there were complications. These included three fractured screws, two screws that missed the medullary canal, and pain in one patient that necessitated screw removal.

Kavanaugh et al also found that several patients treated with non-weightbearing plaster casts (10 to 12 weeks) went on to nonunion, and concluded that plaster immobilization and non–weight bearing was unnecessary. Likewise, Zelko et al concluded that the clinical course did not appear to be influenced by the type of early treatment.

In 1984 Torg et al reported 46 fractures of the base of the fifth metatarsal, distal to the tuberosity, which were treated and followed for a mean of 40 months. They delineated roentgenographic criteria, which were used to define three types of fractures: (1) acute fractures, (2) those with delayed union, and (3) those with nonunion and complete obliteration of the medullary canal by sclerotic bone.

The characteristic features of the acute fractures were no history of previous fracture, although the patient may have had prodromal pain or discomfort; no intramedullary sclerosis; a fracture line with sharp margins and no widening or radiolucency; and minimal cortical hypertrophy or evidence of periosteal reaction to chronic stress (Fig. 1*A*). These roentgenographic features are not characteristic of an acute fracture in the usual sense of the term. Presumably the acute fractures in the series were located at the site of a pre-existing stress concentration or were in the lateral part of the cortex, and became disabling when they extended across the entire diaphysis. Most important was the absence of intramedullary sclerosis.

The distinguishing features of the delayed unions were a previous injury or fracture, or both; a fracture line that involved both cortices with associated periosteal bone; a widened fracture line with adjacent radiolucency due to bone resorption; and evidence of intramedullary sclerosis (Fig. 2*B*).

The features of the nonunions were a history of repetitive trauma and recurrent symptoms; a wide fracture line with periosteal new bone and radiolucency; and a complete obliteration of the medullary canal at the fracture site by sclerotic bone, the hallmark of nonunion (Fig. 3*A*).

Of the 25 acute fractures in the series of Torg et al, 15 were treated with non-weightbearing toe-to-knee casts, and 14 healed in a mean of 7 weeks (see Fig. 1). Only four of the other 10 that were treated with various weightbearing methods progressed to union.

Of 12 of the patients with delayed union, one refused treatment, one was treated with a bone graft, and 10 were treated initially by immobilization of the limb in a plaster cast and weight bearing. Of these 10 fractures, seven healed in a mean of 15.1 months (see Fig. 2) and three eventually required grafting for nonunion.

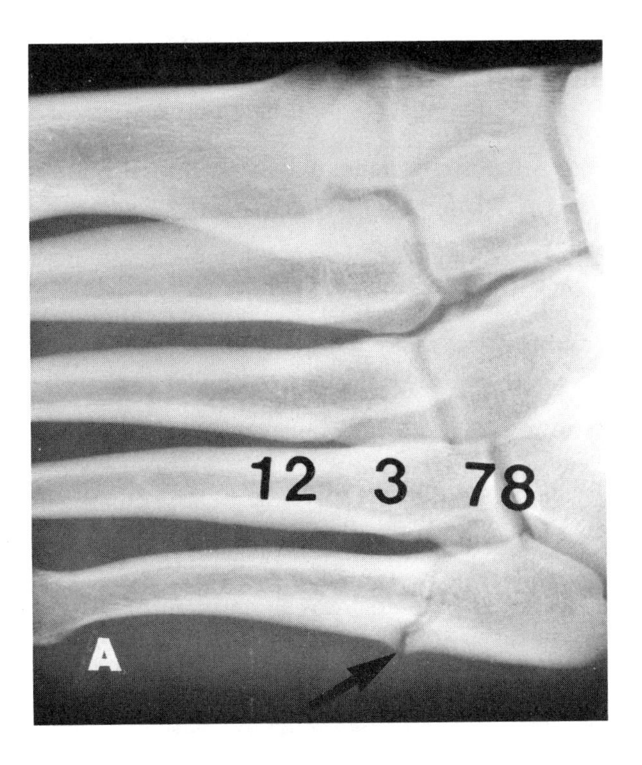

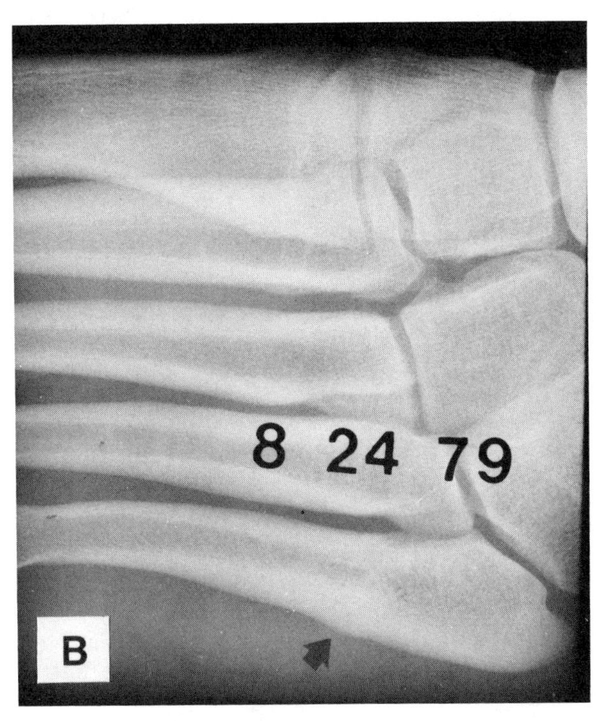

Figure 1 *A*, Oblique roentgenogram of the fifth metatarsal, demonstrating an acute fracture distal to the tuberosity. There is some cortical hypertrophy, an indicator of chronic stress, but the line is narrow, involves both cortices, and (most important) is not associated with intramedullary sclerosis. *B*, After treatment in a non-weightbearing toe-to-knee cast for 6 weeks, there was complete healing. A roentgenogram made 9 months after the initial injury shows maintenance of fracture healing.

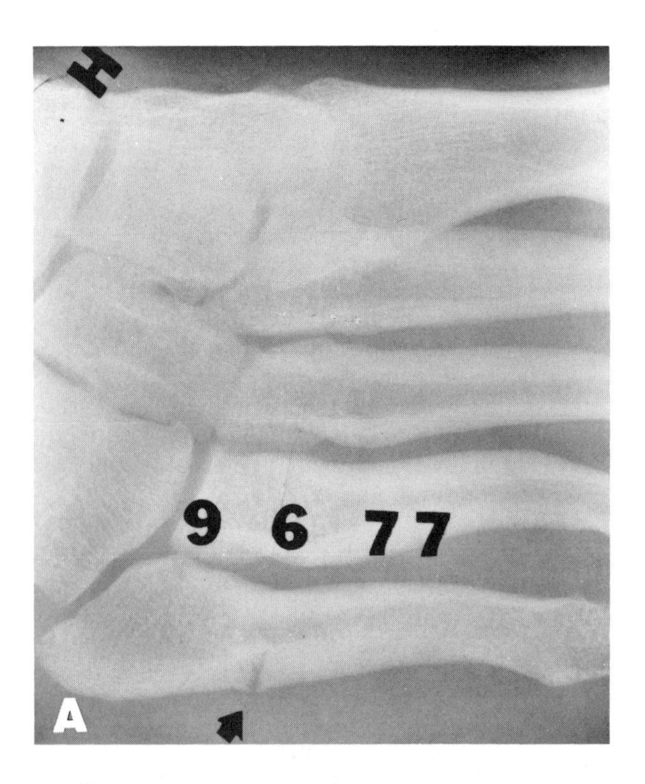

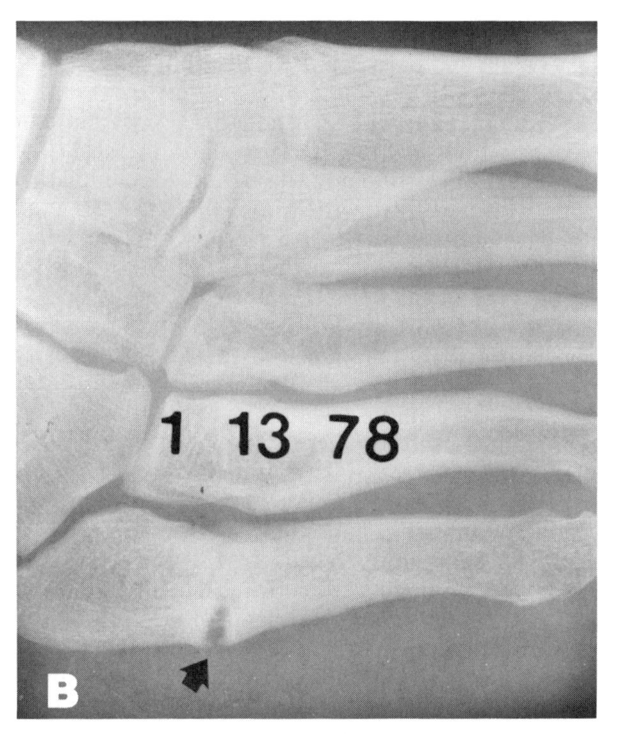

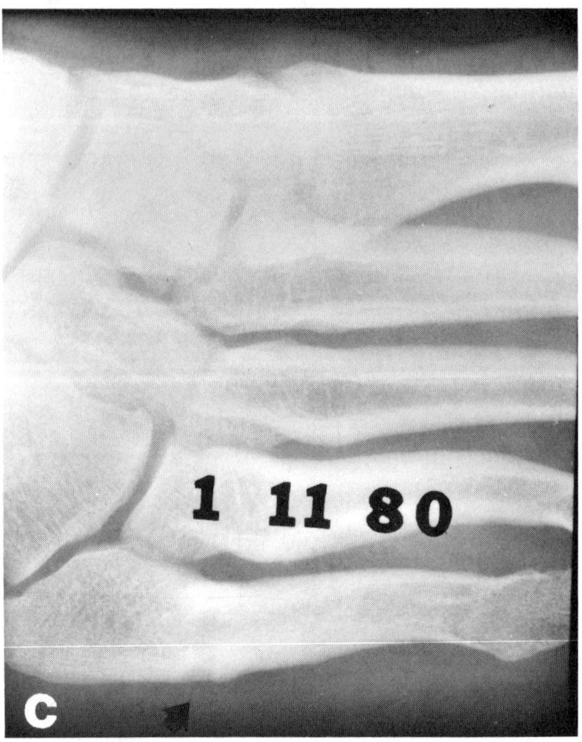

Figure 2 *A*, Oblique roentgenogram of the fifth metatarsal, demonstrating an acute fracture distal to the tuberosity. The patient was initially treated with a walking cast for 6 weeks. *B*, Four months after injury, the fracture line is seen to involve both cortices, and there is some angular deformity, a moderate degree of intramedullary sclerosis, and widening of the fracture line. *C*, Two years later, complete healing of the fracture line has occurred with minimal deformity, and there is recanalization of the medullary canal.

Of the nine nonunions in this series, which were treated primarily with medullary curettage and bone grafting, eight healed in a mean of 3 months (see Fig. 3).

Twenty fractures were treated surgically with curettage of the sclerotic bone that obliterated with intramedullary cavity and inlaid autogenous corticocancellous graft. Of these 20, 19 progressed to complete healing and one to asymptomatic nonunion. No other complications were associated with the procedure of Torg et al.

These authors concluded that the treatment of choice for acute fractures is immobilization of the limb in a toe-to-knee cast with non–weight bearing. Fractures with delayed union may eventually heal if they are treated conservatively, but in an active athlete with delayed union, medullary curettage and bone grafting are indicated. Surgery is also indicated for fractures that have progressed to symptomatic nonunion.

DeLee et al reported on 10 patients with stress fractures of the fifth metatarsal shaft. They defined stress fracture as a "spontaneous fracture of normal bone which resulted from summation of stresses, any of which, by themselves, would be harmless." Their criteria included (1) a history of prodromal symptoms over the lateral aspect of the foot prior to the acute episode that precipitated the patient's seeking medical care; (2) roentgenographic evidence of stress phenomenon in the bone, a radiolucent fracture line, periosteal reactions, excessive callus on the lateral cortical margin, and intramedullary sclerosis that obviously preceded the acute episode of pain; and (3) no history of pre-

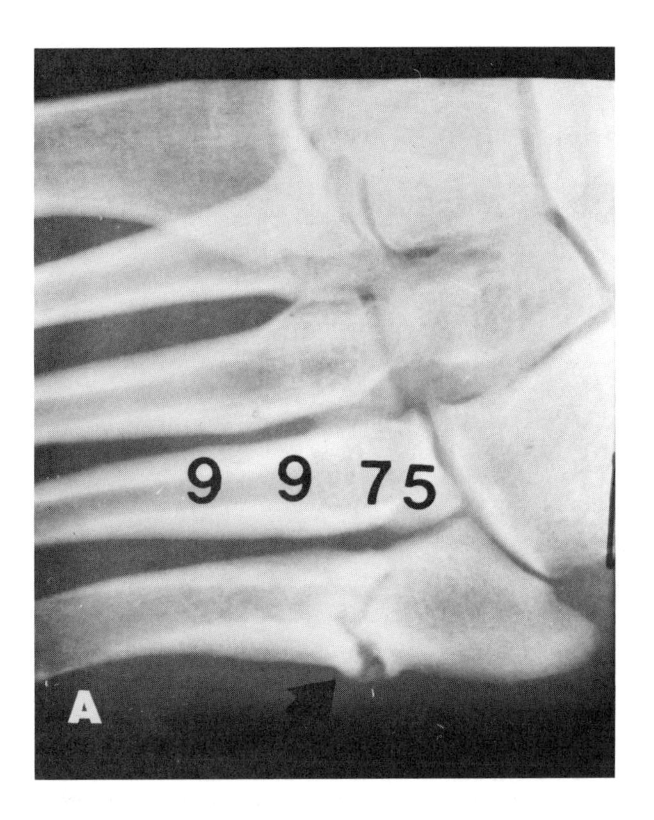

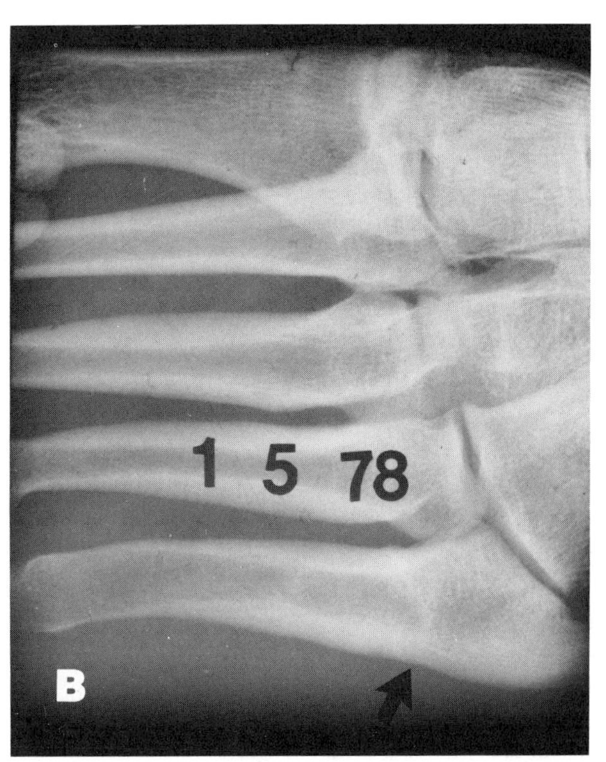

Figure 3 *A*, Oblique roentgenogram demonstrating nonunion. Note the widening of the fracture line, cortical hypertrophy, and dense intramedullary sclerosis completely obliterating the medullary canal. *B*, The fracture had demonstrated clinical and roentgenographic healing at 7 weeks. Follow-up roentgenogram 2½ years postsurgery demonstrates persistence of healed state.

vious treatment for a fracture of the fifth metatarsal.

All patients in the series of DeLee et al underwent internal fixation of the fracture by insertion of a screw in the intramedullary canal of the fifth metatarsal. The average period of follow-up was 14.5 months. The authors defined clinical union as the absence of tenderness and the ability to bear weight. The average time to union was 7.5 weeks, with a range of 6 to 8 weeks. They reported no wound infections or other operative complications.

Three patients complained of tenderness over the head of the screw, and five patients complained of pain under the head of the fifth metatarsal. Four of these five patients were able to obtain relief by wearing a metatarsal pad.

DeLee et al explained this metatarsal pain as an alteration in metatarsal stiffness and/or axial alignment due to the screw. No cases of refracture were reported.

The average time to return to competitive athletics was 8.5 weeks, with a range of 7 to 14 weeks. Seven of the 10 patients required shoe modification.

Surgical procedures for delayed or nonunion fractures of the base of the fifth metatarsal distal to the tuberosity are (1) medullary curettage and inlay bone grafting and (2) closed axial intramedullary screw fixation.

MEDULLARY CURETTAGE AND INLAY BONE GRAFTING

Torg et al described obliteration of the medullary canal by dense sclerotic bone along the margins of the fracture; this bone has a tendency to progress to a nonunion. The authors describe the purpose of the surgical procedure as being to reestablish the continuity of the medullary canal by removing the sclerotic bone, and to facilitate healing by insertion of an inlay bone graft.

Surgical Procedure

The base of the fifth metatarsal is approached through a curvilinear dorsolateral incision. The fracture site is exposed subperiosteally, and a rectangular section of bone measuring 0.7 by 2.0 cm, centered over the fracture, is outlined by four drill holes (Fig. 4*A*) and removed with a sharp osteotome (Fig. 4*B*). The medullary cavity is then curetted or drilled until all the sclerotic bone has been removed and the continuity of the medullary canal has been reestablished (Fig. 4*D*). An autogenous corticocancellous bone graft measuring 0.7 by 2.0 cm is then removed from the anteromedial aspect of the distal end of the tibia through a second incision, with care taken to contour the graft with a high-speed burr so that the cortical portion of the graft fits accurately

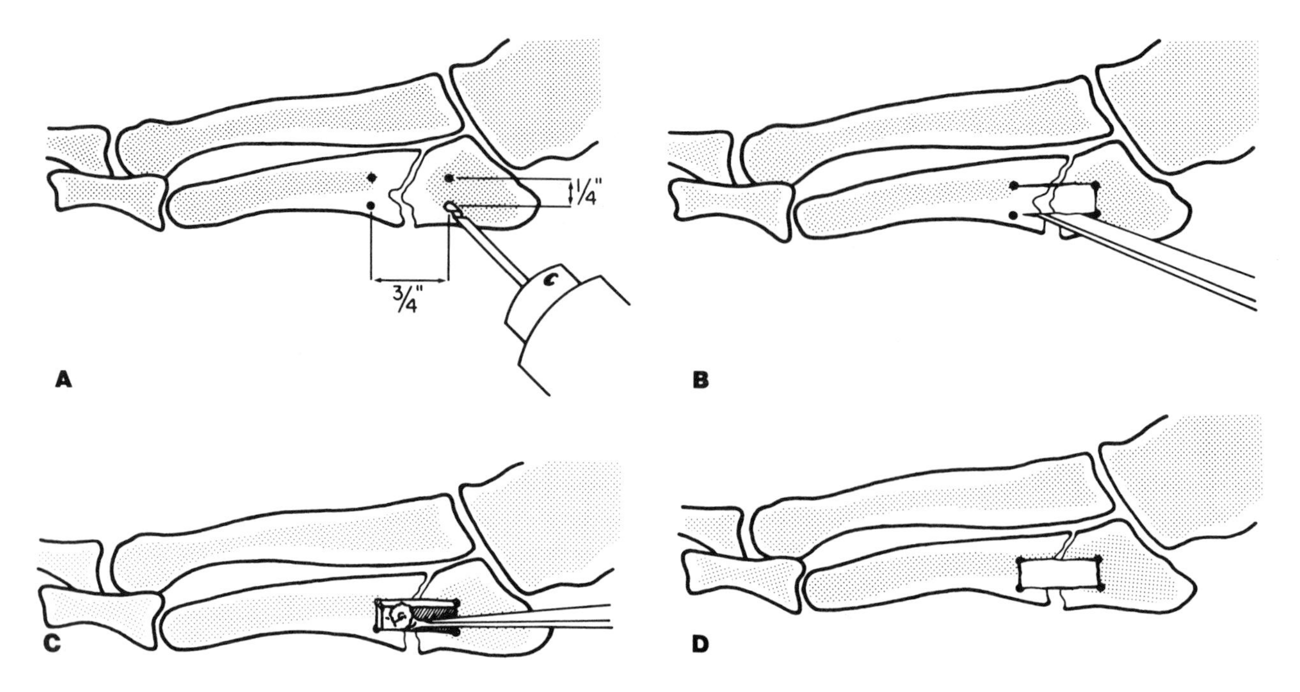

Figure 4 *A*, Subperiosteal exposure of the base of the fifth metatarsal, distal to the tuberosity, through a dorsolateral curvilinear incision reveals the fracture line and associated cortical hypertrophy. A rectangular piece of bone measuring approximately 0.7 by 2.0 cm, centered over the lateral aspect of the fracture, is outlined with four drill holes. *B*, The outlined cortical fragment is then excised with an osteotome. *C*, To reestablish the continuity of the medullary canal, the sclerotic bone in the medullary canal is removed with a curet or drill, or both. *D*, An autogenous cortical graft, obtained from the anteromedial aspect of the distal part of the tibia, is carefully contoured with a high-speed burr and placed in the previously created defect. The periosteum, subcutaneous tissues, and skin are then closed in layers, and immobilization in a non-weightbearing toe-to-knee cast is continued for 6 weeks.

into the rectangular cortical defect and does not protrude into the medullary canal and occlude it (Fig. 4*C*). The periosteum, subcutaneous tissue, and skin are closed sequentially in layers, and attention is turned to the graft site in the tibia. To prevent the formation of a stress raiser, the section of bone removed from the fracture site is placed in the tibial defect before the periosteum, subcutaneous tissue, and skin are closed. A non-weightbearing plaster boot is applied, and immobilization is maintained for 6 weeks.

CLOSED AXIAL INTRAMEDULLARY SCREW FIXATION

DeLee et al reported an alternative surgical technique that does not open the fracture site and as a result of which 10 patients obtained union in an average of 7.5 weeks. These fractures met the criteria of a history of prodromal symptoms before the acute episode; radiographic evidence of a stress phenomenon (periosteal reaction, radiolucent fracture line, and intramedullary sclerosis); and no history of previous treatment. These fractures can be classified as acute injuries with an underlying stress weakness, and would be acute fractures or delayed unions according to Torg's classification.

Surgical Procedure

All patients underwent internal fixation of the fracture by the insertion of a screw into the intramedullary canal of the fifth metatarsal. After substantial changes, the technique that has evolved is as follows:

A straight incision, parallel to the plantar aspect of the foot, is used to approach the tuberosity of the fifth metatarsal. The interval between the peroneus longus and peroneus brevis is located, and the tuberosity of the fifth metatarsal is isolated (Fig. 5*A*). A Kirschner wire is then inserted into the tuberosity in an effort to locate the axis of the medullary canal of the fifth metatarsal (Fig. 5*B*). After this insertion, the location of the wire is checked roentgenographically (either with standard anteroposterior and lateral roentgenographs or under image intensification). Once correct placement of the Kirschner wire is confirmed, a sterile marking pencil is used to mark the skin in order to set the direction for screw insertion (Fig. 5*C*). Next, a 3.2-mm Association for Study of Internal Fixation (ASIF) drill is inserted into the medullary canal in the same direction as the Kirschner wire, using the skin mark as a guide (Fig. 5*D*). The final position of the drill in the intramedullary canal is checked roentgenographically. At this point, an ASIF malleolar screw is

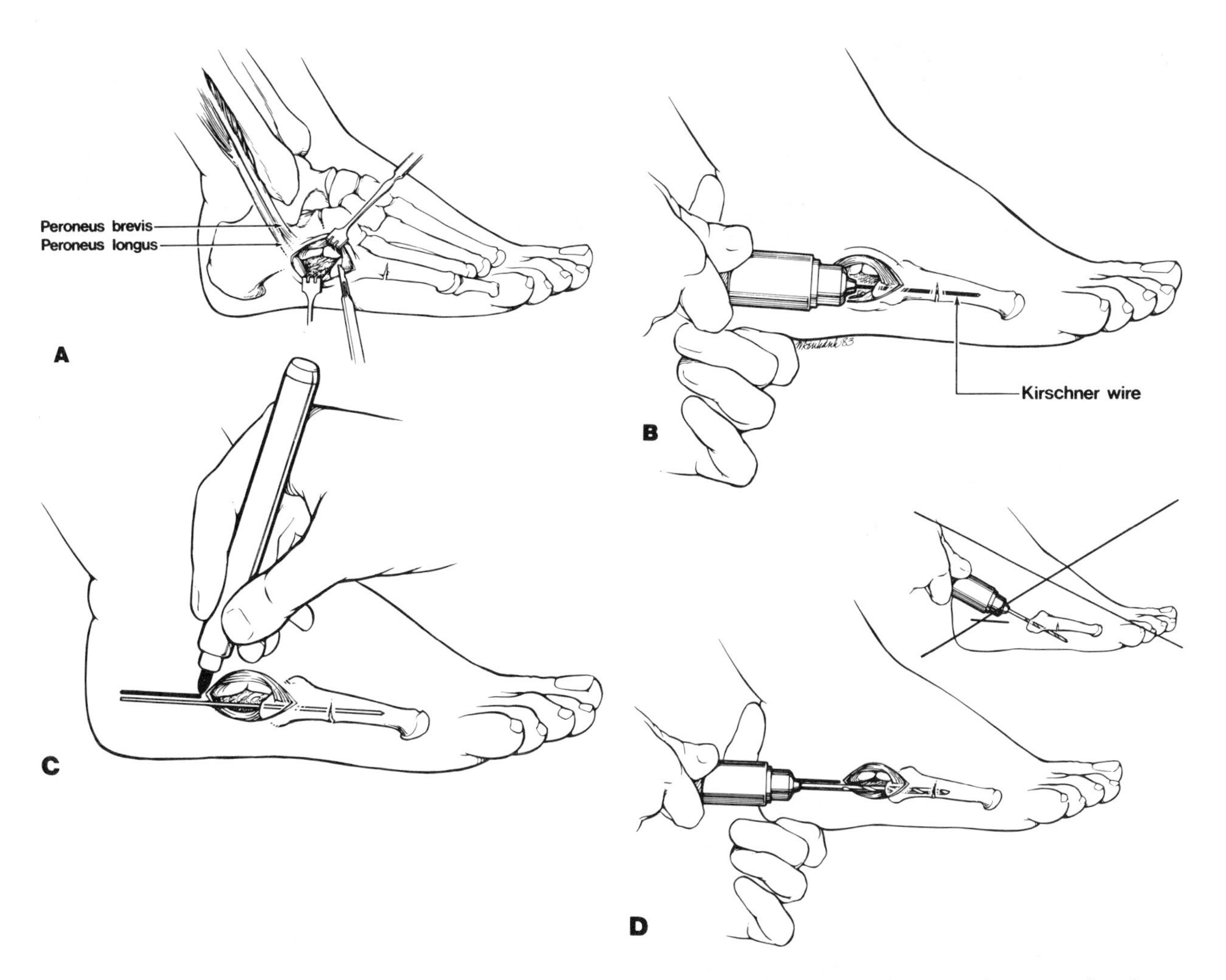

Figure 5 *A*, Surgical exposure of the base of the fifth metatarsal between the peroneus longus and peroneus brevis tendons. Minimal elevation of the peroneus brevis improves exposure. *B*, Insertion of a Kirschner wire (0.0625) into the medullary canal of the metatarsal. Adduction of the forefoot is beneficial for accurate insertion. The position is confirmed roentgenographically. *C*, A sterile marking pen is used to mark the direction of the Kirschner wire on the skin of the foot. This mark is used as a guide for insertion of the drill. *D*, Using the entrance hole of the Kirschner wire and the skin mark for alignment, a 3.2-mm ASIF drill is inserted into the fifth metatarsal. If the skin mark is not followed, the drill will penetrate the metatarsal. The drill's position is confirmed roentgenographically. An ASIF malleolar screw is inserted so that the threads do not cross the fracture site.

inserted down the axis of the fifth metatarsal (Fig. 6). The longest screw that fits into the medullary canal of the individual metatarsal is selected. Care is taken to (1) countersink the screw head so that a prominence is not present and (2) ensure that the screw threads do not cross the fracture site. At no time during the operation is the fracture site exposed or bone grafting performed.

Alternatively, a Leinbach screw is used in the medullary canal in three of the patients. The technique for insertion is similar to that used for the ASIF malleolar screw.

Following screw insertion, the patients are placed in a short-leg nonwalking cast or slipper cast for 2 weeks. The cast is then removed and the foot placed in a hard-sole shoe. Either a wooden shoe of the postbunionectomy type or a standard tennis shoe with a semiflexible steel sole insert is used to protect the foot. Gradual progression of weight bearing is begun. The patients are allowed to return to competitive sports when pain over the fifth metatarsal and the incision is gone. The range of time to return to sporting activity in this series was 7 to 14 weeks.

Upon returning to activity, seven of the 10 patients used a soft shoe insert with a protective area of padding over the lateral border of the foot at the base of the fifth metatarsal, to prevent pressure on the screw head or under the fifth metatarsal head. Three patients did not require this protection.

In review of the surgical technique, the intramedullary screw procedure has the advantages of not opening the fracture site, being a shorter procedure and one that decreases healing time. This pro-

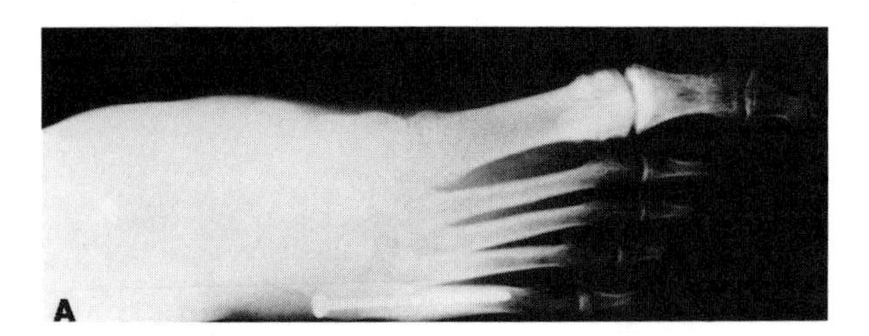

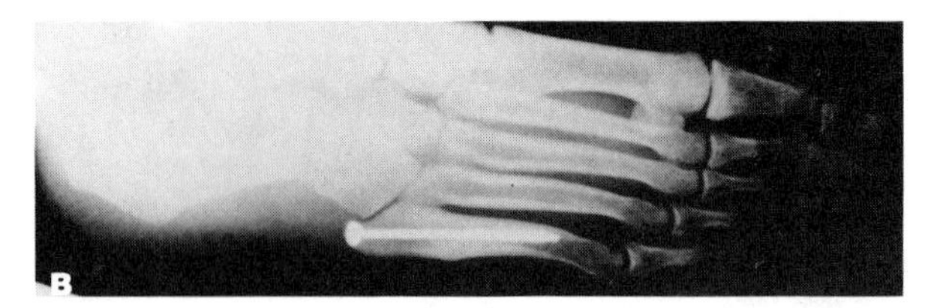

Figure 6 *A,* Anteroposterior and *B,* oblique roentgenograms of the patient 7 weeks after internal fixation. Note the trabeculae crossing the fracture site.

cedure is not without complications. Placement of the screw is critical and not always easily accomplished. Kavanaugh et al reported a 45 percent complication rate, which included screw fracture, missing the medullary canal, and complaints about the screw heads (Fig. 7). DeLee et al also reported that seven of 10 patients required shoe modification.

In conclusion, the treatment of the fracture of the base of the fifth metatarsal distal to the tuberosity should be tailored to the classification. Acute fractures should be immobilized in a non-weightbearing plaster boot. Fractures with delayed union can be treated with non-weightbearing in a cast, but will experience a prolonged period until union. In competitive athletes, fractures with delayed union should be treated operatively, using the surgical technique with which the physician feels most competent and has experience. All fractures with nonunion should be treated operatively.

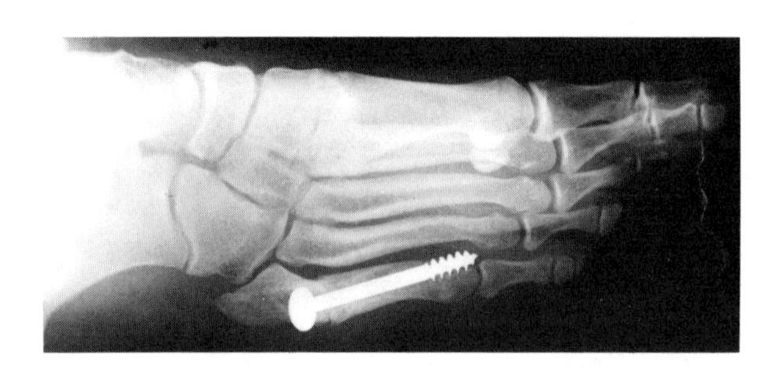

Figure 7 Complications of intramedullary screw fixation are noted and are due to failure to adhere strictly to technique. An incorrect screw is used (6.5 cancellous rather than malleolar); it is placed too distal and is too long, thereby penetrating the distal cortex.

SUGGESTED READING

Carp L. Fractures of the fifth metatarsal bone, with reference to delayed union. Ann Surg 1927; 86:308–320.

Dameron TB Jr. Fractures and anatomical variations of the proximal portion of the fifth metatarsal. J Bone Joint Surg 1975; 57-A:788–792.

DeLee JC, Evans JP, Julian J. Stress fractures of the fifth metatarsal. Am J Sports Med 1983; 5:349–353.

Jones R. Fracture of the base of the fifth metatarsal bone by indirect violence. Ann Surg 1902; 35:697–700.

Kavanaugh JH, Brower TD, Mann RV. The Jones' fracture revisited. J Bone Joint Surg 1978; 60-A:776–782.

Lehman RC, et al. Fractures of the base of the fifth metatarsal distal to the tuberosity: a review. Foot Ankle 1987; 7:245–252.

Stewart IM. Jones' fracture: fracture of the base of the fifth metatarsal. Clin Orthop 1960; 16:190–198.

Torg JS, et al. Fractures of the base of the fifth metatarsal distal to the tuberosity. J Bone Joint Surg 1984; 66-A:209–214.

Zelko RR, Torg JS, Rachun A. Proximal diaphyseal fractures of the fifth metatarsal: treatment of the fractures and their complications in athletes. Am J Sports Med 1979; 7:95–101.

HAGLUND'S SYNDROME

HELENE PAVLOV, M.D.
JOSEPH S. TORG, M.D.

In 1928 Patrick Haglund established a connection between posterior heel pain, a visible and palpable "pump bump" (Fig. 1), the shape of the posterior superior border of the os calcis, and the wearing of rigid low-back shoes. He particularly emphasized the high incidence of this condition among the "Kulturmenschen" (cultured people) who wore stiff low-back shoes when playing golf or hockey.

For the purpose of this discussion we will (1) describe the clinical and radiologic findings of Haglund's syndrome, (2) introduce an objective method for determining prominence of the bursal projection, and (3) differentiate Haglund's syndrome radiographically from other causes of posterior heel pain, including local conditions such as isolated retrocalcaneal bursitis or superficial Achilles tendon bursitis, and systemic conditions such as rheumatoid arthritis or Reiter's syndrome. Haglund's syn-

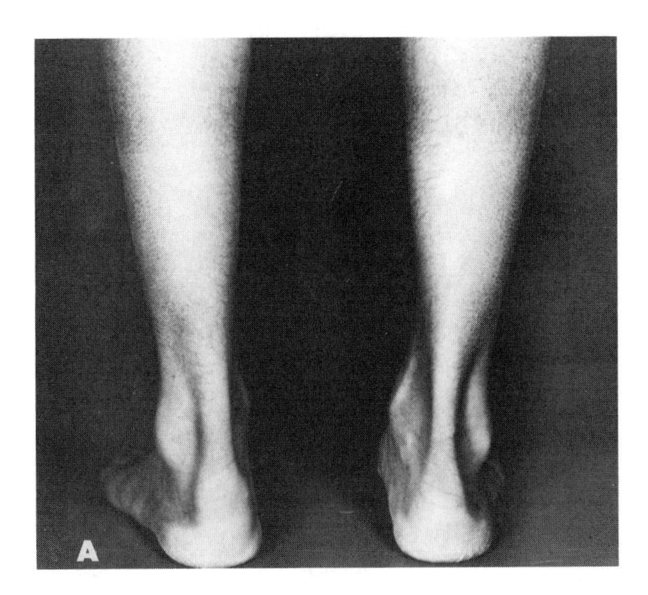

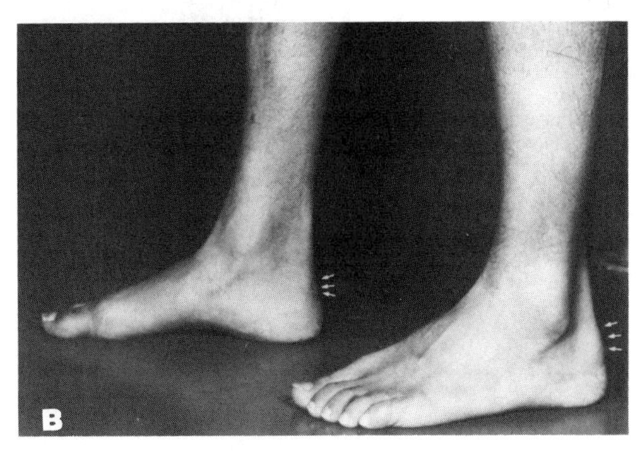

Figure 1 *A*, Clinical presentation of Haglund's syndrome. The posterior view of both heels demonstrates a soft tissue bulge at the Achilles tendon insertion on the left, compared with the normal right side. *B*, Lateral views of both feet demonstrate a pump bump on the left foot, a convexity of the superficial soft tissues.

drome is a cause of pain in the posterior heel characterized clinically by a painful pump bump or thickening of the soft tissues at the insertion of the Achilles tendon (Fig. 1). Patients with Haglund's syndrome range in age from young adults to the elderly, are of either sex, and have varying patterns of daily activity. The syndrome is characterized radiographically by retrocalcaneal bursitis, a loss of the lucent retrocalcaneal recess between the Achilles tendon and the bursal projection; Achilles tendinitis, an Achilles tendon measuring over 9 mm, 2 cm above the bursal projection; superficial Achilles tendon bursitis, a convexity of the soft tissues posterior to the Achilles tendon insertion; a cortically intact but prominent bursal projection; and a positive parallel pitch line (PPL).

The clinically detected pump bump is not diagnostic of Haglund's syndrome. In a controlled population, Pavlov and colleagues reported 15 patients with a pump bump that was determined radiographically to be caused by isolated superficial Achilles tendon bursitis in five patients, and by the posterior displacement of the soft tissues posterior to the bursal projection in 10 patients. In these latter 10 the pump bump was located at a higher level than that associated with Haglund's syndrome, posterior to the bursal projection rather than to the Achilles tendon insertion. The bursal projection was prominent, a positive PPL, in all 10 patients. These patients are predisposed to irritation of the pump bumps depending on their shoe selection.

Pump bumps also occur in association with certain systemic inflammatory articular disorders, such as Reiter's syndrome. In these patients the pump bump is more diffuse, is posterior to the Achilles tendon insertion and the bursal projection, and results from a superficial Achilles tendon bursitis and a retrocalcaneal bursitis, respectively. The cortex of the bursal projection can be eroded by the inflamed retrocalcaneal bursa; these erosions, when present, are diagnostic of an inflammatory articular process. In these patients, trauma to the external soft tissues and prominence of the bursal projection are not responsible for the pump bump, and the swelling occurs despite negative PPLs.

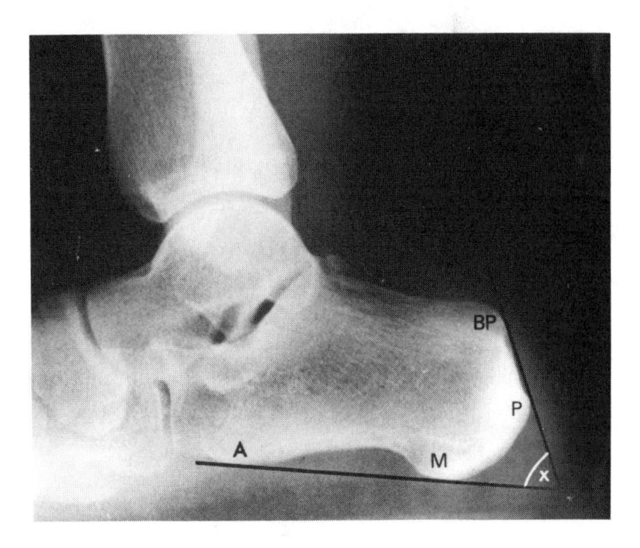

Figure 2 Quantitative evaluation of the shape and pitch of the os calcis. The posterior calcaneal angle (x) of Fowler and Philip is the angle formed by the insertion of the baseline tangent to the anterior tubercle (A) and the medial tuberosity (M) with the line tangent to the posterior surface of the bursal projection (BP) and the posterior tuberosity (P).

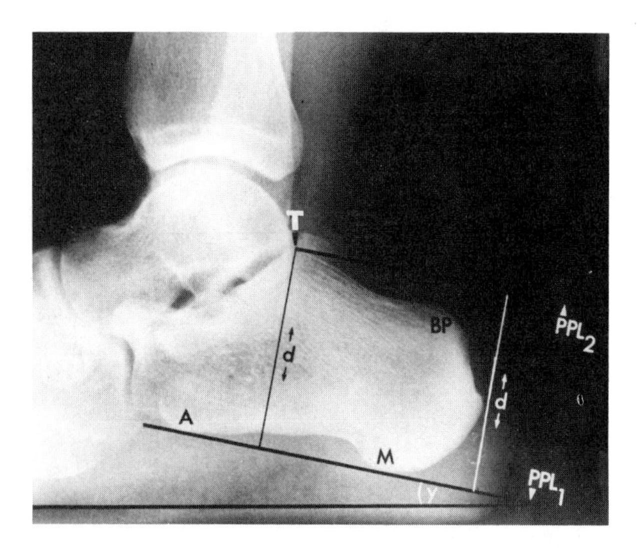

Figure 3 The parallel pitch lines (PPL) determine the prominence of the bursal projection (BP). The lower PPL (PPL_1) is the baseline, constructed as for the posterior calcaneal angle. A perpendicular (d) is constructed between the posterior lip of the talar articular facet (T) and the baseline. The upper PPL (PPL_2) is drawn parallel to the base of the distance (d). A bursal projection touching below the PPL_2 is normal, not prominent, a negative PPL. The pitch angle (y) is formed by the insertion of the baseline (PPL_1) with the horizontal.

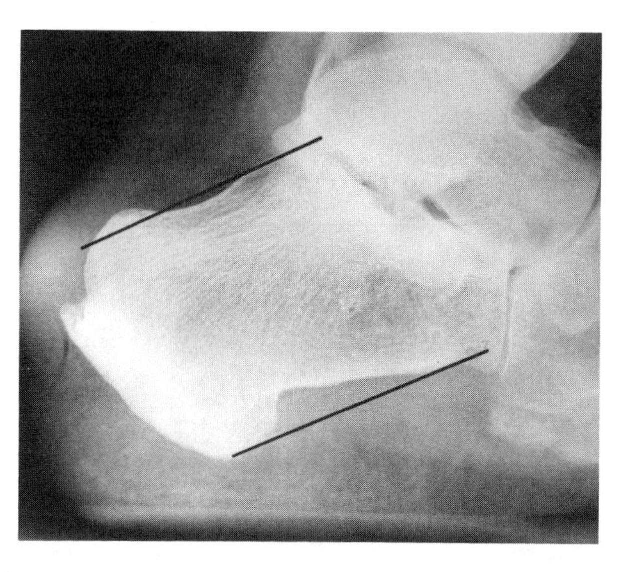

Figure 4 Haglund's syndrome is diagnosed on the lateral view of the heel by a positive PPL; a cortically intact bursal projection; loss of the retrocalcaneal recess, indicating retrocalcaneal bursitis; thickening of the Achilles tendon, measuring over 9 mm at 2 cm above the bursal projection; loss of the sharp interface between the Achilles tendon and the pre-Achilles fat pad, indicating Achilles tendinitis; and convexity of the posterior soft tissues at the level of the Achilles tendon insertion, indicating superficial Achilles tendon bursitis. Clinically, this latter finding presents as a pump bump.

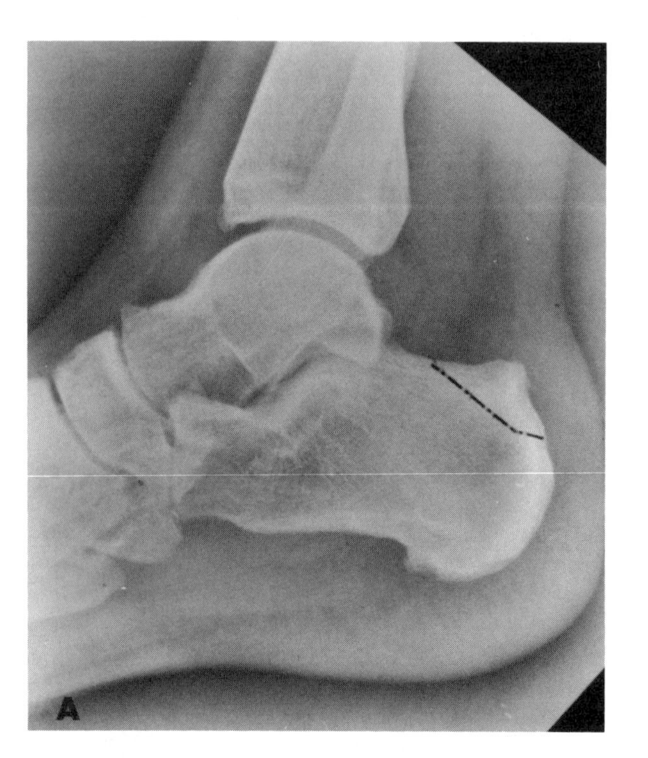

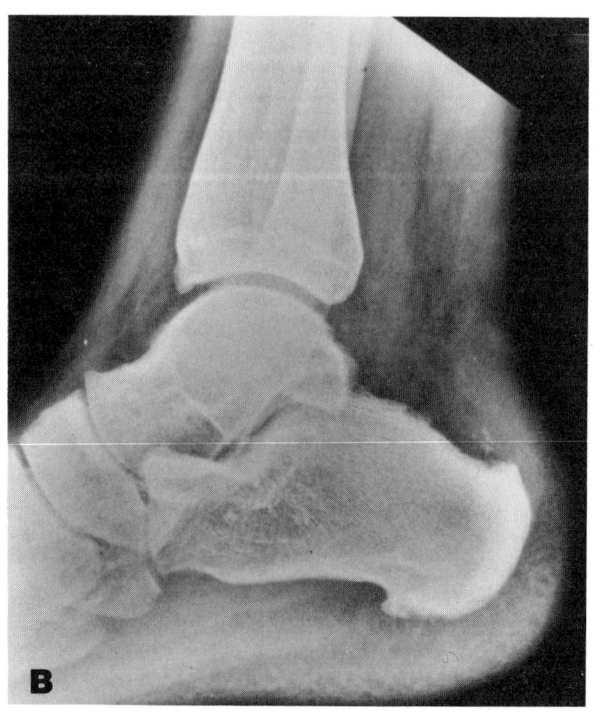

Figure 5 Preoperative (*A*) and postoperative (*B*) lateral roentgenograms of the foot, demonstrating the extent of resection of bursal projection.

Determining the location of the pump bump and the prominence of the bursal projection is essential in the diagnosis and differential diagnosis of posterior heel pain. Prominence of the bursal projection is determined radiographically either by the posterior calcaneal angle (an angle greater than 75 degrees) (Fig. 2) or by the parallel pitch lines (a negative PPL) (Fig. 3). Using the PPLs, the incidence of a positive PPL was increased in patients with plantar osseous projections as compared with patients with normal plantar surfaces. A similar observation was not made by using the posterior calcaneal angle. In the series of Pavlov and colleagues, symptoms correlated statistically with a positive PPL but not with an abnormal posterior calcaneal angle. This latter discrepancy was also reported by Keck and Kelly.

The causes of a pump bump and/or heel pain at the point of contact between the heel and the shoe counter can result from Haglund's syndrome, an isolated inflammation of the superficial Achilles tendon bursa, a posterior displacement of normal soft tissues because of a prominent bursal projection, or systemic articular disorders such as Reiter's syndrome. The key to correct diagnosis is fourfold: (1) a high index of clinical and radiographic suspicion, (2) a lateral radiograph of the heel cord demonstrating soft tissue detail, (3) a careful evaluation of the cortex of the bursal projection, and (4) a working knowledge of the parallel pitch lines (Fig. 4).

Initial management of symptomatic Haglund's syndrome consists of shoe modification, heel lift, and steroid injection into the bursa. Also, an Achilles tendon stretching program is an important component of corrective management. In patients unresponsive to such a program and unable to participate in vigorous activities, surgical excision of the bursal projection may be considered (Fig. 5).

SUGGESTED READING

Keck SW, Kelly PJ. Bursitis of the posterior part of the heel. J Bone Joint Surg 1965; 47:267–273.

Nielson AL. Diagnostic and therapeutic points in retrocalcaneobursitis. JAMA 1921; 77:463.

Pavlov H, Heneghan MA, Hersh A, et al. The Haglund syndrome: initial and differential diagnosis. Radiology 1982; 144:93–98.

Resnick D, Feingold ML, Curd J, et al. Calcaneal abnormalities in articular disorders. Radiology 1977; 125:355–366.

ORTHOTIC DEVICES: INDICATIONS

CHARLES R. BULL, M.D., B.Sc. (Med), F.R.C.S.(C), F.A.C.S., F.I.C.S.

During the past decade, running has become popular. With this explosion in the number of runners came sports clinics, podiatrists, orthotists, brace makers, and pedorthists, and the number of running shoe companies went from three to probably 50. Currently, almost anyone with discomfort in the feet, ankles, knees, hips, or back now wears an orthosis.

Ortho is derived from the Greek word "orthos," denoting straight. Thus, orthotics means a pursuit of straightening or correcting. An orthotic device, or orthosis, is similar to a brace or splint, but connotes an attempt to limit, straighten, or assist the body in an alignment problem. Orthotic devices for the feet attempt to align the entire lower extremity structurally in order to take pressure off the foot, ankle, shin, knee, hip, and possibly back. The orthotist spends as much time trying to line up the knees and hips as he does correcting the abnormality of the feet. Thus, if he can line up the great toe, patella, and anterior superior spine and have uniform spacing between the ankles and knees, he feels successful. An attempt is made to toe out the foot slightly by 15 degrees. This is accomplished through the foot rather than through external rotation of the tibia, and a correction of the valgus or inturned heel is also attempted when the orthotic device is made. The exact location of the mechanical axis of the ankle corresponding to the subtalar joint, allowing for tibial torsion, is a key factor in fashioning orthoses.

These orthoses are basically inserts that can be interchanged from shoe to shoe, but more positive control is possible with caliper bracing, ankle joint stirrups, and spring-loaded rods with a ring attachment to the knee.

Orthoses can be prefabricated (ready-made off the shelf) or tailor-made. Most are made of plastic or a Neoprene type of material, although they have been made of metal, stainless steel and aluminum, hard plastic, hard and soft rubber, and stiffened felt components. Prices vary from a few dollars to as much as $400. The orthoses made by an orthotist under the direction of a physician and molded to the patient's foot at the time of fabrication are inexpensive and continue to be effective for at least 2 years. The podiatrist's orthoses are more sophisticated and more expensive, and they tend to be more effective in difficult cases. They are smaller and better fit the running shoe.

The ready-made orthotics from Spenko or Dr. Scholl (soft, rubbery-type material) can be satisfactory, although they usually are not. The more substantial plastic skeleton types are better, but do not naturally correct all types of foot abnormalities. The soft, tailor-made orthotic with Sorbothane or PVT tends to be a little bulky. It needs a deeper shoe to hold the orthosis and to keep the wearer from falling out of the shoe, but it usually does a very satisfactory job.

The podiatrist's orthosis made by Langer Laboratories of Deerpark, New York can be made from a casting of the runner's foot. The cast is made with care to maintain the foot in neutral position and align with the hind foot in a similar neutral position, with some pressure under the fourth and fifth metatarsal heads and the talonavicular joint. This creates a negative impression of the plantar surface of the foot; Langer then makes a positive plaster cast and fashions the plastic orthosis to that cast. An acrylic heel and anterior post are bonded to this case, and the initial pronation or longitudinal abnormality is corrected. More posting or correction can be done once the orthosis is fitted to the runner by the podiatrist.

We have compared video tapes of runners running with normal foot structure and pronated feet with tapes of runners wearing custom-made orthoses that (1) fit correctly, (2) are undercorrective, or (3) are overcorrective. It is difficult to draw an accurate conclusion from this type of study, but the correction of the pronation usually has to be very accurate or the running gait is made appreciably worse by an incorrect orthotic device.

The orthotic device is of most benefit for foot, ankle, and knee overuse problems such as fasciitis and tendinitis. We doubt that it does much for a true hip problem, and the effect on the back certainly is minuscule. Commonly the patient has pronated feet and valgus heels and knees.

Overweight, poor running style, inexperience—all contribute to an altered footplant. The constant repetitive incorrect plant in running causes accumulated stress on the entire lower limb. Runners made up 58 percent of the patients receiving orthoses in our sports clinic.

It is important to see an abnormal wear pattern on the running shoe. I set the running shoe itself on a flat surface to see how much it is falling inward. The ideal running shoe should either be neutral or fall outward slightly if the runner plants properly.

I also have patients stand facing me with feet parallel and approximately 1 foot apart to see how much of an arch there is and then have them turn around to see how much valgus deformity there is to the heels. The Achilles tendon should be completely vertical when the patient is standing relaxed. Then the patient lies face down with heels out over the end of the bed and again the degree of valgus deformity is measured, and forefoot and rearfoot pronation are noted.

The mere presence of flat feet does not necessitate orthotic correction. There are hundreds of runners with flat feet and no symptoms, many of whom have won every major race in the United States. It may be a racial or ethnic factor—most blacks and North American Indians tend to have flat feet, for instance. These people do not need correction unless they are having symptoms of overuse.

PLANTAR FASCIITIS

The plantar fascia is an inflexible band of tough tissue that is prone to inflammation where it originates from the calcaneus. The point is a central focus for maximal stress, and the inflammation often is localized.

Initial treatment with a felt pad or heel lift or with a Sorbothane heel lift is often beneficial, but if the patient has significant pronation that causes an increased stretching and strain on the plantar fascia, suitably designed orthoses probably help decrease the problem. Elevation of the heel in this type of correction distributes more of the forces toward the forefoot. Initially, we were taught that the pressures were distributed, with 50 percent of the force of walking or running taken in the heel, and then that the force fanned out, the hallux taking two units of force and each of the other four metatarsals taking one. This concept has changed as a result of biomechanical sensor studies. The consensus is that the heel actually takes more than 50 percent of the weight, and the load transfers down through the second and third metatarsals, leaving less weight or pressure on the first, fourth, and fifth metatarsal areas. Thus, the dynamics of correcting plantar fasciitis involve getting a lot of that weight off the heel or area of plantar fascia origin. These patients should be encouraged to wear their orthoses all day long. In difficult cases appropriate physiotherapy, medications, injections, and even surgery are indicated along with the orthosis.

ACHILLES TENDINITIS

This inflammation, which accounts for approximately 11 percent of all the running injuries seen in our clinic, is attributed to microtears in the tendon causing inflammation of the adjacent tendon structures (i.e., the vestigial sheath), which can become chronic and even calcifies in rare cases.

Initial treatment consists of rest, cycling, and swimming (but no running); anti-inflammatory agents; and elevation of the heel with felt or Sorbothane pads. The wearing of moderately high heels, such as cowboy boots, may help by (1) causing relative shortening of the Achilles tendon, (2) causing absorption of forces transmitted to the tendon, and (3) resting the tendon and allowing the microtears to heal.

Varus deformities of the feet have been recognized in runners by the use of high-speed films. The average runner lands on the outer heel, and the forces transfer to the outer side of the foot through the midstance phase. If he or she overpronates through this phase, the Achilles undergoes a "whip-like" action in its sequence. Obviously this initiates, aggravates, and perpetuates the tendinitis. Orthotic correction reduces this type of motion. The gait has more of a light productive force, and less stress is transferred to the Achilles.

Once the tendinitis has subsided, the tendon is stretched and the gastrocnemius-soleus complex is strengthened. With this additional strength and flexibility, the runner should be able to plant better and, after a year or two, dispense with the orthosis. I want to emphasize that many orthoses can be used temporarily. At least 6 months is required to settle an acute problem, and many people improve their running style, strength, and flexibility and thus can dispense with the orthosis after a year or two. This is particularly true in the mature, high-quality runner who has functioned for years without injury; the orthotic device can be used on a temporary basis, and eventually a shoe with a good support, especially a strong heel support, will suffice.

TIB POSTERIOR TENDINITIS

This inflammation occurs at the junction of the posterior tibial muscle and tendon in the midportion of the medial aspect of the leg. It is the most common type of "shin splint" and its most likely cause is "pronated feet." "Shin splints" or inflammation of the shin area (common in runners) can occur in the tib posterior or the periosteum overlying the free tibial border (the classic location), or in the anterior (lateral) compartment. All three types usually benefit from the use of orthotics.

The muscle functions to help maintain the arch of the foot and to supinate the foot so that it can roll out after footplant. A pronated foot stretches the tendon and muscles, and as the foot pronates through the midstance phase an increased force is transmitted to the musculotendinous junction and into the muscle origin along the tibia. Microtears result and create inflammation (tendinitis).

An orthotic device shortens the muscle tendon complex and lessens the need to maintain the arch and supinate the foot. Thus, there is less strain as the foot pronates through the midphase of the running motion. Correction of foot pronation is probably the most important step in relieving the initial inflammation and preventing recurrence. In some cases, if it is left uncorrected, the condition progresses to periostitis, a compartment syndrome, or even a stress fracture.

PATELLOFEMORAL SYNDROME

This is the most common problem seen in our sports clinic. The etiology, reason for pain, management, response to treatment, and long-term sequelae are all controversial.

The most realistic cause is a "malalignment phenomenon." The patella travels in the femoral groove, and as the knee flexes beyond 135 degrees or a quarter squat, the compression between surfaces increases.

Ideally the patella tracks symmetrically, but in chondromalacia there appears to be asymmetry. This causes abnormal wear and tear on the patellar surface and thus a softening or roughening, which is manifested clinically by a grating when the patella is moved on the femoral surface. This situation is particularly uncomfortable when the patella is held against a strong quads contraction. What is incomprehensible is that some of the worst clinical cases exhibit minimal signs arthroscopically. Other clinical signs are a widened Q angle, noticeable infacing or squinting of the patella, a broad pelvis, femoral antiversion, genu valgus, external tibial rotation, and pronated feet. A correction of the pronated feet by an orthosis will alter the alignment of the leg. This is relative, similar to eyeglasses correcting shortsightedness. Basically, the malalignment returns when the orthoses are not used. Thus, tracking is more efficient, causes less irritation on the patellar articular surface, and thereby reduces the pain. Adjunctive treatment includes vastus medialis strengthening and the use of a knee brace for patellar stabilization.

OTHER KNEE PROBLEMS

Pes tendinitis is an inflammation of the pes, which is a confluence of three tendons on the medial aspect of the knee. Because these tendons mesh together so congruently at the knee, they are relatively prone to tendinitis, particularly in the presence of genu valgus. An orthotic device tends to transfer the forces laterally and take the pressure off this medial compartment of the knee. Conversely, ileotibial band and popliteus tendinitis are helped by a lateral wedge, which eases the lateral forces in the knee. In many cases, an orthotic device makes this type of problem worse.

VAGUE KNEE PAINS

The best treatment for fat pad syndrome, synovitis, plicae, internal derangement of the knee (IDK), and patellar tendinitis is alteration of the running schedule, i.e., decreased hills, decreased speed, new shoes, quadriceps-hamstring exercises to correct an imbalance, increased flexibility, and anti-inflammatory medications.

In a resistant case it is worthwhile to watch patients run. If they tend to pronate, throw their feet in or out, or have a heavy wide-track Pontiac style, orthoses may help. It is hard to correct the running style in a master athlete. The orthotic devices alter the style subtly and thereby help to decrease the problem.

CAVUS FOOT

This is almost a contraindication to running. The relatively spastic, high-arched foot is very uncomfortable with ordinary walking. It can become unbearable with running. An orthotic device can cushion the impact but usually cannot create a good mobile running foot.

SUCCESS RATE AND COMPLIANCE

In our study of soft orthotic devices in which 100 patients were reviewed after 1 year, 89 percent felt that the orthoses were of definite benefit; 38 percent limited the use of their orthoses to sports shoes only, while the rest used them in all their shoes; 21 percent stopped using them because the problem had been solved; 69 percent were still using them after 1 year; 10 percent stopped using them because they were of no benefit; and 47 percent returned for a check of their orthoses. It is important to check these at the 3- or 4-week point and again after 3 or 4 months to ascertain that correction is satisfactory. Minor adjustments can make the world of difference in their use. In the same series, 9 percent sought the advice of a podiatrist after receiving their orthoses. Probably 10 to 20 percent of runners use orthotic devices. We have prescribed over a thousand in the past 10 years. We wanted to know (1) whether this was necessary and (2) whether the patient used them. In our series, 69 percent of the 100 patients still used them after 1 year, and 21 percent discarded them because their problem was solved. Thus, we feel orthoses have been beneficial.

Soft orthotic devices are much less expensive than those prescribed by the podiatrist and can be more comfortable. We believe they can be used on a long-term basis to correct a biomechanical problem.

Studies of the hard orthotics prescribed by the podiatrist often cannot delineate a correction of pronation when the runner is filmed or studied biomechanically. However, orthotic devices do work. Podiatrists have been a definite boon to the runner, often eliminating the pain experienced in running. Obviously, the development of quality running shoes has also helped to prevent running injuries.

Orthotics can be applied to other sports. Certainly the use of orthoses in ski boots has been helpful in some cases. Ski boots can also be canted extrinsically to correct a pronated foot. This basically serves the same purpose as an orthosis. Most stop-and-start sports, such as squash and tennis, do not require an orthosis, as the unremitting footplant that occurs in running creates a more serious problem. Thus, orthotic devices are used in racquet sports, but are not as necessary or popular.

The principle of orthosis construction, patient selection, and the biomechanical studies of different sports will change markedly in the next few years. Orthotic devices can be beneficial for specific problems, but should be used in conjunction with other methods of treatment. Certainly, strengthening programs for the entire lower limb should be instituted when the orthoses are prescribed. In my experience, careful patient selection is the key to proper orthosis use. If patients are made aware of the exact indications for orthoses and are observed closely and instructed in their use, the vast majority should improve. It is only the rare patient with a cavus foot, for instance, who continues to have disability after using the orthoses and cannot tolerate them. Old-time runners from the 1950s and 1960s, who had one pair of shoes that they discarded when the sole fell off, were guaranteed to have blisters, missing toenails, and general aches and pains, which they did not acknowledge to anyone. Modern runners complain if the workout is less than 100 percent. They make use of sports clinics, podiatrists, orthoses, and coaches, and probably run a lot longer, farther, and faster in comfort. In many cases this is because of the use of orthotic devices.

ORTHOTIC DEVICES: FABRICATIONS

JOSEPH S. TORG, M.D.

Overuse injuries involving either the feet or other areas of the lower extremities can often be effectively treated with orthotic devices. Orthotics can correct "biomechanical abnormalities" that, when combined with overtraining, create excessive or unusual stress on various weightbearing structures.

The purpose of these devices is to place the subtalar joint in its neutral position during the midsupport phase of the running cycle. This usually consists of maintaining both the forefoot-heel alignment and the leg-heel alignment. Forefoot-heel alignment is normal when the forefoot, at the metatarsal level, is perpendicular to the heel. Leg-heel alignment is present when the subtalar joint is in neutral and the heel is parallel to the distal one-third of the leg.

When these alignments are not "normal," the variations can cause stress on various parts of the musculoskeletal system. If the plane of the forefoot shifts so that the medial side lifts above the neutral plane, supination, or varus (inversion, abduction, and plantar flexion), is observed. Pronation, or valgus (eversion, adduction, and dorsiflexion), occurs when the medial side drops below the neutral plane. Pronation and supination can stress structures of the foot as well as those of the lower leg and knee.

Orthotics are indicated for the treatment of symptomatic pronation, plantar fasciitis, "runner's knee" (chondromalacia), popliteal tendinitis, posterior tibial tendinitis, "shin splints," and Achilles tendinitis.

Plantar fasciitis is an example of injury to the foot caused by either abnormal pronation or supination. In the case of excessive pronation or pes planus, the plantar aponeurosis stretches and causes fascial strain. Orthotics will correct this. For pes cavus, orthotics alleviate the "windlass" effect in which the fascia is tight and there is strain on the calcaneal insertion. If untreated, the stress on plantar fascia can lead to the formation of calcaneal bone spur. Orthotics serve to maintain the subtalar joint in neutral and the midtarsal joint in stable pronated position.

Abnormal pronation is also a contributing factor to the development of "runner's knee." With this injury the relationship between a biomechanical problem in the foot and an injury elsewhere in the body is evident. The patellofemoral joint receives an unusual amount of stress when, owing to abnormal pronation in the foot, there is excessive internal rotation of the entire leg. Lateral displacement of the patella can occur and chondromalacia develops.

A similar scenario is observed in the case of popliteal tendinitis. Hyperpronation causes excessive internal rotation, which stresses the lateral compartment of the knee and the femoral attachment of the popliteal tendon.

A fourth injury resulting from excessive pronation is posterior tibial tendinitis. Krissoff located the pain characterizing this injury behind the medial malleolus and on the posterior medial border of the tibia. Orthotics are the most effective means of treating this injury.

Anterior and posterior "shin splints" develop when various muscles in the leg become overused through attempts to compensate for biomechanical problems. In the case of anterior shin splints the tibialis anterior can be overused if there is forefoot imbalance. This muscle works as a decelerator during heel strike and prevents "heel slap" during the midstance phase. Abnormal pronation can place excessive demands on the posterior tibial longus, flexor digitorum longus, and flexor hallucis longus units, and posterior shin splints can develop. Fatigue tears of the fibers of the tibialis posterior muscle at its insertion into the periosteum of the tibia are common.

Stress reactions and stress fractures are other overuse injuries in which biomechanical difficulties are contributory factors. Supination can lead to tibial stress fractures, and pronation to fibular stress fractures.

Orthotics can also be used to treat Achilles tendinitis. Smart reviewed the etiologic mechanism involved in this condition. The biomechanical factor designated is also that of prolonged pronation. Slow-motion, high-speed cinematography has enabled researchers to identify a whipping action or bowstring effect of the Achilles tendon produced by prolonged pronation, which could possibly lead to microtears. It is speculated that degenerative changes of the tendon are related to torsional forces transmitted through the tendon during pronation. Orthotics work to shorten the phase of pronation during the support phase of running.

A variety of ready-made arch supports are available in shoe stores and sporting goods stores. However, the erudite and sophisticated runners of today usually settle for nothing less than a pair of custom orthotic devices, which cost approximately $275 for their prescription and fabrication.

The semirigid and rigid runner's orthosis requires positive plaster casting or mold of the patient's foot taken with the subtalar joint in neutral position. Presumably, this occurs when the talonavicular joint and forefoot are also in a neutral relationship; i.e., no eversion and no inversion should be present (Figs. 1 and 2). Leg-heel and forefoot-heel alignments, described previously, should also be assessed, and corrections for any deviations from neutral made. The plaster positive mold is then sent to the orthotic laboratory. From the positive casting, a

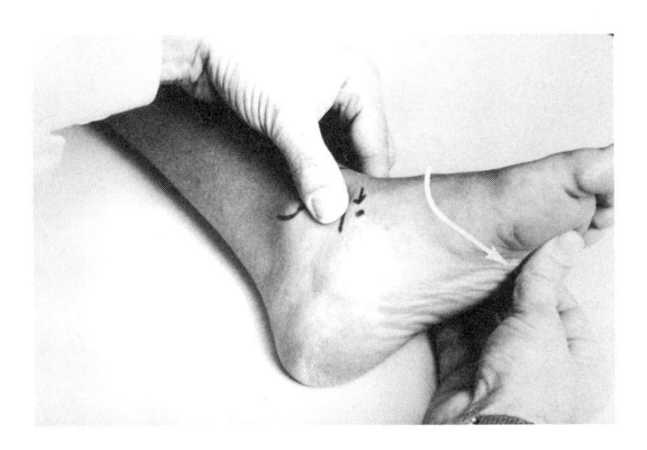

Figure 1 Positive casting for running orthotics should be taken with the subtalar joint in a neutral position; i.e., no eversion and no inversion should be present. Presumably, this is determined by ascertaining talonavicular joint congruity. This is done by palpating the medial and dorsolateral aspects of the talonavicular joint with the thumb and forefinger of one hand, then supporting the forefoot in a neutral position with pressure under the fourth and fifth metatarsal heads as demonstrated.

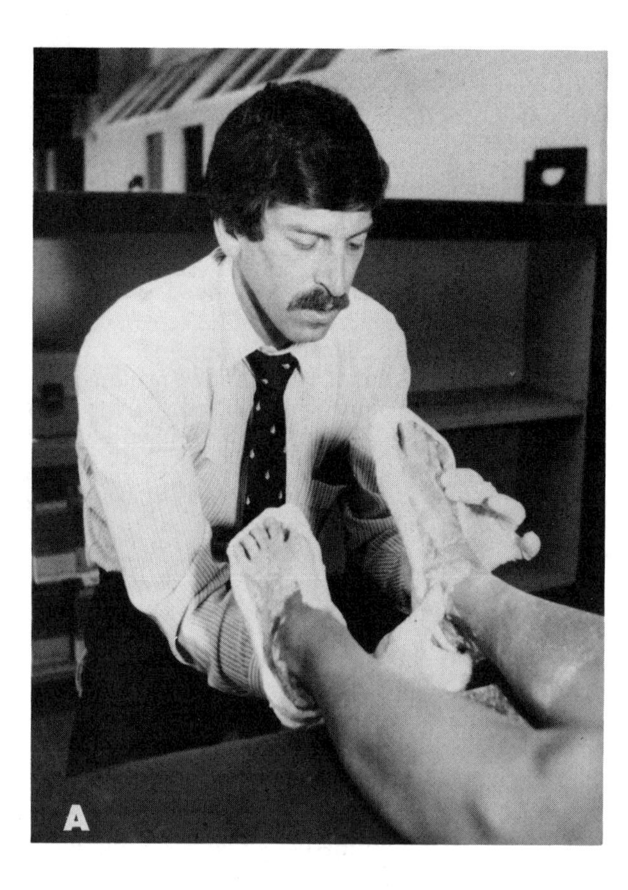

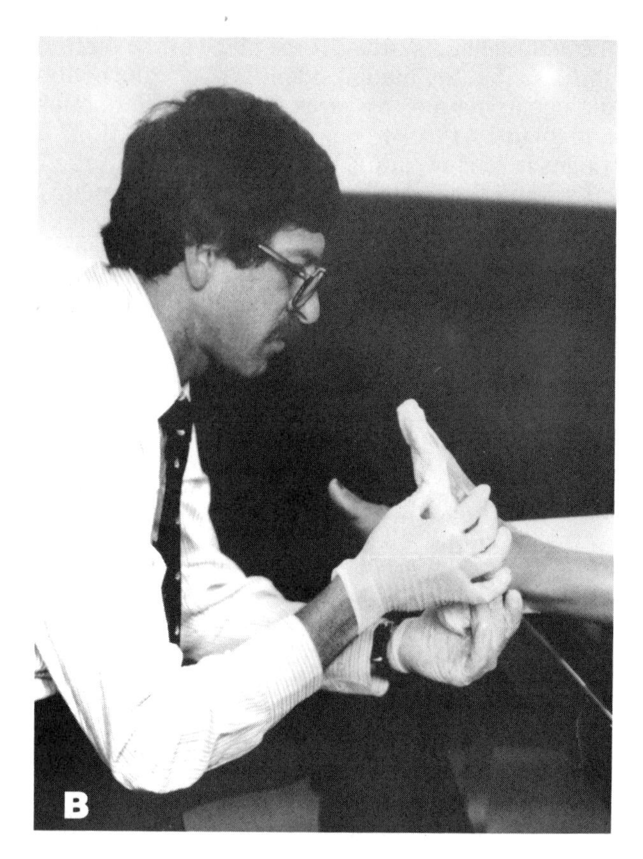

Figure 2 *A*, Casting for runner's orthotics necessitates palpating the talonavicular joint and maintaining it in a neutral position. *B*, With congruity of the talonavicular joint, the forefoot is maintained in a neutral relationship with the hindfoot by exerting pressure under the fourth and fifth metatarsal heads.

negative impression of the configuration of the plantar surface is obtained. From this, an acrylic rigid orthosis is fabricated (Figs. 3 and 4). The orthosis, in addition to providing rigid support for the medial arch and midfoot, is "posted" anteriorly and posteriorly in such a manner as to support the subtalar joint in a neutral position (Fig. 5).

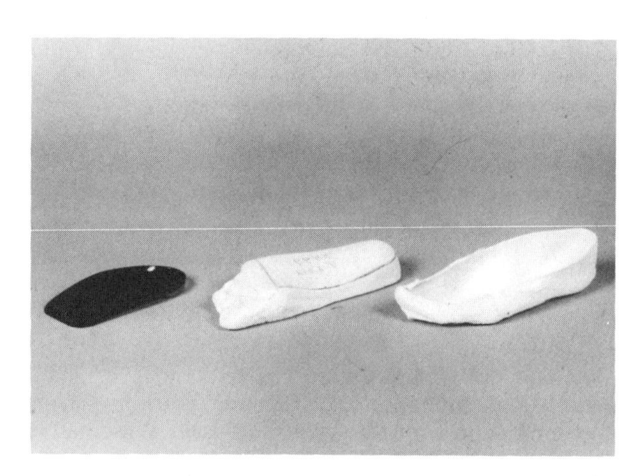

Figure 3 From the positive casting (*right*), a negative impression of the plantar surface of the foot is obtained (*center*). From this an acrylic rigid orthosis is fabricated (*left*).

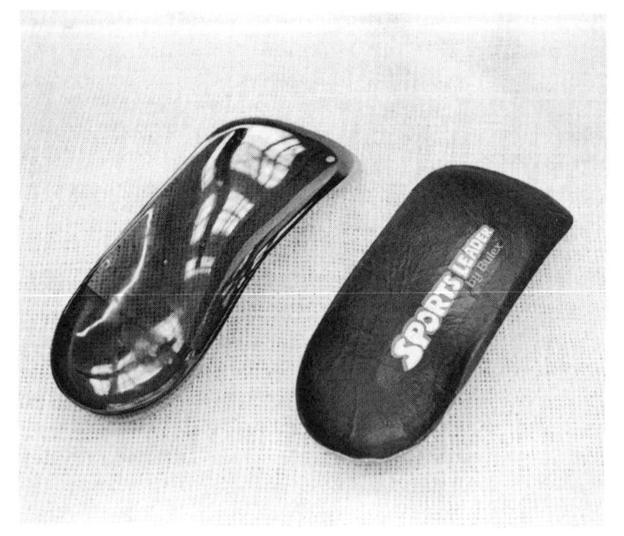

Figure 4 A rigid orthotic (*left*) is used primarily in nonathletic footwear. The sport orthotic (*right*) is more flexible and used for athletic participation.

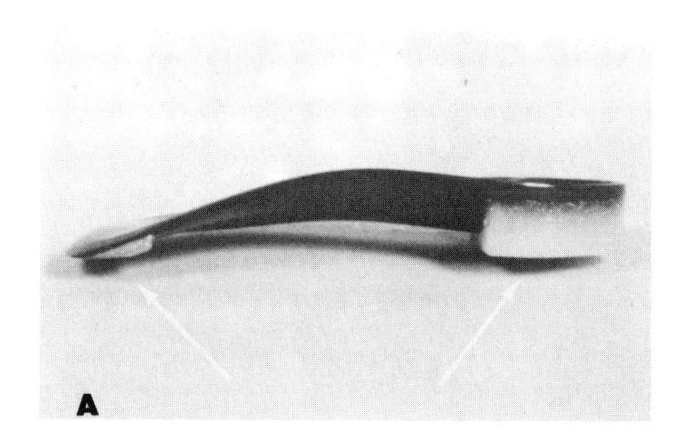

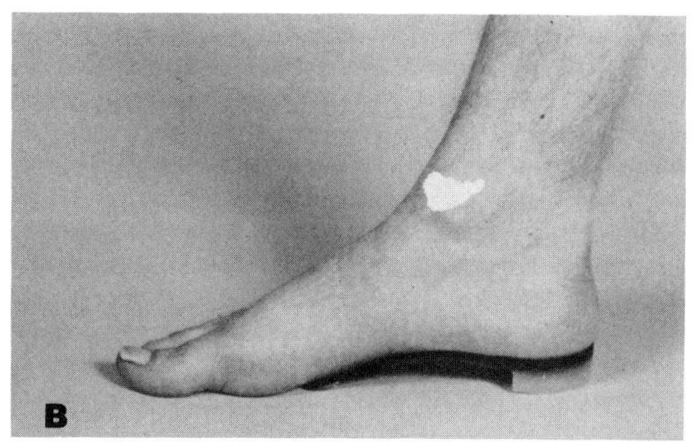

Figure 5 *A*, Viewed from the medial aspect, an anterior and heel post is bonded to the acrylic member. *B*, The runner's orthotic serves two functions: it presumably maintains the subtalar joint in a neutral posture, and it provides support for the medial longitudinal arch.

I ANKLE

DISORDERS AFFECTING TENDON STRUCTURES

R. PETER WELSH, M.B., Ch.B., F.R.C.S.(C), F.A.C.S.
BRUCE R. HUFFER, M.D.

ACHILLES TENDINITIS AND RETROCALCANEAL BURSITIS

The morbidity of this syndrome has not always been appreciated, and treatment efforts have not been rigorous enough to prevent the chronicity of what is a most disabling condition to the athlete involved in any running or jumping sport. Indeed, in a review of 50 track and field athletes engaged in competitive athletics who were afflicted with this syndrome for more than 3 months despite treatment measures, 28 (56 percent) never returned to competitive athletics at their preinjury level, and nine (18 percent) had to give up all sports participation completely.

This condition must be taken seriously and treated much more aggressively than it has been in the past if prolonged morbidity is to be reduced.

Pain occurring about the heel may be a result of several pathologic conditions, often making it difficult to distinguish the exact cause. These can be divided into pathologic conditions directly involving the tendon or the peritendon, and painful bursitis about the calcaneal tuberosity.

Achilles Tendon Disease

The Achilles tendon, unlike other tendons such as the peroneals, is not invested by a true synovial sheath but instead by a film-like peritenon. The tendon itself is made of dense fibrous tissue with little vascularity, but the peritenon is a loose connective tissue with abundant vascularity, prone to an inflammatory response. Achilles tendon disease can be classified into two types: (1) pure peritendinitis and (2) peritendinitis with tendon degeneration. In pure peritendinitis, only the peritendinous structures are inflamed and thickened (the term tenosynovitis should be reserved for tendons with true synovial sheaths). If the tendon itself is also involved, not only with an inflammatory reaction but also in a degenerative process, the tendon appears thicker, softer, and a deeper yellow; it loses its normal collagen configuration and shows areas of focal cyst formation. This classification is histologic and clinically it may be difficult to differentiate the exact pathology, but the etiology is common and appears to be related to problems with tissue vascularity. The blood supply to the Achilles tendon is from two sources. One from the muscle proximally passes distally in the tendon to meet in a watershed area some 2 to 3 cm above the tendon insertion, with vessels coursing upward from the calcaneus. With activity the Achilles tendon is subject to repetitive stretching and compression of the tendon and its blood supply in this critical watershed area. Here a relative abnormal vascularity persists, predisposing to tendon degeneration, with the association peritendinous inflammatory response characterizing the clinical presentation.

Bursitis About the Calcaneus

Although numerous bursae have been described about the Achilles tendon and calcaneus, the only consistent anatomic bursa is the retrocalcaneal bursa between the posterior superior surface of the calcaneus and the Achilles tendon. This bursa may become inflamed and hypertrophied in runners, as can that associated with a prominence of the tuberosities of the calcaneus, so-called pump bumps. On rare occasions a bursitis may develop between the Achilles tendon and the skin.

Symptoms

Pain is the symptom that brings the athlete to seek medical attention. It may be located anywhere from the attachment of the Achilles tendon to the calcaneus to the musculotendinous junction several centimeters above the tip of the superior calcaneal tuberosity. Initially, pain may occur only early in the run, but in chronic cases pain may be constant. Particularly troublesome is stiffness on rising in the morning, which may take some hours to "loosen up."

Physical Examination

Tenderness may be noted anywhere along the length of the Achilles tendon. Nodular thickening may be noted and peritendinous soft tissue swelling may be present. Retrocalcaneal bursitis can often be diagnosed if pain occurs while squeezing the bursal region between the calcaneus and the Achilles tendon. Patients are often noted to have tightness of the Achilles tendon and the entire gastrocnemius-soleus complex, and this should be tested for and compared with the noninjured side. Roentgenographic examination is rarely of use, although on occasion a prominence of the superior tuberosity or calcific deposits within the tendon may be noted.

Treatment

As in most overuse syndromes resulting from repetitive stress, reduced loading of the injured part must be imposed. Runners must decrease their distance and should eliminate hill work. Sprinters and jumpers must refrain from all springing and bounding, and if the tendon is persistently tender, a switch to walking, cycling, or swimming is advised. Soft padding in the hindfoot region of the running shoe may decrease the impact of running on the Achilles tendon, and a slight lift placed into the heel may decrease stress on the tendon. One of the most important aspects of treatment involves the diligent stretching of the triceps surae mechanism before running. Local ice friction treatment can be extremely helpful, and a limited course of ultrasonography should be tried (10 to 12 treatments). Further treatments are unlikely to be of enhanced benefit. Anti-inflammatory medicine can be prescribed, but steroid injections are never used because of their weakening effect on tendinous tissue with a likely predisposition to rupture.

A small percentage of patients do not respond to conservative treatment and require exploration. At surgery it is important to precisely define the pathology; in cases of peritendinitis alone a simple tenolysis is effective. However, if the tendon is degenerate, the yellowish necrotic areas of tendon should be excised through a longitudinal incision into the tendon. Revascularization appears to be encouraged by such a procedure, and recovery generally is most favorable. In cases of a chronically inflamed retrocalcaneal bursa, excision of the bursa and underlying bony prominence is usually effective, but it is very important to leave a negative bony impression where there was previously a prominence if recurrence is to be avoided.

Protected weight bearing with crutches, but with early mobilization of the ankle, is practiced postoperatively. Return to sport may be delayed, and diligent calf-stretching exercises should be practiced throughout the recovery phase.

SUBCALCANEAL PAIN FROM PLANTAR FASCIITIS AND SEVER'S DISEASE

Plantar Fasciitis

Pain originating in the subcalcaneal region is not uncommon in athletes engaged in running and jumping sports. The condition has been given a variety of names including plantar fasciitis, painful heel syndrome, and calcaneal spurs. Pain may arise at the calcaneal tuberosity and origin of the plantar fascia as well as from the subcalcaneal bursa or the heel pad itself, which consists of a thick layer of fibrous septa and fat. Pain may also arise in the tendinous origins of the intrinsic foot muscles at their calcaneal attachment, or from trauma to the medial heel branches of the calcaneal nerve.

Etiology

The cause of plantar fasciitis is not well understood, but in the athlete the process most likely begins as a strain of the plantar fascia, either as a single injury or, more likely, as a result of repetitive trauma at the point of fascial attachment to the calcaneal tubercle. In the early stages a fibrositis of low chronicity takes place, with tendinous degeneration and an ongoing low-grade inflammatory response that never succeeds in adequately repairing the injury. The calcaneal spur may be part of this response, but it is more generally seen as a physiologic local response of the bone to tension stresses in the plantar fascia.

Occasionally, another cause of pain in this area may be entrapment of or trauma to a branch of the medial calcaneal nerve. This branch has been shown to be vulnerable to pressure from calcaneal spurs as well as local irritation and inflammation.

Diagnosis

In general the diagnosis is not difficult to make. The athlete complains of pain when the heel strikes the ground during walking or running, a continuous low-grade pain during the day, and pain and stiffness after use and particularly on rising in the morning.

Clinically one can usually only demonstrate tenderness locally at the attachment of the plantar fascia to the medial process of the tuberosity. Such tenderness is exquisite, aggravated with weight bearing, and occasionally aggravated by hyperpronation of the forefoot as the plantar fascia is put on stretch.

Treatment

The aggravating insult must be reduced if the athlete is to overcome this condition. Thus, impact loading of the heel area must be avoided, which for the running athlete may mean a switch to cycling or swimming.

Strengthening the intrinsic muscles of the foot as well as the tibialis posterior muscle helps in the support of the longitudinal arch and in reducing tensions in the plantar fascia and intrinsic musculature.

A soft orthosis may be of great help, but its design should (1) relieve the pressure on the tender area, (2) support the arch, and (3) control the heel. To these ends a simple foam cushion can be used, as can a "doughnut" with a hole in the center to reduce loads on the heal area. However, it is better to build this into a heel cup with a varus tilt to direct the heel plant to the outer border of the foot and at the same time reduce tension in the plantar fascia.

Local physiotherapy measures with ultrasonography can be strikingly beneficial, and anti-inflammatory medication in high doses for a 2- to 3-week course is often helpful. If a major response is not seen with these measures in the first 2 weeks, the local infiltration of corticosteroid into the tender focus should be undertaken. This can be repeated on two further occasions at 6-week intervals. On rare occasions if symptoms persist to the point at which continued sports participation is impossible, consideration may be given to surgical treatment.

The preferred surgical approach utilizes a 3-cm incision placed medially at the junction of the thick plantar skin with the medial aspect of the heel. Dissection must not damage the heel pad, but must separate the tendinous muscle attachment and plantar fascial origin from their calcaneal attachment. A segment of tendon and fascia is excised together with the calcaneal spur if present. Postoperatively, a compressive dressing is applied, the wound always drained, and weight bearing is restricted with crutches until weight can be borne comfortably on the heel. A very gradual return to activity is allowed; recovery can take as long as 3 to 4 months.

Sever's Disease (Os Calcis Apophysitis)

In the adolescent, maturation of the calcaneus apophysis, to which the Achilles tendon makes its attachment, may be associated with a dysvascular degeneration with fragmentation of the apophysis. This process, one of the osteochondroses, is akin to Osgood-Schlatter disease seen about the knee at the insertion of the patellar tendon, and is similarly associated with local pain and sensitivity to pressure and loads.

Presenting usually in the 11- to 13-year-old age group, the condition is self-limiting, but nonetheless troublesome through the active phase until growth maturation of the calcaneus is completed in the early teens. Pain with running and jumping and a constant aching after activity, particularly at night, may necessitate simple anti-inflammatory analgesic treatment with aspirin. Heel cushions and modification of the sports program are necessary until symptoms subside. Confirmation of the process is shown radiographically, with fragmentation of the heel apophysis early and marked sclerosis later as new bone is laid down and the process matures.

FLEXOR HALLUCIS LONGUS STENOSING TENOSYNOVITIS AND OS TRIGONUM SYNDROME

Pain in the posterior aspect of the ankle and hindfoot is relatively common in athletes. Although the symptoms are most commonly attributed to the Achilles tendon, two other conditions cause pain in this area and may be misdiagnosed as "Achilles tendinitis." These conditions are inflammation and stenosis of the tendon of the flexor hallucis longus and the os trigonum syndrome.

Flexor Hallucis Longus Stenosing Tenosynovitis

Tendinitis of the flexor hallucis longus is extremely common in ballet dancers, although it is occasionally seen in other sports as well. The flexor hallucis longus tendon, called the "Achilles tendon of the dancer's foot," is often strained as it traverses its fibrous and osseous tunnel on the posterior aspect of the talus between the medial and lateral tubercles. The os trigonum is the name of a separate ossicle in relation to this tendon about which progressive inflammation can lead to a stenosing tenosynovitis. If scarring is severe over time, a "pseudo hallux rigidus" can develop. Partial rupture of the flexor hallucis longus tendon has also been reported. Symptoms of tendinitis include recurrent pain, tenderness, and swelling behind the medial malleolus of the ankle, and sometimes triggering or crepitus. A misdiagnosis of tendinitis of the posterior tibial tendon is often made, and indeed such a condition may coexist with disease of the flexor hallucis longus.

Physical examination reveals localized tenderness over the sheath of the flexor hallucis longus behind the medial malleolus. Sometimes, nodules within the tendon can be palpated. Rarely, with an abnormal distal insertion of the muscle fibers on the tendon, a "functional hallux rigidus" can result when the muscle fibers become pulled down into the fibrosseous tunnel. This condition must be differentiated from a posterior impingement syndrome. The pain is usually behind the lateral malleolus in this condition and caused by plantar flexion.

Treatment

Treatment in the early stages consists of rest, anti-inflammatory medication, ice applications, and gentle stretching. Activities that reproduce symptoms should be avoided. Although most cases eventually become asymptomatic with conservative treatment, symptoms occasionally progress and become severe and disabling. In these patients, tenolysis of the flexor hallucis longus should be suspected.

Os Trigonum Syndrome

The os trigonum represents the ununited lateral tubercle on the posterior aspect of the talus and occurs in 8 to 13 percent of the general population. Pain originating at the os trigonum is rare in nonathletes, but relatively common in ballet dancers. When the dancer attempts to force plantar flexion beyond its range, the os trigonum is caught between the posterior tip of the tibia and the calcaneus. This may result in contusion, extrusion, or fracture of the os trigonum.

The diagnosis is suggested when a dancer complains of pain and tenderness posterolaterally in the ankle, whereas with flexor hallucis longus tendinitis pain and tenderness are medially based. The condition may be misdiagnosed as chronic peroneal tendinitis. However, on careful examination the location of the tenderness is found to be behind the peroneal tendons, and forced passive plantar flexion reproduces the symptoms. Lateral roentgenograms with full plantar flexion reveal the os trigonum. Relief of symptoms with locally injected lidocaine (Xylocaine) confirms the diagnosis.

Treatment

In the dancer the most important aspect of treatment is avoidance of any motion that places the ankle in extreme plantar flexion in which posterior impingement occurs. Mild anti-inflammatory medicine and physical therapy, as well as local steroid injections, may be helpful in dancers who are not helped by conservative therapy. Surgical excision may be warranted.

On occasion, stenosing tenosynovitis of the flexor hallucis longus tendon and the os trigonum syndrome occur together. In such situations, when conservative treatment has not been beneficial, combined tenolysis of the flexor hallucis longus as well as os trigonum excision should be carried out. Although surgical treatment can lead to good results, the dancer should be cautioned that full recovery can take as long as 8 months.

PERONEAL TENOSYNOVITIS; TIBIALIS POSTERIOR TENDINITIS AND TENOSYNOVITIS

Stenosing tenosynovitis of the peroneal tendons on the lateral side of the ankle and tibialis posterior on the medial side may be the cause of considerable morbidity in the running and jumping athlete.

Anatomy

The tendons of the peroneus longus and brevis enter a common sheath 4 cm proximal to the lateral malleolus. This sheath encloses them as they pass behind and into a shallow groove in the posterior portion of the fibular malleolus. The brevis tendon continues to its insertion into the tuberosity at the base of the fifth metatarsal, while the longus tendon passes under the cuboid into a second sheath formed by the long plantar ligament and cuboid groove. It inserts into the lateral side of the base of the first metatarsal. The peroneals are active evertors of the foot. They contribute to final pronation and push-off in the second stage of walking and also contribute considerably to the stability of the ankle joint. The tibialis posterior passes posterior to the medial malleolus in company with the long flexor tendons to the toes. As it does so, it is enveloped by a synovial sleeve and retained by a thick retinaculum before passing to its insertion into the tubercle of the tarsal scaphoid.

Post-traumatic Peroneal Tendinitis (Stenosing Tenosynovitis)

Limitation of normal excursion of the peroneal tendons at the level of the peroneal trochlea after trauma can cause lateral tarsal pain. The etiology can be secondary to trauma to other ankle structures, i.e., calcaneal fractures, ankle sprains, subtalar fractures, or fractures of the lateral fibular ridge; acute injury resulting from forced dorsiflexion and inversion may be the initiating cause. The diagnosis is suspected in the patient who complains of pain localized to the lateral aspect of the heel or external malleolar area following injury. The patient notes accentuation of pain when walking barefoot or on rough terrain. On examination there is an antalgic gait, limitation of subtalar motion, and point tenderness over the peroneal tendons. Forced plantar flexion in inversion accentuates the symptoms. Injection of several milliliters of local anesthetic into the tendon sheath with relief of symptoms strongly suggests the diagnosis. Peroneal tenography shows either a complete block or constriction of the peroneal tendon sheath at the level of the inferior peroneal retinaculum.

The tibialis posterior may be similarly involved, but with a similar symptom pattern referrable to the medial aspect of the ankle.

Conservative Treatment

Conservative treatment includes anti-inflammatory medication and stretching of the parent muscle groups, icing and ultrasonography at the local area of inflammation, reduction in the provocative activity, and substitution of a noninjurious exercise program.

Orthotic support can be of great help, but must be carefully customized, the objective being to unload the offended tendon in each case. Thus, with a peroneal tendon problem the ankle should usually be tilted into valgus; with a tibialis posterior problem the heel should be tilted in varus. However, if local tendon compression is believed to be an etiologic factor, reverse wedges are required. Great care must be exercised in using such devices lest the symptoms be further aggravated.

Local steroid infiltration into the tendon sheath is effective if performed before the condition becomes chronic. The tendon itself must not be injected and a limit of three injections must be imposed, for rupture of either of these tendon groups can be disastrous.

Surgical Treatment

Peroneal Tenosynovitis. Surgical decompression of the peroneal tendons is rarely required. If localized tenolysis is carried out, care must be taken to preserve the retinaculum in order to prevent subsequent tendon subluxation or dislocation.

Tibialis Tenosynovitis. Simple tenolysis is most effective for refractory cases. With release of structures behind the medial malleolus, freedom for the tendons to glide ensures relief of pain.

Accessory Tarsal Scaphoid Syndrome

Localized tendinitis of the tibialis posterior may be associated at its insertion with the persistent nonunion of an accessory ossicle—the accessory tarsal scaphoid. Generally this condition responds to orthotic support of the long arch and an intensive course of intrinsic and tibialis-strengthening exercises, as well as the general local measures of ice and ultrasonography.

On occasion, however, symptoms prove unresponsive and local excision of the accessory ossicle is indicated. It is essential to carefully incise the tendon longitudinally and shell out the loose bone, leaving the tendon insertion intact. Cast protection is unnecessary, but protected weight bearing and an arch support are continued until comfort is achieved. Return to sports may take 3 to 4 months.

Dorsal Tenosynovitis

The extensor tendon complex may be involved in dorsal tenosynovitis both anterior to the ankle and over the dorsum of the foot. On occasion, midtarsal osteophytes may be associated with early arthritic change and be a predisposing factor.

If the usual conservative measures, especially avoidance of footwear compression dorsally, are ineffective, a localized tenolysis can be performed. If midtarsal osteophytes are noted in the older athlete, a localized debridement should complement the procedure.

Acute and Chronic Luxations of the Peroneal Tendons

Traumatic dislocation of the peroneal tendons may be seen secondary to skiing accidents. Skiing requires that the peroneal muscles be contracted forcefully whenever the skier is making a turn or is traversing a hill. In such a situation, forced supination of the foot greatly enhances the risk of dislocation. The usual mechanism of injury is the ankle being forced into severe dorsiflexion with the foot slightly inverted, followed by a violent reflex contraction of the peroneals. For the dislocation to take place, the peroneals must go into a violent reflex action. Should the ski tip dive into the snow and become fixed, the patient is thrown forward, causing a dorsiflexion of the ankle, and acute dislocation of the peroneal tendons may ensue.

In the acute situation the diagnosis is suggested by swelling and ecchymosis in a region of the superior peroneal retinaculum, with sharp tenderness in the sulcus as well as along the distal fibula. Because the tendons spontaneously relocate, examination must attempt to reproduce the injury or the diagnosis may be missed. This is done by plantar flexion, eversion, and dorsiflexion against resistance, which will elicit pain and often dislocation.

Chronic subluxation or dislocation is often misdiagnosed as a chronic ankle sprain, with the patient complaining of a sense of uneasiness, giving way, or snapping in the lateral aspect of the ankle. The diagnosis is confirmed by demonstrating tendon displacement about a stable ankle mortise. Roentgenograms sometimes show an avulsion fracture of the lateral ridge of the lateral malleolus.

Treatment

In the presence of acute or chronic subluxation, a trial of conservative treatment is advised. Ankle taping and an elastic ankle support generally suffice, and most patients who have subluxation only will have little functional loss. Surgery is rarely needed in these situations.

Complete dislocation, either acute or chronic, is more difficult to treat. For the acute situation, conservative treatment consists of a below-knee weight-bearing cast for 6 weeks. Surgery is reserved for those in whom the condition recurs.

Surgical stabilization is effected by elevating a periosteal flap and folding it posteriorly to envelop the reduced peroneal tendons, thus reconstructing the peroneal retinaculum. It is important to hinge this flap along the posterior margin of the fibula and prevent any anterior glide of the tendon. The stretched retinaculum and sheath can be enfolded superficially, reinforcing the repair, which is cast protected for 6 weeks.

SUGGESTED READING

Anderson E. Stenosing peroneal tenosynovitis symptomatically simulating ankle instability. Am J Sports Med 1987; 15:258–259.

Crawford AH, Gabriel KR. Foot and ankle problems. Orthop Clin North Am 1987; 18:649–666.

Kleiger B. The posterior tibiotalar impingement syndrome in dancers. Bull Hosp J Dis Orthop Inst 1987; 47:203–210.
Pöll RG, Duijfjes F. The treatment of recurrent dislocation of the peroneal tendons. J Bone Joint Surg 1984; 66-B:98.
Riegler HF. Orthotic devices for the foot. Orthop Review 1987; 16:27–37.
Schepsis AA, et al. Surgical management of Achilles tendonitis. Am J Sports Med 1987; 15:308–315.
Wojtys EM. Sports injuries in the immature athlete. Orthop Clin North Am 1987; 18:689–708.

LIGAMENT INSTABILITY

BERNARD G. COSTELLO, M.D., F.R.C.S.(C)

Considering the frequency with which one encounters ankle ligament injuries, ankle instability should be one of the better understood disorders of the entire musculoskeletal system. It is surprising, therefore, that there are still some areas of disagreement on the subject of ankle injuries. This review provides a practical approach to the problem.

From the moment the athlete sustains an injury to the ankle, a pathophysiologic process is set in motion that must be identified, graded, and treated appropriately, in as short a time as possible, to achieve an optimal result.

The vast majority of ankle ligament injuries occur on the lateral aspect of this region. When deltoid (medial) injuries are present, they are commonly associated with lateral malleolar fractures or with major capsular and/or distal tibiofibular ligament injuries.

When an ankle inversion injury takes place, a predictable series of events occurs. With the initial twist injury, if the ankle is immediately righted by the individual, little or no injury occurs. If the corrective response to inversion is unsuccessful, the lateral collateral ligaments (anterior talofibular, calcaneofibular, and posterior talofibular) sustain injury to some extent (grades I to III), and the peroneal muscle group, forced to perform an extremely vigorous isometric contraction against a relatively fixed foot, also is often injured. Failure to recognize and treat this injury is an important cause of chronic "pseudo"-instability of the ankle. Finally, proprioceptive conduction seems to be delayed after these injuries, and this can also lead to an apparently unstable ankle. Even in the absence of significant ligament instability, some athletes report recurring inversion injuries. The likely reason, in the absence of clear ligamentous instability, is that when inversion occurs, not only is the proprioceptive pathway too slow, but when the message finally reaches the peroneal muscle group to correct the inversion, the muscle itself is too weak to comply.

CLASSIFICATION OF ACUTE INJURY

Ankle sprains are conventionally classified as grade I, II, or III. Grades I and II represent minimal and moderate injuries to the ligaments, with variable amounts of pain, swelling, ecchymosis, and loss of function. Neither of these renders the ankle unstable. Grade III injuries, on the other hand, are major disruptions of the ligamentous structures on the lateral aspect of the ankle and produce certain instabilities, which must be identified early in the course of the injury if treatment is to be successful.

HISTORY

In most of these injuries, the athlete clearly identifies the mechanism as being inversion and frequently notes that there was a "pop" or snapping sound at the time of the injury. Loss of function is variable in each of the three grades and is not fully reliable as an indication of severity of injury.

PHYSICAL EXAMINATION

The physical examination of the injured ankle requires careful and methodical assessment and is not meant to be a random exercise in palpation. Some of the critical areas that must be carefully palpated are the tip of the lateral malleolus, the anterior talofibular ligament area, the calcaneofibular ligament, at least the lateral half of the anterior joint capsule, and finally the base of the fifth metatarsal. It is equally important to detect tenderness over the tibiofibular ligaments, and over the distal interosseus membrane. On the basis of this physical examination, it is usually possible to grade the injuries accordingly, using the following criteria:

1. Grade I: No instability, full range of motion, minimal pain on weightbearing.
2. Grade II: Little or no ankle instability, or the presence of a very mild anterior drawer sign. There is a moderate decrease in range of motion as well as moderate pain and swelling. Weightbearing is usually more difficult than in grade I.
3. Grade III: The joint is clearly unstable. There usually is severe pain and swelling, with ecchymosis, significant loss of range of movement, and the inability to bear weight.

Apart from the general findings of ligamentous injury, the single most important aspect of the physical examination is the method used to demonstrate the presence of instability. The lateral instabilities of the ankle can be in either an anterior direction (a drawer sign) or a varus instability of the hind foot. The drawer sign is performed by holding the ankle in a neutral position and, with the fingers placed behind the heel, drawing the foot forward in an attempt to sublux the talus slightly in a forward direction. The presence of such a sign indicates disruption of the anterior talofibular ligament. The test for varus instability is performed again with the ankle in a neutral position and the hand placed on the lateral aspect of the heel. The foot is then inverted. If a feeling of instability is present, or if a "clunk" can be identified as the talus returns to its normal position upon removal of the varus stress, a strong suspicion of varus instability due to injury of the calcaneofibular ligament must be entertained.

RADIOLOGIC INVESTIGATION

A number of radiographic studies are available for ankle ligament injuries, but a frequent dilemma is to utilize these various investigations appropriately. In all but the most minor ankle injuries, routine views should be obtained, including a mortice view of the ankle. If there is clinical suggestion of lateral instability, varus stress views and a lateral view while the drawer sign is being elicited should be obtained. An anterior subluxation of the talus under the tibia is indicative of a disruption of the anterior talofibular ligament. Interpretation of the varus stress test is slightly more complex; however, a tilting of the talus within the ankle mortice of 0 to 7 degrees of varus is indicative of a disruption of the anterior talofibular ligament. A tilt of 7 to 30 degrees indicates increasing severity of injury, up to the point at which all the lateral collateral ligaments are damaged.

Contrast studies are of some value in evaluating the integrity of the lateral collateral ligaments of the ankle. Ankle arthrography, as reported, has failed to provide consistently useful information in identifying significant injuries of the lateral collateral ligament system of the ankle. A more recent modification of this technique utilizes a peroneal sheath arthrogram to identify major ligament injury to the lateral aspect of the ankle. If the dye is confined to the peroneal sheath, or if a small amount escapes through the sheath but does not enter the ankle joint, this study is considered negative. When the calcaneofibular ligament is torn, the dye passes through the defect in the sheath into the ankle joint, and then, because the anterior ligament capsule also is often torn, the dye may also pass from the joint itself. If doubt persists after stress views are taken, peroneal sheath arthrography may provide a more accurate assessment than ankle arthrography.

PITFALLS

A number of alternative diagnoses should be considered during the course of evaluation of ankle ligament injury. A fracture of the base of the fifth metatarsal may be entirely missed, particularly if routine views of the ankle are ordered without including the foot. Many radiographers exclude the metatarsal bases from an ankle view, and if such a fracture is present and has not been clinically identified through accurate palpation, it will be missed. Osteochondritis dissecans of the talus (osteochondral dome fractures), have been described and should be searched for, as many of them follow an inversion injury. Ankle sprain patterns may coexist with or be confused with a soft tissue injury to the distal interosseous membrane and/or tibiofibular ligament. This is usually a "spreading" mechanism of the ankle mortise, due to talar rotatory movement, in the absence of a fracture.

TREATMENT

Grade I Injuries

Grade I injuries of the lateral collateral ligaments of the ankle are considered, for the most part, to be minor injuries. The all too frequent routine of an elastic compression bandage, crutches, and advice to elevate the foot, often administered in hospital Emergency Departments, is completely unsatisfactory. The most appropriate treatment program for these injuries is the combination of rest, ice, compression, and elevation (RICE). This program is initiated immediately and followed usually for 72 hours, after which the patient is returned to early range of motion and weightbearing, and as rapid a return to normal activity as possible. The use of an adjustable air stirrup splint can be helpful in these cases, particularly in the early stages of return to activity.

Grade II Injuries

The best results for partial tears are obtained by early aggressive management. Again, the RICE program is most appropriate, followed by the early use of appropriate physiotherapy modalities to aid in resolution of the soft tissue damage. Range-of-motion exercises and isometrics are begun as soon as pain allows, usually within 48 hours, and the patient is begun on partial weightbearing at about 1 week. Many of these injuries are better supported by the use of taping or one of many prefabricated ankle compression and support devices on the market (stirrups, etc.). Standard taping techniques are frequently employed, generally using a Gibney basket weave with a heel lock, after swelling has maximized. If taping is initially employed in the management, it must be an open weave for at least 72 hours to avoid constriction should further swelling occur. The use of a plaster cast for grade II injuries should be avoided in most instances. It provides little advantage and does impose upon the injury its own set of consequences (muscle atrophy, stiffness, swelling, and occasionally disuse osteoporosis).

Grade III Injuries

Ligament injuries to the lateral aspect of the ankle resulting in instability involve either the anterior talofibular ligament alone or both the anterior talofibular and calcaneofibular ligaments. Although there may be some place for consideration of nonsurgical management (a plaster cast) in major tears of the anterior talofibular ligament alone, grade III injuries to the ankle usually are treated surgically. After direct open repair, a plaster cast is applied for 10 days followed by a functional splint, which will allow limited motion in the sagittal plane, until 6 weeks have passed. This is followed by a rehabilitation program similar to that used for grade II injuries.

Chronic Instability

Chronic lateral instability of the ankle is a disabling problem. Although nonsurgical methods have been used to stabilize the ankle in these cases, involving lateral heel wedges (unsuitable for athletic footwear) or various forms of stabilizing ankle wraps, the instability remains a problem.

Various surgical techniques have been employed to reconstruct chronic lateral instabilities of the ankle. The Watson-Jones method reconstructs the anterior talofibular ligament only, whereas the Evans procedure utilizes a peroneal tenodesis, again incompletely replacing the damaged structures.

The most logical approach is to perform an operation designed to replace both the anterior talofibular and the calcaneofibular ligaments. The modified Elmslie (Chrisman-Snook) procedure serves well in this regard. One-half or occasionally all of the entire peroneus brevis tendon is freed proximally and reflected distally, attaching the peroneus brevis muscle belly to that of the peroneus longus. The tendon is then woven through a tunnel in the area of the damaged anterior talofibular ligament, continued posteriorly through a drill hole in the distal fibular and then distally, and attached to the os calcis on its lateral surface, either by a staple or through a tunnel.

In a series reported in 1981, 22 modified Elmslie reconstructions were reviewed. All patients returned to their original choice of activity after surgery. In the author's hands, this operation similarly has proved very satisfactory in reducing or eliminating both the varus and the anterior drawer instability of the ankle. Postoperatively there is loss of inversion, but this recovers to a limited extent within 1 year and does not appear to be a major problem for patients.

SUGGESTED READING

Drez D Jr, Young JC, Waldman D, et al. Nonoperative treatment of double lateral ligament tears of the ankle. Am J Sports Med 1982; 10.

Evans GA, Hardcastle P, Frehyo AD. Acute rupture of the lateral ligaments of the ankle: to suture or not to suture. J Bone Joint Surg 1984; 66-B.

Smith RW, Reischl SF. Treatment of ankle sprains in young adults. Am J Sports Med 1986; 14.

Snook G, Chrisman OD, Wilson TC. Long-term results of the Chrisman-Snook operation for reconstruction of the lateral ligaments of the ankle. J Bone Joint Surg 1985; 67-A.

Stormont D, Morrey BF, Kai-Nan A, Cass JR. Stability of the loaded ankle: the relation between articular restraints, and primary and secondary static restraints. Am J Sports Med 1985; 13.

LATERAL ANKLE RECONSTRUCTION FOR CHRONIC INSTABILITY

GEORGE A. SNOOK, M.D.

Chronic lateral ligament instability of the ankle is a condition resulting from inadequate healing of tears of the lateral ligaments of the ankle, specifically the anterior talofibular ligament (ATFL) and the calcaneofibular ligament (CFL). The situation arises because of the anatomic characteristics of the ankle and a casual attitude toward treatment of the original sprain.

ANATOMY—MECHANISM OF INJURY

The ankle is an inherently stable joint with support provided by the bony buttresses of the medial and lateral malleoli and the medial and lateral collateral ligaments. The support, however, is unequal, since the medial malleolus is short and does not completely embrace the talus, while the longer lateral malleolus extends to the subtalar joint. The opposite is true of the ligaments, since the medial collateral ligament is the wide, strong deltoid ligament, while the lateral collateral ligament consists of three thin, well-spaced bands: the ATFL, the CFL, and the posterior talofibular ligament (PTFL). The PTFL provides little or no support for varus instability of the ankle.

A varus force applied to the ankle, therefore, is resisted by the short medial malleolus and the relatively weak lateral ligaments. If the force is severe enough, the foot rolls over the medial malleolus and the ligaments rupture. A valgus force, on the other hand, is resisted by the larger lateral malleolus and the stronger deltoid ligament. If the force is too great in this direction a more serious fracture of the lateral malleolus occurs with rupture of the deltoid ligament.

The basic problem in the development of chronic lateral instability of the ankle is that, unlike the knee joint, the ankle is an inherently stable joint because of the bony supports. After a severe sprain the foot returns to its normal position and some healing of the ligaments takes place. The patient is soon able to walk, but if the joint is not protected the ligaments are subjected to constant motion and stretching, and they either heal elongated or are replaced with a mass of scar tissue. With the loss of integrity of the ligament supports, the ankle becomes unstable and subject to recurrent sprains.

DIAGNOSIS

The history usually is relatively simple. The patient complains of repeated sprains of the ankle, usually initiated by a major sprain on the first occasion. There is apprehension when walking on an uneven surface, and there are occasional sprains even on level terrain or when stepping off a curb.

The physical examination findings may be innocuous depending on the duration of time since the last injury. There may be tenderness over the ATFL. The most constant sign is a positive anterior drawer sign tested when the patient has no pain or tenderness. It is performed with the patient seated on an examining table and the knee flexed at 90 degrees. The lower leg is stabilized with one hand while the other hand grasps the foot at the heel and midfoot. With the foot at a right angle, it is drawn forward. A greater excursion in the injured ankle than in the normal ankle represents a positive anterior drawer test.

Roentgenograms should be taken, especially to determine the presence or absence of osteoarthritis or loose bodies.

Stress roentgenograms may be helpful when compared with similar films of the uninjured side. These must be considered only as an aid, because the results are variable and much depends on the position of the ligaments. The ATFL and the CFL form an arc. This arc makes the CFL the primary restraint when the ankle is at a right angle, while the ATFL is the primary restraint with the foot in plantar flexion. The ATFL is always torn in these injuries, while the CFL is torn in 20 to 90 percent of injuries depending on the investigator. Thus, stress roentgenograms may show normal results with the foot at a right angle, while the anterior drawer sign should always be positive.

The differential diagnosis should include neuromuscular weakness, osteoarthritis, loose bodies, and the impingement syndrome. This syndrome results from recurrent trauma to the joint capsule, synovial membrane, and articular cartilage. It can give the same clinical picture as recurrent ligament sprains, except that the anterior drawer sign is negative. Magnetic resonance imaging (MRI) of the ankle may be of great assistance in making this diagnosis.

NONSURGICAL TREATMENT

Nonsurgical treatment of this condition consists of support, muscle strengthening, and development of position sense. Strengthening of the peroneal muscles is essential to this treatment regimen. This can be performed by resistance exercise of the ankle against rubber bands in abduction and plantar flexion. Development of position sense and protective reflexes can be done on a roller board or tilt table. The simplest form of support is a ¼-inch outer heel wedge in the shoe, which can be quite valuable on even surfaces although useless on uneven ground.

Although taping or ankle wraps can be used for athletic contests, they are not practical for everyday wear. Various types of laced or Velcro-fastened supports are available commercially.

SURGICAL TREATMENT

Surgical treatment is directed toward restoring stability to the lateral ankle while retaining a full range of motion to the joint.

Two types of procedures are currently in use: a direct repair of the ATFL as advocated by Brostrom and a replacement of the lateral ligaments by a tendinous substitute. The latter procedure can be further divided into those procedures that replace only the ATFL and those that replace both the ATFL and the CFL.

The repair procedure is the simplest of these operations: it does not sacrifice tendons and uses a smaller incision. When successful, it restores the normal anatomy. The author finds, however, that separating the ligament from the mass of scar tissue is not easy, and in very old cases the ligament is too short to repair and the surgeon is repairing only scar tissue. A second objection is that it does not solve the problem of the CFL. This operation is preferable for patients whose injury is no more than 6 months old.

There are a variety of reconstruction operations in current use. All of them use a portion or the whole of a tendon to replace the function of the injured ligaments. The peroneus brevis is the one most commonly used. Most of these operations replace the ATFL, and a few replace both ligaments.

The author prefers the Chrisman-Snook procedure, which utilizes one-half of the peroneus brevis tendon and effectively replaces both the ATFL and the CFL.

Procedure

With the patient in the lateral position and the affected ankle uppermost, an incision is made starting at the base of the fifth metatarsal and extending proximally in a curved manner behind the lateral malleolus and up the leg for a distance of about 15 cm. The subcutaneous tissue is divided, hemostasis obtained, and a careful search made for the sural nerve. In most cases it is found alongside the proximal limb of the incision. It is carefully mobilized and retracted. A skin flap retaining the subcutaneous tissue is then mobilized anteriorly to expose the lateral malleolus. The sheaths of the peroneal tendons are opened throughout their length and the tendons mobilized. The peroneus brevis tendon is split longitudinally from its insertion at the fifth metatarsal to the musculotendinous junction. It is best to continue this split up along the tendon fascia that embraces the muscle, to ensure adequate length. One-half of the tendon is then detached proximally but left attached at the insertion. The graft is wrapped in a saline sponge and preserved. A drill hole is placed in the lateral malleolus from front to back at its widest part, starting with a small hole that is gradually enlarged until it is easy to pass the graft through it. Using the same drill bit that was employed in the lateral malleolus, a tunnel is created on the lateral side of the os calcis just below the peroneal trochlea. This is done by making two holes in a "V" direction about 1 cm apart and then enlarging the holes with a curet.

The graft is next passed through the malleolar hole from front to back (Fig. 1). The foot is held in a neutral position while a tacking stitch is placed through the graft and periosteum to maintain the foot in this position against gravity. The peroneal tendons are replaced in their grooves, and the graft is brought inferiorly and through the os calcis tunnel and then proximally to be sutured to itself just in front of the lateral malleolus (Fig 2). The ankle should be held in maximal dorsiflexion when anchoring the graft to itself.

The peroneal sheath is next closed behind the lateral malleolus to guard against subsequent subluxation of the peroneal tendons. The sural nerve is replaced and the wound closed. A short-leg nonweightbearing cast is applied.

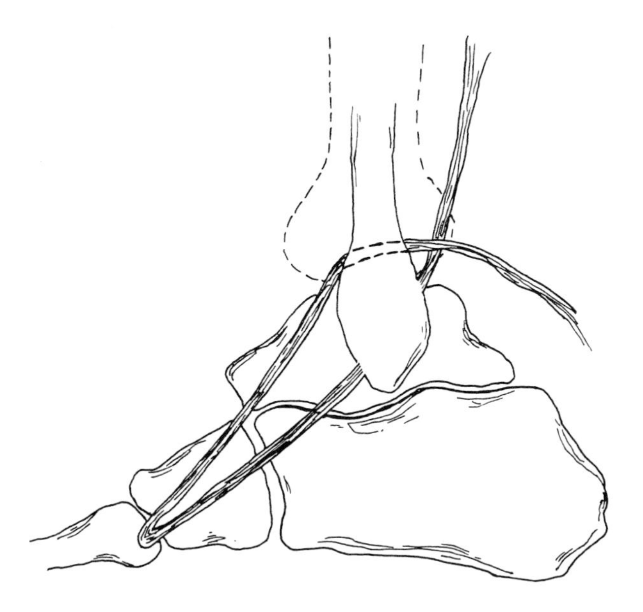

Figure 1 The free end of the divided peroneus brevis is passed through a drill hole in the distal fibula.

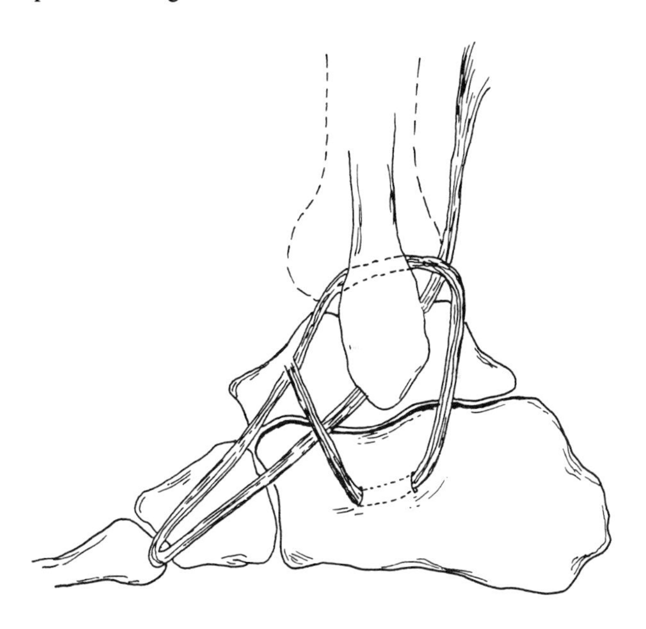

Figure 2 The free end of the tendon of the peroneus brevis is passed through a drill hole in the lateral wall of the os calcis and sewn back to itself to complete the ligament repair.

POSTOPERATIVE CARE

The cast is worn for 3 weeks and a walking cast is then substituted for ambulation, with full weight bearing as tolerated for 5 more weeks. The skin sutures are removed at the 3-week interval. Upon removal of the second cast the patient may start weight bearing using crutches for support for as long as necessary, usually 2 days to 1 week.

Range of motion in dorsiflexion, plantar flexion, and eversion return rapidly, but it may take several months before the final limit of inversion is reached. There may be a slight loss of full inversion but seldom more than 10 degrees. Physical therapy with whirlpool and joint mobilization can be helpful in regaining motion.

COMPLICATIONS

Aside from the complications common to any lower extremity operation (infection, thrombophlebitis), the patient should be warned about the risk of sural nerve neuritis and possible division of the nerve producing diminished or absent sensation along the lateral border of the foot. Neuritis is usually transient, and except for the rare tender neuroma the loss of sensation has not been troublesome to those few patients who have experienced it.

The incision just behind and below the lateral malleolus is apt to heal slower than the rest of the incision, and therefore the skin sutures should remain in place for 3 weeks.

One must be careful not to evert the ankle forcefully when performing the reconstruction, otherwise the patient may have trouble regaining inversion. Some athletes have experienced difficulty with a loss of dorsiflexion caused by making the second and third limbs of the reconstruction too tight. This can be prevented by placing the foot in maximal dorsiflexion and neutral rotation when suturing the third limb to the first at the last stage of the operation. This complication can be corrected by a Z-plasty lengthening of the second and third limbs of the graft.

RESULTS

In a long-term follow-up (4 to 24 years) of 48 operations, all but three patients had good or excellent results. The two patients with fair and the one with poor results experienced severe reinjury of the ankle with presumed damage to the reconstruction.

SUGGESTED READING

Brostrom L. Sprained ankles. III. Clinical observations in recent ligament injuries. Acta Chir Scand 1965; 130:560–569.

Cox JS, Hewes TF. "Normal" talar tilt angle. Clin Orthop 1979; 140:37–41.

Evans DL. Recurrent dislocation of the ankle. A method of surgical treatment. Proc R Soc Med 1953; 46:343–348.

Mandelbaum BR, Bartolozzi AR, Finerman GA, Padilla P, Meyerson M. The anterior capsular impingement syndrome in the ankle of the athlete: methods of diagnosis and treatment. Paper presented at the 13th Annual Meeting of the American Orthopedic Society for Sports Medicine, Orlando, FL, June 29, 1987.

Rubin G, Witten M. The talar tilt angle and the fibular collateral ligaments. J Bone Joint Surg 1960; 42A:311–326.

Ruth CJ. The surgical treatment of injuries of the fibular collateral ligaments of the ankle. J Bone Joint Surg 1961; 43A:229–239.

St Pierre R, Allman F Jr, Bassett FH III, Goldner JL, Flemming LL. A review of lateral ankle ligamentous reconstructions. Foot Ankle 1982; 3:114–123.

Snook GA, Chrisman OD, Wilson TC. Long-term results of the Chrisman-Snook operation for reconstruction of the lateral ligaments of the ankle. J Bone Joint Surg 1985; 67A:1–7.

Stormont DM, Morrey BF, Kai-Nan A, Cass JR. Stability of the loaded ankle. Relationship between articular restraint and primary and secondary static restraints. Am J Sports Med 1984; 13:295–300.

Watson-Jones R. Fractures and joint injuries. 4th ed. Baltimore: Williams & Wilkins, 1955:821.

NONOPERATIVE MANAGEMENT OF ANKLE INJURIES

JOSEPH J. VEGSO, M.S., A.T., C.

It is a well-accepted fact that the ankle is the most frequently injured joint in athletes, representing 10 to 30 percent of all injuries. Although the incidence of injury to the ankle is high, relatively few patients come to surgery. It is therefore the intent of this chapter to present an approach to nonoperative management of ankle injuries.

An accurate diagnosis is the obvious first step in the management of any ankle sprain. The standard grading system of I, II, and III is appropriate in defining the extent of ligamentous instability. In addition, a functional clinical grading system (Table 1) to supplement the instability classification has proved extremely helpful in instituting an appropriate course of treatment.

Grade III injuries in most situations are considered surgical problems, so this chapter focuses on grades I and II.

TABLE 1 Functional Clinical Grading System for Ankle Sprains

Grade I	Minimal pain and swelling Stable joint Full range of motion Pain-free weight bearing Heel and toe walking
Grade II	Moderate pain and swelling Subtle joint or minimal anterior drawer Decreased range of motion Difficulty in weight bearing and ambulation
Grade III	Severe pain and swelling Unstable joint Minimal range of motion or inability to flex dorsally Inability to bear weight

The ankle is an inherently stable joint: nonweightbearing treatment is rarely appropriate and in fact may be detrimental. The common emergency room plan of crutches, Ace wrap, and advice to "stay off it for a while" may prolong the symptoms. The foot is held in the plantar flexed-inverted position, which places the injured ligaments under tension in an elongated position, and the foot is in a dependent position without the benefit of muscle action to increase venous and lymphatic return. Heat is also routinely prescribed after 24 hours, which by increasing the amount of swelling makes healing take longer. One must be primarily concerned with the prevention of swelling in soft tissue injuries because increased swelling is directly related to loss of range of motion and an increase in recovery time. Therefore, heat should never be used in the acute or subacute phases of recovery. Individuals charged with the care of ankle injuries should not only encourage the use of ice but also strongly discourage the use of heat.

The appropriate initial treatment regimen consists of ice, compression, and elevation; this is easily recalled by the mnemonic "ICE" as mentioned by Brown. The use of cold in the acute and subacute stages of healing in athletic injuries is well documented by Kalenak and colleagues and McMaster.

Physiologically, cold causes vasoconstriction, thereby decreasing blood flow and hemorrhage, with a resulting decrease of edema. Additionally, cold acts as a local anesthetic, which aids in the control of pain and secondarily to relieve muscle spasm. Ice is contraindicated for individuals with rheumatic conditions, decreased sensation, or vascular problems.

Frequently, grade II and even grade I sprains develop effusions that require aspiration, often of up to 5 ml of synovial fluid or blood. In addition to the aspiration, a single injection of a corticosteroid such as Kenalog-10 (triamcinolone acetonide) into the joint has been found to be extremely effective in controlling the inflammatory response.

IMMOBILIZATION

The need for support or immobilization is dependent on the individual's ability to bear weight. In cases of mild disability the individual is best supported by an adhesive strapping, an open Gibney in the acute stage followed by a closed Gibney boot.

The open Gibney is used to support the lateral and medial structures of the joint. However, it also allows freedom of movement in plantar flexion and dorsiflexion. It is left open along the dorsal aspect of the foot and ankle to allow normal circulation. The closed Gibney provides the same lateral and medial support, but is used in the subacute stage once edema and hemorrhage have begun to subside.

In individuals who require slightly more rigid support, an Unna boot made of Dome-Paste bandage (Dome Laboratories, West Haven, CT) is utilized. The Dome-Paste bandage is made of 3- or 4-inch wide gauze impregnated with a mixture of zinc oxide and calamine. It is applied like an elastic bandage directly to the skin, with an elastic wrap over it. The bandage becomes semirigid within 24 hours and may be left on for 7 to 10 days. Weightbearing is permissible. This method of support is an ideal compromise between an adhesive strapping and a rigid cast. Crutches may be used to allow partial weight bearing with either method of support.

Rigid casting is reserved for individuals who are unable to bear weight following a grade II injury. Typically, a short-leg weightbearing cast is applied for 1 to 3 weeks. When a rigid cast is used the foot must be placed as much in dorsiflexion and eversion as possible. During cast immobilization, strength in the upper leg and hip of the injured limb will decrease. Therefore, an exercise program designed to maintain strength must be instituted.

It is important to remember that cold therapy can and should be continued while the ankle is immobilized. Cold will penetrate tape, Dome-Paste, and plaster or fiberglass casts.

REHABILITATION

Ankle injuries are too often inadequately rehabilitated. Allman states that "the susceptibility of the ankle to ligamentous injury in athletics necessitates complete rehabilitation following surgery . . . and inadequately treated or poorly rehabilitated ankle injuries often result in instability." "On the other hand," say Klafs and Arnheim, "many sports physicians and trainers maintain that the best method is the moderately active approach, in which the athlete returns to competition much sooner than with the conservative treatment and completes his therapy through activity." Such is the dilemma facing the physician called upon to treat an athlete with an ankle injury.

Adequate healing must be guaranteed before the athlete may return to activity, and such activity must be without limitation in order that the individual may function safely and effectively. Therefore, a program with time constraints that meet these two objectives is warranted.

An accurate diagnosis followed by appropriate first aid are significant steps in the rehabilitation process. Standard first aid after ankle sprains includes ice, compression, and elevation simultaneously for 20 to 30 minutes. This procedure should be repeated four to six times daily for 48 to 72 hours. It is the author's opinion that heat should never be used as an independent modality in the treatment of ankle sprains.

Overnight treatment should consist of repeated cold therapy, in conjunction with an open Gibney strapping, a soft foam horseshoe, and a loosely applied elastic bandage. The athlete should also be placed on crutches with instructions to bear as much weight as pain and range of motion permit. It is better to have athletes ambulate in a normal gait pattern with crutches than to allow them to limp. A 1/4- to 3/8-inch heel lift often permits athletes to ambulate more comfortably in the acute stage. The open Gibney strapping procedure should be continued as long as the possibility of further swelling exists, usually for 48 to 72 hours. Crutch-assisted ambulation should continue until pain-free, normal ambulation is possible. Treatment protocols for ankle sprains by grade are outlined in Table 2.

Range-of-motion exercises for dorsiflexion may be initiated within 24 hours, depending on the severity of the injury. This should be done actively or in an active-assisted manner by having partial body weight provide the assistance, as shown in Figure 1*A*. A wedge board may also be used to perform this exercise (Fig. 1*B*). Calf stretching is also permitted as tolerated. Plantar flexion, inversion, and eversion should be avoided in the early treatment phase in order to permit healing.

It is important that non-weightbearing activities designed to maintain strength and cardiorespiratory conditioning be implemented during the early phases of rehabilitation. Suggested activities include strength training on equipment such as Nautilus (Nautilus Sports-Medical Industries, Deland, FL) or Universal Gym (Universal, Inc., Cedar Rapids, IA); any other strength training equipment that does not require weight bearing; and swimming or arm cycling on a stationary bicycle.

TABLE 2 Treatment Protocol of Ankle Sprains by Grade

Grade I
Accurate diagnosis
ICE* (4 to 6 times daily)
Aspiration and/or injection
Taping or Unna boot for support or immobilization (3 to 5 days)
Cardiorespiratory conditioning and total body strengthening
Agility and functional activities
Grade II
Accurate diagnosis
ICE* (4 to 6 times daily)
Aspiration and/or injection
Unna boot or cast (1 to 3 weeks)
Cardiorespiratory conditioning and total body strengthening
Range of motion and strengthening exercises
Agility and functional activities
Grade III
Accurate diagnosis
Surgical repair
Cardiorespiratory conditioning and total body strengthening
Range of motion and strength
Agility and functional exercises

*Ice, compression, elevation.

Once swelling is controlled or begins to subside and the athlete is able to ambulate pain free, the second phase of the rehabilitation program may be initiated. This may begin as early as 24 to 48 hours after injury. Again, the time frame is dependent on the severity of the injury. Ice treatments should continue as described previously. Support of the injured ankle for all nonathletic activities should be continued if necessary during this phase. This is best accomplished through the use of a loosely applied, closed Gibney strapping, which should be worn during all waking hours. If it is possible to have the ankle

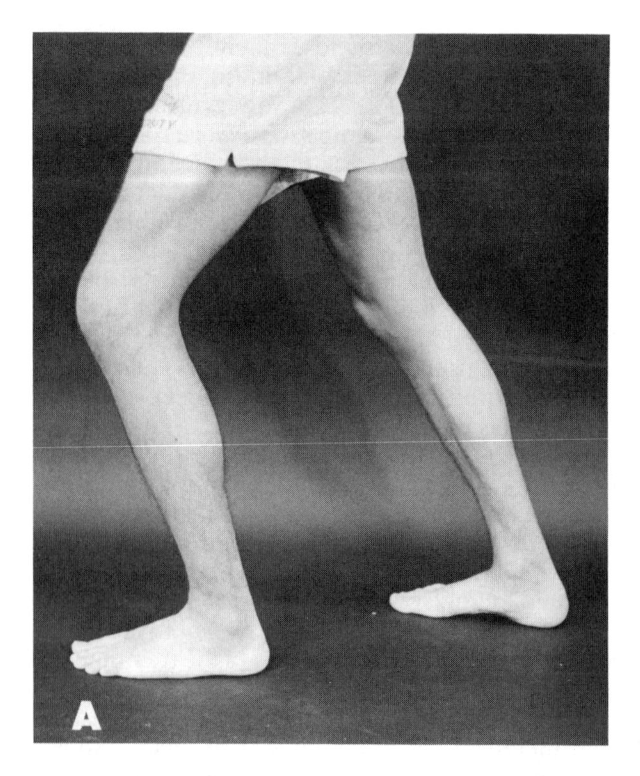

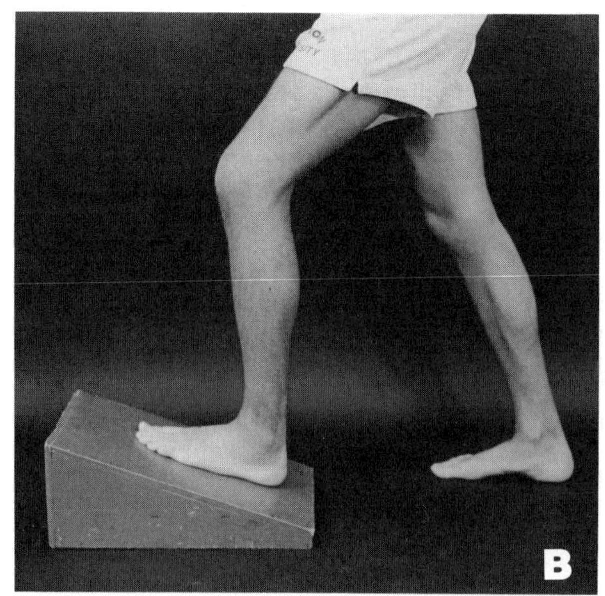

Figure 1 *A,* Ankle range of motion (dorsiflexion) is shown. The left ankle and the knee are flexed, and the foot is flat on the floor. *B,* Ankle range of motion on a wedge board (dorsiflexion) is shown. The left ankle and knee are flexed.

restrapped every day, the strapping should be removed and replaced by a loose-fitting elastic wrap overnight. If this is not possible, the strapping should remain on the ankle 24 hours a day for up to 3 days. However, the athlete must be cautioned with regard to possible tingling, numbness, blue toes, or constant, severe itching. Any of these signs warrant immediate removal of the tape.

Exercises in phase 2 are utilized to increase uniplane range of motion at the ankle joint and muscle strength in the lower leg. Exercises to increase plantar flexion are added to those performed in phase 1. Activities that would cause excessive inversion and eversion must still be avoided.

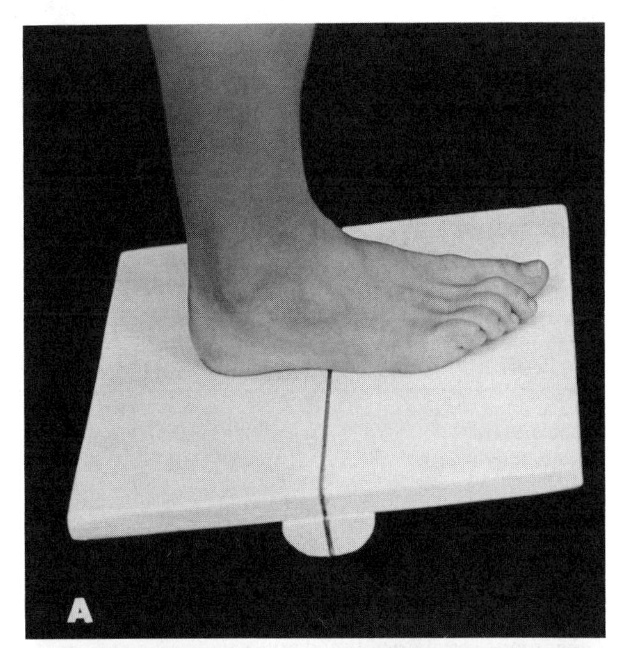

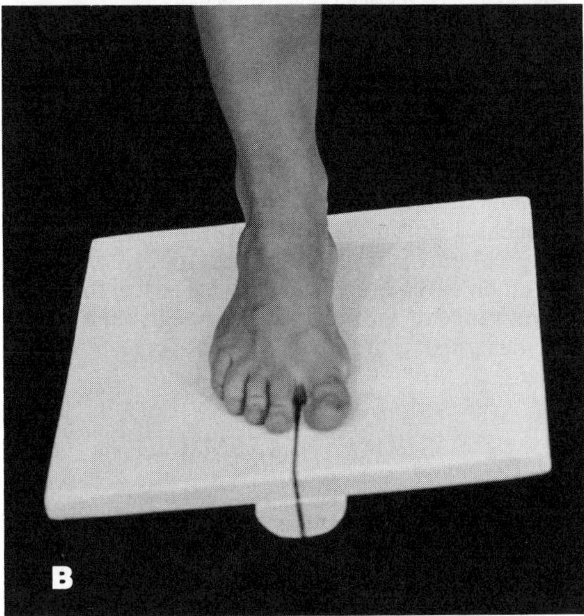

Figure continues on following page.

Toe raises are performed to increase strength in the posterior muscle group. They should be done on a wedge board, stool, or step so that the muscles work through a full range of motion. Heel and toe walking are also performed to improve muscular strength and endurance and neuromuscular function. The position of the feet should be changed so that they are inverted and everted while the heel and toe walking are performed. Dorsiflexion, inversion, and eversion strength can be increased through the use of surgical tubing, manual resistance, or isometric exercises at various angles.

A variety of other methods are employed to increase range of motion, strength, and muscular endurance of the ankle. The Elgin Ankle Exerciser (Elgin Exerciser Appliance Co., Sandwich, IL) and the Cybex II (Cybex-Division of Lumex, Inc., Ronkonkoma, NY) have proved extremely effective in rehabilitating injured ankles.

REINJURY

The most common reason for chronic pain and reinjury following an ankle sprain, in my experience, is decreased dorsiflexion. A simple method for determining whether an athlete has decreased motion is as follows: First, have the athlete place both feet (without shoes) on the floor, hip width apart and parallel. Next, instruct the athlete to bend both

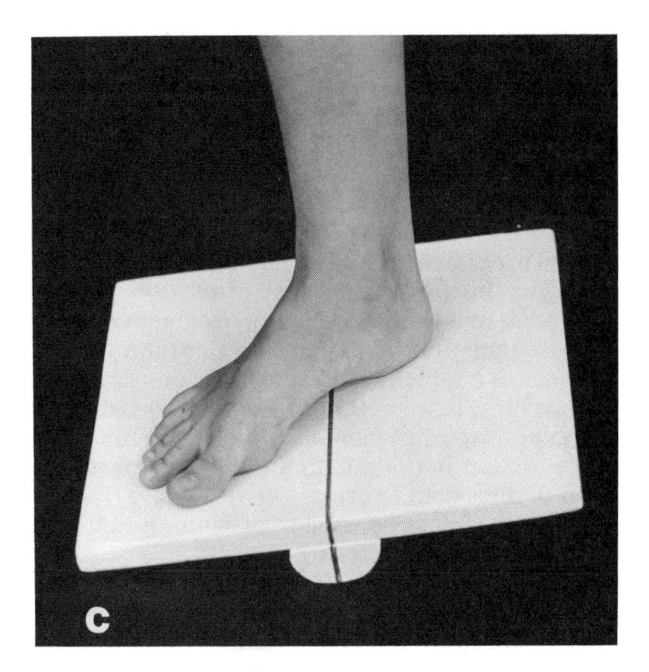

Figure 2 The wobble board for uniplane, proprioceptive exercises is shown; it is made of 15 × 15 × ¾–inch plywood with a 2-inch dowel. The athlete is instructed to rock back and forth in a controlled manner for up to 3 minutes in each direction. *A,* The wobble board position for plantar flexion and dorsiflexion is shown. *B,* Positioning for inversion and eversion. *C,* Position for pronation and supination at 45 degrees of external rotation.

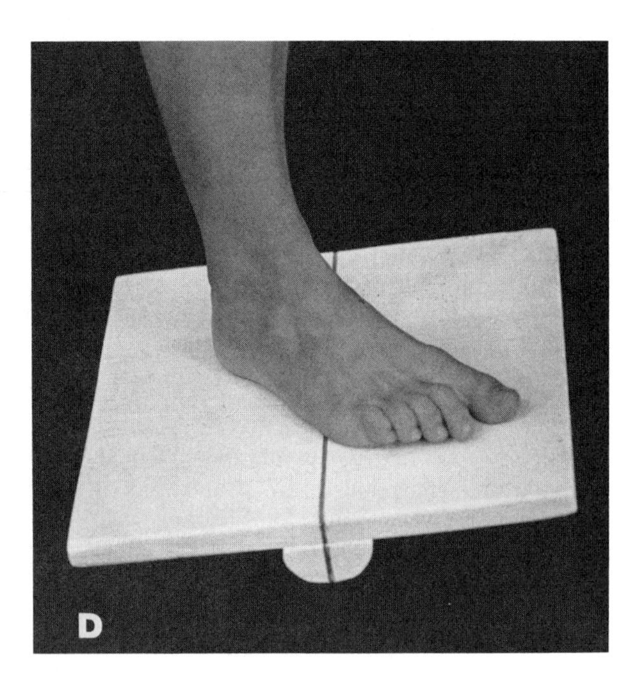

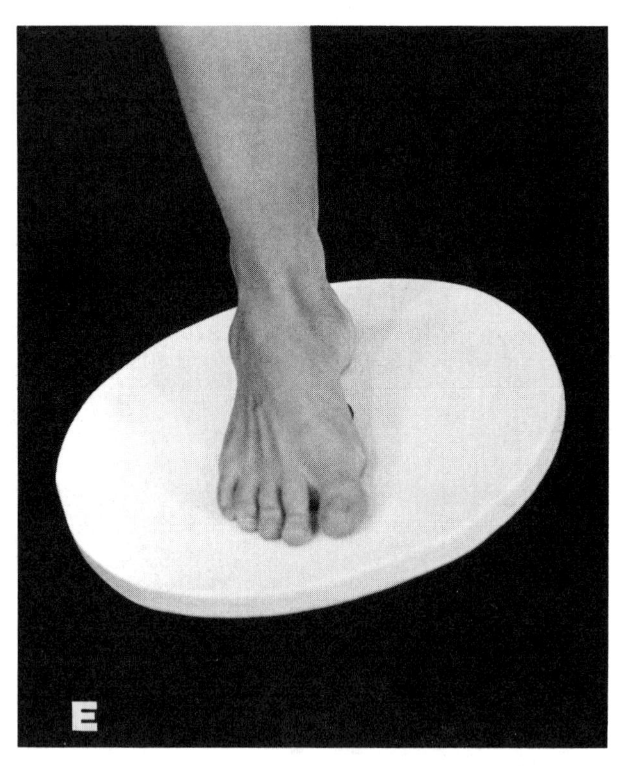

Figure 2 (Continued) *D,* Position for pronation and supination at 45 degrees of internal rotation. *E,* Multidirectional wobble board for proprioceptive exercises.

knees and both ankles while keeping the feet flat on the floor. Then, observe for a difference in motion. This test is an excellent indicator of the need for continuing or reinstituting a rehabilitation program.

Fiore and Leard, Freeman and colleagues, and others emphasize the importance of proprioceptive and neuromuscular function of the ankle joint. This aspect of rehabilitation is left to chance when the athlete is permitted to return to participation before functional, multiplane, and high-speed activities are incorporated into the rehabilitation program. Allowing this important aspect of rehabilitation to take place in the uncontrolled environment of practice or competition needlessly subjects the athlete to reinjury. It is therefore recommended that activities such as those listed in Table 3 should be used to redevelop proprioceptive and neuromuscular functions and to determine the athlete's ability to perform at a level necessary to return to activity safely (Fig. 2). The ankle should be supported with an adhesive strapping for these activities.

Once athletes are capable of performing all their sports-specific activities to the physician's, athletic trainer's, and coach's satisfaction, they are permitted to return to participation. An adhesive strapping should be used for participation following injury and should be continued throughout the season.

It is difficult and unwise to put time constraints on the rate of recovery or specific aspects of recovery. One may find that an athlete who suffers a grade I inversion sprain progresses through the entire rehabilitation program in 3 days; conversely, a nonsurgical grade II or greater inversion sprain may take up to 8 weeks before complete recovery is achieved. It seems, therefore, that a combination of the approaches recommended by Allman and by Klafs and Arnheim is appropriate. Emphasis should be placed on early and continued use of ice, the return to full range of motion, and the inclusion of activities designed to reintegrate neuromuscular function.

TABLE 3 Agility and Proprioceptive Activities

Heel and toe walking
Wobble board
Rope skipping
Straight ahead jogging
Straight ahead running
Backward running
Running circles: clockwise, counterclockwise, backward, and forward (5-yard diameter)
90-degree cuts while running
Running figure eights
Other sports-specific agility and skill activities

SUGGESTED READING

Allman FL. Rehabilitation following athletic injuries. In: O'Donoghue D, ed. Treatment of injuries to athletes. 4th ed. Philadelphia: WB Saunders, 1984.

Blyth CS, Mueller, FO. An epidemiologic study of high school football injuries in North Carolina 1968–1972. Final report. Washington, DC: Consumer Products Safety Commission.

Brown A. Physical medicine in rehabilitation. Md State Med J 1970; 19:61.

Fiore RD, Leard JS. A functional approach in the rehabilitation of the ankle and rear foot. Athl Train 1980; 231–235.
Freeman MA, et al. The etiology and prevention of functional instability of the foot. J Bone Joint Surg 1965; 47B:678.
Garrick JG. The frequency of injury, mechanism of injury and epidemiology of ankle sprains. Am J Sports Med 1977; 5:241.
Jackson DW, Ashley RL, Powell, JW. Ankle sprains in young athletes—relation of severity and disability. Clin Orthop 1974; 101:201.
Kalenak A, et al. Athletic injuries: heat vs. cold. Am Fam Physician 1975; 12:131.
Klafs EC, Arnheim DD. Modern principles of athletic training. 4th ed. St Louis: CV Mosby, 1977.
Mack RP. Ankle injuries in athletics. Athl Train 1975; 10:94.
McMaster WC. A literary review of ice therapy on injuries. Am J Sports Med 1977; 5:124.
Stanford Research Institute: National Football League 1974 Injury Study. Menlo Park, CA, June 1975.

OPERATIVE MANAGEMENT OF LIGAMENTOUS INJURIES

ROBERT L. BRAND, M.D.

Injuries to the lateral ligaments of the ankle are the most common joint injury in sports. They occur in athletes of all ages, and are precipitated by an inversion injury with the ankle in plantar flexion. In the author's experience, the most severe injuries occur in jumping sports, so that basketball is the sport that produces the most common severe injury to the lateral ligaments of the ankle.

ANATOMY

The important lateral ligaments of the ankle are the tibiofibular, the anterior talofibular, and the fibulocalcaneal. The posterior talofibular is little involved in the clinical stability of the ankle. Significant disruption of the tibiofibular ligament is a rare sports injury and beyond the scope of this chapter. The prime ligaments involved in this type of injury are the anterior talofibular and the fibulocalcaneal ligaments.

DIAGNOSIS

The diagnosis of severe injury to the ligaments of the ankle is based on the history, physical examination, confirmatory tests. The history involves an inversion injury often arising from an individual's being involved in a jump or landing from a jump. Often the injured athlete can recall feeling one to three "pops." He or she will have been disabled from further participation if the injury is of significance. The findings at physical evaluation vary, depending on the length of time after the injury. If a significant time has elapsed since the injury, there will be a considerable amount of swelling. This initially begins over the area of the ligaments but can spread on to the foot as time passes. Ecchymosis develops along the lateral aspect of the foot and follows the extensor tendons out on to the toes. There is tenderness over the area of the anterior talofibular and fibulocalcaneal ligaments. However, as time elapses and swelling increases, the localization of this tenderness becomes less and its reliability as an indicator of single or double ligament tears is lessened. The competency of the anterior talofibular ligament is tested by an anterior lateral drawer test. This is performed by placing one hand in the supramalleolar area of the tibia; the hand on the lateral aspect of the ankle cups the heel and draws forward as counterforce is applied with the hand on the tibia. This test is reliable only with the foot in equinus and with the patient relaxed. I have found this to be best performed with the patient's leg over the edge of the examining table flexed at the knee and the foot allowed to hang in a gravity equinus. A sensation of the laxity to inversion stress can be performed in a similar manner, the stress being applied toward inversion with counterforce applied over the medial malleolar area of the distal tibia. With experience, the laxity can be graded mild, moderate, or severe.

Confirmatory tests should include routine roentgenograms of the ankle joint, including anteroposterior, mortis, and lateral views. Assuming there is no fracture, an inversion stress test of the ankle is performed and documented on roentgenography. It is generally possible to perform this test without anesthesia, the knee being flexed over a bolster to produce approximately 20 degrees of flexion at the knee. The foot must be in equinus for the test to be accurate. Anterior drawer stress roentgenography can be performed, but this test is of little help for a diagnosis leading to a recommendation for surgical repair.

I participated in the development of peroneal sheath arthrography, but have not found this test to be of practical use in a clinical situation. The test requires fluoroscopic control, which is cumbersome in an office setting; the stress test is just as reliable. When necessary, peroneal nerve block or local anesthesia can be used to help control the discomfort produced by the examination. On the basis of the studies of Almquist, Bonnin, Cox, and my own experience, talar tilts of over 20 degrees appear to indicate a double ligament tear. A tilt of 15 degrees indicates at least complete disruption of the anterior talofibular ligament.

INDICATIONS FOR SURGERY

I rarely recommend surgery for talar tilts of less than 25 degrees in a primary injury. As the talar tilt increases above this, the surgical approach can be more aggressive. It is more common to find the fibulocalcaneal ligament in a position that is very unlikely to heal as the talar tilt increases toward 40 degrees.

An avulsion fracture of the lateral malleolus with a talar tilt of 15 degrees portends a poor result if treated conservatively and therefore is one indication for surgery.

Functional instability in a patient with a recent injury is an indication for surgery. These persons normally have had numerous sprains and frequently sustain a mild sprain of the ankle stepping off the curb, on a rock, or in a small hole that normally would not produce a sprain. In such individuals with "weak ankles," surgery with minimal talar tilt is recommended.

Surgery is also advisable in those in whom an osteochondral fracture of the talus is identified.

NONSURGICAL TREATMENT

Athletes whose ankle sprains are not severe enough for surgery or who decline a recommendation for surgery are treated in a functional manner. Based on experience, treatment with tape results in a more rapid return to functional status than does cast immobilization. The tape method prevents atrophy of the calf muscles; it allows for early motion, which apparently increases the strength of the healing fibrous tissue; and it perhaps leads to earlier orientation of the fibroblast into ligamentous-appearing tissue.

SURGICAL REPAIR

Surgery is usually carried out under general anesthesia, but spinal or epidural anesthesia is also satisfactory. The hip on the involved side is elevated to produce slight internal rotation, and the calf of the leg is placed on a 5-inch plaster box.

An oblique incision is made following Langer's lines just below the tip of the lateral malleolus. Care is taken to avoid the lateral branch of the superficial peroneal nerve, and the incision is ended short of the area of the sural nerve. The subcutaneous tissue can be bluntly dissected. In fresh injuries, the area of hemorrhage leads quickly to the torn capsule and the lateral aspect of the tibiotalar joint.

After suctioning, blood is aspirated from the joint and a quick inspection is made for osteochondral fragments. The anterior talofibular ligament is identified. The peroneal tendons are then retracted using a Cushing retractor, and the fibulocalcaneal ligament is identified. Most commonly it is torn from its attachment on the calcaneus, but it can be torn from either end or in mid-substance.

If the fibulocalcaneal ligament is torn from its calcaneal attachment, the calcaneus is roughened slightly with a curret. A suture is placed through the distal portion of the fibulocalcaneal ligament, brought out from the peroneal tendons, and tagged with a hemostat to be tied later. The anterior talofibular ligament is then repaired; it also may be torn from either end or in mid-substance. When it is torn from the talar neck, a suture is passed through the heavy periosteum on the talar neck and through the ligament. In mid-substance, the limbs are overlapped with one or two synthetic, absorbable sutures. Before these sutures are tied, the foot is placed in a 90-degree, plantar grade position and held for the remainder of the procedure. When the ligament is torn from the lateral malleolus, the latter is roughened slightly; small drill holes made with a 5th 64 Steinmann pin are placed in the lateral malleolus and a synthetic absorbable suture is passed through these and through the ligament. If an avulsion fracture has occurred, the ossicle is excised and the ligament is approximated to the lateral malleolus. Almost always there is sufficient length to accomplish this.

When the patient has functional instability and there is a good deal of scar, it may be necessary to reinforce the repair. The anterior talofibular ligament usually attaches itself to a portion of the capsule and can be identified, dissected, and repaired. The advantage of performing the repair and reconstruction following an acute injury is that the reinjury most often occurs through the previous scar tissue.

When the tissue is insufficient, the technique of Brostrom is used. Dissection is carried out, the talocalcaneal ligament is identified, and approximately two-thirds of the structure is taken, leaving the portion attached to the talus and sutured through a drill hole to the lateral malleolus. Rarely this ligament cannot be identified; in individuals in whom functional instability has been a problem and the talocalcaneal ligament cannot be identified, the Chrisman-Snook procedure is carried out (see the chapter *Lateral Ankle Reconstruction for Chronic Instability*).

Closure is performed using a subcuticular suture of synthetic absorbable material, reinforced with Steri-Strips. The ankle is immobilized in a short-leg cast for 5 weeks. Full weight bearing is allowed. Currently, about one-half of the individuals undergoing these procedures are able to do so as day surgery patients.

REHABILITATION

After 5 weeks the cast is removed, motion is encouraged, and full weight bearing is continued. The athletes are instructed in heel cord stretching and peroneal exercises. Recently Theraban has been used as an aid in the later exercises.

As soon as full motion in the ankle and strength in the calf muscles have been regained, a return to sports is allowed. Athletes are encouraged to use protective devices such as tape or an air splint during these activities.

SUGGESTED READING

Almquist G. The pathomechanics and diagnosis of inversion injuries to the lateral ligaments of the ankle. J Sports Med 1974; 2:109.

Brand RL, Collins MD, Templeton T. Surgical repair of ruptured lateral ankle ligaments. Am J Sports Med 1981; 9:40–44.

Brostrom L. Sprained ankles. III. Clinical observation in recent ligament ruptures. Acta Chir Scand 1965; 130: 5-60 to 5-69.

Brostrom L. Sprained ankles. VI. Surgical treatment of "chronic" ligament ruptures. Acta Chir Scand 1966; 132:551–565.

Cox JS, Hewes TF. "Normal" talar tilt angle. Clin Orthop 1979; 140:37–41.

Staples OS. Ruptures of the fibular collateral ligaments of the ankle. J Bone Joint Surg 1975; 57A:101–107.

Staples OS. Results—study of ruptures of lateral ligaments of the ankle. Clin Orthop 1972; 85:50–58.

SELECTED LESIONS AROUND THE TALUS

DAVID COLLINSON REID M.D., M.C.S.P., F.R.C.S. (C), M.Ch. (ORTH)

This chapter deals with a group of entrapment and impingement syndromes around the talus that may have the common features of a history of trauma, aggravated by activity and relieved by rest. Most of these are uncommon and some are rare; all have a high incidence of delayed diagnosis. Awareness of these potentially disabling conditions may lead to prompt, effective treatment. The most common of these is the osteochondral lesion of the talar dome. As with the other conditions, the presence of the lesion does not always mean that this is the cause of the symptoms. Caution must be observed at the outset concerning early aggressive surgical treatment, unless other causes of the symptoms have been ruled out. The very existence of some of these syndromes has been questioned, but in highly active individuals these otherwise quiescent lesions can prejudice the chances of successful treatment. The meniscal lesion at the ankle, the anterior impingement syndrome, and the anterolateral corner compression syndrome all give intra-articular signs. The posterior talar compression syndrome is often peculiar to the ballet dancer or soccer player, while the tarsal tunnel syndrome is a neural entrapment phenomenon, but their proximity makes a discussion under the single heading of "selected lesions around the talus" reasonable.

TRANSCHONDRAL FRACTURES OF THE TALUS (OSTEOCHONDRITIS DISSECANS)

Osteochondral lesions of the talar dome are uncommon, accounting for only 4 percent of all osteochondritic lesions and 0.9 percent of all fractures. The true incidence is unknown since usually only symptomatic lesions are detected, and surprisingly even these are not always made obvious by standard diagnostic techniques.

Etiology

In 1959 Berndt and Harty suggested that trauma was the only significant factor in the development of these lesions, and the term "transchondral fracture" has been adopted. In cadaver studies, these authors reproduced lateral lesions with inversion and dorsiflexion and medial lesions with inversion, plantar flexion, and lateral rotation of the tibia on the talus (Fig. 1). Most authors accepted this explanation. Nevertheless, some authors still support the idea of a separate clinical entity of osteochondritis dissecans on an avascular basis. Many lesions are not visible on initial films in review and there is probably a spectrum of pathophysiology with acute shear fractures occurring at one extreme, as well as traumatic injury leading to injury to the subchondral vessels, resulting in delayed avascular collapse or separation. Perhaps at the

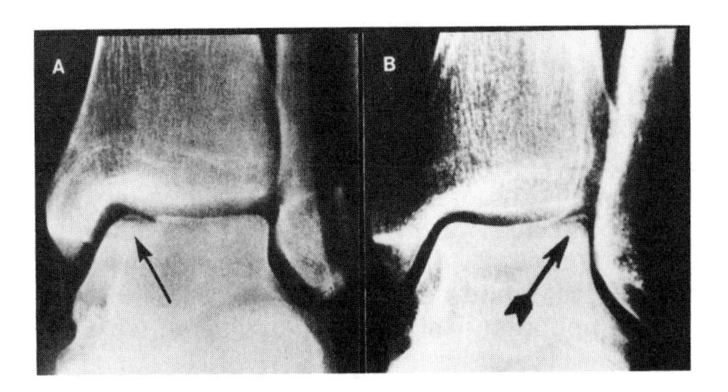

Figure 1 The most frequent sites of transchondral fractures are *A* posteromedial and *B* anterolateral. (Republished with permission from Pavlov H, Torg JS. The running athlete. Chicago: Year Book Medical Publishers, 1987.)

other end of the scale are cases of idiopathic avascular necrosis of systemic and local causes, among other factors. Inasmuch as careful scrutiny has not shown that these lesions heal differently from others, further speculation as to cause is not warranted, and the lesion must be dealt with de novo, according to the symptoms. The undoubted association with trauma, in many cases, means that a high index of suspicion is important in considering the differential diagnosis of chronic ankle pain after injury. This may help reduce the unacceptable delay in diagnosis of from 3 months to 16 years, frequently discussed in the literature.

Signs and Symptoms

The major symptoms include a deep aching or pain aggravated by exercise, and ankle swelling, and occasional crepitus, clicking, true locking, or a catching sensation. The clinical signs include synovial thickening, effusion, and sometimes joint line tenderness and stiffness manifested as loss of range in one or both directions. In all cases, symptoms seem to be magnified by activity. In most people, there is a history of an inversion sprain or ankle fracture; occasionally, the lesion is associated with true or functional instability.

Radiologic Examination

Radiographically the lesions typically can be seen to be anterolateral or posteromedial on the dome of the talus (see Fig. 1). These have been classified further as to the degree of separation (Fig. 2). Normally these lesions can be visualized in the routine ankle views, particularly in the internal oblique projection. However, an overpenetrated view of the plantar flexed ankle (x-ray at 1 m with 70 kV) sometimes facilitates vision of the early posteromedial lesion. Tomography or computed tomography allows accurate surgical planning if insufficient data are obtained from the plain films.

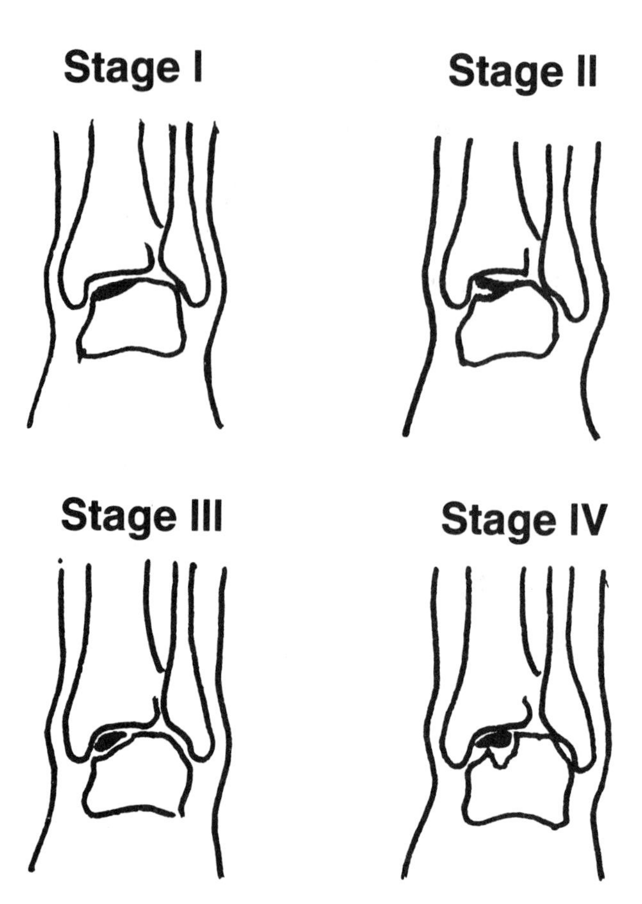

Figure 2 The four stages of osteochondral lesions according to Berndt and Harty. Stage I, a small area of compression. Stage II, a partially detached osteochondral fragment. Stage III, a completely detached fragment but remaining in situ. Stage IV, a detached, displaced fragment.

Treatment

The silent nature of many of these lesions means that all definitive surgical treatment must be preceded by a reasonable attempt at nonoperative therapy. The grades I and II lesions may do well with some protected weight bearing and nonsteroidal anti-inflammatory drugs (NSAIDs). In the series of Hagmeyer and van der Wurff, the stage I lesions treated nonoperatively were graded good, whereas the stage II lesions were mostly assessed fair to poor; the good results in stage II were from surgery. Symptomatic lesions of grade III are less likely to settle, but a trial of NSAIDs plus activity modification is worthwhile. If this is unsuccessful, surgery should be recommended. If the patient is reluctant to undergo surgery, a patella-bearing, weight-relieving ankle brace, worn for 6 weeks to 6 months, usually allows the symptoms to resolve. Alternatively a below-knee, non-weightbearing cast may be used, but this obviously has the disadvantage of more muscle wasting and joint stiffness for the competitive athlete. If a cast is worn, the period of immobilization should not exceed 6 to 8 weeks. The symptoms may return, however, with increased activity. Canele and Belding felt that medial stage III lesions were more likely to settle with nonoperative treatment than the lateral stage III lesions. The displaced type IV lesion should be operated on promptly if symptomatic, particularly if it is causing joint locking, since it may damage the joint surface and predispose to osteoarthritis.

When explaining the surgical options to patients with grades I to II lesions, it is important to bear in mind the work of McCullough and Venngopal, who reported surprisingly few complications and very little evidence of joint degeneration in a 10-year follow-up; however, this series, like most in the literature, was small. Nevertheless, modification of activity may be a viable, preferable, and acceptable option for some young athletes. The degree of symptoms, level of competition, and ultimate athletic goals obviously all govern the decision whether and when to operate.

Surgical treatment may be directed at removing an undisplaced loose fragment, drilling an in situ fragment, or removing a displaced fragment and performing debridement. Depending on the size and position of the lesion, arthroscopic treatment is possible. The anterolateral lesion is the more amenable and it may even be possible to drill the bed. It should be stressed, however, that a well-performed arthrotomy procedure is preferable to a poorly executed arthroscopy.

Surgical Approaches

The position of the fragment determines whether the joint should be approached via an anterolateral, an anteromedial, or a posteromedial exposure.

The Anterolateral Lesion. With the patient in the supine position, a large sandbag or wedge under the ipsilateral hip, and the leg supported on a well-padded box, the anterolateral ankle is easily exposed (Fig. 3). This is an excellent position for exposure of both medial and lateral ankle and can be used for most ankle surgery, including arthroscopy. An incision is made starting 5 cm proximal to the ankle joint, just medial to the crest of the fibula, curved down to approximately the level of the sinus tarsi. It is unfortunate that such a large exposure is usually necessary to perform this procedure well. The subcutaneous dissection is kept medial to the peroneus tertius, which is retracted laterally. Care must be taken to avoid damage to the cutaneous branch of the superficial peroneal nerve, which is retracted medially, along with the extensor digitorum tendons. The capsule is opened longitudinally, and since the malleolar and lateral tarsal arteries are usually divided, it is important to cauterize them before capsulotomy, in order to minimize postoperative hemorrhage. Blunt dissection and periosteal elevation of the capsule usually allow good visualization of the anterolateral lesion, which is facilitated by inversion and plantar flexion of the ankle. The lesion can be drilled or removed, and the edges trimmed. Attempts to secure the lesion with a bone peg or screw usually are not successful, and surprisingly offer little in the way of improved functional outcome over removing the loose fragment and drilling the base.

The Anteromedial Lesion. Thompson and Loomer advocate a medial incision that permits both an anteromedial and a posteromedial deep exposure, avoiding the need for osteotomy of the medial malleolus. An approach using a malleolar osteotomy provides an excellent view and is safe, but a longer recovery period is needed and therefore a soft tissue exposure is probably preferable in com-

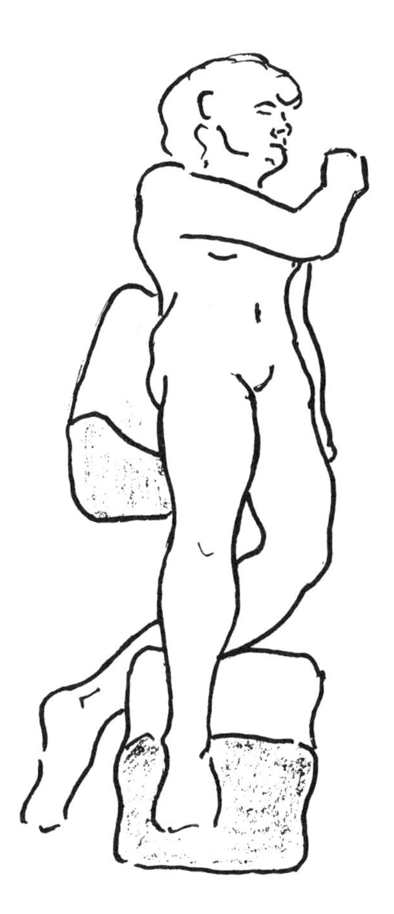

Figure 3 Patient positioned in the lateral decubitus position with the body tilted onto a support, giving access to both sides of the ankle by rotating the hip (after Parisien JS).

petitive athletes. It also eliminates the need for subsequent screw removal.

With the patient in the lying position, a 10-cm incision is curved posteriorly just posterior to the medial malleolus (Fig. 4). The anteromedial capsule and medial ligament are exposed. A 2-cm incision opens the capsule just anterior to the medial ligament. By maximal plantar flexion, the superomedial rim of the talus can be seen. If the medial talar lesion is too far posterior to be visualized, a second incision is made by retracting the tibialis posterior tendon anteriorly. The deep surface of the flexor retinaculum can be divided and the remaining contents of the proximal tarsal tunnel carefully retracted posteriorly. It is not necessary to expose these structures separately to do this. At this point, maximal dorsiflexion usually allows access to the posteromedial half of the talus.

Arthroscopy. The supine position with a large wedge under the hip and the leg in a well-padded box, as previously described, usually permits access to the anterior, posterior, and lateral aspects of the ankle by rotation of the hip. The joint is distended with 10 to 15 ml of Ringer's lactate before the blunt probe is inserted. There are three anterior and one

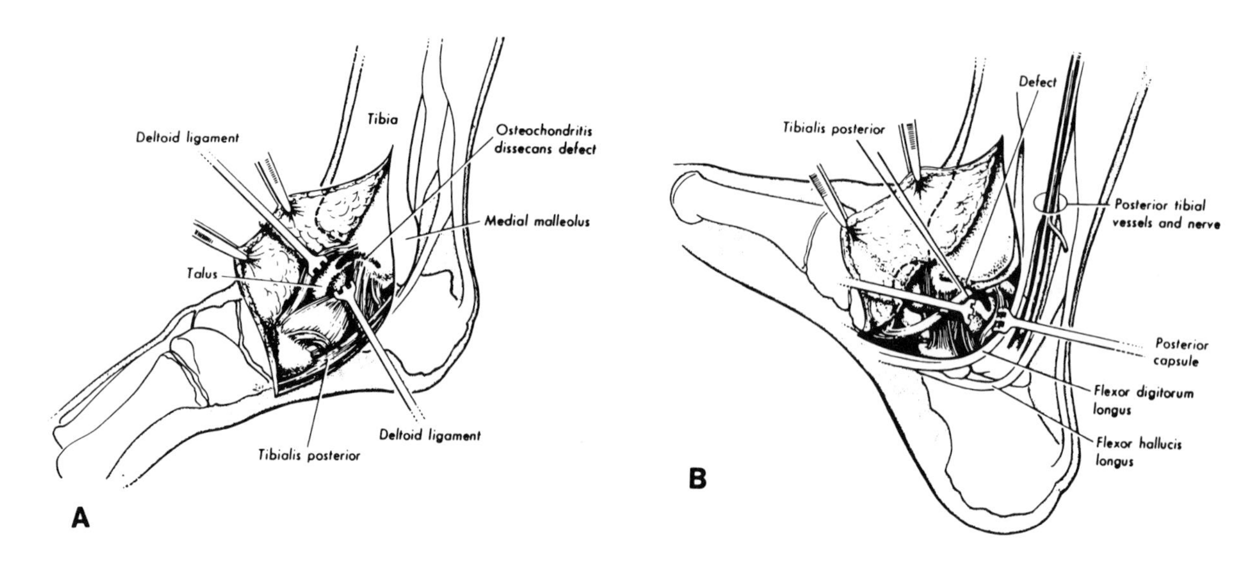

Figure 4 *A,* The anteromedial talus exposed in maximal plantar flexion. *B,* The posteromedial talus exposed via the same skin incision. (Republished with permission from Thompson JP, Loomer RL. Osteochondral lesions of the talus in a sports medicine clinic—a new radiographic technique and surgical approach. Am J Sports Med 1984; 12:460–463.)

posterolateral portals, through which most lesions can be visualized. The anteromedial portal is medial to the tendon of the tibialis anterior, just lateral to the junction of the medial malleolus with the anterior joint space.

The anterocentral portal is lateral to the extensor hallucis longus, and care is needed to avoid the anterior tibial artery and deep peroneal nerve. The anterolateral portal is lateral to the peroneus tertius and the extensor digitorum longus tendons. Care is needed to avoid damage to the two terminal branches of the superficial peroneal nerve. The posterolateral portal is lateral to the Achilles tendon and approximately 2 cm above the tip of the lateral malleolus. The sural nerve and the short saphenous vein are vulnerable. It is rarely necessary to use the more dangerous posteromedial portal behind the flexor hallucis longus, and in very close proximity to the posterior tibial artery and nerve.

Once the scope is in the joint, a partial synovectomy may be necessary to visualize the more anteriorly placed fragment. The loose fragment is often best grouped with a small curved hemostat, the edges curetted and abraded with hand instruments. It may also be possible to drill the bed of an anterolateral lesion, but this is not a simple procedure.

TALAR ANTERIOR IMPINGEMENT SYNDROME

The talar anterior impingement syndrome is related to osteophytes on the neck of the talus or, more frequently, the anterior tibia. Dorsiflexion results in impingement of the bony spurs along with trapping and pinching of hypertrophied and chronically swollen synovium (Fig. 5).

These lesions occasionally are seen after repeated ankle inversion injuries and also are particularly associated with football linemen, in whom chronic repeated impingement stresses of the bony surfaces in dorsiflexion play a role in the etiology. Alternatively, the osteophytes may correlate with the tibial and talar attachments of the anterior capsule, and may relate to chronic traction stresses seen in runners and soccer players (see Fig. 5).

The athlete may simply complain of ankle pain and swelling proportional to the amount of activity. In mild cases this happens only with activities requiring sudden starts and stops or changes in direction, but in severe cases the symptoms occur with simple running or jogging. The feeling of pinching can be reproduced by forced dorsiflexion, and pain is experienced with palpation along the anterior talocrural joint line. Dorsiflexion is eventually limited by bony impingement as well as pain. Plain lateral radiographs help confirm the diagnosis. Support for the theory of chronic traction or compression stresses is lent by the usual absence of degenerative changes within the joint. For this reason,

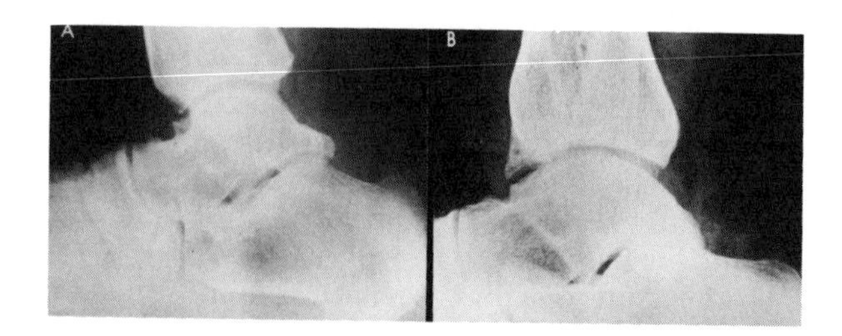

Figure 5 *A,* Hypertrophic spurs on the dorsal talus at the capsular insertion with normal joint space. *B,* Anterior tibial spur also associated with a painful limitation of dorsiflexion. (Republished with permission from Pavlov H, Torg JS. The running athlete. Chicago: Year Book Medical Publishers, 1987.)

removal of the anterior synovium and resection of the osteophytes is usually all that is needed to relieve symptoms, and most athletes can return to full activity. With a small spur, it may be possible to do this arthroscopically, but it is usually necessary to open the joint for successful excision of adequate amounts of bone.

MENISCOID LESIONS OF THE TALOFIBULAR COMPONENT OF THE ANKLE

Wohlin and colleagues in 1950 described a series of patients who experienced chronic pain and swelling over the anterior and anterolateral ankle with activity. Often this is accompanied by a subjective feeling of instability and occasionally actual giving way. There is always a history of a moderately severe ankle injury.

There are two possible causes. This lesion may be secondary to traumatic synovial thickening, with incomplete resorption of the associated exudate. A small portion of inflammatory infiltrate persists between the fibula and the talus and eventually becomes hyalinized secondary to pressure, giving rise to these symptoms (Fig. 6). Other authors have suggested that these meniscoid lesions are tears of the anterior tibiofibular ligament in which the torn fragment becomes interposed between the talus and the lateral malleolus.

These lesions are rare, but it is important to consider the possibility of their presence in athletes who have persistent pain and swelling after inversion sprains, and in whom all roentgenographic and other diagnostic tests are negative.

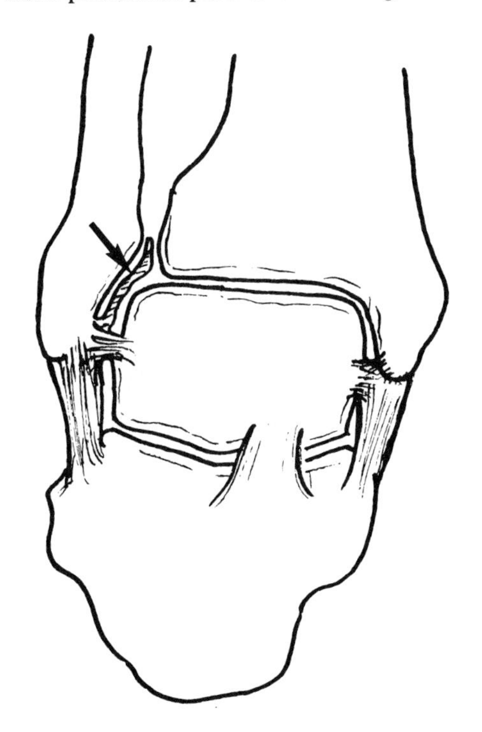

Figure 6 Schematic cross section of the talocrural joint showing a meniscoid lesion that may be related to the lateral ligament (after McCarrol JR).

Arthroscopy will reveal the lesion and the hyalinized, meniscoid-like band, and any redundant synovium may then be removed. Excision should cure the symptoms and prevent further joint irritation.

ANTEROLATERAL CORNER COMPRESSION SYNDROME OF THE ANKLE

Waller reported a syndrome that may be included in the spectrum of the previously described meniscoid lesion of the ankle. The athlete complains of pain located over the anteroinferior aspect of the fibula and the associated anterolateral talus, and the joint line. There is usually a history of inversion injury. The suspected etiology is a post-traumatic chondromalacia of the lateral wall of the talus, with associated synovial reaction.

It is suggested that pain and compression at foot strike makes the athlete, usually a runner, tighten the tibialis posterior and anterior tendons, and inhibits the peroneal tendons. This makes the runner susceptible to multiple inversion strains. The addition of a medial heel and inner sole wedge to the shoe may relieve impingement sufficiently to allow restoration of balanced inversion and eversion muscle action, and relieve symptoms. Walter claims that the symptoms are relieved in a matter of days in most cases. If the condition does not settle with modified activity, an orthosis, and a course of NSAIDs, arthroscopy should be considered to rule out other causes of the pain.

POSTERIOR TALAR COMPRESSION SYNDROME

Pain in the posterior ankle region may be incapacitating in ballet dancers and soccer players when due to impingement of an os trigonum or Stieda's process. This may be a diagnosis of exclusion in many instances, after Achilles tendinitis, peroneal tendinitis, and flexor hallucis longus tendinitis have been ruled out.

First described in 1804 by Rosenmuller, the os trigonum is present in at least 5 percent of feet, and as many as 38 percent of the adult population have an enlarged lateral process in the posterior surface of the talus (Fig. 7). It therefore is frequently present as an asymptomatic structure. Caution is warranted in oversubscribing symptoms to this normal anatomic variant. McDougall proposed three mechanisms for development of the os trigonum: (1) failure of fusion of the secondary ossification center, (2) repeated minor trauma with impingement against the posterior margin of the tibia, and (3) an acute fracture due to forced plantar flexion, occasionally in association with avulsion of the posterior band of the lateral ligament.

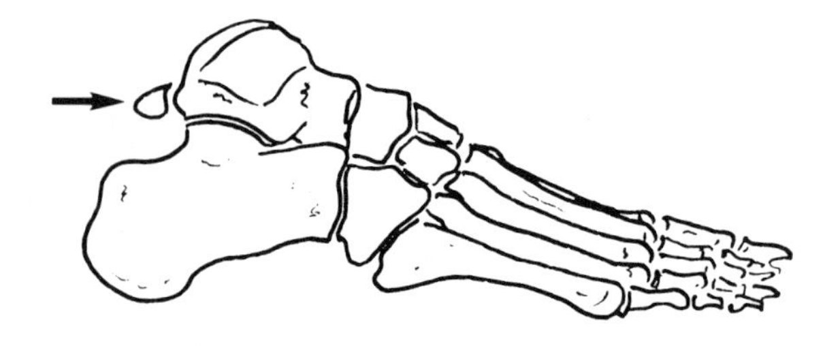

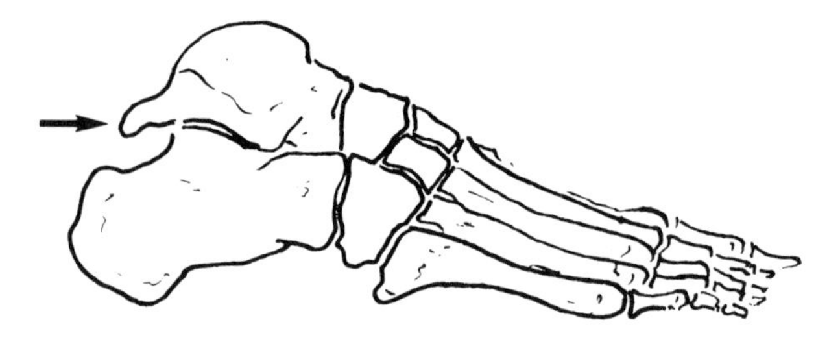

Figure 7 Lateral view of the foot showing an os trigonum and a Stieda's process.

In the posterior talar compression syndrome, there usually is tenderness over the posterolateral aspect of the talus between the Achilles tendon and the peroneal tendons. The pain generally is reproduced by forced plantar flexion. The lack of tenderness over the peroneal tendons should help exclude the diagnosis of peroneal tendinitis.

A bone scan may be positive, but this is not mandatory to confirm the diagnosis. Forced plantar flexion radiography confirms the painful impingement, and temporary relief may be provided by infiltration of the area with 1 percent lidocaine (Xylocaine).

If modified activity and NSAIDs fail to relieve symptoms, excision of the os trigonum or Stieda's process, with adjacent release of the tendon sheath of the flexor hallucis longus, usually allows resumption of activities in about 1 month.

MEDIAL TARSAL TUNNEL SYNDROME

The medial tarsal tunnel syndrome represents a compression neuropathy of the tibial nerve or its terminal branches, the medial and lateral plantar nerves. The impingement frequently occurs in the distal two-thirds of the fibro-osseous canal, which has ill-defined limits. It begins a few centimeters proximal to the tip of the medial malleolus where the crural fascia starts to condense, forming a relatively unyielding roof, the flexor retinaculum. It ends where the medial and lateral plantar nerves enter or pass deep to the abductor hallucis. The anatomy is highly variable with regard to (1) the site at which the tibial nerve divides into the medial calcaneal, the medial plantar, and the lateral plantar nerves; (2) its terminal branches; and (3) the method by which it exits from the canal. The medial and lateral plantar nerves leave through separate fibrous openings or, on occasion, contiguously in one canal, sometimes piercing the abductor muscle (Fig. 8).

Etiology

A variety of factors may lead to compromise of the nerve, and these may present in slightly different ways, contributing to a delay in diagnosis (Table 1).

Anatomic Factors. These include variations in the fibrous septa, areolar tissue, and retinaculum,

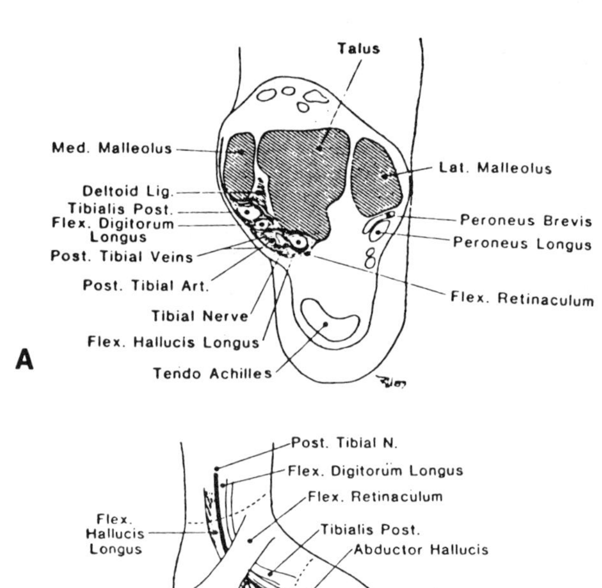

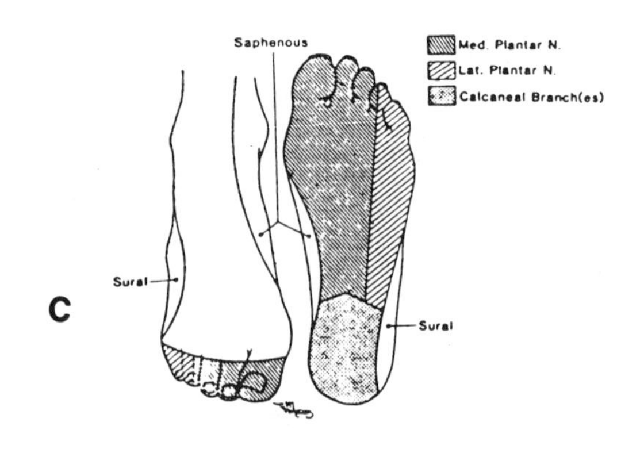

Figure 8 The relationship of the tendons and nerves of the tarsal tunnel (*A*) in cross section and (*B*) from the medial side. (*C*) The sensory areas supplied by the posterior tibial nerve terminal branches (after Kushner and Reid.)

TABLE 1 Etiology of Tarsal Tunnel Syndrome

Anatomic	*Tumor*
Septa	Neuroma
Areolar tissue	Lipoma
Retinacular	Synovial cyst
Vascular anomalies	Tendon tumors
Muscular variations	Neurolemmoma
Valgus alignment	
Trauma	*Inflammatory*
Fractures	Rheumatoid arthritis
Contusions	Ankylosing spondylitis
Postsurgical adhesions	Tenosynovitis
Sprains	Thrombophlebitis
Laceration	
Post-traumatic edema	
Post-traumatic adhesions	
	Miscellaneous
	Footwear
	Overuse syndrome
	Aging
	Fluid retention

which may be fibrous, may scar, or may swell with edema, limiting the space available for the contents of the tarsal tunnel. These may be secondary to trauma, aging, or repeated stresses. The nerve also may be compressed by dilated and engorged veins, and occasionally an arterial arch may cause symptoms. Variations in the anatomy of the abductor hallucis, including anomalous or accessory muscle, may involve the nerve distally. In athletes the repetitive stresses of running may unmask these variations, particularly in the presence of a valgus heel and associated pronated forefoot, which may tighten the flexor retinaculum, the arch of the abductor hallucis, and the calcaneonavicular ligament.

Trauma. The tarsal tunnel syndrome can occur as a complication of ankle, calcaneal, or metatarsal fractures. In a review of 500 os calcis fractures, 10 percent developed tarsal tunnel syndrome and over one-fourth of these required surgical decompression. The syndrome also occurs with ankle sprains, tight casts, or hamstring injuries or postoperatively after osteotomies of the first ray or release of the Achilles tendon. All these causative conditions may have edema and secondary fibrosis as a common factor.

Tumor. In athletes, ganglion and post-traumatic synovial cysts constitute the most common neoplasms causing pressure in the canal. The symptoms may be intermittent, since such tumors swell with activity.

Miscellaneous. Chronic synovitis, ill-fitting footwear, inappropriate training surfaces, poorly graduated and planned training, fluid retention, pregnancy, and weight gain may all play a role. In addition, neuropathic conditions from a variety of systemic causes may precipitate the symptoms.

Clinical Picture

There appears to be no sex predilection and the onset is usually insidious. The most common complaint is of burning pain and paresthesia in the plantar aspect of the foot. Pain is exacerbated by activity and diminished by rest. The usual site is the great toe, followed in descending order of frequency by the remaining toes and the distal sole of the foot (Table 2). Symptoms occasionally occur in the medial plantar surface of the heel. Athletes may also report a "swollen or tight" sensation, as if there is an impending cramp in the arch of the foot. For some individuals the pain may be worse at night, and they report that pain is relieved by hanging the foot out of bed, moving it, rubbing it, or getting out of bed and walking around.

Sensory signs include hypoesthesia to pinprick, diminished two-point discrimination, and a positive Tinel's sign (see Fig. 8). Sustained direct pressure reproduces or exacerbates the symptoms. It is difficult to detect associated weakness.

The definitive test is the nerve conduction study, of both the abductor digiti minimi and the abductor hallucis. Latencies of more than one standard deviation above the normal for the particular laboratory carrying out the test are considered positive, although evaluation of evoked sensory and motor potentials may be a more sensitive indication of a pathologic condition (see Table 2).

Treatment

Nonoperative

Modification of Activity. Advice should be offered with regard to the intensity of training, the building up of mileage, the impact of the terrain, the distance covered, and the spacing of training sessions.

Modalities. Most physiotherapeutic modalities should be aimed at reduction of edema and scarring. These may include the use of ice after activity, ultrasound, interferential therapy, lasers, and short wave diathermy. These may be successful when symptoms are recently acquired, but they rarely are of use for an established neuropathic condition.

Footwear and Orthoses. In view of the highly associated valgus heel and pronated forefoot, a trial of a medial arch support or medial heel wedge may be considered. Extremely tight lacing of shoes or skates may exacerbate the condition, as will shoes worn down at the lateral heel. Occasionally, when edema features highly in the etiology, support hose may be helpful.

Medication. Orally administered NSAIDs are most successful in acute-onset situations associated with tenosynovitis. Occasionally a trial of local injectable steroid is successful, but care should be taken to avoid direct injection into the vessel and nerve. Furthermore, skin atrophy can be trouble-

TABLE 2 Clinical Data on Eight Patients with Medial Tarsal Tunnel Syndrome

Age	Sex	Sport	Occupation	Side	Duration (Mo)	Foot Alignment	Symptoms	Sensory	Motor	EMG	Conservative Treatment	Findings at Surgery	Results
25	F	Runner, 40 mi/wk	Student	L	17	Normal	Pain into great toe after running	Hyperesthesia of great toe and medial foot Tinel +	None	+	US Injection	Constriction by fibrous band in superior tunnel	Relief by 24 hr
35	M	Runner, 60 mi/wk. Chronic tenosynovitis of tibialis posterior over 3-yr period	Teacher	L	38	Valgus heel Pronated forefoot	Numbness and paresthesia Nocturnal pain	Impaired pinprick Tinel −	None	+	US TNS Injection	Thickening of nerve and fibrosis	Relief by 3 mo
22	F	Runner, 45 mi/wk	Student	R	15	Valgus heel Pronated forefoot	Burning sensation in great toe	Hyperesthesia Tinel +	None	+	US Orthototic	Fibrosis of nerve	Relief in 1 mo
43	M	Runner, 65 mi/wk	Lawyer	R	5	Valgus heel Pronated forefoot	Burning sensation	Impaired pinprick Tinel −	None	+	Orthotic	Fusiform thickening of nerve	Relief by 36 hr
19	F	Skater (skate pressure?)	Student	L	16	Prominent calcaneus	Burning sensation	Impaired pinprick Tinel −	None	+	Modification of skates	Normal appearance	Relief in 24 hr
22	M	Soccer (postcontusion)	Phys. ed. teacher	L	8	Normal	Intense burning Nocturnal pain	Decreased pinprick over entire medial plantar nerve distrib. Tinel −	None	+	US SWD Injection Mobilization	Dense scarring	Relief at 1 mo
33	M	Ice hockey (postfractured calcaneus)	Construction worker	R	14	Broadened heel	Intense burning Nocturnal pain	Paresthesia in foot and toes Tinel +	None	+	Wax baths US Injection Mobilization	Dense scarring Neuroma	Relief at 6 wk
29	F	Runner, 80 mi/wk	Student	L	7	Valgus heel Pronated forefoot	Intense burning after running	Decreased tactile sensation Tinel −	None	+	Orthosis US	Scarring near abductor hallucis muscle	Relief at 24 hr

EMG, electromyogram; US, ultrasound; TNS, transcutaneous nerve stimulation; SWD, shortwave diathermy.

some in this situation; this can be minimized by a deep injection of steroid with only about 1 ml of accompanying lidocaine.

Operative

Surgical release may provide rapid relief from the symptoms of the compression neuropathy, although with denervation in established cases some signs may persist. Since it is difficult to localize the exact site of compression, the entire canal is released. The flexor retinaculum is completely divided and the posterior tibial nerve freed from encompassing fibrous tissue. The branches are explored where possible to mobilize them as far distal as the abductor hallucis muscle. Each hiatus for the medial and lateral plantar nerves is checked and released; if there is an accessory abductor hallucis, it is excised. Care is taken not to disrupt the fine calcaneal branches, since damage to these creates heel numbness. If there are tortuous veins present, they should be ligated proximally and distally and then excised. Even with careful dissection, it is impossible to identify unequivocal pathologic condition in about 25 percent of the cases; however, if previous neurophysiologic testing has confirmed the site of compression, relief can be obtained.

Partial weight bearing or limited walking with full weight bearing for 2 weeks is advised. By 3 weeks, more aggressive activity may be undertaken, including balance board work and running. It usually takes 4 to 6 weeks before a full return to sporting activities is possible. Recurrence of symptoms in a well-decompressed nerve is rare, and the only significant, but rare, long-term complication is subluxation of the tibialis posterior tendon.

This syndrome is not usually recognized early, which is unfortunate, since it often resolves promptly with nonoperative treatment in the early stages. For this reason, the variation in presentation and the multitude of etiologic factors have been stressed in this chapter in the hope that this syndrome will be included more often in the differential diagnosis of sources of medial talar, calcaneal, and medial foot pain.

SUGGESTED READING

Alexander AH, Lichtman DM. Surgical treatment of transchondral talar dome fractures. J Bone Joint Surg 1980; 62A:646–652.

Andrews JR, Drez DJ, McGinty JB. Symposium: Arthroscopy of joints other than the knee. Contemp Orthop 1984; 9:71–100.

Berndt AL, Harty M. Transchondral fractures (osteochondritis dissecans) of the talus. J Bone Joint Surg 1959; 41A:988–1020.

Brodsky AE, Khalil MA. Talar compression syndrome. Am J Sports Med 1986; 14:472–476.

Campbell CJ, Rangwat CS. Osteochondritis dissecans: the question of etiology. J Trauma 1986; 6:201–221.

Canele ST, Belding RH. Osteochondral lesions of the talus. J Bone Joint Surg 1980; 62A:97–102.

Cedell CA. Rupture of the posterior talotibial ligament with avulsion of a bone fragment from the talus. Acta Orthop Scand 1974; 45:454–461.

Distefano V, Sack JT, Whittaker R, Nixon JE. Tarsal tunnel syndrome. Clin Orthop 1972; 88:76–79.

Drez DM, Suhl JF, Gollehan DL. Ankle arthroscopy—technique and indications. Foot Ankle 1985; 2:138–143.

Flick AB, Gould N. Osteochondritis dissecans of the talus (transchondral fractures of the talus)—review of literature and new surgical approach for medial dome lesions. Foot Ankle 1985; 5:165–185.

Fu R, Delisa JA, Kraft GH. Motor nerve latencies through the tarsal tunnel in normal adult subjects: standard determinations for corrected temperatures and distance. Arch Phys Med Rehabil 1980; 61:243–248.

Hagmeyer RH, van der Wurff M. Transchondral fractures of the talus on an inversion injury of the ankle: a frequently overlooked diagnosis. J Orthop Sports Phys Ther 1987; 8:362–367.

Hontas MJ, Haddard RJ, Schlesinger LC. Conditions of the talus in the runner. Am J Sports Med 1986; 14:486–490.

Kaplan PE, Kernahan WT. Tarsal tunnel syndrome. J Bone Joint Surg 1981; 63A:96–99.

Keck C. The tarsal tunnel syndrome. J Bone Joint Surg 1962; 44A:180–182.

Kushner S, Reid DC. Medial tarsal tunnel syndrome: a review. J Orthop Sports Phys Ther 1984; 6:39–45.

Langan P, Weiss CA. Subluxation of the tibialis posterior tendon: a complication of tarsal tunnel decompression. Clin Orthop 1980; 146:226–227.

Lindholm TS, Osterman K, Vankka E. Osteochondritis dissecans of elbow, ankle and hip: a comparison survey. Clin Orthop 1980; 148:245–250.

McCarroll JR, Schrader JW, Shelbourne KD, Rettig AC, Bisesi MA. Meniscoid lesions of the ankle in soccer players. Am J Sports Med 1987; 15:255–257.

McCullough CJ, Venngopal V. Osteochondritis dissecans of the talus: the natural history. Clin Orthop 1979; 144:264–268.

McDougall A. The os trigonum. J Bone Joint Surg 1955; 37B:257–265.

O'Farrell TA, Costello BG. Osteochondritis dissecans of the talus: the late results of surgical treatment. J Bone Joint Surg 1982; 64B:494–497.

Parks JC, Hamilton WG, Patterson AH, et al. The anterior impingement syndrome of the ankle. J Trauma 1980; 20:895–898.

Partisien JS. Arthroscopic treatment of osteochondral lesions of the talus. Am J Sports Med 1986; 14:211–217.

Roden S, Tillegard P, Unander-Scharin L. Osteochondritis dissecans and similar lesions of the talus. Acta Orthop Scand 1953; 23:51–66.

Thompson JP, Loomer RL. Osteochondral lesions of the talus in a sports medicine clinic—a new radiographic technique and surgical approach. Am J Sports Med 1984; 12:460–463.

Waller JF Jr. Hindfoot and midfoot problems of the runner—symposium on the foot and leg in running sports. St Louis: CV Mosby 1982:64.

Wohlin I, Glassman F, Sideman S. Internal derangement of the talofibular component of the ankle. Surg Gynecol Obstet 1950; 91:193–200.

I LEG

CHRONIC EXERTIONAL COMPARTMENT SYNDROME

A. AMENDOLA, M.D.
CECIL H. RORABECK, M.D., F.R.C.S.(C).

Chronic exertional compartment syndrome is an exercise-induced condition characterized by local pain and swelling and, less commonly, dysesthesia in the territory of the nerve transgressing the affected compartment. A number of apparent synonyms have been used in the past to describe this entity, including anterior tibial pain syndrome, medial tibial stress syndrome, march synovitis, shin splints, and recurrent compartmental syndrome. All of these most likely should be looked on as a form of chronic exercise-related compartment syndrome. There are also many other causes of leg pain in athletes, including periostitis of the tibia, inflammatory conditions, stress fractures, arteriovenous (AV) malformations, venous disorders, and spinal cord radiculopathy. With an understanding of the pathophysiology, the clinical presentation, and the diagnostic studies available, a rational approach to leg pain and exertional compartment syndromes in athletes may be developed.

PATHOPHYSIOLOGY

It was Volkmann in 1881 who originally described the acute form of compartment syndrome; he believed that the cause was prolonged blockage of arterial blood flow associated with simultaneous venous stasis. Subsequently, others have defined it more clearly as a condition in which increased tissue pressure within a limited space compromises the circulation and the function of the contents of that space.

The existence and importance of chronic exercise-induced compartment syndrome was not appreciated until the publications of Horne and Hughes. These authors noted the development of compartment syndrome in army recruits after unaccustomed strenuous activity, and used the term "march gangrene" to describe it. Mavor and numerous other authors later confirmed the existence of these exercise-induced compartment syndromes.

The underlying cause of pain in a patient with a chronic compartment syndrome is not entirely understood. Although the acute syndrome has been well defined through clinical observations in experimental models, the pathophysiology of chronic compartment syndromes remains obscure. Most authors have suggested that the pain an athlete experiences during exercise is probably related to muscle ischemia secondary to an increase in compartment pressure. They base this observation on the fact that symptoms rapidly subside after cessation of activity. Observations from normal muscle physiology have been extrapolated into an understanding of exertional compartment syndromes. Numerous authors have stated that isometric or isotonic muscle contractures cause an increase in intramuscular pressure. Others have noted a 20 percent increase in muscle volume with exercise, secondary to an increase in blood volume. Postexercise swelling may be due to increased blood flow and muscle fiber swelling and fluid retention. Also, chronic exercise results in muscle hypertrophy, and thus an increase in muscle volume.

These observations relate to normal muscle, but there appears to be a group of patients who have relatively tight unyielding fascia such that, when a muscle expands during a normal contraction, tissue pressure is raised within that muscle. The hypothesis is that the symptoms of chronic compartment syndrome are caused by insufficient perfusion of muscle tissue during exercise due to elevated pressure. Exercise-induced leg pain is a common problem in athletes. In some authors' and our own experience, not all patients suspected of having a chronic exertional compartment syndrome on a clinical basis alone have elevated compartment pressures. Therefore, other factors may be contributing to the development of these syndromes, such as the production of metabolic breakdown products within the muscle itself.

Compartment syndrome has been described in other anatomic locations, but the exercise-induced syndrome is usually reserved for the leg. Classically it has been accepted that the leg is divided into four separate osseofascial muscle compartments: anterior, lateral, superficial, and deep posterior. In the literature the anterior and lateral compartments are the most commonly reported locations of exertional compartment syndrome. In general, most reports have found it difficult to demonstrate elevated pressures in the deep posterior compartment, and so some have questioned the existence of compartment syndrome in this area. Other authors have performed fasciotomy of the deep posterior compartment and found that patients had relief from pain, although the pressures were not significantly altered by the surgery. The tibialis posterior muscle has been shown to be contained within a separate muscle compartment. Knowledge of this fifth compartment has been helpful since, in certain situations, it may be an unrecognized cause of compartment syndrome, or a failure of the "conventional" four-compartment fasciotomy.

CLINICAL PRESENTATION

In exertional compartment syndrome the athlete's leg pain is always induced by repeated or vigorous activity. Symptoms dissipate with rest, usually within minutes but sometimes taking hours. Patients present when the symptoms are so severe that they cannot complete their activities. If there is rest or night pain associated with the exercise-induced pain, the physician should be alerted to the other possible causes of leg pain. History and physical examination should include an assessment of the lumbar spine, lower limb alignment, and knee, ankle, and foot biomechanics.

Patients with chronic exertional compartment syndrome present clinically with symptoms related to either the anterior compartment, the anterior and posterior compartments, or the posterior compartment alone. Thus, there are three modes of clinical presentation. Patients presenting with chronic anterior compartment syndrome give a history of pain centered diffusely over the anterior compartment and occurring at variable periods on initiation of the activity, which usually is running. Pain is frequently, although not always, bilateral. It usually radiates down toward the ankle and is associated with a feeling of swelling in the leg or dysesthesia on the dorsum of the foot. Results of physical examination of these patients are invariably normal. Usually, patients are unable to "run through" the pain they are experiencing.

The second group of patients include those who have symptoms of pain involving both the anterior and posterior compartments of the leg. The pain they experience is again activity related. The anterior pain is in the same location as described above, and the posterior pain typically occurs along the posteromedial border of the tibia. It generally occurs in the middle or distal third and is spread out over an area several centimeters in length. It begins at a variable period after exercise, may or may not be bilateral, and is often associated with a sensation of swelling as well as dysesthesia on the medial or plantar aspect of the foot.

In the third group of patients, those with posterior pain alone, the pain is located along the posterior border of the tibia, usually radiating down toward the ankle. The posterior pain pattern is identical to that described above. Once again, patients are usually unable to "run through" their pain, and the posteromedial pain they experience is of sufficient severity to prevent them from carrying out their activity.

Results of clinical assessment of all three groups are variably normal, with the occasional exception of some discomfort felt deeply along the posteromedial border of the tibia. The differential diagnosis includes a stress fracture, deep venous thrombosis, or periostitis in this situation.

ROLE OF TISSUE PRESSURE MEASUREMENT

Patients presenting with an appropriate history compatible with a clinical diagnosis of chronic compartment syndrome should undergo tissue pressure studies. Most authors would agree that the hallmark for the diagnosis of chronic anterior compartment syndrome of the leg remains a sound clinical history and physical examination. Although the clinical symptoms and signs, in particular the symptoms, are important, diagnosis on a clinical basis alone would result in an overdiagnosis of chronic exertional compartment syndrome. It was noted by some authors that only 14 to 27 percent of patients suspected of having the syndrome show elevated or abnormal pressure in studies. An accurate diagnosis of chronic exertional compartment syndrome can be made with the adjunct of tissue pressure measurement.

A number of techniques are available for intramuscular pressure measurements; most were originally designed to measure pressure at rest, usually in the context of the acute syndrome. Some of these techniques have been modified for static and dynamic pressure monitoring during exercise. Each system has its strengths and limitations, but in the hands of an experienced technician the limitations should be minimized.

Patients who are referred for pressure studies have their pressures measured at rest, during exercise, and immediately after exercise; we use the Slit catheter system. The history will direct the investigator toward the most symptomatic compartment or compartments to be studied. Pre-exercise baseline pressures are recorded. A treadmill is used to exercise the patient until there is a reproduction of symptoms. Dynamic peak-to-peak pressure and mean muscular pressure are recorded. Once symptoms are reproduced, treadmill exercise is stopped and the patient lies supine. Postexercise pressure is recorded immediately and then at 5-minute intervals thereafter for 25 minutes. Normal baseline values should be achieved within 15 minutes after exercise.

Dynamic pressures have been found by some authors to be important in the diagnosis of chronic compartment syndromes. We have found elevated immediate postexercise pressure and a sluggish return to pre-exercise baseline values to be more significant in an accurate tissue pressure diagnosis.

ROLE OF MAGNETIC RESONANCE IMAGING

There are certain inherent disadvantages to the use of intramuscular pressure measurement in the diagnosis of chronic exertional compartment syndrome. Apart from the technical variables, it is an invasive technique, and generally only one compartment can be measured, although there are four or five muscle compartments in the leg. Also, there are other causes of leg pain (as pointed out previously) that may require radiographs, bone scans, or contrast studies to be performed for diagnosis.

Magnetic resonance imaging (MRI) provides a noninvasive, safe method without ionizing radiation for investigating exertional leg pain. Detailed cross-sectional or coronal images are produced to view the soft tissue and bone anatomy. Exercise-induced changes can also be monitored with MRI since it really provides physiologic information. One of the possible causes mentioned previously for chronic exertional compartment syndrome is the production of metabolic byproducts, and MRI appears to be a more appropriate method of investigating these changes. Studies are currently under way to determine the usefulness of MRI in these exertional syndromes.

MANAGEMENT

Once the diagnosis of exercise-induced chronic compartment syndrome has been established and the other possible causes of leg pain have been excluded by history, examination, and appropriate diagnostic studies, treatment can be instituted. Many patients with chronic compartment syndrome feel much more comfortable simply by understanding their condition. Some are willing to modify their activity to avoid recurrence of symptoms. Others may occasionally benefit from a change in footwear or a modification with orthotics. A course of physiotherapy with education regarding an effective warm-up and flexibility program may be helpful. Icing or short courses of nonsteroidal anti-inflammatory drugs may be beneficial during more symptomatic periods.

More dedicated athletes, however, are usually unable to modify their activity level and usually obtain no benefit from conservative measures. The indications for surgery, therefore, are for patients who have failed to respond to nonoperative treatment and in whom pressure studies are abnormal. Both these prerequisites should be met before surgical decompression is advised.

Fasciotomy is carried out according to which compartments is symptomatic for the patient. Two vertical incisions anterolaterally are used to decompress the anterior or lateral compartments. The deep posterior compartment is released through a posteromedial incision, which includes decompression of the tibialis posterior.

Postoperatively, patients are begun on an icing and exercise program immediately in the recovery room. Activity is increased as tolerated, with the guidance of a physiotherapist. Rehabilitation time varies from 6 weeks to 3 months in most patients.

SUGGESTED READING

Anrep GV, Blalock A, Samaan A. The effect of muscular contraction upon blood flow in skeletal muscle. Proc R Soc Lond (Biol) 1934; 114:223–245.

Ashton H. The effect of increased tissue pressure on blood flow. Clin Orthop 1975; 113:15–26.

Barcroft H, Dornhorst AC. The blood flow through the human calf during rhythmic exercise. J Physiol 1949; 109:402.

Barcroft H, Millen JLE. The blood flow through muscle during sustained contraction. J Physiol 1939; 97:17–31.

D'Ambrosia RD, Zelis RF, Chuinard RG. Interstitial pressure measurements in the anterior and posterior compartments in athletes with shin splints. Am J Sports Med 1977; 5:127–131.

Davey JR, Rorabeck CH, Fowler PJ. The tibialis posterior muscle compartment: an unrecognized cause of exertional compartment syndrome. Am J Sports Med 1984; 12:391.

Grant RT. Observations on the blood circulation in voluntary muscle in man. Clin Sci 1938; 3:157–173.

Hill AV. The pressure developed in muscle during contraction. J Physiol 1948; 107:518–526.

Honig CR. Modern cardiovascular physiology. Boston: Little, Brown, 1981: 225.

Horne CE. Acute ischemia of the anterior tibial muscle and the long extensor muscles of the toes. J Bone Joint Surg 1945; 27A: 615–622.

Hughes JR. Ischaemic necrosis of the anterior tibial muscles due to fatigue. J Bone Joint Surg 1948; 30B:581–594.

Jacobsson S, Kjellmer I. Accumulation of fluid in exercising skeletal muscle. Acta Physiol Scand 1964; 60:286.

Leach R, Hammond G, Stryker W. Anterior tibial compartment syndrome (acute and chronic). J Bone Joint Surg 1967; 49A:451–463.

Linge B van. Experimentele spierhypertrofie bij de rat. Assen: Van Garkum, 1959.

Matsen FA, Winguist RA, Krugmire RB. Diagnosis and management of compartmental syndromes. J Bone Joint Surg 1980; 62A:286–291.

Mavor GE. The anterior tibial syndrome. J Bone Joint Surg 1956; 38B:513–517.

Mubarak SJ, Gould RN, Lee YF, et al. The medial tibial stress syndrome: a case of shin splints. Am J Sports Med 1982; 20:201.

Mubarak SJ, Hargens AR. Compartment syndromes and Volkmann's contracture. Philadelphia: WB Saunders, 1981.

Qvarfordt P, Christenson JT, Eklof B, et al. Intramuscular pressure, muscle blood flow, and skeletal muscle metabolism in chronic anterior tibial compartment syndrome. Clin Orthop 1983; 179:284.

Renemann RS. The anterior and lateral compartment syndrome of the leg. The Hague: Mouton, 1968: 176.

Rorabeck CH, Bourne RB, Fowler PJ, et al. The role of tissue pressure measurement in diagnosing chronic anterior compartment syndrome. Am J Sports Med 1988; 16:143–146.

Rorabeck CH, Macnab I. The pathophysiology of the anterior tibial compartment syndrome. Clin Orthop 1978; 113:52.

Sejersted OM, Hargens AR. Regional pressure and nutrition of skeletal muscle during isometric contraction. In: Hargens AR, ed. Tissue nutrition and viability. New York: Springer-Verlag, 1986: 263.

Sheridan GW, Matsen FA. An animal model of the compartment syndrome. Clin Orthop 1975; 113:36.

Slocum DB. The shin-splint syndrome: medical aspects and differential diagnosis. Am J Surg 1967; 114:875.

Styf JR, Lorner LM. Chronic anterior compartment syndrome of the leg. J Bone Joint Surg 1986; 68A:1338.

Veith RG, Matsen FA, Newell SG. Recurrent anterior compartment syndromes. Phys Sports Med 1980; 8:11:80.

Volkmann R von. Die ischaemischen Muskellahmungen und Kontrakturen. Zentralb Chir 1881; 8:801–803.

Wells HS, Youmans JB, Miller DG Jr. Tissue pressure (intracutaneous, subcutaneous, and intramuscular) as related to venous pressure, capillary filtration and other factors. J Clin Invest 1938; 17:489–499.

Whitesides TE, Haney TC, Morimoto K, Harada H. Tissue pressure measurements as a determinant for the need of fasciotomy. Clin Orthop 1975; 113:43–51.

Wright S. Applied physiology. 10th ed. London: Oxford University Press, 1961.

STRESS FRACTURE OF THE LOWER EXTREMITY

JOHN H. OLIVER, M.D., F.R.C.S.(C)

When the forces of daily participation in a sport become excessive, reaction to the accumulated stress can develop in the athlete's anatomic structures. The stress reaction that develops in bones has been termed a "stress fracture." The weightbearing bones of the lower extremity are common sites of stress fractures in athletes who participate in sports that require the repetitive actions of running or jumping.

Stress fracture is a term describing the reaction to injury in the bone. The fracture is a local manifestation of a syndrome of accumulated stress in the anatomic tissues. As the bone develops a fatigue area of injury, new bone forms in reaction to the fatigue. Besides the reaction in the bone, there is usually reaction in the soft tissue support structures, such as the muscle and tendon aponeuroses. The stress reaction in the bone must be considered part of this overall reaction in the local tissues.

Frequent sites for stress fractures are the areas of the lower one-third of the tibia and fibula, and the shafts of the metatarsals. However, stress reactions can occur in any area of the lower extremity bones and have been reported in the femoral neck, in the femoral diaphysis, and in the bones of the foot, the talus and calcaneus.

Proper management of an athlete with a stress injury depends on an accurate diagnosis. Early appropriate steps toward treatment ensure an optimal rate of recovery.

The history of the athlete's activity program often provides clues to the causative factors leading to the injury. The athlete frequently describes symptoms of pain, located at one specific area in the lower extremity, that develops during participation in a certain activity, such as running or jumping. Usually, the athlete has been overtraining or performing the sport activity repetitively. A careful evaluation of the training program or activity routine often provides the clue to the cause of the stress injury. In a sport such as running, the athlete may have inadvertently trained too aggressively over a short period. This is frequently the case when a runner increases distances before a marathon. Occasionally, an athlete may experience a sudden onset of symptoms after a particularly excessive performance; this is often seen in dance-related injuries. A careful review of the athlete's schedule of activities before the onset of the symptoms will point to changes that may have occurred in the training program. The athlete may have adjusted the training environment. Common examples of this are a change from flat terrain to hills, soft running surface to hard pavement, or soft wood floors to a hard concrete surface. Inadvertently, the athlete may have adjusted training schedules by increasing the time spent at daily practices. On occasion, a change in the sports activity can produce the stress reaction, as seen when an athlete takes up a sport for the first time without adequate guidance or preparation.

DIAGNOSIS

The cardinal sign is pain experienced with activity. The pain is localized to one area of the lower extremity and occurs whenever the athlete performs the stressful activity. In runners, the pain of a stress fracture usually is experienced soon after they begin running; the pain only remits when the activity is stopped. The area of sensitivity is usually in the exact region of the stress reaction in the bone. When this area is palpated or pressed, the athlete experiences pain. If the stress reaction has been present for a few days, swelling may be noted in the region, especially in stress fractures of the metatarsals or distal fibula or tibia. Occasionally, the tissues over the stress area may feel warmer to the touch. Pain on weight bearing on the affected leg may cause the athlete to develop an "antalgic" type of limp.

Generally, by the time an athlete seeks medical advice the diagnosis of stress fracture may be evident on the basis of the history and clinical features. An x-ray examination of the involved bone may reveal a site of increased density, but in the early stages of a stress reaction the radiograph may show little, if any, noticeable change. In such instances, a technetium polyphosphate bone scan may reveal a site of increased uptake on the scan in the region corresponding to the site of pain. In many instances, the bone scan shows a site of reaction before a change is noticeable radiographically.

MANAGEMENT

After the initial assessment of the injury, the management program for an athlete with a stress fracture involves a treatment plan customized for the athlete and the sport. First and foremost, the athlete must be educated regarding the cause of the stress fracture and the benefit of modified rest to permit healing of the fracture. In most cases, the pain forces a modification or curtailment of activities. Occasionally, the athlete persists at sport and inadvertently prolongs the healing course of the stress reaction.

The mainstay of any treatment program is to remove the stressful activity from the program. Most athletes require a substitute program of activity to provide a daily cardiorespiratory workout. Swimming or cycling programs are useful alternatives. Application of ice directly to the stress area diminishes local swelling and pain. Ultrasound application may promote healing of the injured area.

Each situation in which an athlete has developed a stress reaction must be individually evaluated. The cause of the stress fracture may have been an error in training. If this error is not corrected, the stress fracture often recurs when the athlete returns to the same activity.

Occasionally, the stress fracture has developed in an athlete who has an anatomic predisposition toward injury. Individuals with a particular alignment of the lower legs, such as bow legs or knock knees, may have a tendency to develop stress fractures. Assessment of shoewear patterns may reveal peculiarities that necessitate correction of the shoe or possibly the use of an orthotic device. The properly fitted orthosis adjusts the forces directed on the lower extremity, evenly distributing these forces. An all-purpose, ready-made orthosis may be adequate, but a custom-fitted orthosis is usually required for the individual with a persistent problem of stress fracture.

When weight bearing causes pain, the athlete should avoid stressing the affected limb, perhaps by using crutches. Occasionally, it is necessary to immobilize the lower leg in a cast. A light-weight, removable plastic splint-orthosis can achieve proper protection and at the same time permit joint motion.

Ultimately, the goal of all parts of the treatment plan is to return the athlete to sports as quickly and as safely as possible. The timing of the return must be carefully judged so as to avoid recurrence of the injury. If proper precautions of rest and protection from continued stress are followed, 8 to 10 weeks are required to permit healing of the bone injury.

There are specific guidelines to help determine when the athlete can return to sports. First, the athlete must no longer perceive local pain in the region of the stress reaction or feel discomfort when the area is palpated. Swelling, redness, and warmth should have disappeared. When scheduling the return to the sport, it is wise to advise the athlete to start with a very relaxed training schedule. For a runner, this may mean a schedule that consists of running on a soft surface, such as a track, for 15 to 30 minutes at a reduced pace, two to three times a week. If there is no pain, the runner may increase the time increment by 10 minutes each run per week for 2 to 3 weeks. Ultimately, the frequency of runs may increase. The aim of the program is to increase the running schedule over a 2- to 3-month time frame.

In a schedule of return to sports involving jumping, the athlete should spend most of the first 2 weeks in a program that mainly consists of running. If running is pain free, the jumping activities may be attempted for periods of 20 minutes per day. These practice periods can be gradually increased at a weekly rate with the aim of returning the athlete to the original program over 2 months.

It is important to inform athletes that stress injuries can recur. On any occasion that they perceive a return of symptoms, the activity level must be adjusted back to a level at which there is no discomfort. If the symptoms return, a careful reassessment of the athlete and the training program is necessary.

EXAMPLES OF STRESS FRACTURES

The most common sites of stress fractures are the diaphyses of the metatarsal bones of the foot. Common symptoms are pain on weight bearing and swelling over the dorsum of the foot. Ice application over the forefoot and elevation helps decrease the swelling, and the use of crutches is advisable to decrease all stress of weight bearing. These stress fractures must be treated with respect. If the athlete returns to activity too soon, the reaction recurs in many cases. A minimum of 6 to 8 weeks is usually required for adequate healing.

Stress fractures of the *distal fibula* often occur at a site just proximal to the level of the ankle joint or at the distal tip of the fibula. These fractures sometimes occur after sudden excessive stress, as when the athlete twists the foot or receives a direct blow to the area. Once the initial symptoms of pain and swelling have diminished, activities that do not involve repetitive stress (e.g., running) may be permitted. Many athletes can return to their sports in less than 8 weeks, particularly if they avoid sudden or repetitive stresses.

Stress fractures of the *tibia* generally occur in the diaphyseal shaft at the level of the middle or distal third. Usually, these fractures develop over a period of a few weeks. The typical case is that of the athlete who has been training aggressively for a competition and often has ignored the early painful symptoms. Palpation over the skin area is particularly painful, and in many cases roentgenograms show evidence of increased density in the region of the stress reaction. Treatment should be aimed at reducing all stress on the site of the injury by the use of crutches and, if necessary, a lightweight plastic below-knee walking orthosis. Fractures in the distal tibia heal readily, usually in 2 to 3 months, if the area is protected from further stress.

Stress fractures of the *femur* are rare, but they do occur in athletes who practice competitively with a daily routine of several hours. The site of the stress reaction is usually the inferior neck of the femur. Symptoms may be subtle at first, consisting only of a dull, diffuse ache in the region of the hip joint or groin. Frequently, these athletes have perceived the symptoms to reflect a "simple muscle strain" and have continued the stressful activity. Other symptoms are a decreased range of motion of the hip joint on the affected side and mild discomfort on palpation. Radiographic views, both anterior and lateral oblique, of the affected hip and the opposite hip should be compared. A stress fracture may be visible in the region of the inferior neck, or (as is often the case) the only visible sign may be increased bone density in the region of the neck. If no abnormality is obvious on a conventional radiograph, a bone scan should help to demonstrate increased activity if there is a stress fracture. Treatment involves close supervision of the athlete and total cessation of all stress-provoking activities. If walking is painful, crutches should be prescribed. Usually, swimming does not aggravate the symptoms and is therefore a good alternative exercise activity.

Although extremely rare, *deformity* of the femoral neck has been known to result from a stress fracture. Examination may reveal a measurable actual leg length discrepancy and an obvious limp, and radiographs show deformity of the femoral neck-shaft angle when compared with the opposite asymptomatic hip. The treatment depends on the extent of deformity. If the measurable leg length difference exceeds ¾ inch and the femoral neck-shaft angle has been altered significantly, surgical correction may be advisable. Fortunately, deformity with a stress fracture rarely occurs. The symptoms of pain usually alert the athlete before accumulated stress causes the bone to become deformed.

SUGGESTED READING

Delee JC, Evans JP, Julian J. Stress fractures of fifth metatarsal. Am J Sports Med 1983; 11:349.

Greaney RB, et al. Distribution and natural history of stress fractures in U.S. Marine Recruits. Radiology 1983; 146:339–346.

Pavlov H, Torg JS, Frieberger RH. Tarsal navicular stress fracture. Radiology 1983; 148:641–645.

RUPTURE OF THE ACHILLES TENDON

JOHN M. SULLIVAN, M.B., Ch.B., F.R.A.C.S.

In a top-class athlete, rupture of the Achilles tendon can herald demotion to a lower class of performance. However, early recognition of the problem and the institution of a rational treatment program can allow the athlete to return to previous peak function. However, recovery may take 12 to 18 months.

Within the sporting world the group at greatest risk is the middle-aged athlete in the fourth decade. The younger supremely fit athlete can be affected, but the pathogenesis is quite different. No sport is particularly spared, and the emphasis on certain sports in some reviews represents often the geographic preponderance of those sports. The more mature racquetball or basketball player is the most vulnerable. In any series of ruptures reviewed, we see skiers, skaters, runners, jumpers, football players, gymnasts, and soccer players. Females are featured to a lesser degree and the incidence on average is about 10 percent that of males. As more females are accepted into the ranks of professional athletes, the percentage will increase.

PATHOGENESIS

The rupture is usually sudden and unexpected; in some instances it is preceded by a period of discomfort or pain. The exercising athlete is usually about to thrust forward or upward, fully weight bearing, with the ankle joint changing from a position of dorsiflexion to plantar flexion. As this occurs, the knee joint passes into an extended position, placing the calf muscles on maximal stretch as they are about to contract explosively. Often the athlete is retreating or decelerating, and the contracted or contracting calf is further loaded by a sudden change in direction. Examples of the foregoing mechanisms are (1) the unconditioned athlete coming out of the blocks at the start of a race; (2) the basketball player changing direction, jumping, and intercepting the ball; and (3) the racquetball player lunging for a passing ball. An extreme example of forced dorsiflexion against a contracting calf occurs when the athlete lands awkwardly after a jump or lands unexpectedly in a hole.

A less common situation occurs when a direct blow is received to a taut Achilles tendon. Steroid injected into the tendon or immediate region may precede the rupture. The site of rupture is regularly 2 to 8 cm above the insertion of the Achilles tendon. A study by Largergren and Lindholm demonstrated that the area of poorest blood supply falls within this section. The rupture may be complete or partial.

COMPLETE RUPTURE

The athlete complains of pain that diminishes over the succeeding hours. Often he describes the sensation of having been "kicked" in the back of the heel, and some may even hear the tendon rupture or describe its tearing. Walking is possible, albeit with a flatfooted gait.

Diagnosis

Diagnosis is aided by the history and completed by a careful examination. With a fresh rupture a defect can be seen and palpated. If some hours have elapsed since the rupture, there is swelling, possibly ecchymosis, tenderness, and a palpable defect (through soft hematoma) 2 cm or more above the calcaneus. The patient may be able to plantar flex the foot by using the toe flexors. The "squeeze" test of Thompson and Doherty is diagnostic. To perform this test, the patient is placed prone or asked to kneel on a stool with the leg relaxed. Squeezing the normal calf produces plantar flexion of the foot. Squeeze applied to the affected leg fails to produce plantar flexion, and this constitutes a positive test result.

A roentgenogram should be taken. This will show alteration of the soft tissues, but more importantly rules out any bone injuries. On the rare occasion, an avulsion flake may be seen and dictates a different form of management.

Management

Nonoperative management will not be discussed as there is no place for this in the treatment of an athlete. Early, (i.e., before surgery) the limb should be elevated and ice applied to the region.

Operative Treatment

The operative procedure is short. Either regional or general anesthesia is employed. The patient is placed prone with a soft roll in front of the ankle. A tourniquet is used.

A medial longitudinal incision is made. The midline should not be crossed in a sinuous manner, and the lateral aspect is avoided to prevent scarring and sural nerve tethering in this area. Full-thickness flaps are raised after incising the deep fascia, and the paratenon is incised longitudinally to allow later closure.

The rupture is exposed and most often is 2 to 8 cm above the calcaneus. The fragmented ends are not excised. The area is irrigated free of blood clot, and with the foot in full plantar flexion the frayed ends of the tendon are meshed together. The suture technique preferred involves the insertion of four separate looped Dexon sutures (No. 1). Two are placed proximally and two distally (Fig. 1), three to four loops in each suture engaging a varying amount of tendon. These are then tied, and several opposing sutures supplement the repair across the central tendon. This produces an extremely strong repair and

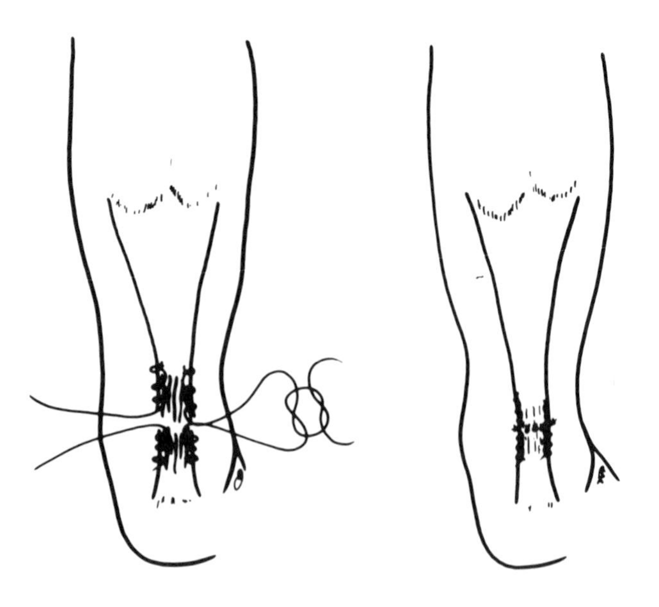

Figure 1 Suture technique.

can justifiably allow early passive mobilization without cast immobilization and without weight bearing. Work on this particular aspect is ongoing (author), and for the present, protected repair will be described.

Argument may be proffered regarding the effect this suture may have on tendon vascularity. To date it has not been seen as a problem. What is achieved is excellent control of the tendon ends, institution of a durable repair, and the best possible scaffold for healing.

The paratenon is closed with 3–0 Dexon. The tourniquet is deflated and bleeding is controlled by diathermy. The skin is closed with interrupted 4–0 nylon. Suction drainage is sometimes used, and its routine use would never be condemned.

The leg is placed in a split, padded, below-knee cast with the foot in plantar flexion just short of the maximum. After 3 days in bed with the leg elevated, mobilization is begun with crutches. At 2 weeks the cast is removed, sutures are removed, and a new cast is applied in a gravity equinus position. A walking platform is applied to level the sole, and partial weight bearing is allowed with the use of crutches. At a total of 6 weeks, the cast is removed and the patient equipped with a 2-cm heel raise.

Rehabilitation

The patient is instructed to wear a raise at all times for the next 4 weeks. Particular stress is placed on caution going upstairs, standing on chairs, or climbing ladders. A specific reminder is given to wear the raised shoe if it is necessary to get up in the night.

Early therapy is aimed at mobilizing the ankle gently and painlessly. Hot whirlpool exposure is extremely beneficial. Swimming and exercycle use with the foot flat on the pedal are subtle encouragements to mobilization. When a heel-toe gait is realized at about the 4-week stage, the raise is removed and passive stretching can be incorporated into the program. Throughout this period, ultrasonography and calf muscle stimulation from the physiotherapist hasten progress. At about 3 months the athlete is usually able to commence running. At about 6 to 9 months near-normal function is achieved, but it may take 12 to 18 months to regain peak power take-off. The program does not end here, and the athlete must be instructed about careful warm-up and stretching procedures for both legs.

NEGLECTED COMPLETE RUPTURE

Because of motivation to return to previous peak performance after injury, and a better level of care for the athlete, late diagnosis is not usually a problem. Nonetheless, it does occasionally occur, and its management will be discussed.

Diagnosis

The history tells the story, and the diagnosis is never in doubt. The calf is wasted and the ankle region thickened and tender. The gait is flatfooted and the "squeeze" test markedly positive.

Operative Treatment

The patient is positioned and the tourniquet applied as for treatment of complete rupture. A posteromedial incision is made from the junction of upper and middle thirds of the calf to the posterior and medial side of the tendon insertion at the calcaneus. The deep fascia is divided and the paratenon opened. The rupture is identified and inspected. The very terminal disorganized scar tissue at the tendon ends is excised. Excision is not carried back to normal tissue, as suggested by some authors, as this leaves a very large defect. Once continuity has been reestablished, this scar will remodel under tension with the realignment of collegen fibers.

It is unusual to be able to oppose and suture the ends, even with the foot in maximal plantar flexion. However, if this can be achieved, the repair is simple. Otherwise, a sheet of fascia from the gastrocnemius is fashioned (Fig. 2), 10 to 15 cm long and about 4 cm wide proximally. It is carefully stripped off the gastrocnemius by sharp dissection, an attempt being made to leave some fascia covering muscle proximally. This is carried down to 2 cm above the distal end. It is turned over and brought anterior to the distal stump of tendon and rolled around this as a tube. Using 0 Dexon, the tube is closed, and the proximal end where this flap hinges is sutured. It is unusual to be able to close the donor defect completely, but this is done if possible. If plantaris is present, it is divided distally, opened as a sheet, and placed over the repair as an added sheath to assist in gliding.

The immobilization is as for complete rupture, except that the cast is required for 8 weeks. The re-

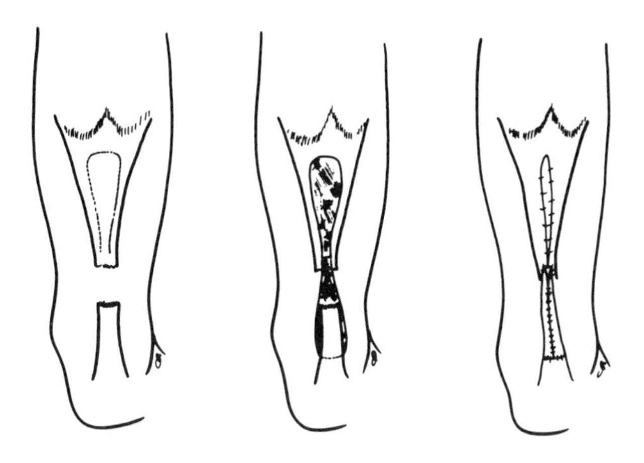

Figure 2 Reconstruction for neglected rupture.

habilitation is similar but more prolonged. Significant morbidity is associated with neglected complete rupture, and a normally functioning unit is difficult to achieve.

PARTIAL RUPTURE

The pathogenesis, as already discussed, must apply in some circumstances. However, partial rupture probably represents an overuse syndrome that occurs in the poorly trained recreational athlete as well as in the intensely trained top athlete.

Pain is the common complaint. It is shooting or tearing in nature (sometimes burning) and is worsened by activity. There may be complaints of stiffness and soreness in the region in the mornings.

Diagnosis

A careful examination is critical. Thickening and nodular formation are often observed. The ability to stand on tiptoes is unimpaired, except by pain. Importantly, there is a negative "squeeze" test. Palpation demonstrates further the thickening, nodules, and point tenderness. If the problem is longstanding, calf wasting and weakness can be demonstrated.

Management

In the very acute stages, before disability develops, conservative treatment is worthy of trial. Three weeks in a walking below-knee cast, followed by physiotherapy with decreased activities for a further 1 month, may achieve a good result. Unfortunately, for a large percentage of patients this regimen fails and the condition becomes chronic.

Operative Treatment

Partial ruptures that have failed conservative treatment and have become chronic are treated surgically. The set-up is as described for a complete rupture. The paratenon is split, and this may be thickened and adherent. In some circumstances it is best excised. The tendon is palpated and the thickening or nodules delineated. In the area of the rupture a longitudinal split is made in the tendon. This reveals altered structure with loss of the normal tendon sheen and fibrous strand appearance. Depending on the duration of the rupture, there may be hemorrhage with early granulation tissue, there may be yellow streaks or patches of yellow soft tissue interspersed with normal tendon, there may be white firm fibrinoid material blending into normal structure.

The abnormal tissue is excised. If only a small amount of pathologic tissue is excised, the tendon can be closed side to side with absorbable sutures. In these circumstances, white 0 Dexon is used. If a large amount of abnormal tissue is removed but continuity is maintained, the area is reinforced with plantaris. If a section has to be excised, a formal repair and reconstruction is performed.

Postoperatively, a below-knee cast with the foot in neutral is applied when a minimal excision is performed. After 1 week, the cast is removed and mobilization is begun. If a large resection is performed or continuity is disrupted, the casting and rehabilitation is as for complete rupture.

I KNEE

PERIARTICULAR OVERUSE SYNDROMES

R. PETER WELSH, M.B., Ch.B., F.R.C.S.(C), F.A.C.S.
CHRISTINE HUTTON, M.B., Ch.B.

Periarticular knee pain can be troublesome to the athlete, diminishing performance and blunting the training effort. With athletic effort, overload or overuse syndromes are common. Symptoms may arise from the patellar mechanism, from the quadriceps tendon or the ligamentum patella at its origin and insertion, from the stabilizing retinacula, from the fat pads deep to the supra- and infrapatellar tendons, or from the synovial lining where it forms plicae or folds that run medially beneath the extensor mechanism and distally along the medial border of the patella to the distal fat pad. In addition, bursae may be aggravated not only in the prepatellar area but also deep to the infrapatellar tendon, as well as beneath the pes anserinus tendons on the medial side and the iliotibial tract on the lateral side. Any of these structures may be involved in the genesis of periarticular overuse syndromes around the knee.

Extensor Mechanism Dysfunction

The most common presenting symptom is that of pain in or around the knee associated with running, jumping, or kicking activities, or with kneeling or crouching. Discomfort is commonly aggravated on ascending and descending stairs; a sensation of instability or crepitus may also be noted. On examination the only positive findings may be tenderness to palpation around or over the patella and its tendons, or to compression of the patella against the femoral condyles. It should be noted that there are no signs of internal derangement and there is no effusion, no loss of range of motion, and no ligamentous instability. There may be some mild quadriceps wasting and occasionally some retropatellar crepitus, but most commonly the examiner is unable to demonstrate major abnormality. This can lead him to discount the significance of the patient's complaints or to erroneously label the condition "chondromalacia." Both these approaches do the patient a gross disservice. A specific diagnosis should be made in every instance.

Patellar Tendinitis (Jumper's Knee)

Inflammation of the distal tendon of the quadriceps muscle (suprapatellar tendinitis), of the origin of the infrapatellar tendon (infrapatellar tendinitis), and of the insertion of the infrapatellar tendon (Osgood-Schlatter disease) are all overuse syndromes associated with running and jumping activities. Pain and tenderness are usually localized to the inflamed area. The discomfort tends to develop during the course of the activity and often persists afterward.

Initial treatment consists of physiotherapy with local ice frictions and ultrsonography, and strengthening and, more particularly, stretching of the quadriceps muscle in conjunction with oral nonsteroidal anti-inflammatory medication for 10 to 15 days. As with all tendinitis, aggressive treatment in the early stages is more successful than later treatment in the chronic established condition. The athlete is reassured that no harm is being done to the knee joint and is permitted to continue with sporting activities, but in modified form. If the provocative exercise involves springing and bounding, these must be discontinued and running or cycling exercises substituted. In all cases the intention should be to maintain the athlete's basic fitness while the condition is allowed to recover without continuing provocative stimuli.

In cases refractory to this regimen, local injection of steroid around the tendon and into the underlying bursa may be indicated. The injection of steroid can have a direct, deleterious effect on the collagenous structures. Injection, particularly of the infrapatellar tendon, should be limited to a maximum of two injections spaced at least 6 months apart lest the weakening of the tendon predispose to its rupture.

Surgical Treatment. On occasion the patellar tendinitis may become so pernicious that the athlete is forced to give up the chosen activity. Under such circumstances, when all conservative treatments have been exhausted, localized tenolysis has been most successful in reestablishing athletic capability.

In this minor procedure through a transverse skin incision, the ligamentum patella is split longitudinally along the direction of its fibers right at the lower pole of the patella. With a sharp dissection the ligamentum is reflected off the lower pole of the patella over an area of about 2 cm, retaining adequate supporting tissue on both the medial and lateral sides. The tendon may be degenerate, with granulation in the substance of the tendon; this degenerate tendon segment, which is usually quite small, is excised and sent for histologic examination. The exposed portion of the lower pole of the patella is then decorticated with an osteotome and the bed drilled with a fine drill point. Access to the infrapatellar fat pad is also gained; if this is hypertrophied, the redundant tissue is excised. A simple oversewing of the tendon is carried out with resorbable sutures, and the limb is protected in a soft dressing. Splint protection is afforded for 2 weeks; after suture removal, a light exercise program including hydrotherapy and bicycle exercises is begun. Isometric quadriceps and hip flexor-abductor exercises are maintained; return to running activity is allowed at 6 weeks.

The condition is not a common indication for surgery, but this simple procedure has been effective in athletes who have proved refractory to all other measures.

Osgood-Schlatter Disease

Osgood-Schlatter disease is a tendinitis in adolescents in which the tibial apophysis is involved. Pressures on the sensitive growth area evoke a local discomfort that can become very disabling. The conventional treatment of this condition has included complete immobilization in a cylinder cast in full extension for 6 weeks. However, in most instances one need not resort to such treatment; the use of an infrapatellar strap worn across the tendon during activity may decrease the pull on the tendon or the tubercle, as happens when a forearm band is used for tennis elbow. The mainstay of management of this condition involves restriction of jumping or bounding activities while the athlete is acutely tender, the use of local ice friction treatments, and diligent application to quadriceps stretching routines. By decreasing the pull on the quadriceps mechanism and making the quadriceps muscle more flexible, the load on the infrapatellar tendon and thus the impact on the tibial tubercle can be greatly reduced. Most athletes can continue their sports activity, but Osgood-Schlatter disease tends to be episodic, and there may be occasions for weeks at a time when restriction of activity becomes necessary. Most adolescents grow through this condition in the course of 2 to 3 years. However, the condition may continue into late adolescence or adulthood, with continuing problems around the tibial tubercle insertion. Local steroid injections may settle symptoms, but there are other instances when surgical treatment becomes necessary.

Surgical Treatment. X-ray review of patients with persistent symptoms around the tibial tubercle often reveals an ossific loose body in the tendon substance where the tibial tubercle apophysis has fragmented and one of the islands of bone has not united with the parent tibia. This local irritation is remedied by the excision of the loose fragment. A transverse incision at the tibial tubercle insertion followed by a longitudinal split in the tendon identifies the loose body; all fragments and any bursal reactive tissue are excised. The tendon is then oversewn and the leg protected in a soft dressing. Return to activity is allowed as symptoms dictate, but it usually takes 6 to 8 weeks before jumping and bounding activities can be recommended.

Bursitis

Prepatellar Bursitis

Prepatellar bursitis (housemaid's knee) presents with pain and swelling in the bursal tissue over the anterior surface of the patella resulting from either direct trauma or repetitive irritation. A fluctuant swelling can be aspirated, local steroid injected, and a compression dressing applied. Follow-up care with anti-inflammatory medication and a therapy program with ultrasonography settles most cases. In long-standing cases, it may be necessary to consider surgical excision of the bursa.

Surgical Treatment. A transverse incision enables the prepatellar bursa to be completely shelled out and peeled off the surface of the patella. The tissues often are very extensively scarred and thickened; removal leaves a large space for potential hematoma formation. To control this, the prepatellar subcutaneous tissues should be sewn down to the fascia over the patella to close this space. A suction drain should be left in situ for 24 hours and a compression bandage applied for 2 weeks.

Infrapatellar Bursitis

Infrapatellar bursitis is a common accompaniment of infrapatellar tendinitis, associated also with the infrapatellar fat pad syndrome. Local steroid injection into the bursa through the ligamentum patella usually settles an infrapatellar tendon bursitis satisfactorily. At the time of surgery for infrapatellar tendinitis, this area should be thoroughly inspected for its possible involvement in the pathology.

Iliotibial Band Bursitis

Iliotibial band bursitis is a troublesome inflammation of the bursa underlying the distal portion of the iliotibial tract on the lateral aspect of the knee. It results from the friction forces associated with repetitive knee flexion and extension associated with impact loading of the knee, as in jogging. This is a perplexing condition that presents in an athlete with no previous indication of harm or injury. It may suddenly smite the athlete even in the course of a race event with a sharp pain over the lateral femoral condyle, and become so painful within a space of 100 yards that the athlete is forced to discontinue the activity completely. On walking the knee seems to improve spontaneously, but as soon as attempts are made to run again the sharp pain returns. On endeavoring subsequently to run, athletes find that they can often run for a short distance only to find the pain appear as suddenly as it had initially. This condition is often confused with internal derangements. Runners must recognize that with this condition they cannot persist in running farther than the threshold of discomfort allows. Maintaining a steady activity level over a reduced distance (even at an increased pace) often sees the condition disappear as mysteriously as it occurred. Ice friction treatments, ultrasonography, stretching and strengthening exercises, and oral anti-inflammatory medication are all adjunctive therapies often necessary to help alleviate this troublesome condition. On occasion, local steroid injection into the bursa may be indicated and surgical treatment may become necessary.

Surgical Treatment of Iliotibial Band Bursitis. There are class athletes whose condition fails to respond to local measures, modification of activity, and attention to the footwear and gait pattern. Their condition may warrant surgical release of the iliotibial tract and excision of the bursa.

A longitudinal incision is made over the lateral femoral condyle parallel to the upper border of the iliotibial tract. The fascia is incised longitudinally in the direction of its fibers, marking the upper margin of the iliotibial tract and releasing distally to the point of the femoral condyle and proximally for 2 inches. On flexion and extension of the knee, the fascial band is seen to have been freed and the bursa clearly revealed on flexion. Redundant bursal tissue can then be excised. Sutures are required only in the subcutaneous tissues and skin; a soft dressing is then applied. Light activity can commence when the sutures have been removed, with a return to running activity as symptoms allow.

Pes Anserinus Bursitis

Pes anserinus bursitis is an inflammation of the bursa underlying the sartorius, gracilis, and semitendinosus tendon complex on the medial aspect of the knee. This troublesome condition, which affects cyclists, runners, and swimmers, is treated locally with ultrasonography and ice frictions, these being the mainstays of therapy. Oral anti-inflammatory medication and local steroids may be necessary. Attention to footwear may be required, with particular concern for overpronation in runners. In swimmers, this bursitis can be very troublesome and associated with a medial ligament tendinitis; unless there is modification of the kick technique, this condition may prove refractory and jeopardize the athlete's ability to continue successfully in competitive swimming.

Retinaculitis

Inflammation of the medial and lateral supporting structures presents with pain and tenderness over the retinacula where they play over the underlying femoral condyles, pinching the synovium and evoking pain from this source as a consequence of repetitive loading of the knee. It is important to distinguish this state from a true chondromalacia, for the prognosis is much different. Urgent attention to flexibility exercises, particularly stretching out the quadriceps, is essential to relieve pressures over the femoral condylar margins.

In the genesis of a tighter retinaculum and extensor mechanism, one must comment on the overzealous closure of the knee after arthrotomy. If the capsule is tightened unduly following a surgical arthrotomy of the knee, there can be a marked increase in the pressures over the condylar margins, increasing pressures on the patella as well. Postsurgical knee pain often stems from this tightening of the capsule, and postoperative stretching exercises for the quadriceps mechanism are therefore a very important adjunct to any surgical intervention in the knee.

Fat Pad Impingement Syndromes

Impingement of the patellar fat pads or the synovium can be either acute or chronic in nature. Acute impingement can occur with sudden forced extension of the knee where the structures are caught between the patella or its tendons and the underlying femoral condyle. The mechanism of injury is elicited from the history, with pain and tenderness noted clinically medial and lateral to the patellar tendons or within the joint. The natural course of the injury is full recovery without intervention.

Chronic impingement syndromes often develop without specific history of trauma. With repetitive activity, the fat pad and synovium hypertrophy and become pinched between the patella and femur, where they are subject to repetitive low-grade trauma and become persistently symptomatic. This condition is often confused with chondromalacia patella because of the associated crepitus that is sometimes present. Careful examination differentiates the area of involvement from the patella, which remains completely smooth and uninvolved. Haffa's syndrome can become troublesome to the athlete and may even require surgical excision of the hypertrophied tissue for satisfactory resolution.

At the outset, it is important to reduce patella loads with a program of flexibility exercises for the quadriceps muscle group. Avoidance of provocative overloading is most important, and discontinuation of springing activity may be necessary. The athlete with a fat pad syndrome is often found to be engaging only in intermittent activity. It is vital to even out the athletic effort and continue a program of regular, daily activity at a reduced but consistent level of performance. Local ultrasonography and ice frictions are sometimes of help; a steroid injection may be tried but is usually ineffective. On occasion, surgical treatment may become necessary.

Surgical Treatment. Arthroscopy of the knee should be performed to rule out completely any associated internal derangement or involvement of the articular surface of the patella. It is possible by arthroscopic technique to trim the infrapatellar fat pad to reduce the impingement between the lower pole of the patella and the femoral condyle. At the same time, a lateral retinacular release should be carried out and is best made through a separate 2-cm incision, exposing the retinaculum on the lateral side. A compression dressing is applied for 5 days before a light exercise routine is begun. Before the advent of arthroscopic surgical technique, an open fat pad excision was carried out, making a small arthrotomy and completely excising the infrapatellar fat pad. Should arthroscopic excision of the fat pad be inadequate, this treatment is still recommended. It should be emphasized that it is only in very rare instances that the fat pad need be excised; however, on occasion the symptoms can be extreme, as in the case of a pianist who had to give up her chosen profession because of fat pad sensitivity while operating the foot pedals. After excision of the fat pad, she returned to her "sport" without further problems.

SUGGESTED READING

Crenshaw AH, ed. Campbell's operative orthopaedics. St. Louis: C.V. Mosby, 1984.

Terry GC, Hughston JC, Norwood LA. The anatomy of the iliopatellar band and iliotibial tract. Am J Sports Med 1986; 14:39–45.

Kujala UM, Kuist M, Heinonen O. Osgood-Schlatter's disease in adolescent athletes. Am J Sports Med 1985; 13:236–241.

PATELLOFEMORAL ARTHRALGIA, PATELLAR INSTABILITY, AND CHONDROMALACIA PATELLA

R. PETER WELSH, M.B., Ch.B., F.R.C.S.(C), F.A.C.S.
CHRISTINE HUTTON, M.B., Ch.B.

PATELLOFEMORAL ARTHRALGIA

Of all knee maladies, the patellofemoral derangements pose the greatest difficulty in management. Running and jumping sports put great demands on the patellar mechanism where seemingly trivial imperfections can seriously compromise the athlete's optimal performance. Overt pathology is usually not evident; the spectrum of normal anatomy and physiology is so wide that determining the variants predisposing to pain and dysfunction poses a true dilemma to the clinician. The site and origin of pain are often obscure.

Essential to an understanding of the patellofemoral arthralgias are the concepts of abnormal patellar pressures and abnormal patellar excursion.

The patella is a sesamoid bone lying in the quadriceps apparatus that provides enhanced mechanical advantage to the muscles during extension. The anatomy of the extensor mechanism is such that the patella is subject not only to the forces directed along the line of the quadriceps muscles and the infrapatellar tendon, but also to the resultant vectors of these forces.

Factors leading to increases in quadriceps load result in abnormal patellar pressures. The resulting pain is believed to be due to stimulation of nerve endings in the underlying subchondral bone, but may also relate to strain in the retinacula or impingement of the fat pad or the synovium, which are both richly endowed with nerve elements.

Abnormal Patellar Pressures

Inflexibility of the quadriceps muscles is probably the most common cause of primary abnormal patellar pressures. During the adolescent growth spurt, bone growth may outstrip the rate at which muscle fibers stretch, causing abnormal muscle tightness and excessive compressive forces across the patella. Juveniles are particularly susceptible to derangement of this type, accounting for many instances of patellofemoral arthralgia in teenagers.

Muscle injury from trauma with hematoma and scar formation may similarly cause abnormal muscle tightness, as can surgical intervention. Indeed, overzealous capsular closure after arthrotomy may significantly tighten the capsule, thereby increasing the patellofemoral pressures, a state likely to worsen with subsequent surgery, and producing more scarring. Likewise, with patellar stabilization procedures these forces may be increased. Lateral retinacular release is therefore an essential adjunct to all surgery performed to reduce these pressures.

Abnormal Patellar Excursion

The line of force of the quadriceps is basically along the line of the shaft of the femur. The physiologic valgus of the knee gives an angle Q between the pull of the muscle and that of the infrapatellar tendon. In the normal knee the natural tendency of the patella to displace laterally is resisted by the medial stabilizing structures, the distal fibers of the vastus medialis and the medial retinaculum, and lateral excursion is further limited by the prominent lateral femoral condyle. Genu valgum, excessive external tibial torsion, and pes planus effectively increase the Q angle and the lateral force.

Failure of the medial structures, i.e., lax retinaculum or weak quadriceps, shortening or tightness of the lateral stabilizing structures, and bone anomalies such as a flattened lateral femoral condyle also predispose to force imbalance, resulting in lateral tilting or lateral excursion (subluxation or dislocation) of the patella. It is claimed that minimal but persistent recurrent subluxation of the patella is a major contributing factor in the development of chondromalacia patellae. A true degenerative change in the articular cartilage may result from alterations in patellar excursion, but patellofemoral pressures and trauma are also important in the pathogenesis of this condition.

The misnomer chondromalacia patella has in the past been applied indiscriminately to cases of patellofemoral arthralgia. This diagnosis should be applied only when there is actual patellar articular cartilage degeneration.

Iatrogenic Arthralgia

Too often the diagnosis of patellar subluxation has led to overzealous orthopaedic treatment of patients with patellofemoral arthralgia, even though these individuals were not shown to suffer from proved instability of the patellar mechanism. The result can be an aggravation of the discomfort, or worse, a true deterioration of the status of the articular surfaces.

Procedures that tighten the medial structures or draw the patella down also significantly increase patellar pressures, and therefore increase the shear forces interacting between the articulating surfaces. The reversal of these changes can be very difficult and may combine articular debridement, retinacular release, and patellar tendon transposition.

Clinical Features

The different forms of patellofemoral arthralgia can be specifically defined. It is important to separate the entities clinically, because the prognosis and treatment are often different. A clear definition of the condition is essential in order to distinguish these states from true internal derangement.

Quadriceps wasting may occur, and an effusion may be present but is unusual unless there is an associated reactive synovitis. Range of motion and stability of the knee are never affected. Specific sites of pain should be elicited and any local swelling noted. Signs of abnormal patellar excursion and pressure should be documented, noting the overall limb alignment: the Q angle and patella position as well as the tightness of the retinacula and the quadriceps muscle group. Crepitus may be from the patella itself but can also arise from the retinacula and fat pads; care should be taken to determine its exact site of origin.

Finally, the status of the feet with regard to heel varus or valgus and the degree of pronation of the forefoot should be noted; these may have an important bearing on patellar responses on load bearing.

Management

Conservative Treatment

Nearly all these syndromes respond to a conservative approach. On occasion, the provocative activity must be modified; i.e., sport must be carried out at a reduced level, coupled where necessary with alterations in technique and form. A change of activity, e.g., from running to cycling, may be necessary, the emphasis being on maintaining basic fitness until the natural history of the process runs its course.

Although physiotherapy treatments with shortwave diathermy and ultrasonography are often symptomatically helpful, an intensive individual program of exercise therapy must be maintained. Isometric quadriceps setting and straight-leg raising, followed by progressive resisted exercise over the final 5 to 10 degrees of knee extension, are emphasized. Resisted exercises through the full range of motion are avoided because of the excessive compressive forces they apply across the patella. Sequential faradism can be applied if muscle bulk is significantly reduced. Stretching must be equally emphasized in an effort to reduce the loads across the joint and at the same time enhance the strength capability of the muscle group. Orthotics aimed at correcting pes planus and heel valgus may be helpful in cases where such a condition is contributing to abnormal patellar mechanics, particularly in association with genu valgum.

Surgical Treatment

Intensive conservative management for at least 6 months should precede any surgery; the patient should have been disabled to the point of nonparticipation in work or sport before such treatment is contemplated.

Retinacular Release. The lateral retinaculum is a capsular structure. It is extra-articular, and therefore an intra-articular arthroscopic procedure makes no sense at all. However, arthroscopy is an essential prelude to this procedure, not only to scan the joint but also to deal with any intra-articular pathology that may be encountered. Once the surgeon has been reassured that the interior of the joint is normal, retinacular release should be carried out extra-articularly in order to preserve the integrity of the synovium.

A skin incision 1 cm in length is made over the lateral aspect of the knee at the junction of the upper and middle third of the patella. Dissection is continued subcutaneously to expose the capsule and fascial elements. A careful incision of the retinaculum is made and the capsule is separated from the underlying synovium. The retinaculum and lateral capsule are then released proximally and distally over a 10-cm length, avoiding completely the synovium. Simple skin closure and a pressure dressing are added, and the patient is able to begin an active rehabilitation program 2 days after surgery.

Fat Pad Excision. With repetitive activity, the fat pad and synovium hypertrophy and become pinched between the patella and femur, where they are subject to repetitive low-grade trauma and become persistently symptomatic. This condition is often confused with chondromalacia patella because of the associated crepitus that can sometimes be elicited. Careful examination differentiates the area of involvement from the patella, which is completely smooth and uninvolved. Haffa's syndrome may require surgical excision of the hypertrophied tissue for satisfactory resolution.

The fat pad is a very substantial structure, and although it is possible to nibble away at this with basket forceps and other arthroscopic instruments, this can be very time consuming and often incomplete. As a first-line treatment it is commendable because it carries a low morbidity rate. However, if arthroscopic excision of the fat pad proves inadequate, open excision should be considered. A short medial arthrotomy offers excellent visualization of the fat pad, which can be excised in its entirety. Because a prearthrotomy arthroscopy has been carried out, it is not necessary to explore the joint further, but zealous cauterization of the bleeding points in the base of the excised area is essential, for the fat pad is an extremely vascular structure.

Synovial Excision. In the suprapatellar area at the superior margin of the intercondylar articular groove, synovial impingement can become extremely troublesome, and local excision of the excessive synovial tissue becomes necessary. Given that preliminary arthroscopy has excluded other pathologic conditions, localized synovectomy using arthroscopic instrumentation is relatively easy.

PATELLAR INSTABILITY

Acute Patellar Dislocation

Traumatic dislocation of the patella is an injury that must be treated as any other ligamentous derangement of the knee. It requires a full evaluation to determine the extent of the instability and any other associated injury to the joint. The hemarthrosis should be aspirated before the knee is further carefully evaluated. X-ray studies should include skyline views of the patella and should be carefully evaluated to determine whether there is any associated damage to the articular surfaces, since portions of the articular cartilage and osteochondral fragments may be sheared off when the patella is forcibly dislocated.

Arthroscopy and Conservative Treatment

Arthroscopy should be carried out if there is doubt about the presence of a loose body. By arthroscopic technique, such fragments may be removed from the joint before a stovepipe cast is applied in full extension. After 4 weeks in cast, during which time quadriceps setting exercises and faradic stimulation are instituted, protection is further offered with a patella-restraining brace. Knee mobilization is commenced at this time; return to sports activity can be allowed only when full range of motion and full function of the quadriceps, with particularly full flexibility, has been restored.

Open Surgical Treatment

Occasionally, traumatic dislocation is so severe as to shear off a major portion of the articular surface and/or produce a major disruption of the medial retinacular structures. Under these circumstances, it is better to open the knee formally, remove the loose body, and debride the damaged joint surface by shaving the margins and drilling the base. A formal arthrotomy is made medially, releasing the patellar mechanism sufficiently to evert the patella and obtain adequate visualization of the undersurface to deal with any local pathology. An extra-articular lateral release must be carried out, preserving the synovium but relaxing completely the lateral retinaculum and associated capsule along a line parallel to the iliotibial tract, distally to the ligamentum patella and proximally outside the vastus lateralis.

Medial capsular plication should reconstitute the medial side without overzealous tightening that would unduly increase pressure on the patella. The repair must be fully tested through a full range of motion and, under direct vision, be seen to be sound and without excessive tension on the repaired area. Hinge-brace protection allowing a 0- to 30-degree range is practiced for 4 weeks, during which time an ongoing program of selective quadriceps faradism to the vastus medialis and isometric quadriceps exercises is initiated. After removal from the hinge-brace, a patella-restraining support is utilized for 4 weeks as therapy intensifies with range-of-motion and flexibility exercises.

Patellar Subluxation

The diagnosis of patellar subluxation is too readily applied to patients with patellar symptomatology and varying presentations of patellar mechanics. The extremely wide variation of patellar tracking and anatomic variance of the Q angle seen in athletes often makes it difficult to decide where true "normal" lies. Patellar subluxation should be confirmed only in patients with demonstrably unstable patellae and a positive apprehension sign.

Nonoperative Treatment

Efforts at rehabilitation are directed in two areas for those with patellar subluxation. Attention must be paid to the overall limb alignment and foot mechanics. In patients with undue genu valgum or a tendency to overpronation, orthotic support should be considered with a medial heel wedge in a shoe with a firm heel counter, the forefoot being aided further with a scaphoid pad and first metatarsal mound.

The knee itself then becomes the focus of further support with a simple, elasticized patella-restraining brace for use during sports activity. The exercise program has a twofold thrust: to develop the strength in the muscle groups, and supplement this with faradic stimulation selectively applied to the vastus medialis. However, quadriceps flexibility is the key to reducing pressures on the patella, and a diligent program of stretching exercises must be undertaken if the quadriceps is to function as a better shock absorber. With reduced tensions in this muscle group, there is less tendency for the patella to subluxate laterally, and the clinical situation is greatly enhanced.

Surgical Stabilization for Patellar Subluxation

For patients with patellar instability without true dislocation who are symptomatically limited in their sports endeavors by a knee that gives way, stabilization by soft tissue reconstruction should suffice. There should be little need for meddling with the tibial tubercle insertion of the ligamentum patellae unless there is frank dislocation or true chondromalacic degeneration of the patella.

Arthroscopy of the knee should precede patellar stabilization to ensure that no other internal derangement is overlooked. A combination of a lateral retinacular release and medial capsular plication with vastus medialis advancement will secure the patella without undue tension. The vastus medialis is released as a tongue in its distal portion; after plicating the capsule in a double-breasted fashion, the muscle is sewn down at its fascial margin, overlapping slightly the capsular repair. The repair should be completely sound, with the knee capable of being passed through a full range of motion before closure. The lateral side is left completely open with an extrasynovial lateral retinacular capsular release. Hinge-brace protection is afforded for 4 weeks allowing a 0- to 30-degree excursion within the brace. Weight bearing should be protected with crutches during this time. The ongoing rehabilitation program is then similar to that for the patient managed conservatively. Return to sport is allowed when optimal range and strength have been achieved.

Patellar Dislocation

True dislocation of the patella requires a major stabilization if the athlete is to return to competitive activity. However, few conditions in orthopaedic surgery are associated with greater morbidity than that seen in patients who have been subjected to unnecessary and injudicious stabilization procedures for supposed instability of the patella. If the patellar mechanism is overtightened or if the patella is drawn down to an unphysiologic location, impaired function with inevitable, rapid, articular deterioration will be the result. The objective of a patella stabilization procedure must be to secure the patella without interfering unduly with the patellar mechanics by tightening the capsule and increasing patellar pressures.

Surgical Stabilization

The essential features of stabilization are a release of the lateral structures and a realignment of the distal insertion of the ligamentum patellae.

A good view of the patella can be obtained through a lateral skin incision. This allows for an adequate debridement of any articular irregularity and the drilling of roughened bone areas if necessary. The lateral retinaculum and lateral capsule are released proximally lateral to the vastus lateralis and distally to the ligamentum patellae.

The tendon insertion is now gently elevated on a 3-mm-thick sliver of bone freed proximally but hinged distally; it can be eased medially in the manner of Elmslie and Trillat on a 3×1.5 cm pedicle of bone. The bed should be prepared medially by gentle decortication with an osteotome and the transposed tendon insertion impacted before being secured with a single screw. Only the lateral synovium is closed; the capsule is left open. A soft dressing is all that is necessary; early mobilization is encouraged, with active range of motion and full weight bearing with crutches beginning on the third postoperative day.

CHONDROMALACIA PATELLA

True chondromalacia patella, in which the articular facets of the patella are degenerate with ragged fronded surfaces, can be a difficult condition to handle.

Conservative Treatment

Avoidance of provocative overload is essential. Therefore, for the chondromalacic patient, jumping sports such as basketball and gymnastics are ruled out. Jogging and skiing are also troublesome, and for many athletes much of their training will have to be modified to avoid compounding the insult. Supplemental training with cycling and swimming may be the only way of maintaining form. An enthusiasm for exercise therapy with quadriceps strengthening must be tempered in such individuals, for overloading the quadriceps may well aggravate the condition. It is vital to avoid all resisted exercises, crouches, and deep knee bends. Particularly to be condemned are the traditional quadriceps exercises using weight resistance with the knee extending from a flexed position.

Anti-inflammatory medication can be of help if there is a reactive synovitis, enteric-coated acetylsalicylic acid being favored because of the chronic nature of the condition. Steroid injection may occasionally help if recurrent effusions prove troublesome, but if the athlete is troubled to this degree it may be necessary to consider some form of surgical intervention.

Surgical Treatment

Arthroscopic Debridement and Retinacular Release. A lateral retinacular release should be combined with any intra-articular debridement and may even precede or follow the joint surgery. The role of arthroscopic debridement has yet to be defined, but certainly with fine scissors, basket forceps, and articular shavers it is possible to smooth off much of the superficial roughness. Arguments about the genesis of the chondromalacic state abound, and many authors contend that such superficial treatments do not address predisposing mechanical abnormalities. This is true, but they certainly offer a great advance over open articular debridement, which is mentioned only to be condemned because of its attendant morbidity in terms of the much longer time required for recovery.

Open Debridement and Maquet Patelloplasty. Open debridement alone offers no advantage over a closed procedure. However, when other measures have failed, open debridement combined with an elevation of the tibial tubercle insertion of the ligamentum patellae can favorably alter the clinical course of patients suffering from chronic chondromalacia patella.

The approach recommended utilizes a lateral skin incision and complete retinacular and capsular release as described for the patella stabilization procedure. The patella is everted and a careful debridement is carried out. Full-thickness lesions should be demarcated with vertically cut edges and the malacic cartilage excised. The bed should be drilled through the subchondral plate. Superficial and fibrillated lesions should be shaved down to smooth substance but sound adjacent cartilage should not be interfered with in any way.

The elevation of the tibial tubercle is carried out with sharp osteotomes in a manner similar to that employed for stabilization procedures. The tendon, along with a 3-mm-thick sliver of bone, is elevated on a pedicle 1.5 cm wide by 3 cm long. A wedge-shaped bone block, 1.5×1 cm, is easily taken from the lateral flare of the tibia adjacent to the tibial tubercle insertion. The bone graft is then impacted beneath the elevated tendon, where it remains fully secure and needs no extra fixation. Because there is no tibial osteotomy as such, fasciotomy is not required, but the closure is left completely open on the lateral side after the synovium is closed. The elevation of the tibial tubercle by 1 to 1.5 cm appears to be sufficient to redistribute forces on the patella. The results of this procedure have greatly surpassed those achieved previously by debridement alone. Because the graft is secure beneath the ligamentum, early mobilization can be instituted. It is essential to maintain motion after the patellar debridement; cast immobilization is contraindicated. Weight bearing is protected with crutches for 4 weeks until the graft has consolidated.

SUGGESTED READING

Crenshaw AH, ed. Campbell's operative orthopaedics, Vol. 3. St. Louis: C.V. Mosby, 1987.

Ficat RP, Hungerford DS. Disorders of the patellofemoral joint. Baltimore: Williams & Wilkins, 1977.

Hungerford DS, Barry M. Biomechanics of the patellofemoral joint. Clin Orthop 1979; 144:9–15.

PATELLAR PAIN SYNDROME: INSTABILITY AND LATERAL RETINACULAR RELEASE

S. C. CHEN, F.R.C.S.

Patellar pain in the young patient is usually due to chondromalacia patellae. This condition can arise as a result of:

1. Direct trauma causing a contusion of the articular cartilage.
2. Increased stress on the patellofemoral compartment in strenuous sporting activities.
3. Patellar malalignment, due to an increased Q angle, patella alta or baja, or an abnormal femoral condylar ridge.
4. Patellar instability such as recurrent subluxation or dislocation. Patellar malalignment or instability can cause chondromalacic changes due to abnormal pressure.

The earliest change in chondromalacia is edema of the articular cartilage that progresses to softening, fibrillation, and fissuring. The area affected may extend from a small isolated area to the whole of the articular surface. The areas most affected are the contact areas of the patella, usually the lateral facet, and less often the medial facet. The depth of cartilage affected can vary from the surface layer to the basal layer. Chondromalacia patellae does not necessarily progress to osteoarthritis unless the articular cartilage is eroded down to bone.

There are two types of patellar instability. In one there is an underlying pathologic condition such as an abnormal patella, a high or low patella, a deficient lateral femoral condyle, a lateral attachment of the ligamentum patellae, genu valgum, genu recurvatum, or contracture of the lateral patellar retinaculum and capsule. The other is a normal knee that has suffered an acute dislocation of the patella. The medial patellar retinaculum and capsule heal with undue laxity, so that the patella subsequently can dislocate or subluxate easily.

It is very common for patellar instability and chondromalacia to coexist. Insall maintains that patellar malalignment is primarily responsible for patellar pain and that the chondromalacic changes are a consequence of this.

CLINICAL FEATURES

A careful history taking will reveal any direct blows on the patella in sporting activities, such as kicks or falls on the knee. A feeling of giving way may be due to pain that results in sudden quadriceps inhibition or patellar instability. There may be a history of momentary locking due to maltracking of the patella. The knee may become swollen owing to associated synovial congestion and effusion. There may be a history of acute dislocation, recurrent dislocation, or subluxation of the patella.

Clinical examination reveals wasting of the vastus medialis. Tightness of the lateral and medial retinaculum is assessed by side-to-side movement of the patella. The patella may be tilted slightly laterally and during knee movement this lateral maltracking may be more obvious, especially during the last stages of extension. There may be patellofemoral tenderness during passive knee movement. It may also be present during quadriceps contraction while the patella is pressed against the lower femoral condyle. The undersurface can be palpated by pushing the patella to one side and then to the other; this may elicit tenderness. The apprehension test may be positive, indicating patellar instability.

The Q angle is measured, and if it is more than 20 degrees (normal = 14 degrees), there is lateral placement of the patella.

The height of the patella and the length of the ligamentum patellae are measured. Normally they should be the same. In patella alta, the ligament is longer than the height of the patella; in patella baja, the reverse is the case.

RADIOGRAPHY

Plain anteroposterior, lateral, and skyline views of the patella are taken. The anteroposterior view is taken with the knee extended. The lateral views are taken with the knee extended and flexed to 90 degrees. Measurements of the height of the patella and the ligamentum patellae are made in the knee-extended view. In the 90-degree flexed view, a line drawn across the front of the femoral shaft should skim over the top of the patella. If the patella is above this line, patella alta exists. Skyline views of the patella are taken at 30, 45, and 90 degrees of flexion. These will show lateral maltracking during flexion, if present (Fig. 1).

TREATMENT

Conservative treatment consists of (1) rest from sporting activities for at least 6 weeks and (2) physiotherapy, which should include shortwave diathermy or laser therapy and static quadriceps exercises with the knee in extension, so that the vastus medialis is strengthened and the patella is not subjected to increased pressure. It is important to note that the vastus medialis comes into play only in the last few degrees of knee extension.

Anti-inflammatory drugs, particularly aspirin-based agents, are given during this period. Compression bandages on the knee are discouraged because they increase pressure in the patellofemoral

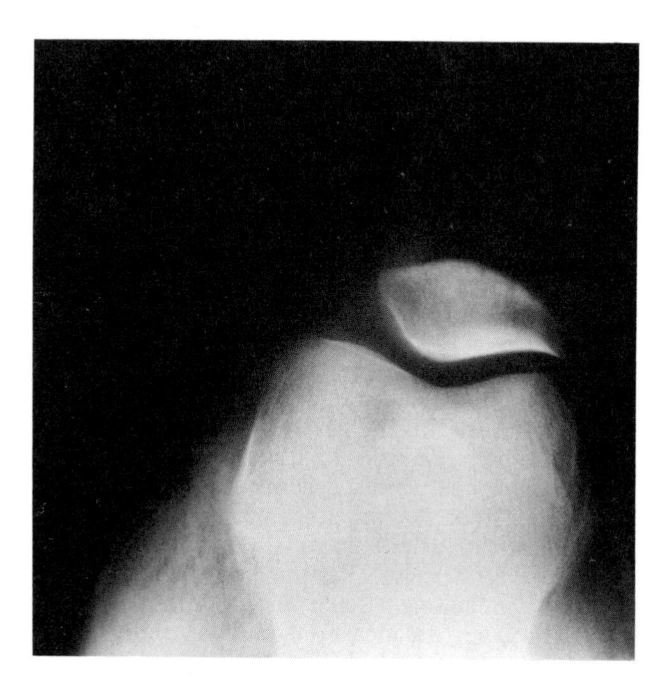

Figure 1 Skyline view of the patella with the knee flexed to 45 degrees to show a slight lateral malalignment.

compartment. Intra-articular steroid injections are inadvisable since they can lead to increased degradation of articular cartilage.

In about 75 percent of patients with chondromalacia patellae, symptoms resolve after conservative treatment. If conservative measures fail and symptoms persist after 3 months, surgical treatment is undertaken.

RATIONALE OF SURGICAL TREATMENT—LATERAL RELEASE OF PATELLA

The object of surgical treatment is to decrease the pressure on the patellar surface and to correct any malalignment. Lateral release of the patella achieves both objectives, by releasing the tethering effect of the patellar retinaculum and lateral capsule. It also interrupts the nerve supply to the patella from the lateral side, as neuromatous degeneration can cause symptoms. It is a simple procedure with a low morbidity rate, first described as an open procedure by Evans.

Procedure

A preliminary arthroscopic examination is carried out to confirm the diagnosis and to exclude any other pathologic condition. The arthroscope is introduced via an anterolateral portal. The same stab incision in the skin is employed in carrying out the lateral retinacular release with a Smillie knife. This knife comes in pairs, mirror images of each other, and both are necessary (Fig.2).

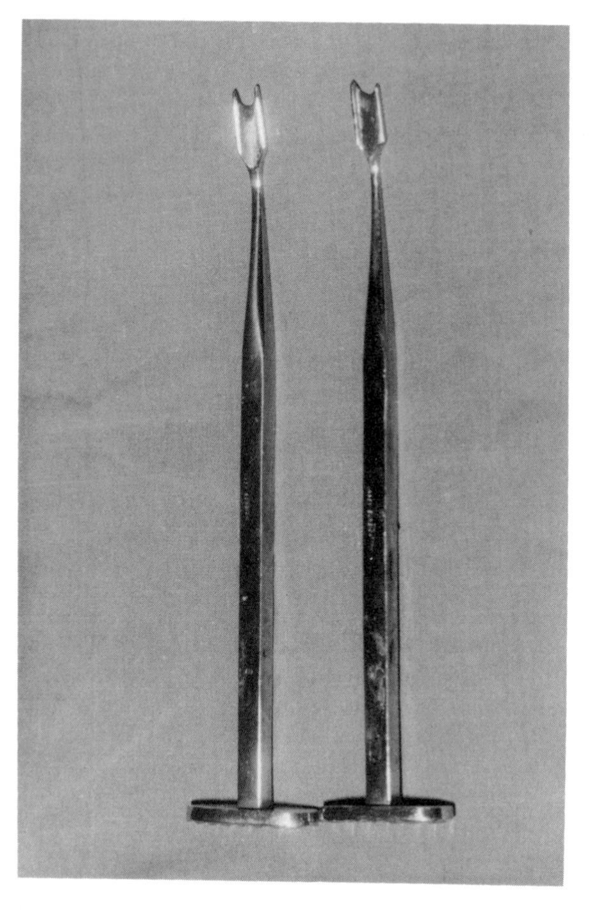

Figure 2 A pair of Smillie knives to show the curve of the blade and the two prongs of differing lengths.

The knee is kept fully extended during the closed lateral release to avoid damage to the intra-articular structures. The tibial tubercle, lateral border of the patella, and lateral joint line are identified by palpation. With the knee still distended with the Ringer's fluid after the arthroscopic examination (which helps in tensing the lateral retinaculum and lifting it from the lateral femoral condyle), the Smillie knife, with its tip curved outward, pointing upward, and the longer prong nearer the skin, is introduced through the stab incision (Fig. 3). The longer of the two prongs of the knife is inserted deep to the puncture wound in the retinaculum that was made during arthroscopy. The correct Smillie knife is used, to avoid cutting the retinaculum too medially and damaging the quadriceps muscle. A firm resistance is felt if the Smillie knife is astride the retinaculum. The knife tip is palpated through the skin and is guided upward and outward when pushed. By deviating laterally, the vastus lateralis muscle and lateral genicular vessels are avoided. The retinaculum is divided for a distance equal to twice the height of the patella. Since the knee is fully extended during the procedure, the joint is closed anteriorly and therefore cannot be damaged (Fig. 4).

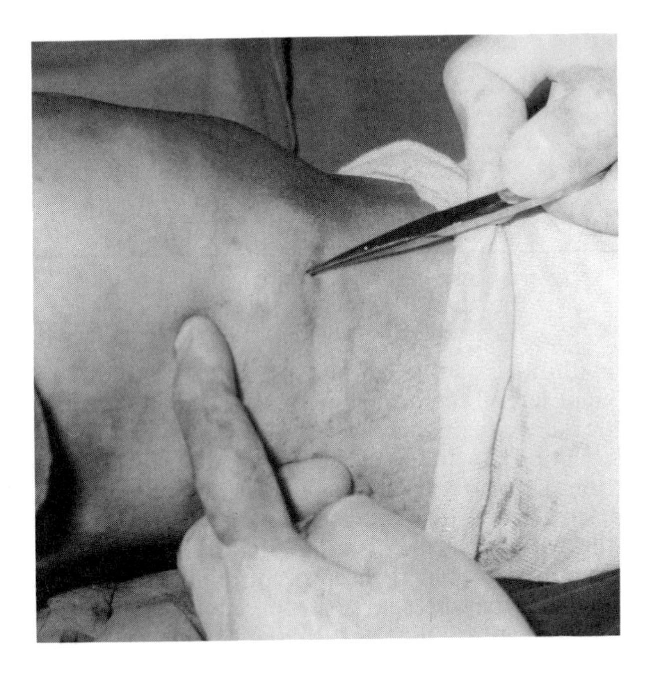

Figure 3 The Smillie knife is astride the lateral retinaculum. Note the finger palpating the knife through the skin, ascertaining its position as it is pushed along.

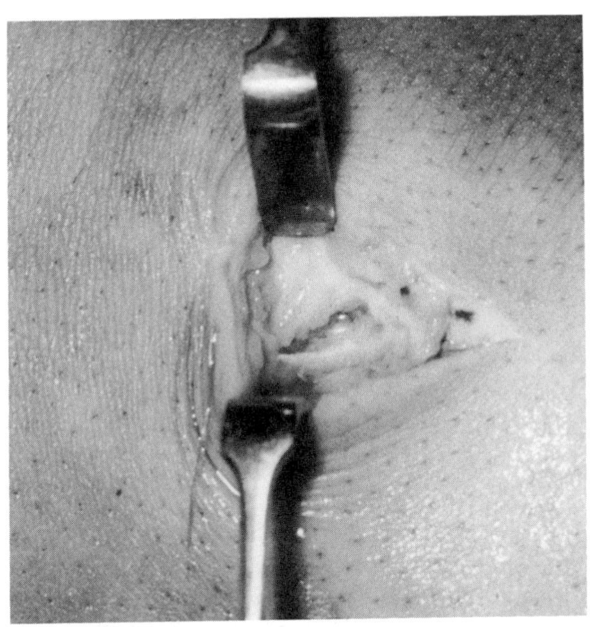

Figure 4 The lateral retinaculum has been exposed after a closed lateral release to show the incision made by the Smillie knife.

The knife is removed. The other Smillie knife is then introduced with its tip curved outward, pointing downward, the longer prong nearer the skin. With the cutting edge astride the retinaculum, it is pushed down lateral to the ligamentum patellae. The patella is displaced medially to check that it is adequately released. The knee is also flexed and extended to ensure that the patella is tracking correctly. When the lateral retinaculum is divided adequately, a sausage-shaped bulge is seen along the lateral side of the patella, caused by the fluid distending the subcutaneous tissues and skin (Fig. 5). This usually disappears in about 3 months. The synovial membrane is not incised, and therefore the lateral femoral condyle cannot be damaged by the Smillie knife (Fig. 6). One absorbable stitch is used for the skin wound (Fig. 7).

Patients are allowed out of bed the day after surgery, and full weight bearing is permitted. During the first week they walk with the operated knee extended to prevent any effusion developing. They are discharged 2 days after surgery with instructions to carry out static quadriceps exercises and gentle mobilizing exercises for up to 30 degrees of flexion during the first week, and intensive quadriceps strengthening and knee mobilizing exercises are then instituted. By the end of the second week patients can return to work.

RESULTS

Ninety-three percent of patients with chondromalacia patellae responded well to a lateral release (Table 1). In patellar instability the incidence of excellent or good results was 81.5 percent in recurrent dislocations, 90 percent in recurrent subluxations, and 87 percent in acute dislocations (Table 2). There have been no complications in either series.

A simple closed lateral release procedure is carried out even if there is an underlying cause for the

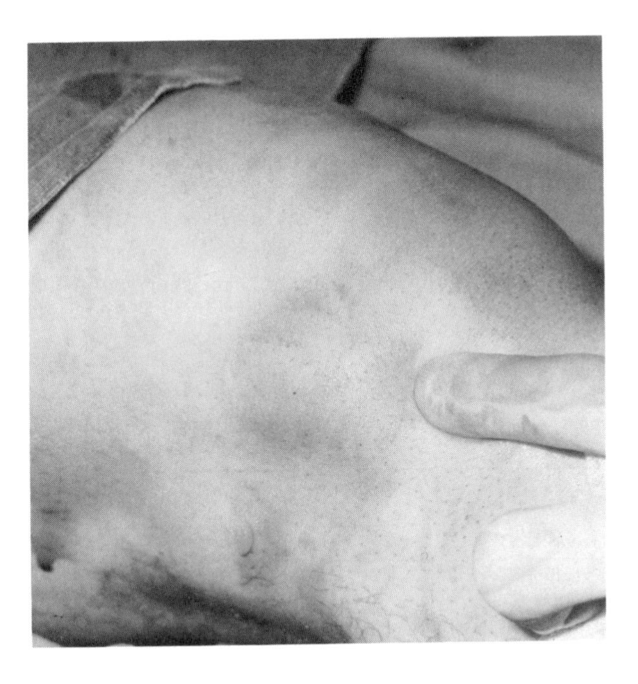

Figure 5 Sausage-shaped bulge on the lateral side of the patella following an adequate retinacular release.

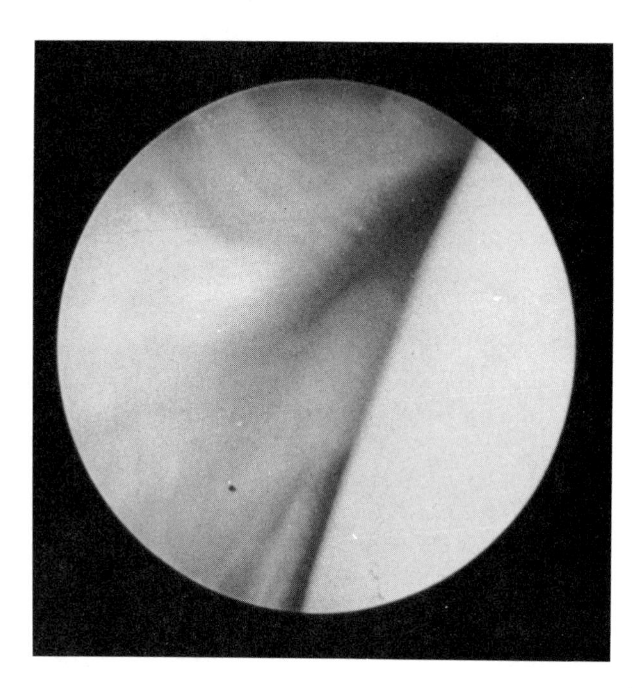

Figure 6 Arthroscopic view of the Smillie knife superficial to the synovial membrane.

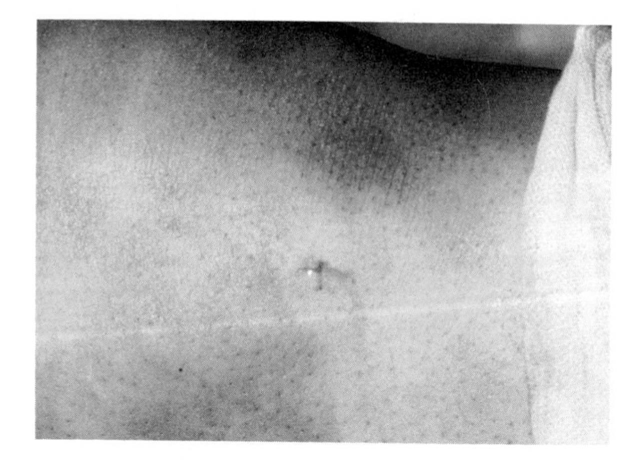

Figure 7 One absorbable stitch for the skin wound.

TABLE 1 Lateral Retinacular Release in Chondromalacia Patellae*

	No. of Patients	*Relief from Symptoms*	*Failures*
Male	24	23	1
Female	20	18	2
Total	44	41	3

*Average age, 23 years (range 9 to 57 years)

condition, such as an increased Q angle or a deficient lateral femoral condyle, since a large proportion of patients may have no further symptoms. A small proportion may require an additional operation such as a medial tibial tubercle transfer through a small transverse skin incision, or a patellectomy if the patellar surface is grossly affected with severe chondromalacia. If the procedure is staged, many patients may be spared unnecessary surgery, prolonged immobilization, and possible complications. Furthermore, an unsightly scar is avoided.

Other forms of surgical treatment include proximal realignment, such as advancement of the vastus medialis if the Q angle is less than 14 degrees. The classic Hauser operation, which consists of lateral retinacular release, medial capsular reefing, and medial transfer of the tibial tubercle, is a major procedure involving at least 4 to 6 weeks in a plaster cast; the complete form may not be necessary. Furthermore the procedure can increase the pressure on the patellofemoral compartment and cause an unsightly large scar.

Chondroplasty, or shaving of the affected articular cartilage, is useful for severe forms of chondromalacia. It can be performed arthroscopically with a chondrotome. Multiple drilling of the shaved areas helps the regeneration of fibrocartilage. This can be combined with lateral release of the patella.

Elevation of the tibial tubercle can decrease pressure on the patellofemoral compartment, but can lead to greater instability if congenital abnormalities, such as patella alta or baja or a deficient femoral condyle, are present. It is a major procedure that may produce complications such as wound breakdown and a prominent anterior bone swelling below the knee.

TABLE 2 Lateral Retinacular Release in Patellar Instability*

	Recurrent Dislocation	*(n=16)*	*Recurrent Subluxation*	*(n=10)*	*Acute Dislocation*	*(n=15)*
Grade	*Knees*	*Percent*	*Knees*	*Percent*	*Knees*	*Percent*
Excellent or good	13	81.5	9	90	13	87
Fair or poor	2	12.5	1	10	2	13
Worse	1	6	0	0	0	0

*Average age, 20 years (range 13 to 35 years)

Primary patellectomy for severe chondromalacia may prove necessary, but should be undertaken only when other measures have failed. In this context, lateral retinacular release serves a useful role as a preliminary stage in the treatment. Patellectomy can lead to slight weakness due to loss of the lever action provided by the patella. This loss of quadriceps power, however slight, may not be acceptable in individuals engaging in sporting activities.

SUGGESTED READING

Bentley G. Chondromalacia patellae. J Bone Joint Surg 1970; 52A:221–232.

Chen SC. Closed lateral retinacular release of the patella. J Orthop Surg Tech 1986; 2:49–53.

Chen SC, Helal B, King J, Roper B. Lateral retinacular release in chondromalacia patellae. Proceedings of S.I.C.O.T., Copenhagen, 1976.

Chen SC, Ramanathan EB. The treatment of patellar instability by lateral release. J Bone Joint Surg 1984; 66B:344–348.

Evans D. Lateral patella release. Proceedings of British Orthopaedic Study Group (1969–1987), 20th anniversary edition, 1970.

Fulkerson JP, Tennant R, Jaivan JS, Grunnet M. Histologic evidence of retinacular nerve injury associated with patellofemoral malalignment. Clin Orthop 1985; 197:196–205.

Goodfellow J, Hungerford DS, Woods C. Patellofemoral joint mechanics and pathology. 2. Chondromalacia patella. J Bone Joint Surg 1976; 58B:291–299.

Insall J. Patellar malalignment syndrome. Orthop Clin North Am 1979; 10:117–127.

Insall J, Falvo KA, Wise DW. Chondromalacia patellae. A prospective study. J Bone Joint Surg 1976; 58A:1–8.

Insall J, Salvati E. Patella position in the normal knee joint. Radiology 1971; 101:101–104.

Maquet PGJ. Biomechanics of the knee. New York: Springer-Verlag, 1976: 134.

Zimbler S, Smith J, Scheller A, Banks H.H. Recurrent subluxation and dislocation of the patella in association with athlete injuries. Orthop Clin North Am 1980; 11:755–770.

PATELLOFEMORAL DYSFUNCTION

FRANK NOFTHALL, M.D., F.R.C.S.(C)

Patellofemoral derangements are among the most common and most frustrating problems seen by orthopaedic surgeons. Activities of daily living (e.g., going up and down stairs) place great demands on the patellar mechanism, let alone athletic activities. Although symptoms are often severe, overt pathology often is not evident.

Essential to an understanding of the patellofemoral arthralgias are the basic biomechanics of the patellofemoral joint, including patellar pressures and patellar excursion.

The patella increases the efficiency of the extensor mechanism by as much as 50 percent. The compressive force or joint reactive force of the patellofemoral joint is the resultant vector of the pull of the quadriceps mechanism and the resistance of the patellar tendon. The compressive force across the joint may be three to four times the body weight when a person goes up and down stairs, and is increased as flexion of the knee increases.

Another function of the patella is to translate the divergent forces of the quadriceps mechanism and transmit these to the patella tendon. Patellar excursion is determined by the resultant of these force vectors. Any anatomic, physiologic, or pathologic factor that alters this patellar function will affect the excursion of the patella and may lead to pain syndromes. Patellar excursion is affected by many factors. One of the most important is the so-called Q angle, which is formed by the line of pull of the quadriceps muscle and the line of the patellar tendon. This is normally a valgus angulation. The natural tendency is for the patella to displace laterally. This is resisted by the prominent lateral femoral condyle and trochlear groove, the fibers of the vastus medialis distally, and the medial retinaculum. Any tightening laterally, laxity medially, or deficiency of the bone structures laterally increases the tendency of the patella to displace laterally.

Any factor that increases the Q angle also increases the tendency for the patella to displace laterally. Genu valgum, excessive external tibial torsion, and pes planus effectively increase the Q angle.

Clinical Features

Patients with patellofemoral disorders generally have complaints when the patella is in a position of maximal compressive forces (again, during stair climbing and descending). They also complain of sensations of giving way, a feeling of instability or insecurity, and "locking" or catching sensations.

On examination there often is quadriceps atrophy. Effusions are not common but occasionally are seen. Stability test results are all normal in the patient with isolated patellar pain. Retro-or parapatellar pain sites can be elicited in most cases. Crepitus is often palpable but this may also be found in patients without any pain syndromes. The patellar excursion should be visualized throughout the range of extension to full flexion and back to extension, to observe any tendency toward lateral displacement or variation from the normal sinusoidal motion. Overall limb alignment, the Q angle, and finally the heel and foot position should be documented.

Radiologic Investigation

The radiologic investigation of patients with patellofemoral pain consists of plain film radiography including anteroposterior, lateral, intercondylar, and most important tangential (axial) views of the patella. Various techniques have been described for taking the axial view, and each has its own advantages and disadvantages. I believe that the techniques with the knee in 20 to 60 degrees of flexion probably are the most useful. The most important factors are consistency and reproducibility.

In recent years, computed tomographic (CT) scanning has been used increasingly to assess the patellofemoral joint. New and useful information has been provided, but for the most part this has been of investigational use only to this point. This modality will undoubtedly increase in usefulness in the future, especially in refractory cases.

Radionuclide scanning is also being used but at present is still mostly in the investigational stages.

Source of Pain and Management

Over the years, various theories have been put forward regarding the source of pain in patients with patellofemoral arthralgias; many of these are difficult to prove or disprove. Stimulation of nerve endings in subchondral bone, neuromatous degeneration in retinacular nerves, stretching and straining of the retinaculum and capsule, and impingement of the fat pad and/or synovium are among a few of the suggested sources of patellofemoral pain. The source of the pain in fact is actually not too important in this entity; it seems that regardless of the source, most cases of patellofemoral pain respond to conservative management, and only a few require surgical intervention.

The first step in management consists of modification of the provocative activity. The duration or intensity of the activity may have to be diminished. Sometimes a change of activity is necessary. The important point is that fitness must be maintained during the treatment process.

Physiotherapy is the mainstay of treatment of patellofemoral disorders, regardless of their cause. Strengthening exercises have to be explained appropriately, because certain exercises may actually aggravate the pain. Isometric quadriceps setting and straight leg raising, followed by progressive resisted exercises over the final 10 degrees of knee extension, are emphasized. Resisted exercises over the full range of motion are discouraged because of the excessive compressive forces generated and the tendency to intensify symptoms. Stretching of the quadriceps and hamstring groups is as important as strengthening. Shortwave diathermy and ultrasound techniques may be beneficial, especially in times of acute inflammation, but should not take the place of strengthening and stretching exercises. Faradic stimulation may also be helpful in selected patients. Orthotics aimed at correction of foot problems such as pes planus and heel valgus may be helpful when these conditions are contributing to abnormal patellar mechanics.

Anti-inflammatory medications have a limited role in the treatment of patellofemoral pain. They may provide some relief for patients experiencing acute exacerbations of pain or in whom there is evidence of inflammation or recent injury. They should be used over short periods in relatively high doses for maximal effect.

Two important points about patellofemoral pain need stressing. First, despite the presence at times of very significant symptoms, the majority of patients cause themselves no special harm or damage if they "play through" their pain. Second, before conservative management is to be considered a failure, it is necessary to be sure that patients have complied with the recommended therapy.

Surgical Treatment

Conservative management should be continued for at least 6 months. The patient should be disabled to the point of nonparticipation in work or sport.

Arthroscopy should be performed in all patients with patellofemoral pain who have reached the point of surgical intervention. The entire knee joint can be assessed and most of the pathology identified and initially dealt with.

The initial success of and enthusiasm for lateral retinacular release has not been sustained. The use of this relatively minor procedure should be reserved for patients having tight or contracted lateral structures, excessive lateral pressure, or radiographic evidence of lateral displacement or tilting of the patella. Avoidance of hematoma is mandatory, and patients should begin active rehabilitation early in the postoperative period. Again, as in conservative management, excessive loading of the patellofemoral joint must be avoided.

Fat pad hypertrophy and fibrosis may be one of the causes of patellofemoral pain identified at arthroscopy. The fat pad becomes impinged between the patella and the femur. Hoffa's syndrome is a definite entity, and arthroscopic excision is a very good form of initial surgical management. The fat pad is a substantial structure, and frequently a small medial arthrotomy is required to debride the structure adequately. Again, hemostasis is mandatory because of the very vascular nature of the fat pad.

Synovial hypertrophy and impingement may occur in the suprapatellar region. Arthroscopic excision in this region tends to be more satisfactory than with fat pad excision owing to greater accessibility and (usually) the smaller volume of tissue involved.

The medial plica syndrome can also be addressed arthroscopically. It is important not only to disrupt the continuity of the plica but to excise a segment, since it has been documented that the plica may heal and become symptomatic once again.

CHONDROMALACIA PATELLAE

One of the reasons for confusion with patellofemoral pain syndromes is that many similarly symptomatic disorders have been labeled as chondromalacia patellae. This led to much unnecessary surgery for minor conditions that did not warrant such aggressive therapy. True chondromalacia is a relatively rare entity and, comparing the number of patients with patellofemoral pain with those who actually undergo changes in the articular surface, the latter are in the minority.

The pathology of articular cartilage changes is well described. There are four stages: in stage I there is swelling and softening of the cartilage, in stage II fissuring, in stage III surface breakdown known as fasiculation, and in stage IV osteoarthritis.

As with any other condition affecting the patellofemoral joint, the first step in treating patients with chondromalacic changes is conservative. Physiotherapy aimed at quadriceps strengthening must be tempered with caution, for overloading the quadriceps may well aggravate the condition. It is important, however, to keep the quadriceps in good condition. All resisted exercises, deep knee bends, and crouches are to be avoided, as is any exercise involving knee flexion.

Obviously, any jumping, running, or squatting during sports activities may aggravate the condition; this is unavoidable. Maintenance of physical fitness may have to be supplemented by swimming or by cycling with the seat elevated. An athlete's training may have to be modified to avoid the intensification of symptoms. Anti-inflammatory agents may be helpful in acute exacerbations or if synovitis is present. Steroid injection is controversial and should probably be avoided in younger patients.

After an adequate trial of conservative management (at least 6 months), any patient who still has incapacitating symptoms may be considered for operative intervention. The first step is arthroscopic examination of the joint. This procedure allows the condition to be diagnosed and rules out other intra-articular pathology. Debridement of the joint can be accomplished, albeit sometimes with difficulty, using manual or mechanical devices. However, this does not address the underlying disorder causing the chondromalacia patellae. At the same time, if there is any evidence of excessive tightening of the lateral structures, a lateral retinacular release can be performed; if there is no such evidence, this will probably be unsuccessful.

The definitive procedure for the treatment of chondromalacia patellae unresponsive to less aggressive measures is elevation of the tibial tubercle. The true Maquet procedure is rarely performed today, because the original operation carried an unacceptably high degree of major complications, mainly skin breakdown and infections. This was attributed to the 2 cm of elevation initially described along with poor skin coverage. A number of modifications of the Maquet procedure have been reported. Most recommend 1 to 1.5 cm of elevation and no distal transfer of the tubercle. If any maltracking laterally or dislocation is present, this elevation can be combined with a medial transfer. Through elevation of the tibial tubercle, the patella gains mechanical advantage and becomes more efficient. This decreases patellofemoral pressure and reduces the joint reactive forces. A 1-cm elevation can produce approximately a 33 percent increase in efficiency, which is thought by most authors to be sufficient. The incidence of wound breakdown is markedly diminished but not completely eliminated.

Tibial tubercle elevation is usually combined with lateral retinacular release and frequently with open debridement. Degenerated cartilage should be excised, and any subchondral bone exposed should be drilled. If possible, early motion should be instituted. Undoubtedly, continuous passive motion will be used more frequently in the future in cases involving subchondral drilling. The patella should not be actively loaded during the postoperative period for at least 4 weeks. Depending on the technique, internal fixation can be avoided and early motion instituted if the bone graft is secure.

PATELLAR INSTABILITY

Patellar Subluxation

In the past, patellar maltracking and subluxation was too readily ascribed to patients with patellar symptomatology. It is undoubtedly the cause of patellar problems in many cases, but it has been overdiagnosed. This leads to the indiscriminate use of lateral retinacular release, and predictably poor results. Patellar maltracking is often difficult to diagnose except in the most obvious cases. Subluxation is often diagnosed on the basis of static x-ray films when it is a dynamic process. The biomechanics leading to maltracking and lateral subluxation have been described earlier.

Conservative treatment consists of anatomic and dynamic considerations. Foot alignment must be addressed, as pronated feet may cause an increased Q angle and lead to lateral subluxation of the patella. An orthotic to place the heel and foot in a more neutral or slight supinated position may be all that is necessary.

Patella-stabilizing braces have been used with reasonable success. The major problem with braces as well as orthotics is patient compliance. Orthotics generally are custom made, while patella-stabilizing braces are usually off the shelf and mass produced. There are a number on the market, most having a patellar groove that helps stabilize the patella from displacement while not putting any pressure directly on the patella. These tend to be useful only in very severe cases.

Physiotherapy concentrates on strengthening the vastus medialis portion of the quadriceps while increasing the flexibility of the quadriceps group; the latter is probably the more important. By a diligent stretching program, pressure on the patella is reduced and the muscle acts as a better shock absorber. With reduced tensions in this muscle group, there is less tendency for the patella to subluxate laterally.

Operative treatment is reserved for patients who have exhausted a comprehensive conservative program. Arthroscopy is performed to rule out other unsuspected intra-articular pathology. If this is discovered, it is dealt with first and the patient is observed to see if any improvement occurs. Patients should be markedly impaired in their activities to warrant surgical intervention.

Soft tissue procedures should suffice in most cases of true lateral subluxation. Since arthroscopy has been performed, a formal arthrotomy is unnecessary, and this decreases postoperative morbidity. A lateral retinacular release is performed either through a small incision in a semiopen fashion or through a formal incision. This may or may not be combined with a medial capsular plication and vastus medialis advancement. In most cases there is no need to transpose the tibial tubercle medially.

PATELLAR DISLOCATIONS

Acute Patellar Dislocation

When this occurs in the athlete it is a painful, worrisome, and potentially career-ending injury. As with any other dislocation, early reduction is of the utmost importance. Usually, simple extension of the extremity affects reduction and the injured person feels immediate relief. Most often the joint is reduced before the individual is examined. The history can be confused with that of an acute anterior cruciate injury. The physical examination usually gives the experienced examiner enough information to differentiate between the two conditions. Both, however, may show a painful hemarthrosis, but patients with an acute patellar dislocation have exquisite tenderness along the medial aspect of the patella, which intensifies on flexion of the knee. The anterior cruciate ligament (ACL) stability tests should be normal.

X-ray films should be carefully examined to rule out osteochondral fractures; the lateral and skyline views are the most useful. If there is any doubt, arthroscopy should be performed. Small fragments should be removed, but an attempt at repair should be made for large osteochondral fragments with large areas of articular cartilage; this is often difficult.

Simple cast immobilization in a stovepipe cast with the knee in full extension and molding to displace the patella medially is prescribed for from 4 to 6 weeks. During this time, quadriceps setting exercises are performed in conjunction with faradic stimulation if available. After cast removal, a patella-stabilizing brace can be used. Mobilization of the knee is begun. Return to sports activities is allowed only when full range of motion and full quadriceps rehabilitation, particularly flexibility, have been restored.

Recurrent Patellar Dislocation

With recurrent dislocations, soft tissue procedures are generally insufficient. However, before skeletal maturity there is no choice, as any operation that damages the proximal tibial growth plate could prove disastrous. Conservative treatment would consist of physiotherapy concentrating on medial quadriceps and a patella stabilizing brace. If conservative treatment fails, soft tissue plication medially with a lateral retinacular release and medial displacement of the tibial tubercle should be considered. Tibial tubercle displacement should only be done in the skeletally mature individual. This can be a very troublesome procedure, since internal fixation is required to hold the tubercle medially displaced, and if the soft tissue medial reconstruction is too tight it can lead to patellar problems postoperatively.

The medial displacement of the tibial tubercle can be combined with an elevation of the tubercle if chondromalacia patellae is present. This can be difficult to manage postoperatively: with chondromalacia it is important to institute motion as soon as possible, but because of the sometimes tenuous fixation of the tubercle it is often necessary to hold patients back from early motion until bone healing is secure.

SUGGESTED READING

Carson WC, et al. Patellofemoral disorder: parts I and II. Clin Orthop; 185:165–186.

Kettelkamp DB. Management of patellar malalignment. J Bone Joint Surg; 63-A:1344–1348.

Insall J. Patellar pain. J Bone Joint Surg 65-A:147–152.

Patello femoral pain. Orthop Clin North Am. April 1986.

PATELLAR DISLOCATION, SUBLUXATION, AND THE ELMSLIE-TRILLAT PROCEDURE

DAVID E. BROWN, M.D.

Patellar subluxations and dislocations occur frequently in athletes. The wide range of normal alignment patterns, the subtle misalignments that lead to symptoms, and the many causes of malalignment make the evaluation and management of these injuries difficult. Therefore, the clinician must first understand the etiology before an individualized treatment plan can be formulated.

Patellar malalignment may be caused by abnormalities occurring anywhere in the lower extremity. Excessive femoral anteversion, deficient or weak vastus medialis obliquus (VMO), tight vastus lateralis, abnormal insertion of the vastus lateralis, excessive genu valgum, shallow femoral trochlea, external tibial torsion with lateral insertion of the ligamentum patellae, and pes planus with hindfoot valgus are the most frequent factors leading to malalignment. Generalized joint laxity or trauma may exacerbate any of these factors.

EVALUATION

Complete patellar dislocations are easy to diagnose when the patient recalls the frightening sensation of displacement of the patella. It is more difficult to determine whether the patient is actually experiencing subluxations of the patella. However, episodes of buckling, momentary giving way, and "catching" are often symptoms of patellar instability. These may be associated with pain, swelling, and grinding.

The physical examination should include evaluation of rotational deformities of the hip and tibia and standing alignment of the hindfoot. Excessive femoral anteversion, external tibial torsion, and hindfoot valgus result in elevation of the quadriceps (Q) angle. Flexibility of the thigh musculature, particularly the vastus lateralis and iliotibial band, should be determined.

Knee examination should isolate the deficient VMO or tight lateral retinaculum, determine abnormal patellar mobility or tilting, and make a gross assessment of patellar tracking. The patellar apprehension test, if positive, is extremely helpful in isolating the cause of the patellar instability. I believe it essential to measure the quadriceps angle, in full knee extension. Normal values are generally considered to be 10 degrees for males and 15 degrees for females. When the Q angle is elevated, the patella tends to displace more laterally with active quadriceps contraction.

Other causes of knee pain and instability must be diligently sought, as they may coexist with patellar instability.

Radiographic evaluation should include one of the axial patellar views described by Merchant and Laurin and their colleagues. Nonstandardized axial views, especially if obtained in more than 30 degrees of knee flexion, rarely demonstrate patellar malalignment. The lateral view is evaluated for patella alta by the method of Insall and Salvati. Fulkerson described a computed tomographic (CT) method that allows evaluation of patellar position from full extension to 30 degrees of knee flexion, a range that may be more sensitive than that in the axial radiographs, since it correlates with the range of patellar instability. The CT scan is also the method of choice for quantifying femoral anteversion.

NONSURGICAL TREATMENT

Nonsurgical treatment should be given for 3 to 6 months unless evidence of an intra-articular loose body is seen. The vast majority of subluxators respond to an appropriate regimen aimed at alleviating or compensating for the cause of malalignment.

Rehabilitation of the deficient vastus medialis is nearly always required. Isometric quadriceps setting, straight leg-raising exercises, and progressive resistive exercises near terminal extension are emphasized. Bicycling (with the seat elevated) and swimming with a kick board are useful in developing quadriceps strength without irritating the patellofemoral articular surface. Stretching of the quadriceps and hamstring muscles and mobilization of the patella to relieve a tight lateral retinaculum may reduce contact pressures in the patellofemoral joint. All these modalities are initially supervised by a physical therapist, but the patient must be willing to continue a maintenance program two to three times a week once the symptoms are alleviated.

A patella-stabilizing brace helps to control mild lateral tracking or hypermobility. The brace additionally functions to keep the knee warmer during activity, often reducing the sensation of stiffness that most patients experience. When hindfoot valgus is present, a medial heel wedge and a shoe with a firm heel counter reduce overpronation and the resultant internal torsion of the knee. If relief of symptoms is obtained, a custom orthotic can be ordered.

SURGICAL TREATMENT

Surgical treatment should always include arthroscopy to complete the evaluation of patellar tracking, perform superficial chondroplasty, and evaluate the remainder of the knee for any pathologic condition. If possible, arthroscopy is performed under local anesthesia, without a tourniquet, to evaluate patellofemoral alignment under dynamic conditions and without the potential errors induced by tourniquet compression of the quadriceps muscles. An inferolateral portal immediately adjacent to the patella tendon and the superolateral portal are used to demonstrate lateral patellar subluxation or tilt.

Once this evaluation is complete, surgical realignment can be tailored to the needs of the patient. Surgical options include proximal soft tissue reconstruction (medial capsule imbrication and/or lateral retinaculum release), distal realignment (tibial tubercle or patella tendon transfer), and anterior displacement of the tibial tubercle. On rare occasions, femoral and tibial derotation osteotomies are required to correct severe rotational deformities.

TABLE 1 Treatment Regimen for Chronic Patellar Instability

Diagnosis	*Arthroscopic Findings, Radiographic Findings, Q Angle*	*Treatment Protocol*
Subluxation	Patella tilt alone	Lateral release
Subluxation or	Subluxation + tilt Q angle < 15 degrees or Open physes	Proximal realignment Medial capsule reefing Lateral release
Dislocation	Q angle ≧ 15 degrees	Elmslie-Trillat
	Grade II–III chondromalacia	Elmslie-Trillat + Further anteriorization with local bone graft

Acute Patellar Dislocation

After the patella is reduced, the joint is aspirated, examination is carried out, and a complete set of radiographs are obtained. Any suspicion of an intra-articular loose body warrants arthroscopic examination. If excessive lateral subluxation is present, lateral release is performed. When the vastus medialis is avulsed from the superiomedial pole of the patella, an open repair is indicated. Postoperatively or after the injury, the knee is immobilized in extension, and weight bearing is allowed as tolerated. Within the first week, the patient is expected to perform active and passive motion in the first 30 to 40 degrees of flexion while wearing a patella-stabilizing brace.

This limited range-of-motion and quadriceps rehabilitation is prescribed to be carried out four times a day; extension immobilization is continued throughout the rest of the day for 4 weeks. The stabilizing brace is then worn for another 4 weeks while range-of-motion and more aggressive quadricep exercises are instituted.

Acute Patellar Subluxation

Short-term immobilization is occasionally necessary, but motion, rehabilitation, and resumption of activity are instituted as soon as possible. A careful search is performed for correctable causes of malalignment. High-intensity activities are delayed until complete quadriceps function returns and the patellar apprehension sign is negative.

Chronic Patellar Instability

Surgical reconstruction is indicated if there is failure to improve after 3 to 6 months of conservative therapy. Before surgical intervention, the surgeon must be able to confirm the clinical impression of subluxation or dislocation by radiography, arthrometry, or arthroscopy, much the same as for tibiofemoral or lateral ankle ligamentous reconstructions. Table 1 describes a treatment regimen based on the clinical diagnosis, objective findings, and radiographic findings.

Elmslie-Trillat Procedure

Diagnostic and therapeutic arthroscopy are completed, if not previously performed. A long, lateral parapatellar incision is made and a medially based skin flap is developed, exposing the medial retinaculum, tibial tubercle, and quadriceps tendon. Lateral release is accomplished from the insertion of the vastus lateralis to the tibial tubercle. The vastus medialis insertion is released and imbricated in a vest over pants fashion using multiple, absorbable mattress sutures. Distal advancement of the VMO may be required if the original insertion was too proximal.

An incision is then made on both sides of the tibial tubercle and the periosteum is elevated. The lateral side must be developed well, exposing at least 1 cm of the steep lateral tibial metaphysis. The interval between the patella tendon and fat pad is developed and a wide, curved osteotome inserted at a 45-degree angle to the horizontal, inclining to the medial side. The initial depth is 6 to 8 mm, gradually diminishing as the osteotome is driven distally 5 to 10 cm, leaving only a distal periosteal hinge. The tubercle is transferred medially 6 to 10 mm until the intraoperative Q angle is 10 degrees. This will result in 4 to 5 mm of anterior displacement. If additional anteriorization is desired, a local bone graft can be obtained from the lateral side of the tibial tubercle. A 10-cm osteotomy is necessary to improve the cosmetic appearance of the anteriorized tubercle. The tubercle is then held in its transferred position with a 3.2-mm drill bit, and the patellofemoral alignment is observed throughout the range of motion.

Frequently adjustments are made to the imbrication of the VMO, ensuring that the patella is centralized and does not tilt. Once the alignment is deemed satisfactory, the drill bit is replaced with a 40-mm malleolar screw. The tourniquet is released, alignment is reexamined, and meticulous hemostasis is obtained. The lateral side is left open and routine closure is accomplished over closed suction drainage. The knee is immobilized in a hinged knee brace in 0 degrees of flexion, and weight bearing is allowed as tolerated. Flexion to 40 degrees is begun at 2 weeks and increased to 90 degrees at 4 weeks. The brace is discontinued at 6 weeks. Quadriceps rehabilitation is begun immediately after the operation.

SUGGESTED READING

Brown DE, Alexander AH, Lichtman DM. The Elmslie-Trillat procedure: evaluation in patellar dislocation and subluxation. Am J Sports Med 1984; 12:104–109.

Cox JS. Evaluation of the Roux-Elmslie-Trillat procedure for knee extensor realignment. Am J Sports Med 1982; 10:303–310.

Ferguson RB, Brown TD, Fu FH, et al. Relief of patello-femoral contact stress by anterior displacement of the tibial tubercle. J Bone Joint Surg 1979; 61A:159–166.

Fulkerson JP. Anteromedialization of the tibial tubercle for patellofemoral malalignment. Clin Orthop 1983; 177:176–181.

Insall J, Salvati E. Patella position in the normal knee joint. Radiology 1971; 101:101–104.

Laurin CA, Dussault R, Levesque HP. The tangential x-ray investigation of the patellofemoral joint. Clin Orthop 1979; 144:16–26.

Merchant AC, Mercer RS, Jacobsen RH, et al. Roentgenographic analysis of patello-femoral congruence. J Bone Joint Surg 1974; 56A:1391–1396.

Schutzer SF, Ramsby GR, Fulkerson JP. Computed tomographic classification of patellofemoral pain patients. Orthop Clin North Am 1986; 17:235–248.

QUADRICEPS AND PATELLAR TENDON RUPTURES

CHRISTOPHER W. SIWEK, M.D.

Injuries to the extensor mechanism of the knee have been recognized and described since the times of Galen. Samuel of England is credited with the first published case of quadriceps tendon rupture in English literature, in 1838. Treatment of these injuries consisted of immobilization and limited weight bearing until Lister in 1878 first practiced suture of the knee extensor. Charles McBurney reported the first successful repair of the quadriceps tendon in North America in 1887. McMaster in 1933 published his experimental studies on ruptures of tendons and muscles in animals. He concluded that ruptures of the quadriceps and patellar tendons rarely occur through their substance, but rather are sustained at the musculotendinous junction or insertion of the tendon into the bone. During the last half-century, several different methods have been described, dealing with repairs and reconstruction of neglected, delayed ruptures of extensor mechanism of knee joint.

MECHANISM AND LEVEL OF RUPTURE

Continuity of the extensor mechanism of the knee is disrupted as a result of sudden, powerful contracture of quadriceps muscle against the weight of the body applied to the affected extremity. The actual moment of tearing occurs when the knee is in a mild flexion, the patella firmly held against the femoral condyles by the pull of quadriceps muscle and the force continuing.

The mechanism of rupture for quadriceps as well as patellar tendons is the same. The level of rupture is determined by predisposing factors.

It appears to me that the single most important factor is the individual's age. The natural physiologic aging process "favors" patellar tendon ruptures in individuals younger than 40 years of age and quadriceps tendon ruptures in those above that age. Males sustain injuries six times more often than females, according to my study. Other predisposing factors include diabetes, rheumatoid arthritis, gout, psoriatic arthritis, hyperparathyroidism, systemic lupus erythematosus, and nephritis. Ruptures of patellar tendons in athletes following multiple knee injections with steroids have also been documented.

EXAMINATION

Ruptures of the quadriceps and patellar tendons are uncommon considering all the trauma that occurs about the knee. The severe hematoma that often accompanies the acute rupture may conceal the important diagnostic signs. Much too frequently, these ruptures are misdiagnosed in the acute stage of knee injury. In my study, 39 percent of ruptures have been missed on the initial examination. Testing of the extensor mechanism should be an essential part of the total comprehensive knee evaluation. It is of utmost importance that an early diagnosis be established in order to ensure good final results. During examination, one must look for loss of active knee extension or inability to maintain a passively extended joint against gravity. If the rupture does not extend through medial and lateral retinacula, the patient may have limited, weak, active extension, but still is not able to maintain the completely extended knee joint against gravity. Lack of complete active extension, accompanied by local tenderness and hemarthrosis, strongly suggests at least a partial tear. Complete ruptures are always associated with a palpable soft tissue defect. The rent is easily identifiable in quadriceps tendon, owing to a larger mass of the tissue. However, it may be difficult to palpate a rent in the patellar tendon at the time of swelling and hemarthrosis. In this situation, one should examine the joint while the patient is sitting on a table with his or her legs hanging down. Examination is done by comparing both patellar tendons. The examiner sits in front of the patient, identifies both patellar tendons by placing his thumbs on them, and asks the patient to slowly extend both knees. The examiner should immediately feel "sudden tension" under the thumb that is over the normal patellar tendon, but this tension is absent on the affected side. Proximally (patellar tendon rupture) or distally (quadriceps tendon rupture), a displaced patella may also be observed clinically or radiographically. Old untreated ruptures with partial return of function may be a diagnostic problem. Although partial return of quadriceps function in these cases may occur several weeks after the injury, the disability remains.

QUADRICEPS TENDON RUPTURES

Occurrence

As noted previously, this lesion usually occurs in individuals who are past the fifth decade in age. I have reviewed 117 cases, published from 1880 to 1978, in which the age of the patient was given. There were 69 quadriceps tendon ruptures, and all but four occurred in patients 40 years of age or older. In my own study, 78 percent of quadriceps tendon ruptures occurred in the fifth decade of life or later.

The tears are transverse in nature and begin in the central portion of the rectus femoris, traversing its entire thickness. Only on rare occasions is the tear limited to the rectus femoris; usually it extends laterally and medially, implicating the fibrous expansions of the vastus lateralis and medialis for varying distances. Most of the injuries are observed at the level of the quadriceps tendon attachment to the patella. The margins of the tear are ragged, and tissues are infiltrated with blood. Intratendinous tears do not occur so frequently, and once such a tear is found a "pathologic tear" should be suspected. Systemic diseases, as previously mentioned, or prior steroid infiltrations should be included in the differential diagnosis.

Microscopic examination of tissue from the rupture site shows local degenerative changes, including a decreased level of collagen in fibers of the tendon, fibrotic degeneration, and infiltration.

Diagnosis

The diagnosis is made readily, provided that correct interpretation is given to the clinical features. Frequently the true nature of the lesion is overlooked because the examiner does not suspect the possibility of a rupture of the quadriceps tendon and depends too heavily on roentgenographic findings, which are not always helpful. The clinical findings are directly related to the extent of the tear and the degree of separation of fragments. The cardinal clinical features are a history of stumbling, with severe pain above the knee and subsequent inability to extend the joint.

In complete tears, including synovial membrane, a large hemarthrosis is present. Upon flexion of the knee, the bloody content of the joint is displaced into the suprapatellar pouch and is easily observed as an "abnormal" bulge at the level of rupture. One can palpate a soft tissue defect above the patella. The patella itself may be displaced distally, and it has increased side-to-side motion when compared with the unaffected leg. Roentgenograms may reveal a distally displaced patella, and soft tissue technique may demonstrate the rent itself. If the tear occurs at the tendo-osseous junction, small fragments of avulsed superior pole of the patella appear to be displaced proximally, being retracted with the rectus femoris.

Small tears within the rectus femoris alone may be difficult to diagnose. This may be especially true in obese individuals. These patients still have active extension against gravity, but never complete extension. The examiner may reverse the test: rather than asking the patient to extend the joint, he should bring the knee to complete extension and ask the patient to maintain it. In cases of tear, one always notices a "drop" of the leg of varying degrees. During the examination, the patient complains of increased pain in the suprapatellar region owing to quadriceps tension. In some of these diagnostically difficult cases, a computed tomographic (CT) scan has been helpful in identifying the rupture, its extent, and its location.

Proper diagnosis of small tears can be easily missed. I have observed that this incorrect diagnosis is most often made in the emergency room. Usually the history and physical examination fit into a pattern of "sprained knee," and the patient is given some kind of knee splint. Because the knee support allows some mobility, reasonable comfort, and noticeable steady improvement, the patient may continue this incorrect therapy for several weeks. Disappointment comes when the patient cannot regain full quadriceps strength and is unable to climb stairs or walk on an inclined plane without risk of falling. Return to even mild recreational sport activity is impossible.

Treatment

Repair of the defect should be achieved by surgical intervention in all cases of tear of the extensor mechanism. Adequate assessment of the tear should be made in order to achieve proper and lasting repair. Treatment is generally divided into early and late repair. Distinction between these two phases is made more by the amount of retraction of quadriceps, by difficulty of end-to-end approximation, and by the amount of scar tissue formation than by the actual time from rupture to repair. These findings vary from case to case. In the past I have used 2 weeks as a cut-off time between early and late repairs, but in many instances I was able to make primary repairs with end-to-end suture in tears as old as 3 weeks, and in small tears even older. I would suggest that we use the term "late repair" when, because of time loss, surgical treatment is more extensive and requires additional reinforcement of suture, other than just end-to-end repair. In my experience, no additional reinforcement has been necessary in early repairs or in cases in which end-to-end approximation is achieved without significant strain and tension.

Preferred Methods for Early Repairs

Techniques of repair may vary according to the level of rupture. If the tear is intratendinous and an adequate amount of tissue is available for approximation, an end-to-end suture repair is sufficient. In cases in which the quadriceps tendon is avulsed from patellar attachment, longitudinal holes have to be drilled in the patella for placement of sutures to secure the repair.

Surgical Technique (End-to-End Repair)

A midline anterior longitudinal skin incision is begun about 10 cm proximal to the superior pole of the patella. In tears involving large portions of medial and lateral retinaculum, the incision may have to be extended proximally for an additional 5 to 7 cm. Distally, the incision ends at the joint level. After subcutaneous and fatty tissues are dissected, the rupture is exposed with its hematoma and ragged edges. All clots are removed and the cavity is well irrigated. The entire quadriceps tendon and the suprapatellar pouch area are examined and damage is assessed. The edges of the tendon are trimmed of all devitalized and frayed strands of tissue. If the synovial membrane of the suprapatellar pouch is torn, it should be repaired first. If there is difficulty in approximation, a towel clip should be placed in the rectus femoris tendon at the proximal side of the wound and traction applied distally. A rent in the quadriceps tendon should be closed with heavy, absorbable horizontal mattress sutures. Deep layers are closed first; suturing is continued outward through the middle layers of the vastus medialis and lateralis to the most anterior tendon of the rectus femoris. The suture line is tested under direct vision. The knee is passively flexed to 90 degrees and the repair carefully examined. Subcutaneous and skin closure is done with the knee in 45 degrees of flexion to avoid tight suturing and future tissue contractures, which may delay recovery of range of motion. The entire procedure is done without tourniquet control. The tourniquet is applied, but used only if necessary; an inflated tourniquet causes additional retraction of the proximal fragment and distorts the anatomy of the thigh muscles. Meticulous hemostasis is done to avoid hematoma formation.

Surgical Technique (Tendon-to-Bone Repair)

The technique differs slightly in cases of avulsion of the tendon from the superior pole of the patella. An avulsed rectus is less frayed than with an intratendinous rupture. There is always a good thick stump of tendon to work with. Attention should be directed toward debridement and preparation of the patella for acceptance of the tendon, and proper placement of holes drilled through the body of the patella. By means of a small curette, the edge of the superior pole is "cleaned" from remaining fragments of tendon and sclerotic bone; damage to articulating surface is avoided. With a drill sized 3/32, three holes are made in the following fashion. A sponge is placed onto the floor of the defect to prevent bone fragments from falling into the knee joint. The first hole is drilled centrally, starting at the proximal pole of the patella just superior to the articulating surface. The drill should exit at the lower portion of the body of the patella, making the hole at least 2 cm long; otherwise, fracture may occur. A small guide wire may be placed into the hole to ensure parallel placement of two additional holes. The lateral holes should be at least 1 cm away from the central one, but well within the body of the patella. Two separate heavy sutures are placed through the holes and the rectus femoris (Fig. 1). Additional reinforcing sutures are placed through the superior layer of the rectus femoris. The remaining portion of tear within both vastus muscles are closed as described previously. The use of more than three holes in the patella is unnecessary and may weaken the bone. Occasionally, I use Bunnell's pull-out wire to secure the repair for the period of healing.

Late Repair

Neglected cases exhibit marked disability because of lack of stability in the affected extremity.

Many of these patients must depend on a cane or a brace in order to walk. The quadriceps muscle becomes contracted and extensive adhesions develop. The edges of ruptured tendon become thickened and sclerotic.

Debridement and excision of devitalized tissue should be the first step in surgical repair. All necrotic tissues at the rupture site must be evacuated in order to have vital substances for approximation. Failure to achieve this may result in poor delayed healing and possible re-rupture. Release of adhesions, mainly between the quadriceps and the femur, may allow for additional distal displacement of the stump. Meticulous hemostasis must be achieved. If good approximation is possible, I prefer to repair by means of the tendon-to-bone technique already described. Sutures passed through drilled holes make the repair more secure. At this point, after the rent itself is closed, routine testing of suture line by knee flexion is done, and about 90 degrees of flexion should be possible. The surgeon has to bear in mind that excessive tension of the extensor mechanism will cause limited range of motion and may produce painful patellar symptoms, particularly in active sports-oriented individuals.

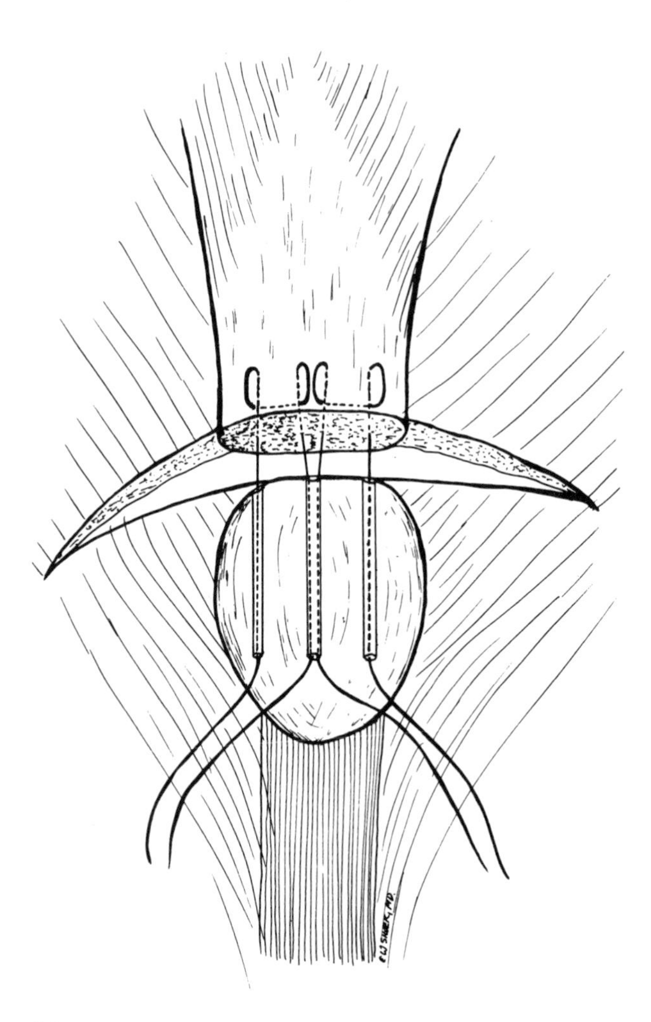

Figure 1 Tendon-to-bone repair of quadriceps tendon rupture. Two separate heavy sutures are placed through the holes in the patella and the rectus femoris.

The next step in late repairs of the quadriceps tendon is reinforcement of the rupture. The least traumatic and most adequate repair is achieved by means of the Scuderi-type inverted V-flap, taken from the rectus femoris and crossed over the suture line. The triangular flap is based 2 cm above the side of the rupture, and it covers the entire width of the rectus. A height of 6 to 8 cm is sufficient for the triangle. An even thickness of 3 to 4 mm (about one-third the full thickness of the tendon) is stripped, starting from the apex of the triangle and ending 2 cm above the rupture level. The flap is inverted and tacked down to the distal portion of the extensor mechanism covering the rent. Depending on the quality of the repair, an additional pull-out wire can be used for protection and may remain in place throughout the healing process. In late repairs, I prefer to anchor the pull-out wire to the transverse tibial pin rather than place the pin through the patella. In the latter case, demineralization of the patella occurs owing to prolonged disuse, and additional transverse holes may dangerously weaken the patella, subjecting it to fractures.

One further step is taken in the repair of a neglected quadriceps tendon rupture when, despite releases, approximation of the edges of the rent is not possible. A lengthening of the quadriceps tendon by the "sliding" method of Codivilla is used. Occasionally, I have reinforced the suture line with a wide strip of fascia lata obtained from the same side. This is used instead of the Scuderi inverted V-flap in cases in which the area is already weakened by a quadriceps-lengthening procedure. The reinforcing strip is sutured to the vastus muscles above, and to the patella and its medial and lateral retinacula below.

Postoperative Management

After the operation the knee is maintained in complete extension. Compression dressings and a conventional knee splint are applied. In less reliable patients, a long leg cast is preferred. Routine wound care is given to the operated site. The patient uses crutches and is allowed "toe touch" for balance only. Quadriceps setting and leg raising with assistance are initiated as soon as postsurgical pain and soreness permit. Two weeks after surgery, sutures are removed. The leg is placed in a brace with adjustable hinges at the knee level. Passive range of motion starts 3 weeks after repair and does not exceed 60 degrees until the fifth postoperative week. The patient is allowed partial to full weight bearing as tolerated, beginning the third postsurgical week. Quadriceps stimulation is used if necessary. The brace is discontinued between the fifth and the seventh week. Judgment regarding the optimal time to discontinue the immobilization is based on the size of the tear and the "soundness" of the repair. Range of motion is continued since full recovery seldom is obtained at this point. Strengthening exercises should include a comprehensive program to regain complete balance of all muscle groups in the leg.

Mild, recreational, noncontact sports activity may be initiated 3 to 4 months after surgery, depending on the severity of the tear. Competitive sports should not be allowed until the full strength of the quadriceps muscle is achieved.

Results

Early repair of the quadriceps tendon, with adequate postoperative physical therapy, gives excellent results. Thirty patients whom I studied regained quadriceps strength comparable with that of the opposite leg, and range of motion measured 120 degrees (in older patients) or more.

Late repair greatly diminishes the chance of regaining satisfactory function postoperatively. In my study, the main obstacle to better results was limited range of motion. Of six patients who underwent delayed repair, only one regained more than 90 degrees of knee flexion. Five of them had persistent quadriceps atrophy.

Since quadriceps tendon ruptures occur in the older population, the timing of physical therapy after repair is very important. In patients with adequate secure repairs, strengthening exercises and range of motion should begin soon after surgery. In motivated patients, complete recovery can be expected.

PATELLAR TENDON RUPTURES

Occurrence

Rupture of the patellar tendon is very rare and occurs mostly in individuals below the age of 40. In a group of 33 patients whom I studied, only one sustained injury after the age of 40 (the patient was 47); the remaining 32 were under 40. The incidence of patellar tendon rupture is about equal to that of quadriceps tendon rupture, and the mechanism is the same.

Most commonly, the lesion comprises complete avulsion of the tendon from the inferior pole of the patella, and the tear extends into both medial and lateral retinacula. Occasionally, small fragments of bone are avulsed from the patella. A healthy patellar tendon does not rupture through its substance, and if such a lesion is found one should suspect underlying causes other than the injury. Effects of injudicious steroid injections in young athletic individuals have to be included in the differential diagnosis. Bilateral simultaneous ruptures also are suspect for systemic diseases. There is no mention of such a case in the literature, all reported simultaneous, bilateral ruptures being associated with a variety of "predisposing factors."

I have seen cases in which some longitudinal fibers of the patellar tendon have been detached from the patella and others from the tibial tubercle (Fig. 2), causing severe shredding of the tissue. This "spaghetti-like" effect makes direct suturing impossible, and fascia lata graft is necessary to restore continuity.

Injuries to the distal portion of the patellar tendon are usually associated with avulsion fractures of the tibial tubercle, often preceded by Osgood-Schlatter disease.

Diagnosis

A detailed history helps to recreate the actual moment of injury, which should strongly suggest rupture of the extensor mechanism. The cardinal sign—lack of active extension—is always present. Proximal migration of the patella is easily noted clinically and radiographically. In more difficult cases, one can make comparisons with the opposite knee. If swelling obscures the pathology, a test of

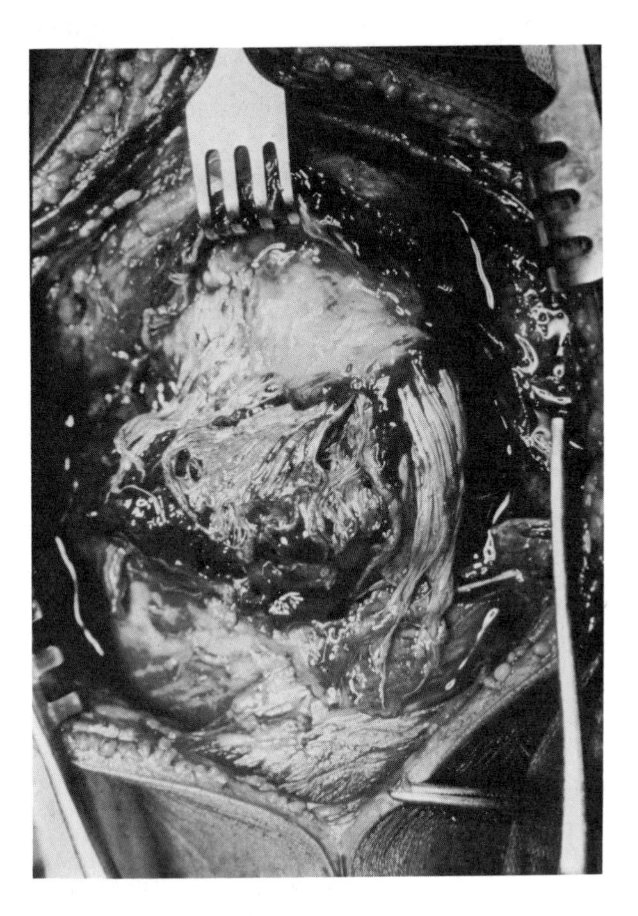

Figure 2 Patellar tendon rupture. Some longitudinal fibers have been detached from the patellar tendon and others from the tibial tubercle, causing severe shredding of the issue.

"sudden tension," as described previously, may be of value.

Treatment

Ruptures should be repaired at the earliest opportunity. In early repairs, surgical technique differs according to the level of injury. Delayed suturing may require additional preoperative or intraoperative procedures. Regardless of the type of injury and the surgical technique used, gentle handling of the tissues is important. The fat pad should remain undisturbed and its normal contact with the patellar tendon preserved, since it serves as a very important blood supply to the tendon. Any debridement at the rupture site must be adequate, but careless excision of tissue should be avoided. Functionally disabling patella baja may result if an excess of tendon is removed.

Actual repair of the patellar tendon, as opposed to quadriceps tendon repair, does not give a sense of "soundness" and security. The patellar tendon is susceptible to longitudinal separations of its fibers, and placement of sutures under excessive traction may cause additional shredding of the tendon. Sutures have to be passed through "tight" healthy portions of tendon in a manner that will not cause strangulation of tissue. I routinely use pull-out wires to avoid tension on the suture line and weakening of the repair.

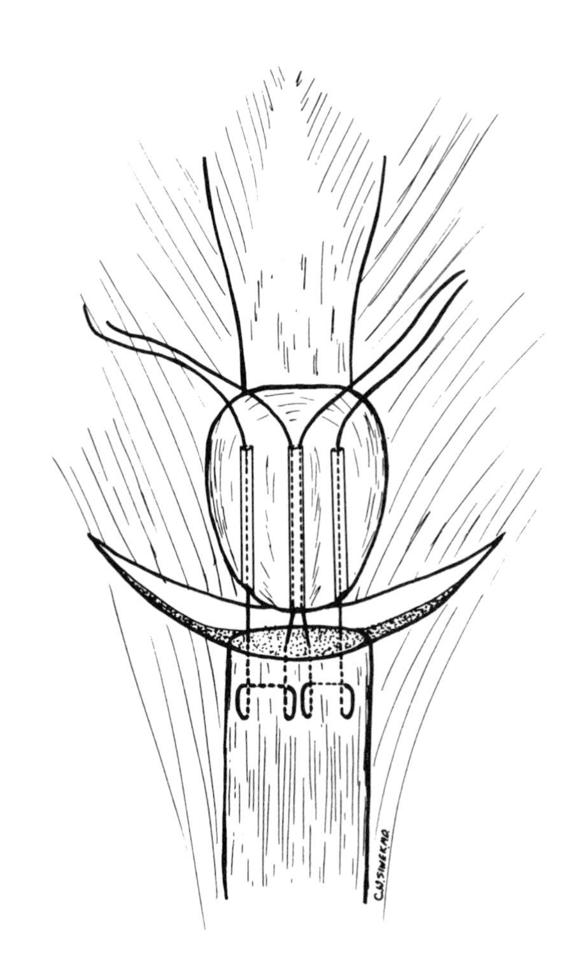

Figure 3 Bone-to-tendon repair of patellar tendon rupture. The main supporting sutures are opposed (see text).

Preferred Methods

Bone-to-Tendon Technique

This repair is a mirror image of the technique described for quadriceps tendon avulsion from the superior pole of the patella.

The skin incision extends from 5 cm above the superior pole of the patella to the tibial tubercle in straight anterior fashion. The entire patellar tendon is exposed and the quality of tissue noted. The avulsed end of the tendon is debrided by sharp transverse dissection, removing enough frayed fragments to leave a thick wide stump for repair. The main supporting sutures are opposed (Fig. 3). The same technique may be used in cases of fracture of the inferior pole of the patella when comminuted fragments are excised.

Tendon-to-Tendon Technique

As already mentioned, one should suspect "pathologic" rupture when a tear has occurred transversely through the substance of the tendon. In these patients direct mattress suturing is not strong enough to maintain continuity of the tendon, even with the leg immobilized in full extension. Quadriceps contractures may cut the sutures through fragile tendon, causing separation of fragments. On the other hand, more vigorous and more bulky suturing may strangulate the tissue.

I reinforce the suture line with a strip of fascia lata obtained from the same side. The strip has to be three times the length of the ruptured tendon and 1.5 cm wide in order to be sufficient for repair. Two tunnels are made, one at 1.5 cm to 2 cm above the inferior pole of the patella and the second 1 cm below the attachment of the patellar tendon to the tibial tubercle. A high-speed air drill with a 3-mm burr is excellent for shaping the edges of the tunnels. When this instrument is used, chipping of bone and fractures is easily avoided. One has to ensure that edges of both tunnels are smooth and round to prevent them from cutting into a fascia lata graft. Before final repair is made, a pull-out wire is passed through the superior pole of the patella, and sufficient distal traction is applied. Wires are anchored to the transverse tibial pin. Excessive traction on the patella is avoided since it may result in a patella baja. The graft is rolled into a cord and passed through both tunnels (Fig. 4). The entire graft is tucked down to both sides of the patellar tendon. The wound is closed in the usual manner.

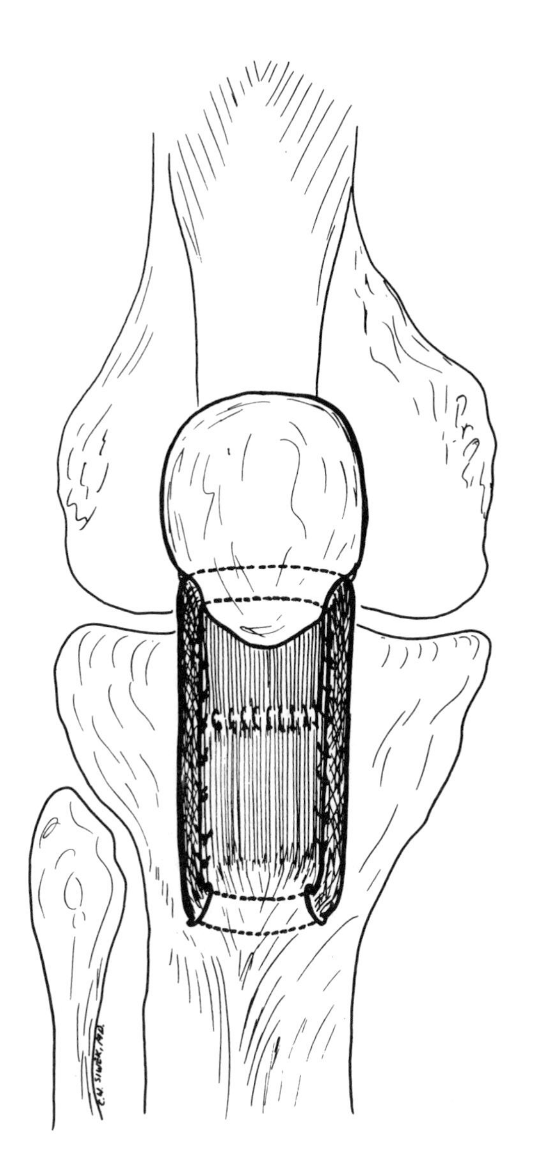

Figure 4 Tendon-to-tendon repair of patellar tendon rupture. The graft is rolled into a cord and passed through both tunnels (see text).

Delayed Repairs

Despite delay, primary approximation of fragments is possible in many cases. These ruptures can be treated by one of the techniques described above. In severely neglected cases, preoperative skeletal traction may be necessary to overcome contractures and adhesions of the quadriceps mechanism. The following are indications for preoperative traction: (1) marked clinical and radiographic proximal displacement of the patella, (2) an inability to move the patella manually to its anatomic position, and (3) a loss of free passive side-to-side motion of the patella (indicative of severe adhesions).

Traction is applied through a 9/64-inch Steinmann pin placed transversely into the patella. The size of the pin largely depends on the size of the patella. To avoid skin tension, the skin is displaced proximally before pin insertion, and a maximum of 2 kg of weight is applied. It may take a few days to 2 weeks before adequate displacement is obtained. Progress of the traction is checked clinically or radiographically. During the period of traction, the knee is engaged in passive range of motion. This is done most comfortably with the patient lying on the unaffected side.

When satisfactory distal displacement of the patella is achieved, surgical repair follows. After routine exposure of the lesion, a second Steinmann pin is inserted into the proximal tibia. The patella is brought to its anatomic position and maintained there by wiring both Steinmann pins together. Actual repair of the patellar tendon is made by means of the tendon-to-tendon technique already described.

A patellar tendon that is not performing its function because of rupture quickly undergoes disuse, degeneration, and disintegration. In these severe cases, one may have to reconstruct the entire patellar tendon, and I prefer to use the distal tendinous portion of the semitendinosus muscle as a substitute for the patellar tendon. The tendon is looped through transverse tunnels in the patella and proximal tibia and then sewn onto itself. After wound closure, a long leg cast is applied, incorporating both pins.

Postoperative Care

For early repairs with good strong approximation, postoperative management is the same as for early repairs of quadriceps tendon ruptures.

In delayed repairs of the patellar tendon, judgment of postoperative management is based on the extent of rupture, the quality and availability of tissues for approximation, and the actual strength of the suture line at the conclusion of surgery. If pins and wires have been used, they should be maintained for 4 to 5 weeks. Cast immobilization with the knee in full extension is continued for 7 to 8 weeks postoperatively.

In early repairs, mild, recreational, noncontact sports activity may be initiated 3 to 4 months after surgery. Prolonged recovery in delayed repairs may extend this time to 6 months.

Results

In my study, 25 patients underwent early repairs of patellar tendons. Twenty of them obtained excellent results with full range of motion and strength of quadriceps muscle equal to that of the opposite leg. Four patients were unable to obtain full active extension, even though passive extension was possible. One patient re-ruptured his patellar tendon 8 weeks after the original repair, while attempting to play football on a recreational level.

Results of seven late repairs in my study were directly related to but he had other medical problems that did not allow him to receive a proper course of therapy. In the remaining five ruptures, motion ranged from full extension to 130 degrees of flexion. Good quadriceps strength was regained despite persistent atrophy of thigh muscles.

SUGGESTED READING

Feagin J, Jackson D. Quadriceps contusion in young athletes. J Bone Joint Surg 1973; 55A:95–105.

Grenier RE, Guimont A. Simultaneous bilateral rupture of the quadriceps tendon and leg fractures in a weight lifter: a case report. Am J Sports Med 1983; 11:145.

Kamali M. Bilateral traumatic rupture of the infrapatellar tendon. Clin Orthop 1979; 142:131.

McCouister Evarts C. Surgery of the musculo skeletal system. New York: Churchill Livingston, 1983: 195.

Rao J, Siwek K. Bilateral spontaneous rupture of the patellar tendons. Orthopaedic Rev 1978; 7:5.

Siwek C, Rao J. Rupture of the extensor mechanism of the knee joint. J Bone Joint Surg 1981; 63A:932–937.

OSTEOCHONDRITIS DISSECANS, OSTEOCHONDRAL FRACTURES, AND OSTEOARTHRITIS

JOHN C. CAMERON, M.D., F.R.C.S.(C)

OSTEOCHONDRITIS DISSECANS

Osteochondritis dissecans of the knee is a condition in which a fragment of bone, adjacent to the articular surface of the knee, is deprived of its blood supply and undergoes avascular necrosis. As new blood vessels invade the necrotic bone, it is gradually replaced by creeping substitution. During this period, the overlying articular cartilage, nourished by the synovial fluid, remains viable. If repeated impact or joint motion causes micromovement of the fragment, the progress of invading vessels is hindered, and the avascular bone fragment may displace and form a loose body within the knee joint, leaving a defect in the articular cartilage.

The symptoms of osteochondritis dissecans usually occur in the second decade. The most frequent symptom is pain, with associated swelling as well as locking and instability. The symptoms are generally related to physical activity. Many of the patients present with pain associated with an effusion, with no specific history of injury, and on physical examination little is found other than the effusion. Radiographic studies are essential for diagnosis. The lesion can occur (in decreasing order of frequency) in the lateral aspect of the medial femoral condyle, lateral femoral condyle, femoral groove, and patella.

There are many theories regarding the cause of the lesion, from abnormal secondary centers of ossification in younger patients to impingement against an enlarged anterior tibial spine. Wilson devised a clinical test for osteochondritis dissecans. He noted that patients with this condition walked with the tibia in external rotation. In carrying out his test with the patient supine, the knee is flexed through 90 degrees and the tibia is internally rotated. The knee is then gradually extended, and at 30 degrees of flexion sharp pain is elicited. External rotation of the knee immediately relieves this pain.

The management of the lesion in the individual patient is determined by the age of the patient and the size and location, as well as the radiographic appearance, of the fragment. Most lesions in younger patients have a favorable prognosis. The skeletally immature patient has a much greater potential for revascularization of the avascular fragment before any damage to the overlying articular cartilage occurs. When patients develop symptoms in the latter part of the second decade, operative intervention is often unavoidable.

The operative management of the condition is determined to a large extent by the integrity of the articular cartilage. If the fragment has separated at an early stage, the defect often fills in and is hardly noticeable on arthroscopic examination. In these cases the symptoms are generally due to the loose osteochondral fragment, and can usually be managed by arthroscopic removal of the fragment.

A more difficult decision is necessary in a symptomatic individual with a large lesion and an intact articular surface. If there is a very dense sclerotic margin on the femoral side of the lesion, we carry out a retrograde curettage through a large drill hole starting from the extra-articular surface of the medial femoral condyle. By palpation of the articular cartilage at the time of curettage, we can avoid damage to the articular surface. We curette out as much of the avascular bone and sclerotic margin as possible and replace this with a local bone graft from the femoral metaphysis. This bone graft is packed solidly up to the articular surface in order to provide support. The patient is then kept non–weight bearing on crutches for 3 months with quadriceps rehabilitation and range-of-motion exercises.

In a patient with osteochondritis dissecans and an intact joint surface with minimal sclerosis about the lesion, internal fixation is utilized. Smillie pins provide fixation for shearing forces, but do not provide any compression across the line of cleavage between the fragment and the distal femur. We are now using scaphoid screws with cancellous threads crossing the cleavage plane to achieve compression of the fragment. Often it is possible to keep the screw placement so that the screw head is off the major weightbearing portion of the condyle, adjacent to the intercondylar notch. The screw head should also be countersunk in the articular cartilage. Results with this treatment have been excellent, and again these patients are kept non–weight bearing for 3 months. X-ray examination at 3 months is generally not helpful in assessing union, but patients have remained asymptomatic with progressive weight bearing after this period.

In most of these patients we have carried out arthroscopic examination under local anesthesia to probe the lesion, and to determine the stability of the repair and its support of the articular surface. To date, these examinations have shown maintenance of articular cartilage viability and congruence, as well as restoration of subchondral bone support. Progressive activity, based on absence of symptoms and joint effusion, is then carried out, with a gradual return to normal activities.

OSTEOCHONDRAL FRACTURES OF THE KNEE

One of the more serious causes of acute hemarthrosis of the knee is an osteochondral fracture. The patient presents after a knee injury with a hemarthrosis of rapid onset. If a diagnostic aspiration is carried out, it should be performed under sterile conditions and the aspirate should be examined for evidence of fat droplets. There are three reasons for carrying out aspiration of the knee: (1) to establish a diagnosis, i.e., whether the fluid is blood or excess synovial fluid; (2) to relieve pressure that is causing excessive pain, and (3) if swelling restricts movement of the knee to less than 90 degrees.

Hemarthrosis due to an osteochondral fracture usually recurs rapidly after aspiration.

All knee injuries resulting in acute hemarthrosis must undergo x-ray examination. The specific injuries in which diagnosis should be made early are major knee ligament disruption, and intra-articular fractures, including osteochondral fractures. One should be able to diagnose the first group on physical examination. If a satisfactory examination cannot be carried out because of pain, an examination under anesthesia should be considered. In the group of patients with intra-articular fractures, roentgenograms should be taken in multiple planes, anteroposterior, lateral, two obliques, and a 30-degree skyline patellofemoral view. In many cases one may see only a small osseous fragment, while the associated articular cartilage fragment is very large.

Most osteochondral fractures occur with patellar dislocation. As the patella rides over the lateral femoral condyle, a portion of the articular surface of the patella or the lateral femoral condyle is sheared off and forms an osteochondral loose body within the knee. The amount of bone seen on x-ray examination is often deceptive with regard to the size of the fragment. Occasionally, fragments may be avulsed from the medial border of the patella, and as they remain attached to the patellar retinaculum they are stable and are not considered loose fragments. Unfortunately this often cannot be determined unless arthroscopic examination is carried out.

The size and source of the osteochondral fragment also may be determined by arthroscopic examination. When the patient is asleep, physical examination of the knee may demonstrate marked crepitus in the area of the lesion. Treatment of the injury depends on the location, size, and comminution of the osteochondral fragment. In general, the smaller and the more comminuted fragments should be removed, and the larger intact fragments should be put back in their bed and internally fixed. The larger the fragment of bone involved, the greater the likelihood of subsequent union. The most troublesome lesions are the highly comminuted fractures occurring on a major weightbearing surface, such as the patella. Our results with excision and debridement and early continuous passive motion have been encouraging. On repeat arthroscopic examination, most of these lesions are seen to have filled in with fibrocartilage. However, most patients remain symptomatic with pain and effusion when they stress their knee, and seldom do they return to their preinjury level of function. Rehabilitation of the lower extremity muscles is very important, and consideration should be given to surgical correction of any underlying predisposition to patellar dislocation. Our approach is to rehabilitate the knee after the acute injury before considering elective surgical procedures.

We believe that immobilization of a knee with an osteochondral fracture is detrimental to articular cartilage, and that procedures for patellar tendon transfer, which require immobilization of the knee, should be avoided. At the time of anesthesia for the acute injury, accurate documentation of patellar instability should be made and any patellofemoral or lower extremity malalignment noted. In many cases, quadriceps rehabilitation is all that is required for dynamic patellar stabilization. The return of the patient to sporting activities must be slowly progressive and determined primarily by symptoms, such as pain and instability, and physical signs, such as swelling.

OSTEOARTHRITIS OF THE KNEE

Osteoarthritis of the knee in the athlete usually falls into one of several categories: (1) associated with ligamentous instability, (2) postmeniscectomy, or (3) post-trauma (secondary to joint surface injury).

Knee ligament instability, particularly anterior cruciate instability, places the meniscus and joint surface under conditions of shear stresses, for which they do not function well. The resultant meniscal tears and joint surface damage often lead to a rapid downgrading in knee function. Because the ligamentous instability must be considered the underlying pathologic condition, it is often necessary to deal with this in order to preserve knee function. In many cases the patient's symptoms are initially due to the ligamentous instability, but with progressive joint surface damage the later symptoms may be due to degenerative arthritis. The treatment, either knee ligament repair or osteotomy, is dependent on the stage of progression of the disease. We believe that early ligamentous reconstruction in a patient who is symptomatically unstable usually halts further progression of articular surface damage. The rehabilitation necessary to regain a high level of physical performance is considerable, but many of these patients function surprisingly well in spite of significant joint surface damage. The task of the treating physician or surgeon is then to determine what the primary source of the disability is, whether knee ligament instability or degenerative osteoarthritis.

Consider the following common scenario. The patient with chronic anterior cruciate instability, whose instability goes unrecognized, subsequently has a meniscectomy that may relieve some of the discomfort initially, but does nothing to stabilize the knee. Then, over the course of several years, he or she develops increasing pain in the knee and, on physical and radiographic examination, demonstrates osteoarthritis.

The patient with posterior cruciate instability who develops patellofemoral degenerative changes will deteriorate functionally. However, we have found that maintenance of quadriceps function and strength allows many of these athletes to continue to function at very high levels. In assessing the disability in a particular athlete, it is necessary to consider the particular sport. Many sports that involve straight-ahead movement only, without any lateral movement or pivoting, can be carried out without significant problems in patients with anterior cruciate instability. Therefore, to take athletes who are functioning at a very high level and subject them to a ligamentous reconstruction is of questionable value. On the other hand, athletes who are involved in sports such as soccer, which involves rapid lateral movement and pivoting, are generally significantly disabled by their instability and, in spite of rehabilitation of the quadriceps and hamstring muscle groups, are unable to regain their former function after anterior cruciate injuries.

A postmeniscectomy patient who has unicompartmental joint surface wear in association with either valgus or varus alignment may be treated by osteotomy. This realignment often transfers sufficient weight to the undamaged compartment of the knee, so that excellent function is restored. Lesser degrees of disability require only continued muscle rehabilitation and anti-inflammatory medications. Unfortunately, joint surface wear in this type of patient tends to progress more rapidly when subjected to excessive loads. It has therefore been our policy to discourage patients with osteoarthritic changes from participating in activities that involve repetitive heavy loading or impact of the damaged knee.

A similar approach is taken in dealing with patients who have post-traumatic arthritis secondary to joint surface injuries, such as intra-articular fractures. In many cases, tibial plateau fractures, if well managed, return to a high level of activity, but one can expect a progressive downgrading in performance with increasing surface damage. As these patients progress in their rehabilitation, we often carry out outpatient arthroscopic examinations under local anesthesia in order to determine a prognosis at 6 months and 1 year following any injury, and also to give patients some idea of the activity level toward which they should aim. There is not much doubt that continued impact loading on a damaged articular surface will lead to gradual deterioration. However, if the articular cartilage is relatively undamaged or is restored, and on arthroscopic examination appears relatively normal, we encourage these patients to gradually increase their activity level, again depending ultimately on the symptoms and signs.

SUGGESTED READING

Aegerter E, Kirkpatrick JA. Orthopedic diseases. 4th ed. Philadelphia: WB Saunders, 1975: 302.

Hughston JC, Hergenroed PT, Courtenay BG. Osteochondritis dissecans of the femoral condyles. J Bone Joint Surg 1984; 66:1340–1348.

Muborak SJ, Carroll NC. Juvenile osteochondritis dissecans of the knee: etiology. Clin Orthop 1981; 157:200–211.

Pappas AM. Osteochondritis dissecans. Clin Orthop 1981; 158:59–69.

INJURY TO THE ANTERIOR CRUCIATE LIGAMENT

R. PETER WELSH, M.B., Ch.B., F.R.C.S.(C), F.A.C.S.

Rupture of the anterior cruciate ligament constitutes a major handicap to people who are athletically inclined. A knee so injured is vulnerable to episodes of "giving way" that may not only seriously compromise athletic performance but also render the knee subject to further major articular insult with meniscal disruption and articular surface breakdown.

It is imperative to identify all such lesions and afford appropriate advice, counsel, and treatment. This does not imply that all ruptures of the anterior cruciate ligament should be surgically treated per primum, since not all cruciate-deficient knees become manifestly unstable. However, athletic performance after injury to the anterior cruciate ligament may well have to be modified, and if instability of the knee becomes an ongoing problem, late stabilization may be necessary. The incidence of secondary articular injuries (meniscal derangement, 54 percent, and serious articular lesions, 38 percent) encountered in a series of 125 late reconstructions followed up over a 5-year period leads me to conclude that a more aggressive surgical approach should be undertaken in the athletically active individual.

ACUTE RUPTURE OF THE ANTERIOR CRUCIATE LIGAMENT

An athlete who, propping to cut or leaping to make a shot, feels a sudden "pop" in the knee and an associated sensation of "the knee coming apart" is probably experiencing a tear of the anterior cruciate ligament. This can also occur from direct trauma as in skiing falls or in contact sports such as football or hockey where the impact of an opponent provides a disruptive external force. However, these injuries are more dramatic and the injury is less likely to be overlooked than in the first group of individuals in whom a seemingly innocuous noncontact presentation is often the catalyst. Both instances present athletes with disruptions of the anterior cruciate ligament that deserve close attention.

Hemarthrosis almost always accompanies such injuries, and the presence of blood in the knee may make the joint difficult to examine. The hemarthrosis should always be aspirated; if necessary, the instillation of local anesthetic (20 ml of 1 percent lidocaine [Xylocaine]) can often aid further evaluation of the joint. Under such circumstances, it should be possible with the Lachman test to identify most lesions of the anterior cruciate ligament.

The Lachman test should be carried out gently with the knee in 15 degrees of flexion, grasping the thigh and leg and drawing the tibia gently forward. The Macintosh test provides further confirmation: the pivot shift can be elicited in all cases of anterior cruciate rupture. The key again is gentleness in examination, the examiner cradling the leg with the knee in 15 degrees of flexion; as the patient relaxes the hamstrings, the tibia will subluxate forward from the femur. If the examiner maintains a gentle valgus pressure on the limb and flexes it slightly, a reduction of the tibia will occur. The key to confirmation of anterior cruciate ligament rupture is the initial subluxation of the tibia; attempts to force a "pivot shift" should not be pursued, as these may be resisted by the patient with an acutely injured knee. The major fault in examining the acute knee is the exertion of too great a valgus stress or the overzealous loading of the limb with longitudinal pressure, causing the hamstring to go into spasm and totally preventing the tibia from subluxating forward on the femur.

Traumatic rupture of the anterior cruciate ligament, associated soft tissue injury to other structures about the knee, and possible rupture of the medial collateral ligament may make clinical examination difficult without anesthesia. When there is any clinical doubt, examination under general anesthesia should be carried out, with the Lachman and Macintosh tests confirming the diagnosis of anterior cruciate ligament rupture and determining the status of other ligamentous structures.

If a general anesthetic proves necessary, it should be standard practice to arthroscope the knee at the same time. Arthroscopic evaluation is carried out not to confirm the tear of the anterior cruciate ligament but to define whether there is any other associated intra-articular pathologic condition either to the menisci or to the joint surfaces. This may require patient irrigation of the joint in order to clear the hemarthrosis and make possible effective visualization. However, it can be extremely misleading to try to define tears of the ligament by direct visualization. With trauma to the tissues in the intercondylar area and to the synovium and fat pad, definition of a cruciate tear may be very difficult. It is emphasized that confirmation of anterior cruciate ligament deficiency is a clinical observation that should be confirmed by Lachman and Macintosh testing, not by an endeavor to interpret the tangled mess that so often obscures the view within the acutely injured knee.

Management

Having defined a tear of the anterior cruciate ligament, a definite plan of action should be outlined for each athlete based on the injury, the patient's sporting aspirations, and his or her work and social circumstances.

Indications for Primary Repair

1. Rupture of the medial collateral and anterior cruciate ligaments is an absolute indication for reconstruction of both ligaments in all athletic patients.
2. All ruptures involving avulsion of the tibial tubercle attachment of the anterior cruciate ligament should be repaired per primum.
3. Repair of an isolated anterior cruciate ligament should be undertaken in any competitive athlete with a manifestly unstable knee, i.e., with a grossly positive pivot shift instability.
4. Primary repair is indicated for ruptures in young athletes who wish to pursue a competitive sports program, and in older athletes whose work or family commitments allow the time for surgery and full rehabilitation without too great a disruption of their normal lifestyle.

The grayer zone arises when the ligament is torn but the knee is not grossly unstable. If there is an associated meniscal injury, consider an arthroscopic surgical treatment of the meniscal pathology, and pursue a watch-and-wait policy with regard to the ongoing stability of the knee. If stability proves unsatisfactory, the knee may be stabilized electively as a late procedure.

Timing of Repair

Recent experience seems to indicate that if an athlete with an acute knee ligament injury is first to rehabilitate the knee from the initial traumatic episode, a speedier rehabilitation can be achieved. The compounding of traumas when surgical treatment is imposed in the first week or so is greater than if it is delayed 6 to 8 weeks and carried out on a semielective basis. The quality of the repair will not have been jeopardized, as borne out by the results from the same procedure for late stabilization, and problems with stiffness and patellofemoral pain appear to be obviated.

With an acute ligament injury, early diagnosis is essential. Evacuation of the hematoma should be followed by early mobilization of the knee, with range-of-motion exercises starting as soon as the acute swelling has subsided. Splint support should be offered with or without hinges, and weight bearing must be protected on crutches with just light touch. Isometric strengthening exercises can be started early and a light resisted program added.

When the knee has regained motion and the swelling completely subsided, semielective surgery can then be undertaken 4 to 6 weeks after the injury.

Conservative Management

Surgical treatment of the acute anterior cruciate ligament lesion involves a certain commitment on the patient's part. After the procedure a period of cast and brace protection and non–weight bearing on crutches is required. It may be 3 months before the patient can place the foot to the ground for effective weight bearing, and even then a cane may be required for another month or more. For the young athlete or student, this is not too great a hardship. For the older person, work and family commitments may make such limitation of daily activity a social and economic hardship, leading one to consider pursuing a conservative course with a view to undertaking a late stabilization should the knee prove unstable in the long term.

Therefore, an alternative to primary reconstruction must be offered. If primary surgical repair is not chosen or if individuals do not present within the first month after injury (beyond which time a primary reconstruction is no longer feasible owing to contraction of injured ligament structures), a definite program of rehabilitation should be mapped out. After the immediate injury, rest with splint support is recommended for 3 days. During this time, ice pack application controls swelling, eases pain, and paves the way for an early, active rehabilitation program. Physiotherapy is instituted on the fourth day with heat, pool therapy, and gentle mobilizing exercises. The use of the exercise bicycle is encouraged as strength develops. Strengthening exercises are added, emphasizing the hip flexors and abductors and the hamstrings. Quadriceps building is done with isometric strengthening and quadriceps faradism, but resisted exercises are not encouraged. Weight bearing is allowed as comfort permits; by 6 weeks, full mobilization should have been achieved, allowing a graduated return to sporting activity. As the athlete returns to sport, an elasticized knee support is often of great help; it offers support for the stabilizing muscle groups of the thigh and leg and greatly aids proprioceptive feedback, which is often disrupted in ligamentous injuries of this type.

Positive guidance should be given to patients with a known cruciate ligament injury who are returning to a sports program. Sports such as running, cycling, and swimming will cause few problems; skiing, skating, and hockey may be fine because the knee is maintained in flexion. However, sports involving jumping, leg extension, and propping and cutting may cause problems. Basketball, tennis, and baseball may pose difficulties and can predispose to further injury if repeated episodes of "giving way" occur. Under these circumstances, sports should be discontinued and consideration given to late surgical stabilization if an active sporting career is to be further pursued.

I have not found stabilizing braces to be totally effective for the knee suffering from cruciate deficiency. If the knee becomes unstable, a brace only protects the knee from further extraneous insult, as in contact sports, but it cannot control the inherent instability enough to allow propping and cutting activities. These patients must consider a late stabilization procedure and then may use a brace to prevent the knee from being further traumatized by extraneous insult.

Primary Surgery

When the anterior cruciate ruptures, it usually suffers an intersubstance tear, with avulsion of a portion of the ligament from its femoral attachment and propagation of the tear through the body of the ligament, usually to its midportion. In so doing, the rupture causes a complete disruption of the blood supply from the posterior geniculate artery, so that direct primary suture of the anterior cruciate is a totally ineffective and futile surgical gesture, mentioned only to be condemned.

Reinforcement is an essential component of primary anterior cruciate ligament repair. It is essential to provide a supporting scaffold for the replication of the original structure. The only exception is an avulsion of the tibial tubercle attachment of the anterior cruciate ligament. Here, direct accurate relocation of the avulsed fragment is totally successful because the blood supply of the ligament is not jeopardized. During open arthrotomy it is imperative to relocate the avulsed ligament completely and accurately, impacting the bone into its bed after drawing it into place with two stout sutures. These sutures are passed through two drill holes directed from the proximal tibia up through the bed of the avulsed area; tied in place, the ligament will consolidate in place. Consolidation of its bony insertion takes only 4 to 6 weeks with brace protection.

Most cruciate ligament disruptions involve intersubstance tears and necessitate graft reinforcement. The modified Macintosh technique has been used with great success and is my preferred treatment. In a series of 80 repairs carried out over a 5-year period, only six unsatisfactory results were encountered. This procedure can be commended as effective and reliable, provided certain technical points are closely adhered to.

The quadriceps patellar tendon over-the-top reconstruction is a variation of the Jones repair and can be recommended. The lateral one-third of the patellar tendon is used, taking only partial thickness of the quadriceps tendon above the knee, widening out over the patella to gain sufficient tissue, and then taking only limited tissue below. This is formed into a tube graft with a longitudinal running suture to facilitate later drawing through the knee. Minimizing the interference with the quadriceps mechanism above the knee obviates difficulties from overzealous harvesting of tissue and tightening of the suprapatellar tendon complex. Such tightening otherwise interferes severely with patellar function and can account for postoperative patellofemoral pain, knee stiffness, and impaired range of motion.

The tendon graft is next passed through a drill hole in the proximal tibia, the line of the graft passing up through the bed of the torn ligament. The remnant of the torn ligament is taken as a separate entity on a further suture enfolding the new graft, which acts as a scaffold for tissue reconstitution. Beyond 3 to 4 weeks from the time of injury, this stump of original ligament has usually shrunk. It is essential always to use a supplemental graft. Ligament suture alone will fail.

Macintosh emphasized that the correct positioning of this graft should replicate that of the original ligament, which inserts not into but around the back and over the top of the lateral femoral condyle. A drill hole is then passed from the lateral femoral condyle to the over-the-top point in the intercondylar notch, and the graft on its drawer suture is drawn up through the tunnel. It is further tightened and the knee is cycled from full flexion to full extension to ensure its isometricity before being secured with suture and staple.

A compression dressing and splint are employed in the first 2 days postoperatively before early range-of-motion exercises are initiated. Thereafter, the splint alone is employed, maintaining 15 degrees of flexion at rest. Weight bearing is protected with crutches for 6 weeks, only light touch being permitted during this time.

The early mobilization following surgery greatly assists recovery and avoids postoperative stiffness and patellofemoral problems, which were occasionally of concern after prolonged cast immobilization. Even so, a 5-degree flexion tendency is often seen at 6 months, and return to active sports should be delayed for a further 3 months.

Brace protection may be offered for individuals in contact sports such as football and hockey to prevent reinjury, but otherwise brace use has been unnecessary. In the original series of 80 patients undergoing acute repair, only eight had any problems with persistent instability in a follow-up period now exceeding 10 years.

CHRONIC ANTERIOR CRUCIATE LIGAMENT INSTABILITY

Chronic anterior cruciate ligament instability seriously compromises an athlete's performance and poses a threat to the knee in that persistent episodes of uncontrolled subluxation must inevitably lead to internal derangement, including meniscal tears and articular insult. In its fulminant form, progressive degeneration ensues with bicompartmental post-traumatic arthritis, the arthropathy of cruciate neglect.

Clinical Features

In patients presenting for late stabilization, the time lapse between acute injury and reconstructive surgery may be many years. In a series of 155 late reconstructions, the time lapse ranged from 1 to 22 years, with a mean of 3½ years. In many such instances, the acute episode may be forgotten or at best remain ill defined in the patient's memory. In many cases all that can be recalled is a severe knee strain that occurred "some years ago." After a somewhat prolonged recovery phase, in most instances the athletes return to active sports, and it is only over a period of time that their problem becomes manifest. Many individuals seem able to cope adequately for several years, with only the occasional episode of "giving way." Gradually, however, the knee becomes more insecure, until it finally decompensates and becomes critically unstable not only for sports activities but for everyday life.

It is often at this stage that surgical control is sought; brace control, although it may be adequate for certain sports activities, cannot generally be applied if the knee is unstable at work or in everyday activity. Unfortunately, by this stage further irrepairable articular insult may have occurred. In our series of 155 late reconstructions, 38 percent showed major articular lesions, and 54 percent had meniscal tears requiring meniscectomy.

It is essential at this stage to identify the nature of the knee derangement, defining the cruciate deficiency and any associated meniscal or articular disorder, so that a rational program of management can be planned.

The Lachman test and Macintosh pivot shift test, as described earlier, form the basis for the clinical confirmation of an anterior cruciate deficiency. Both tests demonstrate the anterior subluxation of the tibia beneath the femur, but the Macintosh test can be quantitatively more helpful in the chronic situation. The degree of tibial subluxation should be documented, noting if possible whether the lateral plateau presents the more obvious subluxation or whether the medial plateau presents with equal prominence. This has great significance in defining whether a lateral substitution repair alone will suffice if the instability is predominantly a lateral phenomenon. When the tibia presents as a whole with major medial subluxation as well, a repair based on the lateral aspect alone will be inadequate, and further reinforcement, both intra-articularly and medially, should be contemplated.

A further examination of the knee should include an assessment of the status of the menisci and articular surfaces and any derangement of patellar mechanics. Finally, it is worth noting the general body type of a patient; those who are loose jointed and hyperflexible offer a greater challenge in achieving stability than do the "tight" body types.

Conservative Management

It is obvious that not all individuals with a disruption of the anterior cruciate ligament require stabilization. Many people can cope adequately in everyday life or modify their work and recreational activities so that their knees are never functionally unstable. It is important to counsel individuals against pursuing recreation that may be unsuitable to their situation. Thus, athletes who are involved in jumping sports such as basketball, football, or baseball find that when they land with their leg in extension or pivot from the affected side, their knee gives way; these patients should consider giving up that sport or having the knee stabilized. Brace control may be tried, but there is no brace that adequately controls many of these situations, which demand loading in extension or pivoting from the affected side.

Surprisingly, sports such as skiing, skating, or squash may be possible. As long as a flexed attitude of the knee is sustained, the knee will not subluxate, and sports participation may be continued as long as further internal derangement is not evident.

For those whose knees are insecure, redirection into less provocative sport activities may therefore be a viable alternative. Even so, active strengthening of the knee should be a part of the serious athlete's exercise program. Although quadriceps drills are important for strength and durability, these should not overload the patellar mechanism, and if anything, extra emphasis should be given to overdeveloping the hamstrings as well as the hip flexors and abductors.

Bracing does have a definite role and can offer a threefold benefit: (1) controlling the knee so that it does not extend fully, thus avoiding potentially unstable situations; (2) protecting the compromised knee from extraneous forces as in contact sports, thus preventing the superimposition of further insult, which might damage further other ligament structures; and (3) enhancing the proprioceptive feedback and muscle control of the extremity, which in turn further enhances the protective responses of the body. The prototype brace and the benchmark against which all other imitations must be compared remains the Lennox-Hill derotation brace. Such braces should endeavor to build in cruciate control restraints and control extension so that the hamstrings remain the effective dynamic group acting across the joint, restraining the tibia in its tendency to anterior subluxation, thus substituting for the deficiency of the anterior cruciate ligament.

However, should a cruciate-deficient knee prove unstable in everyday life, as in stepping down off a curb or turning about, surgical stabilization becomes mandatory. Similarly, for many individuals engaged in sports in whom the anterior cruciate knee proves unsatisfactory, and for whom alternative treatments have been exhausted, consideration should be given to surgery, particularly if other internal derangement is apparent.

Age should not be considered a limiting factor in the management of anterior cruciate ligament lesions, either acute or chronic. Repair should be offered on the basis of disability, and excellent repairs have been achieved in patients in their fifth and sixth decades.

Surgical Management

It is essential in evaluating the clinical status that the nature of the instability pattern be fully appreciated before surgical repair is undertaken. The Macintosh is the single most important test in defining whether the repair can be confined to the lateral aspect of the joint or whether an intra-articular or medial reinforcement is required.

If subluxation of the whole tibia is apparent, restraint with three-point fixation must be offered if a durable repair is to be achieved. The difference between the acute injury and the late situation is that in the chronically unstable knee the secondary periarticular capsular and tendinous restraints, as a consequence of repeated episodes of subluxation, have been stretched out and attenuated to the point where they no longer support the knee and require substitution.

In devising a reconstruction for a particular patient, examination under anesthesia before surgery affords an opportunity to reaffirm the pattern of instability present. Arthroscopic evaluation permits a thorough inspection of the interior and detection of any intra-articular disorder that may need concurrent surgical remedy.

Lateral Compartment Pivot Instability

If the instability is one of anterior cruciate ligament deficiency with a lateral pivot shift alone and no medial subluxation, a lateral substitution repair will stabilize the knee completely. Here the objective is to secure the posterolateral corner of the knee. Although it is possible to use three structures — the popliteus, the biceps, or the fascia lata — the modified Macintosh technique is preferred.

Modified Macintosh Technique of Lateral Substitution Repair. Examination under anesthesia confirms the pattern of instability with a purely lateral pivot shift phenomenon, and any intra-articular disorder is treated before surgery by arthroscopic surgical technique.

A long lateral incision exposes the iliotibial tract, allowing a strip graft 2 cm in width and 20 cm in length to be mobilized. The graft is left attached distally at Gerdy's tubercle, but is folded side to side on itself and fashioned into a tube with a longitudinal running suture, which is left long at the end to act as a drawstring.

The tube graft is now passed deep to the lateral ligament, deep to the popliteus, and deep to the arcuate complex in the posterolateral corner of the knee. A subperiosteal tunnel is fashioned up the back of the lateral femoral condyle and the graft passed in this deep to the intermuscular septum. While the knee is maintained in external rotation and flexion, the ligament graft is secured to the lateral ligament, popliteus, arcuate tendon, and posterolateral capsular structures. The free end of the graft is now passed deep to the arcuate tendon and lateral ligament, paralleling the original course before being folded back on itself and sewn into the posterolateral capsule as further reinforcement. It is possible to close the fascial defect distally, but often the defect must be left wide open proximally.

Postoperatively the patient is maintained in a hinged brace allowing 90 degrees of flexion with restriction to 20 degrees of extension. Four weeks of protection is offered for patients under 30 years of age, 3 weeks for those aged 30 to 40, and 2 weeks only for those over 40.

Pivot Instability with Complete Tibial Subluxation

In major degrees of anterior cruciate ligament insufficiency, the whole tibia can be subluxated forward on Macintosh testing. In this case, control of the instability must be offered not only laterally, but also internally with a graft substitution through the knee.

The through-the-knee graft can be formed with fascia lata, semitendinosus, or patellar tendon. However, the preferred technique is to use the patellar tendon in exactly the same manner as practiced for the acute repair.

Experience now extends over 4 years with this procedure in the chronic situation, and the results equal those achieved in primary repair. So encouraging are the results that delayed primary repair and late repair can be recommended to all but the more serious competitive athletes who require early return to sports activities and may choose to undergo repair at an earlier stage.

Surgery for Failed Anterior Cruciate Repair

When the knee remains unstable despite previous attempts at repair, the major instability pattern must be clearly identified and dealt with.

Even after previous surgery for which fascia lata has already been utilized, it is usually possible to harvest enough fascia lata to carry out a lateral substitution repair and tighten up the posterolateral corner. A patellar tendon graft must be used to reconstitute the intra-articular restraint, the technique employed again being similar to that described for the acute repair. However, it is for the knee that has undergone multiple operations yet has continuing marked instability that artificial ligament grafts may be used to reinforce the repair. At this time, experience with these repairs is limited but most encouraging.

Technique with Leeds-Keio Dacron Graft. The Leeds-Keio Dacron graft is a loosely woven mesh tape that is used to reinforce the Macintosh patellar tendon graft. The patellar tendon is harvested as a 1- to 1.5-cm strip, a partial-thickness graft only above the patella in the quadriceps tendon and a full-thickness graft down the lateral aspect of the patella. It is left attached distally at the tibial tubercle where the Leeds-Keio tape is sewn into the body of the tendon, starting at the insertion. As the patellar tendon is folded on itself to form a tube, so the Dacron tape is enclosed in the center and secured with each suture. The cord at the end of the Dacron tape is ideal to draw the complete graft of Dacron mesh enclosed in patellar tendon through the prepared drill holes. The tension is adjusted in the graft before it is secured on the outer aspect of the lateral femoral condyle with a Stone staple. The knee should be moved through full range and stress tested on the table for stability before the graft is secured and before closure is undertaken.

Early mobilization is encouraged, and a Universal splint support is offered for 4 weeks with 15 degrees of flexion built into the splint to prevent full extension. The device can be removed for exercise or shower activity, but weight bearing other than the lightest touch is not allowed for 6 weeks.

Postoperative Rehabilitation

After the brace or splint has been removed, patients are allowed 3 weeks to loosen the knee on their own and are encouraged to mobilize the extremity freely, using where possible a spa or whirlpool.

Active physiotherapy is then instituted, with emphasis on first mobilizing the knee with hydrotherapy, cycling exercises, and gentle passive stretching.

Strengthening exercises are subsequently added, emphasizing the hip flexors, hip abductors, and hamstrings, using initially only isometric and faradic stimulation for the quadriceps. Until knee extension is achieved, resisted quadriceps exercises are minimized in order to reduce loading of the patellar mechanism, because the development of patellar pain after a period of immobilization will only be aggravated by overzealous quadriceps loading. For similar reasons, crutch walking is continued until the knee extends to 10 degrees, usually by the end of the third month, and from this time on more aggressive strengthening can be undertaken.

Return to sport is allowed when full range and strength have been achieved and a normal running gait pattern has been established.

Brace protection is offered to those who wish to return to heavy contact sports, but otherwise is not routinely employed.

SUGGESTED READING

Butler DL, Noyes GR, Grood ES. Ligamentous restraints, anterior-posterior drawers in the human knee: a biomechanical study. J Bone Joint Surg 1980; 62A:259–270.

Galway HR, MacIntosh DL. The lateral pivot shift sign of anterior cruciate ligament insufficiency. Clin Orthop 1980; 147:45–50.

Jakob RP, Hassler H, Stäubli HU. Observations on rotary instability of the lateral compartment of the knee: experimental studies on the functional anatomy and the pathomechanism of the true and the reversed pivot shift sign. Acta Orthop Scan 1981; 52 (Suppl): 191.

Jakob RP, Stäubli HU, Deland JT. Grading the pivot shift: objective tests with implications for treatment. J Bone Joint Surg 1987; 69B:294–299.

ARTHROSCOPICALLY ASSISTED RECONSTRUCTION OF THE ANTERIOR CRUCIATE LIGAMENT

ALEXANDER A. SAPEGA, M.D.

Any individual with chronic, symptomatic anterior cruciate ligament (ACL) deficiency unresponsive to knee rehabilitation and bracing, or any active athlete with acute disruption of the ACL, is a potential candidate for ligamentous reconstruction. One surgical option for these patients that is rapidly becoming the treatment standard in the field of athletic trauma surgery is arthroscopically assisted ACL reconstruction. Simply stated, this represents intra-articular ACL reconstruction without an open arthrotomy. It is properly referred to as "arthroscopically assisted" because extra-articular incisions, although limited, are still needed for graft harvesting and/or bone tunnel drilling. It therefore is not strictly an arthroscopic procedure. The basic surgical method can be applied to the placement of any ACL graft or substitute that can be placed through tibial and femoral bone tunnels, with only slight modification for prosthetic ligaments that require femoral "over-the-top" placement.

There are some obvious clinical advantages to this surgical method, such as lower perioperative morbidity, easier institution of voluntary joint motion, less intra-articular scar formation, and improved cosmetic results. Technical advantages include better visualization of the landmarks within the intercondylar notch before graft placement and the ability to evaluate the ACL substitute critically once it is in place to check for osseous contact-abrasion or impingement with knee motion. Controlled distention of the joint and lavage with the arthroscopic irrigant solution often allow the arthroscopic portions of the procedure to be performed with the limb tourniquet deflated, thus cutting ischemia time by 75 percent or more. Perhaps the only disadvantages relative to traditional open surgery are the greater dependence on surgical instrumentation and the fact that a good deal of patience and technical skill with the arthroscope are necessary.

ANATOMIC CONSIDERATIONS

The ACL is a broad, ovoid-sectioned ligament that, when viewed in extension, is composed of a continuum of parallel fibers (Fig. 1), with no detectable physical boundaries between different fiber "bundles" (Odensten and Gillquist, 1985; Sapega et al, 1989). Different portions of the ligament's macrostructure are therefore best referred to as "fiber regions," which are arbitrarily distinguished by their geographic area of insertion on the tibia (Sapega et al, 1989; Girgis et al, 1975). Because of its noncylindric shape and its broad osseous insertional areas (maximal diameter, 17 to 30 mm), it is not yet technically feasible to reconstruct surgically the entire macrostructure of the normal ACL. A reasonable surgical alternative is to reconstruct the most functionally significant portion of the ACL in as anatomic a manner as possible. Given the limited diameter (6 to 12 mm) of the tibial and femoral bone tunnels generally employed for graft placement during ACL reconstruction, the surgeon can only direct the ACL substitute through approximately one-half of each anatomic insertional area. In choosing which half of the ACL fibers to reconstruct (anterior, central, or posterior), biomechanical factors come into play.

BIOMECHANICAL CONSIDERATIONS

Arms and colleagues (1984) consider that the anterior or, more specifically, the anteromedial fiber region should be the choice for selective reconstruction. Graf (1987a) stated that the anteromedial fibers are the most isometric of any in the ACL. My own laboratory studies have confirmed Graf's conclusion (Sapega et al, 1988, 1989), and also demonstrate that the anterior fibers of the ACL act as the principal restraint to anterior tibial translation at both 15 and 90 degrees of flexion (Figs. 2 and 3). This is consistent with the original observations of Rosenberg and Rasmussen (1984) and the recent data of Hollis and associates (1988). Based on the weight of available experimental evidence as well as clinical experience, the author actively attempts to reconstruct the anteromedial fiber region as anatomically as possible during surgery rather than the central fiber core of the ACL. This involves the use of intra-articular landmarks as well as intraoperative "isometry" testing, as described later.

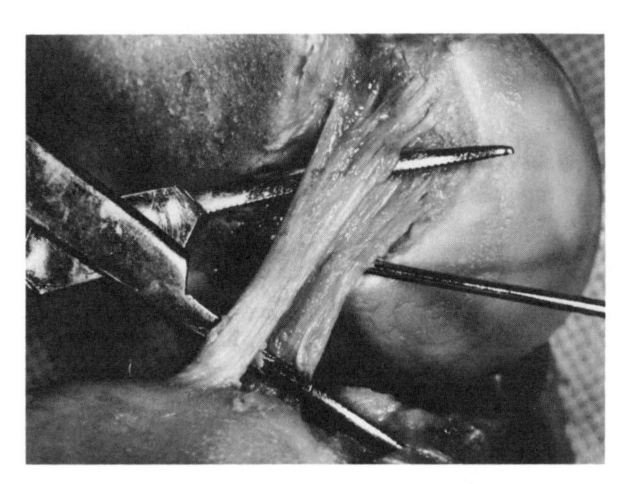

Figure 1 Fiber-splitting dissection shows that, aside from a limited degree of proximal and distal fiber fanning, the parallel arrangement of fibers seen on the medial surface of the ACL (knee in extension) is maintained throughout the ligament's substance. No anatomically separate fiber "bundles" are visible.

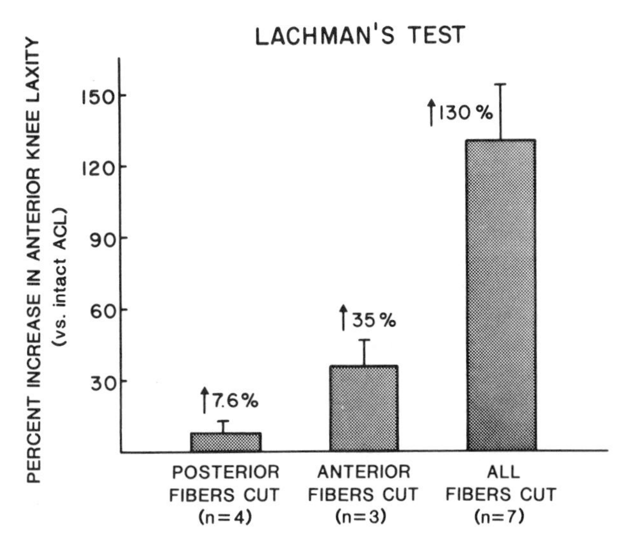

Figure 2 The results of standard manual Lachman's testing before and after selectively cutting the anterior and posterior 50 percent of the ACL fibers in seven fresh knee preparations, instrumented as described by Sapega and colleagues (error bars = SEM).

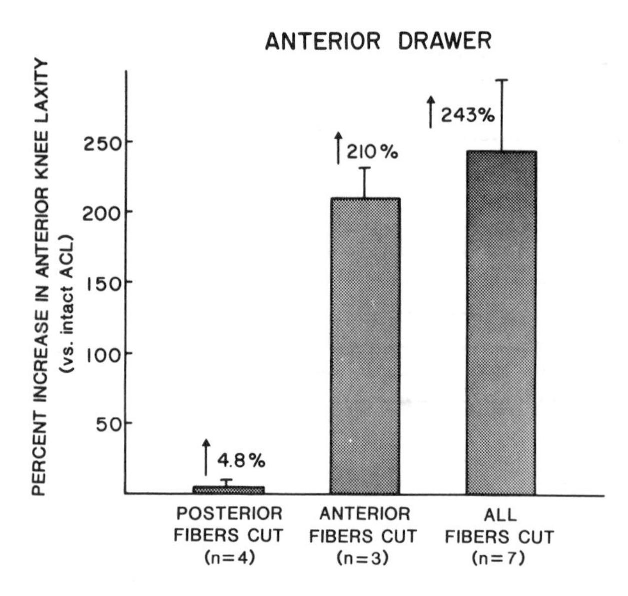

Figure 3 The results of standard manual anterior drawer testing before and after selectively cutting the anterior and posterior 50 percent of the ACL fibers (same knee preparations as in Figure 2).

My current personal preference for the ACL substitute is a combined semitendinosus and gracilis autograft. According to the data of Noyes and colleagues (1984), the combined strength of these two tendons (approximately 120 percent of normal ACL strength) compares favorably with the calculated strength of a 9.5-mm (10-mm bone tunnel) patellar tendon graft (100 percent of normal ACL strength). The tensile strength of the semitendinosus and gracilis tendon tissue, in terms of load capacity *per unit cross-sectional area*, is almost twice that of patellar tendon tissue (Noyes et al, 1984); thus, considerable overall tensile strength can be packed into an osseous tunnel of limited diameter (6.5 to 7.5 mm). This permits precise, selective fiber region reconstruction and theoretically minimizes inhomogeneous loading within the graft caused by differential fiber length behavior within the graft as the knee moves through its range of motion. Harvesting the semitendinosus and gracilis tendons involves a minimum of operative morbidity, leaves the extensor mechanism undisturbed, and produces no detectable loss of leg strength in either knee flexion or internal tibial rotation (Lipscomb et al, 1982). Leaving the natural distal osseous attachments of these tendons intact provides satisfactory tibial fixation and avoids troublesome hardware irritation under the distal incision. My recent use of a double fold-over stapling technique (three staples, incorporating two 180-degree folds of the graft within a rectangular cancellous bed) on the femoral side has thus far allowed immediate postoperative weight bearing as tolerated, without any detectable loss of stability. Clinically, the long-term biologic fixation of this soft tissue graft has not been observably different when compared with bone-block grafts.

Regardless of the type of ACL autograft or allograft employed, there is a theoretical place for the use of a ligament augmentation device (LAD) (Roth et al, 1985) to reinforce the waning tensile strength of the graft at or later than 4 weeks after surgery, when the patient is beginning to resume normal daily activities with only a brace for support. Owing to United States governmental restrictions regarding the use of the current, commercially available polypropylene LAD, since 1986 I have empirically employed six heavy strands of nonabsorbable suture (three woven into each tendon) for graft augmentation. No known complications have resulted. From a biologic standpoint, this technique should be no different than open primary repairs of the ACL with nonabsorbable suture material. The mechanical efficacy of this particular technique, however, has not been evaluated in any controlled studies.

SURGICAL TECHNIQUE

The technique described here represents my currently preferred method of arthroscopically assisted ACL reconstruction. Although the choice of available drill guide instruments and the means of performing intraoperative "isometry" testing (if this is desired) necessarily create variations in technique, the basic steps are generally similar for all methods employing tibial and femoral bone tunnels. The addition of a supplemental lateral extra-articular procedure is considered optional, in accordance with the preference of the surgeon. I generally do not employ lateral, extra-articular "back-up" procedures for simple anterolateral rotatory instability, but will perform a supplemental posteromedial capsular reefing and gastrocnemius-semimembranosus tenodesis for patients exhibiting significant chronic anteromedial rotatory instability.

To obtain a consistently high degree of surgical precision and accuracy in the intra-articular placement of the tendon grafts, intraoperative "isometry" testing is quite helpful (Graf, 1987b). I employ a drill guide system that combines the technical capabilities of drill guide instruments with those of an isometer gauge system, to allow the performance of intraoperative isometry testing without the need to drill pilot holes in the tibia or femur (Graf, 1987b) (Kinemetric Drill Guide System, Dyonics, Inc., Andover, MA). This permits the testing of as many prospective bone tunnel sites as needed to achieve ideal graft placement, with little time expenditure, before any guide pin placement or tunnel drilling.

All required arthroscopic meniscus–articular surface work is generally completed before the intra-articular reconstruction is begun. Tourniquet use is minimized. With adequate joint distention, tourniquet inflation can generally be avoided whenever

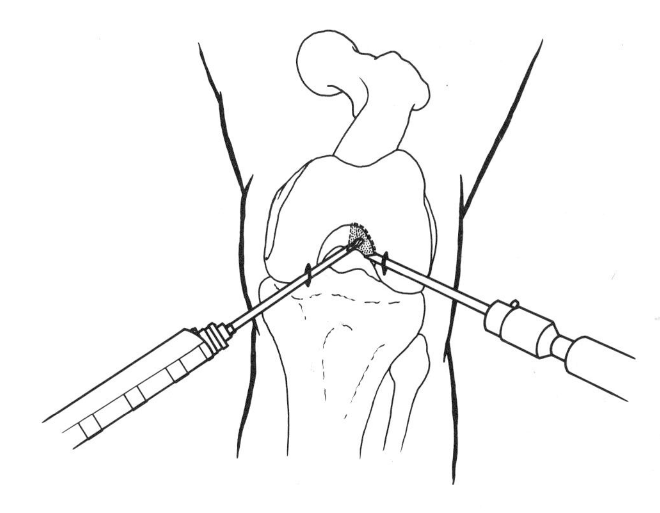

Figure 4 Using anterolateral and inferomedial portals, clearance of obstructive ACL remnants followed by widening of the intercondylar notch ("notchplasty") is performed with a high-speed resector and/or burr. (Reproduced with permission from ACL Drill Guide Instructional Manual. Andover, MA: Dyonics, Inc.)

the arthroscope is in use. Only two portals are required for the procedure, a low anteromedial (inferomedial) portal and an anterolateral portal. The use of a suprapatellar medial or lateral portal for placement of an inflow cannula is helpful, but optional.

Intercondylar notch preparation begins with clearance of soft tissue scar and obstructive anterior cruciate remnants, followed by intercondylar notch widening ("notchplasty") with a high-speed motorized burr or resector (Fig. 4). The degree of widening needed depends on the degree of intercondylar notch stenosis secondary to the cruciate insufficiency, if chronic. Good visualization and clearance for ACL substitute placement must be obtained, from the anterior inlet of the intercondylar notch to its posterior outlet, directly adjacent to the "over-the-top" position.

A 1½-inch extra-articular incision is made over the tibial insertion of the semitendinosus and gracilis tendons. These are identified and detached proximally at their musculotendinous junction in a closed fashion with a tendon stripper. The distal tibial insertions are left intact. A 2- to 2½-inch lateral extra-articular incision is made to expose the metaphyseal flare of the femur. Both incisions serve as drill guide access points and external bone tunnel exit sites.

The drill guide–isometer gauge system is set up as shown in Figure 5. Maintaining the arthroscope in the lateral portal, the tips of the drill guides' aimer arms are initially positioned by visual judgment into what appear to be the areas of greatest isometry, corresponding to the anatomic attachment areas of the ACL's anteromedial fibers. The femoral guide employs a posterior, "over-the-top" approach for the introduction of its aimer arm. The tibial guide has a cannulated aimer arm, through which passes a heavy monofilament suture that spans the intra-articular distance between both aimer arm tips. It is tied to the femoral aimer tip and slides freely in and out of the tibial aimer arm tip as the distance between these two tips changes with knee motion. Within the body of the tibial guide, the suture is fixed to a spring-loaded "isometer" (suture excursion) gauge, which registers the changes in intra-articular suture length on an external read-out scale.

The knee is then passively flexed to at least 100 degrees and brought back out to full extension (see Fig. 5). The changes in read-out scale position followed by the suture excursion marker indicate, in millimeters, the changes in linear distance between the tips of the tibial and femoral aimer arms (prospective bone tunnel sites) as the knee is brought through its range of motion. If the initially selected sites on the tibia and femur yield what is thought to be an optimal separation distance profile through the range of motion, the intra-articular tips of the guide's aimer arms are left in place and 3/32-inch guide pins are drilled (from outside to inside) through the guide pin sleeves clamped to the tibia and femur.

If the excursion profile yielded by the gauge indicates that a nonoptimal or unacceptable graft

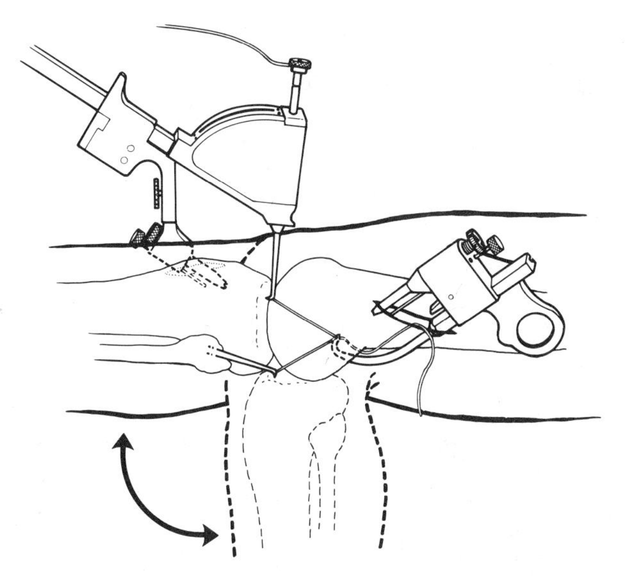

Figure 5 The drill guide–isometer instrument system used by the author. Operative isometry testing is performed with both guides in place, without the use of any pilot bone tunnels. The isometer gauge is located within the body of the tibial drill guide; it measures the changes in length of the segment of suture in between the two guide arm tips as the knee is passively brought through a range of motion. (Reproduced with permission from ACL Drill Guide Instructional Manual. Andover, MA: Dyonics, Inc.)

length change profile would be provided by the tibiofemoral points selected, either the femoral or tibial guides may be unclamped and their aimer arm tips maneuvered to a different site on the femur or tibia. The testing process is then repeated as described above. This is continued until the optimal tibial and femoral points are found. When the tibial aimer arm is properly positioned at the anteromedial fiber insertion area, an isometer gauge reading that indicates only aimer arm tip *separation* as the knee is flexed generally indicates that the femoral aimer arm has been positioned "anterior" (arthroscopist's perspective) to the normal attachment site of the anteromedial fibers. A gauge reading that demonstrates *only* aimer tip *approximation* with knee flexion, with *no reseparation* back toward the starting distance by 100 degrees of flexion, generally indicates that the femoral aimer arm has been positioned "posterior" (arthroscopist's perspective) to the anatomic anteromedial fiber insertion area.

Under simulated intraoperative isometry testing conditions, cadaver studies have shown that the anatomic centers of the anteromedial fiber region's osseous insertion areas naturally exhibit a small (1.5 to 3-mm) deviation from true isometry, demonstrating a characteristic pattern of decreasing tibiofemoral distance from zero to 30 degrees of flexion, followed by reseparation with further flexion through 120 degrees (Sapega et al, 1988, 1989). The anatomic central and posterior fiber attachment sites demonstrate somewhat similar patterns but with a greater deviation from isometry (Sapega et al, 1988, 1989). Although the ideal suture excursion gauge measurement to search for intraoperatively has not yet been definitively established, I believe that deviations from true isometry greater than 1.5 mm should be evaluated in terms of their *pattern* (i.e., directions) of change in tibiofemoral distance over the range of motion. If sites demonstrating absolute changes of 1.5 mm or less cannot be found, deviations from isometry up to 3 mm should prove acceptable as long as the directional profile of the deviation follows a relatively anatomic (or what might be termed a "physiometric") pattern.

Once the final tibiofemoral tunnel sites are selected and the guide pins drilled, the latter will be seen to exit the tibia and femur at intra-articular locations that either match, or are slightly offset from, the points occupied by the tips of the tibial and femoral aimer arms. This will depend on whether or not the drill guides were preset to provide an intentional guide pin offset (see below). The drill guides are removed and the guide pins are then overreamed with an appropriately sized cannulated bone drill. The internal entrances of the bone tunnels are meticulously radiused with an internal radiusing tool or arthroscopic bone tunnel rasps.

The tendon grafts are drawn up the tibial bone tunnel, across the joint, and out of the femoral tunnel. With tension placed on the grafts external to the femoral tunnel, the knee is brought through a range of motion while the degree and pattern of tendon excursion in and out of the femoral tunnel are observed externally. This should match the isometer gauge reading obtained just before the guide pins were drilled.

The intra-articular span of the graft is observed arthroscopically while the knee is brought through a full range of motion. It must be seen that no impingement of the graft by the roof of the intercondylar notch occurs in knee extension, and that no significant lateral (notch) wall contact abrasion occurs during knee motion. If either of these phenomena is observed, supplementary notch clearance is performed.

With firm manual tension on the grafts, they are fixed to the femur by the previously described stapling technique. The knee joint angle selected for graft tensioning and fixation depends on the graft excursion profile observed, as described above. With a perfectly isometric graft, the joint angle does not matter. With a "physiometric" graft length profile, i.e., one that matches the normal, slight deviation from isometry exhibited by the anteromedial fibers, a joint angle of 80 to 90 degrees of flexion is generally selected. This allows full knee extension without excessive graft tension.

Standard wound closure procedures are followed. Drains usually are not needed. A sterile electrical muscle stimulation electrode is placed over the distal vastus medialis, followed by application of a compression dressing. A long-leg rehabilitation brace is applied, its hinges generally set to allow joint motion from 20 to 90 degrees of flexion.

ECCENTRIC (OFFSET) GUIDE PIN PLACEMENT

As originally observed by Clancy and colleagues (1982), ACL substitutes tend to lean toward the leading edges of their intra-articular bone tunnel entrances, producing an undesired shift in the effective fixation points of the graft. This effect is magnified when a radius is put on the tunnel entrance to minimize graft abrasion (Fig. 6). Tests in my laboratory using simulated bone tunnels and a variety of actual fresh tendon preparations have indicated that the degree of this graft shift error depends on the relative match between graft and tunnel diameters; well-fitted cylindric grafts shift the least and loosely fitted and/or flat (e.g., patellar tendon) grafts shift the most (Fig. 7). Special corrective graft positioning within the bone tunnel is often possible with bone-block grafts, but otherwise one or both of the bone tunnels must be drilled in a slightly offset or eccentric location to the desired graft center points, to compensate for this error (Clancy et al, 1982).

The drill guide system that I employ provides for a variable degree of eccentric guide pin (tunnel

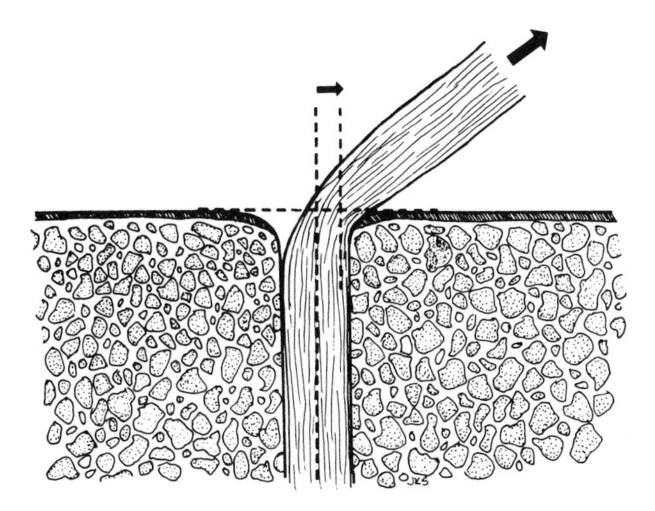

Figure 6 Schematic illustration of how the central fiber of a tendon graft shifts off center at an intra-articular bone tunnel entrance. (Reproduced with permission from ACL Drill Guide Instructional Manual. Andover, MA: Dyonics, Inc.)

center) placement. A 3-mm offset is selected for the semitendinosus-gracilis graft. The orientation of the tibial guide's aimer arm, when positioned properly in the knee through the inferomedial portal, provides that its offset is in the desired anteromedial direction (Clancy et al, 1982). When the femoral guide is properly placed in the knee, its orientation provides that its offset is in the "posterior" (arthroscopist's perspective) direction. No superior offset (toward the middle of the roof of the notch) is

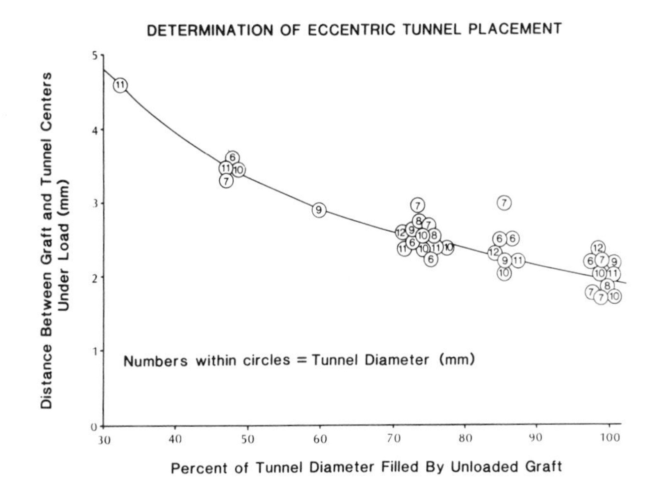

Figure 7 Graph of measured off-center tendon shift versus the relative size match between the graft and its tunnel. The more snugly a tendon graft is fitted in its tunnel, the less is the eccentric shift. The absolute tunnel diameter does not matter nearly as much as the relative fit of the graft within it.

provided because this only applies to the *flexed* knee position, and tends to reverse itself in extension. In contrast, the posterior offset is applicable through the greater part of the functional range of knee motion.

POSTOPERATIVE REGIMEN

Electrical muscle stimulation (2 hours per day) and active range-of-motion exercise is begun within 72 hours. If no chondroplastic or meniscal repair work has been performed, weight bearing and careful ambulation are allowed as tolerated. Transfer from the long-leg rehabilitation brace to a functional ACL brace, stationary bike exercise, and isokinetic quadriceps work (limit, 30 degrees from full extension and using an "antishear" device) are generally instituted by the end of the third postoperative week. The rehabilitation regimen becomes progressively more active over time, straight running being allowed at 6 months and return to sport at 10 months.

REFERENCES

Arms SW, Pope MH, Johnson RJ, et al. The biomechanics of anterior cruciate ligament rehabilitation and reconstruction. Am J Sports Med 1984; 12:8–18.

Clancy WG, Nelson DA, Reider B, et al. Anterior cruciate ligament reconstruction using one-third of the patellar ligament. J Bone Joint Surg 1982; 64A:352–359.

Girgis FG, Marshall JL, Al-Monagem ARS. The cruciate ligaments of the knee joint. Clin Orthop 1975; 106:216–231.

Graf B. Biomechanics of the anterior cruciate ligament. In: Jackson DW, Drez D, eds. The anterior cruciate deficient knee. St Louis: CV Mosby, 1987a:55.

Graf B. Isometric placement of substitutes for the anterior cruciate ligament. In: Jackson DW, Drez D, eds. The anterior cruciate deficient knee. St. Louis: CV Mosby, 1987b:102.

Hollis JM, Marcin JP, Horibe S, et al. Load determination in ACL fiber bundles under knee loading. Trans Orthop Res Soc 1988; 13:58.

Lipscomb AB, Johnston RK, Snyder RB, et al. Evaluation of hamstring strength following use of semitendinosus and gracilis tendons to reconstruct the anterior cruciate ligament. Am J Sports Med 1982; 10:340–342.

Noyes FR, Butler DL, Grood ES, et al. Biomechanical analysis of human ligament grafts used in knee-ligament repairs and reconstructions. J Bone Joint Surg 1984; 66A:344–352.

Odensten M, Gillquist J. Functional anatomy of the anterior cruciate ligament and a rationale for reconstruction. J Bone Joint Surg 1985; 67A:257–261.

Rosenberg TD, Rasmussen GL. The function of the anterior cruciate ligament during anterior drawer and Lachman's testing. Am J Sports Med 1984; 12:318–322.

Roth JH, Kennedy JC, Lockstadt H, et al. Polypropylene braid augmented and nonaugmented intra-articular anterior cruciate ligament reconstruction. Am J Sports Med 1985; 13: 321–336.

Sapega AA, Moyer RA, Schneck C, et al. Intraoperative "isometry" testing during anterior cruciate ligament reconstruction: anatomical and biomechanical considerations. Submitted for publication.

Sapega AA, Moyer RA, Schneck C, et al. The biomechanics of intra-operative "isometry" testing during anterior cruciate reconstruction. Trans Orthop Res Soc 1988; 13:130.

SYNTHETIC LIGAMENTOUS REPLACEMENT

FREDERICK C. BALDUINI, M.D.

Although in the past, it was generally believed that the long-term prognosis for anterior cruciate ligament insufficiency could be broken into thirds, with only one-third requiring replacement surgery, it now appears that perhaps only 25 percent of individuals can truly be classified as "cruciate-independent," with the remainder ultimately suffering recurrent episodes of buckling, meniscal damage, and the hastened development of articular chondral changes. As the orthopedic community has come to a better understanding of the critical function of this ligament as it relates to knee stability and meniscal preservation, the philosophy of dealing with its deficiency has changed. Credit goes to the many biomechanicians who have enlightened us about our errant conceptions.

THE ANTERIOR CRUCIATE LIGAMENT

If one is to synthesize and replace the anterior cruciate ligament (ACR), it seems only logical that the anatomy, biomechanics, and function of the normal structure be closely followed. Problems that are common to all the synthetics to be discussed include wear particle generation, stiffness, strength, and placement isometry.

Anatomy

Girgis et al and Norwood and Cross generally receive the credit for our present conception of the gross anatomy of the anterior cruciate ligament. Their findings of a structure composed of two integrated bands are generally accepted. These two bands, the anteromedial and posterolateral are named for their respective tibial insertions (Fig. 1).

The femoral attachment (the more critical of the two when reconstruction is involved) is on the medial aspect of the lateral femoral condyle. It is a semicircular arrangement inclined 25 degrees from the vertical axis of the femur. Its posterior-most attachment is approximately 4 mm from the "over-the-top" position of the posterior condyle (Fig. 2). The tibial insertion is noted to be slightly anterolateral to the medial tibial eminence, beginning 15 mm from the anterior tibial margin. The ligament extends 30 mm posteriorly from that point in an ovoid insertion (Fig. 3).

Difficulty arises when one attempts to simulate these insertion points with synthetics. The greatest problem that occurs is the abrasion that occurs around the femoral tunnel. This is partly due to the

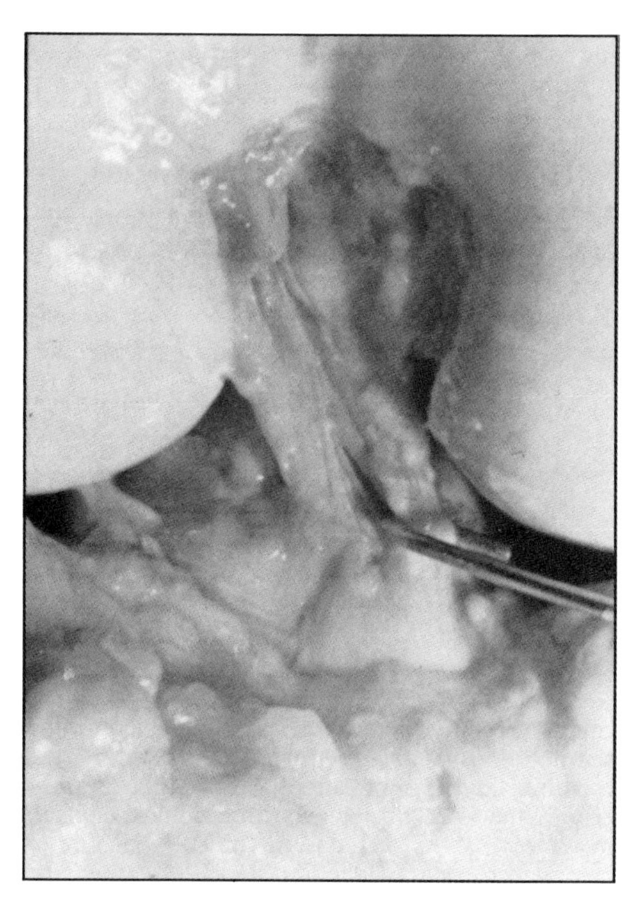

Figure 1 Anteromedial and posterolateral bands of ACL. (Republished with permission from Balduini FC, Clemow AJT, Lehman RC. Synthetic ligaments: scaffolds, stents, and prostheses. Thorofare, NJ: Slack, Inc., 1986:12.)

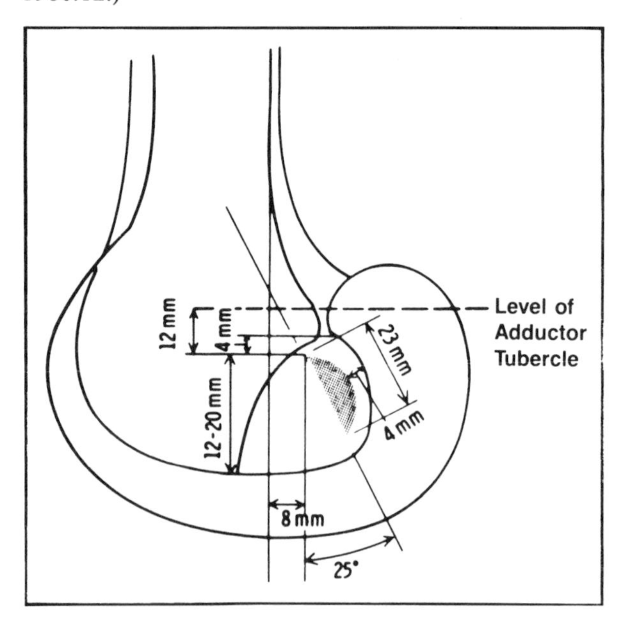

Figure 2 Femoral insertion of ACL. (Republished with permission from Balduini FC, Clemow AJT, Lehman RC. Synthetic ligaments: scaffolds, stents, and prostheses. Thorofare, NJ: Slack, Inc., 1986:11.)

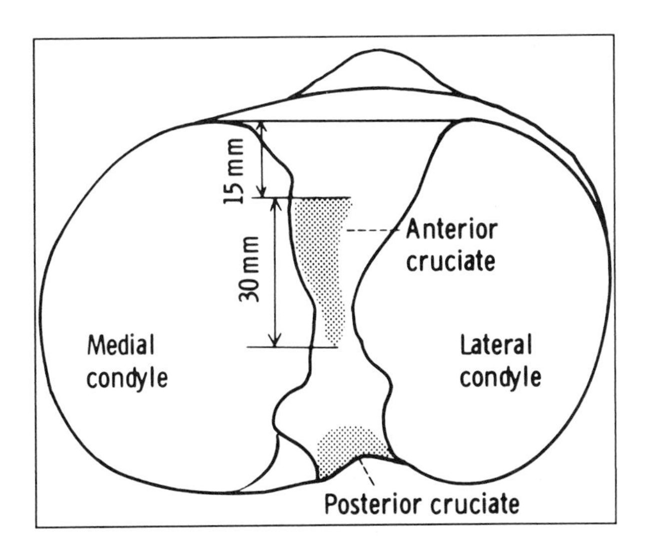

Figure 3 Tibial insertion of ACL. (Republished with permission from Balduini FC, Clemow AJT, Lehman RC. Synthetic ligaments: scaffolds, stents, and prostheses. Thorofare, NJ: Slack, Inc., 1986:10.)

TABLE 1 Relative Autogenous Tissue Strengths

	Noyes	*Kennedy*
Anterior cruciate	1,730 N	626 N
Patellar tendon-bone	2,900 N	589 N
Semitendinosus	1,300 N	473 N
Gracilis	847 N	449 N
ITB, 18 mm	657 N	834 N
ITB, 25 mm	920 N	N/A
Fascia lata, 16 mm	622 N	N/A
Fascia lata, 45 mm	1,760 N	N/A

Republished with permission from Balduini FC, Clemow AJT, Lehman RC. Synthetic ligaments: scaffolds, stents, and prostheses. Thorofare, NJ: Slack, Inc., 1986:21.

stiffness of the presently available synthetics and secondarily to the centrode of motion occurring at the femur. Because abrasion cannot be avoided when a bony femoral tunnel is chosen, in all devices but one the "over-the-top" femoral position for placement is used. This results in a stable knee during extension, but leads to a significant anterior displacement when the knee is subjected to stress in flexion.

Biomechanics

Because of the viscoelastic behavior of tissues, the ultimate strength to failure and failure mode of the ACL are dependent on strain rate. At lower strain rates, failure occurs by avulsion from bone, whereas at higher rates, midsubstance failure occurs, with this mode tending to correlate with clinical findings.

Noyes demonstrated ultimate failure of a bone-tendon-bone complex to be 1,725 Newtons (N) when strained at 100 percent per second; however, this was in individuals 16 to 25 years of age (Table 1). That strength dropped to 734 N in individuals older than 50 years of age. Noyes has further shown that the ACL elongates as much as 60 percent before ultimate failure, with microscopic failure and significant weakening commencing when elongation is greater than 10 percent, the upper limit of strain seen under physiologic loading. The strain at the yield point of the normal (where permanent plastic deformation occurs) is approximately 25 percent.

None of the synthetics have this viscoelastic behavior. Yield-point strains in the synthetics vary from a low of 1 to 5 percent in carbon and Gore-Tex to a maximum of 15 to 20 percent in the Stryker-Meadox and LAD devices. Whereas stiffness may impart a degree of strength, it also exposes the graft to a greater risk of failure due to bending and cyclic fatigue.

Particle Formation

It has been known virtually from the onset of synthetic material usage that wear particles are generated. The experience with Teflon in artificial hips and knees and the recent problems with silicone synovitis should serve as warnings about the potential problems that can develop. Olson and Fu deserve the credit for enlightening us as to the problems associated with wear particles generated by synthetic cruciate replacements (Fig. 4). Although their study does not report on the wear particle generation of autologous bone-tendon-bone preparations, it nonetheless serves as a guideline for awareness.

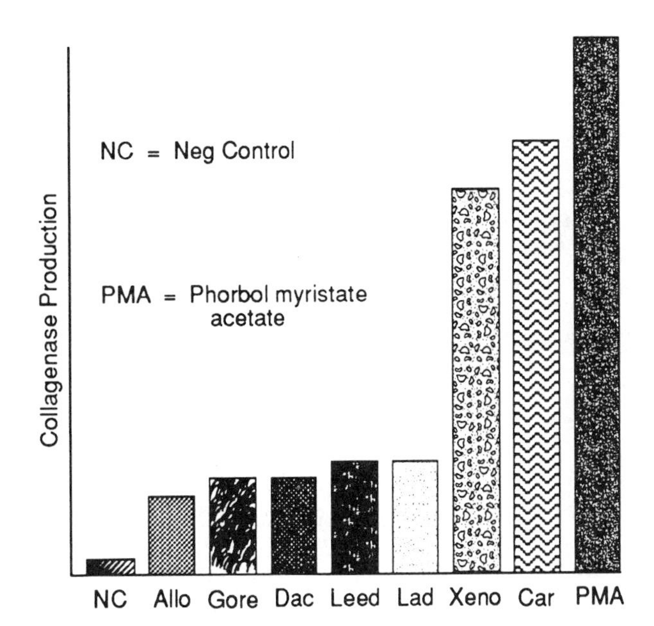

Figure 4 Enzyme production secondary to wear particle generation. (Adapted from Olsen.)

Furthermore, it is not yet known what level of collagenase is significant for cartilage degradation. Although any increase over a baseline level must be considered detrimental to the joint, the long-term effects of a minimal elevation are unknown. It may very well be that there is a greater collagenase activity associated with recurrent pivot-shifting than there is with some of the synthetic, allograft, or autologous materials.

THE SYNTHETICS

The ideal synthetic ligament should permanently restore all the functions of the normal ACL. However, there has not yet been any success in meeting this ideal. The problems associated with material failure, anatomic positioning, and abrasion are made painfully conspicuous each time another "synthetic" fails. Nonetheless, technology and techniques continue to evolve and presently there appear to be some reasonable substitutes. I say "appear to be" because sufficient time has not elapsed for the long-term results to be fully evaluated. In the past, one needed to wait only 2 to 3 years to know the dismal failure rate of some of the earlier devices. It is to the engineers' credit that the newer devices are lasting as long as they do.

Depending on their respective functions, the devices currently being tested and marketed can be divided into three basic groups: scaffolds, stents, and prostheses. Scaffolds are intended to act as a lattice framework upon which new fibroblasts and collagen can grow. Stents function by providing interval strength to tissue considered too weak to tolerate functional loads. They are intended to bear load while the autologous tissue has an opportunity to regenerate, revascularize, and strengthen. Prostheses are designed to be inherently strong and durable with no intention of neocollagenization.

Scaffolds

This represents the largest group of synthetic devices. The attractiveness of biologic ingrowth may well be why the industry has devoted much of its efforts here. The bulk of the devices are designed to fail mechanically after providing initial support for collagen ingrowth. At this time, research continues on the development of truly absorbable scaffolds, but as yet, none have been approved. The three scaffolds with the greatest clinical experience are Carbon (Integraft/Versigraft), Dacron (Leeds-Keio), and Dacron-Velour (Stryker-Meadox). Of these, only the Dacron-Velour graft has been recommended for approval by the FDA. Carbon approval in the United States has been rejected on more than one occasion and experience with the Leeds-Keio ligament has been confined abroad. The Xenotech bovine tendon was originally thought to act as a scaffold, and although initial studies appeared to show collagen ingrowth, closer examination has shown it to fail in that regard. It will therefore be considered as a prosthesis.

Carbon

No material has received as much attention nor generated as much controversy as carbon. Literally hundreds of articles have been written concerning its use, with the bulk of these being positively oriented. Nonetheless, it is the significant number of ambivalent and frankly negative articles that have provided fuel for the controversy.

The original work performed by Jenkins dealt with an uncoated carbon material. This device was extremely brittle and difficult to handle. As a result, there tended to be early breakage (mechanical degradation as some would prefer to call it) with the development of articular debris and synovial staining. Those flaws accepted, it did possess some desirable mechanical characteristics and proved to be nonimmunogenic.

In an effort to cope with the difficult handling characteristics of carbon, experimentation with biologic coatings led to the development of two devices. The first of these, Plastifil is a unidirectional device with 40,000 tow of carbon each possessing a strength of 0.15 N with an ultimate device strength of 600 N. The entire device is coated with gelatin to improve handling. Lafil is a braided device coated with either collagen or dura, once again, to protect the fragile carbon fibers. Presently, the most commonly used formulation utilizes a polymeric coating of polylactic acid and polycaprolactone. This polymer has been demonstrated to biodegrade at approximately the same rate that neocollagenization progresses, thereby protecting the carbon fibers until they are invested in a soft tissue coating.

The greatest concern with the use of carbon filament has been the finding of synovial staining, articular cartilage staining, and the presence in some animal studies of carbon particles in peripheral lymph nodes. Further criticism has revolved around the diversity of indications and techniques that were used in evaluating this device. Many times extra-articular reconstructions were combined with intra-articular substitution, making it difficult to compare results and assess the value of the device as an ACL adjunct alone.

Leeds-Keio

The Leeds-Keio ligament is a tubularized Dacron graft that has been used extensively in Europe and Japan (Fig. 5). One of the biggest attributes of the Leeds-Keio device is that it enables one to place the graft isometrically through femoral as well as tibial bone tunnels. The designers of this system have seemingly overcome the problems of femoral tunnel abrasion by providing a unique means of harvesting bone plugs which seat tightly into an ex-

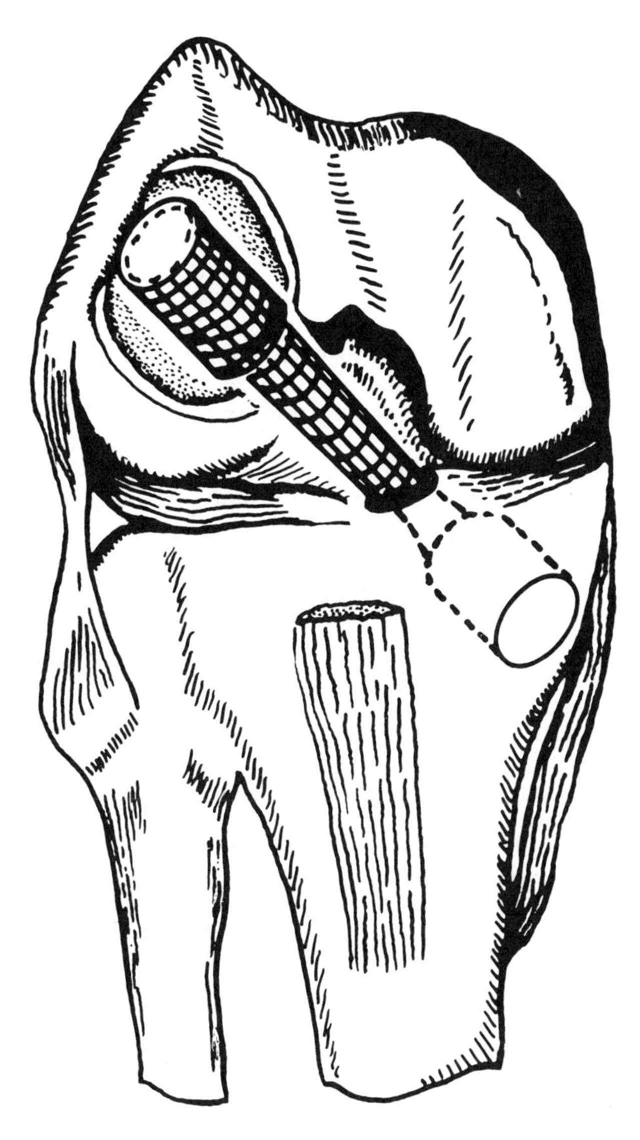

Figure 5 Concept of anchoring method for Leeds-Keio ligament.

panded pocket of the device, thereby minimizing graft abrasion.

The Leeds-Keio ligament possesses a 2,000-N strength to failure which approximates that of the normal ACL. Although it is intended to serve as a scaffold, inducing collagen ingrowth, the quality of this collagen must be suspect since because of the stress shielding that occurs as a function of the dual bony fixation, there was a 9 percent failure rate of the construct in the initial 80 intra-articular reconstructions. When an extra-articular extension of the graft was included in the reconstruction, the failure rate diminished to 1 percent.

Stryker-Meadox

The Stryker-Meadox graft evolved from the company's original Dacron graft designed for acromioclavicular reconstruction. That graft did not have enough strength to be used effectively as an intra-articular graft and was altered by the addition of four cross-beams, thereby increasing the strength and stiffness. Ultimate strength is 3,000 N. The Dacron portion of the graft is covered with velour to minimize abrasion and induce collagen ingrowth.

In a report on 58 patients followed for as long as 4 years, there was an improvement in both Lysholm scores and Tegner activity levels. However, there are also some alarming numbers in this initial report. There were seven graft failures during the initial 36 months, a far greater number than would be predicted based upon the cyclic failure testing performed. This represents a 12 percent early failure rate for the device. More worrisome is the significant increase in laxity over time, noted especially during the first 3 months after surgery. This could be caused by the technique of passing the graft in the "over-the-top" position and subsequent soft tissue adaptation or necrosis, or perhaps by the technique of stapling used to fix the graft to the bone. At 48 months, there was a return to the original laxity values, with a mean of 3 mm side to side difference. The authors (Giluist et al) justify this by stating that the normal side must be becoming more lax in order to have a mean of only 3mm. However, what has actually occurred is that the initial 2-mm initial post operative difference has been carried over to the longer-term follow-ups.

Stents

The only stent device presently approved by the FDA for use is the Kennedy Ligament Augmentation Device (LAD). This is a braided polypropylene device that is attached by nonabsorbable sutures to the patellar fascia harvested during a standard McIntosh reconstruction. It is intended to provide added strength to the otherwise weak patellar fascia and thereby reinforce the overall construct. Much like the Stryker-Meadox and Gore-Tex grafts, this device is also intended for an "over-the-top" positioning. In an effort to prevent stress shielding, it is attached to bone at one end only.

The mechanical characteristics of the graft reveal an ultimate strength of 1,700 N. This further supports the rationale for tethering the graft at one bone only.

The LAD has been studied in extensive experimentations with both humans and animals. Most of the animal studies were performed in goats. In these studies, several interesting biomechanical data came forth. The time-zero failure strengths were much lower than the failure strength of the graft itself, indicating failure at the graft-patellar fascia suture line. At 24 months postoperatively, there was a significant decrease in the strength of the nonaugmented reconstructions, which does not make sense in view of our present understanding of collagen maturation.

In the human studies, there are no biomechanical data for the obvious reasons. KT-1000 testing, pivot-shift tests, and subjective criteria have been evaluated in a series of 82 patients undergoing LAD augmentation and compared with those of a small "control" group of 12 patients with Eriksson "over-the-top" procedures. Results were generally good in the LAD group, with an improved overall function and reduced degree of swelling, although objective criteria such as Lachman's sign, pivot-shift, and KT-1000 were similar in the two groups.

Prostheses

Two devices head the list of prostheses: (1) Gore-Tex and (2) Xenotech (bovine ligament and tendon). Research continues in this area and there is one report on a Swiss polyethylene ligament.

Xenotech

As it became understood that many of the autologous tissues transplanted for ACL reconstruction functioned predominantly as scaffolds or lattice work for neocollagenization, it was only a matter of time before xenografts (similar tissues from different species) would be utilized—especially in view of the long-term success of porcine heart valves.

As with other xenograft material, the Xenotech bovine tissues were treated with glutaraldehyde for: antisepsis, reduction of immunogenicity, and the strengthening and stiffening caused by increased collagen cross-linking. For the purposes of preservation, the materials were shipped in vials bathed in a glutaraldehyde solution and were to be bathed for 30 minutes before implantation. Although the theory seemed good, there were problems with the xenografts from the outset.

Since the time of the last report (1985), more than 400 Xenotech implants have been used, 250 of which were for intra-articular ACL reconstructions. Early experiences revealed an unacceptably high complication rate, with 12 percent graft-related problems (synovitis or graft rupture), 5 percent infections, and 12 percent failure due to "nongraft-related" occurrences. Moreover, favorable clinical scores tended to decrease by 50 percent at the time of the 24-month follow-up (Fig. 6).

In studies designed to explain the high incidence of synovitis associated with usage of this particular device, Arnoczky demonstrated that the elution of deeply embedded glutaraldehyde as bony abrasion exposed the inner core of collagen. Glutaraldehyde has been shown to be highly toxic to synovial tissue and articular cartilage. With Xenotech, the grafts began to be subsequently bathed in saline when shipped, in an effort to reduce the concentration of glutaraldehyde, but the evolution of other synthetics and allografts ultimately led to the demise of xenografts for ACL substitution.

Gore-Tex

Gore-Tex has undergone the most intensive biomechanical, animal, and human investigation of all the prostheses and is second only to carbon in overall usage. As such, it has come under critical scrutiny and was approved by the FDA for general usage in 1986. However, there is a caveat: Gore-Tex is to be used only as a salvage device in knees where previous autologous reconstruction has failed. Gore-Tex should not be used for failed allografts and failed ACL staplings. In defense of Gore-Tex, the manufacturer has always reflected this policy in their instructional courses and continues to develop the product and instruct surgeons in its proper usage and surgical technique.

Gore-Tex is a braided polytetrafluorethylene (PTFE) device (Fig. 7). This material still concerns some surgeons because of its rather notorious failure when used in total hips and knees. It is constructed with a molded eyelet at each end for tibial and femoral bony fixation. It possesses an ultimate strength of 5,300 N, but has a bone pull-out strength closer to 2,000 N. It is considerably stiffer than the normal ACL, with a modulus of elasticity of 3,000 mPa. Projected lifetime is 6 times 10^8 cycles, with the average human knee being exposed to 4 times 10^6 cycles per year.

To date, the Gore-Tex graft has been implanted in more than 3,000 knees. As of January 1986, there have been 1,000 implanted in the United States alone. Results have been generally good, but not without compromise or complication. The overall complication rate as reported by H. Royer Collins in a 1986 study of 187 prostheses implanted between 1982 and 1984 revealed a device failure of 6 percent with infections in another 2.7 percent and sterile effusions in 5 percent. In the 1,000 patients, the overall complication rate was 14.3 percent with 4 percent of patients requiring graft removal.

The Gore-Tex graft is also designed to be placed in the "over-the-top" position. This is necessary because of its stiffness, which exposes it to the risk of abrasion when placed through acute femoral tunnels. The manufacturer has gone to the extent of developing special tools to facilitate this placement and further reduce the effects of abrasion. Because of this anatomic positioning, the graft must be placed and tensioned with the knee in extension. As a consequence, the knee tends to display laxity in flexion with a proportionately greater anterior drawer test than Lachman's sign.

When one looks at Collins's favorable data on the results of Lachman's sign and anterior drawer testing, it should be understood that 72 of 187 intra-articular substitutions were also accompanied by extra-articular procedures. It is generally accepted and understood that an "over-the-top" position—whether Gore-Tex, Stryker-Meadox, or LAD—results in clinical and sometimes functional laxity in

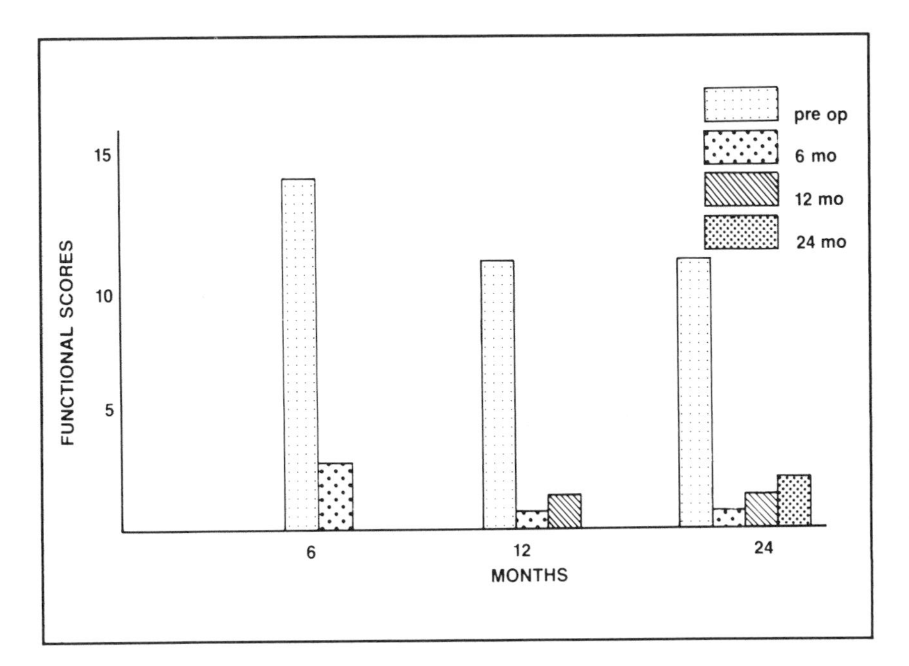

Figure 6 Functional results after Xenograft reconstruction. (Republished with permission from Balduini FC, Clemow AJT, Lehman RC. Synthetic ligaments: scaffolds, stents, and prostheses. Thorofare, NJ: Slack, Inc., 1986:46.)

flexion. With Gore-Tex, in which case the device is intended for salvage use only, this appears to be an acceptable shortcoming.

Allografts and Absorbables

Although allografts do not fall into the category of "synthetics," a brief mention is deserved. It now appears that allografts will provide a tissue capable of acting as an isometric, intra-articular scaffold of high-strength, without some of the problems inherent to the synthetics. Early use of allografts met with poor results, which have been traced to the use of freeze-drying and ethylene oxide sterilization (the latter performed to minimize disease transfer). More recent reports in which sterile harvesting and fresh frozen allograft have been used appear favorable. Yet no long-term studies of this technique exist, and there is still the stigma of potential vial transfer, despite testing.

Rodkey has discussed the merits of absorbable scaffolds and has provided insight into some of the early failures. Nonetheless, this still seems to be an ideal technique by which the temporary strength during the period of neocollagenization could be provided by an absorbable device. A further benefit of this type of device would be the potential graduated stress-sharing that would occur during reabsorption. Investigation continues in this area, and it is hoped that these materials will be forthcoming shortly.

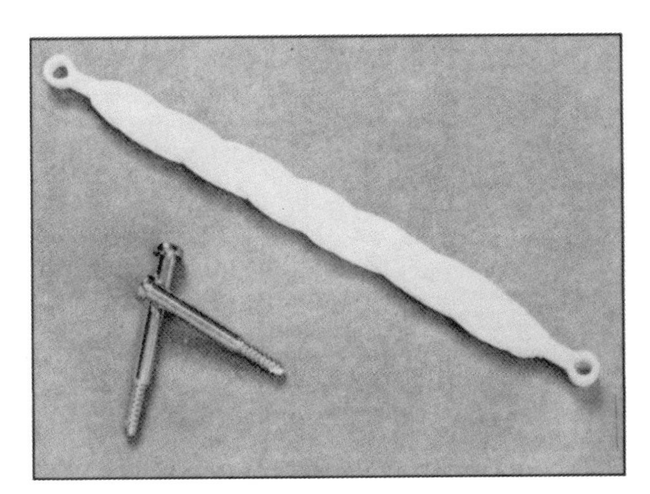

Figure 7 Gore-Tex prosthetic ligament. (Republished with permission from Balduini FC, Clemow AJT, Lehman RC. Synthetic ligaments: scaffolds, stents, and prostheses. Thorofare, NJ: Slack, Inc., 1986:60.)

SUGGESTED READING

Arnoczky S. Presented—University of Pennsylvania, 1985.
Bhate AP, et al. Visoelastic characterization of Stryker-Dacron ligament prosthesis. Presented at Advances in cruciate ligament reconstruction of the knee. Palm Springs, FL, 1988.
Bolton CW, et al. The Gore-Tex expanded polytetrafluoroethylene prosthetic ligament: an in vitro and in vivo evaluation. CORR 1985; 196:202.
Chen EH, Black J. Materials design analysis of the prosthetic anterior cruciate ligament. J Biomed Mater Res 1980; 14:567.
Claes L, Neugebauer R. Investigation of long-term behavior and fatigue strength of carbon fiber ligament replacement. CORR 1985; 196:77.
Collins HR. Clinical results of Gore-Tex implantation. Presented at Advances in cruciate ligament reconstruction of the knee. Palm Springs, FL, 1985.
Fowler P. Braided polypropylene as an augmentation device. Presented at Advances in cruciate ligament reconstruction of the knee. Palm Springs, FL, 1988.

Fujikawa K. Clinical study on ACL reconstructions with the Leeds-Keio artificial ligament. Presented at Advances in cruciate ligament reconstruction of the knee. Palm Springs, FL, 1988.

Giluist J. Presented at Advances in cruciate ligament reconstruction of the knee. Palm Springs, FL, 1988.

Girgis FG, et al. The cruciate ligaments of the knee joint. CORR 1975; 106:216.

Indelicato P. Presented at Joint Meeting, New York, New Jersey, and Pennsylvania Orthopaedic Societies. Aruba 1988.

Jenkins DHR. The repair of cruciate ligaments with flexible carbon fiber. J Bone Joint Surg 1978; 60B:520.

McMaster WC, et al. Properties and clinical applications of bioprosthetic tendons and ligaments. Presented at Prosthetic ligament reconstructions of the knee. Palm Springs, FL, 1985.

McPherson GK, et al. Experimental mechanical and histological evaluation of the Kennedy Ligament Augmentation Device. CORR 1985; 196:186.

Mendes DG, et al. Histologic pattern of biomechanical properties of the carbon fiber-augmented ligament tendon: a laboratory and clinical study. CORR 1985; 196:51.

Norwood LA, Cross MJ. Anterior cruciate ligament: functional anatomy of its bundles in rotatory instabilities. Am J Sports Med 1979; 7:23.

Noyes FR, et al. Biomechanics of anterior cruciate ligament failure: an analysis of strain-rate sensitivity and mechanism of failure rates in primates. J Bone Joint Surg 1974; 56A:236.

Olson EG, et al. Wear particles in artificial ligament surgery. Presented at Advances in cruciate ligament reconstruction of the knee. Palm Springs, FL, 1988.

Rodkey WG. Laboratory studies of biodegradable materials for cruciate ligament reconstruction. In: *The crucial ligaments.* New York: Churchill Livingstone, 1988:535.

Roth JG, et al. Polypropylene brain augmented and nonaugmented intra-articular anterior cruciate ligament reconstruction. Am J Sports Med 1985; 12:321.

Seedhom BB, et al. The Leeds-Keio artificial ligament for replacement of the cruciate. Inst Mech Eng 1984; 200:99.

Weiss AB, et al. Ligament replacement with an absorbable copolyman carbon fiber scaffold: early clinical experience. CORR 1985; 196:77.

THIGH, HIP, AND PELVIS

SOFT TISSUE INJURY TO THE HIP AND THIGH

CHARLES R. BULL, M.D., B.Sc. (Med), F.R.C.S.(C), F.A.C.S., F.I.C.S.

HEMATOMAS

In hockey the missed hip check resulting in a thrust of the knee at a fleeting opponent can often inflict an unpenalized and unrecognized serious injury. The blow taken on the central lateral midthigh area produces a hematoma with moderate initial pain. The injured player is often able to continue to participate and in so doing effectively pumps more blood into the hematoma. He can even take an additional injury, compounding the problem. Then, after the 10-minute intermission, he is unable to walk or skate. Untreated, this injury may lead to the complication of myositis ossificans, which may leave the individual sidelined with a partially mobile knee for as long as 1 year in some cases.

Initial Management

The measures that constitute immediate local management—RICE (spelled by the first letter of each measure)—are as follows:

1. *Rest* (R) with the leg on a bench or on pillows at 90-90-degree position of hip and knees. The important thing is to have the foot elevated well above the heart.
2. *Ice pack* (I) in a towel over the hematoma, on the area of maximal pain because there is not usually any bruising initially. The ice pack should be removed every 20 minutes for 20 minutes and then reapplied (20 minutes on, 20 minutes off), and continued to a lesser extent for at least 72 hours. *Do not apply heat.*
3. *Compression* (C) with two or three 6-inch, tightly applied tensor bandages. Be careful not to compromise the circulation; monitor the circulation by checking the peripheral pulses frequently. Just elevate the leg. Do not massage it or otherwise exercise it.
4. *Elevation* (E), with the foot elevated well above the heart, for 72 hours. The patient should remain totally off the feet for this period.

Medications

The use of Papase (*Carica papaya* enzymes) has never been proved effectual and should be abandoned.

Anti-inflammatory medications should be given as early as possible, particularly within the first 24 hours, to reduce the swelling and muscle spasm. The antiprostaglandins, such as Anaprox (naproxen sodium), are probably the most effective preparations—two tablets immediately and then one tablet three times daily for 7 to 10 days. Antiprostaglandins are recommended because a large amount of prostaglandin is released immediately at the time of injury, and this is a major factor in causing the initial swelling. Muscle relaxants do not work and theoretically can cause more bleeding in the relaxed muscle. (Alcohol is also contraindicated for the same reason.)

The most important initial management is recognition of the serious nature of the problem. Thus, rest, crutches, bed rest, ice, and elevation should be followed by a surgical assessment.

An initial soft tissue radiograph delineates a hematoma in one-third of the cases and is worthwhile. One should probably try to grade these hematomas as first, second, and third degree, as determined by pain, lack of mobility, degree of swelling, and response to rest.

First- and second-degree hematomas permit 90-degree movement and straight leg raising. Third-degree hematomas restrict movement to less than 90 degrees and permit *active* knee flexion, but not straight leg raising. These patients have severe pain in spite of medication and should be hospitalized.

The very serious third-degree injuries usually are fairly obvious. There is severe pain, immobility of the knee in particular, as well as the hip, and swelling that increases by 1½ to 2 inches (4 to 5 cm) the girth of the quadriceps by actual measurement. A very tense, large swollen area, 6 to 8 inches in diameter (15 to 20 cm), can often be felt bulging beneath the fascia lata. It feels "different," not truly fluctuant but much tenser than normal muscle, and there is often an associated large, tense synovial effusion in the knee. This can be mistaken for an intrinsic knee problem, but is actually a sympathetic response and the knee itself is normal.

Wydase (hyaluronidase), steroids, or local anesthetics have been injected into these hematomas in the first 72 hours, but this practice is contraindicated because of (1) increased tendency to infection and (2) their alteration of the defense mechanism and production of collagen fibers, which in essence would delay healing rather than enhance it.

At 72 hours the repair stage starts, and patients with first-degree hematoma should be fairly comfortable. Some swelling is noted, but there should be moderately good mobility and, at this stage, fairly extensive bruising in the classic cases.

The muscle fibers are crushed or torn and the hematoma can be very extensive. The most frequent problem is an *inter*stitial or *inter*muscular hematoma in which the muscle sheath ruptures and the blood and bruising tracks up or down the leg. These are the "good ones," although they do look bad because of extensive bruising.

The "bad ones" are the *intra*muscular hematomas, in which the muscle sheath remains intact and thus the hematoma remains isolated. Absorption is much more difficult. In these cases the periosteum also is often damaged and osteoblasts become available to convert the subperiosteal or intramuscular hematomas into myositis ossificans.

Physiotherapy can push the "good ones" (intermuscular), but the "bad ones" have to rest to prevent further bleeding and enlargement of the hematomas. Cool whirlpool, range-of-motion exercises, light cycling, light weights, springs and pulleys, and early walking progressing to light jogging and early skating can be instituted in the good ones.

The third-degree injuries are worse at the end of 72 hours, with unremitting severe pain and increasing immobility, and these should be operated on. Under general anesthesia, a satisfactory 4-inch (10-cm) incision is made laterally through the fascia lata. Careful probing with a Kelly hemostat is then undertaken, and as soon as blood and clot are released the incision is opened more widely by blunt dissection.

The hematoma usually lies right on top of the bone and can be evacuated and completely removed with the assistance of copious irrigation with gentamicin sulfate (Garamycin) solution. The fascia lata, the subcutaneous tissue, and the skin are then closed and a Jones bandage is applied from toes to groin. Once the clot has been evacuated, treatment can be the same as for a first-degree injury over the next 7 to 10 days—physiotherapy, ice, sound, progressing to range of motion, but no massage.

Second-degree injuries are puzzling, but when in doubt they should be treated as third-degree injuries. A long 16- or 14-gauge needle introduced into the hematoma in an attempt to aspirate blood seems a sensible procedure, but is not. It is usually hard to find the exact fluctuant area, and often the clot cannot be aspirated. Furthermore, the needle is likely to introduce an infection; once the hematoma is infected, a systemic problem exists, requiring surgical drainage and systemic antibiotics and increasing the danger of long-term complications. Therefore, the hematoma is either decompressed satisfactorily in the operating room or treated conservatively.

A missed third-degree injury may come to light at the 7- to 10-day mark, as indicated by a swollen painful thigh and an immobile hip and knee. These injuries are often treated with hot baths and are the most likely to develop into myositis ossificans.

I still surgically explore these on occasion. I also prescribe physiotherapy to try to mobilize these people with gentle pool therapy, ultrasonography, and management to decrease the swelling, but again no massage, no faradism to stimulate the muscle or increase bleeding, and no isokinetic or isotonic weight program.

The first radiologic signs of ossification, the typical "sandstorm" appearance, are visible about 3 weeks after the injury. As this matures, an anvil-shaped lesion appears. The full-blown myositis ossificans, verified radiographically (Fig. 1), needs no treatment other than rest. Swimming and cycling are permitted, but no running, skating, and the like.

It can take up to 6, even 12, months for this problem to settle completely. I never operate on a fully developed myositis ossificans (fully calcified) because the ossification tends to recur.

The fully developed quiescent case of myositis ossificans allows a normal return to unlimited sports.

Prevention consists of

1. *Better conditioning* to avoid the missed hip check.
2. *Better warm-ups.*
3. *Stretching exercises* starting from the neck and working down literally to the Achilles tendon, feet, and toes. These form part of the basis of a sensible warm-up program.
4. *Equipment* that fits properly; this should be used even during light practice. The Cooperall reduces hematomas because of its uniform fit and total body padding (Fig. 2).
5. *Following the rules.* Kneeing, spearing, and crosschecking rules all have to be enforced by the coach as well as the referee.
6. *Protective taping or adhesive,* tensor bandage, or bracing. This is beneficial on a weakened joint or limb. In current use are "pro" type neoprene sleeves

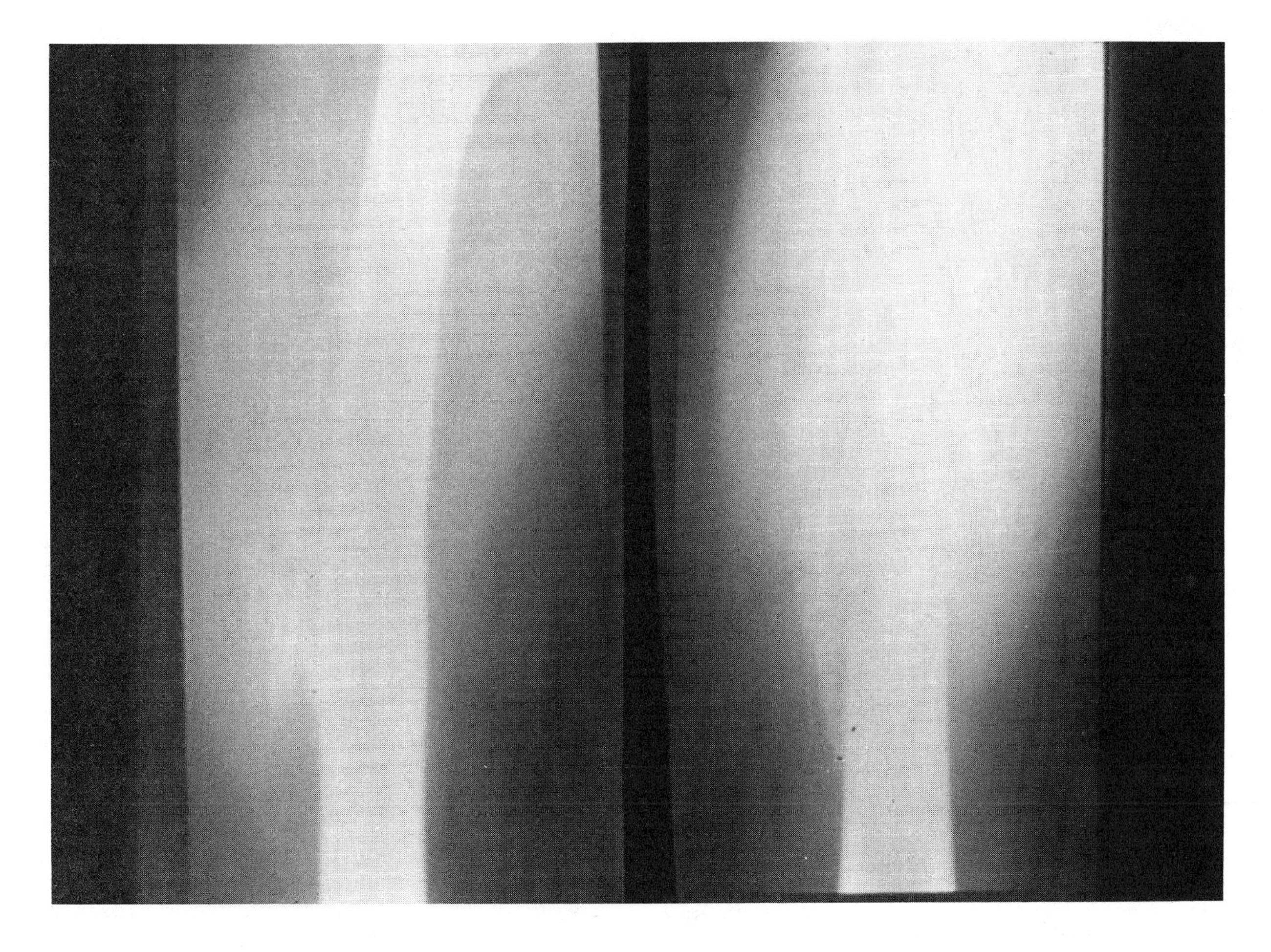

Figure 1 Myositis ossificans subsequent to thigh hematoma.

or even pantaloon leg sleeves, for thigh hematomas in particular, which are effective but expensive.

7. *Cautious return.* Beware of further trauma. Basically, the player can skate in a straight line at first, but must not push, twist, or pivot; gradually he progresses to these activities as strength returns.

8. *Caution regarding massage.* Trainers, physiotherapists, and masseurs must be very careful in the active phase not to prolong or initiate bleeding or augment tissue damage.

9. *Avoiding other methods* of treatment. Ethylchloride spray (which is probably of no benefit), analgesic balm, and DMSO are contraindicated as they only remove the pain. Pressure or trigger point injection, acupuncture, and TNS Probe are advocated by some and may have some benefit, although to date this has not been proved.

10. *Strengthening.* After severe injury it takes at least 6 weeks to get into the remodeling phase with additional strength. This can be graded clinically from 1 to 6 by the physiotherapist or physician, but it is more realistically graded by Cybex isokinetic equipment. This gives a computerized assessment of the exact strength deficiency and compares it with the opposite leg, as well as quadriceps to hamstrings and fast-twitch to slow-twitch muscle strength. In our clinics, results of these Cybex tests should be 90 percent of normal before the patient returns to the sport.

11. *Additional overall strength training.* Isokinetic training is best, and in the case of the thigh it should be not only the gastrocnemius and hamstrings, but also the adductors and abductors, evertors and invertors with stereotactic training (jumping over sticks or boxes), and thus the athlete is less apt to restrain the injured limb. This is different from conventional weight training, which is strictly isotonic. The isokinetic strengthening also develops the fast-twitch fibers and creates more overall strength in the limb. This type of training has not been emphasized enough in the past.

HIP POINTERS

Hip pointers are more likely to be self-inflicted by a fall into the boards or goalpost or, less often, a hard crosscheck, in lacrosse for instance. Specifically, a collection of blood forms beneath the periosteum in the area adjacent to the iliac crest, and involves the muscles and soft tissues above the crest.

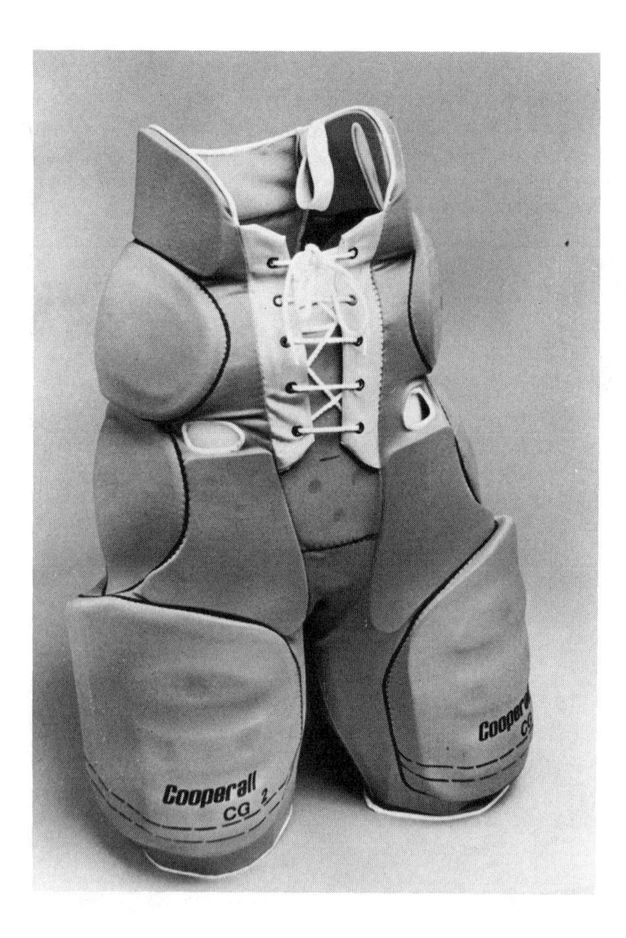

Figure 2 Protective equipment, such as the Cooperall, greatly reduces the incidence of thigh hematoma.

The hip pointer is a very painful localized swelling with significant localized bruising. However, it is never as serious on a long-term basis as the previously discussed hematomas.

Because long-term problems are very unusual, treatment can be a little less aggressive. However, the same principles apply: (1) RICE and (2) immediate physiotherapy with sound or interferential, no injections, and usually no operation.

X-ray studies should be performed to rule out a fracture or displaced epiphyseal fracture, which requires a much longer immobilization process (6 to 8 weeks). In an uncomplicated hip pointer, a large protective doughnut-type pad can be fashioned over the hip, and in many cases the player can return in 7 to 10 days, although I have known some to take as long as 2 months.

Better warm-up and conditioning are the best preventive measures, and better equipment (e.g., the Cooperall) is second in importance.

MUSCLE STRAINS

Muscle strains can result from indirect or direct injuries. Muscles commonly affected are antagonist or checking muscles, such as the hamstrings or adductors, and the condition can occur anywhere in the muscle tendon unit. It is most likely to affect the muscle origin or insertion, but a muscle tendinous junction, muscle belly, or tendon sheath can be involved.

The resultant inflammatory response (tendinitis), in the case of the adductors, causes the "pulled groin." Psoas and rectus muscle involvement are alternative forms of the "pulled groin." In the hamstrings the tendinitis-periostitis picture at the ischial tuberosity characterizes the "pulled ham."

The isolated inner-body muscle strain in the midportion of the hamstrings or adductors is usually more responsive to treatment, and with successful therapy athletes return to their sport in approximately half the time. The same principles of early recognition and caution regarding reaggravation apply. The cause is often some new stretching exercise or a sport or drill unrelated to the major sport, e.g., off-ice drills such as dancercize or running as an adjunct to hockey. The essential management is to stop the off-ice activities.

Physiotherapy is the key here, and a good physiotherapist (massage therapist) can initially decrease a lot of the muscle spasm. Then, a strong rehabilitation strengthening program with springs, pulleys, surgical tubing, stair stepping, and side stepping should be added. Progress in the final remodeling-strengthening phase through isokinetic equipment is very worthwhile. (The adductor-abductor machine, for instance, can be used for both speed and endurance.)

Aquabics or pool therapy—running in water, doing the alphabet in water, kicking in water—is quite worthwhile in early phases, but should be followed by a return to short-stride activities such as skating without stretching out the stride or slow running without lifting the leg. *Pain should be your guide,* and obviously anything that hurts should be avoided.

Muscle strains are endemic in quality runners, and are usually due to the drills. Hard interval training, such as repeat 50s, 100s, and 200s with unsatisfactory rest breaks, is the culprit. Many national sprinters warm up for 1 hour before doing their interval work.

The A and B drills, which require a hard goose-step kicking out very quickly, or a high-stepping, very quick knee elevation like that of a majorette, can cause these muscle strains and should be done only after a 20-minute basic warm-up, and deemphasized when any type of injury has been sustained.

These muscle and ligament strains can also be satisfactorily classified as first, second, and third degree. The first-degree strains, particularly in sprinters, are often just a type of muscle spasm or strain, and in some cases the sprinter can compete the same day. Calcium lack is a possible cause, and calcium (Sandoz, 4 ml or 1 teaspoon daily) is sometimes a good prophylactic medication.

The second-degree strain is usually an overuse, overtraining injury that can respond quickly to a training alleviation or alteration, e.g., substituting cycling and swimming for running.

The third-degree conditions give the athlete pain before, during, and after the sport. They interfere with lifestyle and everyday activities and are probably associated with a true tear in the muscle, muscle tendon junction, or insertion into the periosteum. Treatment consists of complete rest for as long as 6 to 8 weeks, and in cases of severe adductor or hamstring tendinitis, some quality athletes are kept away from sport as long as 3 to 6 months; running is prohibited, but judicious cycling and swimming are allowed.

Return to competition should be determined by leg strength. Cybex evaluation can indicate when drills such as cuts, pivots, figure-of-eights, hard striding, jumps, and full stretching work-outs can be resumed.

A person who is subject to repeated muscle strains needs to have the training schedule reevaluated. Some athletes experience a "true overuse syndrome," in which the resting pulse is elevated. They are agitated and restless, literally owing to total body exhaustion. They are prone to muscle strains and pulls.

Complete blood work, a zeta sedimentation rate (ZSR) and serum ferritin determination may show altered chemistry and should be repeated in athletes who are trying to "peak" and are not succeeding.

Principles

1. *It is hard to strain a hot muscle.* Therefore, warm up. Olympic sprinters warm up for more than 1 hour to run a 50- or 100-meter run.

2. *You cannot tire a young athlete.* Some of the tennis greats can run for half an hour, skip for half an hour, and play for half an hour before the match. A proper warm-up will not tire you; it enhances performance and prevents injuries.

3. *Sensible drills.* The only person who has to do Olympic weight training is an Olympic weight lifter. Thus, sensible drills to strengthen and tone up muscles with realistic weights—three sets of 10 or three sets of 30—are indicated. Isokinetic work-outs, beating the clock (for instance, 20 times in 20 seconds), are also good, but the muscle has to be exercised short of excess fatigue or exhaustion. There is no point in wearing out a muscle. The principle is to strengthen it.

4. *The best training is the sport itself.* Skating is for hockey players, gymnastics for gymnasts. They are most apt to get hurt in alternative sports or repetitive drills, e.g., repetitive jumping and dunking in basketball or running with ankle weights on.

5. *Routine medications and diet supplements.* Vitamin C is probably needed by individuals in hard training to improve the biochemical environment and regeneration of constantly strained muscles. Calcium can be used in certain cases to decrease muscle cramps. Emphasize a balanced diet, and no other regular medications or supplements are needed.

6. *Avoid muscle overload.* Strengthen muscles, reduce load, alter equipment, improve style.

7. *Chronic problems.* Heat before playing, aspirin before playing, massage with liniment, ultrasonography, whirlpool as necessary.

8. *Trigger points* for massage. Good athletic trainers can often remove some of the muscle knots and spasms before competition.

9. *Stretch throughout the day,* four times daily for 10 to 15 minutes, to keep muscles relaxed and in tone.

10. *Bone scans* can be used to elucidate the magnitude of the muscle-periosteal injury in some cases, but usually are not indicated.

11. *Other medications.* Spreading or dispersal agents and oral proteolytic enzymes are ineffective. Muscle relaxants usually have no place in muscle strains of the hip and just tire a young athlete. Local anesthesia to freeze the area of muscle strain or spasm to allow the athlete to play is too risky. It is almost guaranteed to increase the injury (to convert a first-degree to a third-degree injury).

12. *Steroids.* Local steroids can be used if there is an isolated trigger point or a localized point, such as the adductor tendon origin strain. The steroids are then injected around the pubic tubercle and cautiously instilled beneath the spermatic cord. Steroids should not be introduced into the tendon itself or into the cord, but injected judiciously along the periosteum with a small 25-gauge needle. This can be done in resistant cases and repeated on three occasions 1 month apart. This must be augmented by physiotherapy. Oral steroids basically are never used in my practice. Topical agents are ineffectual. However, some benefit may be derived from iontophoresis with 5 percent hydrocortisone cream and 5 amps of electronic stimulation placed over a gauze pad for 20 minutes, administered at 2-day intervals.

13. *Anabolics.* Oral anabolics are considered to have some effect in the healing of a torn muscle, but they are used so indiscriminately for muscle strengthening and training that these nontherapeutic uses of anabolic steroids, or even growth hormones, make their therapeutic use questionable. Thus, even if therapeutic uses are beneficial, one should probably avoid these medications.

14. *Surgery.* I have operated on the adductor tendon to release it from its insertion into the pubis. This is a full adductor tendon release; it is similar to

a tennis elbow release in that it allows the pressure to be removed from that area, but results have not been proved. In my hands it has been beneficial in the long-term, very resistant case.

Differential Diagnosis

Lumbar disc herniation with resultant nerve root irritation and sciatica may be mistaken for muscle strain, as may stress fracture of the pubic ramus. Strained rectus femoris muscles can be confused with a stress fracture of the femur or an intrinsic pathologic condition in the hip joint itself.

Around the hip joint two major bursal complexes are subject to inflammation in response to athletic activity. The gluteal bursa in the buttock, and the trochanteric bursa over the greater trochanter, may both be the sites of a very troublesome bursitis.

The trochanteric bursa is inflamed from repetitive slipping back and forth across the trochanter of the tensor fascia lata. Common in runners, dancers, and gymnasts, it may also trouble racquet sports players with pain during activity; local tenderness to pressure may prevent lying on the affected side. The deep gluteal bursae when inflamed are associated with a deep-seated buttock discomfort, which may simulate referred pain from the back and has to be distinguished from a lumbar disc problem or piriformis syndrome in which the sciatic nerve is irritated at its emergence through the greater sciatic notch.

Modification of activity is the mainstay of treatment; physiotherapy with deep heat or ultrasonography, anti-inflammatory medication, and local steroids also has a place. Occasionally, surgical release of the tensor fascia is necessary in refractory cases of trochanteric bursitis, and on occasion a piriformis release is necessary in patients with a piriformis syndrome, but care has to be taken to rule out a lumbar spine problem absolutely.

PARTICIPANT CHARACTERISTICS AND SPORTS PARTICIPATION

Guidance in the selection of a suitable sport for an individual should be an important factor in pregame physicals. Obviously, people who are much too stiff and inflexible should not be allowed to participate in sports in which pulled muscles and tendons are a problem. Similarly, individuals with undue joint laxity may be at risk in contact sports. Judicious guidance to the player from the coach, doctor, or parent may help prevent many of these injuries. There should also be avenues for immediate medical referral and satisfactory physiotherapy of an immediate nature, followed by long-term complete rehabilitation and counseling regarding reinjury if the morbidity rate of these common soft tissue injuries is to be reduced.

FRACTURE OF THE PELVIS AND FEMUR

JAMES F. KELLAM, B.Sc., M.D., F.R.C.S.(C)

THE PELVIS

Before dealing with the specifics of pelvic fractures, an understanding of the pelvis as a functional unit is needed. The pelvis is composed of two innominate bones and the sacrum. These bones in isolation represent no stability. In order for the pelvis to perform its function, it is necessary for the innominate bones to be firmly fixed to the sacrum and to themselves. This fixation is obtained posteriorly with the anterior sacroiliac ligaments and the posterior sacroiliac ligaments. The posterior sacroiliac ligaments running from the posterior tubercle of the ilium to the sacrum are the largest and strongest ligaments in the body. The anterior structures of the ilium and the two innominate bones are joined through the symphysis pubis, which is a strong fibrous junction. Pelvic stability is also maintained by strong ligaments running from the sacrum to the ischial tuberosity (the sacrotuberous ligament) and to the ischial spine (the sacrospinous ligament). The lumbar spine also participates in pelvic stability with the iliolumbar ligaments, which run from both transverse processes of the fifth lumbar vertebra to the posterior iliac spines. With these ligaments intact, the pelvis is thus a stable structure able to withstand the forces of weight bearing through the acetabulum, up the strong thick cancellous and cortical bone of the posterior ilium, and through the sacrum and along the vertebral column. The anterior structures, the pubic rami and ischial rami and symphysis, do not participate significantly in the weightbearing forces, but act as a strut to maintain the pelvis in its normal anatomic configuration and to protect the pelvic contents. It is important to remember the pelvic contents in massive pelvic disruptions because they are frequently injured and can lead to bladder, urethral, nerve, and (particularly) acute hemorrhagic problems.

Pelvic stability is defined as the ability of the pelvis to withstand physiologic forces applied to it.

This means that the posterior ligamentous complexes must remain intact. Pelvic instability represents disruption of the posterior osseous ligamentous complex. This may occur by fractures through the sacrum, sacroiliac dislocations, or a combination of fracture-dislocations of the ilium and sacroiliac joint as well as fractures through the posterior iliac wing. This stability can be represented as a spectrum and must be assessed in each individual case.

Stress fractures appear to occur more commonly in women than in men. This may be due to the fact that female bones are somewhat more slender and the pubic symphysis shallower, and to several other anatomic differences that really do not effectively explain this difference. Gait differences between male and female during running may account for some mechanistic differences. The female runner tends to rely on hip extension forces to a greater extent than does the male, so that the female pelvis would be more acceptable to tensile stresses. It is interesting to note that stress fractures in the pelvis appear to be secondary to exposure to tensile stress rather than compression stress. This is because of the medial position of the fractures in the pubic or ischial ramus where muscle pulls are occurring during hip extension. This would account for a single fracture occurring in a winglike structure. The other interesting difference in pelvic stress fractures is that they do not appear to be associated with the usual changes in technique, equipment, or surfaces of running. They do appear to occur within a specific time after high-intensity activities, which may represent failure from excessive repetition of muscle contraction.

Incidence of Pelvic Fractures

In order for major pelvic disruptions to occur, high energy must be transmitted through the pelvic ring. This is normally seen in motor vehicle and motorcycle accidents in the civilian population. It may also be noted after falls from heights. Sports are not known for the production of major pelvic disruptions. It is obvious that such high-energy sports as motorcar racing, motocross, and rodeo lead to the potential for major pelvic disruptions. However, in most sports the participant is well protected and does not suffer massive pelvic disruption. Stress fractures or stable pelvic fractures are more common.

Clinical Presentation

Pelvic fractures can be divided into two groups: stress fractures and major pelvic fractures.

With the major pelvic fracture, the mechanism of injury is obviously one of a high-velocity, high-energy transfer. This acute injury occurs as a sudden event. When first seen, the patient generally is unable to bear weight and is in significant pain in the region of the pelvic girdle. The history should point to the mechanism of injury. Pelvic fractures occur from anteroposteriorly directed forces, forces directed laterally to the pelvis such as a blow over the buttock or greater trochanteric region, and the vertical shear forces that occur in falls. Further questioning of the patient should bring to light symptoms of associated intra-abdominal or intrapelvic injuries, such as abdominal pain, an inability to void, and neurologic symptoms of numbness, tingling, or weakness in the lower extremities.

Stress fractures generally occur as a sudden onset of discomfort, usually related to the pelvic region. They are seen in runners or people who are doing repetitive activities that place significantly high stresses across the pelvis over a prolonged period. It is important to inquire into the training regimen of the athlete: whether there has been a sudden increase in mileage, a change in technique, or a change in training surfaces and location. It is also important to know when the discomfort occurs: whether with weight bearing such as walking or only during the athletic event or training.

Physical examination of the pelvis determines the stability of the injury as well as associated injuries. It is imperative to remember that the acute pelvic fracture is often accompanied by hypovolemic shock. The initial evaluation of the patient requires the physician to remember the priorities of resuscitation. Examination of the airway, breathing, and circulatory status of the patient should be done before the pelvic examination. Stabilization of the patient in hypovolemic shock or with airway problems is imperative. Intra-abdominal bleeding should also be evaluated.

The assessment of the pelvis begins with inspection. One should look for areas of swelling and bruising. Major pelvic disruptions are noted in patients with large flank hematomas, scrotal hematomas, and large hematomas posteriorly over the sacroiliac complex. Deformity of the lower extremity may also be noted. A lateral compression pelvic fracture causes an internal rotation deformity of the lower extremity, and an anteroposterior displaced fracture results in increased external rotation of the lower extremity. A vertical shear fracture causes a discrepancy in leg length, the shorter side being on the fracture side. Palpation of the pelvic ring, both posteriorly over the posterior sacroiliac complex and anteriorly over the pubic rami and symphysis, is imperative to determine areas of tenderness and discomfort. Manual compression of the pelvis by placing the hands on the anterosuperior iliac spines and forcing the pelvis inward will reveal an instability or discomfort posteriorly or anteriorly, depending on the fracture; forcing the pelvis outward also shows instability. The urethra is inspected for blood, an indication of urethral disruption. In addition, a rectal examination is made in males to determine the position of the prostate. A high-riding prostate or one that is mobile is another indication of urethral tears. Catheterization should not be attempted in these patients until cystourethrography has been performed to evaluate the urethra. If it is intact, a catheter may then be passed. Further evaluation of the lower extremities for neurologic involvement and vascular involvement should also be done at this time.

Investigations

In order to assess the pelvis radiographically, three views are required. The pelvis is approximately 40 degrees oblique to the long axis of the body. Consequently, an anteroposterior (AP) film of the pelvis represents an oblique view of the pelvis. This view is necessary to provide an overview of the pelvis and its structures. Two further views at right angles to each other can be obtained. The inlet view is done with the patient supine and the x-ray beam directed from cephalad to caudad at 45 degrees to the long axis of the body. This view permits assessment of posterior displacement, of rotation (whether internal or external), and of the sacrum for fractures. The outlet view, or tangential view, is done at 45 degrees to the long axis of the body with the tube directed from caudad to cephalad. This view allows assessment of the sacrum, sacral foramina, and superior rotation as well as superior migration of the pelvis. These two views, at right angles to each other, fill the criteria of fracture evaluation, especially that of stress fractures. Because of overlap in the AP view, it may be difficult to determine the exact structure that is injured in a stress fracture with only the AP view.

Bone scanning is particularly useful in the athlete who complains of a potential stress fracture. The bone scan is particularly sensitive to areas of increased bone turnover, as occur in stress fracture. If radiographs do not demonstrate a fracture, bone scanning is the next step. The stress fracture is demonstrated on the scan as a well-localized area of increased activity in the area of fracture.

Computed tomography (CT) is another useful technique for assessing the pelvis and its displacement, but more so in acute pelvic fractures than in stress fractures.

Tomograms of the pelvis may also be useful in the delineation of stress fractures.

Management

Once a pelvic fracture is diagnosed in an athlete, the major decision in management concerns the stability of the pelvic ring. Stability depends on the degree of disruption of the posterior bony, ligamentous complex of the pelvis. A clinical impression of instability can be verified radiographically. Significant displacement posteriorly in the femoral sacral arch around the sacroiliac joint region of greater than 5 mm to 1 cm represents significant instability. Evidence of avulsion fractures of the transverse process of L5, of the spinous process of the ischium, and occasionally of the origin of the sacrotuberous and sacrospinous ligaments from the sacrum also represents potential instability. The type of fracture pattern is also helpful in determining instability. Impacted fractures in cancellous bone represent a stable situation, whereas a shear fracture or a fracture through cancellous bone in which a gap is noted is potentially unstable. Stable pelvic fractures can be managed on bed rest until comfort is achieved. At this point the patient may be mobilized on crutches, non–weight bearing on the involved side. During this period, functional rehabilitation involving the cardiovascular system and the uninjured side may be carried out within the limits of discomfort for the patient. Pelvic fractures take approximately 6 to 8 weeks to become relatively solid, so that partial weight bearing may occur. This time period should be judged clinically with the assessment of each individual athlete. A stable pelvic fracture may be well united and early rehabilitation of the athlete may be possible within 6 weeks in some circumstances, provided lower extremity deformity, such as rotation or shortening, is not significant.

In the unstable pelvic fracture, anteroposterior compression injuries disrupt the symphysis and open the pelvis like a book. With less than 2.5 cm of disruption through the symphysis, these fractures remain relatively stable and may be managed with some method of closing the book—by internal fixation, external skeletal fixation, or a pelvic sling. A minimum of 6 weeks (more likely 3 months) is required for union to occur with this type of treatment. External skeletal fixation of the pelvis in an anteroposterior stable compression injury is ideal in that it allows functional rehabilitation. The patient may be up with crutches, non–weight bearing on the involved side, and be able to participate in upper extremity activities. Most lateral compression injuries are stable and may be managed with appropriate bed rest and mobilization. The vertical shear injury is an unstable injury. The end point of all mechanisms results in an unstable fracture that follows the pattern of a vertical shear injury. With a posterior instability, evaluation must be made as to how significant this is. Control of posterior instability is not possible with external skeletal fixation frames, but requires open reduction and internal fixation of the posterior bony ligamentous complex. This type of internal fixation of the pelvis is not without complications. Infection, gluteal muscle necrosis, and impingement of the sacral roots with internal fixation devices into the sacrum have occurred. This type of surgical intervention should be done by a surgeon experienced in pelvic fracture treatment. Other methods of treatment of the unstable fracture are combinations of external skeletal fixation and traction. This type of treatment usually requires a 3-month period of bed rest, with 6 to 8 weeks of traction followed by another 6 weeks of recumbency for union of the fracture to occur.

Stress fractures are managed symptomatically. If they occur during weight bearing and walking, crutch walking or pool therapy may be helpful. If they occur during training, this must be either slowed down or abandoned and other forms of maintenance of the athlete must be instituted. Evaluation of technique, environment, and equipment should be undertaken by consultation among physician, coach, and athlete in order to ascertain why this occurred and what can be done to correct it. The presence of a stress fracture should alert one to other potential problems, such as primary or secondary malignant disease.

Athletes should not return to competitive sports until they are pain-free and have regained strength, endurance, and agility. Otherwise, they are at significant risk for recurrent or new injury.

THE FEMUR

Fractures of the femur are a serious problem to an athlete. The femur, the largest bone in the body, is subject to the greatest stress and is surrounded by the major musculature of the lower extremity. At either end of the femur are the two major weight bearing joints required in all athletic activities: the hip and the knee. The hip is important in that stress fractures of the femoral neck may occur in athletes and thus lead to significant problems if missed or treated inadequately. If femoral shaft fractures are not treated properly, the thigh musculature cannot be maintained in good condition and ultimately affects knee function, through weakness, fibrosis, or secondary joint stiffness. Fractures in or above the knee are discussed elsewhere in this text.

Fractures of the femoral neck, which usually are stress fractures but may be incurred during high-energy sporting activities, can lead to several difficulties, the most serious being the development of avascular necrosis of the femoral head. This blood supply to the femoral head comes from a circle of vessels around the greater trochanteric region, courses up the posterior retinaculum of the femoral neck, and dives into the femoral head at the articular cartilage margin. Fractures of the femoral neck may disrupt this blood supply and thus lead to avascular necrosis and its attendant complications if late segmental collapse of the femoral head occurs. Nonunions and malunions also may occur. The hip requires an anatomic reduction in order that the biomechanics of gait, particularly for running, are maintained. Therefore, if a nonunion or malunion does occur, the athlete will be hindered.

The femoral shaft is enclosed within the major musculature of the lower extremity. Anteriorly the quadriceps, the major extensor of the knee as well as one of the major components of the patellofemoral mechanism, can be injured. Posteriorly, the hamstring groups of muscles are also involved as well as the sciatic nerve. Thus, femoral shaft fractures involve some form of muscle injury, particularly anteriorly to the quadriceps, and ultimately lead to knee problems through the weakness or loss of function of the quadriceps. Depending on the treatment of femoral shaft fractures, knee stiffness may result. This stiffness, along with shortening and malunion, may be a particular problem to athletes who require their lower extremities for repetitive and power activities. In addition to fractures of the femoral shaft caused by high velocity, stress fractures of the shaft, neck, and proximal area have been reported.

Incidence

Femoral fractures in athletes are extremely uncommon. The usual causes of stress fracture are overuse and change, particularly in marathon runners. It generally occurs in the beginning of training or after a sudden intensification of activity, such as a long run. Nonstress fractures or acute fractures of the femoral shaft have been documented in different contact sports. In a series of hockey injuries, only one of 108 fractures reviewed was to the femur. In other reviews, contact sports or high-velocity sports do not involve significant femoral shaft fractures, although they do occur sporadically.

Clinical Presentation

The acute femoral neck fracture or femoral shaft fracture usually occurs in isolated incidents with the sudden onset of acute discomfort and pain after a significant transfer of energy to the extremity. This may be through contact or can occur simply through twisting activities. The patient is unable to bear weight and complains of pain at a specific site.

Stress fractures of the femoral neck or medial aspect of the proximal femur usually are gradual in onset. The patient develops pain and discomfort, normally during activity or during a long run. This pain persists and is aggravated by increased activity. It is relieved by rest or non–weight bearing. This fracture occurs as an acute episode and is not preceded by chronic discomfort. Pain in the knee region, particularly on the medial aspect of the knee, may be indicative of hip joint disease. It also appears that stress fractures of the femur occur in the early part of a training routine, because increased stress is placed on the bone before the bone is able to withstand it.

Physical examination of an acute fracture usually shows the patient lying with an externally rotated leg, with acute pain and discomfort on motion and crepitus at the fracture site. With femoral shaft fractures, significant blood loss may occur, although it is uncommon. In a patient with a stress fracture, the leg usually has normal alignment, but on range-of-motion examination of the hip there are decreases in the range owing to pain with rotation and flexion. Pain usually occurs at the extremes. There may be tenderness at the region of the fracture.

Investigations

The first study consists of an anteroposterior and lateral roentgenogram of the hip or femur. It is important that both the joint above and that below the fracture be examined radiographically, particularly in the acute fracture. Because a stress fracture may not be visible on initial examination of the films, a high index of suspicion is necessary. One should also be aware of other diagnoses that may cause pain in this region (tumors or infection). A stress fracture may be one of two types and it is important to make the distinction. The compressive type, which usually is noted at the lower border of the femoral neck, is demonstrated radiographically as increased radiodensity along the fracture site or sclerosis at the fracture line. This type of fracture is rarely displaced unless continued stresses are placed on it. The second type of stress fracture, the distraction fracture, is transverse in direction, is seen in older individuals, and usually occurs at the superior aspect of the neck with a radiolucency. The fracture line develops at right angles to the line of stress, and displacement is common.

Acute fractures of the femoral neck are obvious. It is important to determine the amount of displacement. The greater the displacement of the femoral neck fracture, the greater is the risk of avascular necrosis and the greater the necessity for an accurate anatomic reduction.

Acute fracture of the femoral shaft should also be assessed. It is important to determine the type of comminution present and thus whether the fracture is stable or unstable. Fractures of the femoral shaft that have more than 50 percent of the cortex intact on both the distal and proximal fragment are stable fractures. The two fragments can be lined up to prevent any axial displacement such as shortening. Comminution is particularly important in the proximal and distal portions. Although 50 percent of the cortex may be intact in the distal fracture, comminution may allow the fracture to slip, depending on the treatment, and thus shorten. If there is less than 50 percent cortical contact between both fractures, the fracture is considered unstable.

Bone scan may be indicated. Radionuclide images of the femoral shaft or femoral neck may be diagnostic in individuals in whom stress fractures are expected but not visualized on the plain radiographs. Tomography may also be necessary to delineate the fracture. This study may be necessary for diagnosis or to determine the extent of the fracture, particularly in the femoral neck, i.e., whether the fracture is completely across the neck or incomplete.

Management

In managing the acute fracture, one should initially ascertain that the patient is stabilized. If this fracture has occurred in a high-velocity situation, other associated injuries may be present. Priorities of resuscitation should be honored before treatment of the fracture is begun. This is not a particular problem with stress fractures.

Treatment of a stress fracture involving the femoral neck is based on the nature of the fracture. Compression fractures of the femoral neck, as mentioned, rarely cause displacement if the stresses are removed by appropriate non–weight bearing, either by crutches or by bed rest. The distraction stress fracture of the femoral neck usually is displaced and should be internally fixed. Any displaced fracture of the femoral neck should undergo internal fixation to allow for anatomic reduction. Most stress fractures are minimally displaced or may be reduced anatomically by means of a closed method using a fracture table. After this maneuver, they may be internally fixed by means of an appropriate device. Fractures in which anatomic reduction cannot be obtained should be considered for open reduction.

There are many techniques for the fixation of femoral neck fractures. The principle of internal fixation of these fractures requires a technique that allows for controlled impaction of the fracture, usually by means of a sliding compression screw system. Multiple pin fixation, using smooth pins or cancellous screws, is also a useful technique for the minimally displaced or anatomically reduced stress fracture of the femoral neck. After reduction and internal fixation of the fracture, the vascularity of the femoral head should be evaluated. It is probably best done at this time by a bone marrow scanning technique using technetium-99m sulfur colloid. It may also be adequately performed with one of the currently used bone scanning agents incorporating technetium-99m. If the femoral head is viable, no further treatment should be considered. However, if the bone scan demonstrates an avascular head, consideration should be given to a muscle pedicle bone graft using the quadratus femoris–based bone-block technique. This may increase the chances of revascularization of the femoral head and fracture union.

After operative or nonoperative treatment, weight bearing should not be allowed for approximately 6 weeks. This should be guided basically by the radiographic evidence of fracture union. As the fracture unites, gradual weight bearing may be reinstituted. Cardiovascular fitness may be maintained by activities that do not allow stresses to be placed across the femur (e.g., swimming or waist-deep water walking or running). These should be incorporated into the treatment as the clinical course permits. Most patients with stress fractures of the femoral neck can resume activities about 6 months after injury.

The treatment of acute femoral shaft fractures should preserve and encourage as much functional return as possible as quickly as possible. The technique of closed intramedullary nailing of long bone fractures is ideally suited for this fracture. This technique, developed by Gerhard Küntscher, is based on his principles of fracture care. The first and foremost principle was the restoration and preservation of function, which is imperative in the athlete. This was accomplished by a technique that allowed for fracture immobilization until healing occurred, but at the same time avoided assault on the fracture site, thus eliminating significant muscle dissection and devascularization of fracture fragments. This technique also encouraged healing by secondary bone union, particularly with its own internal bone graft from reamings.

The technique is performed with a closed reduction of the femoral shaft fracture. When this has been completed on the fracture table, through a small incision over the greater trochanteric region, the greater trochanter is entered in line with the axis of the medullary canal, a guide wire is passed across the fracture site, and the medullary canal of the femur is reamed with reamers of progressively increasing size. This allows for the internal aspect of the medullary canal to be made into a tube of a specific size, to permit passage of a nail large enough to immobilize the femur without bending and to allow for impingement between the nail and the internal aspect of the femur. This elastic impingement, which occurs as the nail is driven into the bone, provides the stability if associated with a stable fracture pattern. However, only fractures that are transverse or short oblique in nature are amenable to this closed technique because the nail is a weightsharing device. It allows the fracture to participate in bone healing and weightbearing stresses. Because it is close to the central axis of the femur, very few stresses are placed on the nail as far as tension or bending are concerned. There is minimal change in the cortical bone of the femur, and thus the problems of removal of the nail are minimal for recovery.

Recently, the indications for this technique have been extended by the development of a locked intramedullary nail which is a cloverleaf nail that has holes at the proximal and distal ends. Through specially designed siting devices, these holes may be filled with locking screws. Fractures that do not have stability (i.e., comminuted fractures, fractures in the distal and proximal third of the femur) may also be treated by the closed intramedullary nailing technique, as may any fracture of the shaft of the femur from within approximately 2 to 3 cm of the lesser trochanter to within 5 cm of the adductor tubercle.

This method of treatment of femoral shaft fractures allows for immediate mobilization of the athlete. The first day postoperatively the athlete may begin quadriceps setting exercises and be encouraged in straight leg raising. Once straight leg raising has been accomplished, there is sufficient quadriceps control for the patient to be mobilized onto crutches in a non-weightbearing or partial weightbearing mode, depending on fracture stability. If a locking nail has been used and it has been necessary to lock this at both ends, i.e., a static locked nail, weight bearing is delayed until bridging callus is noted between the fracture fragments. This usually occurs at 3 months, at which point one of the sets of screws may be removed and full weight bearing may be commenced to mature the callus. Range-of-motion exercises of the knee are begun immediately. Usually by 3 weeks 90 degrees of motion has been obtained, and in stable fractures full weight bearing may be commenced. Union is rapid with this technique. During the initial 6 weeks, cardiovascular fitness may be obtained by non-weight bearing exercises such as swimming, walking in waist-deep water, and bicycling. Once the fracture has consolidated adequately, further rehabilitation may be started. Usually by 12 months the fracture has fully consolidated and healing has matured to allow removal of the nail. Nail removal should be undertaken in patients under the age of 50. This is a simple operation requiring several days of hospital admission. After this, the patient may recommence activities in a protected fashion until comfortable, usually within 3 to 6 weeks. Removal of the implant should be timed with the sporting activities. As long a period as possible should be observed between nail removal and the recommencement of highly stressful activities. Usually in 6 to 9 months the femur has regained its strength and full activities can be allowed.

Recent reports of the closed intramedullary nailing technique have shown that a 99 percent union rate with a less than 1 percent infection rate in closed femoral shaft fractures has been obtained. These results are similar to the early results of the locked intramedullary nailing technique. Other methods of femoral fracture treatment are associated with problems that may be particularly difficult for the athlete to overcome. The treatment of femoral shaft fractures in traction is usually associated with significant quadriceps atrophy and weakness, as well as a decrease in the range of motion of the knee. Cast bracing of fractures may, as with traction, allow for some decreased quadriceps power, range of motion of the knee, and occasional shortening and malunions. Plate fixation of femoral fractures allows for an anatomic reduction, but requires an open procedure with stripping of the muscle, particularly the quadriceps, which may lead to decreased range of motion and quadriceps weakness. Plate fixation is also associated with refracturing, particularly at the time of plate removal. Although the incidence of this is low if the fracture is united, there is evidence that the bone underneath the plate may undergo cancellization or become weakened owing to the weight-relieving aspects of a plate. To avoid this requires protection of the patient for a 12-month period before stressful activities are resumed.

With femoral shaft fractures, knee ligament injuries and internal derangements of the knee may also occur. This has been noted in up to 25 percent of patients with femoral shaft fractures. Once the fracture has been stabilized, examination of the knee is imperative. If significant knee injuries have occurred, these should be treated appropriately. In this situation, it is imperative that the femoral fracture be fixed in order that a knee reconstructive procedure and rehabilitation can be undertaken.

Finally, as far as treatment is concerned, return of athletes to full activity depends on their ability to regain strength, endurance, and agility.

I SPINE

INJURIES TO THE CERVICAL SPINE

JOSEPH S. TORG, M.D.

Of the variety of injuries that can occur in the athlete, those involving the head and neck are the most difficult to evaluate and manage on the field. Because of the actual or potential involvement of the nervous system, risks can be high and consequently the margin for error is low. The initial clinical picture frequently may be misleading. Patients with significant intracranial hemorrhage may at first present with minimal symptoms, only to follow a precipitous downhill course. On the other hand, short-lived conditions such as neurapraxia of the brachial plexus may at first present with paresthesia and paralysis, raising the question of a significant spinal injury, only to resolve within minutes so that the individual returns to activity. Fortunately, the more severe injuries that can occur to the neck are infrequent. As a result, most team physicians and trainers have little, if any, experience in dealing with them.

Management of the unconscious athlete or one suspected of having sustained significant injury to the cervical spine is a process that should not be performed hastily or haphazardly. The best way to prevent actions that could convert a reparable injury into a catastrophe is to be prepared to handle the situation.

Thus, the single most important point to remember is, *prevent further injury.* Adequate preparation will alleviate indecision and second-guessing. Immediately immobilize the head and neck, and check first for breathing and then for level of consciousness.

If the victim is breathing, simply remove the mouth guard, if present, and maintain the airway. Once it is established that the athlete is breathing and has a pulse, simply maintain the situation until transportation is available, or until the athlete regains consciousness. If the athlete is face down when the ambulance arrives, change his position to face up by logrolling him onto a spine board. Make no attempt to move him except to transport him or perform cardiopulmonary resuscitation (CPR) if necessary.

The transportation team should be familiar with handling a victim who has a cervical spine injury. It is important not to lose control of the care of the athlete. Therefore, prior arrangements with an ambulance service should be made.

Lifting and carrying the injured athlete require five individuals: four to lift and the leader to maintain immobilization of the head.

The same guidelines apply to the choice of a medical facility as to the choice of an ambulance: be sure it is equipped and staffed to handle an emergency neck injury. There should be a neurosurgeon and an orthopaedic surgeon to meet the athlete upon arrival.

NERVE ROOT–BRACHIAL PLEXUS NEURAPRAXIA

The most common cervical injuries are the pinch-stretch neurapraxias of the nerve roots and brachial plexus. The key to the nature of this lesion is its short duration and the presence of a full, pain-free range of neck motion. Although most of these injuries are short-lived, they are worrisome because of the occasional plexus axonotmesis that occurs. However, the youngster whose paresthesia completely abates, who demonstrates full muscle strength in the intrinsic muscles of the shoulder and upper extremities, and (most important) who has a full, pain-free range of cervical motion may return to activity.

The occasional athlete who experiences recurrent episodes of root or plexus neurapraxia should undergo cervical spine roentgenography and electromyographic studies. If the results of these, as well as the physical findings, are negative, an intensive isotonic neck muscle–strengthening program should be initiated. It takes several months for the benefits of such a program to be realized. The susceptible individual should continue the program on a year-round basis, and wear a cervical neck roll.

If the electromyogram demonstrates involvement of the deltoid, infraspinatus, supraspinatus, and biceps, the lesion should be considered an axonotmesis.

Persistence of paresthesia, weakness, or limitation of cervical motion requires that the individual be protected from further exposure and that he undergo neurologic, electromyographic, and roentgenographic evaluation. Athletes demonstrating evidence of associated axonotmesis should be withheld from contact sports until they have achieved full muscle strength, and show evidence of axonal regeneration upon repeat electromyography. This usually takes a minimum of 4 to 6 weeks. In addition to protection from further injury, treatment consists of a neck and upper extremity muscle-strengthening program with emphasis placed on the involved muscles. A neck roll should also be worn.

ACUTE CERVICAL SPRAIN SYNDROME

Acute cervical sprains are frequently seen in contact sports. The patient presents with limitation of cervical spine motion and without radiation of pain or paresthesia. Neurologic examination is negative and roentgenographic results are normal.

Stable cervical sprains and strains eventually resolve with or without treatment. Initially, the presence of a serious injury should be ruled out by a thorough neurologic examination and determination of the range of cervical motion.

The athlete with less than a full, pain-free range of cervical motion, persistent paresthesia, or weakness should be protected and excluded from further activity. Subsequent evaluation should include appropriate roentgenographic studies, including flexion and extension views to demonstrate fractures or instability.

In general, treatment of athletes with "cervical sprains" should be tailored to the degree of severity. Appropriate measures include immobilization of the neck in a soft collar, application of heat, and use of analgesics and anti-inflammatory agents until there is a full, spasm-free range of neck motion. Individuals with a history of collision injury, pain, and limited cervical motion should undergo routine cervical spine roentgenography. Lateral flexion and extension roentgenograms are also indicated after the acute symptoms subside. If the patient has pain and muscle spasm of the cervical spine, hospitalization and head-halter traction may be indicated.

CERVICAL VERTEBRAL SUBLUXATION WITHOUT FRACTURE

Axial compression-flexion injuries incurred by striking an object with the top of the head can result in disruption of the posterior soft tissue supporting elements with angulation and anterior translation of the superior cervical vertebrae. Fractures of the bony elements are not demonstrated on roentgenograms, and the patient will have no neurologic deficit. Flexion-extension roentgenograms reveal instability of the cervical spine at the involved level manifested by motion, anterior intervertebral disc space narrowing, anterior angulation and displacement of the vertebral body, and fanning of the spinous processes. Demonstrable instability on lateral flexion-extension roentgenograms in a young, vigorous individual requires vigorous treatment. When soft tissue disruption occurs without an associated fracture, it is likely that instability will develop despite conservative treatment. When anterior subluxation greater than 20 percent of the vertebral body is due to disruption of the posterior supporting structures, a posterior cervical fusion is recommended.

CERVICAL FRACTURES AND DISLOCATIONS: GENERAL PRINCIPLES

Fractures or dislocations of the cervical spine may be stable or unstable, and may or may not be associated with neurologic deficit. When fracture or disruption of the soft tissue supporting structure immediately violates or threatens to violate the integrity of the spinal cord, implementation of certain management and treatment principles is imperative.

The first goal is to protect the spinal cord and nerve roots from injury through mismanagement. Second, the malaligned cervical spine should be reduced as quickly and gently as possible to decompress the spinal cord effectively. When dislocation or anterior angulation and translation are demonstrated roentgenographically, immediate reduction is attempted with skull traction, using Gardner-Wells tongs. These tongs can be easily and rapidly applied under local anesthesia, without shaving the head, with the patient in the emergency room or the hospital bed. Since these tongs are spring-loaded, it is not necessary to drill the outer table of the skull for their application. The tongs are attached to a cervical-traction pulley, and weight is added at a rate of 5 lb per disc space or 25 to 40 lb for lower cervical injury. Reduction is attempted by adding 5 lb every 15 to 20 minutes and is monitored by lateral roentgenograms.

Unilateral and bilateral facet dislocations, particularly at the C3–C4 level, are not always reducible by skeletal traction. In such instances, closed skeletal or manipulative reduction under nasotracheal anesthesia may be necessary. The expediency of early reduction of cervical dislocations is emphasized.

It has been proposed that a bulbocavernous reflex indicates that spinal shock has worn off and that, except for recovery of an occasional root at the injury, neither the motor nor the sensory paralysis will resolve regardless of treatment. The bulbocavernous reflex is produced by pulling on the urethral catheter. This stimulates the trigone of the bladder, producing a reflex contraction of the anal sphincter around the examiner's gloved finger. Although a bulbocavernous reflex is generally a sign that there will be no further neurologic recovery below the level of the injury, this is not always true. The presence of this reflex does not give the clinician license to handle the situation in an elective fashion. The cervical spine malalignments and dislocations associated with quadriparesis should be reduced as quickly as possible, by whatever means necessary, if maximal recovery is to be expected.

In most instances in which a vertebral body burst fracture is associated with anterior compression of the cord, decompression is logically effected through an anterior approach with an interbody fusion. Likewise, traumatic intervertebral disc herniation with cord involvement is best managed through an anterior discectomy and interbody fusion. In cervical fractures and dislocations, posterior cervical laminectomy is indicated only rarely when it is necessary to excise foreign bodies or bone fragments in the spinal canal. Realignment of the spine is the most effective method for decompression of the cervical cord.

Indications for surgical decompression of the spinal cord have been delineated. A documented increase in neurologic signs is the clearest mandate for surgical decompression. Further observation, expectancy, and procrastination in this situation are contraindicated. Persistent partial cord or root signs, with objective evidence of mechanical compression, are also an indication for surgical intervention.

Management of cervical spine fractures and dislocations requires the generous use of parenteral corticosteroids (dexamethasone) to decrease the inflammatory reactions of the injured cord and surrounding soft tissue structures. Initially, 100 mg of dexamethasone should be given intravenously in a single bolus followed by 1 mg per kilogram per day intravenously in divided doses for 10 days. Drugs that inhibit norepinephrine synthesis or deplete catecholamines have been advocated to prevent autodigestion of the cord, but there is no evidence as yet that this is of value in improving the prognosis for cord recovery. Procedures such as durotomy, myelotomy, and rhizotomy require extensive laminectomy (adding further instability) and are contraindicated.

The third goal in managing fractures and dislocations of the cervical spine is to effect rapid and secure stability, thus preventing residual deformity and instability with associated pain and the possibility of further trauma to the neural elements. The method of immobilization depends on the postreduction status of the injury. Indications for nonsurgical and surgical methods for achieving stability may be summarized as follows:

1. Patients with stable compression fractures of the vertebral body, undisplaced fractures of the lamina or lateral masses, or soft tissue injuries without detectable neurologic deficit can be treated adequately with traction and subsequent protection by a cervical brace until healing occurs.
2. Stable, reduced facet dislocation without neurologic deficit can also be treated conservatively in a halo jacket until healing has been demonstrated by negative lateral flexion-extension roentgenograms.
3. Unstable cervical spine fractures or fracture-dislocations without neurologic deficit may require either surgical or nonsurgical methods to ensure stability.
4. Absolute indications for surgical stabilization are an unstable injury without neurologic deficit and late instability following closed treatment.
5. Relative indications for surgical stabilization in unstable injuries without neurologic deficit are anterior subluxation greater than 20 percent, certain atlantoaxial fractures or dislocations, and unreduced comminuted vertical compression injuries.
6. Cervical spine fractures with complete cord lesions require reduction followed by closed or open stabilization as indicated.
7. Cervical spine fractures with incomplete cord lesions require reduction followed by careful evaluation for the need of surgical intervention.

The fourth and final goal of treatment is rapid and effective rehabilitation started early in the treatment process.

Transient Quadriplegia

An infrequently occurring and not well documented phenomenon is that of transient quadriplegia. This characteristically occurs to an athlete, most often a football player, who sustains either forced hyperextension or hyperflexion to the neck and cervical spine. A painless paralysis ensues, which may manifest as weakness or complete absence of motor function in all four extremities. The episode is brief, lasting 5 to 10 minutes. The involvement of sensory function has not been established. Roentgenograms do not demonstrate acute trauma to the cervical spine, but examination of the lateral films reveals either a congenital fusion or a developmental decrease in the sagittal diameter of the spinal canal, which is shown to be increased on lateral flexion and extension roentgenograms.

There is no evidence that patients who experience one or more episodes of transient quadriplegia are prone to more severe injury, namely, permanent quadriplegia. However, they are susceptible to recurrence of the transient episodes, and therefore it is recommended that they avoid certain contact activities.

Cervical Spine Instability

The spectrum of late cervical spine instability following an injury is a necessary diagnostic consideration when an athlete is injured. If possible, it is well to avoid subsequent permanent or transient narrowing of the spinal canal with compression of the neural elements. For each particular injury, it is not possible to predict accurately whether late instability will result in structural malalignment with or without neurologic deficit. However, the recent work of White, Southwick, and Punjabi in establishing guidelines regarding this problem is noteworthy.

These authors performed a series of cadaver studies in which the various supporting structures were systematically cut, and resulting spinal instabilities were noted. The supporting structures of the lower cervical spine can be divided into two groups, anterior and posterior. The anterior group includes both soft tissue supporting structures anterior to and including the posterior longitudinal ligament: these are the anterior and posterior longitudinal ligaments, the intervertebral disc, and the annulus fibrosus. The posterior group consists of the facet capsular ligaments, the ligamentum flavum, and the interspinous and supraspinous ligaments. White and colleagues have devised a check list for the diagnosis of clinical instability of the lower cervical spine. If point values are assigned to the elements in Table 1 and the points total 5 or more, the spine should be considered clinically unstable. Evaluation of the first two entities, the status of the anterior and posterior elements, is based on clinical history, evaluation of radiographs, and interpretation of flexion-extension films.

TABLE 1 Check List for Diagnosis of Clinical Instability in Lower Cervical Spine*

Elements	*Point Value*
Anterior elements destroyed or unable to function	2
Posterior elements destroyed or unable to function	2
Relative sagittal plane translation >3.5 mm†	2
Relative sagittal plane rotation >11 degrees‡	2
Positive stretch test	2
Spinal cord damage	2
Nerve root damage	1
Abnormal disc narrowing	1
Dangerous leading anticipated	1

*Total of 5 points or more = unstable.
†As measured on lateral flexion-extension films.
‡As measured on lateral films.
From Spine 1976; 1:15.

ACTIVITY RESTRICTIONS

Physicians involved in the management of athletes who have sustained significant cervical spine injuries are ultimately faced with the question of whether or not the patient can return to sports activity. Since few, if any, attempts have been made to address this question formally, the following guidelines are offered, based on clinical experience.

Youngsters who have been diagnosed and successfully treated for cervical sprains, intervertebral disc injuries without neurologic involvement, and stable wedge compression fractures may return to all activities when they are symptom free, have a full range of cervical motion, have full muscle strength, and show stability of the cervical spine on flexion and extension radiography.

Patients with lesions of the cervical spine resulting in subluxation without fracture should be precluded from further participation in contact sports despite lack of motion on lateral flexion-extension films. Flexion and extension films are a static demonstration of stability and not an adequate measure of the stability of the spine when it is subjected to the forces involved in contact sports.

Individuals who have undergone a successful one-level anterior interbody decompression and fusion for herniated nucleus pulposus or anterior instability may return to all activities provided they have a full range of motion and strength. However, they should be fully apprised of the possibility of intervertebral disc herniation at an adjacent level.

Patients who undergo more than one-level anterior fusion or posterior fusion for cervical spine injury should be evaluated on an individual basis with regard to return to *noncontact* sports. However, these individuals should not be permitted to return to contact activity regardless of how "solid" the fusion appears on roentgenograms. Altered biomechanics of the cervical spine with more than a two-level fusion presents several problems. The decrease in motion will, in itself, deprive the spine of its capability of dissipating force through motion. Also, there is a higher risk of injury because of the increased torque on the lever arm on the level above and below the fusion mass. The effect of cervical fusion as a precipitating cause of degenerative disease at other levels is another question that may be unanswered but should be considered.

SUGGESTED READING

Torg JS. Athletic injuries to the head, neck and face. Philadelphia: Lea & Febiger, 1982.

CERVICAL SPINAL STENOSIS WITH CORD NEURAPRAXIA AND TRANSIENT QUADRIPLEGIA

JOSEPH S. TORG, M.D.

Characteristically, the clinical picture of cervical spinal cord neurapraxia with transient quadriplegia involves an athlete who sustains an acute transient neurologic episode of cervical cord origin with sensory changes that may be associated with motor paresis involving both arms, both legs, or all four extremities after forced hyperextension, hyperflexion, or axial loading of the cervical spine.

Sensory changes include burning pain, numbness, tingling, or loss of sensation; motor changes consist of weakness or complete paralysis. The episodes are transient and complete recovery usually occurs in 10 to 15 minutes, although in some cases gradual resolution does not occur for 36 to 48 hours. Except for burning paresthesia, neck pain is not present at the time of injury. There is complete return of motor function and full, pain-free cervical motion. Routine x-ray films of the cervical spine show no evidence of fracture or dislocation. However, a demonstrable degree of cervical spinal stenosis is present.

There is sparse documentation in the literature of the incidence of cervical spinal stenosis. Payne and Spillane reported the association between developmental stenosis of the spinal canal and the development of myelopathy. They recognized that a decrease in the sagittal diameter is further accentuated by encroachment of osteophytes, degenerative disc disease, or vertebral subluxation. Moiel and colleagues subsequently reported on the significance of a congenitally narrow cervical canal in the absence of degenerative osteoarthritic changes. Narrowing of the sagittal diameter of the cervical spine may occur secondarily to either a diffuse developmental condition or an acquired stenosis, predicated on spondylolytic changes. Several investigators have observed that symptoms may be associated with both types of stenosis of the spinal canal.

PENNING'S PINCER MECHANISM

When considering cervical stenosis, it is important to note how it is affected by motion; this will indicate whether stenotic individuals are at risk during athletic activities. Penning measured the sagittal diameter of the cervical canal as it is affected by flexion and extension. He measured the sagittal diameter of the spinal canal from the inferior portion of the superior vertebral body to the closest point on the spinolaminar line of the inferior vertebra. Penning called this the pincer mechanism (Fig. 1), whereby the cord is pinched between the process of the two opposing bodies. The degree of pinching of the spinal cord is dependent on the sagittal diameter of the spinal canal and on the degree of extension. The degree of compression of the cord is compounded by the presence of spondylitic degenerative spurs. Penning noted that if the sagittal diameter is less than 11 mm in extension, there should be a strong suspicion of compression of the spinal cord. In other words, individuals with cervical stenosis are at risk of greater cord compression with extension.

DETERMINATION OF SPINAL STENOSIS: METHOD OF MEASUREMENT

In order to identify cervical stenosis, a method of measurement is needed. The standard method, the one most commonly employed for determining the sagittal diameter of the spinal canal, involves measuring the distance between the middle of the posterior surface of the vertebral body and the nearest point on the spinolaminar line. Using this technique, Boijsen reported that the average sagittal diameter of the spinal canal from the fourth to the sixth cervical vertebra in 200 healthy individuals was 18.5 mm (range, 14.2 to 23 mm). The target distance he used was 1.4 m. Kessler noted that values of less than 14 mm are uncommon and fall below the standard deviation for any cervical segment. Other measurements reported in the literature vary greatly. It is the variations in the landmarks and the methods used to determine the sagittal distance, as well as the use of different target distances for roentgenography, that have resulted in inconsistencies in the so-called normal values. Therefore, the standard method of measurement for spinal stenosis is a questionable one.

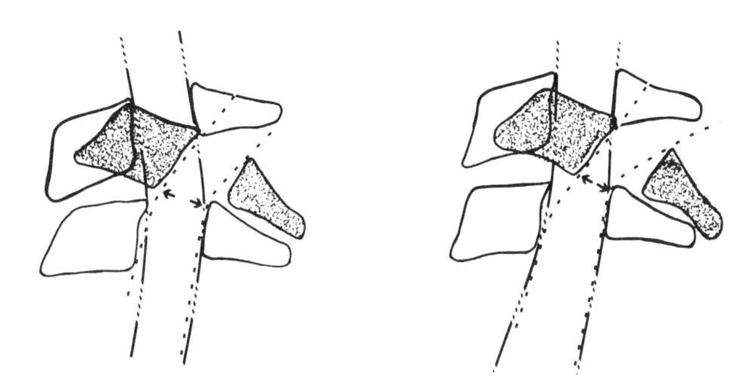

Figure 1 The pincer mechanism described by Penning occurs between the posterior inferior aspect of the vertebral body and the anterior superior aspect of the spinolaminar line of the subjacent vertebra.

THE RATIO METHOD

An alternative way to determine the sagittal diameter of the spinal canal was devised by Pavlov and is called the ratio method. It compares the standard method of measurement of the canal with the anteroposterior width of the vertebral body at the midpoint of the corresponding vertebral body (Fig. 2). The actual measurement of the sagittal diameter in millimeters, as determined by the conventional method, is misleading both as reported in the literature and in actual practice; this is because of variations in the target distances used for roentgenography and in the landmarks used for obtaining the measurement. Using the standard method, the actual measurement of the canal in our observations has occasionally been within the acceptable normal range. The ratio method compensates for variations in roentgenographic technique because the sagittal diameter of both the canal and the vertebral body is affected similarly by magnification factors. The ratio method is independent of variations in technique, and the results are statistically significant. Using the ratio method of determining the dimension of the canal, a ratio of the spinal canal to the vertebral body of less than 0.80 is indicative of significant cervical stenosis. We believe that the ratio of the anteroposterior diameter of the spinal canal to that of the vertebral body is a more reliable way to determine cervical stenosis (Fig. 3).

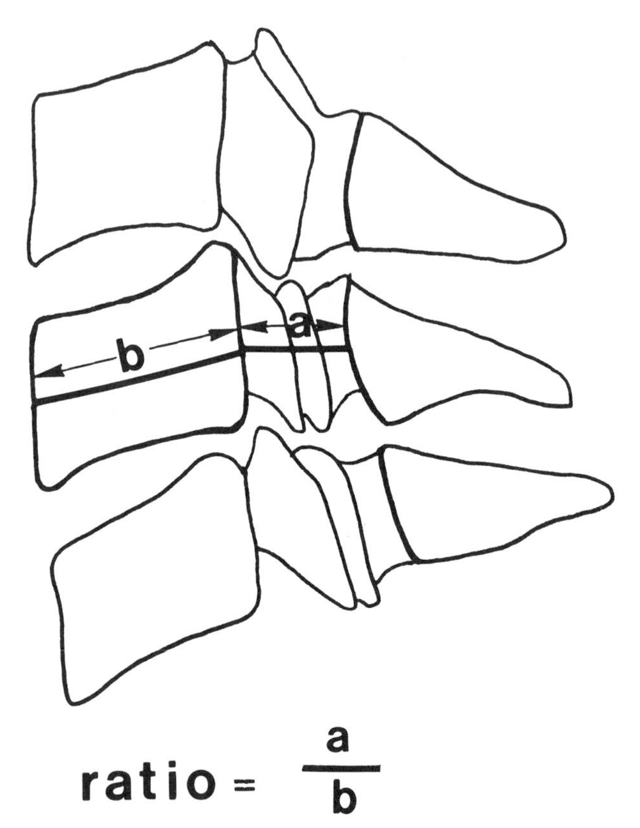

Figure 2 Pavlov's ratio. The spinal canal to vertebral body ratio is the distance from the midpoint of the posterior aspect of the vertebral body to the nearest point on the corresponding spinolaminar line (*a*) divided by the anteroposterior width of the vertebral body (*b*).

On the basis of these observations, it may be concluded that the factor identified that explains the described neurologic picture of cervical spinal cord neurapraxia is diminution of the anteroposterior diameter of the spinal canal, either as an isolated observation or in association with intervertebral disk herniation, degenerative changes, posttraumatic instability, or congenital anomalies. In instances of developmental cervical stenosis, forced hyperflexion, or hyperextension of the cervical spine, a further decrease in the caliber of an already stenotic canal occurs, as explained by the pincer mechanism of Penning (see Fig. 1). In patients whose stenosis is associated with osteophytes or a herniated disc, direct pressure can occur, again with the spine forced in the extremes of flexion and extension. It is further postulated that with an abrupt but brief decrease in the anteroposterior diameter of the spinal canal, the cervical cord is mechanically compressed, causing transient interruption of either its motor or its sensory function, or both, distal to the lesion. The neurologic aberration that results is transient and completely reversible.

A review of the literature revealed that few reported cases of transient quadriplegia occurred in athletes. Attempts to establish the incidence indicate that the problem is more prevalent than expected. Specifically, in the population of 39,377 exposed participants, the reported incidence of transient paresthesia in all four extremities was six per 10,000, whereas the reported incidence of paresthesia associated with transient quadriplegia was 1.3 per 10,000 in the one football season surveyed. From these data, it may be concluded that the prevalence of this problem is relatively high and that an awareness of the etiology, manifestations, and appropriate principles of management warranted.

Characteristically, after an episode of cervical spinal cord neurapraxia with or without transient quadriplegia, the first question raised concerns the advisability of restricting activity. In an attempt to address this problem, 117 young athletes have been interviewed who sustained cervical spine injuries associated with complete permanent quadriplegia while playing football between the years of 1971 and 1984. None of these patients recalled a prodromal experience of transient motor paresis. Conversely, none of the patients in this series who had experienced transient neurologic episodes subsequently sustained an injury that resulted in permanent neurologic injury. On the basis of these data, it is concluded that a young patient who has had an episode of cervical spinal cord neurapraxia with or without quadriplegia is not predisposed to permanent neurologic injury because of it.

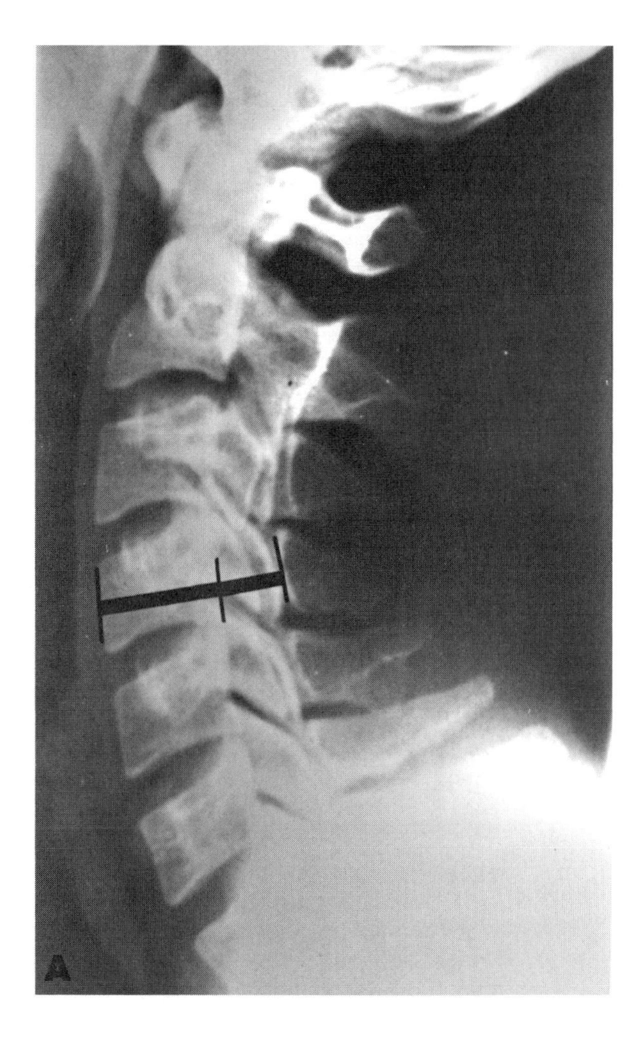

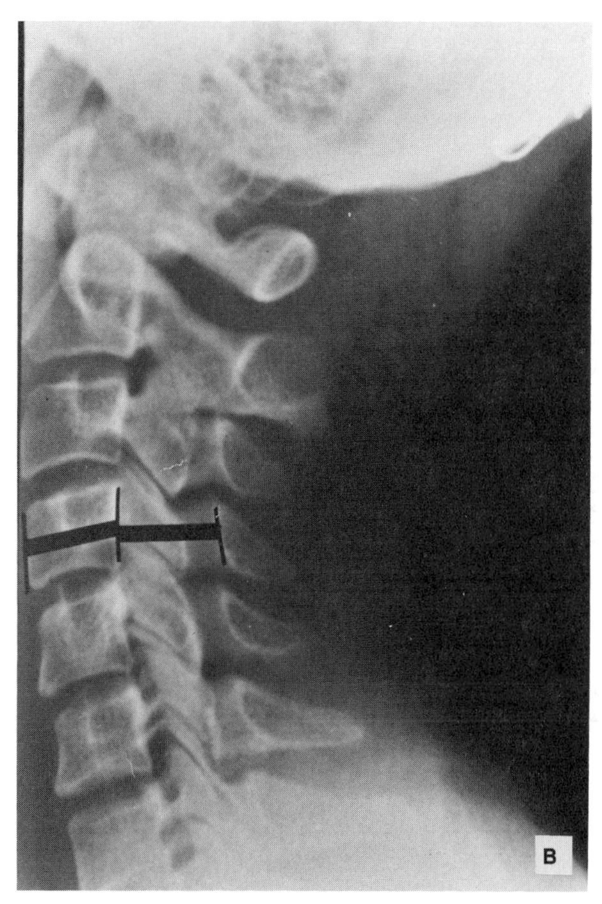

Figure 3 A comparison between the ratio of the spinal canal to the vertebral body in a stenotic patient and that in a control subject is demonstrated on lateral roentgenograms of the cervical spine. The ratio is approximately 1:2 (0.50) in the stenotic patient (*A*) compared with 1:1 (1.00) in the control subject (*B*).

With regard to restrictions in activity, no definite recurrence patterns have been identified to establish firm principles in this area. However, athletes who have this syndrome associated with demonstrable cervical spinal instability or acute or chronic degenerative changes should not be allowed further participation in contact sports. Athletes with developmental spinal stenosis or spinal stenosis associated with congenital abnormalities should be treated on an individual basis. Of the six youngsters with obvious cervical stenosis who returned to football, three had a second episode and withdrew from the activity, and three returned without any problems at 2-year follow-up. The data clearly indicate that individuals with developmental spinal stenosis are not predisposed to more severe injuries with associated permanent neurologic sequelae.

SUGGESTED READING

Boijsen E. The cervical spinal canal in intraspinal expansive processes. Acta Radiol 1954; 42:101–115.

Funk FF Jr, Wells RE. Injuries of the cervical spinal spine in football. Clin Orthop 1975; 109:50–58.

Grant TT, Puffer J. Cervical stenosis: a developmental anomaly with quadriparesis during football. Am J Sports Med 1976; 4:219–221.

Pavlov H, et al. Cervical spinal stenosis: determination with vertebral body ratio method. Radiology 1987; 164:771–775.

Payne EE, Spillane JD. The cervical spine: an anatomicopathological study of 70 specimens (using a special technique) with particular reference to the problem of cervical spondylosis. Brain 1957; 80:571–596.

Penning L. Some aspects of plain radiography of the cervical spine in chronic myelopathy. Neurology 1962; 12:513–519.

Torg, et al: Neurapraxia of the cervical spinal cord with transient quadriplegia. J Bone Joint Surg 1986; 68-A:1354–1370.

BACKACHE

IAN MACNAB, M.B., Ch.B., F.R.C.S., F.R.C.S.(C)

REFERRED PAIN

A major factor that has clouded and confused the diagnosis of soft tissue lesions of the back is the phenomenon of referred pain. When a deep structure is irritated, whether by trauma, disease, or the experimental injection of an irritating solution, the pain resulting may be experienced locally, referred distally, or experienced both locally and radiating to a distance. It is important to recognize that tenderness may also be referred to a distance, as has been shown by the injection of hypertonic saline into the lumbosacral supraspinous ligament. Under such circumstances, pain not only may radiate down the leg but also may be associated with tender points, which are commonly situated over the sacroiliac joint and the upper outer quadrant of the buttock (Fig. 1).

The complaint of pain and the demonstration of local tenderness may obscure the fact that the offending lesion is centrally placed and may lead the clinician to believe erroneously that the disease process underlies the site of the patient's complaints. This false belief may apparently be confirmed by the temporary relief of pain on injection of a local anesthetic when in reality there is no local problem at all. These points must be borne in mind when considering the site and nature of soft tissue injuries giving rise to low back pain; a failure to do so will lead to diagnostic and therapeutic errors.

MYOFASCIAL SPRAINS OR STRAINS

Partial tears of the attachment of muscles may occur, giving rise to local tenderness and pain, generally of short duration. There is always a history of specific injury, either a blunt blow or a forceful movement, usually rotation. The pain and tenderness are always away from the midline. This is a young man's injury with strong muscles guarding a healthy spine. A similar injury sustained by an older man with weaker muscles and with degenerate discs is much more likely to result in a posterior joint strain.

These lesions heal with the passage of time despite, rather than because of, treatment.

Injections of local anesthetic (with or without the addition of local steroids) in and around the area of maximal tenderness certainly afford temporary relief of varying duration, but it is doubtful whether they speed the resolution of the underlying pathologic condition. The symptoms may persist for about 3 weeks in varying degree, during which time the patient is well advised to avoid provocative activity. If symptoms persist beyond this period, the problem should be carefully reassessed lest some more significant underlying lesion be overlooked.

TENDINITIS

Tendinitis by custom has come to be associated with athletic activities. However, it must be remembered that tendinitis is just a clinical syndrome, the pathologic basis of which is inadequately defined. Clinically, it is recognized that well-localized areas of tenderness may develop at the attachment of tendons, fascia, or ligaments to bone, anywhere in the body.

In the spine, breakdown changes of this nature may occur at the attachment of muscles to the sacrum or iliac crest, or the supraspinous ligaments may give rise to pain after having been subjected to moderate to mild trauma. On examination, the areas of breakdown present a small but well-localized area of tenderness. Pressure over the area

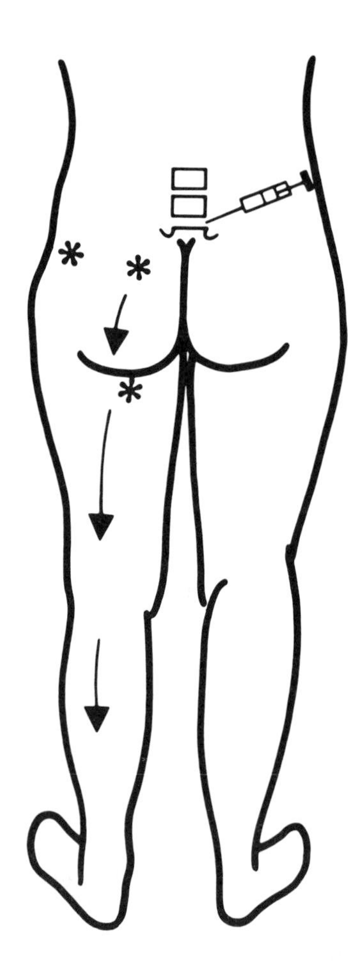

Figure 1 The injection of hypertonic saline into the supraspinous ligament between L5 and S1 gives rise to local pain and pain referred down the back of the leg in sciatic distribution. Usually, this does not extend below the knee, and there are points of tenderness in the lower limbs, most commonly noted at the sites marked by the asterisks.

not only elicits tenderness, but when maintained reproduces the symptoms.

The pathologic basis of this syndrome is probably a local area of tendon breakdown or degeneration, which invokes an inflammatory or autoimmune response. It is possibly the vascular reaction associated with localized edema that accounts for the pain and tenderness. Empirically, it has been found that gratifyingly rapid relief of pain can be obtained by the injection of steroids.

KISSING SPINES: SPRUNG BACK

Approximation of the spinous processes (kissing spines) and the development of a bursa between them have been indicted as a cause of low back pain after hyperextension injuries. "Sprung back" is a term coined by Newman to describe rupture of the supraspinous ligament following a sudden flexion strain applied to the spine with the pelvis fixed, as in falling on the buttocks with the legs outstretched. It is doubtful whether either of these entities is of itself a cause of low back pain (Fig. 2) in the absence of disc degeneration allowing excessive movement at the segment.

With a normal disc, extension of a segment is limited by the anterior fibers of the annulus, and at the limit of normal extension the spinous processes do not come into contact. Contact between the spinous processes is seen only with abnormal mobility associated with disc degeneration. Although apposition of the spinous processes and the development of a painful bursa may aggravate and intensify the symptoms derived from segmental instability associated with degenerative disc disease, these are never the sole source of symptoms. Tearing of the supraspinous ligament, thought to be the basis of "sprung back," can occur only in the presence of disc degeneration allowing an abnormal degree of flexion, or with an injury severe enough to disrupt the posterior fibers of the annulus and the capsule of the posterior joints.

Separation and apposition of the spinous processes when symptomatic are indicative of segmental instability associated with disc degeneration, and the treatment of such lesions is therefore that of the associated disc degeneration.

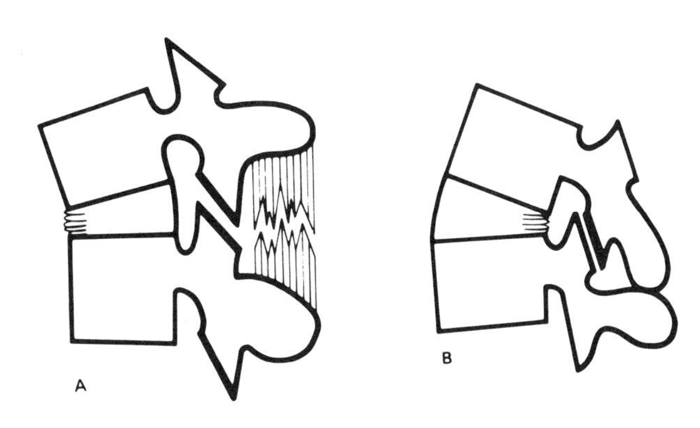

Figure 2 *A*, An acute flexion injury of the spine may produce a tear of the supraspinous ligament. This lesion has been referred to as a "sprung back." It is unlikely, however, that this lesion can occur in the absence of gross disc degeneration, which by itself is probably the source of the patient's complaint. *B*, The radiologic demonstration of apposition of the spinous processes has been referred to as "kissing spines." This anatomic disposition of the spinous processes cannot occur in the absence of an unstable disc segment. In the balance of probabilities, it is the associated disc degeneration rather than the bony apposition of the spinous processes that is the cause of the symptoms.

DISC DEGENERATION

It is necessary to discuss briefly the changes associated with disc degeneration and the manner in which they predispose to symptoms after minor to moderate injury.

The intervertebral discs are composed of a combination of the annulus, the nucleus pulposus, and the hyaline cartilage plate, which makes for a very efficient coupling unit, provided that all the structures remain intact. Normally, the vertebral bodies roll over the incompressible gel of the nucleus pulposus, whose structural integrity is maintained by the annulus, with the posterior joints guiding and steadying the movement. Once degenerative changes involve any one of the components of the disc, such as inspissation of the nucleus pulposus, a tear in the annulus, or a rupture of the hyaline cartilage plate, the smooth roller action is lost and the movement between adjacent vertebral segments becomes uneven, excessive, and irregular. Although these changes occur most commonly at about the age of 40, they may affect younger age groups, especially when there is a family history of low back pain.

Normally, on flexion of the spine, the discal borders of the vertebral bodies become parallel above the level of L5. This is the maximal movement permitted. In the stage of segmental instability, excessive degrees of extension and flexion are permitted and a certain amount of backward and forward gliding movement also occurs (Fig. 3). This abnormal type of movement can be shown clinically by roentgenograms taken with the patient holding the spine in full extension and in full flexion. One problem posed by motion studies is the fact that when a patient is in pain, the associated muscle guarding does not permit adequate flexion and extension films to be taken. However, there are two radiologic changes that are indicative of instability, the Knuttson phenomenon of gas in the disc and the "traction spur."

The traction spur differs anatomically and radiologically from other spondylophytes in that it projects horizontally and develops about 2 mm

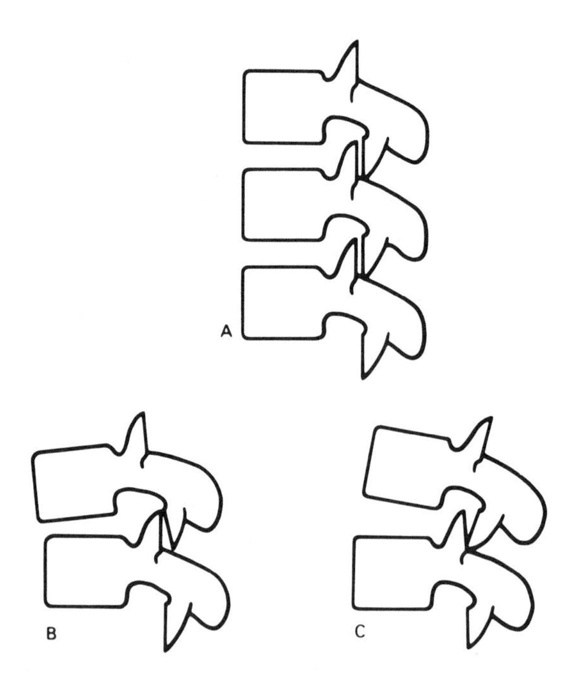

Figure 3 In the early stages of degenerative disc disease, excessive degrees of flexion and extension are permitted at the involved segment. This abnormal mobility is associated with rocking of the posterior joints (*B* and *C*).

above the vertebral body edge (Fig. 4). It owes its development to the manner of attachment of the annulus fibers. With abnormal movements, an excessive strain is applied to the outermost annulus fibers, and it is here that the traction spur develops. It is a small traction spur that is clinically significant in that it is probably indicative of present instability.

Segmental instability by itself is probably not painful, but the spine is vulnerable to trauma. A forced and unguarded movement may be concentrated on the wobbly segment and produce a posterior joint strain or a posterior joint subluxation. Repeated injuries may indeed produce osteochondral fractures and loose bodies in the posterior joints.

In the next stage of disc degeneration, segmental hyperextension occurs. Extension of the lumbar spine is limited by the anterior fibers of the annulus. When degenerative changes cause these fibers to lose their elasticity, the involved segment or segments may hyperextend (Fig. 5). A similar change may be seen in the next stage of disc degeneration, disc narrowing. As the intervertebral discs lose height, the posterior joints must override and subluxate (Fig. 6). In both segmental hyperextension and disc narrowing, the related posterior joints in normal posture are held in hyperextension, and this postural defect is exaggerated if the patient has weak abdominal muscles or tight tensors.

When the posterior joints are held at the extreme of their limit of extension, there is no safety factor of movement, and the extension strains of everyday living may push the joints past their physiologically permitted limits and thereby produce pain.

On the premise that most backaches occur before the age of 40, the roentgenograms of 300 40-year-old laborers, who had been engaged in heavy work all their lives, were reviewed. Of these, 150 denied any history of low back pain and 150 were under treatment for backache at the time of the review. A careful statistical analysis of the films

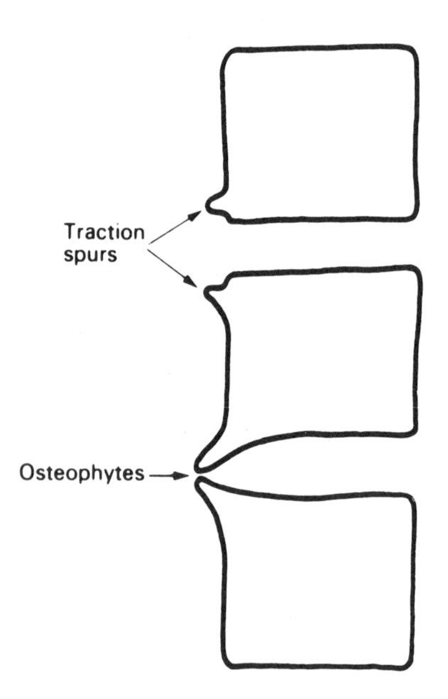

Figure 4 The traction spur projects horizontally from the vertebral body about 1 mm away from the discal border.

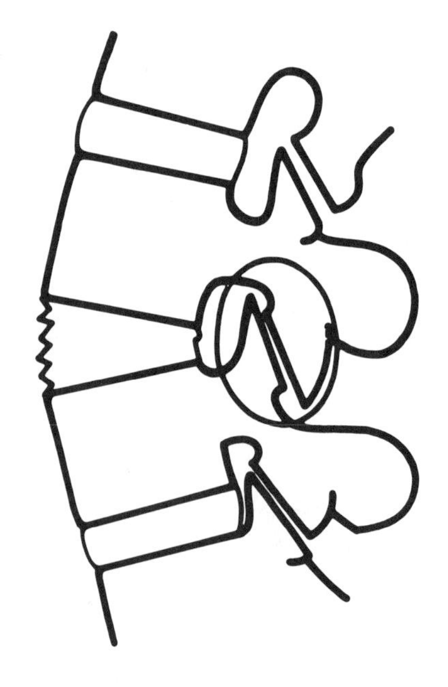

Figure 5 When the anterior fibers of the annulus lose their elasticity, the involved segment falls into hyperextension, permitting subluxation of the related posterior joint.

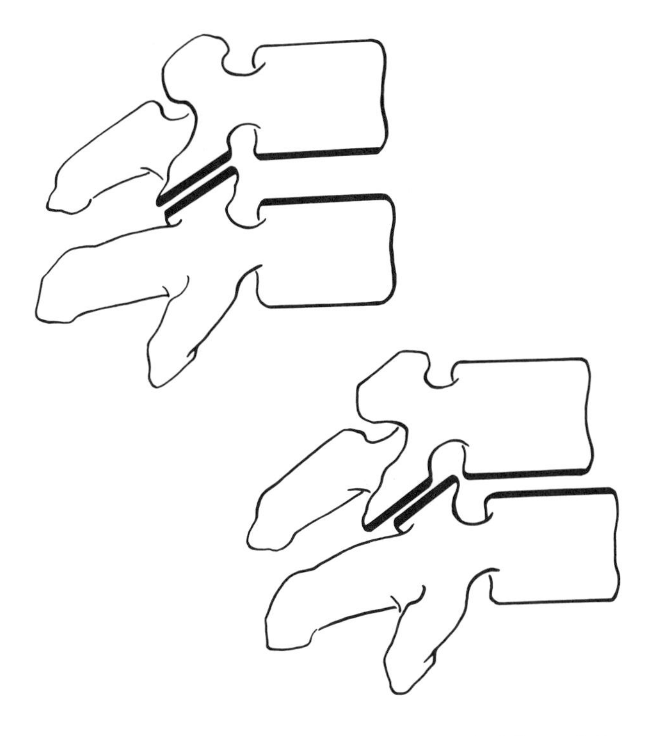

Figure 6 As the intervertebral discs lose height and the vertebral bodies approach one another, the posterior joints must override and assume the position normally held in hyperextension. It is to be noted that owing to the inclination of the posterior joints, as the upper vertebral body approaches the vertebral body beneath it, it is displaced backward, producing a retrospondylolisthesis. This posterior displacement of the vertebral body, indicative of posterior joint subluxation, is readily recognizable on routine x-ray examination of the lumbar spine.

showed no difference in the incidence of anatomic variants and the incidence of degenerative changes in the two groups studied. This is important because the mere demonstration of an anatomic anomaly or a minor pathologic change is no reason to prevent the athlete from continuing with sports activities.

With our present state of knowledge regarding disc degeneration, only the following may be stated: (1) disc degeneration may occur and may remain asymptomatic; (2) disc degeneration may be associated with changes within the disc itself, which may be productive of pain; and (3) disc degeneration may give rise to mechanical instability that renders the spine vulnerable to trauma, as a result of which pain may arise from ligamentous or posterior joint damage.

The pain experienced may remain localized to the back; there may be both local pain and referred pain; or there may be referred pain only.

DISC RUPTURES

An intervertebral disc separating two vertebral segments may be likened to the old-fashioned motorcar tire, with a hard, outer fibrous casing and an inner tube—in this case filled with jelly. A ruptured disc may occur in one of two forms: either similar to a blister in the motorcar tire with a weakening of the outer casing, or on occasion as a complete blowout (sequestration) of the inner tube through the hole in the outer fibers of the annulus.

In 1934 Mixter and Barr suggested that sciatic pain could result from irritation of a lumbar nerve root by a prolapsed intervertebral disc. Although skeptically received at first, this concept soon became universally accepted and founded the "dynasty of the disc," during which time the complaint of sciatic pain tended to become uncritically equated with a diagnosis of disc herniation. Surgical exploration of patients with evidence of lumbar nerve root irritation revealed that there are indeed several sources of nerve root compromise, of which a ruptured intervertebral disc is but one example.

A ruptured intervertebral disc produces nerve root pressure and this presents as radicular pain, i.e., pain radiating from the buttock to the ankle, associated with paresthesia, associated with signs of root tension, and on occasion with evidence of impairment of root conduction. This lesion does not commonly result from a sports-related injury.

If the person has a mechanically insufficient spine and sustains a vigorous strain, the symptoms resulting, as stated previously, may be backache with pain *referred* down the leg in sciatic distribution. This referred pain rarely goes below the knee; it is not associated with paresthesia; it is not associated with signs of nerve root tension, such as limitation of straight leg raising; and it is never associated with any evidence of impairment of root conduction, as reflected by changes in reflex activity, sensory appreciation, or motor power.

If patients are just about to suffer from a prolapsed disc, they may well sustain the prolapse while going down a ski slope, but the sport of skiing is not of itself commonly associated with the production of a ruptured disc. The back injuries associated with athletics are the injuries of joint sprains and associated muscle and fascial damage. The pain resulting from this varies in severity. Characteristically, while patients are carrying out normal activities in sports, they are suddenly seized with back pain and cannot move ("I was paralyzed with pain"). The lumbar spine is splinted rigidly, and patients can move only with painful caution, clutching their back and walking with the trunk leaning forward, keeping the hips and knees slightly bent.

Examination reveals that all movements of the spine are limited by pain and muscle spasm, but there is no evidence of nerve root tension. The clinical picture is explosively dramatic and threatening to the patient. Physicians must not overreact, but constantly remind themselves that even if they elected to treat the patient by rolling peanut butter on each buttock, in the balance of probabilities the patient would get well fairly quickly.

In most such cases the patient is suffering from a "sprain" of one of the zygoapophyseal joints. When trying to rationalize treatment, one should compare the lesion with a severely sprained ankle in a patient who has only one leg and who is unable to wear a prosthesis. There is only one way to treat a sprained ankle in such a patient: the patient has to be put to bed. Theoretically, the patient with an acute low back strain should also be treated by strict bed rest. However, theoretical treatment must be tempered by reason, and reasoning must be tempered by the patient's reaction to therapeutic suggestions.

Let me repeat: you are treating a patient and not a spine, and the experience of the lay world is that many (in fact, most) get better by just creeping around with the pain mollified by analgesics. Some patients, however, cannot cope; their pain is too severe. In such instances, if they cannot do their normal daily work, they should be sent to bed.

A patient with pneumonia is ill and defeated, and happy to go to bed. Patients with severe low back pain feel well in themselves and do not want to go to bed. They are mad at their affliction, and your insistence on bed rest will increase their frustration unless you take time to explain in detail the purpose of this apparently neglectful form of management. It is advisable to give patients some literature explaining in detail the probable underlying pathology and the rationale of treatment by bed rest. You must advise them about toilet facilities. Using a bedpan at home is an impractical acrobatic feat. Crutches make it easier for patients to get to the bathroom, and the purchase of a high toilet seat is essential.

To relieve the pain, local ice application has definite merit for the first 48 hours. Local application of ice over a muscle probably acts on the muscle's spindle system. A muscle that retains its extensibility through its normal resting length is usually pain free. When it does not retain its extensibility, it is considered to be in "spasm" and a source of pain. Ice applied to the overlying skin probably sends impulses to the cord that "compete" with the pain, producing impulses that are conveyed by much slower fibers. The ice-produced impulses temporarily cause a refractory period in the other impulses, and the muscle spasm is momentarily relieved. Stretch of the muscle is now possible, which decreases the spasm. If ice is applied for too long a period, the muscle may become literally chilled, and this increases muscle spasm and adds to the pain.

There are very few orally administered muscle "relaxants" that have any effect on skeletal muscles. If they were truly effective, the eye muscles would also be grossly relaxed, and the patient would develop nystagmus. Their major action is as a tranquilizer. Analgesics in sufficient doses can be given, but they must be given on a time-dependent basis and not on demand. These patients must not be allowed to pop pills for pain; otherwise the physician is just inducing a habituation. In the vast majority of patients, after 2 or 3 days the "smoke clears away" and they can get around each day with increasing comfort.

If on neurologic examination there is neither evidence of nerve root compression or irritation nor of impairment of root conduction, the resolution of symptoms may be speeded by a flexion manipulation (Fig. 7). The patient lies on the back and the physician raises the patient's legs, maintaining the knees in flexion. By applying pressure on the heels, the physician then pushes the patient's knees toward the shoulders; this is done very slowly. The degree of flexion obtained is determined by the discomfort the patient experiences. The movement is then repeated slowly and rhythmically over a period of 5 minutes. In most cases the range of movement that can be achieved by this passive manipulation gradually increases, and at the conclusion of the manipulation the patient is instructed to flex his knees fully and allow his feet to come down to the bed, soles first.

The patient then carries out a series of passive flexion manipulations of his spine once an hour. He

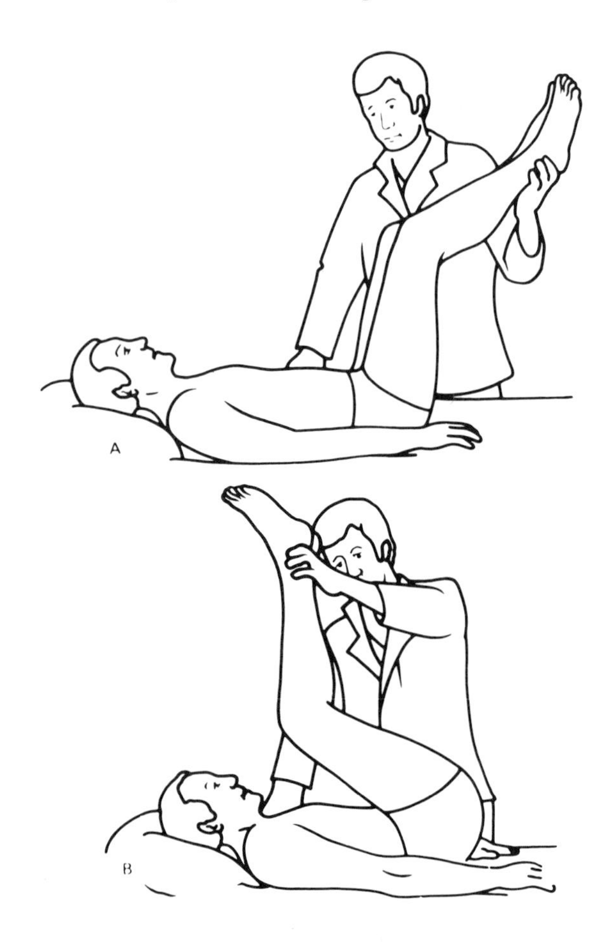

Figure 7 *A*, Flexion manipulation by the physician, who raises the patient's legs, maintaining the knees in flexion. *B*, By applying pressure to the heels, the physician then pushes the patient's knees toward the shoulders.

does this by lying on his back and pulling his knees slowly up to his chest (Fig. 8). He should maintain this position for 5 minutes. In very acute attacks with severe pain, the patient may find it easier to assume the same position lying on his side. By the second day the patient should be able to carry out the flexion manipulations of his back himself (Fig. 9).

Once the attack is over, the patient and the physician are now faced with the difficulty of trying to prevent recurrent episodes. Adequate trunk muscles are the major guardians against repeated attacks. It must be remembered that the spinal column is not a self-supporting structure. If the trunk and abdominal muscles are paralyzed, as in infantile paralysis, the spine collapses. The spine is supported by muscle action in much the same way the mast of a ship is supported by stays (Fig. 10). In addition to this, the abdominal cavity acts as a hydraulic sac, dissipating loads by pressing upward on the diaphragm and downward on the pelvic floor, thereby unweighting the spine (Fig. 11). Because of this, the tone and strength of the abdominal muscles are of vital importance in protecting the spine against weight bearing and extension strains.

The exercise program is started by pelvic tilting. This is best carried out with the patient lying supine on a firm surface. The patient lies in a comfortable position with the hips and knees flexed, keeping the soles of both feet flat on the bed or floor. The patient now presses the lower back down flat against the floor so that the lumbar lordosis is obliterated. This movement is achieved by a combined contraction of the abdominal muscles and the glutei. In order to help the patient get into this habit, it

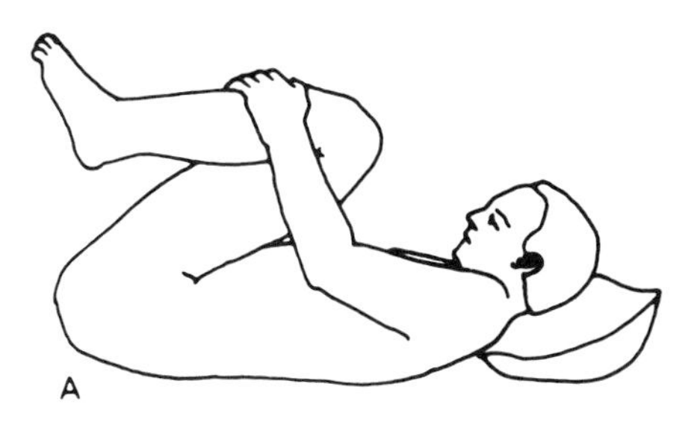

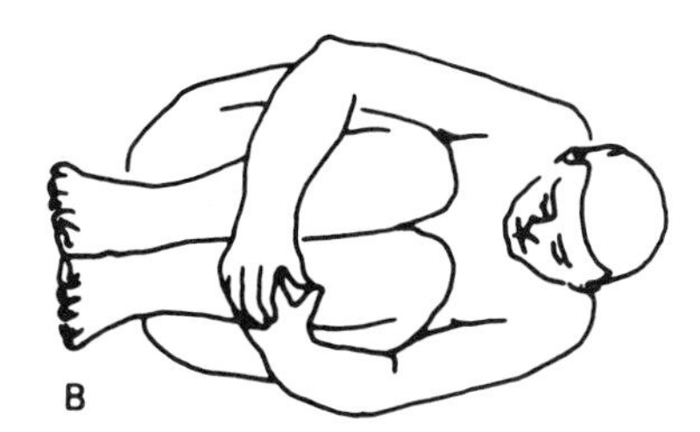

Figure 8 A patient may abort an acute episode of low back pain by lying on his back and pulling his knees slowly up to his chest. *A*. He should maintain this position for 5 minutes. If pain is severe, the patient may find it easier to assume the same position lying on his side (*B*).

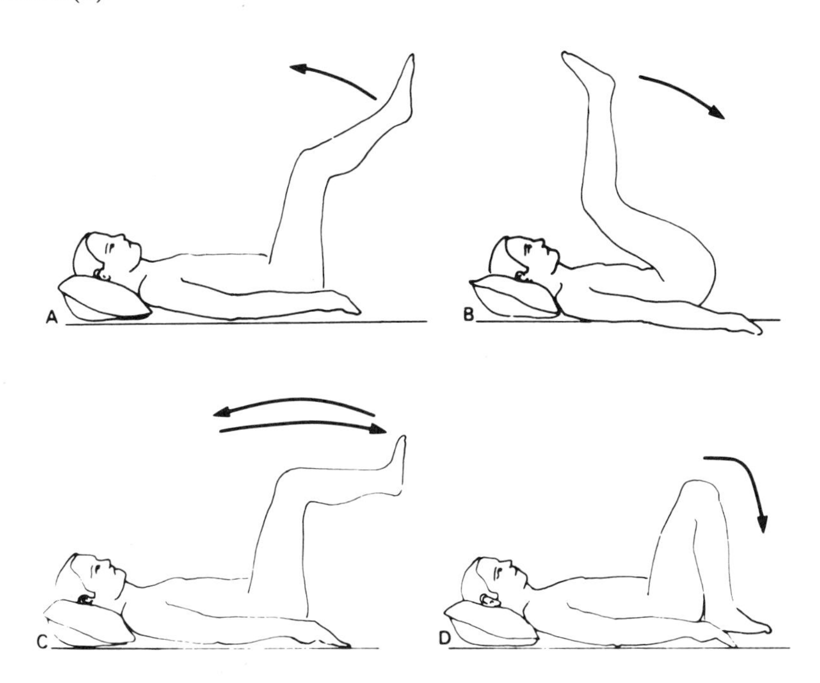

Figure 9 Flexion exercise-manipulation of the lumbar spine. The patient lies on the bed with his head supported by a pillow. *A*, The hips are flexed to 90 degrees and the knees slightly flexed. *B*, The patient now attempts to kick his feet over his head, raising the buttocks approximately 6 inches off the bed. *C*, After each "kick-up" the patient returns to the starting position. *D*, After five kick-ups, the patient rests by lowering his legs with the knees fully flexed, thereby putting his feet on the bed, soles first. It is very important not to lower the legs with the knees fully extended because this places a painful hyperextension strain on the spine.

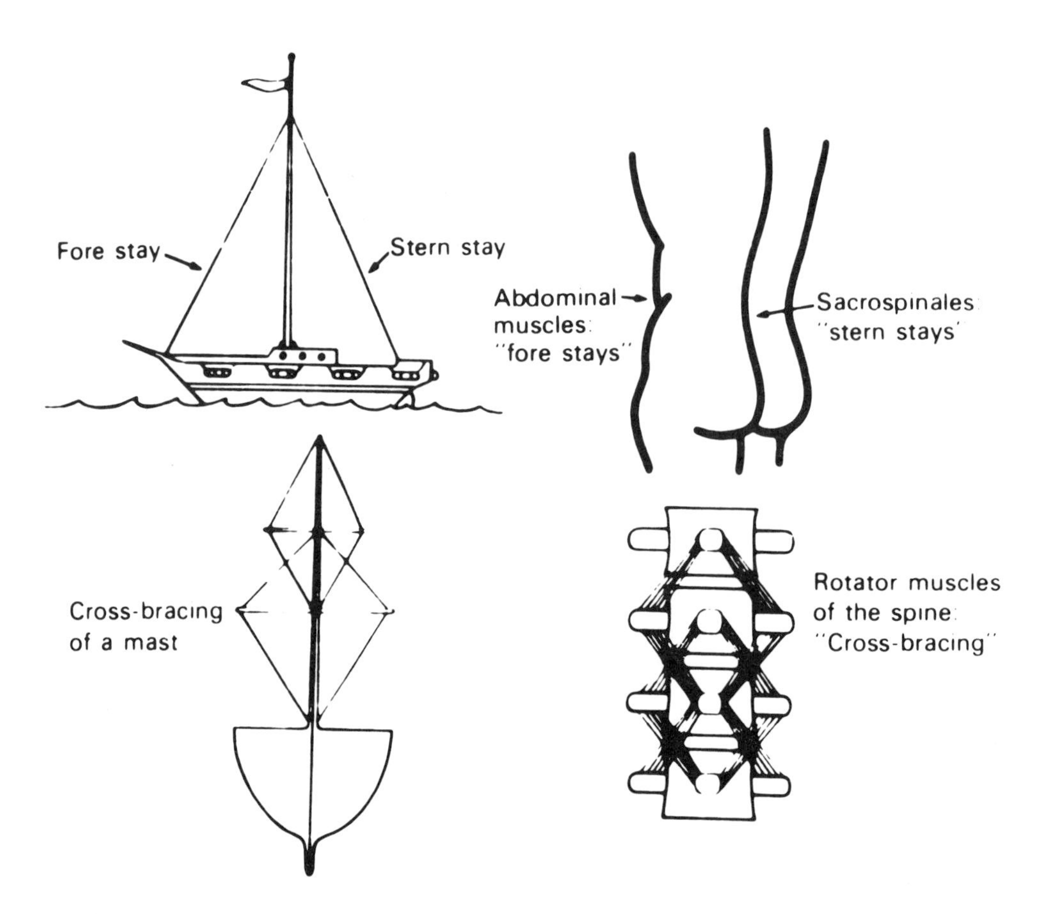

Figure 10 It is interesting to note the similarity between the bracing used to support the mast of a ship and the muscular bracing of the human spine.

is often easier to ask him to put his hands behind his back and press his spine back onto his hands.

Once the lumbar spine is pressing against the floor, the pelvis is rotated by raising the buttocks from the floor. As the buttocks are being raised, the lower back must not be permitted to leave the floor.

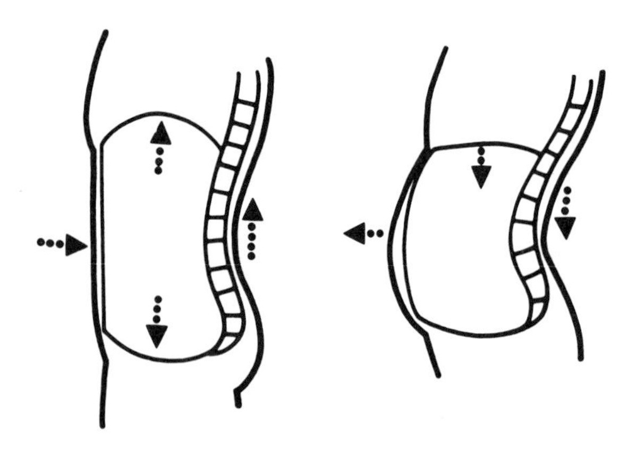

Figure 11 The abdominal cavity acts in a manner similar to a hydraulic sac. By increasing intra-abdominal pressure, the diaphragm is pushed up and the pelvic floor is pushed down. This tends to "elongate" the lumbar spine, thereby taking some of the weight off the discs and the posterior joints.

Raising the buttocks away from the floor reverses the lumbar lordosis. Patients may find it easier if they put one hand on the symphysis pubis and the other on the xyphoid process and then try to bring their hands together while doing the exercises. As patients become more adept at this exercise, they should practice the movement rhythmically, initially with the hips and knees flexed before trying the same exercise with the hips and knees flat.

Pelvic tilting can also be practiced with the patient standing with his back flat against the wall and his feet about 2 feet away from the wall. Holding his lumbar spine flat against the wall (checking this with a hand placed between his spine and the wall), he then gradually brings his heels toward the wall and tries to straighten his knees. To begin with this is difficult, but when he can achieve this easily he has managed to learn the art of pelvic tilting in a manner that will overcome a tendency to hyperlordosis.

When flexion exercises are started, the patient should lie on his back with his hips and knees bent and his feet *supported.* He should put his hands forward to touch his thighs and then gradually crawl up his thighs until his hands are on the top of his knees. He should then take his hands away from his knees and let his back fall gently into the supine position. Flexion exercises should never be performed with the patient holding his knees fully extended. The only way it is possible to get up with the knees extended is to whip the back up, because the weight of the trunk is greater than the weight of the legs. A person has to put an extension strain on the lower back to begin the movement and then the rest of the spine is flung forward, as with a whiplash.

At this stage it is necessary, in the prevention of recurrence of back pain, to test for the flexibility of the hamstrings and the heel cords. The supine position is again used. One leg is fully flexed at the hip with the knee and thigh against the chest. The leg undergoing the stretching of the hamstrings is maintained in full extension. The patient now tries to sit up slowly and reach toward the toes of the extended leg. The fixed, flexed leg prevents the occurrence of hyperlordosis during the act of sitting up. If the heel cords are found to be tight, the extended leg should be placed in such a manner that the sole of the foot is flat against the wall. The heel cords can also be stretched by leaning forward against the wall, keeping the feet flat on the floor, and the force applied to the heel cords can be increased by getting the patient to squat down.

On occasion, a tight tensor fascia femoris causes anterior pelvic rotation, which increases the lumbar lordosis. This needs passive stretching by a physiotherapist.

As in all therapeutic exercises, a few specific exercises are initially directed toward the lesion being treated, but once the discomfort starts to subside it is of vital importance that the patient engage in a general controlled physical exercise program.

FURTHER INVESTIGATION

The question is often asked, "When should you take an x- ray?" Probably the following criteria are adequate:

1. Severe back pain following significant trauma.
2. Incapacitating back pain.
3. Excessively anxious patients. In such people, an x-ray examination is an essential part of treatment; they cannot be reassured by clinical examination alone.
4. Patients in whom the history and examination are suggestive of an early ankylosing spondylitis. A specific request should be made for oblique views of the sacroiliac joint.
5. Patients with clinically apparent spinal deformity.
6. Patients with significant root tension and patients presenting with evidence of impairment of root conduction. It must be remembered that being very athletically inclined does not prevent these young people from having a tumor of the cauda equina.
7. If severe pain persists for longer than 2 weeks despite treatment, an x-ray examination is indicated, not only to exclude the possibility of some obscure spinal abnormality, but also to reassure patients that they are not suffering from a serious progressive disease.

On occasion the radiograph reveals a spinal anomaly. Of the spinal anomalies once believed to cause back pain, such as sacralization of L5, spina bifida occulta, the ossicle of Oppenheimer, and a unilateral iliotransverse joint, all are now recognized as being incidental findings that have no influence on the development of low back pain.

There remains just one bone anomaly that gives rise to concern. If the radiograph reveals a spondylolysis of L5 with or without a listhesis, the question always arises whether this defect in the pars interarticularis developed as a result of repeated trauma on the football field or whether the patient had this defect before he started playing football.

It has been reported, and convincingly demonstrated radiographically, that linebackers may develop in the course of the season, as a result of the vigorous hyperextension strains they place on each other, a stress fracture through the pars interarticularis, giving rise to a spondylolysis. Without specific therapy and certainly without surgery, over the course of the next 6 months, these stress fractures heal by themselves and will not be the source of further disability.

In patients in whom a routine x-ray examination reveals a spondylolisthesis of grade I or more, the question is always raised whether it is safe to let the young athlete continue with contact sports. There is no evidence that vigorous physical contact will cause an increasing slip. These patients may have a pain derived either from the subjacent disc, from the syndesmosis at the site of the isthmic defect, or most probably from degenerative disc changes occurring at the level above the slip. Any one or all three of these factors may be responsible for repeated episodes of discomfort during play and may markedly interfere with the patient's competence.

In these patients, there are two choices. Either they must give up contact sports or, if this is going to be their profession, the question is raised whether they should be admitted to the hospital for more detailed analysis of the source of the discomfort, to see whether it is possible to stop abnormal movement at the level of the defect and stabilize the degenerative disc above the slip by a localized intertransverse fusion. It must always be remembered that it will take at least 9 months to 1 year before this young person returns to competitive sports.

In the diagnosis and management of a patient presenting with low back pain, orthopaedic surgeons must play many roles: family practitioner, internist, radiologist, physiatrist, orthotist, psychiatrist, social worker, and friend. They should rarely find it necessary to play the role of their chosen avocation— orthopaedic surgeon.

CONSERVATIVE BACK CARE

HAMILTON HALL, M.D., F.R.C.S.(C)

Much of the management currently offered for low back pain is primarily passive in nature and requires no active patient participation. This approach is particularly unsuitable for the athlete with back trouble. Most passive forms of treatment provide short-term pain relief and have no impact on long-term control. The athlete whose primary concerns are a prompt return to competition and the maintenance of a superior performance level requires a more aggressive back care program.

Passive modalities are usually intended to accelerate recovery through a reduction in inflammation and control of edema. Most deliver some type of thermal or mechanical stimulus. These therapies can shorten a necessary period of immobility but are rarely indicated in chronic situations. To be effective, treatment should be applied as soon as possible after the onset of an acute episode as determined by the logistics and economics of the situation. Because passive therapies are intended to provide only symptomatic relief, a definite diagnosis of the cause of the back pain is not usually required before treatment begins. The benefit of the treatment is measured in the rate of recovery and the speed of return to competition.

The value of any specific form of treatment for back pain in the athlete is difficult to assess. It is, after all, therapy applied to a condition with a high percentage of spontaneous remission. Although it may be difficult for many athletes to accept, almost 90 percent of acute back attacks subside completely in 3 months or less with no treatment at all. Anecdotal accounts of miraculous cures and dramatic testimonials for new treatment methods may reflect nothing more than the application of an ineffective technique to back pain already beginning spontaneous recovery. Valid prospective studies to compare the effect of a single passive modality against an appropriate control group are not yet available.

Particularly in the athlete with back injury, passive treatment programs risk producing dependence. Because of their level of expectation and extreme focus on musculoskeletal discomfort, athletes who gain temporary pain relief may give a treatment more credit than it deserves. This is particularly true when the therapy comes highly recommended and possesses an aura of advanced technology. High-level athletes see themselves as special people with special needs, which may not be satisfied by lengthy and mundane treatment. More than most, competitive athletes require and expect an immediate result. The current emphasis on science in the training program translates into a demand for science in the treatment of back pain.

The problem is complicated by the prevalence of the complaint: 80 percent of the adult population in North America will at some time suffer an attack of back pain, and athletes are no exception. With so many "experts" speaking from personal experience, it is difficult to establish standards for good conservative care.

Because the precise nature and location of most back pain is poorly understood, misconceptions abound. Regretfully, these mistaken beliefs are often fostered by those with a financial incentive to provide the cure. Although discs never slip, athletes may be given sessions of spinal manipulation that purport to return the disc to its proper location. When this manipulation does produce pain relief, probably through the temporary elimination of paraspinal muscle spasm, the erroneous concept of the slipped disc gains unwarranted credence. It becomes a small step to belief in the necessity of a maintenance manipulation program to preserve normal spinal alignment. The lack of any scientific proof for this approach is no longer a factor. Similar problems exist with many of the conventional passive therapies. The relief of pain is tied to physiologically impossible principles, which in turn are used as the basis for unjustified long-term treatment.

Back care and the treatment of back pain are often classified as invasive or noninvasive. Since the degree of invasiveness is limited, however, this division is usually unimportant. A more useful classification differentiates between the active and passive therapies and further subdivides each group according to its principal effective component.

Active treatment is the key to successful back care in the athlete. It contains two major factors: education and exercise. Because of the widespread fear and misunderstanding that envelop the subject of back pain, education must be an integral part of any long-term management. The athlete who is afraid that the back may suddenly go out of place is unlikely to take part in a vigorous rehabilitation program. The impact of back problems on future performance, the risks of returning to competition, and the relationship between hurt and harm must be addressed directly. The athlete who appreciates the strength and durability of the spine and recognizes the essentially benign nature of most back pain will be more willing to resume training than the athlete who has failed to understand that back pain is not synonymous with back injury.

To avoid dependence on temporary pain-relieving measures, it is necessary to develop a self-reliant approach. Effective education that reduces fear, restores confidence, and provides a clear picture of the spine's enormous potential for recovery is necessary before the athlete can begin an independent routine of therapeutic back exercise. Although the exact role of exercise remains controversial, recent work suggests that the previously reported lack of benefit resulted most often from an inadequate amount of physical effort. What was prescribed as back exercise in the past bears little resemblance to the routines in use today. A better knowledge of muscle physiology and function, equipment that allows the selective strengthening of individual muscle groups, and a focus on exercise patterns that simulate specific athletic endeavors have enhanced the value of back exercise programs.

The current trend is a balanced approach based on the pain source as a means of determining the pattern of treatment. When the back pain is aggravated on repetitive forward bending, a program will begin with extension exercise. Conversely, when the pain is increased with extension, the exercises begin with abdominal strengthening and pelvic tilt. Ultimately, most athletes require a combination of flexion and extension. To allow better protection of the back, there is also increased emphasis on strengthening the arms and legs in accordance with the demands of the particular athletic activity.

Stretching as well as strengthening has become a goal for back exercise. Although there is no evidence that increased spinal flexibility reduces the risk of back injury, there is a correlation between restoring normal movement and reducing pain after injury has occurred. The timing of an active exercise routine is as important as the exercises chosen. The schedule must be advanced or reduced in accordance with the athlete's functional response. To aid motivation, the rehabilitation must be oriented clearly and openly toward a return to competitive activity.

Active treatment should be initiated as soon as symptoms permit, generally much earlier than is commonly anticipated. Athletes can begin an exercise routine within days of an acute attack even in the presence of continuing back muscle spasm. The duration of active treatment is usually self-imposed. Although a return to an acceptable level of competition marks the end of the recovery process, a maintenance program of protective back care is still required. Ideally, this routine is self-administered without the need for medical supervision. The problem of excessive participation is of greater importance in the athlete than it is in the general back patient population. Either too much or too little exercise for a recovering back may retard the return to competition.

Recognized surgical pathology, particularly that involving acute nerve root irritation, is a contraindication to active treatment and requires a period of passive therapy. An acute episode of back pain and muscle spasm is a relative contraindication. In both instances, the athlete should realize the importance of returning to active participation as quickly as pain and the diagnosis permit. The initiation of an active routine and the continued use of passive pain-relieving modalities are not mutually exclusive.

While active participation is the ultimate goal, immediate pain relief is an important aspect of back care in the athlete. To the motivated individual, reducing or eliminating pain through passive measures means the opportunity to resume training and return to competition. For the most part, these measures do not attack the primary back problem but act instead on the secondary features of inflammation, edema, and awareness of pain. Because they have no curative function, the value of passive procedures is determined by their ability to relieve pain. It makes no sense to continue to employ these agents when there is no pain reduction or when they produce an increase in the symptoms. They are contraindicated in situations in which they may become the only source of pain control and may create dependence. For this reason, passive modalities should not be continued as the only form of therapy for more than a few months.

Passive therapies include many physical modalities, therapeutic injections, and medications. The physical treatments can be classified as thermal, mechanical, movement restricting, and those that modify the perception of pain. Therapeutic injections involve trigger points, facet and sacroiliac joints, nerve roots, and the epidural space. Medication includes narcotic and non-narcotic analgesics, anti-inflammatory drugs, tranquilizers, and antidepressants.

Thermal therapy describes the application of liniments, hot packs, ice packs, heat lamps, and deep heat. Although there are claims for specific therapeutic value, this group of therapies appears to act primarily as a counterirritant, a physical means to retard or reduce edema and a method of producing muscle relaxation. Heated pools, mineral baths, saunas, and steam rooms are part of this list. Thermal treatments remain the most popular method of rapid pain control for the athlete. They are readily accepted and often provide psychological as well as physical comfort.

Traction, manipulation, mobilization, therapeutic massage, chiropractic adjustment, whirlpools, and hydrotherapy are all forms of mechanical treatment that can produce sudden dramatic pain relief. If this coincides with the start of further spontaneous remission, the athlete can easily attribute value to the treatment that it does not deserve. There is no evidence that mechanical modalities produce any lasting effect, but athletes who derive short-term benefit can become rapidly dependent on this form of passive pain relief.

Bed rest is the simplest and most frequently prescribed method of restricting movement. A few days of rest have been shown to accelerate the subsequent return to athletic activity. Prolonged bed rest creates a significant catabolic effect and a psychological deterioration that extend the athlete's period of disability far beyond the acute episode. The rationale for reduced movement is the reduction of inflammation. It is therefore inappropriate to recommend bed rest in cases of chronic mechanical back pain aggravated only by specific movements or activities. Careful instruction and modified training to reduce or avoid the pain-producing maneuvers are more beneficial. Restricting movement with a brace or back support can shorten the painful episode or allow continued athletic participation. External protection without continuing exercise, however, can lead to a lowering of performance and the creation of psychological or physical dependence through the loss of abdominal or paraspinal muscle tone. The continuous use of a brace should be avoided.

Classic acupuncture is the prototype of physical pain modification treatment. Most studies ascribe its action to the release of endorphins within the brain. Treatments claiming the same mode of action include acupressure, cold laser therapy, and electrical stimulation of the acupuncture needles. Because the mechanism of endorphin release is not fully understood, the value of most of these treatments remains unproved. However, transcutaneous electrical nerve stimulation (TENS) has a well-established role in short-term pain control. Self-administered and without adverse physical effects, TENS can be used by the athlete for extended periods. Unfortunately, repetitive application for back pain leads to increasing resistance to the stimulation, requiring greater current flow and more frequent applications.

Therapeutic injections are seldom indicated for athletic back pain. Trigger points are uncommon without chronic pain, and the behavior disorders of a chronic pain syndrome are rarely found in the active athlete. When present, a trigger point can be injected with local anesthetic to produce excellent short-term pain relief. Like other passive modalities, this treatment may coincide with or even precipitate an extended pain-free interval. Facet or sacroiliac joint injections, root blocks, or epidural anesthesia are usually reserved to treat prolonged or disabling back pain. Therapeutic steroid injections can control acute joint or dural inflammation, but the potential complications limit their use in most attacks of back pain, which subside within 12 weeks.

Because back pain in the athlete is usually mechanical, medication plays a secondary role. Pain relief is usually possible with one of the physical modalities. Narcotic analgesics are almost never indicated and even in extreme cases should be discontinued after a few days. Non-narcotic medications may have a short-term role, but although the potential for abuse is less, the long-term use of any analgesic should be avoided.

Anti-inflammatory medications are useful to treat acute low back pain. In many cases they can substitute for analgesics or minor tranquilizers and are often the only medications required. There are various classes of nonsteroidal anti-inflammatory drugs (NSAIDs) and the response of the individual athlete to a specific medication is impossible to predict; several may be tried before one is found that will reduce the pain. Similarly, a single NSAID may not be equally effective in two athletes suffering the same type of back problem. In some circumstances, pain relief is achieved even when the drugs are not taken on a regular basis. In these instances the anti-inflammatory agents may be used intermittently as dictated by the symptoms.

Tranquilizers and antidepressants affect athletic performance. Their use is limited to cases in which a high level of anxiety or depression is judged a significant contributory factor to the back pain. The use of these drugs indicates the diagnosis of a behavioral disorder and implies treatment beyond that required solely for low back dysfunction.

Successful conservative back care in the athlete depends on (1) the rapid formulation of a non-threatening diagnosis to avoid the creation of unnecessary fear, (2) early and active mobilization to prevent physical and psychological decompensation, and (3) a minimum of passive pain-relieving modalities to reduce dependence. Progressive competition simulation is an effective guide in the preparation for actual athletic pursuits. The ability of the athlete must be matched to the demands of the game, and the treatment program must be tailored to the specific needs of the situation. A return to competition is advisable only when the risks of reinjury are understood and the barriers to performance have been eliminated.

SUGGESTED READING

Haldeman S. Spinal manipulative therapy in sports medicine. Clin Sports Med 1986; 5:277.

Jackson C, Brown M. Is there a role for exercise in the treatment of patients with low back pain? Clin Orthop 1983; 179:39.

Mayer TG, Gatchel RJ. Functional restoration for spinal disorders: the sports medicine approach. Philadelphia: Lea & Febiger, 1988.

Nachemson A. Advances in low back pain. Clin Orthop 1985; 200:266.

Videman T. Connective tissue and immobilization: key factors in musculoskeletal degeneration? Clin Orthop 1987; 221:26.

Wiesel SW, Rothman RH. Acute low back pain. An objective analysis of conservative therapy. Spine 1980; 5:324.

Zylbergold RS, Piper MC. Comparative analysis of physical therapy treatments. Arch Phys Med Rehabil 1981; 62:176.

SPINAL DEFORMITIES

LYLE J. MICHELI, M.D.
ELLY TREPMAN, M.D.

The physician dealing with sports-related injuries must have a working knowledge of both normal spinal contour and structural spinal deformities. The importance of the spine in normal function cannot be overemphasized. It is the structural centrum from which extremity motion initiates, and it contains important elements of the central nervous system and the origin of the peripheral nerves. Spinal deformities may increase the potential for spinal injury or compromise spinal function during athletic activities.

The four major issues pertaining to spinal deformities are

1. Detection of spinal abnormalities that may render sports participation ineffective or even dangerous for a child.
2. Early detection of spinal deformity in the child athlete, with the initiation of ongoing assessment or bracing.
3. Effective management of relatively mild spinal deformities with bracing or electrical stimulation techniques and directed exercises while a child continues to participate in sports.
4. Determination of the level of athletic participation that is safe and effective for a child who has required a spinal fusion.

THE NORMAL AND ABNORMAL SPINE

The spine consists of a series of seven cervical, 12 thoracic, and five lumbar vertebrae perched upon the sacrum, and is designed for both stability and movement. In the sagittal plane, this semirigid column has a normal thoracic kyphosis (convex posterior angulation) and lumbar lordosis (convex anterior angulation). The cervical spine is capable of a wide range of motion, but normally is postured in a position of slight lordosis (Fig. 1).

The degree of angulation of the spine is determined by the Cobb technique (Fig. 2). The angle subtended by the top of the most tilted vertebra above, and the bottom of the most tilted vertebra below, is defined as the angle of curvature.

The range of normal magnitude of these angulations is controversial. In general, when a person is standing, the normal range of thoracic kyphosis is 20 to 50 degrees; deviations outside these limits are either hypokyphosis (<20 degrees) or hyperkyphosis (>50 degrees). Similarly, the range of normal lumbar lordosis is 20 to 50 degrees (see Fig. 1).

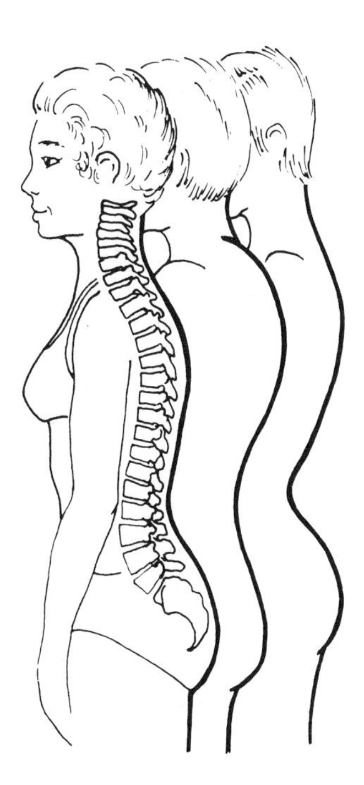

Figure 1 The normal range of thoracic kyphosis and lumbar lordosis is 20 to 50 degrees.

The incidence of dorsal (thoracic) hyperkyphosis may be increased among athletically active adolescents, especially males. This condition, known as Scheuermann's kyphosis, is defined as a dorsal kyphosis of more than 50 degrees in which there is at least 15 percent wedging of at least three

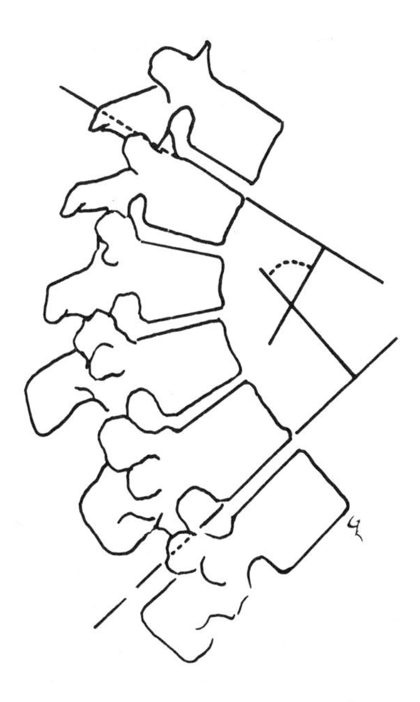

Figure 2 The Cobb angle, a quantitative measure of spinal curve, is the angle between the top of the most tilted vertebral body at the superior limit of the curve and the bottom of the most inferior vertebral body.

vertebral bodies, narrowing of the disc spaces, and irregularity of the vertebral body end plates. The condition may have a genetic predisposition, or it may be acquired, secondary to repetitive microtrauma on the anterior aspects of the vertebral bodies of the dorsal spine, with resultant wedging. A tight lumbar lordosis may contribute to the problem by preventing adequate forward flexion of the lumbar spine; as a result, with forward flexion, more flexion must occur in the thoracic spine, leading to injury of the anterior aspect of the vertebral bodies, with secondary structural changes and dorsal roundback deformity.

Any curvature of the spine in the coronal plane is defined as scoliosis. This condition is abnormal and is therefore considered a deformity, even though 10 percent of the population may have a mild scoliosis (up to 10 degrees) in some portion of the spine.

Scoliosis may be functional—the result of muscle spasm, postural angulation of the spine, or extraspinal factors such as limb length discrepancy or pelvic obliquity. In functional scoliosis, there is no fixed deformity of the spine, and when the causative factor is corrected the spine becomes straight.

In contrast, structural scoliosis is a fixed deformity of the spine, although it may be partially corrected with mechanical techniques such as pulsion pressure or traction. The causes of structural scoliosis include (1) paralytic disorders such as poliomyelitis or myelodysplasia, (2) congenital abnormalities of the spine, or (3) idiopathic scoliosis.

Idiopathic scoliosis, the most common type of scoliosis in North America, is often familial, with a fivefold increased risk in family members. It may become apparent at a specific time in the growth and development of the child. The classification of idiopathic scoliosis includes (1) infantile-onset scoliosis, which is evident during the first year of life; (2) juvenile-onset scoliosis, which begins during the prepubescent period; and (3) adolescent-onset scoliosis, which can develop rapidly and progressively once adolescence begins.

Most conditions that cause scoliosis occur during childhood or adolescence. Therefore, it is important to consider the possibility of spinal deformity in childhood participation in sports, because (1) the deformity may influence the child's ability to engage in sports safely and effectively, and (2) the sports environment, particularly that of organized team sports, provides an excellent opportunity for early detection of a developing spinal deformity. The preparticipation physical examination, which should be performed annually for any child involved in organized sports, should include an assessment and careful measurement of the posture and contour of the body, with special attention to the spine, torso, and pelvis. The child who exhibits symmetric posture on examination may the following year show signs of progressive scoliosis or early kyphosis (dorsal roundback).

Abnormalities of posture and contour are carefully assessed in school screening programs, which are currently mandated in more than half of the United States as well as in Canada. These programs are at least 85 percent effective in the early detection of spinal abnormalities. In combination with an effective bracing or electrical stimulation program, they can often prevent the progression of spinal deformity and the need for surgery.

DIFFERENTIAL DIAGNOSIS

Spinal deformities or structural abnormalities, congenital or acquired, may significantly increase the risk of injury from sports participation.

Certain congenital conditions, such as Down's or Morquio's syndrome, are associated with an increased incidence of instability of the upper cervical spine. This is of particular concern for Special Olympics competition. In these children, lateral radiographs in flexion and extension are recommended to rule out measurable mechanical instability of the cervical spine. An excursion greater than 5 mm of C1 on C2 is a sign of ligamentous instability or laxity. In cases of detected instability, opinions vary regarding the indications for prophylactic fusion, but there is general agreement that contact sports and head-impact activities, such as heading the ball in soccer, are absolutely contraindicated.

Klippel-Feil syndrome, characterized by shortness of the neck or webbing, may be associated with congenital abnormalities of the cervical spine. In these cases, plain radiographs and, if indicated, lateral flexion and extension views of the cervical spine may also be necessary to confirm the mechanical stability of the spine before allowing such activity.

In the lumbar spine, spondylolysis or spondylolisthesis may result in postural deformity or scoliosis. An athlete with either of these conditions may have increased tightness of the hamstrings, relative flattening of the lumbar spine with posture, and pain on hyperextension of the spine. Radiographs of the lumbar spine, including oblique views, are usually diagnostic (Fig. 3).

If a frank lack of continuity of the neural arch is detected at the pars interarticularis, a standing lateral radiograph of the lumbar spine is recommended to determine the amount of instability at this site, if any, and the coexistence of spondylolisthesis. In our experience, symptomatic spondylolysis or grade I spondylolisthesis in young athletes appears to be a stress fracture of the lumbar spine, and rarely progresses to frank instability.

Spinal deformity may be the presenting sign of more significant disease, such as localized spinal infection, discitis, or spinal tumor. These conditions

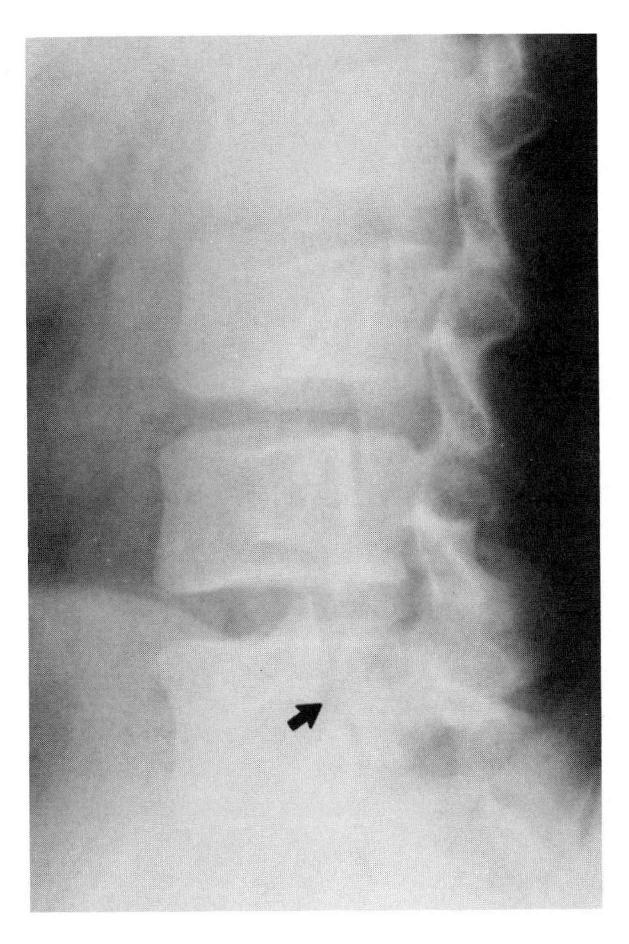

Figure 3 Spondylolysis, a defect in the pars interarticularis of the vertebra, is best visualized on the oblique radiograph.

are more common in the young athlete than in the adult, and may present initially with scoliosis. Any spinal deformity or scoliosis that persists beyond 3 weeks and is associated with muscle spasm and pain must be investigated thoroughly, and must not be ascribed to a minor back strain or sports injury.

EARLY DETECTION OF SPINAL DEFORMITY

The preparticipation evaluation provides an excellent opportunity for scoliosis screening. Symmetry of shoulder and pelvic heights, balance in the sagittal or coronal plane, and the symmetry of contour between the two sides of the back or lumbar spine are noted. On forward bending, asymmetry of the height of the torso may be a reflection of idiopathic scoliosis, due to the axial rotation of the spine and torso that occurs in addition to the curvature.

After limb length discrepancies or other causes of functional spinal curvature have been eliminated, cases of coronal or sagittal decompensation are further evaluated by obtaining standing posteroanterior (PA) and lateral radiographs of the thoracolumbar spine. If these reveal a scoliosis curvature of less than 15 degrees, or a dorsal kyphosis of more than 50 degrees, we recommend a program of directed exercises to increase the strength and flexibility of the spine and pelvis. Dorsal extension or asymmetric lateral bend exercises are also instituted for hyperkyphosis or scoliosis, respectively.

It is imperative to continue regular follow-up of any curvature, large or small, because of the risk of progression. The child is initially reevaluated after 3 to 4 months with a repeat clinical examination. If Moiré topographic photography is available, comparison of the initial with the follow-up photograph may help determine any progression of torso asymmetry associated with scoliosis. If this is not available, the clinical examination can determine whether truncal asymmetry has progressed. If spinal asymmetry appears to have increased, a repeat radiograph is obtained; a single view (standing posteroanterior for scoliosis or lateral for kyphosis) is sufficient to evaluate for radiographic progression of the curvature of scoliosis. If this has progressed beyond 15 degrees, and at least 3 degrees since the previous radiograph, corrective bracing or electrical muscle stimulation should be instituted.

NONOPERATIVE TREATMENT OF SPINAL DEFORMITY

Scoliosis

In most cases, spinal bracing is the most effective and the most readily available technique for preventing progression of scoliosis. The Milwaukee brace has been the standard treatment in North America for the management of progressive spinal disorders. However, during the past 10 years several different low-profile orthoses have been developed, which appear to manage scoliosis effectively while allowing a significant increase in function. In our experience, these orthoses can adequately prevent progression of a scoliosis curvature if the apex of the curvature is below T9.

Electrical muscle stimulation for scoliosis must be considered experimental. The techniques being used at present provide obvious advantages for the sports-active child. The treatment, which is applied at night, consists of intermittent pulses that stimulate the muscles in the convexity of the curve. During the day, full sports participation continues unhindered.

Full-time brace treatment has usually been required to prevent progression of the curvature. In our clinic, this consists of 23 hours per day of treatment, including use at night, with 1 hour out of the brace to permit bathing and exercising. The sports-active child is allowed to remove the brace during periods of sports participation or practice, for a maximum of 4 additional hours per day, and no ill effects such as increased rate of progression or brace failure have been noted. Most children can participate in sports while wearing the low-profile brace, and this includes physical education in school and most recreational sports activities such as bicycle riding, climbing, and running.

Most physicians treating juvenile-onset idiopathic scoliosis (in patients aged 6 to 10 years) report a dramatic mechanical response to brace treatment over a period of 3 to 6 months. After this, a part-time bracing regimen is adopted, usually 12 hours per day. Ongoing follow-up is mandatory to determine whether there is loss of correction with this program. We prescribe this part-time bracing program for younger patients with juvenile-onset scoliosis, who must wear the brace until skeletal maturity has been reached, sometimes for 5 to 6 years. This regimen has been successful in allowing an essentially normal lifestyle, while preventing progression of the curvature.

In the fully mature athlete, a scoliosis curve as great as 40 to 50 degrees is not a contraindication to full active sports or dance participation (Fig. 4). It is noted that as many as 25 to 30 percent of serious young amateur or professional dancers in modern dance or ballet have scoliosis curvatures. Despite this, there is no increased incidence of backache or long-term disability in these individuals. When a young, fully mature candidate for dance participation is noted to have a scoliosis curvature, we obtain a standing posteroanterior radiograph of the spine to document the degree of curvature before encouraging full dance or sports activity, in conjunction with a full back exercise program.

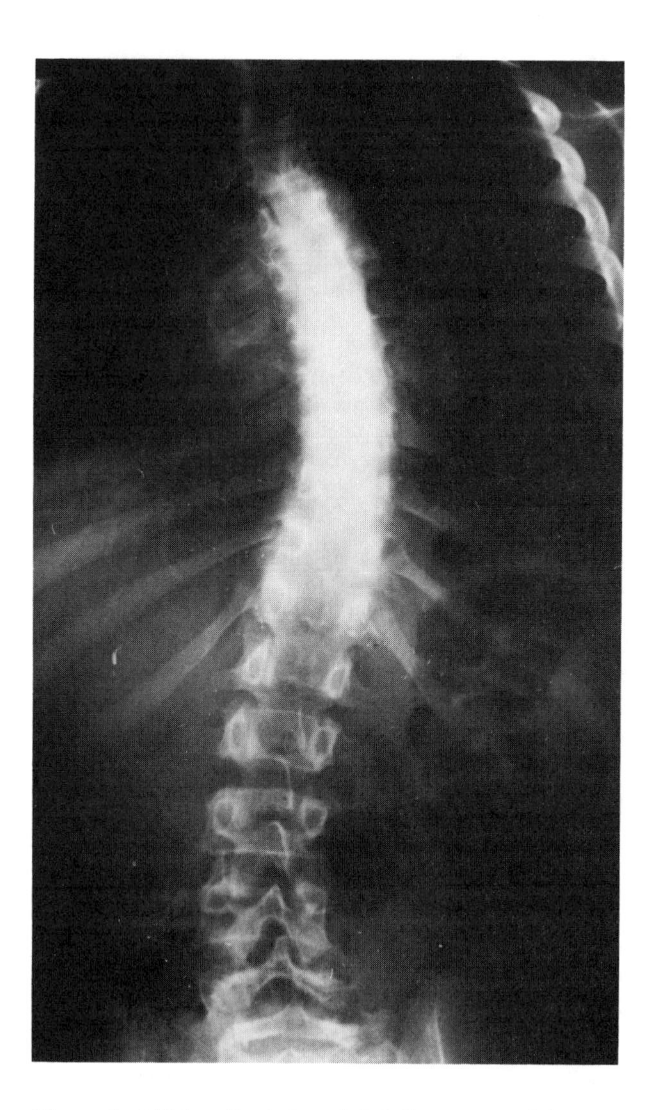

Figure 4 Mild scoliosis in a skeletally mature adolescent is not a contraindication to full sports participation.

Scheuermann's Kyphosis

Early detection of Scheuermann's kyphosis is imperative because of the dramatic reversal that may occur, if growth remains, as a result of prompt and early bracing techniques. Although scoliosis generally requires bracing until growth ceases, Scheuermann's kyphosis can be treated effectively for 9 to 12 months, with reconstitution of anterior vertebral height and restoration of a relatively normal contour of the spine. A disadvantage of the bracing regimen is that it usually requires a full brace with neck ring, especially in the young adult male. The treatment program should include an exercise regimen specifically directed at restoring strength and flexibility of the lumbar spine and hamstrings.

Lumbar Hyperlordosis

Hyperlordotic posturing ("swayback") of the low back may be flexible or fixed. With flexible lumbar hyperlordosis, forward bending causes the lumbar spine to flatten and reverse, and there may be no excessive tightness of the lumbodorsal fascia or hamstrings. The child with this posture is treated with an antilordotic exercise program and reassessed at regular intervals.

For fixed lumbar hyperlordosis, we institute a directed exercise program of antilordotic strengthening, with lumbodorsal fascia and hamstring flexibility exercises. If exercises alone are ineffective, an antilordotic bracing program is added.

Certain sports, such as figure skating, gymnastics, and ice hockey, appear to increase the tendency to develop lumbar hyperlordosis. Participants in these activities should perform prophylactic abdominal strengthening and lumbar flattening exercises, with particular emphasis on the pelvic tilt.

Lumbar hyperlordosis increases the risk of spondylolysis, and continuous or intermittent hyperlordotic posturing may also predispose to disc herniation. Therefore, young athletes who perform hyperlordotic maneuvers should also maintain a prophylactic antilordotic exercise program.

The young athlete with hyperlordosis and back pain should be completely evaluated for spondylolysis, disc problems, or other etiologic conditions, before the diagnosis of mechanical back pain is made. If exercises alone do not relieve the back pain, antilordotic bracing should be considered. The response to such bracing is often dramatic, with progressive reposturing of the lumbar spine, resolution of the pain, and concurrent full participation in sports activity. The young athlete initially wears the antilordotic, low-profile brace during sports activity; when the pain is relieved and the patient remains asymptomatic during sports participation, the brace can be safely removed for sports, but must be worn for the rest of the day. A minimum of 6 months of brace treatment is required to attain satisfactory realignment of the spine.

In contrast, brace treatment for spondylolysis is effective only with full-time wearing of the antilordotic, low-profile brace, which flattens and immobilizes the lumbar spine, and therefore relieves pain and promotes healing of the defect (Fig. 5). A concurrent antilordotic stengthening and flexibility exercise program should be maintained, and the bracing program is continued for a minimum of 6 months. Radiographic healing of the pars defect, in addition to resolution of pain, may be observed. When the child becomes asymptomatic and free of pain, and when hamstring flexibility is increased, participation in sports can be safely and effectively resumed, even while the brace is worn.

SPINAL FUSION

Fusion of the spine may be required in certain cases of severe or progressive spinal deformity such as dorsal roundback and scoliosis. Furthermore, localized fusion may be required for instability due to a previous spinal injury or deformity. The athlete will need recommendations regarding the safety and possibility of returning to sports participation after spinal fusion.

Spinal instrumentation, which is commonly used in conjunction with spinal fusion, has improved our ability to straighten the spine and may increase the rate of fusion from such a procedure (Fig. 6). In some situations, postoperative external casting or brace support may not be required. Nevertheless, it is generally agreed that establishment of a stable, solid spinal fusion takes approximately 12 months after surgery. Vigorous sports activities that involve twisting, turning, or potential impact to the spine should not be resumed earlier than this. We do allow swimming early in the postoperative period, occasionally as early as 6 to 8 weeks after spinal fusion, with a protective plastic brace.

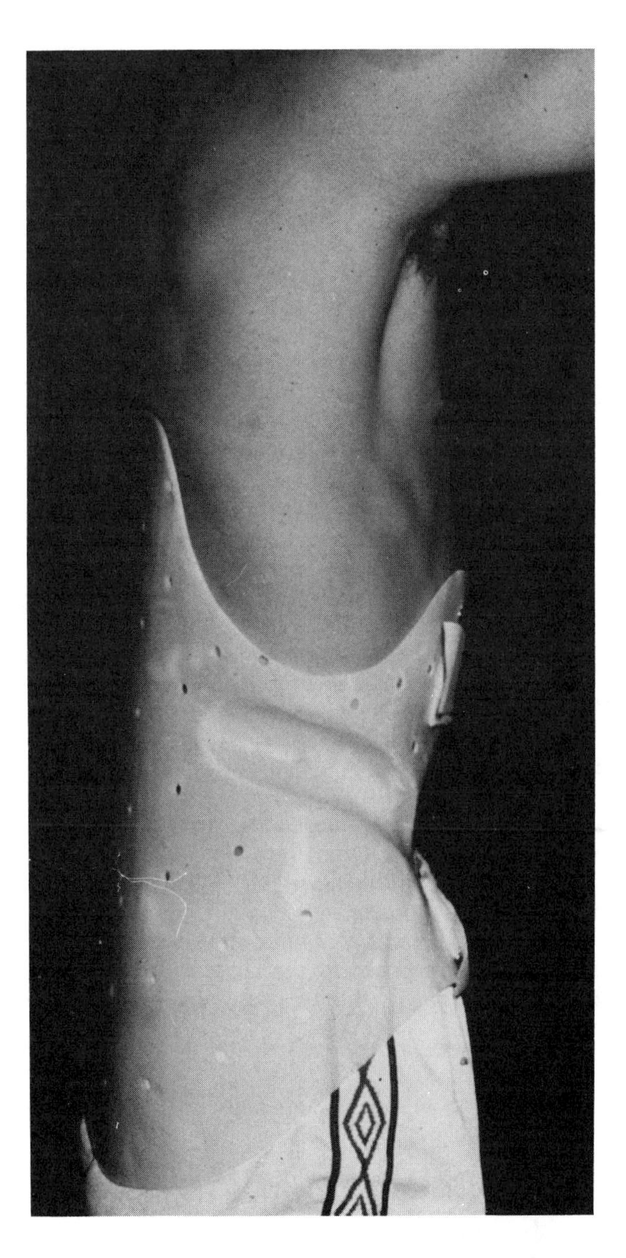

Figure 5 A thermoplastic low-profile brace used to treat spinal deformities or certain cases of low back pain in young athletes.

A child or adolescent who has had spinal instrumentation and fusion of more than two segments of the spine should be strongly counseled against participation in high-impact sports such as gridiron football or rugby, even after solid fusion has been established. However, moderate contact sports such as basketball, soccer, or field lacrosse are generally allowed.

In the case of more localized fusion, such as single-level fusion of the cervical spine for antecedent trauma, or fusion across the lumbosacral junction for spondylolysis, the return to sports partici-

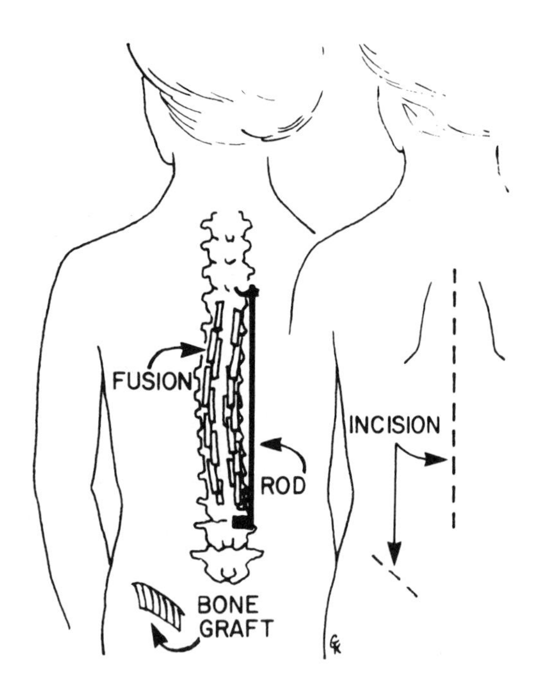

Figure 6 Extensive spinal fusion with instrumentation is a contraindication to contact sports, but many other sports and fitness activities are allowed.

pation must be individualized. With any spine fusion, there is an increased risk of long-term problems due to deterioration of the spinal elements immediately above or below the area of fusion. This deterioration may be hastened by vigorous sports participation, particularly if this includes active impacting or use of the head and neck.

The presence of associated neurologic symptoms or compromise at the time of the initial injury must also be a factor in the decision regarding continued participation in sports activity.

The athlete who has had lumbosacral fusion is generally allowed to return to full sports participation, including contact sports, after 1 year, if it is certain that a stable fusion has been attained and there is no neurologic compromise in the lower extremities. In some instances, with newer techniques of localized instrumentation of the fractured pars interarticularis, return to sports participation has been allowed as early as 3 months after fusion, but this is decided on an individual basis.

SUGGESTED READING

Micheli LJ. Low back pain in the adolescent: differential diagnosis. Am J Sports Med 1979; 7:362–364.

Micheli LJ. Back injuries in dancers. Clin Sports Med 1983; 2:473–484.

Micheli LJ. Sports following spinal surgery in the young athlete. Clin Orthop 1985; 188:152–157.

Micheli LJ. The use of the modified Boston brace system (B.O.B.) for back pain: clinical indications. Orthot Prosthet 1985; 39: 41–46.

Micheli LJ, Hall JE, Miller ME. Use of modified Boston brace for back injuries in athletes. Am J Sports Med 1980; 8:351–356.

Stanish W. Low back pain in athletes: an overuse syndrome. Clin Sports Med 1987; 6:321–344.

Winter RB. Spinal problems in pediatric orthopaedics. In: Lovell WW, Winter RB, eds. Pediatric orthopaedics. 2nd ed. Philadelphia: JB Lippincott, 1986: 569.

RUPTURED LUMBAR DISCS (HERNIATED NUCLEUS PULPOSUS)

JOHN A. McCULLOCH, M.D.

It is a simple matter to treat a ruptured disc. It is an altogether different matter to arrive at the correct diagnosis. Unfortunately, a ruptured lumbar disc is not an obvious diagnosis like a sprained ankle or a limb fracture. In fact, if someone could guarantee the diagnosis of a ruptured lumbar intervertebral disc, spine surgeons would strike a treatment "bonanza."

Problems arise when patient motivational factors are mixed in with the disability. Is someone consciously or unconsciously embellishing the illness to avoid competition? Are there hidden diseases that are fortuitously being brought to light at the moment that symptoms of the disc herniation are noted? An example might be a young male patient with referred buttock discomfort on one side who may appear on the surface to have a disc herniation, but upon closer scrutiny is found to have ankylosing spondylitis. Are we actually dealing with a disc herniation, or is this a problem of mechanical back pain with referred leg pain? If this is a ruptured disc, what is the level? Is it at L4–L5 or is it at L5–S1? Is there an asymptomatic structural lesion present such as spondylolisthesis that is deflecting the diagnosis away from the true cause of symptoms such as a herniated nucleus pulposus (HNP) at another level? So many factors go into the correct diagnosis of a ruptured lumbar disc that it is easy to miss the diagnosis when it is the cause of the leg pain, or to conclude that the diagnosis is a ruptured disc when there is another cause of radiating leg pain.

If this is not enough to confuse the issue, it is apparent to everyone dealing with low back pain that almost all patients with a mechanical low back condition get better with the passage of time. This well-known placebo effect can serve anyone's purpose when reporting expertise with treating low back problems. On the other hand, it is not unusual to read a series on a particular treatment for low back conditions and be told that a success rate of 70 to 80 percent is acceptable. This percentage of success, presented to total joint surgeons, would be a joke! The final common denominator in spine problems is that the aging process gets us all: if you live long enough you will eventually develop degenerative changes in your discs and may even rupture a lumbar disc. By now you have a handle on how difficult it is to make the diagnosis of a ruptured lumbar disc. Therein lies the juggernaut of spine surgery.

DEFINITION

A herniated nucleus pulposus causing sciatica fulfills the criteria listed in Table 1.

There are two different "breeds" of disc herniation. There is the kind that occurs in the young patient, usually in the form of a disc protrusion containing much proteoglycan or nuclear jelly. The second "breed," which occurs in the older patient (above 35), is more collagenous in nature and often is of the extruded or sequestered variety (Fig. 1). It is almost as if we were treating two separate conditions when disc ruptures are considered in age groupings. As with any general rule in medicine, there are exceptions: there are younger patients with older discs and older patients with young discs!

VERIFICATION OF STRUCTURAL LESION AND ANATOMIC LOCATION

History has declared that the gold standard for investigating a patient with a disc rupture is myelography. Times are changing and the standard of investigation today is quickly becoming magnetic resonance imaging (MRI). MRI provides all the information needed to verify the diagnosis of a disc rupture, to determine the anatomic level, and to allow for a "fine-tuned" treatment decision. It is unusual for myelography or even computed tomographic (CT) scanning to be required if good MRI facilities are available. Unfortunately, MRI is an easy test to order and has a reasonably high false-positive rate when interpreted in the vacuum of no clinical information. MRI should be carried out only if the patient fails to respond to conservative treatment and is being considered for surgical intervention.

Table 1 Criteria for the Diagnosis of the Acute Radicular Syndrome (Sciatica Usually Due to an HNP)*

Two Symptoms

1. Leg pain, including buttock discomfort, dominating over the back pain
2. Presence of localizing neurologic symptoms (e.g., paresthesia in a dermatomal distribution)

Two Signs

1. Marked reduction in straight leg-raising ability and/or bowstring discomfort and/or cross-over pain
2. Two of four neurologic signs (wasting, weakness, sensory loss, reflex alteration)

*Three or four of these criteria are required for diagnosis. The exception is the young patient (<25 years) who may have no neurologic symptoms or signs.

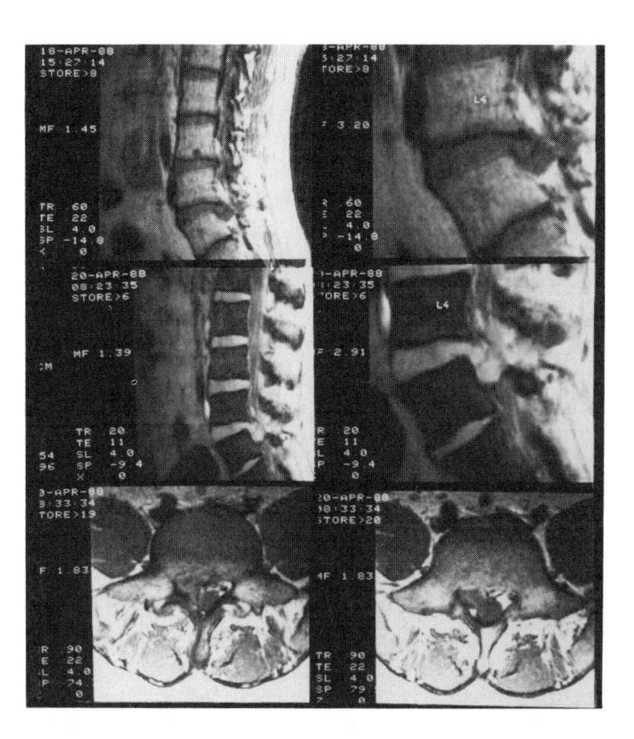

Figure 1 MRI showing a disc extrusion, L4–L5 right. *Top,* Axial T1 weighted images. *Middle,* Axial partial T2 weighted images. *Lower,* Axial views.

ADEQUATE CONSERVATIVE CARE

If the diagnosis of a lumbar disc rupture has been made, what constitutes adequate conservative care? Remember that it is natural for the symptoms of a disc rupture to subside spontaneously. Even while waiting for this spontaneous cure, it is possible to allow patients to function at a reasonable level, provided that they understand that increasing symptoms with increasing activity represent hurt and not harm. Unless patients insist on pursuing a high level of repetitive bending or lifting activities, it is unlikely that effects detrimental to a disc herniation will occur with continuing light activities. Of course, if the sciatic discomfort is so severe that a patient cannot stand on the affected leg, this rule does not apply. This leads to the next consideration in conservative treatment: to match the proposed conservative treatment with the severity of the disability. If a patient cannot swing a nine iron without producing leg pain, it seems unreasonable to prescribe 2 weeks of bed rest to treat the problem. On the other hand, if a patient has severe leg pain and needs crutches to get around, it is absurd to propose exercise treatment intervention. Although these are two extreme examples, a lot of "fine tuning" is needed to determine what constitutes an adequate conservative treatment program.

There are only two useful forms of conservative treatment for a disc rupture. First is rest, which may include complete bed rest, a bed on the patient's back (a corset), weight reduction, job modification, or activity modification. Second is the passage of a reasonable amount of time before one pronounces failure. For the first occurrence of sciatica, it is reasonable to extend conservative treatment for not less than 6 weeks, provided that the symptom is not severely incapacitating. If bed rest is prescribed, how long is long enough? The duration of prescribed bed rest is undergoing dramatic modification in the past few years. In the past, it was not unusual to request 2 weeks of complete bed rest as a standard of care for an acute disc rupture. It is now evident that, at most, 5 days is all that is required, as long as the examiner notes two key parameters: (1) the relief of leg pain and (2) the degree of improvement in straight leg-raising ability. If after 5 days of complete bed rest the patient shows no improvement in leg pain or no improvement in straight leg-raising ability, it is likely that continuing complete bed rest will be fruitless.

Many other therapies have been invoked to cure the so-called ruptured disc, including the various forms of exercises and other treatments such as manipulation, ultrasonography, massage, deep heat, and diathermy. There is no body of scientific evidence to support these forms of treatment as useful in the management of an acute disc rupture.

RESPONSE TO TREATMENT

There are three responses to conservative treatment: (1) the patient is cured; (2) the patient is not cured; or (3) although the patient is initially cured, there is a recurrence of symptoms.

INDICATIONS FOR SURGERY

If a patient fails to respond to conservative treatment or initially responds to such treatment only to have recurrent episodes of sciatica, surgical intervention is indicated. The two other classic indications for surgical intervention on an emergent basis are bladder and bowel involvement and an increasing neurologic deficit. Controversial indications for surgical intervention include a significant neurologic deficit and a significant structural lesion found on investigation. Perhaps the most controversial recommendation is that all patients below the age of 20 to 25 years will almost certainly fail to respond to conservative treatment for a ruptured disc, and should be treated much more aggressively than older patients.

CHOICES OF INVASIVE TREATMENT

There are three invasive options for treating patients who have failed to respond to conservative treatment: (1) chemonucleolysis, (2) surgery, and (3) percutaneous discectomy.

Basic Science Considerations

In trying to decide upon the best form of invasive surgical therapy for a patient with a disc rupture, it is important to determine the nature of the fragment of disc material pressing on the nerve root. There are two components in a ruptured disc fragment: proteoglycan and collagen. The younger the patient, the more likely it is that there is a high proteoglycan content to the disc rupture; the older the patient, the more likely there is to be a high collagen content in the ruptured disc material. Other changes such as calcification and air in the disc cavity or the ruptured disc material are also suggestive of a low proteoglycan content. Finally, a disc rupture that is extremely large, and a disc rupture that has migrated away from the disc space, either up behind the vertebral body above or down behind the vertebral body below, are suggestive of a low proteoglycan content and a higher collagen content. The significance of trying to determine the extent of proteoglycan content in the disc herniation becomes evident in the following section on chemonucleolysis.

Chemonucleolysis

Chymopapain is a proteolytic enzyme that is extracted from the papaya plant. It is a protein foreign to the body and capable of invoking a wide variety of allergic reactions, the most feared being anaphylaxis. When injected into a disc protrusion containing a lot of proteoglycan, the positively charged enzyme is attracted to the negatively charged proteoglycans. It splits off the mucopolysaccharide side chains, interfering with the proteoglycan's ability to hold onto water. In essence, the chemonucleolysis "deflates" a bulging disc, relieving pressure on the nerve root.

Chemonucleolysis should be seen as the last step in conservative care rather than the first step in surgical care. It is a nonsurgical procedure that is accomplished by placing a needle into the offending disc and injecting a small amount of enzyme to dissolve the disc rupture. Obviously, it only affects disc protrusions and only affects discs that have a high proteoglycan content. It does not affect any other conditions of the spine, such as bony root or canal encroachment. There are a number of contraindications to the use of chymopapain, including an allergy to the drug, previous surgery, a previous chymopapain injection, pregnancy, or an associated neurologic diagnosis of unknown etiology such as multiple sclerosis.

Chymopapain is a safe drug when injected into the intradiscal cavity. When injected in error into the subarachnoid space, it has a devastating effect on the basement membranes of the pia-arachnoid vessels. The result is a dissolution of these membranes and a subarachnoid hemorrhage, which can spread to include an intracerebral hemorrhage, a cauda equina syndrome, and a somewhat delayed sinister complication of transverse myelitis. These three severe neurologic complications have actually occurred in chymopapain-treated patients (fortunately not often), but it is my opinion that they are all due to technical errors and not related to any inherent problem with the drug.

The dreaded complication of anaphylaxis has been brought under control with preinjection skin testing. If a patient has a negative skin test, an anaphylactic reaction is highly unlikely, on the basis of my experience with over 1,000 cases.

The procedure is usually performed in the operating room under local neuroleptic anesthesia. Single levels should be injected, since disc ruptures occur at single levels and not multiple levels. The approach to the disc space must not violate the subarachnoid space, and thus the posterolateral approach is necessary (Fig. 2). Following the manufacturer's recommendation to reduce the dose of chymopapain injection to 0.75 to 1.0 ml, the incidence of postinjection back spasm has been reduced.

Patients may leave the hospital on the day of the procedure or a day or so afterward. They are best supported in a light canvas corset for approximately 4 to 6 weeks, after which time an x-ray film should be taken to decide whether there is disc space narrowing. A successful result at this stage is considered to be relief of leg pain, increased straight leg-raising ability, and disc space narrowing on x-ray examination. Failure represents a patient with persistent sciatica or persisting reduction in straight leg-raising ability, with or without disc space narrowing on plain radiograph. If patients fail to respond to a chymopapain injection, a determination should be made within 6 weeks to take them on to surgical intervention.

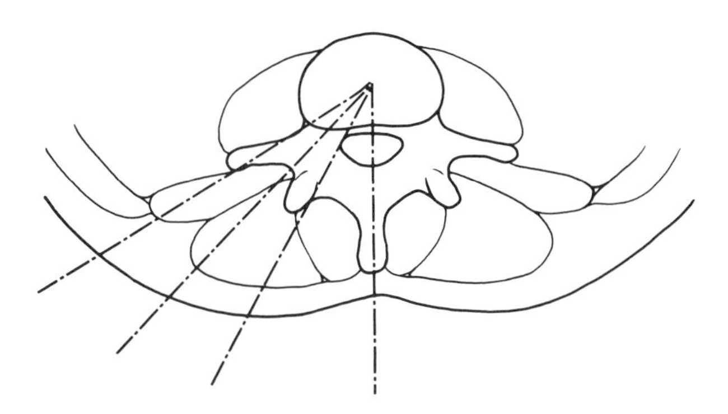

Figure 2 Posterolateral approach.

In young patients (below the age of 25 to 30) with a disc herniation, chemonucleolysis probably represents the best choice of treatment.

Surgical Intervention

It is the author's recommendation that the standard laminectomy-discectomy for surgical management of patients with disc rupture is no longer necessary. Instead, a microsurgical approach can be used, which reduces the size of the skin incision, the extent of the muscular dissection, the size of the postoperative hematoma, and finally the healing by secondary intention (i.e., the formation of scar). The smaller incision decreases the postoperative morbidity significantly, allowing for early ambulation on the day of surgery or the day after. This in turn has a very beneficial effect on the formation of collagen tissue.

The use of the microscope to assist in decompression of a nerve root compromised by a disc herniation represents nothing more than the technical advancement of using the magnification and illumination that are a part of the microscope. Whether or not the magnification and illumination are used to assist the surgeon is not important; what *is* important is that the nerve root is adequately decompressed. If a disc excision is "completed" but the nerve root is still compromised by residual disc material, or if there is another pathologic condition such as bony root encroachment, patients will not be relieved of the sciatic discomfort, regardless of whether or not the microscope was used.

After microsurgical excision of a disc herniation, patients are ambulated the day of surgery or the day after. As with chemonucleolysis, a canvas corset support is recommended for 4 to 6 weeks as a reminder to patients that an operation has taken place. During that time, patients are on routine activity limitations and should perform a stretching exercise of the affected leg (Fig. 3).

There are many causes of failure to relieve sciatic discomfort when using a limited surgical exposure. The most common cause is exposing the wrong level, which is a constant threat to any surgeon performing microsurgery. In addition, if the radiographs have not been interpreted carefully with regard to the exact location and nature of the disc herniation or other root encroachment pathology, it is possible to leave behind fragments of disc material or other root encroachment. Minor complicating features of the limited surgical exposure include bleeding that obscures the field of vision, damage to neurologic structures because of the limited field of work, and finally a slightly increased incidence of disc space infection (because of the presence of

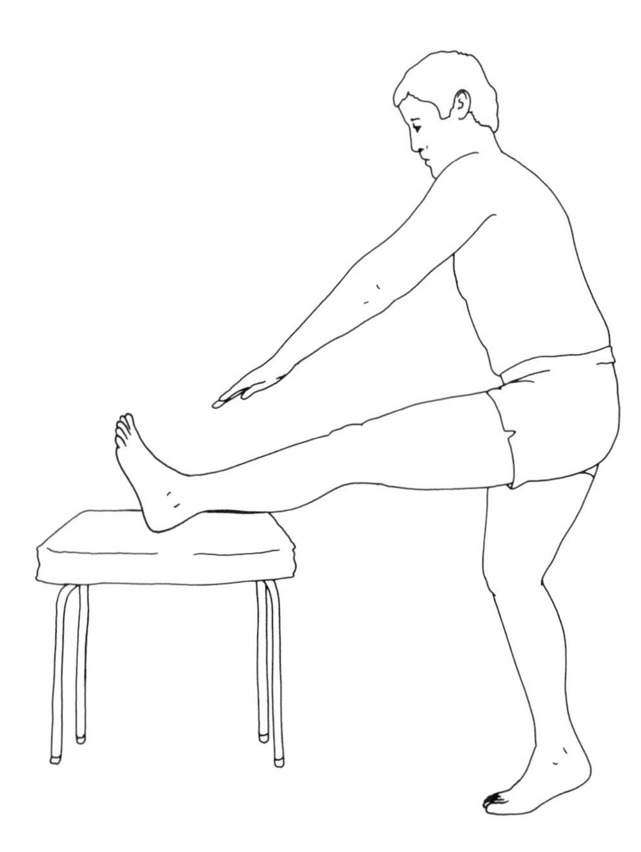

Figure 3 The postoperative stretching exercise.

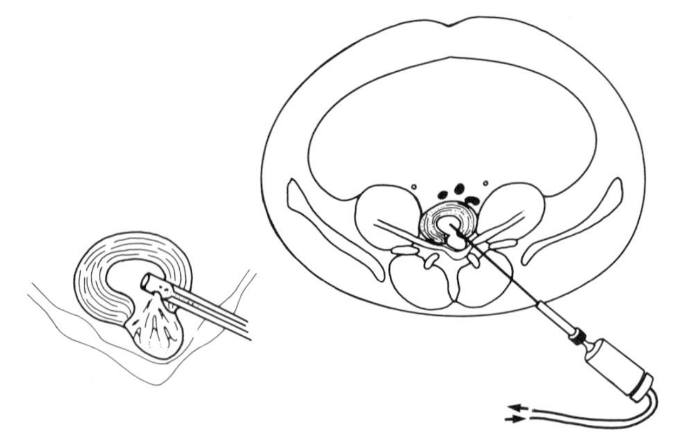

Figure 4 The percutaneous discectomy with the "suction" nucleotome.

some exposed parts of the microscope over the wound).

Percutaneous Discectomy

The technology of managing a disc rupture is in a state of evolution. The original modification to the standard laminectomy-discectomy was chemonucleolysis, which was first proposed in the early 1960s. Next came the microsurgical approach to root decompression, and now there are percutaneous approaches to the disc space with either a suction probe or grasping forceps. This approach is depicted in Figure 4 and is similar to the chemonucleolysis route. However, instead of injecting an enzyme into the disc space, a suction probe or a grasping instrument is used to remove the discal material.

The advantages of percutaneous discectomy are that it is a nonoperative procedure, and thus eliminates a number of complications attendant upon general anesthesia and a surgical wound. The procedure is minor enough to be done under local neuroleptic anesthesia on an outpatient basis. The disadvantages of the procedure are that (1) the technique is somewhat more difficult to learn than chemonucleolysis, (2) it is possible with a larger-bore cannula to injure the nerve root when attempting to enter the disc space, and (3) it is highly likely that if a disc fragment is extruded or sequestered outside the confines of the disc space, it will not be reached with a probe. If the surgeon is unfamiliar with the technique and is somewhat clumsy, the incidence of disc space infection is raised.

Perhaps the most serious concern with percutaneous discectomy is the fact that not all the nuclear material can be reached with the approach and the recurrence rate is likely to be high. The technique is young in its development, and I predict that a higher than acceptable recurrence rate will detract from the advantages.

SUGGESTED READING

Bell GR, Rothman RH. The conservative treatment of sciatica. Spine 1984; 9:54–56.

McCulloch JA, Dolovich G, Canham W. Skin testing for chymopapain allergy: a preliminary report. Allergy 1985; 55: 609–611.

Van Royen BJ, O'Driscoll SW, Dhert WJA, Salter RB. A comparison of the effects of immobilization and continuous passive motion on surgical wound healing in mature rabbits. Plast Reconstr Surg 1986; 78:360–366.

HEAD AND FACE

HEAD INJURIES

LEONARD A. BRUNO, M.D.
THOMAS A. GENNARELLI, M.D.
JOSEPH S. TORG, M.D.

The athlete who receives a blow to the head, or a sudden jolt to the body that results in a sudden acceleration-deceleration force to the head, should be carefully evaluated. If the individual is ambulatory and conscious, the entire spectrum of intracranial damage, ranging from a grade I concussion to a more severe intracranial condition, must be considered. Initial on-field examination should include an evaluation of:

1. Facial expression.
2. Orientation to time, place, and person.
3. The presence of post-traumatic amnesia.
4. The presence of retrograde amnesia.
5. Abnormal gait.

Traumatic injuries to the brain can be classified as diffuse or focal.

The immediate and definitive management of athletically induced trauma to the brain depends on the nature and severity of the injury. Those responsible for managing such injuries must understand these problems from the standpoint of basic pathomechanics.

DIFFUSE BRAIN INJURIES

Diffuse brain injuries are associated with widespread or global disruption of neurologic function and are not usually associated with macroscopically visible brain lesions. Diffuse brain injuries result from shaking of the brain within the skull, and thus are lesions caused by the inertial or acceleration effects of a mechanical input to the head. Both theoretic and experimental evidence points to rotational acceleration as the primary injury mechanism for diffuse brain injuries.

Since diffuse brain injuries, for the most part, are not associated with visible macroscopic lesions, they have historically been lumped together to include all injuries not associated with focal lesions. More recently, however, diagnostic information has been gained from computed tomographic (CT) scanning, as well as from neurophysiologic studies, that make it possible to define more clearly several categories within this broad group of diffuse brain injuries.

Three categories of diffuse brain injury are recognized:

1. Mild concussion. Several specific concussion syndromes involve temporary disturbances of neurologic function without loss of consciousness.
2. Classic cerebral concussion. This is a temporary, reversible neurologic deficiency caused by trauma that results in temporary loss of consciousness.
3. Diffuse axonal injury. This takes the form of prolonged traumatic brain coma with loss of consciousness lasting more than 6 hours. Residual neurologic, psychologic, or personality deficits often result because of structural disruption of numerous axons in the white matter of the cerebral hemispheres and brain stem.

Mild Cerebral Concussion

The syndromes of mild cerebral concussion are included in the continuum of diffuse brain injuries; they represent the mildest form of injury in this spectrum. Mild concussion syndromes are those in which consciousness is preserved, but with some degree of noticeable temporary neurologic dysfunction. These injuries are exceedingly common and, because of their mild degree, often are not brought to medical attention; however, they are the most common brain injuries encountered in sports medicine.

A grade I mild concussion, the mildest form of head injury, results in confusion and disorientation unaccompanied by amnesia. This temporary confusion, without loss of consciousness, lasts only momentarily after the injury. This concussion syndrome is completely reversible and is associated with no sequelae. An individual with a grade I mild concussion is confused and has a dazed look; there may also be mild unsteadiness of gait. However, post-traumatic and retrograde amnesia are not prominent features. This clinical picture is best described by the athletes themselves who say, "I had my bell rung." Usually the state of confusion is short-lived and the athlete is completely lucid in 5 to 15 minutes. When his mind is clear, he may return to the activity under the watchful supervision of the team physician or trainer. However, associated symptoms such as vertigo, headaches, photophobia, and labile emotions should preclude returning to the game.

A grade II mild concussion is characterized by confusion associated with retrograde amnesia that develops after 5 to 10 minutes. Again, this is an extremely frequent event. Athletes may experience a "ding," and although confused may continue coordinated sensorimotor activities after the accident. If examined immediately, these players have total recall of the events immediately before impact. However, retrograde amnesia develops 5 to 10 minutes later, and thereafter they do not remember the impact or events immediately before impact. The amnesia usually covers only several minutes before the injury; it may diminish somewhat, but players always have some degree of permanent, though short, retrograde amnesia despite resumption of completely normal consciousness. The confusion and disorientation totally resolve within minutes.

Individuals manifesting amnesia should not be permitted to return to play that day. These athletes require postinjury evaluation. They may develop the "postconcussion syndrome," characterized by persistent headaches, inability to concentrate, and irritability. In some instances, these symptoms may last for several weeks after the injury, and participation in the sport is precluded as long as symptoms are present.

As the mechanical stresses to the brain increase in the grade III mild concussion, confusion and amnesia are present from the time of impact. Athletes can usually continue to play while having no recollection of previous events. By this stage, some degree of post-traumatic amnesia (forgetting events after the injury) also occurs in addition to retrograde amnesia (forgetting events before the injury). The patient's length of confusion may last many minutes, but then the level of consciousness returns to normal, usually with some permanent degree of retrograde and post-traumatic amnesia.

These three syndromes of mild cerebral concussion have been witnessed frequently and described in detail. Although consciousness is preserved, it is clear that some degree of cerebral dysfunction has occurred. The fact that memory mechanisms appear to be the most sensitive to trauma suggests that the cerebral hemispheres, rather than the brain stem, are the location of the mild injury forces. The degree of cerebral cortical dysfunction, however, is not sufficient to disconnect the influence of the cerebral hemispheres from the brain stem activating system, and therefore consciousness is preserved. No other cortical functions except memory seem in jeopardy, and the only residual deficits that patients with mild concussion syndromes have is the brief retrograde or post-traumatic amnesia. However, since definite alteration of brain function has occurred, athletes who sustain a mild cerebral concussion should not be permitted to participate in the remainder of the contest.

Classic Cerebral Concussion

Classic cerebral concussion is seen in the "knocked-out" player. This individual is in a paralytic coma, usually recovers after a few seconds or minutes, and then passes through stages of stupor, confusion with or without delirium, and finally an almost lucid state with automatism before becoming fully alert. This individual will most certainly have retrograde and post-traumatic amnesia. If the loss of consciousness lasts for more than several minutes or if there are other signs of a deteriorating neurologic state, the patient should be immediately transported to a hospital.

Initial evaluation of the athlete who has been rendered unconscious should involve determining whether he is breathing, whether there is a pulse, and the level of consciousness. If unobstructed respirations and an adequate pulse are present, there is no immediate need to do anything except keep in mind that head and neck injuries are frequently associated. Therefore, the player should be protected from injudicious manipulation or movement.

Such patients frequently remain semistuporous for more than several minutes. They should be carried off the field on a spine board or stretcher rather than be permitted to stagger off. An athlete who has been rendered unconscious for any time should not be allowed to return to contact activity, even if mentally clear. Overnight observation in a hospital should be seriously considered for these such individuals.

Insufficient attention has been given to the precise stages of recovery from classic cerebral concussion. Although, by definition, loss of consciousness is transient and reversible, the sequelae of concussion are commonplace. Some sequelae such as headache or tinnitus may reflect injuries to the head, the inner ear, or other noncerebral structures. However, subtle changes in personality and in psychologic or memory functioning have been documented and must have a cerebrocortical origin. Thus, although most patients with classic cerebral concussion experience no sequelae other than amnesia for the events of impact, some individuals may have other long-lasting, although subtle, neurologic deficiencies that must be investigated further.

Brain Swelling

Brain swelling is a poorly understood phenomenon that can accompany any type of head injury. Swelling is not synonymous with cerebral edema, which refers to a specific increase in brain water. Such an increase in water content may not occur in brain swelling, and current evidence favors the concept that brain swelling is due in part to increased intravascular blood within the brain. This is caused by a vascular reaction to head injury that leads to vasodilation and increased cerebral blood volume. If this increased cerebral blood volume continues long enough, vascular permeability may increase and true edema may result.

Although brain swelling may occur in any type of head injury, the magnitude of the swelling does not correlate well with the severity of the injury. Thus, both severe and minor head injuries may be complicated by brain swelling. The effects of brain swelling are thus additive to those of primary brain injury, and may in certain instances be more severe than the primary injury itself.

Despite the lack of knowledge of the precise mechanism that causes brain swelling, it can be conceptualized in two general forms (Table 1). It should be remembered that many different types of brain swelling exist and that acute and delayed brain swelling represent phenomenologic, rather than mechanistic, entities.

Acute brain swelling occurs in several circumstances. Swelling that accompanies focal brain lesions tends to be localized, whereas diffuse brain injuries are associated with generalized swelling. Focal swelling is usually present beneath contusions but does not often contribute additional deleterious effects. On the other hand, the swelling that occurs with acute subdural hematomas, although principally hemispheric in distribution, may cause more mass effect than the hematoma itself. In such circumstances, the small amount of blood in the subdural space may not be the entire reason for the patient's neurologic state. If the hematoma is removed, the acute brain swelling may progress so rapidly that the brain protrudes through the craniotomy opening. Every neurosurgeon is all too familiar with external herniation of the brain, which, when it occurs, is difficult to treat.

TABLE 1 Brain Swelling

I. Acute swelling
   A. Associated with focal lesions
      1. Acute subdural hematoma—hemispheric
      2. Contusions—focal
   B. Associated with diffuse brain lesions
II. Delayed swelling
   A. Associated with lethargy
   B. Associated with light coma
   C. Associated with deep coma

The more serious types of diffuse brain injuries are associated with generalized, rather than focal, acute brain swelling. Although not all patients with diffuse axonal injury have brain swelling, the incidence of swelling is higher than in patients with either classic cerebral concussion or one of the mild concussion syndromes. Because of the serious nature of the underlying injury, it is difficult to determine the extent of swelling in these patients. The swelling, although widespread throughout the brain, may not cause a rise in intracranial pressure for several days. This late rise in pressure probably reflects the formation of true cerebral edema, and it may be that diffuse swelling associated with severe diffuse brain injuries is harmful because it produces edema. In any event, this type of swelling is different from the type of swelling associated with acute subdural hematomas.

Delayed brain swelling may occur minutes to hours after head injury. It is usually diffuse and is often associated with the milder forms of diffuse brain injuries. Whether delayed swelling is the same as or a phenomenon different from the acute swelling of the more serious diffuse injuries is unknown. However, in less severe diffuse injuries there is a distinct time interval before delayed swelling becomes manifest, thus confirming that the primary insult to the brain was not serious. Considering the high frequency of the mild concussion syndromes and of classic cerebral concussion, the incidence of delayed swelling must be low. However, when it occurs, delayed swelling can cause profound neurologic changes or even death.

In its most severe form, severe delayed swelling can cause deep coma. The usual history is that of an injury associated with a mild concussion or a classic cerebral concussion from which the patient recovers. Minutes to hours later the patient becomes lethargic, then stuporous, and finally lapses into a coma. The coma may be either a light coma with appropriate motor responses to painful stimuli, or a deep coma associated with decorticate or decerebrate posturing.

The key differences between these patients and those with diffuse axonal injury is that in the latter the coma and abnormal motor signs are present from the moment of injury, whereas with delayed cerebral swelling there is a time interval without these signs. This distinction is significant, however, since with diffuse axonal injury a certain amount of primary structural damage has occurred at the moment of impact, but this is not present in cases of pure delayed swelling. Therefore, the deleterious effects of delayed swelling should be potentially reversible, and if these effects are controlled the outcome should be good. However, such control may be difficult. Vigorous monitoring of and attention to intracranial pressure is necessary, and prompt and vigorous treatment of raised intracranial pressure is required in order to control brain swelling. If this is successfully accomplished, the mortality rate from increased intracranial pressure associated with diffuse brain swelling should be low.

FOCAL BRAIN SYNDROMES

In discussing the occurrence of intracranial hematoma resulting from athletic injury, two major points must be emphasized. First, owing to recent developments in the clinical evaluation of patients and correlated animal research, there is a satisfactory understanding of the mechanism of occurrence of focal intracranial hematoma, which is somewhat different from older concepts of patients with head injuries. Second, management of such patients has advanced rapidly and changed dramatically over the last decade from what was accepted medical practice in the past.

The entire spectrum of traumatic intracranial hematomas occurs in sports injuries. These include cerebral contusions, intracerebral hematomas, epidural hematomas, and acute subdural hematomas. The presentation of athletes with head injuries who have had serious trauma is similar in most instances. Management depends on definitive diagnosis, and varies according to the underlying pathologic process.

Intracerebral Hematoma and Contusion

Athletic injuries of this type occur in patients with an impressive intracerebral pathologic condition who have never suffered loss of consciousness or focal neurologic deficit, but who do have persistent headache or periods of confusion after head injury and post-traumatic amnesia. As with any patients who have suffered head injuries, athletes with such symptoms should undergo a CT scan to permit early differentiation between solid intracerebral hematoma and hemorrhagic contusion with surrounding edema.

Epidural Hematoma

With epidural hematoma the middle meningeal or other meningeal arteries are often imbedded in bony grooves in the skull, and skull fractures, crossing this bony groove, frequently tear the blood vessel at that site. Because bleeding in these instances is arterial, accumulation of clot continues under high pressure; as a result, bleeding does not stop early enough to prevent serious brain injury.

The classic picture of an epidural hematoma is that of loss of consciousness at the time of injury, followed by recovery of consciousness in a variable period, after which the patient is lucid. This is followed by the onset of increasingly severe headache, decreased level of consciousness, dilation of one pupil (usually on the same side as the clot), and decerebrate posturing and weakness (usually on the side opposite the hematoma). In our experience, however, only one-third of the patients with epidural hematoma present with this classic history. Another one-third of patients do not become unconscious until late in their course, and the remaining one-third are unconscious from the time of injury and remain unconscious throughout their course.

The absence of a classic clinical picture of epidural hematoma cannot be relied on to rule out this diagnosis, and the best diagnostic test for evaluating these patients is a CT scan.

Acute Subdural Hematoma

Athletic head injuries result from inertial loading that is lower than that in serious head injuries caused by vehicular accidents or falling from heights. Thus, an acute subdural hematoma also occurs much more frequently than epidural hematoma in athletes. In patients with head injuries in general, approximately three times as many acute subdural hematomas occur as do epidural hematomas.

Two main types of acute subdural hematomas have been clearly identified: (1) those with a collection of blood in the subdural space, apparently unassociated with underlying cerebral contusion or edema; and (2) those with collections of blood in the subdural space, but associated with an obvious contusion on the surface of the brain and hemispheric brain injury with swelling. The mortality rate for simple subdural hematomas is approximately 20 percent, but this increases to more than 50 percent for subdural hematomas with an underlying brain injury.

Patients with an acute subdural hematoma typically are unconscious, may or may not have a history of deterioration, and frequently display focal neurologic findings. Patients with simple subdural hematomas are more likely to have a lucid interval following their injury and are less likely to be unconscious at admission than patients with hemispheric injury and brain swelling. It is necessary to obtain a CT scan or angiogram to diagnose an acute subdural hematoma. The size of the subdural clot relative to the size of the midline shift of the brain structures can be evaluated best by CT scan. Of patients with acute subdural hematoma, 84 percent also have an associated hemorrhagic contusion or intracerebral hematoma with associated brain swelling.

The term "acute subdural hematoma" raises the image in most physicians' minds of a large collection of clotted blood in the intracranial cavity, compressing the brain substance and causing compromise due to the space occupied by the hematoma. This is not an infrequent consequence of closed head trauma, but this type of subdural hematoma is more common in adults who have a degree of cortical atrophy.

Young athletes, and especially children, frequently develop only minimal subdural hematomas with underlying cerebral hemispheric swelling. This type of brain injury is not the result of a space-occupying mass from clotted blood causing brain compression, but rather swollen brain tissue causing consequent rises in intracranial pressure. The advent of CT scanning permits accurate differential diagnosis between these two conditions, which frequently cause similar clinical pictures. The modalities of treatment for these two distinct types of acute subdural hematomas are quite different.

TABLE 2 Management of Head Injury

First Aid—Hyperventilation *Diagnosis*—CT Scan	
Surgery	*No Surgery*
Epidural hematoma	Small subdural hematoma
Large subdural hematoma	Confusion
Large intracerebral hematoma	Diffuse injury
	Most intracerebral hematomas
Intracranial Pressure Monitoring and Treatment	
Goal:	Keep ICP less than 15 mm Hg
Modalities:	Hyperventilation (P_{CO_2} 22–30 mm Hg)
	Corticosteroids (1 mg/kg)
	Mannitol (1 g/kg, serum osmolality 330–320 mOsm/L)
	Barbiturates (30 mg/kg loading and 0.5–3.0 mg/kg/hr maintenance)

PRINCIPLES OF MANAGEMENT

As our knowledge of physiology and pathophysiology has increased, so has our ability to resuscitate seriously ill or severely injured people successfully. The 1950s saw the start of successful treatment of acute respiratory and postoperative problems, followed by satisfactory cardiac resuscitation and emergency cardiac care in the 1960s. Innovations in critical care medicine were extended in the form of brain resuscitation in the 1970s. Such care is based on the concept that the degree of permanent neurologic, intellectual, and psychologic deficit after brain trauma with coma is only partly the result of the initial injury, and is certainly in part due to secondary changes, which can be worsened or improved by the quality of the supportive care received. Head injuries, by their very nature, require resuscitation, i.e., therapy initiated after the insult. The proper care of patients with head injuries, athletic or otherwise, depends on the full appreciation and use of brain resuscitation measures in an intensive care setting.

Treatment for focal intracranial hematoma consists of removal of hematoma, and recognition of and treatment for the underlying brain injury. Included in this concept is that of resuscitation of the brain, which is therapy designed to have specific neuron-saving potential once general resuscitation methods and supportive care have begun. Our current management and treatment protocol is outlined in Table 2.

First aid should consist of getting the patient safely into a supine position and determining vital signs and the significance of any associated injuries. Initial treatment should be to establish an adequate and useful airway and begin hyperventilation maneuvers. This can be accomplished by using a manual resuscitation bag with supplemental oxygen, if available. The patient should then be transferred as quickly as possible to a medical facility where diagnosis and treatment of brain injury can begin. Although these measures are important for all patients who have suffered concussion, they are vital for patients who remain comatose after trauma. An initial dose of parenteral corticosteroids is specifically indicated; 100 mg dexamethasone or 1 g methylprednisolone sodium succinate can be administered to the average adult. Once patients arrive in the emergency room and it is determined that their cardiorespiratory status is stable, endotracheal intubation is immediately performed on comatose patients. A CT scan is obtained as soon as possible, to provide an immediate diagnosis of the intracranial condition. Patients are then categorized as either surgical or nonsurgical cases, depending on the size of the intracranial hematoma.

Initial evaluation of all patients with head trauma includes determination of the coma state by numerical ranking on the Glasgow Coma Scale (Table 3). This scale is based on the patient's response to stimulation by eye opening, best motor response, and best verbal response. Scores of 15 to 3, from normal neurologic status to deeply comatose, are possible.

Patients with a Glasgow Coma Scale score of 7 or lower should receive immediate intracranial pressure (ICP) monitoring. Intracranial hypertension, defined as a pressure over 15 mm Hg, is seen in 50 percent or more of patients with severe head injuries. The poor correlation between alterations in ICP and the neurologic status has been well described in the past. Therapy for intracranial hypertension can be given correctly only when the pressure is known. We are firmly convinced of the usefulness of continuous ICP monitoring in the intensive care of patients with severe head injuries. Because intermittent waves of increased pressure, which commonly occur without other signs or symptoms, can be diagnosed and treated before significant neurologic deterioration occurs, ICP monitoring facilitates titration of therapy.

When muscle paralysis or barbiturates are used to control elevated ICP, it is impossible to follow the patient's neurologic state. Other than brain stem–evoked potentials, ICP is the only parameter that can be followed. It would be inappropriate to use muscle paralysis or barbiturates without continu-

TABLE 3 Glasgow Coma Scale

Eyes	Open	Spontaneously	4
		To verbal command	3
		To pain	2
		No response	1
	To verbal command	Obeys	6
To painful stimulus*		Localizes pain	5
		Flexion—withdrawal	4
Best motor response		Flexion—abnormal (decorticate rigidity)	3
		Extension (decerebrate rigidity)	2
		No response	1
Best verbal response†		Oriented and converses	5
		Disoriented and converses	4
		Inappropriate words	3
		Incomprehensible sounds	2
		No response	1
Total			3 to 15

* Apply knuckles to sternum; observe arms.
† Arouse patient with painful stimulus if necessary.

ously recording ICP. Ideally the ICP should be monitored from the earliest possible time after the patient's arrival in the hospital. In our unit, it is usually possible to obtain a CT scan within 1 hour of admission for all severe head injuries. The ICP monitor is usually inserted after the CT scan has been taken and within 2 hours of admission.

However, if any delay in diagnosis is foreseen or if the patient is rapidly deteriorating, an ICP bolt is inserted immediately after emergency resuscitation. This early insertion is especially important in patients showing signs of shock from other injuries that require rapid fluid replacement. In other cases, pressure is monitored in the emergency room with a portable recording system.

The ICP monitoring system must be simple, easily inserted, and reliable. The subarachnoid bolt, which can be easily inserted and maintained and does not require an operating room procedure, can be inserted at the bedside under local anesthesia.

We monitor ICP in comatose patients with head injuries whether they are operated on initially for decompression or not. Surgical intervention to remove contused brain is rare; if ICP can be controlled, the removal of potentially functional brain tissue is unacceptable, since it may limit the patient's recovery. After surgical intervention in patients with hematoma, subarachnoid bolts are routinely inserted and ICP is monitored to determine the need for further therapy.

The following principles of management of patients with head injuries apply to those in whom there are no indications for surgical intervention and to those who have undergone surgery. Management is guided by the monitored variables, and its goals are to prevent three major complications that cause most deaths in patients alive on arrival at the hospital: (1) intracranial hypertension, (2) inadequate cerebral oxygenation, and (3) systemic medical complications. These must be attacked vigorously for optimal results. Treatment for intracranial hypertension is also designed to maximize cerebral oxygenation, and the modalities are those previously listed.

Of all therapies for high ICP, hyperventilation is the first one used and is extremely effective. With the patient intubated, the PCO_2 is kept at 22 to 30 mm Hg and the fall in ICP should be rapid after hyperventilation; in some instances, this is all that is necessary for control.

Corticosteroids in large doses (1 mg per kilogram dexamethasone every 6 hours) are given routinely. Hyperosmotic agents decrease ICP by removing brain water, owing to an induced osmotic gradient from the brain to the intravascular component. Although slightly less rapid in its action, 20 to 25 percent mannitol has largely replaced 30 percent urea in the United States because of the lower rebound after administration. Two forms of hyperosmotic therapy are available: intermittent bolus use and continuous infusion therapy. High-dose bolus therapy, 1 to 2 g per kilogram mannitol, is reserved for initial emergency control of ICP, usually for patients in whom there is a rapid decrease in level of consciousness, dilating pupils, or decerebration. Maintenance therapy can then be carried out with smaller boluses of 0.15 to 0.3 g per kilogram mannitol every 1 to 2 hours or whenever the ICP exceeds 15 mm Hg. Close attention must be given to the serum osmolality so that it does not rise above 320 mOsm per liter. Significant cardiopulmonary and renal complications are frequent and often irreversible when serum osmolality is above these levels. Clinicians employing this therapy should have a thorough understanding of the hyperosmolar state.

The most recent contribution to ICP control is the use of barbiturates. When these were first used to protect the brain by lowering metabolism, it became apparent that reductions of ICP occurred regularly. Although the mechanism of action of barbiturates on elevated ICP is not known, their successful use when other forms of therapy have failed to lower ICP is encouraging. The doses of barbiturates required have varied. Pentobarbital has been the most widely used agent, usually in loading doses of 10 to 30 mg per kilogram; thereafter, infusions of 0.5 to 3 mg per kilogram per hour are maintained. We have been impressed with the wide variation of serum levels obtained by similar doses in different patients, and no longer rely solely on serum levels as criteria. It is preferable to titrate the dose until a burst-suppression pattern is present on the electroencephalographic monitor. Therapy is then closely regulated to keep the burst-suppressions of equal length. At this physiologic end point, the serum pentobarbital level may vary from 2.5 to 5.0 mg per deciliter. Care must be taken to prevent barbiturate cardiac toxicity and subsequent hypotension. This has not been a problem except in older patients, and the cerebral perfusion pressure can be adequately maintained without the use of pressor agents.

For the duration of barbiturate therapy, monitoring must be intensive because neurologic signs are abolished. Spontaneous respiratory activity is not present, and all other neurologic signs are generally absent. Although we have continued barbiturate therapy for as long as 21 days, the usual course is less than 5 days; by this time the ICP rarely rises when an attempt is made to discontinue the barbiturate infusion. Once a patient's ICP is less than 15 mm Hg for longer than 48 hours, we discontinue therapy in a sequential manner, stopping barbiturates first, then decreasing hyperosmolar therapy, and finally ceasing hyperventilation.

The accepted treatment of a patient with acute subdural hematoma remains controversial. Some neurosurgeons believe that most such patients are not helped by surgery and that the major problems are the control of brain swelling and elevated ICP. Others consider that when there is obvious deterioration in the condition of the patient, evacuation of the hematoma, no matter how large or small, improves intracranial compliance and the neurologic state.

In patients whose CT scans show a large localized subdural clot with an equal or large shift of the midline structures, the hematoma is surgically evacuated. In patients with a "smear subdural" a few millimeters thick over the entire lateral aspect of one hemisphere, with the midline shift greater than the thickness of the subdural, we probably would not operate but would aggressively control ICP. Disagreements arise when a state between these two is seen. The argument against surgical intervention is that the major cerebral problem is brain injury, which cannot be helped by an operation. If there is a disruption of the blood-brain barrier with vasogenic edema, craniotomy decreases tissue pressure, increases hydrostatic pressure gradients between capillaries and tissue, and therefore may cause a marked increase in edema in the decompressed hemisphere. Thus, even if the clot is removed, the increased edema may cause swelling of the hemisphere, which rapidly returns the intracranial volume-pressure relationships to where they were before the operation.

If surgery is performed, we recommend a large temporofrontoparietal craniotomy flap with evacuation of the clot and control of the hemorrhage from bridging veins and cortical laceration. Patients with a sizeable subdural hematoma should undergo an operation for evacuation of the clot followed by management of ICP. Patients with a small subdural hematoma along the outside of the left hemisphere are best managed by aggressive treatment of brain swelling and therapy for increased ICP.

The mortality rates for the surgical treatment of acute subdural hematoma reported in the last 10 years range from 42 to 63 percent. One important variable seems to be the level of consciousness of the patient at the time of the operation. We do not believe that surgery is necessary in all patients with acute subdural hematoma, but it is vital that all patients, including those who have undergone surgical intervention, should receive postoperative ICP monitoring and control. Twenty-five percent of deaths after surgical intervention were from uncontrollable elevated ICP. Thus, postoperative ICP monitoring plays a major role in the care of patients with acute subdural hematomas; it improves not only the mortality rates, but also the quality of life.

SUGGESTED READING

Adams JH, et al. Diffuse brain damage of immediate impact type. Brain 1977; 100:489.

Bruce DA, Gennarelli TA, Langfitt TW. Resuscitation from coma due to head injury. Crit Care Med 1978; 6:254.

Bruno LA. Focal intracranial hematoma. In: Torg JS, ed. Athletic injuries to the head, neck and face. Philadelphia: Lea & Febiger, 1982.

Fischer CM. Concussion amnesia. Neurology 1966; 16:826.

Gennarelli TA. Cerebral concussion and diffuse brain injuries. In: Torg JS, ed. Athletic injuries to the head, neck and face. Philadelphia: Lea & Febiger, 1982.

Gennarelli TA, Dzernicki A, Segawa H. Acute brain swelling in experimental head injury. In press.

Ommaya AK, Gennarelli TA. Cerebral concussion and traumatic unconsciousness. Correlation of experimental and clinical observations on blunt head injuries. Brain 1974; 97:633.

Yarnell PR, Lynch S. The "ding": amnestic states in football trauma. Neurology 1973; 23:186.

Zimmerman RA, Bilaniuk L, Gennarelli TA. Computed tomography of shearing injuries of the cerebral white matter. Radiology 1978; 127:393.

OCULAR INJURIES

ROBERT C. PASHBY, M.D., F.R.C.S.(C)
THOMAS J. PASHBY, C.M., M.D., C.R.C.S.(C)

Eye injuries account for 1 percent of the total related to sports. They can end the career of a professional athlete and change the lifestyle and earning power of others. Their prevention is possible, as proved first in hockey and now in racquet sports. When they do occur, they must be recognized, their severity assessed, and treatment instituted. The team physician, trainer, or first aid attendant should have a basic knowledge of eye anatomy and physiology (Fig. 1) and the necessary equipment to carry out on the spot examination. He must decide whether the injury can be treated and the patient released or whether ophthalmologic consultation is necessary.

EXAMINATION

A minimal list of equipment required for ophthalmologic examination includes:

1. Vision card
2. Pen light
3. Sterile fluorescein strips
4. Sterile eye pads
5. Eye shield
6. Tape
7. Sterile Q-Tips
8. Sterile irrigating solution

To determine the severity of an eye injury, a routine eye examination is carried out. By oblique illumination of the eye with a pen light, damage to the conjunctiva, cornea, anterior chamber, iris, pupil, and lens can be determined. Intraocular examination behind the lens requires the use of an ophthalmoscope and the ability to interpret findings.

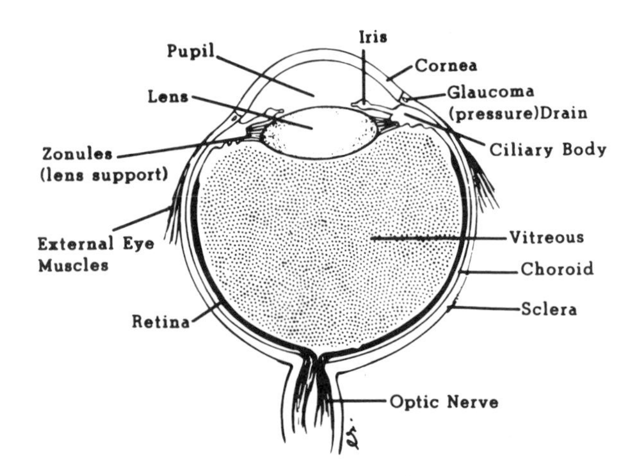

Figure 1 Cross section of the eye.

The steps in the examination are as follows:

1. Inspection of the soft tissues for laceration, bruising, or hematoma.
2. Inspection of the conjunctival sac for hemorrhage, laceration, and foreign bodies. In many cases eversion of the upper eyelid reveals a foreign body, which is easily brushed away. Displaced contact lenses often are found.
3. Examination of the cornea by oblique illumination for foreign bodies, abrasions, and lacerations. Abrasions are readily outlined by a fluorescein strip dipped into the tears exposed as the lower lid is pulled downward.
4. The clarity and depth of the anterior chamber is compared with that of the fellow eye.
5. Pupillary size, shape, and reaction to light are compared with those of the other eye.
6. The iris colors of each eye are compared.
7. Intraocular examination with an ophthalmoscope (if available) may reveal lens, vitreous, and retinal damage.
8. Visual acuity is tested in each eye separately, using a reading card or book; corrected vision less than 20/40 is referred.
9. Peripheral vision is tested by having the patient fix on the examiner's nose and, after occluding the fellow eye, asking for identification of the number of fingers held up in all fields of gaze. A normal visual field extends to 90 degrees temporally, 65 degrees downward, 60 degrees nasally, and 45 degrees upward. Any loss of field demands referral.
10. Ocular movements are tested by having the patient follow a light to his right, then upward, then downward, then similarly to his left. Both eyes should move together. Any diplopia must be referred.
11. Facing the patient, determine whether one eye is sunken (narrowing the palpebral aperture) or proptosed (enlarging it). The former suggests an orbital floor fracture while the latter suggests an orbital hemorrhage. Should there be any doubt about the function of the eye or seriousness of the injury, referral is indicated.

In our series of almost 3,300 eye injuries caused by sports, gathered over the past 12 years, all of which required ophthalmologic care, 11 percent resulted in a legally blind eye (20/200 or less) and most suffered severe intraocular damage.

The sport causing most eye injuries varies from country to country (Table 1). In Canada, hockey has been responsible for most eye injuries, although since the hockey mask was introduced, racquet sports are rapidly catching up (Table 2).

Examining the hockey injuries in more detail proves the benefit of wearing certified protective

TABLE 1 Causes of Sports-Related Eye Injuries in United States and Canada

*Canada (COS Study)**	*Sport*	*United States (CPSC)†*
39%	Hockey (post, mask)	4%
30%	Racquet sports	20%
11%	Baseball	27%
8%	Ball hockey	1%
4%	Football and soccer	7%
1%	Basketball	20%

* Canadian Ophthalmological Society
† Consumer Product Safety Commission

equipment. Before hockey face masks were introduced, an average 272 hockey eye injuries, including 32 blinding injuries, were reported annually. Since masks have been required in minor hockey, the annual average number of eye injuries has dropped to 94 and the number of blinding injuries to 14. No eye injury has been reported to a player wearing a Canadian Standards Association certified mask.

An analysis of 3,295 sports-related eye injuries reveals that over 50 percent are intraocular in type (Table 3).

TREATMENT AND MANAGEMENT

Orbital Hemorrhage

This type of injury usually results from blunt trauma. Bleeding into the orbit causes swelling and proptosis. It is wise to check for intraocular damage before the swelling becomes extensive. Central and peripheral vision, pupils, iris color, and the presence of diplopia must be recorded. Most injuries resorb without treatment, but severe hemorrhage may embarrass the blood supply to the optic nerve and cause visual loss. Such injuries must be referred. Application of an ice pack is suggested.

Corneal lacerations present, again, with similar symptoms. If the eye can be gently opened without undue squeezing and without pressure on the globe, the pupil will appear irregular, the anterior chamber shallow, and the iris probably attached to or prolapsed outside the corneal wound. A sterile eye pad is gently applied, and the patient is referred to the hospital for immediate ophthalmologic repair.

TABLE 2 Number of Eye Injuries According to Sport

Sport	*Injuries*	*Blind Eyes*
Hockey (13 years)	1,578	238
Racquet sports (11 years)	782	34
Baseball	322	18
Ball hockey	219	20
Football	125	5
Golf	35	13
Skiing	22	8
War games (3 years)	43	17
Other sports (11 years)	169	21

Injuries to the Lens

The lens can be injured by blunt trauma interfering with lens metabolism or causing a split in the lens capsule, allowing aqueous to enter the lens, rendering it opaque. The lens may also be involved in penetrating injuries. Cataract changes may occur immediately or develop over weeks or months. The lens is suspended within the eye by radiating zonular fibers attached to the ciliary body. Zonular rupture is not unusual following injury, and this allows vitreous to herniate into the anterior chamber. If the zonular rupture is extensive, the lens may subluxate. The iris will jiggle (iridodonesis).

Removal of the cataractous or dislocated lens and replacement with an implant or the fitting of a contact lens usually restores vision to normal. Lens injuries, or course, demand specialized care.

Traumatic Glaucoma

Intraocular tension often fluctuates above and below normal for days after ocular trauma. If there is no structural damage inside the eye, intraocular tension then settles back to normal. More severe trauma may produce a split in the anterior chamber angle. The ciliary body is damaged, the anterior chamber is deepened, and the aqueous outflow channels are embarrassed. Should the remaining undamaged aqueous outflow channels be unable to handle aqueous production adequately, ocular hypertension ensues. Glaucoma will develop in 10 percent of split angles early or even after many years. Once anterior chamber angle damage has been identified, the intraocular pressure should be followed at regular intervals.

Secondary glaucoma commonly complicates lens dislocation and occurs with hyphemas, especially after secondary hemorrhages. Normalization of pressure is necessary to prevent optic nerve dam-

TABLE 3 Types of Sports-Related Eye Injuries

Soft tissue	34%
Orbital fractures	4%
Corneal injuries	9%
Hyphemas	27%
Other intraocular injuries	23%
Ruptured globes	3%

age and peripheral field loss. Secondary glaucoma complicating hyphema requires early attention to prevent blood staining of the cornea. Evacuation of the blood and blood clots from the anterior chamber is indicated.

Hyphema

Hyphema is a collection of free blood in the anterior chamber. It is a very common ocular sports injury. Over 890 hyphemas are listed in our series. It is important that the person rendering first aid recognize this type of injury, because immediate referral and hospitalization is required. Aspirin should be avoided.

Lid Lacerations

With any lid laceration, damage to the globe, ocular muscles, and orbit must be ruled out. Bleeding can be controlled by direct pressure. Close inspection is necessary to reveal lacerations of the lid margin, of the puncta, or into the lacrimal apparatus. Such lacerations demand meticulous closure to prevent epiphora. Primary repair using the microscope is indicated. Examination of the globe and a record of visual function is necessary.

Conjunctival Injuries

Minor lacerations of the conjunctiva do not require suturing. Foreign bodies may be removed with a moist, sterile Q-Tip. A sterile eye pad is applied for 24 hours when follow-up examination is made.

Foreign bodies commonly lodge under the upper lid margin. Eversion of the upper eyelid will expose them. They too can be wiped away with a moist Q-Tip.

Conjunctival Hemorrhage

Although the bright red blood covering the white sclera is an alarming sight, such uncomplicated injuries are not serious. Eye function is recorded, and if it is normal, no treatment is needed. The redness gradually disappears over 10 days.

Orbital Fractures

These injuries usually result from blunt trauma. The most common fracture occurs to the orbital floor where the bone is thinnest. Blunt trauma forces the eye back into the orbit, increasing the orbital pressure and causing a "blow-out" fracture of the orbital floor. The inferior ocular muscles may be caught in the fracture, causing limitation of upward and downward gaze with resulting diplopia. Enophthalmos is usual. Eye function is recorded, and x-ray studies including tomograms are arranged. Some patients recover spontaneously; others require freeing of the inferior ocular muscles and insertion of a Teflon plate along the orbital floor to cover the fracture. Fractures into the sinuses cause leakage of air into the orbit, producing crepitus, a crackling sound, with finger pressure over the swelling. X-ray examination reveals air in the tissue. Spontaneous resolution is usual. Roof fractures require immediate neurosurgical care because they involve the anterior cranial fossa.

Corneal Injuries

Corneal injuries cause sudden severe pain accompanied by tearing, photophobia, and blepharospasm. Superficial corneal foreign bodies can be irrigated off with sterile solution or brushed off with a moist Q-Tip. Eye function is recorded, a sterile eye pad applied, and the eye reexamined in 24 hours. Embedded foreign bodies will not irrigate or brush off the cornea and require removal by an ophthalmologist using a sterile needle or eye spud under slit lamp magnification. Eye function is recorded, a sterile eye pad applied, and recheck in 24 hours arranged.

Corneal abrasions produce similar symptoms. Fluorescein outlines the denuded area. Should no foreign body be present, visual function is recorded, a sterile eye pad applied, and follow-up examination in 24 hours carried out.

When the injured eye is first examined, the blood appears as a haze in the anterior chamber. The pupil is usually irregular in shape and sluggish in reaction to light. The anterior chamber may be deepened. These diagnostic points are readily appreciated by comparing the injured with the fellow eye. Vision is blurred. On bed rest the blood settles down by gravity and appears the next day as a level in the anterior chamber. Continued bleeding may occur, however, and if this is severe the anterior chamber appears black, the so-called "8-ball eye." Most hyphemas clear in 5 days, but 15 percent suffer secondary bleeds, usually within 2 to 5 days. Prompt recognition and referral is necessary. Conservative treatment includes hospitalization, sedation, and binocular bandages, especially for children. Secondary glaucoma occurs in 50 percent of secondary hemorrhages. Irrigation of the anterior chamber is indicated to relieve the increased intraocular pressure and prevent blood staining of the cornea.

Injuries to the Posterior Pole

These injuries commonly result from a blunt blow to the front of the eye, producing a pressure wave that travels to the posterior pole and crushes the choroid and retina against the tough sclera. This contra-coup force commonly causes a choroidal split or tear. Should the split occur across the macular area, visual acuity is markedly reduced. Less severe contra-coup forces may cause macular edema with reduced visual acuity. Depending on the severity of the blow, resolution may occur, but usually the edema creates a macular cyst, which then may rupture and leave a macular hole. Central vision is then markedly reduced.

Retinal injuries may result in hemorrhages or detachments. One-third of traumatic retinal detachments are sports related. Recovery of visual function depends on early recognition and treatment. Once the detachment involves the macula, normal vision will not be restored, although the retina is successfully reattached.

No outward sign of retinal detachment is evident. Some blurring of vision, when tested, with some loss of peripheral field is diagnostic. For this reason, eye injuries of even moderate degree deserve ophthalmoscopic examination at the time of injury, and certainly on recheck the following day. The patient is warned to report any loss of visual function, especially to the sides, up, or down.

Ruptured Globe

These injuries destroy vision and usually result in removal of the eye. Over 100 such injuries have

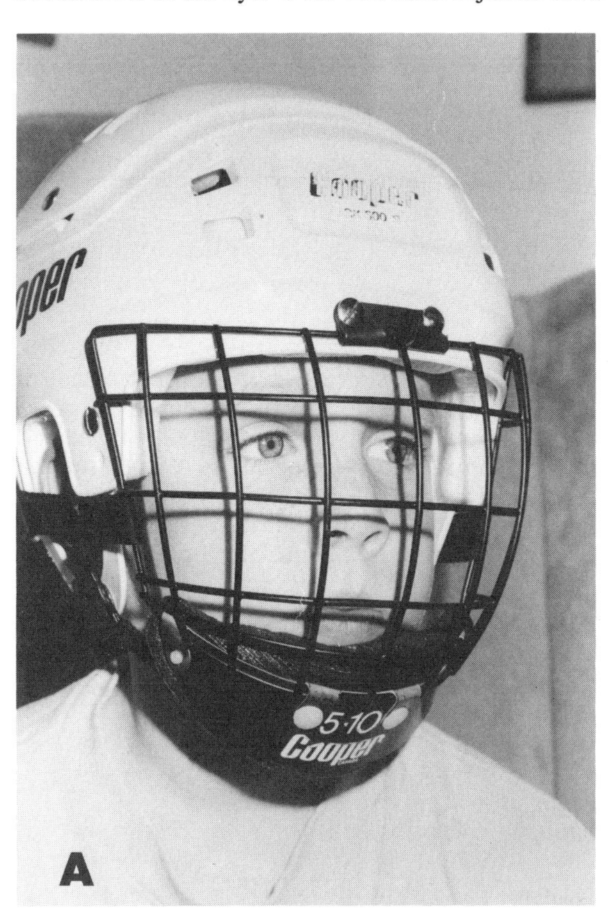

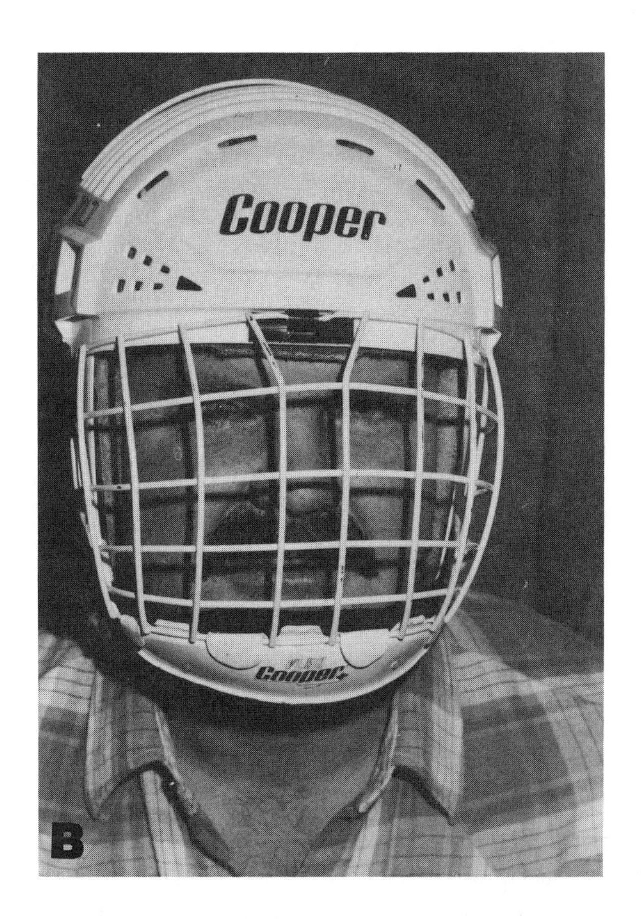

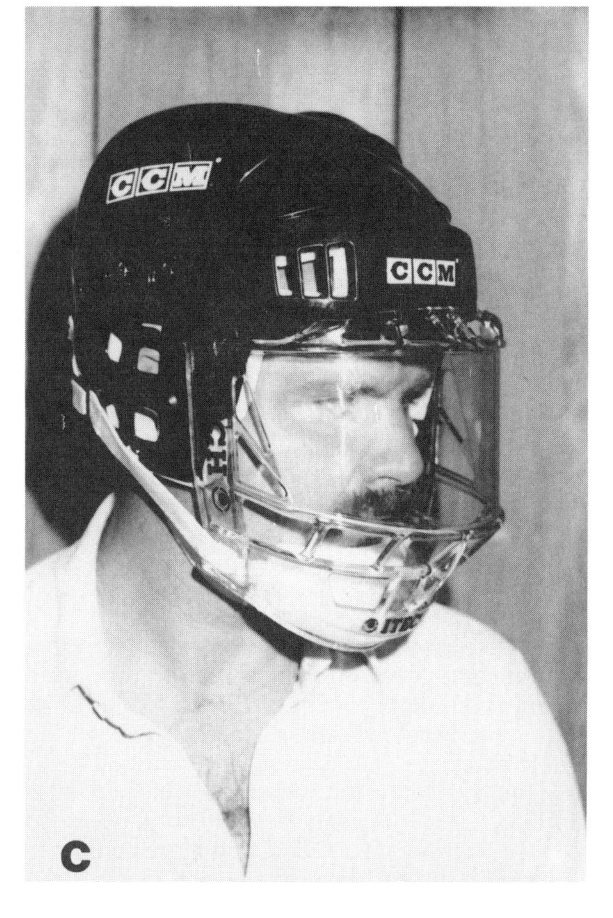

Figure 2 *A,* Certified mask-helmet for 5- to 10-year-old hockey players. *B* and *C,* Certified mask-helmets for older players.

been recorded in our series. The offending weapon is usually a hockey stick or puck, a golf ball or club, a ski tip, a squash ball or racquet, or a tennis ball or baseball. At the time of injury, pain causes orbicularis spasm. If the lids can be gently opened, the eye will appear soft and sunken in the orbit. Vision will usually be reduced to perception of hand movement or light. Treatment requires gentle application of a sterile eye pad and transport to a hospital for immediate ophthalmologic care.

PREVENTION

Prevention is the key. Modifying rules and the wearing of certified protective equipment have done much to reduce the number of eye injuries in Canadian hockey. Racquet sports eye protectors with polycarbonate lenses are saving eyes in squash and racquetball as well (Figs. 2 and 3).

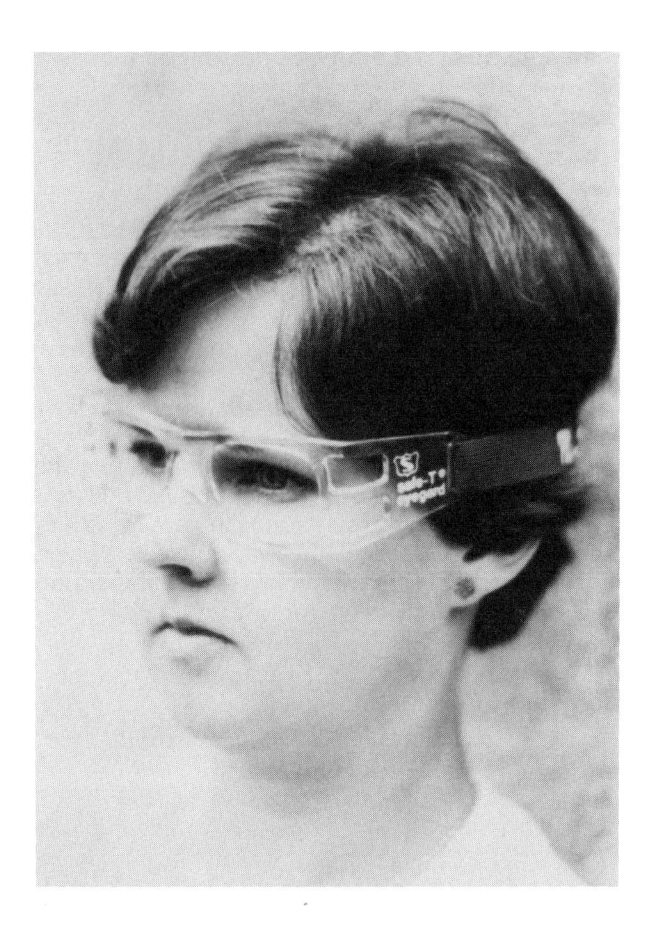

Figure 3 Eye protector for racquet sports participants.

EYE PROTECTORS IN RACQUET SPORTS

MICHAEL EASTERBROOK, M.D., F.R.C.S. (C), F.A.C.S.

The purpose of this chapter is to summarize our experience over the last 10 years with eye protectors, specifically in racquet sports.

BADMINTON

It has been apparent for some time that the badminton shuttlecock is ideally suited to produce an eye injury. Indeed, speeds of 130 to 135 miles per hour have been recorded, using high-speed film (Table 1).

Table 2 demonstrates the increasing percentage of badminton injuries in racquet sports in Canada over a 5-year period, as more and more racquetball and squash players are wearing eye protection.

Although no surveys have been performed in recent years, it appears that the incidence of injuries in badminton is relatively high in doubles. The badminton community is becoming concerned that national and provincial organizations and local clubs may be liable if a strong educational program is not designed to promote the use of eyeguards.

TABLE 1 Ball and Racquet Velocities

	Speeds (mph)
Racquetball	
Ball	85–110
Racquet	85–90
Squash	
Ball	130–140
Racquet	95–110
Tennis ball	90–110
Handball	60–70
Badminton shuttlecock	130–135

C.A. Morehouse, ASTM

TABLE 2 533 Eye Injuries in Racquet Sports in Canada

Year	Number of Injuries	Racquetball and Squash (%)	Badminton (%)	Tennis (%)
1982	90	73	13	14
1983	87	59	22	19
1984	115	58	16	26
1985	82	50	33	17
1986	83	36	35	29
1987	66	38	38	24

Although testing by the Canadian Standards Association (CSA) has not yet been carried out for eye protectors in badminton, it appears that the polycarbonate eye protectors used in squash and racquetball may well suffice to prevent eye injuries in this very active sport.

RACQUETBALL AND SQUASH

Racquetball and squash are ideally suited to produce an eye injury: the balls and racquets either fit exactly or can be compressed to fit into the human orbit (Fig. 1). Table 3 lists some of the injuries seen over a 10-year period in Canada. Table 1 lists the speeds of squash, racquetball, and tennis balls; it is not surprising that eye injuries are occurring on a regular basis.

It is apparent that energy levels in racquet sports are significant (Table 4). To pass the industrial lens safety standard in the United States, a lens must not break after a 1-lb ball is dropped on it from a distance of only 0.6 foot. This is grossly inadequate to resist the enormous energy levels in squash and racquetball. A novice racquetball player hits the ball at 78 miles per hour; an "A" player hits the ball at speeds of 125 to 140 miles per hour.

TABLE 3 Canadian Racquets Survey 1978–1987

Injury	*Squash*	*Racquetball*
Lid hemorrhage	57	42
Lid laceration	36	19
Subconjunctival hemorrhage	31	14
Corneal abrasion	44	32
Corneal lacerations requiring surgery	6	2
Iritis	26	26
Iris tear or dialysis	10	8
Angle recession	18	4
Hyphema	114	106
Secondary hemorrhage	5	4
Cataract	8	6
Vitreous/retinal hemorrhage	17	21
Macular scar	8	5
Retinal detachment	10	3
Orbital fracture	3	1
Number of patients	*393*	*293*

TABLE 4 Energy Levels in Racquet Sports

ANSI Z87 STANDARD (Industrial safety lenses)	0.6 ft/lb
RACQUETBALL	
1.4 oz at 128 mph	29.0 ft/lb
1.4 oz at 78 mph	17.8 ft/lb
SQUASH	
70+: 1.25 oz at 100 mph	23.63 ft/lb
Yellow dot: 0.846 oz at 100 mph	17.76 ft/lb

OPEN EYEGUARDS

A variety of open eyeguards that were unbreakable and did not restrict peripheral vision, but allowed eye penetration, entered the market in the late 1970s (Fig. 2). It was apparent, without formal testing, that squash and racquetball balls readily penetrated these open eyeguards (Fig. 3). Table 5 gives details of the first 80 patients who sustained an injury while wearing open eyeguards.

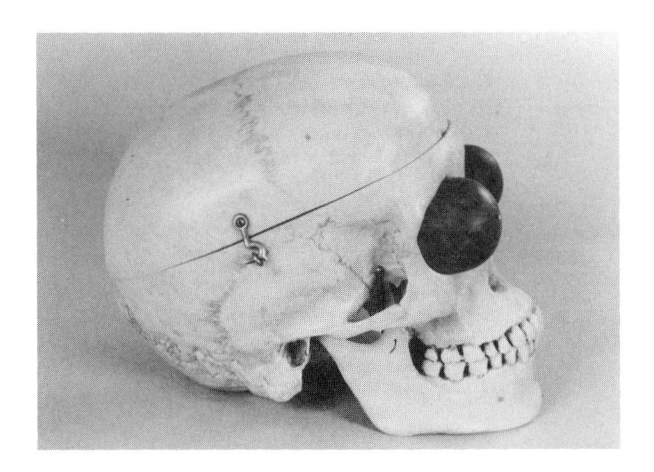

Figure 1 Skull containing an international yellow dot soft ball in the right orbit, and a 70+ American ball in the left orbit.

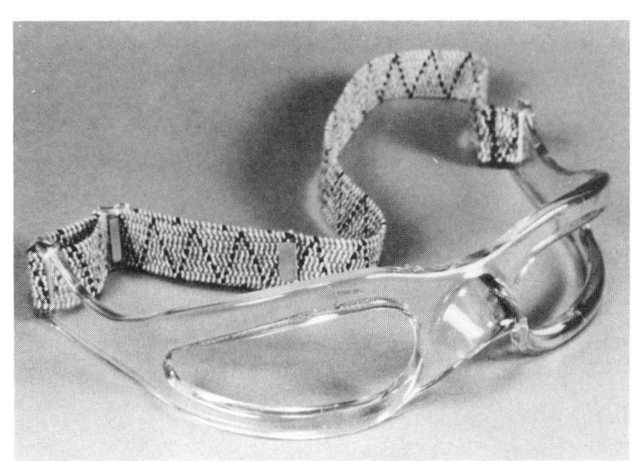

Figure 2 Protec, one of the initial open eyeguards widely distributed for squash and racquetball.

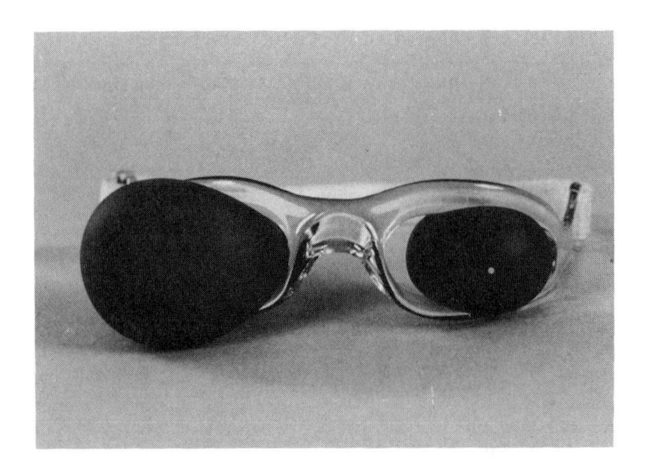

Figure 3 Penetration of an open eyeguard by a racquetball ball and squash ball.

These eyeguards were of no use in racquetball, in which 95 percent of the injuries were caused by the ball. Indeed, players have indicated that they had a false sense of security, since players who feel protected watch the ball more closely. It might be argued that these open eyeguards, being unbreakable, only funnel a compressible squash or racquetball ball directly into the eye, increasing the risk of ocular injury. On the basis of these reports of inadequate eye protection, standards were set in Canada and the United States. Table 6 lists the eyeguards which have passed C.S.A. standard. Table 7 lists the eyeguards that have met the 1985 or 1986 ASTM standard in the United States.

TABLE 5 Injuries Sustained by 80 Athletes Wearing Open Eyeguards:

Injury		
Lid hemorrhage		11
Lid lacerations		3
Corneal abrasions		10
Iritis		8
Hyphemas		56
Mechanism of injury		
Ball		77
Racquet		3
Ball penetrated eyeguard		69
Eyeguard displaced		11
Eyeguard	Squash	Racquetball
Protec	14	22
Ektelon	1	15
Rainbow	5	2
Voit	2	13
Solari	1	2
Champion	1	–
Duraguard	0	2
	24	56

CLOSED EYEGUARDS

The present Canadian and American standards relate to performance, not design. An eyeguard is positioned on a head form (Fig. 4), which is placed in a testing device (Fig. 5) whereby balls are projected at speeds of 90 miles per hour at the lens and at the hinge. If contact is made between the lens and the head form, the eyeguard fails.

In late 1986, several eyeguards passed these standards; these are illustrated in Figures 6 to 15.

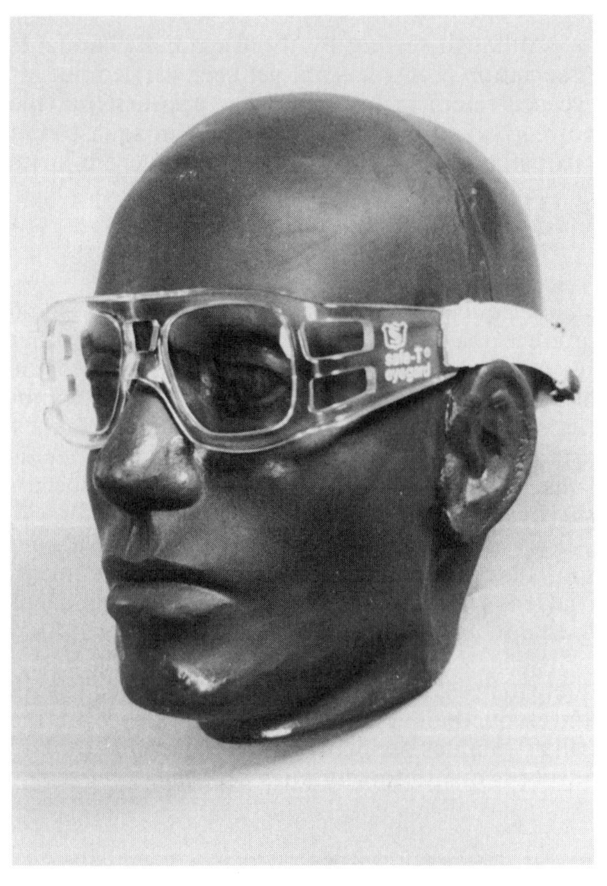

Figure 4 Eyeguard on Alderson head form.

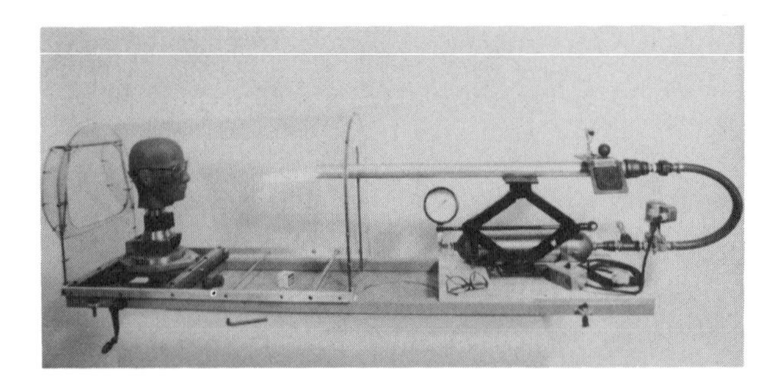

Figure 5 Testing device at Canadian Standards Association.

TABLE 6 Canadian Standards Association Approved Eyeguards, 1989

Model	*Cost (Can $)*	*Manufacturer/ Distributor*	*Address (Canada)*	*Address (United States)*
1. Defender 600	26.00	Peepers	Peepers Inc. P.O. Box 951, Station A 150 Chatham Steel Hamilton, Ontario L8N 3P9 416-525-3369	Peepers International 417 Fifth Ave. New York, NY 10016 212-696-9797
2. CRS 300	29.95	CRS Sports	CRS Sports International Inc. 10021 169th Street Edmonton, Alberta T5P 4M9 403-483-5149	Same address as Canada
3. Sports Scanners	35.40	American Optical	AOCO Ltd. 80 Centurian Dr. Markham, Ontario L3R 5Y5 416-479-4545	American Optical Mechanic Optical Southbridge, MA 01550 617-765-9711
4. Safe-T Eyegard	30.00	Imperial Optical	Imperial Optical Canada 21 Dundas Square Toronto, Ontario M5B 1B7 416-595-1010	Embassy Creations P.O. Box 143 234 Holmes Rd. Holmes, PA 19043 215-586-9640
5. Albany	22.00	Leader	International Forums Inc. (Leader Sports) 1150 Marie Victoria Longuevil, Quebec J4G 1A1 514-651-2300	LST Leader Sports Products Inc. P.O. Box 271 Main Street, Route 22 Essex, NY 12936 518-963-4268
6. New Yorker	27.50	Leader	Same address as no. 5	Same address as no. 5

TABLE 7 United States ASTM: Passed to 1985 and/or 1986 Standard

Model	*Cost (US $)*	*Manufacturer/ Distributor*	*Address (Canada)*	*Address (United States)*
1. Action Eyes	30.00	Viking Sports	Black Knight Enterprises 3792 Commercial Street Vancouver, British Columbia V5N 4G2 604-872-3123	Viking Sports 5355 Sierra Road San Jose, CA 95132 408-923-7777
2. Albany	20.00	Leader	International Forums Inc. (Leader Sports) 1150 Marie Victoria Longuevil, Quebec J4G 1A1 514-651-2300	LST Leader Sports Products Inc. P.O. Box 271 Main Street, Route 22 Essex, NY 12936 518-963-4268
3. New Yorker	25.00	Leader	Same address as no. 2	Same address as no. 2
4. Sierra	20.00	Ektelon	Paris Glove of Canada Ltd. 9200 Rue Meilleur St. #101 Montreal, Quebec B2N 2A8 514-381-8611	Ektelon 8929 Aero Dr. San Diego, CA 92123 619-560-0066
5. Court Goggles	20.00	Ektelon	Same address as no. 4	Same address as no. 4
6. Safety Lites (tested and approved for racquetball, not squash)	22.00	Penn	Same address as US	306 South 45th Avenue Phoenix, AZ 85043 602-269-1492

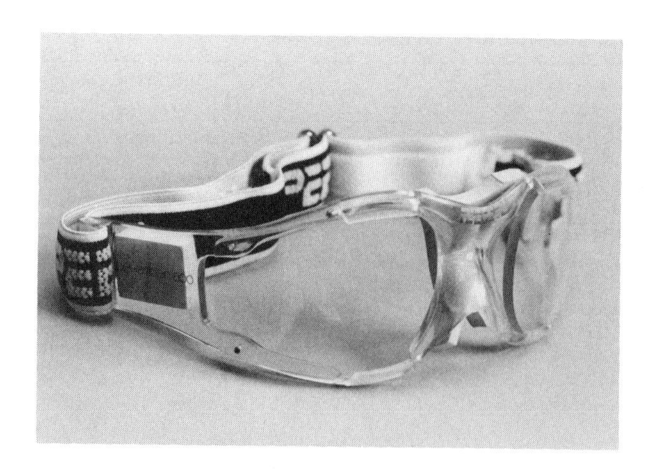

Figure 6 Defender 600 Eyeguard Peepers: CSA approved.

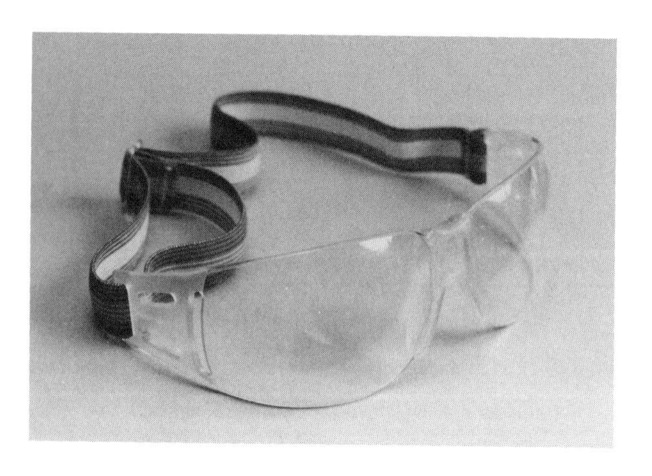

Figure 7 CRS 300 CRS Sports: CSA approved.

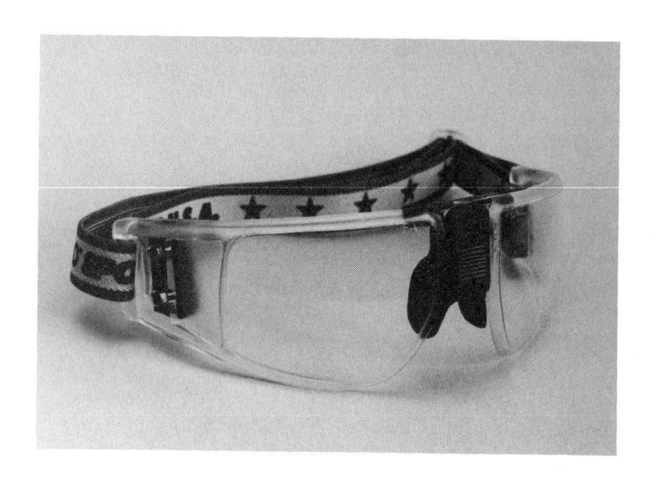

Figure 8 Sports Scanners American Optical: CSA approved.

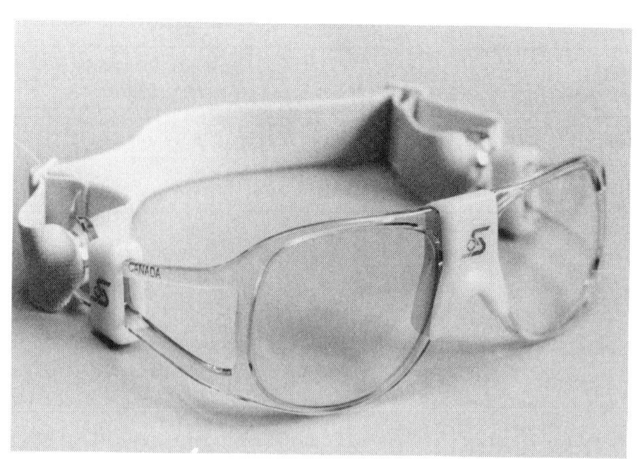

Figure 9 Safe-T-Eyegard Imperial Optical: CSA approved.

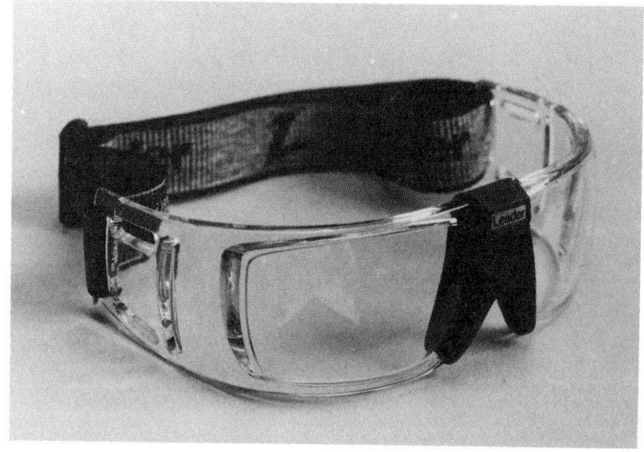

Figure 10 Albany Leader: CSA approved and meets ASTM 1985 or 1986 standard.

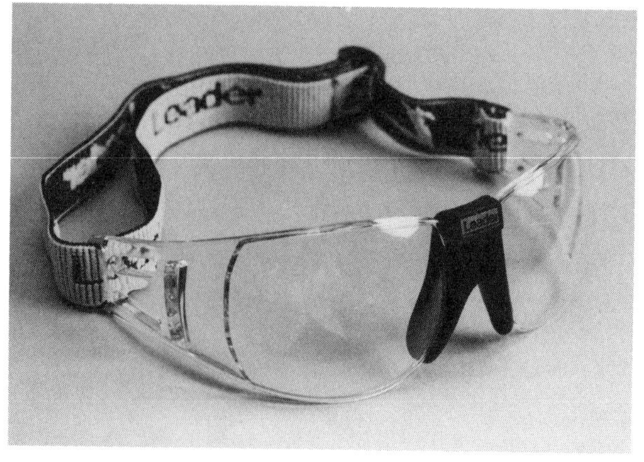

Figure 11 New Yorker Leader: CSA approved and meets ASTM 1985 or 1986 standard.

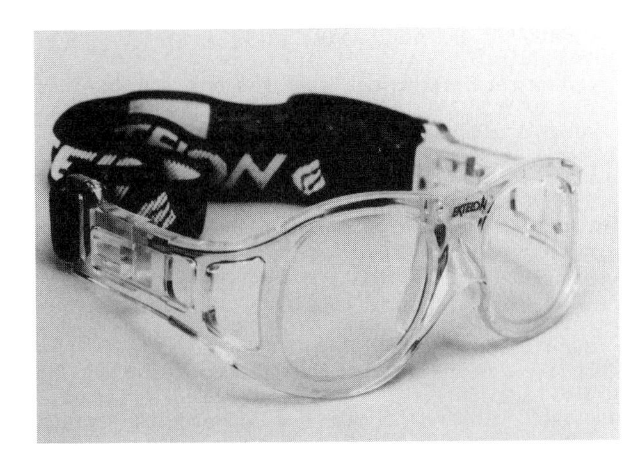

Figure 12 Sierra Ektelon: meets ASTM 1986 standard.

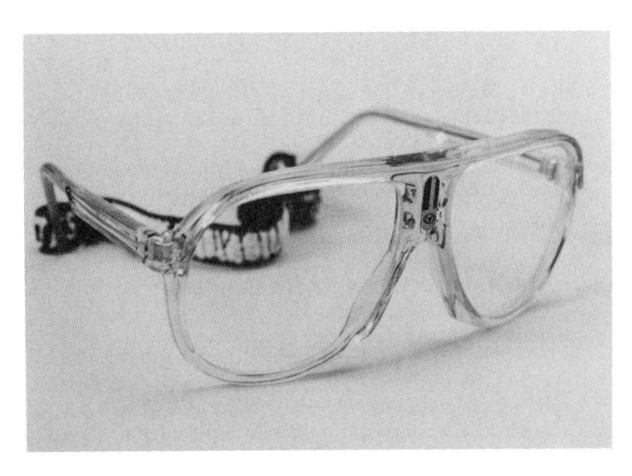

Figure 15 Safety Lites Penn: meets ASTM 1986 standard for racquetball.

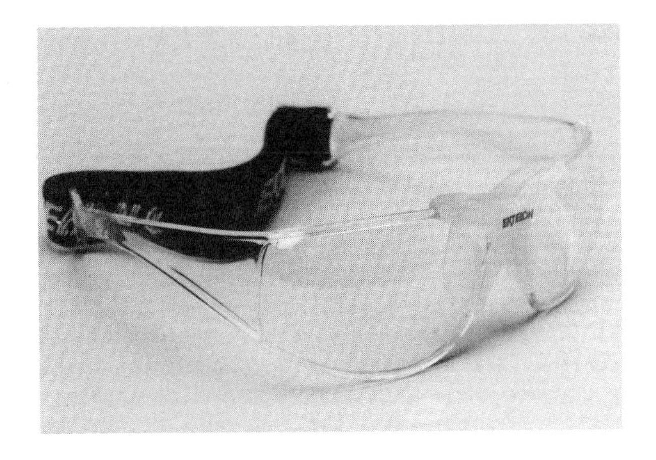

Figure 13 Court Goggles Ektelon: meets ASTM 1986 standard.

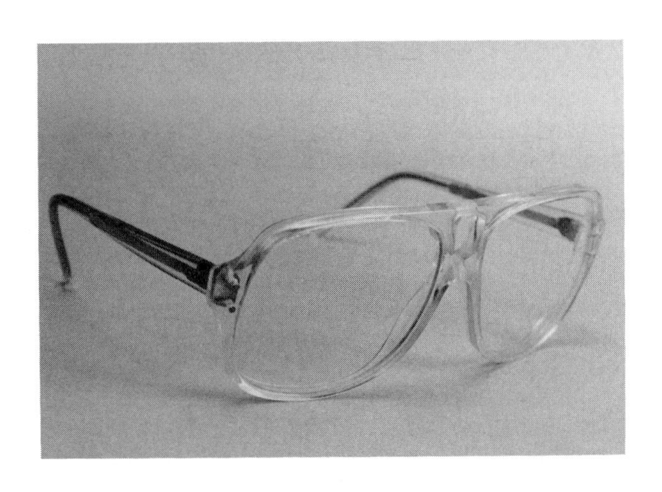

Figure 14 Action Eyes Viking Sports: meets ASTM 1986 standard.

CONCLUSION

Surveys in the late 1970s and early 1980s at squash and racquetball clubs in Canada and the United States revealed a startling increase in eye injuries in recreational squash and racquetball players. In Canada 686 racquetball injuries involving 31 blind eyes were reported at the Canadian Ophthalmological Society over a 10-year period, 1978–1987.

There are eye protectors currently on the market that protect players at speeds in excess of 90 miles per hour. No significant ocular injury has been reported in North America to players wearing polycarbonate eyeguards that meet CSA and/or ASTM 1985 or 1986 standards.

Any player can wear sunglasses; any player can wear a closed eyeguard. Newer eyeguards are meeting standards designed as performance standards. Antifog coating is available on many of the new eyeguards.

Excellent eye protection is now available. It behooves all physicians and those interested in the prevention of vision loss to encourage all recreational racquet players to wear eyeguards certified for competitive racquet sports.

Acknowledgments. I am grateful to the eye surgeons of Canada and the Canadian squash and racquetball players for submitting these data and encouraging us to make safer eye protection. Thanks are offered to the instructional media services of the Wellesley Hospital and to Mrs. Joanne Nathanson for her assistance with the preparation of this chapter. The leadership of Dr. Paul Vinger and Dr. Tom Pashby in their effort to reduce eye injuries in sport cannot be overestimated.

SUGGESTED READING

Barrell GV, Cooper PJ, Elkington AR, et al. Squash ball to eye ball: the likelihood of squash players incurring an eye injury. Br Med J 1981; 283:893–895.

Bishop PJ, Kozey J, Caldwell G. Performance of eye protectors for squash and racquetball. Phys Sports Med 1982; 10:63–69.

Blonstein JL. Eye injury in sport. Practitioner 1975; 215:208–209.

Diamond GR, Quinn GE, Pashby TJ, Easterbrook M. Ophthalmologic injuries. Clin Sports Med 1982; 1:469–482.

Diamond GR, Quinn GE, Pashby TJ, Easterbrook M. Ophthalmological injuries. Primary care. 1984; 11:161–174.

Doxanas MT, Soderstrom C. Racquetball as an ocular hazard. Arch Ophthalmol 1980; 98:1965–1966.

Easterbrook M. Eye injuries in squash: a preventable disease. Can Med Assoc J 1978; 118:298–305.

Easterbrook M. Eye injuries in racquet sports: a continuing problem. Can Med Assoc J 1980; 123:268.

Easterbrook M. Eye injuries in racquet sports; a continuing problem. Phys Sports Med 1981:91–101.

Easterbrook M. Eye injuries in racquet sports. Int Ophthalmol Clin 1981; 21:87–119.

Easterbrook M. Eye injuries in squash and racquetball players: an update. Phys Sports Med 1982; 10:47–56.

Easterbrook M, Cameron J. Sports injuries; mechanisms, prevention and treatment. Schneider RC, et al, eds. Injuries in racquet sports, Baltimore: Wilkins & Wilkins, 1985: 553.

Easterbrook WM. Eye protection in racquet sports: an update. Phys Sports Med 1987; 15:180–186.

Easterbrook M. Eye protection in racquet sports. Clin Sports Med. In press.

Easterbrook M. Eye protection in racquet sports. Int Ophthalmol Clin 1988; 28:232–237.

Editorial. A ball in the eye. Br Med J 1973; 2:195–196.

Feigelman M, Sugar J, Rednock N, Read J, Johnson PL. Assessment of ocular protection for racquetball. JAMA 1984; 250:3305–3309.

Fowler BJ, Seelenfreund M, Newton JC. Ocular injuries sustained playing squash. Am J Sports Med 1980; 8:126–128.

Kennerley-Bankes JL. Squash rackets: a survey of eye injuries in England. Br Med J 1985; 291:1539–1540.

Ingram DV, Lewkonia I. Ocular hazards of playing squash racquets. Br J Ophthalmol 1973; 57: 434–438.

Maberley AL. Retinal detachments and athletic eye injuries. BC Med J 1981; 23:70–73.

Moore MC, Worthley DA. Ocular injuries in squash players. Aust J Ophthalmol 1977; 5:46–47.

Seelenfreund MH, Freilich DS. Rushing the net and retinal detachment. JAMA 1976; 235: 2723–2726.

Vinger P. The eye and sports medicine. In: Duane T, ed. Clinical Ophthalmology, Vol. 1. Philadelphia: Harper and Row, 1985; 1.

Vinger PF, Toplin DW. Racquet sports: an ocular hazard. JAMA 1978; 239:2575–2577.

Vinger PF. Sports eye injuries—a preventable disease. Ophthalmology 1981; 108–113.

Vinger PF. The incidence of eye injuries in sports. Int Ophthalmol Clin 1981; 21:21–46.

FACIAL INJURIES

LEITH G. DOUGLAS, M.D., F.R.C.S.(C), F.A.C.S.

Injuries to the face are common in many sports, particularly those involving body contact. In my experience as team plastic surgeon with the Toronto Maple Leafs of the National Hockey League for some 20 years, I have seen approximately 100 per season. The main instrument of injury has been the hockey stick, accounting for about 80 percent of cases. The puck, the ice, skates, goalposts, the glass surrounding the rink, and fists accounted for the remainder. The incidence has remained approximately the same, but the seriousness of the injuries has decreased now that almost everyone in the National League wears a helmet.

PREVENTION

Body contact sports will always be responsible for some facial trauma. This probably can still be reduced to some degree. The use of properly fitting helmets in hockey and football is mandatory, and their value is self-evident. Face guards may become popular in hockey in the future if they can be made lighter and easier to wear. Penalties for improper use of hockey sticks and deliberate attempts to injure in any way should be increased and will act as a deterrent to violence-minded players. Football goalposts have been made much safer, so consideration might be given to altering the construction of goalposts in hockey. The removal of the deep central tongue of the net and the introduction of the new magnetically seated net are steps in the right direction.

Facial injuries can be broadly classified into those involving soft tissue only and those involving the facial bones.

SOFT TISSUE INJURIES

The types of soft tissue injury are (1) contusions, (2) abrasions, (3) puncture wounds, and (4) lacerations (simple and complicated).

Contusions

Most contusions are simple and require no treatment other than the application of an ice bag. However, some may result in hematoma formation. A small hematoma is completely absorbed in a few weeks, but larger ones that become encapsulated require incision and drainage. Incisions for these should be placed so that the resulting scar is minimized and no vital structures are damaged. Sometimes it is necessary to insert a small Penrose drain in the incision for 24 to 48 hours. It is best to evacuate hematomas at the "currant jelly" stage rather than go on for many weeks waiting for full liquefaction. I have not found proteolytic enzymes given systemically to be of any help in liquefying hematomas.

Hematomas of the external ear must be promptly and properly drained and prevented from reaccumulating or developing a seroma. Failure to do so results in the formation of a cauliflower ear.

Abrasions

Abrasions vary from simple brush burns of the epidermis to those that go through the epidermis and into the dermis. The former require nothing other than cleansing with a good detergent and the application of an antibiotic cream for a few days. With deeper abrasions the area should be fully cleansed and any foreign material removed. The time to do this is at the initial treatment. Foreign material left in a wound not only contributes to the incidence of infection, but may result in traumatic tattooing. It becomes fixed to tissues in about 12 hours and becomes extremely difficult to remove without a formal surgical abrasion procedure. The use of local, and even general, anesthesia may be necessary to permit proper cleansing. A soft brush may be required to remove deeply embedded material. The area should then be covered with an antibiotic ointment and suitably dressed. Most abrasions heal in about a week unless they become infected.

Puncture Wounds

The principles of treatment are the same as for puncture wounds anywhere on the body. The track of the puncture should be followed and the possibility of deep injury to nerves, vessels, or other vital structures ruled out. It is particularly important to determine whether foreign bodies are retained in the wound. X-ray examination should be done as indicated. Narrow puncture wounds are best not sutured, particularly if they are deep and if there is a possibility of the development of infection. The track should be irrigated with saline or hydrogen peroxide and covered with a dry dressing.

Bite wounds are a special type of puncture wound. They may occur when a player strikes his face on an opponent's teeth or, fortunately infrequently, as a result of malicious intent. These are very serious wounds and have a very high potential for infection. They should be copiously irrigated with hydrogen peroxide and saline, getting to the depths of the wound with the liquid. They should be left open in all except the rare case in which a vital function is compromised as, for example, in a complete tear of a lower lip. In these cases, loose closure is done, with definitive repair carried out secondarily or as a delayed primary procedure.

Penicillin and cloxacillin are started immediately in moderately high dosage; cephalosporins are used in patients with penicillin allergy. The wound is reexamined in 24 hours, and may be secondarily closed in a few days if it remains clean. Evidence of developing infection warrants admission to the hospital, where high-dose intravenous antibiotic therapy is administered.

Lacerations

Simple Lacerations

These may be linear lacerations due to hockey sticks and other sharp objects, but are frequently of the bursting type caused by a bony prominence of the face coming in contact with a blunt object. With these there is also an element of contusion.

They should be cleansed with a good antiseptic solution, such as aqueous Hibitane, then irrigated with saline. Needless to say, no material should be used on the face that is poisonous, stains the skin, or is dangerous to the eyes.

Examination of the wound for foreign material and damage to blood vessels and nerves is then carried out. A judicious debridement may be necessary if there are small tags of nonviable tissue or ragged edges in bursting wounds, but this should be very judicious.

The vast majority of simple facial lacerations may be repaired under local anesthesia. I usually use 1 percent lidocaine without epinephrine. Infiltration with a No. 25 or 27 needle through the wound is adequate. Many athletes prefer not to have the area anesthetized, arguing that it swells more and is more prone to infection afterward. I have no evidence to support this claim, but I respect their wishes and have repaired more lacerations in hockey players without anesthetic than with it. The area is usually much less sensitive initially owing to the contusion, and thus it is not really as barbaric as it sounds.

If an adequate clinic room is available at the arena or stadium, most simple facial lacerations can be repaired there without compromising good medical practice. There should be adequate space with a good light and a quiet environment. One must have an assistant to help with the supplying of materials and possibly to cut sutures and sponge as indicated. Antiseptic solutions, saline, gauze dressings, drapes, and sterile instruments are required. I have been using disposable paper drapes with a small window cut out for some time, and they are excellent for this purpose. Instruments needed are a suitable needle holder, Adson forceps, about 6 hemostats, curved and straight iris scissors, the necessary syringes and needles, and suture material.

My choice of suture material for facial lacerations is 5–0 or 6–0 nylon on the surface, sometimes supplemented by deep sutures of 4–0 or 5–0 polyglycolic acid material.

Any small bleeders should be caught and ligated as necessary. Wound closure should be done somewhat more loosely than in a clean surgical wound, because the element of contusion leads to more swelling, causing the sutures to tighten and cut in. Interrupted suture technique is usually employed, although subcuticular closure with a continuous suture may be possible in some clean, incised linear wounds.

Simple lacerations are usually dressed with a small adhesive dressing strip. Sometimes an antibiotic ointment may be applied over the suture line. When there is contusion, the application of ice over the dressing is indicated.

I recommend removal of dressings in 24 hours and gentle daily washing after that. My infection rate in such wounds has been practically zero.

Complicated Lacerations

These include more extensive lacerations requiring more than 10 or 12 sutures as well as those involving specialized structures.

Lacerations of the eyelids and of the alar margin and complex lacerations of the ears are probably best dealt with in the Emergency Department of a hospital rather than in a clinic room. The technique remains the same, i.e., cleansing, anesthetizing properly, very judicious debridement, and accurate closure. Closure of lacerations crossing anatomic boundaries, such as the vermilion border of the lip and the eyebrow, should be done very carefully, in order to restore the anatomy as perfectly as possible. This is not always as easy as it sounds and frequently requires considerable effort. Incidentally, one *never* shaves an eyebrow!

Also included in this group are lacerations with actual soft tissue loss. If this is minimal the wound may be closed by simply advancing the edges. Other more complicated situations with avulsion of flaps should be treated in the hospital and, in rare instances, may require skin grafting to restore the deficit.

The trap door flap or U-shaped laceration is always a problem. The dimensions of the flap may be such that the length-to-width ratio leads to compromising of its circulation. It may therefore be necessary to excise the questionable part and close it by advancing the edges. In curved lacerations, direct closure frequently leads to a pincushion effect with the central part becoming heaped up in relation to the surrounding tissues. This is due to contracture along the line of the scar and sometimes to a degree of edema, which makes it stand out even more prominently. This is particularly true if the flap is in a true U shape based superiorly rather than an inverted U shape, as this tends to act as a barrier to normal lymphatic drainage. Despite this problem, there is no place for Z-plasties and excisions of tissue at the initial procedure. The best plan is simply to close the wound as carefully as possible, revising it later only if necessary. Since it is not possible to predict just how good or how bad a given flap is going to be, it is always wisest to wait.

With simple lacerations the player is usually able to return to the game, but with the more complicated ones it is prudent to give them a chance to heal without danger of further trauma. A simple laceration heals in a few days, sutures being removed at 4 or 5 days. In more complicated ones a few sutures may be left in place for 2 or 3 days more. Lacerations that have transgressed the facial nerve or parotid duct and other such serious injuries are beyond the scope of this discussion. They should be dealt with in the same manner as they would be in nonsports practice.

Antibiotics are employed only when dictated by common sense. In simple lacerations they are not indicated unless there is gross contamination. They should be employed in the more complicated ones, those involving eyelids and ears, and those in which there has been considerable contamination or in which there is a doubt whether the wound has been cleansed adequately.

The patient's tetanus immunization status should be determined and supplemented as indicated.

It is necessary to carry out a proper examination of vital structures, such as the eyes if the eyelids are injured, the internal structure of the nose if the nose is injured, or the teeth and underlying bone if the mouth area is involved. Facial nerve injuries do not occur frequently, but function should be tested if there is any possibility of damage.

The cardinal principles are (1) a full assessment of the injury, (2) thorough cleansing, (3) hemostasis, (4) judicious debridement, and (5) anatomic closure with fine sutures.

FRACTURES OF THE FACIAL BONES

These may be classified as closed (simple) and open (compound) fractures. By far the greater majority are compound. This compounding is from within rather than from without in most cases. For example, nasal bone fractures and fractures of the zygoma and maxilla almost invariably involve tears of the mucoperiosteum of the nasal cavity or the maxillary antrum. Most fractures of the mandible, being through tooth-bearing areas, are also compound. Fractures may be further classified as linear or comminuted, displaced or undisplaced, and stable or unstable.

The Nose

The nose is the most commonly injured bone structure on the face. Fractures may be due to blows from the side or directly end-on. The former type of injury usually produces simple fracturing with deviation to one side, whereas end-on blows may result in comminution of both bone and cartilage.

Diagnosis usually is not difficult. The patient may have heard or felt a crack in the nose at the time of the injury. There is usually epistaxis, which may be profuse, and a clinical deformity of the nose may be obvious to both the patient and the attending physician. Roentgenograms are helpful, but the decision to treat and the assessment of the results of treatment are a matter of clinical judgment.

It may be possible to manipulate a fractured nose quickly back into position in a relatively painless manner if the physician sees the patient immediately after the injury. This has the effect of reducing the bleeding, reducing bruising and edema, and affording considerable comfort to the patient.

A good clinical examination of the internal as well as the external nose is mandatory. If the nasal septum is fractured, it is possible to develop a septal hematoma. The characteristic bluish bulge on the septum should alert the physician, and appropriate drainage with packing should be carried out without delay. The mucoperichondrium may be dissected off the underlying cartilaginous septum by the hematoma. This can lead to resorption of the cartilage and loss of tip support. In some cases, cartilage is laid down as it is in a cauliflower ear, producing a mass that obstructs the airway. Septal abscess formation is also possible. Septal hematomas are of vital importance in children, because loss of cartilaginous tip support in a growing nose may lead to severe "snub-nose" deformity.

Reduction of the fracture, if necessary, may be done under local or general anesthesia after the swelling has subsided—usually within 4 or 5 days. Intranasal packing and plaster splinting are usually necessary in complex injuries involving comminution or septal hematomas, but the simpler fractures may be treated without them.

It is usually inadvisable for players to resume playing for at least a week after a nasal fracture of any consequence. Before they return it is necessary to be sure that there is no significant swelling and no possibility that bleeding will recur, and that the fracture is stable and does not require external support.

An external protective device is usually required for at least 4 weeks after such an injury. The wearing of helmets in hockey facilitates the attachment of a face guard, and in football, of course, it is already worn.

Antibiotics usually are not necessary in the treatment of nasal fractures unless there has been gross comminution or operative intervention such as the drainage of a septal hematoma.

The Zygoma and Orbit

Blows to the prominence of the cheek may result in zygomatic fractures. These may involve only the arch laterally or, more commonly, may cause the classic fracture through the frontozygomatic, zygomaticomaxillary, and zygomaticotemporal suture lines, the zygoma being displaced medially and inferiorly.

Diagnosis may be made by inspection alone when there is obvious flattening of the cheek on the affected side. Patients complain of pain and, frequently, of trismus due to the impingement of the displaced zygomatic arch on the coronoid process of the mandible. They may also complain of diplopia due to displacement of the lateral canthal ligament of the eye, which is attached to the zygoma. There may be loss of sensation on the tip of the nose and the upper lip on the affected side due to impingement of the fracture site on the infraorbital nerve. Unilateral epistaxis is also seen due to the fracture crossing the antrum and thus tearing its mucoperiosteum and causing bleeding, which spills over through the ostium into the nose. In addition to these symptoms and signs, palpation over the fracture sites will reveal the characteristic steps in the bone.

X-ray examination shows the fractures at these three sites, opacification of the antrum due to blood, and an alteration of the contour of the lateral wall of the maxilla.

The majority of these are sufficiently displaced to warrant surgical intervention. Most can be managed by simple elevation, an elevator being passed down behind the zygomatic arch in the temporal area and the bone levered up into normal position. Although this measure is usually sufficient, some of these fractures may be unstable, and interosseous wiring may be required.

Blow-out fractures of the orbital floor also occur. The surrounding bone framework of the orbit itself need not be fractured, and the damage may be confined to the orbital floor. This occurs when a blow to the eyeball forces it backward, compressing the orbital fat so that it finally bursts out through the inferomedial part of the floor, which is its weakest part. Herniation of the orbital contents into the antrum may occur, producing enophthalmos. This constitutes a significant cosmetic deformity and may also produce diplopia. It is also possible for the extraocular muscles to become caught up on the bony margin of the blown-out segment, thereby becoming tethered and limiting upward gaze. The presence of these signs and symptoms should be sought in any player after a blow to the eye. Facial roentgenograms show antral opacity and air in the orbit suggesting the injury, but tomograms are necessary to delineate fully the damage. Surgical exploration is usually required. The defect in the floor may be repaired by replacing the fracture fragments with bone from the anterior wall of the antrum or with a sheet of silicone rubber. Obviously, a full ophthalmologic examination is mandatory in such cases. Sometimes the blow may cause only a small crack between the ethmoid sinus and the orbit. When the patient blows the nose, air is forced back up through this into the orbit, and the eyelids rapidly inflate with surgical emphysema, causing the patient considerable alarm. There is no specific treatment other than to refrain from blowing the nose for 2 weeks or so while the opening closes spontaneously. Antibiotic cover is prescribed. This phenomenon may sometimes be seen in fractures of the zygoma, particularly if the patient has engaged in vigorous nose blowing.

Players with a fractured zygoma or orbit should not engage in contact sports for at least 3 weeks, and then should wear a protective face mask to avoid further injury for at least another 3 weeks.

The Maxilla

Fractures of the maxilla are classically divided into three types:

1. *LeFort Type I.* This extends horizontally across the maxilla at the level of the floor of the nose, thereby shearing off the hard palate and upper dental alveolus.
2. *LeFort Type II.* Also called a pyramidal fracture, this extends obliquely upward and medially through the body of the maxilla toward the apex of the nose on both sides, thereby fracturing out a pyramid-shaped section of bone.
3. *LeFort Type III.* Also called a craniofacial separation. This describes the injury in that the fracture extends from one frontozygomatic suture line across the craniofacial junction to the other side. This shears the facial bones completely away from the cranium. It is usually due to a blow from straight ahead, and the wedge-shaped face is driven posteriorly and downward along the inclined plane of the base of the skull, producing a dish-face deformity or an "equine facies."

Combinations of these types may occur, e.g., LeFort II on one side and III on the other or bilateral II and III. The deformities may be evident on inspection, and palpation of the bones reveals the fracture sites. In most cases mobility may be demonstrated in the fractured segment. X-ray examination confirms the clinical findings.

These are very serious injuries, particularly the craniofacial separation, and require reduction and appropriate interosseous wiring and suspension of the fracture fragments. A tracheotomy is frequently necessary at the time of surgery. The wiring is usually maintained for at least 6 weeks. It may be many months before any consideration can be given to a return to sports following such an injury. Residual deformity is frequent despite adequate surgery. Loss of sense of smell is also common owing to tearing of the olfactory bulbs.

It is obviously possible to suffer an associated craniocerebral injury with fractures of the maxilla or, indeed, with any facial injury. One extremely important finding, which should be sought at the time of the original examination, is the presence of cerebrospinal fluid rhinorrhea, indicating a fracture in the area of the cribriform plate of the ethmoid and tearing of the dura mater. Neurosurgical consultation should be sought in all patients with significant facial trauma whether or not they show signs of head injury.

The Mandible

Fractures of the mandible may be simple or compound. The latter is the rule, since most of them occur through the tooth-bearing area, thus opening a free passage from the mouth down to the root level. They may be unilateral or bilateral, or may have multiple sites. They may also be classified anatomically, i.e., condylar neck, ascending ramus, angle, body, coronoid process, or parasymphyseal.

The diagnosis is usually straightforward. The patient may have actually heard or felt the bone fracturing at the time of the injury. There is usually significant pain. In the case of a compound fracture, bleeding may be noted in the mouth. The patient may complain of malocclusion, and crepitus and mobility may be noted at the fracture site. X-ray examination usually confirms the diagnosis. It is sometimes necessary to employ special x-ray techniques, such as the Panorex view, but this is not common.

Single undisplaced fractures of the condylar neck and the ascending ramus, or of the body in an edentulous patient, may warrant a trial period of conservative management employing only soft diet and avoidance of trauma without wiring of the teeth. This is sufficient if the patient is comfortable. The majority, and certainly all compound fractures, should be immobilized in some way. The simplest form of immobilization for single undisplaced fractures is the application of islet loops with cross-wiring to hold the teeth in occlusion. With instability or displacement, some form of arch is necessary to hold the fragments in place before the teeth are wired into occlusion. A cable arch made up of twisted 24-gauge wire (Risdon's method) or patent arches of the Erich or Winter type may be used. These latter have an added advantage in that elastic band traction may be employed with them and the cross-elastics or wires may be more readily removed for access to the mouth in an emergency. In fractures that are unstable or unfavorable in their angulation, an open reduction with interosseous wiring as well as interdental wiring is done. Patients with partial or full dentures should have them in place to maintain spacing and for stability during the period of immobilization.

The presence of fractures of the roots of teeth is significant, and a dental consultation may be sought to determine whether certain teeth are salvageable and to extract fractured roots. Fragments of teeth, fillings, and dentures should always be sought in the patient's mouth at the time of injury to prevent his swallowing or aspirating them. It is necessary to obtain a chest roentgenogram of a patient with a missing tooth, denture, or tooth fragment to rule out the possibility of its having been aspirated, particularly if he has been unconscious.

Fractures of the mandible may constitute a life-threatening injury under some circumstances, particularly in patients with bilateral, displaced, unstable fractures of the body. The patient, in effect, loses control of the tongue and may be unable to swallow properly. This, plus the presence of blood and saliva, and possibly vomitus in the mouth, may constitute a threat to the airway. Such patients should be cared for initially in the sitting position or, failing this, while prone with their face turned to one side to allow free drainage from the mouth. A tensor bandage around the face under the chin may temporarily hold the mandible immobilized in occlusion, thus affording considerable comfort to the patient and helping him to retain some control over the airway.

Compound fractures of the mandible rarely become infected nowadays, but this is indeed possible. All patients require appropriate antibiotic coverage.

Immobilization of most fractures is required for approximately 6 weeks. In simpler fractures in which an arch bar has been applied to the lower dentition, it may be possible to open the interdental fixation earlier and rely on the arch alone for stability.

Contact sports are out of the question during this 6-week period, and the patient should wear an appropriate face protector for at least a further 6 weeks to prevent another injury.

Maintenance of proper nutrition may be a problem with patients who have their teeth wired into occlusion, particularly those who do not have any gaps due to missing teeth through which solid food can be passed. Food reduced to the fine consistency of baby food by a food processor is required.

Dislocations of the Mandible

These may occur if the patient is struck while the mouth is open wide. They may also result from simply opening the mouth very widely in a shout or a yawn, as in nonsports practice.

To reduce a dislocated mandible, first be seated behind the patient, cradling his head against the chest. Place both *well-padded* thumbs just posterior to the last lower molars. Then, exert downward and posterior traction with the thumbs, at the same time rolling the mandible upward and anteriorly so that the condyles slip back into position.

Some persons have very lax temporomandibular joints and suffer periodic dislocations. Reduction is usually easy in them.

It may be necessary to employ sedation for sufficient relaxation to carry out the reduction in some patients, particularly if they are having a considerable amount of pain or are very apprehensive.

After-care should include resting the mandible and avoidance of maneuvers that might lead to another dislocation.

This has been a brief summary of facial injuries in sports. Many aspects could not be covered because of space limitations. The interested reader is referred to the standard texts for further information.

SUGGESTED READING

Converse JM. Reconstructive plastic surgery. Philadelphia: WB Saunders, 1977.
Schultz RC. Facial injuries. 3rd ed. Chicago: Year Book Medical Publishers, 1988.
Schultz RC, deCamara DB. Athletic facial injuries. JAMA 1984; 252:3395–3398.

EAR, NOSE, AND THROAT INJURIES

J. SIMON McGRAIL, M.D., M.S., F.R.C.S.(C)

The head and neck areas of the body are vulnerable to injury in sports that involve bodily contact. This contact can be with an opponent's head, fist, or other parts of his anatomy, or with a foreign object held by the opponent, such as a hockey stick.

Like injuries from any cause, these can be classified into soft tissue injuries with or without involvement of the underlying bone or cartilage. Soft tissue injuries include injuries to skin, subcutaneous tissue, muscles, nerves, and blood vessels. Each of these must be considered when an injury is being evaluated.

THE NECK

Injuries to the neck are usually blunt injuries and do not involve laceration of the skin and underlying soft tissues. By far the most important structure in the neck to consider is the airway. The larynx can be injured by blunt trauma, e.g., a cross-check from a hockey stick or a karate chop.

In this type of injury the head is usually extended, bringing the larynx closer to the surface where it is much more vulnerable to the assault. Immediately the player complains of discomfort in the neck, but more important, there can be different degrees of airway obstruction. If there is immediate hemoptysis a mucosal tear is present, and with this combination of events the player must be immediately removed from the scene of activity and carefully and thoroughly assessed.

The first consideration is the adequacy of the airway. If his breathing is noisy but he can inflate his chest well, there is time to get this player to a hospital where he can be properly examined. If his breathing is such that he has gross airway obstruction, indicating a badly smashed larynx, an airway has to be secured. Fortunately, most laryngeal fractures involve the thyroid cartilage, and placing an airway into the cricothyroid membrane alleviates most of the obstruction. A hypodermic needle placed in the cricothyroid membrane can act as a very adequate first aid measure until the player can be moved to a hospital. Alternatively, in the past I have employed a stab incision over the cricothyroid membrane and inserted the outer casing of a ballpoint pen, which gives a very adequate airway. Any time a cricothyrotomy is carried out, a tracheostomy must be done later in an orderly manner, but there is no urgency in this, provided that the revision is done within 24 hours. However, in the case of a badly smashed larynx, a tracheostomy almost certainly would be necessary anyway to assist in the rebuilding process.

An alternative cricothyrotomy instrument is the Fisher tube, which is part of a standard intravenous set.

The majority of sports injuries to the neck fall short of this dire emergency, but certainly can be worrisome to the attending physician or trainer. Any player who has received a neck injury and has any degree of airway problem should be sent as soon as possible to the nearest hospital where indirect laryngoscopy can be carried out. The usual finding in such a case is some degree of laryngeal edema, with or without submucosal hemorrhage, the degree of edema being reflected in the amount of airway obstruction present. As the edema is likely to progress for up to 12 to 24 hours, these players should be kept under close observation in a hospital setting until the airway has returned to normal.

Most such injuries do not require surgical intervention. They subside with rest, steam, and reassurance. I do not advocate sedatives in these cases because of their respiratory depressant action, and I find that most players respond well to a full explanation of this, together with the reassurance already mentioned. Most patients need a 3- to 4-day stay in the hospital. As soon as the larynx has returned to normal, the player can resume full normal activities.

If a mucosal tear is suspected because of hemoptysis, nothing further need be done unless the tear can be seen. If it can be visualized on indirect laryngoscopy, the larynx should be carefully assessed under general anesthesia, because a compound fracture of this nature may require an open reduction.

Finally, I would not recommend intubation of a suspected laryngeal fracture until the extent of the injuries can be assessed fully. It is better to establish an airway below the area of fracture, and then assess the degree of damage. Intubation may be difficult because of edema, and also may cause further damage and displacement of laryngeal fragments. If available, Heliox is always useful in the treatment of airway obstruction, but the vast majority of such injuries subside without heroic measures, particularly if a calm reassuring attitude can be maintained.

Sharp injuries (e.g., from a skate blade) can cause significant lacerations to the neck and, if deep enough, can cut the sternocleidomastoid muscle and the underlying jugular vein. Fortunately this type of injury is relatively uncommon, but it is a very dramatic one when it does occur. In one case a jugular vein was cut during a hockey game, and the player's life was saved by the quick action of the trainer, who was able to exert pressure on both sides of the laceration and occlude the jugular vein until this could be surgically repaired.

A more common injury is the superficial laceration, which usually can be primarily sutured. As with all lacerations, care should be taken to clean the wound to ensure that no foreign particles have been left behind.

Lacerations around the upper neck, the ear, and the face may damage the facial nerve. In the immediate evaluation of the injury, it is sufficient to document whether facial nerve function has been affected. If the player is asked to close the eyes tight, wrinkle the forehead, screw up the nose, smile, and whistle, any facial asymmetry should be recognized during these maneuvers. If there is injury to the facial nerve, this should be mentioned so that appropriate exploration and nerve repair can be carried out within a few hours of the injury.

THE MOUTH

Injuries to the mouth include those of the lips, teeth, and tongue.

Injuries to the lip follow the principles that Dr. Douglas outlined in the preceding chapter (*Facial Injuries*), and it is worth noting that most mucosal injuries heal spontaneously, often with minimal morbidity. If a laceration includes skin and mucosa, this must be carefully sutured, preferably in a hospital setting.

Trainers of sports teams are usually taught good first aid procedures, and for a lip laceration the most important measure is to squeeze it tightly on either side of the laceration to cut down on what is often very free bleeding. Having the patient suck an ice cube and placing this next to the laceration also helps. Similar principles apply to lacerations of the tongue, which are not uncommon hockey injuries. They usually occur in a player who, while skating hard with mouth open and tongue out, receives a blow under the jaw to cause a self-inflicted bite injury to the tongue.

These bleed freely, but firm pressure on either side of the cut controls the bleeding until hemostasis can be secured and the tongue sutured. Because of the possible edema that can result from this type of injury, it should be treated in a hospital setting and the player kept under observation for 24 hours to ensure that there is no airway problem.

THE EAR

Injuries to the ear are relatively uncommon, occurring most often in wrestlers. We are all familiar with the classic cauliflower ear of the wrestler and boxer, and this should be an entirely preventable result of injury. It follows from a subperichondrial hematoma that is not treated and finally absorbs the underlying cartilage, resulting in a grotesque abnormality. If a hematoma is recognized in the auricle, the correct treatment is immediate incision. The hematoma is drained, and to prevent its recurrence careful localized packing is placed in the different nooks and crannies of the auricle, and a firm pressure bandage applied over the ear and head. This should be inspected daily until it is clear that the hematoma is not forming again. If this treatment is carried out expeditiously, the ear will suffer no anatomic damage. The patient should be given antibiotics because the danger of perichondritis is high, and this in itself can cause severe deformities.

THE NOSE

Lacerations to the nose are discussed by Dr. Douglas in the chapter *Facial Injuries*. I mention them here only to reinforce the view that a laceration to the nose that involves a through-and-through injury with underlying mucosal damage must be treated in a hospital setting. Treatment consists of careful intranasal mucosal approximation by suturing, followed by suturing of the skin laceration. If this type of injury is neglected, adhesions within the nose can cause significant nasal obstruction in the future.

Perhaps the most important injury of the nose is that affecting the nasal septum. Careful evaluation is necessary to see whether a septal hematoma is forming. If a bulge in the septum is noticed, particularly bilaterally, this must be drained immediately. This is done by a sharp incision through the nasal septal mucosa and suctioning out the blood that is present. Through this incision a small wick is inserted, and the nose is packed fairly firmly to hold the septal mucosa together and prevent recurrence of the hematoma. If a hematoma is overlooked or neglected, a septal abscess is likely to develop, causing loss of bone and cartilage in the nose and leaving a nose that is difficult to correct from both a cosmetic and a functional point of view. Antibiotics should be given when a septal hematoma is diagnosed, in an effort to prevent infection.

Although nasal fractures will be discussed, I will describe here the first aid treatment of the nosebleeds that so frequently accompany nasal fractures.

After any injury to the nose with epistaxis, the player is instructed to sit forward with head down and to gently blow one nostril at a time. This measure is expected to remove clots, allow the vessels to contract and retract, and stop the nosebleed. The nose is then gently pinched, if this is possible (i.e., if there is no associated fracture), and the nosebleed stops quickly, in which case the player can probably resume activity. If there is an associated fracture that prevents pressure from being applied, ice is applied to the back of the neck in the hope of causing a reflex vasoconstriction, and a small amount of packing into both sides of the nose usually helps. When there is an associated fracture, the player is sent to the hospital where a reduction of the fracture can be performed, either within 24 hours or within the next 7 to 10 days, depending on the degree of edema and bruising.

Although most nosebleeds are caused from septal blood vessels, a significant nosebleed can be caused by injury to the anterior ethmoidal artery. This is seen with a blunt injury to the root of the nose and the medial canthal area of the eye, as from a fist or hockey puck. This can result in a brisk hemorrhage, which needs careful and thorough packing in the roof of the nose to control it. This type of bleeding tends to persist even after adequate packing, and it is not unusual to explore the ethmoid sinuses through an external incision and clip the anterior ethmoidal vessel.

I SHOULDER

IMPINGEMENT SYNDROME

EDWARD P. FINK, M.D.
R. PETER WELSH, M.B., Ch.B., F.R.C.S.(C), F.A.C.S.

The shoulder is a loosely constrained joint that is subject to considerable functional demand in sports. Its peculiar anatomy and the complex motions made by athletes make it susceptible to chronic overuse injuries, in particular the shoulder impingement syndrome. This latter is the most common shoulder condition affecting participants in athletic endeavors at all levels. The magnitude of the problem is attested to by the fact that 30 to 60 percent of competitive swimmers and 25 percent of baseball pitchers incur this malady at some point during their careers. The significance of the shoulder impingement syndrome is that if it is allowed to progress to a point at which surgical intervention is required, very few athletes ever return to their preinjury level of competition. Recognition of the syndrome and early nonoperative intervention are essential to a successful resolution and the return of athletes to their accustomed level of performance.

ETIOLOGY

The architecture of the shoulder joint and the vascular supply to this area contribute to the pathogenesis of impingement.

While stability of the shoulder is conferred primarily by the enveloping soft tissues, the capsule, rotator cuff, and the biceps tendon, these structures and the overlying bursa must pass through a relatively unyielding space bounded by the acromion and coracoacromial ligament superiorly and the humeral head inferiorly. In activities in which the arm is elevated in forward flexion above the horizontal plane, the greater tuberosity compresses these soft tissue structures against the anteroinferior acromion and the coracoacromial ligament.

While forward shoulder flexion may predispose to mechanical impingement a tenuous blood supply predisposes to intrinsic degenerative soft tissue changes. Cadaver studies of the microcirculation to the rotator cuff have demonstrated a relatively avascular zone in the supraspinatus near its insertion on the greater tuberosity. In addition, the intracapsular portion of the biceps tendon as it passes over the humeral head near the supraspinatus insertion has a similar zone of decreased vascularity. This precarious vascular supply may predispose to early tendon attrition and degeneration.

The genesis of the impingement syndrome arises from these complementary features of mechanical impingement exerted upon areas of poor blood supply. With repetitive loading of the shoulder, the subacromial bursa becomes irritated, as well as the underlying supraspinatus tendon. Inflammation and thickening of the bursa may ensue, effectively increasing the volume of the soft tissues traversing the fixed subacromial space. Microtears originate in the relatively avascular areas, and partial or complete rotator cuff tears may result.

Although seemingly very different, baseball pitching, hitting an overhead serve in tennis, and several swimming strokes all demand similar shoulder motions that predispose to the impingement syndrome. During a cocking or backswing, the shoulder is extended, abducted, and externally rotated. In this manner the arm is positioned ready for the generation of a momentum force much like a catapult. With forceful contraction of the biceps, anterior deltoid, and subscapularis, the arm is then whipped overhead into forward flexion with varying degrees of internal rotation and adduction. It is during this acceleration phase and the subsequent pullthrough that shoulder impingement occurs.

In swimmers, free style, butterfly, and back strokes produce this overuse syndrome. Weight lifters may complain of pain while performing a military press maneuver but not while performing a bench press. The military press is performed overhead from a sitting position, reproducing the impingement arc, whereas no shoulder flexion above the horizontal plane occurs in the bench press. Gymnasts are also prone to this condition with repetitive work-outs on the parallel bars and rings.

CLINICAL PRESENTATION

The clinical presentation of the impingement syndrome is protean, ranging from mild shoulder discomfort with activities to severe pain even while at rest. Similarly, a spectrum of changes in the soft tissues is encountered, progressing from mild subacromial bursitis to rotator cuff tendinitis and degenerative tears. On the basis of these clinical and pathologic characteristics, three stages of impingement have been described. There may be some overlap between the stages, but their delineation helps to provide guidelines for treatment and long-term management.

Stage one is the most frequently encountered form of the chronic impingement syndrome, occurring in elite athletes as well as weekend tennis aficionados. A dull aching pain about the shoulder not associated with any weakness or restriction of shoulder motion is the most prominent feature. The pain usually develops insidiously after overhead shoulder motion and is usually perceived after the athletic endeavor. This stage corresponds to mild inflammatory subacromial bursitis and inflammatory foci in the rotator cuff and biceps tendons. These lesions are usually reversible if the activities that provoke them are curtailed.

Tenderness may be present over the greater tuberosity at the supraspinatus insertion or over the anterior acromion or biceps tendon. The most important confirmatory sign, however, is the impingement sign, a maneuver that reproduces the pain by compressing the greater tuberosity against the coracoacromial ligament and the anteroinferior acromion. This is performed by forward flexion of the arm with elevation above 90 degrees, and by internally rotating the forward-flexed arm.

Stage two impingement represents the irreversible pathologic changes resulting from repeated insults. The pain is quite similar to that experienced in the previous stage and now is felt during shoulder motion as well. This discomfort may compel the athlete to refrain from the inciting activity, and frequently the pain awakens the patient from sleep. Soft tissue changes consist of edema and thickening of the subacromial bursa with degeneration and fibrosis of the supraspinatus and biceps tendon.

In *stage three* there is a prolonged history of shoulder pain with restriction of active shoulder motion. These chronic changes may be severely disabling to the older individual. The pain is more constant and intense than in stage two, and active shoulder motion becomes restricted primarily because of pain, but sometimes because of muscle weakness from associated rotator cuff tears. Passive range of motion is usually full but often quite painful, and the impingement sign is usually elicited. Partial and complete tears of the rotator cuff may be seen, along with bicipital tendon ruptures.

RADIOGRAPHIC REVIEW

Radiographs are not used primarily to confirm the presence of the shoulder impingement syndrome, because clinical signs and symptoms are sufficiently diagnostic. Indeed, plain radiographs are often normal in stages one and two. Nonetheless, routine views of the shoulder (anteroposterior in internal and external rotation, and an axillary lateral view as well as a view of the acromioclavicular joint) should be obtained to delineate any coexisting pathologic condition.

In late stage two and stage three impingement, radiographs may show degenerative changes about the shoulder with subacromial bone proliferation. Studies have correlated certain acromial shapes with the impingement syndrome, although it is not clear whether the impingement produced these changes or whether the actual shape of the acromion predisposed to impingement. Cysts, flattening, and sclerosis of the greater tuberosity may be present, and degenerative changes in the acromioclavicular joint, including inferiorly oriented osteophytes, may be seen. Arthrograms are generally diagnostic of complete or incomplete rotator cuff tears, and should be obtained as a preoperative study in patients considered for surgery. Ultrasonography is a useful noninvasive tool for diagnosis of complete rotator cuff tears greater than 8 mm, but its sensitivity in diagnosing lesser tears has yet to be proved. Arthroscopy of the shoulder joint or subacromial bursa may also reveal rotator cuff tears.

DIAGNOSTIC CONFIRMATION

The history, physical examination, and provocative tests of impingement usually establish the diagnosis. To confirm the presence of early impingement syndrome, infiltration of 10 ml of 1 percent lidocaine into the subacromial bursa should alleviate the pain. Other entities should be considered if the diagnosis is unconfirmed.

Other Causes of Shoulder Pain

Cervical spine herniated discs at the C4–C5 level may refer pain to the shoulder area, producing pain similar to that of the impingement syndrome. Pain will not be influenced by shoulder positions, and herniated discs are often accompanied by pain with neck motion and other neurologic signs.

Acute traumatic bursitis may result from a direct blow to the shoulder or following a traumatic glenohumeral subluxation or dislocation. The history is of primary importance, and the symptoms should subside with time. A complete tear of the rotator cuff may occur with many types of shoulder trauma, and the competency of the rotator cuff must be aggressively ascertained in all cases.

Calcific tendinitis may occasionally be associated with chronic impingement syndrome. The etiology of this condition where calcium apatite is deposited predominantly in the infraspinatus tendon is obscure, but the rotator is invariably intact. Treatment may require surgical excision.

Acromioclavicular joint pathology may exist concomitantly with the impingement syndrome, but primary acromioclavicular joint degeneration usually occurs after injury. Often a history of a type II or III acromioclavicular separation is elicited, and tenderness occurs primarily over the acromioclavicular joint. The pain is reproduced with shoulder adduction and internal rotation, thereby compressing the diseased acromioclavicular joint. This may be misconstrued as a positive impingement sign.

Entrapment of the suprascapular nerve as it courses over the suprascapular notch can cause vague anterior shoulder pain. Weakness of abduction and external rotation is also present, and atrophy of the supraspinatus and infraspinatus muscles may be discerned in chronic cases. Impingement signs will be absent, and electromyographic changes will confirm this entity.

An isolated rupture of the long head of the biceps tendon without a preexisting pathologic condition is quite rare. Degeneration of the intracapsular portion of the biceps tendon occurs secondarily to chronic impingement, or perhaps as a result of abnormalities in the intertubercular groove or its overlying transverse ligament. Minor trauma to chronically inflamed rotator cuff and biceps tendon may cause tears in both structures. The rotator cuff tear is potentially more debilitating, and with any biceps tendon rupture its presence should be actively considered. Isolated rupture of the long head of the biceps tendon causes few functional disabilities.

Instabilities about the shoulder may become a diagnostic enigma. The common recurrent anterior dislocations usually present no diagnostic difficulties because there is usually a history of the injury and a positive apprehension test, and the range of motion of the shoulder is full and without pain. In other shoulder instabilities the history is often vague and the physical findings nonspecific. Anterior or posterior shoulder subluxation may present with pain only during a particular shoulder motion, associated with a click. Arthroscopy reveals a labral flap similar to a meniscal bucket handle tear, and resection of the flap is often curative.

MANAGEMENT

The treatment for the chronic impingement syndrome is similar to the management of other overuse syndromes. Most athletes and recreational sports enthusiasts present with stage one disease, and conservative treatment will return them to their accustomed level of activity.

A most important tenet of treatment is the avoidance of aggravating activities. For patients with mild to moderate discomfort, activities should be modified until pain subsides. This may necessitate rest or restricted activities. Modification of training techniques and practices may help prevent progression of the condition.

Nonsteroidal anti-inflammatory medications are often efficacious in reducing the inflammation in the bursa and rotator cuff. Since there are five different classes of anti-inflammatory medications based on their varying modalities of action, a change to a different drug category after a failed trial of one type may produce desired effects.

Various forms of physical therapy are used to produce localized effects in the soft tissue. Moist heat, ultrasonography, and diathermy stimulate blood flow to the affected areas and are useful before exercise. The vasoconstrictive effects of ice after exercise decrease edema and hemorrhage.

The injection of steroids into the subacromial space may be beneficial, but the negative effects of these agents should be well recognized. Collagen necrosis and weakening of the tendon may be precipitated if the injection is intratendinous instead of intrabursal. In our shoulder clinic, if conservative management of a person has failed for approximately 4 to 6 months, a corticosteroid injection is offered. If there is a rapid but transient relief of pain, a second injection may be tried 6 weeks later. No response to the first injection or minimal response to the second constitutes a failure of conservative management. Multiple injections should not be undertaken due to cumulative attritional effects on soft tissues.

EXERCISE PROGRAM

With the subsidence of pain, a well-structured exercise program should be implemented to aid rehabilitation and prevent further injury. Stretching exercises should be performed to regain flexibility in musculotendinous units, which may be contracted owing to chronic tendinitis and limited motion due to pain. Strengthening the muscles around the shoulder should emphasize supraspinatus function. The supraspinatus acts as a depressor of the shoulder and plays a pivotal role in rotational control. If the supraspinatus is weak and the deltoid strong, overpowering of the supraspinatus results in impingement. The supraspinatus can be specifically strengthened with a relatively simple exercise, lifting light weights in forward elevation at 30 degrees, that is in the plane of the scapula. By stopping at 90 degrees before the impingement zone is infringed, further aggravation of the inflamed bursa and tendon is avoided.

SURGERY

Surgical intervention for the chronic impingement syndrome is indicated only for refractory cases that do not respond to prolonged conservative management. Surgery is unnecessary in stage one impingement since the pathology is reversible and usually responds to nonoperative treatment. Patients with stage two impingement unrelieved by conservative treatment usually benefit from surgical decompression. However, surgery is no panacea. As noted earlier, a return to full competitive activity at preinjury level is unusual after surgical intervention. Operative treatment is recommended only for athletes who simply cannot continue participation in their activity, having exhausted other forms of therapy. The structures responsible for the impingement, the anteroinferior acromion and the coracoacromial ligament, are resected. Some surgeons advocate simple resection of the coracoacromial ligament, leaving the acromion intact, but this may provide inadequate decompression in those who really need such an undertaking, and recurrence is also possible. Of paramount importance in any surgery around the shoulder is preservation of the deltoid. The deltoid origin is carefully reflected off the acromion as an intact sleeve and repaired simply side to side after the partial acromial resection. There is no place for more radical acromial resection.

As in stage 2, surgical intervention in stage 3 is indicated for chronic pain and inability to continue in athletic participation. However, resection of the anteroinferior acromion and the coracoacromial ligament may need to be supplemented by debridement and partial resection of the acromioclavicular joint. The underlying rotator cuff may show a chronic tear, and debridement of the tear and repair can also be undertaken without extending the exposure. It is very important in the athlete to preserve the integrity of the deltoid.

The postoperative rehabilitation should not be hastened. Early passive mobilization and active assisted exercises are initiated the day after surgery and continued by the patient upon discharge from the hospital. Resisted strengthening exercises should be deferred for 6 weeks, and the temptation to return to sport too soon must be strongly discouraged. Full range of motion, strength, and stamina must first be restored.

Arthroscopic subacromial decompression now offers the possibility of a less radical intervention and a speedier recovery. The same principles apply, however; full function must be regained before competitive activity is undertaken.

SUGGESTED READING

Bigliani LV, Morrison DS, Arpil EW. The morphology of the acromion and its relationship to rotator cuff tears. Orthop Trans 1986; 10, 2:228.

Neer CS, Welsh RP. The shoulder in sports. Orthop Clin North Am 1977; 8:583.

Rathburn JB, Macnab I. The microvascular pattern of the rotator cuff. J Bone Joint Surg 1970; 52B:540.

Tibone JE, Jobe FW, Keslin RK, et al. Shoulder impingement syndrome in athletes treated by anterior acromioplasty. Clin Orthop 1985; 198:134–140.

PRINCIPLES OF SHOULDER ARTHROSCOPY

JAMES R. ANDREWS, M.D.
SCOTT P. SCHEMMEL, M.D.

Advances in equipment, techniques, and individual expertise have resulted in expanded use of arthroscopy in the diagnosis and treatment of intra-articular pathologic conditions.

Initially, the use of arthroscopy at the shoulder was limited to glenohumeral joint evaluation and simple interventional techniques. Currently, however, more complex and more technically demanding surgical procedures are applied to glenohumeral joint disorders. For example, evaluation and treatment of subacromial space and acromioclavicular joint pathology are now possible. These advances have greatly expanded the indications for and use of arthroscopy for the shoulder and have necessitated a redefinition of the term "shoulder arthroscopy."

Arthroscopic evaluation of the shoulder is not complete until the glenohumeral joint and the subacromial space have been inspected. When indicated, the acromioclavicular joint should be evaluated either via the subacromial space or by direct entrance into the joint from above.

The purpose of this chapter is to discuss the principles of shoulder arthroscopy, as employed in the evaluation of glenohumeral, subacromial, and acromioclavicular pathology. Treatment of the various other pathologic entities encountered is discussed elsewhere in this volume.

GLENOHUMERAL JOINT ARTHROSCOPY

Arthroscopic investigation of any joint is an equipment-intense endeavor that must be carried out in a systematic and reproducible manner with minimal variation, while still allowing for adaptive maneuvers when necessary. Before the procedure is begun, the following equipment should be available: one 30-degree and one 70-degree 4.0-mm arthroscope, an 18- or 20-gauge spinal needle, an interchangeable interlocking 4.5- and 5.5-mm cannula system without "side ports," a full-radius synovial resector, a meniscal resector, a burr, and a fluid pump or 3-liter bags of normal saline for joint distention.

Surgical Technique

With the patient under anesthesia, an examination is made to determine shoulder instability and document range of motion. The patient is placed in the lateral decubitus position with the torso supported by a vacuum bean bag. The arm is suspended in a prefabricated wrist gauntlet or a soft wrap secured by Velcro straps. We prefer the arm to be suspended at 70 degrees of abduction and 15 degrees of forward flexion by means of a rope and pulley system attached to the surgical table. Approximately 15 (never more than 20) pounds are necessary for adequate distraction and subsequent visualization. It is important to ensure that the patient's torso does not drift anteriorly as the procedure is carried out, because this would make the procedure technically more difficult and might cause the arm to become extended. The extended arm position should always be avoided, since it results in traction being applied to the brachial plexus. Once adequately and securely positioned, the patient's exposed arm and shoulder region is prepared and draped, and the wrist gauntlet is covered with a sterile towel and a plastic drape.

The surgeon is positioned behind the patient with the surgical technician and necessary equipment toward the patient's feet. Optimally, the video monitor should be placed immediately anterior to the patient and directly across from the surgeon.

Bone landmarks about the shoulder are palpated and outlined with a surgical marking pen. These landmarks include (1) the anterolateral and posterolateral borders of the acromion, (2) the acromioclavicular joint, and (3) the coracoid process. They serve to orient the surgeon in establishing initial portals and additional portals as needed during the procedure. Without such markings, extravasation of fluid can make the later points of entry difficult to identify.

Diagnostic arthroscopy is begun through a posterior portal approximately 2.5 to 3 cm distal and slightly medial to the posterolateral tip of the acromion. This area should correspond to the interval between the infraspinatus and teres minor muscles, which is a palpable "soft spot." An 18-gauge spinal needle is inserted through this soft spot and is directed anteriorly toward the coracoid process. A common error is to direct the needle too horizontally, thus entering into the subacromial space rather than the glenohumeral joint itself. Ten to 15 ml of saline solution is injected into the joint, and free backflow confirms proper needle placement. A total of 40 to 50 ml of saline is then injected into the joint, and the needle is removed. A small skin incision is made at the point of needle entry, and a sharp 4.5-mm trocar and sleeve are inserted, following the same path as the needle. Once the subcutaneous tissues and muscle interval are penetrated, a blunt trocar replaces the sharp one, and the posterior glenoid rim and humeral head are palpated through the capsule with the trocar. The glenohumeral interval is thus identified, and with anterior pressure the trocar penetrates the joint capsule. It is important to "step off" the posterior glenoid rim and to enter the joint as close to the posterior rim as possible, thus avoiding penetration of the infraspinatus tendinous contribution to the rotator cuff. The arthroscope is introduced through the posterior sheath, and inflow is provided through the scope.

It is possible to inspect the joint through a one-portal technique, but distention is limited and thus can hinder thorough examination. Therefore, we prefer to establish an anterior portal for inflow to aid in diagnosis and surgery, inserting an 18-gauge spinal needle into the glenohumeral joint from a point midway between the coracoid process and the anterolateral tip of the acromion. The needle should penetrate the anterior capsule just inferior to the long head of the biceps. Once correct placement of the needle is confirmed by direct arthroscopic visualization, the needle is removed, and a 4.5-mm trocar and sleeve are directed into the joint. A 5-mm skin incision is made at the needle entry point, and the sharp trocar is advanced to the joint, following the same path as the needle. The joint capsule is penetrated, after the sharp trocar is replaced with a blunt one. Once the anterior portal is established, inflow is transferred to this cannula. An infusion pump (or 2- to 3-liter normal saline fluid bags elevated on intravenous poles) will maintain joint distention throughout the procedure. Suction can be placed on the arthroscope to enhance flow or to remove debris.

If intra-articular pathology requires the use of motorized instrumentation, a second anterior portal can be established, optimally placed immediately adjacent to the first anterior portal. We prefer to avoid the use of the supraclavicular portal in whose activities include throwing athletes. This portal, which is established at the junction of the lateral clavicle and scapular spine, penetrates the supraspinatus near its musculotendinous portion. Although it may be quite functional and harmless in many cases, this portal should be avoided in the throwing athlete, because any insult to the supraspinatus structure may already be a source of a pathologic condition.

Arthroscopic Anatomy of Glenohumeral Joint

Arthroscopic evaluation should be conducted in a systematic fashion, identifying and inspecting all structures regardless of the preoperative diagnosis. The biceps tendon is the first structure identified. With the patient positioned as previously described, this structure is orientated approximately 15 degrees away from an imaginary vertical line. The tendon should be visualized from the bicipital groove anteriorly to its insertion into the supraglenoid tubercle at the superoposterior aspect of the glenoid where it is continuous with the glenoid labrum.

Next, the glenoid labrum is inspected. The "12 o'clock" position on the glenoid that corresponds to the biceps tendon labrum continuum is identified. From here the labrum is followed anteriorly; with momentarily increased traction of the arm, the anteroinferior labrum can be seen. With slight retraction of the arthroscope the posterior labrum can be followed inferiorly to superiorly back to the "12 o'clock" position.

The humeral head and glenoid articulation are visualized next. By internally and externally rotating the humerus, the entire articular surface of the humeral head can be inspected. The smaller, pear-shaped glenoid can be seen clearly at this point.

The glenohumeral ligaments, consisting of superior, middle, and inferior structures, are next scrutinized. These ligaments may have capsular origins or sometimes arise distinctly from the labrum itself.

The superior glenohumeral ligament is sometimes hidden behind the biceps tendon and not well seen. However, when identified, it courses from the anatomic neck of the humerus up to the superoanterior glenoid and also sends an attachment to the coracoid process. Although the middle glenohumeral ligament is broad, its middle portion is that which is most identifiable arthroscopically. This portion of the ligament can be seen arising just posterior to the subscapularis tendon and sweeping posteriorly to insert into the anterior border of the glenoid at its middle and inferior third. Occasionally, the middle glenohumeral ligament fuses with the subscapularis tendon. The inferior glenohumeral ligament arises from the inferior aspect of the surgical neck of the humerus and sweeps back to insert into the anteroinferior glenoid.

Subscapularis Tendon and Recess

With the patient's arm in the 70-degree abducted position, the subscapularis tendon can be seen in the anterior aspect of the glenohumeral joint. Arthroscopically, the posterosuperior edge of the subscapularis tendon is visualized. This structure is usually well defined and easily identifiable. However, in some shoulders this tendon may be obscured or may appear to blend with the middle glenohumeral ligament. The subscapularis recess can be found also in the anterior aspect of the shoulder, usually superior but occasionally inferior to the middle glenohumeral ligament.

Rotator Cuff

Examination of the rotator cuff begins by returning to the biceps tendon landmark. The supraspinatus tendon can be seen directly superior to the biceps tendon. The tendinous fibers of the rotator cuff structures can be seen to insert along the articular margin of the humeral head. After visualization of the supraspinatus contribution to the rotator cuff, the arthroscope is retracted slightly and is swept down along the posterior margin of the glenoid. With the arthroscope lens rotated superiorly, the infraspinatus and the teres minor contributions to the rotator cuff can be visualized. It is important to observe these more posterior contributions to the cuff closely for any signs of fraying or obvious tearing.

Superior Recess

The superior recess is located superior and slightly anterior to the superior aspect of the glenoid and to the insertion of the biceps tendon. This recess should be routinely examined for any abnormalities, specifically loose bodies.

Once this systematic evaluation of the glenohumeral joint has been completed from the posterior portal, the arthroscope should be placed through the anterior portal, and the inflow then placed posteriorly. This allows for further evaluation of any previously identified pathology and may reveal abnormalities not noted through the posterior portal. This is particularly important in regard to the posterior rotator cuff structures.

Subacromial Space

Subacromial space pathology can occur either in conjunction with glenohumeral joint pathology or independent of it. Evaluation of the subacromial space as part of a general arthroscopic shoulder examination helps to ensure that concomitant subacromial space pathology is identified and appropriately treated, and that it does not later have a less than satisfactory result when more obvious glenohumeral joint pathology has been corrected. Subacromial pathology, as in the spectrum of the impingement syndrome, should be recognized and treated.

Surgical Technique

After completion of the glenohumeral joint evaluation and treatment, the inflow and arthroscope are redirected into the subacromial space. The previously established anterior skin portal is used to introduce a redirected 5.5-mm cannula. The cannula and blunt trocar are advanced to the anterolateral aspect of the acromion, which is then palpated with the tip of the trocar. The trocar and cannula are advanced through the coracoacromial ligament into the subacromial space directly beneath the undersurface of the acromion. Ideal placement of this cannula is through the coracoacromial ligament itself. Placement of the trocar and cannula medial to the coracoacromial ligament inhibits inflow and limits visualization, making diagnosis and any operative procedure difficult. Once the cannula is seated beneath the acromion, the blunt trocar is removed and inflow is established. Next, a 4.5-mm cannula with a blunt trocar is introduced through the posterior skin portal and redirected toward the posterolateral aspect of the acromion. The posterolateral tip of the acromion is palpated with the trocar, and the trocar is advanced into the subacromial space. The blunt trocar is left within the cannula, and the entire 4.5-mm trocar and cannula are invaginated into the 5.5-mm cannula. This step ensures that both the inflow cannula and the arthroscopy cannula are within the same plane in the subacromial space and not separated by bursal tissue planes. Such separation by soft tissue makes flow within the subacromial space difficult and hinders any further attempts at visualization or instrumentation. The trocar is removed from the 4.5-mm cannula, and the arthroscope is introduced through the sheath. The anterior cannula is then slowly retracted anteriorly until the arthroscope is freed from the 5.5-mm sheath. The inflow portal is then immediately assessed to determine adequate placement through the coracoacromial ligament; once this is confirmed, diagnostic arthroscopy of the subacromial space can continue.

Quite often, especially when bursitis and tendinitis associated with the impingement syndrome are present, visualization of the rotator cuff and the undersurface of the acromion is difficult initially. The bursal tissue may need to be removed with a full-radius synovial resector, which is introduced through a lateral portal. This portal is established through triangulation after introduction of an 18-gauge spinal needle approximately 2 to 3 cm directly lateral from the acromion. This needle passes through the muscle and fascia of the deltoid and into the subacromial space. Once the needle is visualized, a 6-mm skin incision is made at the point of its insertion, and a 5.5-mm blunt trocar and sheath are introduced into the subacromial space. The trocar is removed and, with a full-radius synovial resector, the subacromial bursa is removed and adequate visualization of the important structures is possible.

It is important that continuous flow through the subacromial space be established and subsequently maintained throughout the course of the diagnostic or operative procedure. Because bleeding may be encountered with instrumentation of this space, particularly around the acromioclavicular joint, 1 ml of a 1:1,000 epinephrine solution is added to each 3-liter bag of fluid.

The normal subacromial space is usually well defined, with a thin layer of bursal tissue overlying the rotator cuff tendons. If the bursal tissue is hypertrophic or shows evidence of abrasions, it will be necessary to resect it carefully with a synovial resector from the underlying tendons so that they can be fully inspected for partial-thickness tears or abrasions. By internally and externally rotating the arm, a significant portion of the rotator cuff—particularly the supraspinatus and infraspinatus—can be visualized clearly. The undersurface of the acromion is covered with a relatively thick and continuous layer of fibrous tissue, which should be smooth in appearance. By palpation with a blunt instrument, the anatomic borders of the acromion can be established laterally, anteriorly, and posteriorly. An 18-gauge spinal needle passed through the acromioclavicular joint from above serves to identify the medial border of the acromion. Any fraying of the fibrous tissue on the undersurface of the acromion, particularly when this is combined with inflammation, erythema, or hypertrophy of the subacromial bursa or underlying rotator cuff, indicates an impingement phenomenon. By abducting the arm under direct visualization, an area of fraying on the undersurface of the acromion often corresponds with an area of erythema on the rotator cuff, as these two surfaces are approximated. By removing the soft tissue about the acromioclavicular joint, the undersurface of the clavicle can be identified. The clavicle, which serves as an important landmark in the procedure of subacromial decompression, should be explored to rule out the existence of spurs from the inferior surface of the distal clavicle. The coracoacromial ligament is easily identified, particularly if the anterior cannula was placed appropriately as it pierces directly through this white ligamentous structure. The coracoacromial ligament itself may be frayed, but only rarely are changes within the substance of the ligament indicative of any specific pathologic condition. It is not within the realm of this chapter to discuss fully the technique of subacromial decompression, although by using the lateral portal, a full-radius synovial resector, and a large high-speed burr, it is possible to carry out this procedure systematically and reproducibly.

The acromioclavicular joint can be evaluated through the subacromial space. If necessary, acromioclavicular joint decompression with removal of the joint meniscus and resection of the distal clavicle can be completed. When the acromioclavicular joint is identified preoperatively as the source of the patient's complaints and when no glenohumeral or subacromial pathology is otherwise identified at the time of arthroscopy, we prefer to perform direct acromioclavicular joint debridement and distal clavicle resection. For this we use an arthroscopic technique that involves introduction of the arthroscope and necessary equipment directly into the acromioclavicular joint from above.

The acromioclavicular joint is identified by direct palpation, and two 18-gauge spinal needles are introduced into the joint, one at the most anterior and the other at the most posterior aspect of this interval. Saline is injected through the posterior spinal needle with a 40-ml syringe, and flow through the joint is confirmed by the presence of saline from the anterior spinal needle. At the beginning of this procedure, a third spinal needle should also be introduced directly through the center of the acromioclavicular joint. Outflow should be confirmed through this third spinal needle as fluid is injected through the posterior spinal needle. Once all three needles are determined to be within the acromioclavicular joint, the posterior spinal needle is removed. A small skin incision is made, and a 4.5-mm cannula and trocar (or in a tight joint, a 2.7-mm cannula and trocar) are introduced. An arthroscope of the appropriate size is placed into the joint, and the central and anterior spinal needles are identified. Flow is then established through both the arthroscope and the central spinal needle, and instrumentation is brought in anteriorly once the anterior spinal needle has been removed and a 2.7-mm or 4.5-mm cannula and trocar have been placed. When there is adequate visualization and instrumentation within the joint, debridement of the acromioclavicular joint meniscus and distal clavicular resection, using full-radius synovial resectors and high-speed burrs, can be accomplished. Care must be taken to avoid directing the instrumentation too far inferiorly, thus entering the subacromial space and inadvertently injuring the underlying rotator cuff structures.

SUGGESTED READING

Andrews JR, Carson WG. Arthroscopic anatomy of the shoulder. In: McGinty JB, ed. Shoulder surgery in the athlete: techniques in orthopaedics. Rockville, MD: Aspen Systems Corp, 1985:25.

Andrews JR, Carson WG. Arthroscopy of the shoulder. Orthopedics 1983; 6:1157.

Andrews JR, Carson WG, Ortega K. Arthroscopy of the shoulder: technique and normal anatomy. Am J Sports Med 1984; 12:1.

Caspari RB. Anatomy and portals for arthroscopic surgery of the shoulder. In: Jackson DW, ed. Shoulder surgery in the athlete: techniques in orthopaedics. Rockville, Md: Aspen Systems Corp, 1985:15.

Caspari RB. Shoulder arthroscopy: a review of the present state of the art. Contemp Orthop 1982; 4:523.

Johnson LL. Shoulder arthroscopy. In: Arthroscopic surgery. St. Louis: CV Mosby, 1986.

Lombardo SJ. Arthroscopy of the shoulder. Clin Sports Med 1983; 2:209.

Matthews LS, Terry HL, Vetter WL. Shoulder anatomy for the arthroscopist. Arthroscopy 1985; 1:83.

Matthews LS, Vetter WL, Helfet DL. Arthroscopic surgery of the shoulder. Adv Orthop Surg 1984; 8:203.

Matthews LS, Zarins B, Michael RH. Anterior portal selection for shoulder arthroscopy. Arthroscopy 1985; 1:33.

McGlynn FF, Caspari RB. Arthroscopic findings in the subluxating shoulder. Clin Orthop 1984; 183:173.

ARTHROSCOPIC SUBACROMIAL DECOMPRESSION

HARVARD ELLMAN, M.D.

A method of performing arthroscopic subacromial decompression (anterior acromioplasty) using arthroscopic surgical techniques is described here. The operative goal is to (1) release the coracoacromial ligament, (2) resect the anterior undersurface of the acromion, and (3) when indicated, debride the bursa or cuff and relieve calcareous deposits with a needle technique.

INDICATIONS

The procedure is indicated for

1. Stage II impingement syndrome unresponsive to conservative treatment for at least 6 to 12 months.
2. Selected irreparable rotator cuff tears with intractable pain.
3. Superficial calcareous deposits with chronic impingement.

It is not recommended as a substitute for open repair of routine full-thickness rotator cuff tears.

EQUIPMENT

The procedure involves the use of basic arthroscopic instruments that are readily available, including the following:

Thirty-degree arthroscope.
Powered shaver system.
Synovial resector shaver blade.
Meniscal trimmer shaver blade.
Large arthroplasty burr.
Small open bone curette.
Electrosurgical generator.
Hook electrode for subcutaneous lateral release.
Plastic cannula with diaphragm.

The patient is placed in a lateral recumbent position, and after routine preparation and draping, the extremity is maintained in 15 to 20 pounds of "sky-hook" traction with the arm abducted about 20 degrees. The bone landmarks of the acromion, acromioclavicular joint, and coracoid are outlined (Fig. 1).

The course of the coracoacromial ligament is indicated traveling from the coracoid to insert on the anterior edge of the undersurface of the acromion. The arm should be placed in traction before these landmarks are outlined. The posterior angle of the acromion is identified and two portals are marked. First, the arthroscopic portal (*a*) is marked 1 cm below and 1 cm anterior to the posterior angle of the acromion. A second portal for an accessory fluid ingress cannula (*b*) is marked 1 cm inferior and medial to the posterior angle. Portals are infiltrated with a few milliliters of 0.25 percent bupivacaine with epinephrine, and the subacromial space is distended with 20 ml of normal saline.

Orientation pins are next placed to outline the acromial attachment of the coracoacromial ligament; 18-gauge lumbar puncture needles are used with the stylet left in position. The medial needle is introduced just anterior to the acromioclavicular joint. The more lateral needle is located at the anterolateral angle of the acromion. The arthroscope is introduced to lie directly under the anterior edge of the acromion. When properly positioned, both medial and lateral needles can be visualized. The needles can be wiggled to aid in their identification.

INSERTION OF OPERATIVE CANNULA

A 5-mm plastic cannula with rubber diaphragm is introduced (Fig. 2) into the subacromial space at this point (*c*) 3 to 4 cm from the acromion and in a direct line with the marker pins. A blunt-nosed powered shaver is introduced and the subacromial space is thoroughly debrided to enhance visualization. Both the floor and roof of the bursa should be cleared; this debridement will allow good visualization of the marker pins.

The coracoacromial ligament is then cut with a hooked or right-angled electrosurgical instrument (Fig. 3). The electrosurgical pencil is introduced through the operating cannula and visualized in a trial passage from one pin to the other. In order for

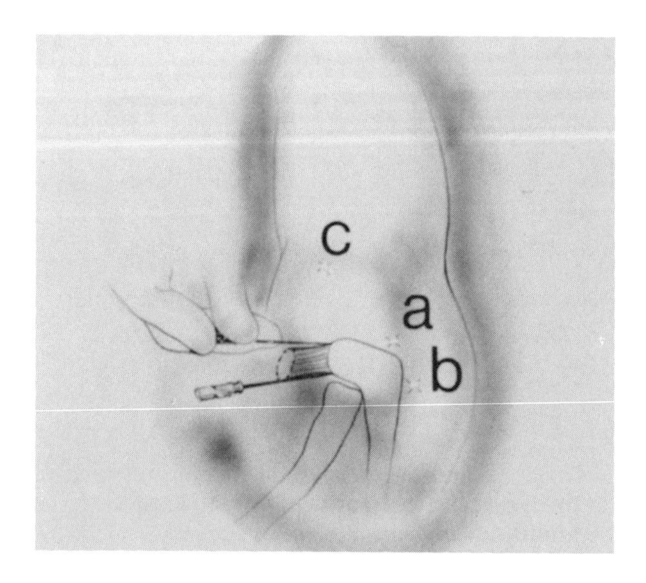

Figure 1 Bone landmarks drawn. Orientation pins outline the coracoacromial ligament attachment. Portals are marked (*a*) arthroscope, (*b*) accessory fluid inflow, and (*c*) operative cannula. (Republished with permission from Takagishi NT. The shoulder. 4th ed. Tokyo: Professional Postgraduate Services, 1987: 192–194.)

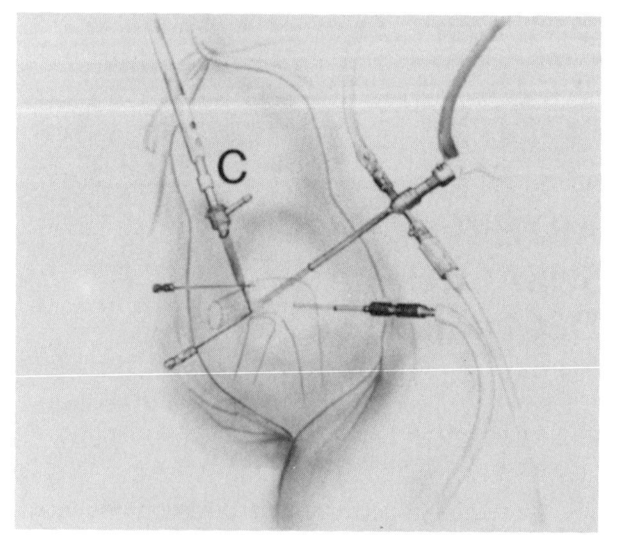

Figure 2 Surgical cannula (*c*) introduced 3 to 4 cm from the acromion in direct line with marker pins. An electrosurgical pencil passes through the cannula. All other instruments are in place. (Republished with permission from Takagishi NT. The shoulder. 4th ed. Tokyo: Professional Postgraduate Services, 1987: 192–194.)

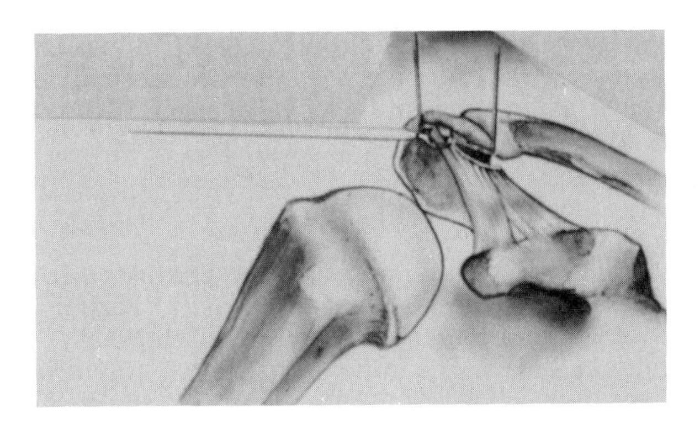

Figure 3 Cut coracoacromial ligament with an electrosurgical pencil from the medial marker pin toward the lateral pin. Distilled water irrigation is required temporarily for electrocautery to function. (Republished with permission from Takagishi NT. The shoulder. 4th ed. Tokyo: Professional Postgraduate Services, 1987: 192–194.)

cautery to occur, the normal saline must be removed from the subacromial space, and sterile distilled water for irrigation must be introduced. Three thorough flushings are necessary to eliminate the normal saline and permit electrosurgical cutting to occur. The cutting current on a specially designed generator is gradually increased until it begins to cut the thickened subacromial bursa, underlying the coracoacromial ligaments. The cut travels from the medial pin in a straight line toward the lateral pin. A surprising amount of thickened bursa must be divided in some cases before the ligament itself is actually cut. The cut is placed adjacent to the acromial attachment of the ligament, thereby minimizing the risk of injury to a branch of the coracoacromial artery. The coagulation current can be utilized when necessary to control bleeding from this artery. Once the ligament is severed, *the distilled water is flushed from the subacromial space and the remainder of the operation is performed with normal saline.* It is important to avoid prolonged instillation of distilled water; 15 minutes should be sufficient.

ANTERIOR ACROMIOPLASTY

The anterior undersurface of the acromion is visualized and the thickened subacromial bursa attached to this area is removed, initially with a small open curet and subsequently with an angled synovial resector. This tissue must be removed for effective use of the burr. The large arthroplasty burr is then placed under the anterior acromion (Fig. 4) and applied to an area where the bone has been exposed. The burr is then used to thin the anterior edge of the acromion to a degree desired by the surgeon. The full width of the acromion should be reduced from the anterior edge to a point about 2 cm posteriorly. Any spurs projecting from the undersurface of the outer end of the clavicle should also be

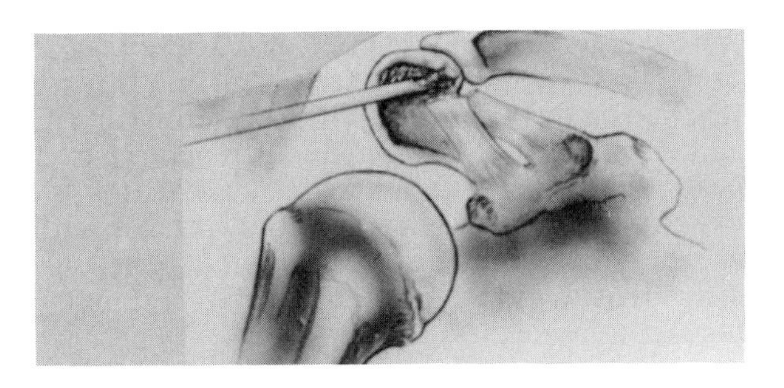

Figure 4 Open curet is used to resect the undersurface of the anterior acromion. (Republished with permission from Takagishi NT. The shoulder. 4th ed. Tokyo: Professional Postgraduate Services, 1987: 192–194.)

removed (Fig. 5). Bleeding from cancellous bone and resected synovium may make visualization difficult. Copious irrigation and distention will permit inspection to confirm the amount of bone removed. Distilled water may be introduced for a short time and the electrocautery unit used to obtain hemostasis. This will facilitate final burring and debridement. Fifteen ml of 0.25 percent bupivacaine with epinephrine is instilled at the conclusion of the procedure, and the portals are closed with 4–0 nylon sutures.

POSTOPERATIVE MANAGEMENT

Patients are encouraged to resume full active range of motion on the evening of surgery. They are instructed to stretch the arm overhead while supine and perform pendulum exercises every morning

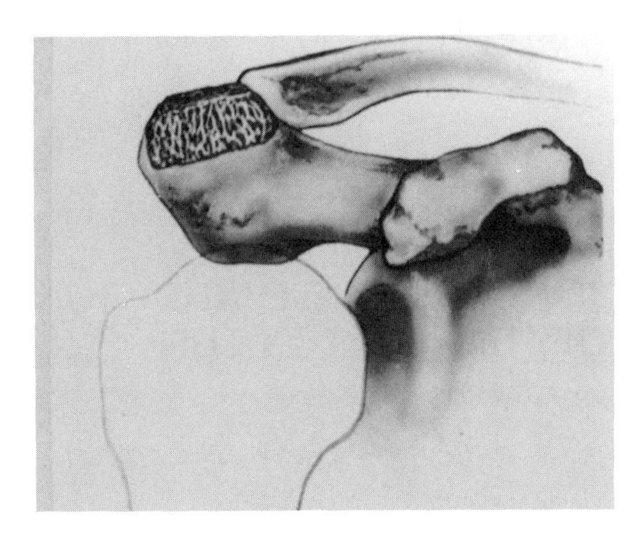

Figure 5 Burring completed. The acromion is thinned across the full width from the anterior edge to at least 2 cm posteriorly. Any spurs beneath the outer end of the clavicle are also resected. (Republished with permission from Takagishi NT. The shoulder. 4th ed. Tokyo: Professional Postgraduate Services, 1987: 192–194.)

and evening for 1 minute in order to prevent adhesion formation. No sling is used, and there is no restriction on daily living activities, including driving and reaching overhead. Strenuous repetitive overhead activity, however, is avoided for at least 4 to 6 weeks; this includes tennis and throwing. Strengthening exercises utilizing surgical tubing are begun at 4 to 6 weeks, and the patient gradually resumes all normal activities as tolerated.

DECOMPRESSION AND DEBRIDEMENT OF ROTATOR CUFF TEARS

The treatment of irreparable or recurrent full-thickness rotator cuff tears with arthroscopic decompression and debridement is carried out in selected patients. The procedure is not performed as a substitute for open repair of the routine cuff tear. Debridement and decompression are reserved for patients in whom an extensive tear has been present for several years, and whose preoperative evaluation suggests that at best a "limited goals result" will be achieved.

CALCIFIED TENDINITIS

Large calcareous deposits in the supraspinatus tendon can be relieved arthroscopically. Calcification generally develops within the tendon, and unfortunately many small and medium-sized calcifications cannot be seen when the cuff is viewed from the surface. An inflamed hypertrophic bursa further tends to obscure visualization. A needle is used to explore the rotator cuff in search of a calcific deposit; probing with the needle into a bed of calcium will liberate "snowflakes" of calcium into the bursa. Further needling, or a small incision in line with the fibers of the tendon, will permit the introduction of a curet, and large calcifications can be subsequently removed. Radiographic control assists in localization of the calcific deposit. The need for decompression in association with removal of calcific deposits is controversial.

RESULTS

This procedure has now been performed in a total of 217 patients during the past 5 years. The overall group contains 65 cases of full-thickness rotator cuff tears. The initial 82 patients in this series have been followed for 2 to 5 years and the results noted as 85 percent satisfactory and 15 percent unsatisfactory.

The results of arthroscopic decompression are comparable with those of open anterior acromioplasty. The procedure is technically challenging. It can be performed as an outpatient procedure and there is minimal morbidity. Patients return to activities of daily living within a few days. Arthroscopic subacromial decompression is an alternative to open anterior acromioplasty in selected cases of advanced stage II or III impingement syndromes.

SUGGESTED READING

Ellman H. Arthroscopic subacromial decompression. Orthop Trans 1985; 9:48.

Ellman H. Arthroscopic subacromial decompression: analysis of 1–3 year results. Arthroscopy 1987; 3:173.

Hawkins RF, Kennedy JC. Impingement syndrome in athletes. Am J Sports Med 1980; 8:151.

Neer CS II. Anterior acromioplasty for the chronic impingement syndrome in the shoulder. A preliminary report. J Bone Joint Surg 1972; 54A:41.

Neer CS II. Impingement lesions. Clin Orthop 1983; 173:70.

Post M, Cohen J. Impingement syndrome—a review of late stage II and early stage III lesions. Orthop Trans 1985; 9:48.

Pujadas GM. Coracoacromial ligament syndrome. J Bone Joint Surg 1970; 52A:1361.

Raggio CL, Warren RF, Sculco T. Surgical treatment of impingement syndrome: 4-year follow-up. Orthop Trans 1985; 9: 48.

SONOGRAPHIC EVALUATION OF THE ROTATOR CUFF

EDWARD V. CRAIG, M.D.

In recent years a number of published reports have examined the potential role of ultrasonography in the evaluation of disease, wear, degeneration, and tearing of the rotator cuff and biceps tendon apparatus. Traditionally, methods of evaluating the soft tissue around the shoulder have been indirect. With the torn rotator cuff, plain radiography often reveals associated bone changes in the area of the greater tuberosity, acromion, and acromioclavicular joint and changes in the acromiohumeral interval. Arthrography, although highly accurate in diagnosing full-thickness tears, provides only evidence of the presence or absence of tearing; it does not indicate the quality of the remaining tendon or the extent and location of the tear. In addition, arthrography is invasive, has some morbidity, has a variable patient acceptance, exposes the patient to radiation, provides little if any information about incomplete-thickness tears of the tendon, and is not a practical means of demonstrating the condition of the contralateral rotator cuff in all patients. Thus, investigations into noninvasive means of imaging the rotator cuff have been viewed with interest by all who treat pathologic conditions about the shoulder.

Ultrasonography is a technology in which images are constructed from echoes produced when high-frequency sound waves are projected into the structure of interest. Although this technique has been used in other areas of medicine, the development of high-resolution, real-time instruments in which small structures could be imaged with a high frame rate made possible its application in examination of more complex structures such as the shoulder. As early as 1977 Mayer introduced the concept of using ultrasound to diagnose problems involving the rotator cuff. Seltzer and co-workers were able to demonstrate effusions about the shoulder, but the analysis of the rotator cuff tendon structures still seemed to be a problem. In 1983 the first sonographic demonstration of rotator cuff pathology was reported by Farrar and co-workers, and the evaluation of their patients has led numerous investigators throughout the world to recommend ultrasonography as a method of evaluating the rotator cuff.

In theory the use of sound waves to image the rotator cuff has many advantages: (1) it is safe and has no known risk, (2) it is noninvasive, (3) it can be done rapidly and inexpensively, (4) both shoulders can be scanned quickly (taking less than 5 minutes per shoulder), (5) the position of the transducer over specific tendons may provide a potential means of precisely localizing tendon pathology, (6) tendinous pathology other than full-thickness tearing may be demonstrated, (7) there is no radiation exposure, and (8) changes in the surrounding bone, biceps, and deltoid muscle may be seen.

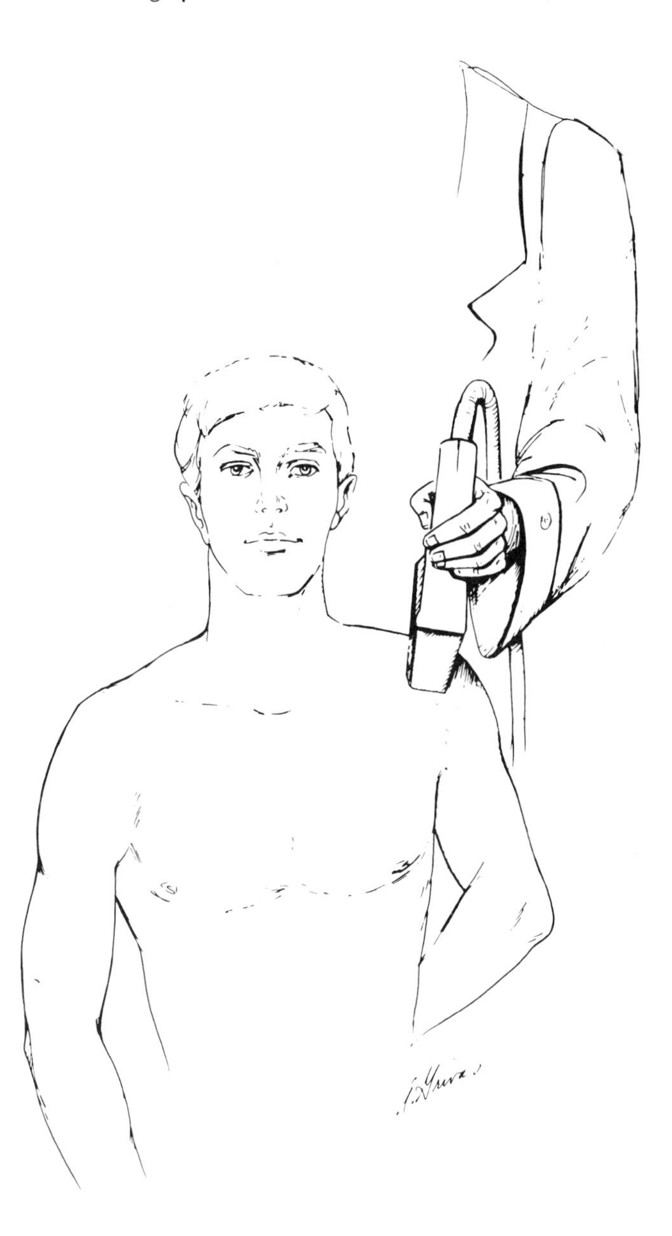

Figure 1 Ultrasound examination of the shoulder is performed as the sonographer, standing adjacent to the shoulder being examined, passes the transducer over the rotator cuff.

TECHNICAL CONSIDERATIONS

The rotator cuff is well suited to sonographic study. Ultrasound is unable to see through bone, so correct patient positioning is critical in order to bring the area of rotator cuff under study into view. The scan is typically made with the patient seated on a rotating stool, and the ultrasonographer standing at the side being examined, the screen in view to both sonographer and patient (Fig. 1). The examination of both shoulders provides comparison for any observed sonographic abnormalities. The position of the patient's arm can enhance the study. Although many authors have suggested studying the rotator cuff with the arm at the side without any rotation, others have found that hyperextension and internal rotation appears to bring more of the supraspinatus and infraspinatus out from underneath the acromion. Active motion of the arm has been suggested as providing a "dynamic study" of the rotator cuff tendon motion, but excellent images of the tendon can be seen without active arm movement.

A number of machines are currently available for scanning the rotator cuff. In most instances a commercially available real-time, high-resolution, small-parts instrument is used. Most sonographers use a 7.5- or 10-MHz scanner to provide the best image. An organized and systematic study of the rotator cuff is essential. The rotator cuff is imaged in two perpendicular planes (Fig. 2). The sagittal plane is one in which the transducer scans the cuff parallel to its fibers; the transverse plane is one in which the transducer is perpendicular to the plane of the tendon fibers.

The following is the suggested order for rotator cuff visualization:

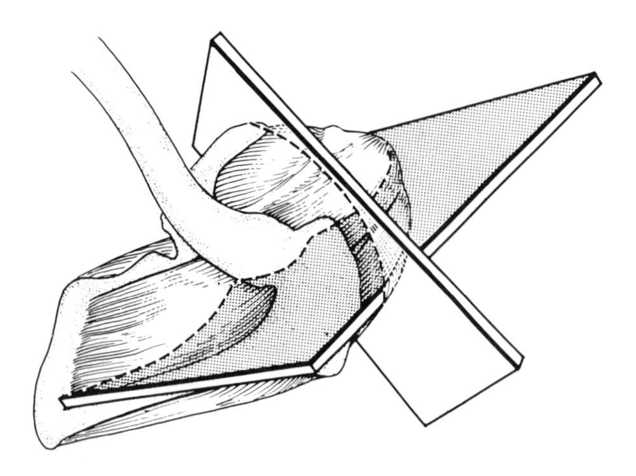

Figure 2 The rotator cuff is imaged in two perpendicular planes. The sagittal plane is parallel to the fiber orientation of the rotator cuff. The transverse plane is perpendicular to the fiber orientation of the rotator cuff.

1. Bicipital groove (transverse). This is the anatomic landmark for orientation when beginning the scan. It provides a key to visualization of the soft tissues around the shoulder.
2. Supraspinatus tendon (transverse). The transducer is moved laterally (posterior) to the groove until the supraspinatus tendon is visualized. The transducer is moved proximally along the tendon to visualize the entire length of the supraspinatus, until the image is obscured by the acromion.
3. Infraspinatus and teres minor (transverse). Although this area is involved less frequently than the supraspinatus tendon in cuff pathology, larger tears often involve one or both of these tendons; thus, they are equally important to visualize. The transducer is moved more posteriorly to image these two tendons. Investigators have reported that this is an area in which imaging is enhanced with passive external and internal rotation using real-time imaging.
4. Subscapularis (transverse). The transducer is brought back to the bicipital groove and moved medially (anteriorly) to visualize the subscapularis attached to the lesser tuberosity. Although this is an unusual site for rotator cuff pathology, it is easily visualized sonographically.
5. Biceps tendon (sagittal). The transducer is returned to the bicipital groove, rotated 90 degrees and the biceps is seen along its longitudinal axis.
6. Supraspinatus (sagittal). The transducer is moved posteriorly approximately 1 cm, again parallel to the fibers of the rotator cuff, and the supraspinatus tendon can be seen parallel to its long axis. Abduction against resistance may help to visualize small tears and asymmetry of muscle action in this tendon.
7. Infraspinatus and teres minor (sagittal). The transducer is moved posterior to the supraspinatus tendon, and the infraspinatus and teres minor are again imaged in the sagittal plane.

NORMAL SONOGRAPHIC ANATOMY

The normal sonographic anatomy consists of three distinct tissue planes: the skin and subcutaneous tissue, the deltoid muscle, and the rotator cuff tendon (Figs. 3 to 6). The skin and subcutaneous tissue layer is seen as a variable white band of moderate echogenicity (increased whiteness). The deltoid muscle is usually of low echogenicity. Its thickness is surprisingly consistent, usually about the same as

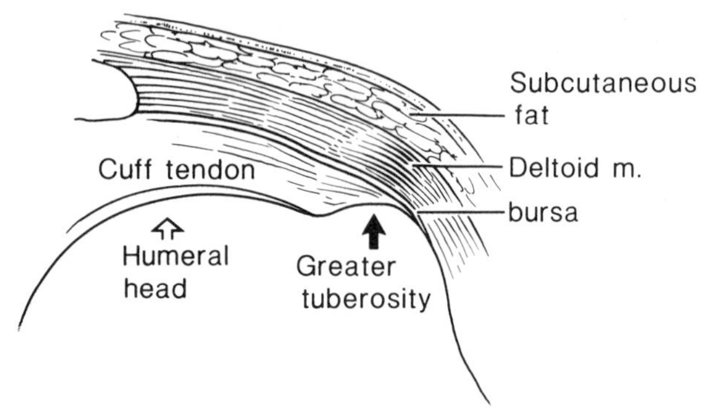

Figure 3 Diagrammatic representation of sagittal ultrasonography. Three distinct layers are seen: skin and subcutaneous fat, deltoid muscle, and the rotator cuff. The rotator cuff is seen to taper to its insertion on the greater tuberosity. Occasionally a bursal line may be seen between deltoid and rotator cuff.

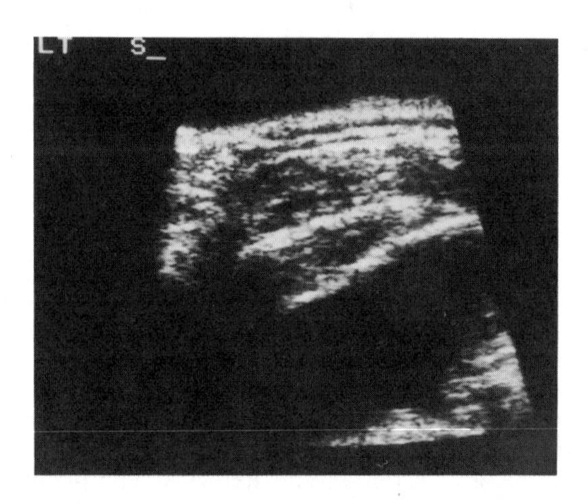

Figure 4 A normal sagittal ultrasound image, with three identifiable layers. The echogenic line between deltoid and rotator cuff represents the layer occupied by the subdeltoid bursa. The black acoustic shadows immediately to the left of the rotator cuff represent the acromion, from beneath which the rotator cuff is emerging. The dark black area immediately inferior to the rotator cuff layer represents the humeral head. In the normal ultrasound image, the rotator cuff layer is homogeneous and well organized, with a low level of echogenicity (increased whiteness).

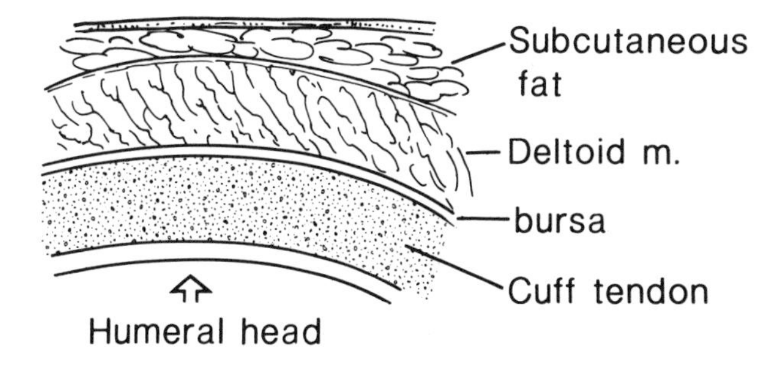

Figure 5 The transverse ultrasound image is seen diagramatically. Because this is perpendicular to the fiber orientation, the rotator cuff layer is not seen to taper. Three distinct layers are again noted.

the rotator cuff when measured 2 cm proximal to the cuff insertion on the greater tuberosity. The average deltoid thickness is approximately 5.9 mm, without any difference between dominant and nondominant arms or left and right shoulders.

The subdeltoid bursa, in its normal nonpathologic state, may not be resolved sonographically as a separate structure. However, when seen it is usually 1 mm or less in thickness. When pathologically thickened, the bursal thickness can be several millimeters. The echogenic line in this area identifies the superficial border of the rotator cuff (see Fig. 4).

The normal rotator cuff is seen as a homogeneous, well-organized layer, with a low level of echogenicity that is typical of healthy tendon. It is often slightly more echogenic than the deltoid muscle. Focal areas of mildly increased echoes are occasionally encountered in asymptomatic patients, but these are usually symmetric compared with the contralateral shoulder. The low-level echogenic cuff tendon is interposed between the echogenic bursal

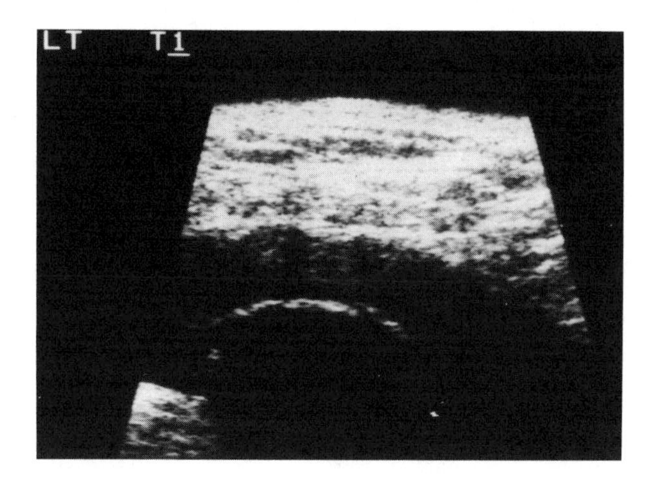

Figure 6 A normal transverse ultrasound image. Again, notice the low level of echogenicity, which is normal in the rotator cuff layer. The thickness of the rotator cuff layer normally approximates that of the adjacent deltoid layer.

plane and the high-level echoes originating from the humeral head. In the sagittal view the cuff is seen to taper gradually toward its insertion on the greater tuberosity (see Fig. 4). The tendon may then be followed proximally until acoustic shadowing from the acromion prevents further visualization. The average thickness of the rotator cuff is approximately 6 mm, and usually no substantial difference is noted between male and female patients or between right and left shoulders.

The echogenic lines, below the cuff layer, resulting from reflections of the proximal humerus, are composed of a convex portion laterally representing the greater tuberosity, a convex portion medially representing the humeral head, and a concave portion between the greater tuberosity and humeral head, which is the anatomic neck. In the transverse sonographic image, the tendon is seen in cross-section. It may have a punctate appearance in this image, and unlike the sagittal image it is not seen to taper (see Fig. 6). Its thickness is relatively constant throughout the tendon in this transverse view.

The biceps groove and tendon have also been thoroughly described sonographically. A transverse scan at the groove level shows the groove as a semicircular depression in the anterior aspect of the proximal humerus, formed by the lesser tuberosity medially and the greater tuberosity laterally. The biceps tendon appears as an echogenic circular structure within the bicipital groove. The intra-articular portion of the tendon is seen as an echogenic ellipse located against the humeral head between subscapularis and supraspinatus. The average thickness of the biceps tendon sonographically is 4.3 mm.

FULL-THICKNESS TEARS

There have been a number of reports on the use of ultrasound to assess full-thickness tears of the rotator cuff. Crass and associates described four sonographic patterns.

Focal Echogenicity

This is the most frequent sonographic pattern in small full-thickness tears of the rotator cuff (Fig. 7). This focally echogenic material may be caused by a combination of frayed and fibrillated tendon edge, fibrinous debris, blood clot, or granulation tissue within the tear. In another report, however, it was suggested that echogenicity was not a good criterion for cuff tear because of its lack of specificity and that, for that reason, ultrasonography could not be considered very sensitive in the diagnosis of rotator cuff tears under 1 cm in diameter. Accuracy for small tears might be improved by using the technique of dynamic scanning (movement of the shoulder during the scanning technique) and observing the echogenic area move. These reports emphasized

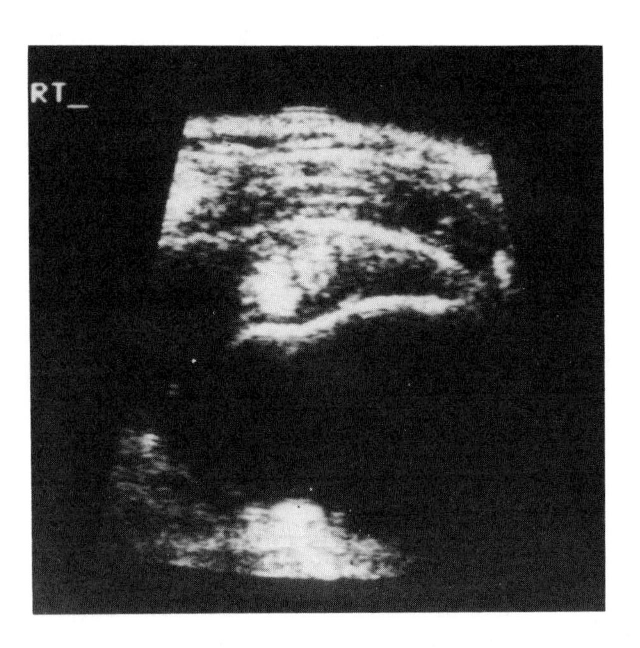

Figure 7 In the rotator cuff layer, there is a focal area of increased echogenicity. In this patient a small full-thickness tear of the rotator cuff was found at surgery. Although this is the most common sonographic abnormality, a focally echogenic area is not considered to be specific for a full-thickness rotator cuff tear.

that disrupted cuff does not move synchronously with normal cuff in a dynamic scan. Since it is generally agreed that increased echoes are the most frequent abnormal finding in rotator cuff sonography, the experience of the sonographer appears to be critical in distinguishing the numerous diagnostic possibilities when there are subtle changes in tendon echogenicity.

Large Defects or Complete Absence of Cuff Layer

This condition is thought to be pathognomonic for a tendon tear. As the tendon tear enlarges, the margins of echogenicity separate, the tendon appears to be pulled away from the greater tuberosity, and an actual defect is seen in the tendon (Fig. 8). The deltoid often appears to fill in the gap created by the retracting rotator cuff. In some ultrasound studies, there may be complete absence of the rotator cuff, the deltoid muscle being seen to rest directly on the humeral articular surface. This sonographic finding generally correlates with a massive rotator cuff tear (Fig. 9).

Thinning of the Rotator Cuff

This finding often corresponds to the tendon defect that is filled in with abnormal and thick bursal tissue (see Fig. 8).

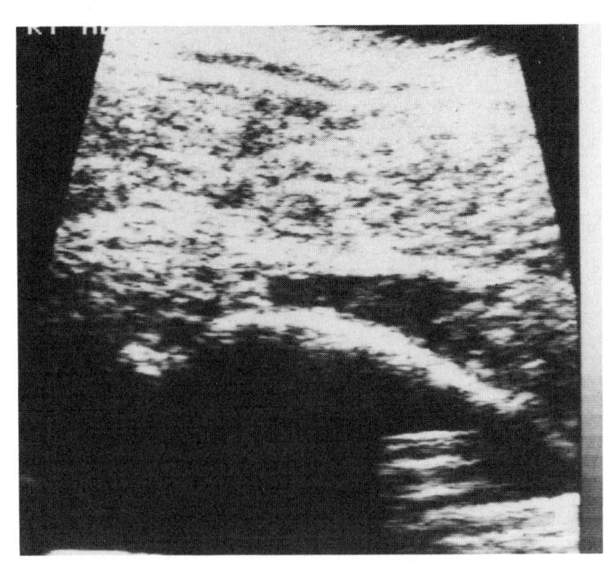

Figure 8 A full-thickness tear of the rotator cuff. An actual gap (dark, sonolucent) region is seen in the rotator cuff layer. Note also the focal area of thinning in this area of the rotator cuff. This is probably sonographically pathognomonic for a full-thickness tear of the rotator cuff.

Thickened Tendon With Irregular Foci of Increased and Decreased Echogenicity

It is not certain what causes these irregular foci of increased and decreased echo changes, but they may be due to associated edema and hemorrhage if the tear is acute.

Middleton and colleagues reported four sonographic criteria for cuff tear:

1. Focal thinning of the cuff, which in their series was the most common sonographic finding and gave 100 percent predictive value for tears of the

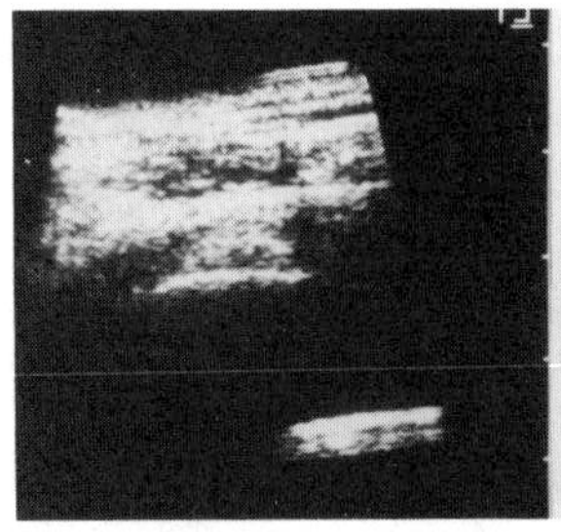

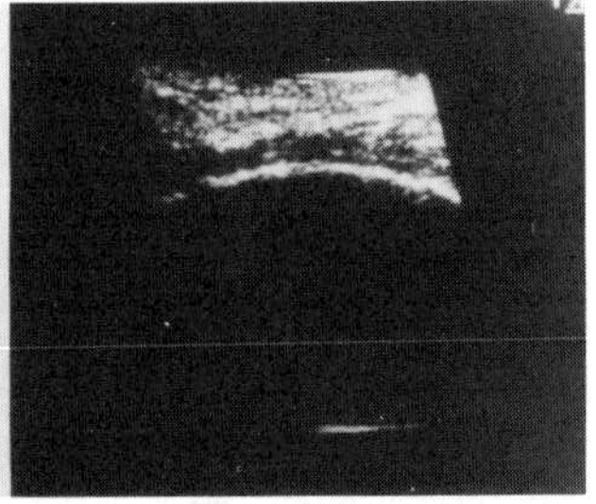

Figure 9 A sonographic study of the left and right shoulders in a patient with symptoms of pain and weakness on the right. Note that in the left study there are still three distinct layers. The rotator cuff layer, though not entirely normal, is certainly identifiable. In the right study the deltoid layer is seen directly adjacent to the humeral head. No rotator cuff is identifiable. This absence of rotator cuff layer is also pathognomonic for a rotator cuff tear and usually represents a massive tear.

rotator cuff. There was usually an abrupt cut-off from normal tendon thickness to the area of focal thinning, and the surrounding rotator cuff tendon was normal.
2. Complete nonvisualization of the cuff. This corresponded to a large cuff tear seen at surgery or arthrographically.
3. Focal discontinuity in the homogeneous rotator cuff without thinning. These authors had several patients in whom there was this sonographic finding but negative arthrograms.
4. A central echogenic band in the region of the rotator cuff.

From the numerous studies evaluating full-thickness tears of the rotator cuff, the following observations can thus be made:

1. Complete nonvisualization of the rotator cuff layer appears to be a pathognomonic sonographic finding corresponding to a large rotator cuff tear.
2. An actual disruption in rotator cuff continuity probably corresponds to a full-thickness tear. Perhaps dynamic use of the ultrasonography can further clarify the area of disruption. If both sides of the disruption do not move synchronously, this almost certainly indicates a full-thickness tear.
3. Significant thinning of the rotator cuff layer, especially if there is an abrupt transition to this thinned tendon, probably corresponds to a full-thickness tear.
4. Echogenicity alone is more difficult to interpret. Although small tears may present as echogenic foci, the lack of specificity makes it impossible to diagnose a full-thickness tear of the tendon by this criterion alone. However, echogenicity does not appear to be normal, and abnormal echoes in the tendon, even if focal, generally represent a pathologic condition in the tendon.

Incomplete-thickness tears of the rotator cuff may be bursal side, joint side, or intratendinous disruptions. In 1985 Craig and Crass reported a series of 17 patients with incomplete-thickness tears of the rotator cuff; in 14 of these there were abnormal sonographic results, including two with purely intratendinous tears. This represented the first abnormal radiographic study in purely intratendinous tears of the rotator cuff, suggesting that ultrasound might be a means of recognizing intratendinous pathology.

However, the most common sonographic abnormality in partial-thickness tears is echogenicity of the tendon. The echogenicity is usually more than that seen in normal tendon, but is not as marked as the echogenicity seen in small full-thickness tears. Thus, it appears impossible at this point sonographically to distinguish small complete- from small incomplete-thickness tears. If differentiation between the two is necessary, arthrography should be considered. Because echogenicity is the most common sonographic abnormality in the incomplete-thickness tear, sonography cannot be considered at this point to be accurate or specific in the diagnosis of this lesion.

CALCIFIC TENDINITIS

A calcific deposit within the substance of the rotator cuff manifests itself as a sono-rich area with a small echolucent focus adjacent to it. Since the calcific deposit can usually be seen on plain radiographs, there is little chance of confusing calcific tendinitis with other causes of abnormal echogenicity in the tendon.

BICEPS LESIONS

Lesions of the biceps tendon often occur in association with rotator cuff abnormalities. The biceps tendon lies anatomically adjacent to the supraspinatus. Any pathologic conditions of mechanical wear or degeneration may thus extend to involve the biceps tendon from the area of the supraspinatus. Groove spurring and other anomalies make the tendon prone to inflammation. Arthrography and plain radiography have traditionally given a limited evaluation of the bicipital groove and biceps tendon. Arthrographically, poor filling of the biceps tendon sheath may be associated with a number of shoulder conditions, including tears and tendinitis. Although arthrography is probably better than sonography in imaging the bone configuration of the groove, the soft tissue and fluid within this space have been reported to be visualized better with ultrasound. In addition, sonography may identify the location of a long head of biceps rupture if the tendon ends have not retracted, while an empty groove may be associated with either rupture or dislocation of the tendon.

POSTOPERATIVE SONOGRAPHIC ANATOMY

The potential for a noninvasive test that may image the rotator cuff has proved particularly exciting with regard to its application to the postoperative rotator cuff. It is known that arthrography may be positive in as many as 20 percent of clinically successful rotator cuff repairs.

In the postoperative shoulder, ultrasound results are always abnormal. There is a loss of soft tissue planes surrounding the rotator cuff tendon and an abnormal increase in echogenicity in the tendon. However, the thickness of the rotator cuff substance is usually well maintained despite the abnormal echogenicity. Nonetheless, the echogenic appearance of small rotator cuff tears may be mimicked by these postoperative changes, which may persist as long as 6 years after a clinically successful rotator cuff repair. However, as the tear enlarges, even in the postoperative patient, a gap or defect can be seen within the cuff tendon, and this appearance allows confident diagnosis of a retear after surgical treatment.

It appears that if the sonographic criteria for cuff tears are altered for the postoperative tendon, this method remains accurate in its ability to identify tendon disruption. However, sonographic tendon disruption does not correlate well with good or poor clinical results after repair of the rotator cuff.

RESULTS

There have now been several reports in the literature detailing the diagnostic accuracy of rotator cuff ultrasonography, and comparing it with arthrography in evaluation of rotator cuff disease. As sonographic technology has improved, particularly with linear array scanners, and as individual sonographers have gained experience, this technique is emerging as a valuable screening tool for the painful shoulder.

The first report by Farrar and associates showed sonography to have an overall accuracy of 83 percent in identifying full-thickness rotator cuff tears; these authors emphasized that while it was particularly accurate for tears larger than 3 cm, it was less reliable for small tears. The first published report in the literature of ultrasound for the diagnosis of rotator cuff tears was by Crass and associates, who described a small series and correlated the sonographic results with surgical findings. This group later published their large experience with ultrasonography in 500 patients who had been referred for the evaluation of a painful shoulder. In this study, ultrasonography proved more accurate than arthrography in identifying the overall pathology of rotator cuff tears. If incomplete-thickness tears were excluded, the accuracy was 91 percent with ultrasonography. It was suggested that sonography could be more accurate than arthrography in evaluating the postoperative patient for recurrent tears. These investigators concluded that ultrasound should be the initial modality for examination of the rotator cuff, if adequate real-time instrumentation is available.

In another large series of patients, Middleton and associates described their wide experience using ultrasound to evaluate the rotator cuff and biceps tendon. In patients who had been referred for arthrography, the sensitivity and specificity of ultrasound in detecting a full-thickness tear was 91 percent. Many of the false-positive and false-negative results could be attributed to lack of experience with the procedure. In Middleton's series, nonvisualization or focal thinning of the cuff had a positive predictive value of 100 percent. These authors concluded that with normal sonography the negative predictive value was high enough to suggest that no further radiology was needed unless the patient failed to respond to conservative treatment. If the sonographic finding was of focal thinning or nonvisualization, the authors again suggested that no further radiology need be performed, since the likelihood was so high that this indicated a full-thickness tear.

Mack and associates published their experience with dynamic ultrasound, using the motion of the humerus to increase the image accuracy of the cuff layer. This report was extremely valuable in identifying the fact that echogenicity alone was not a reliable finding in the diagnosis of a full-thickness tear. Compared with surgery and arthrography, ultrasonography had an overall accuracy of 94 percent. These investigators commented that after a high-resolution linear array scanner was introduced, there were no false-positive or false-negative results in their series. This group now uses ultrasonography instead of arthrography as the routine method for imaging rotator cuff integrity. However, all investigators emphasized that it is vital to use an ultrasonographer experienced with the technique and with its interpretation in order to distinguish between the subtle echo abnormalities that may exist in a variety of normal and abnormal shoulders.

This technique is highly dependent on the quality of the instrumentation, the technique of the sonographer, and above all the skill and experience of the person performing the examination. There does appear to be a significant "learning curve" to the technique. However, the results published to date certainly justify the continued use of ultrasonography to image the rotator cuff. As technology and experience improve, it is anticipated that the uniformity of results and reproducibility of images will also improve.

PITFALLS IN ULTRASONOGRAPHY

Some studies have emphasized that there are pitfalls in interpreting the findings of ultrasonography, as follows: (1) errors of technique, (2) misinterpretation of normal anatomy, (3) errors caused by associated soft tissue abnormalities other than full-thickness tears, and (4) errors caused by bone abnormalities in the glenohumeral joint. If these pitfalls are recognized and avoided, the diagnostic accuracy of the technique is enhanced.

SUGGESTED ROLE OF SONOGRAPHY

Ultrasonography, although an exciting area of investigation, has yet to enjoy widespread use, probably because it has not been proved in all centers to have the accuracy of arthrography.

The suggested role of ultrasound, given a sonographer experienced with the technique and its interpretation, is as follows:

1. An initial screening of the painful shoulder. If this is entirely normal and an adequate study has been performed, no further radiographic investigation need be undertaken. Investigation can focus on other causes of shoulder pain, and the integrity of the rotator cuff may be taken for granted. However, if the usual treatment does not improve the symptoms, further investigation of the cuff with arthrography or magnetic resonance imaging should be considered.

2. If the ultrasonographic examination clearly shows no rotator cuff layer, no further investigation need be made, and a large rotator cuff tear may be assumed to be present. This, of course, may be mimicked by severe muscle atrophy.

3. If there is a focal disruption of cuff, and if the area adjacent to the disruption does not move synchronously on dynamic scanning, a cuff tear can be assumed to be present.

4. Severe thinning or focal thinning in the tendon with the adjacent normal tendon can be assumed to represent a tear.

5. If the only unusual finding is an abnormal increase in echogenicity, the contralateral shoulder should be carefully examined for the same sonographic finding. If the contralateral shoulder is sonographically normal, the abnormality of echogenicity should be considered to indicate abnormal tendon. Whether this represents a small full-thickness tear, an incomplete-thickness tear, late impingement with scarring, postoperative changes, or calcific tendinitis can be determined (if it is important to do so) from the clinical history, physical examination, plain radiography, or shoulder arthrography.

SUGGESTED READING

Ahovuo J, Paavolainen P, Slatis P. Diagnostic value of sonography and lesions of the biceps tendon. Clin Orthop 1986; 202:184.

Bretzke CA, Crass JR, Craig EV, et al. Ultrasonography of the rotator cuff. Normal and pathologic anatomy. Invest Radiol 1985; 20:311.

Calvert PT, Packer NP, Stoker DJ, et al. Arthrography of the shoulder after operative repair of the torn rotator cuff. J Bone Joint Surg 1986; 68B:147.

Collins RA, Gristina AG, Carter RE, et al. Ultrasonography of the shoulder: static and dynamic imaging. Orthop Clin North Am 1987; 18:351.

Craig EV. Incomplete thickness tears of the rotator cuff. Presented at the Annual Meeting of the American Association for Sports Medicine, New Orleans, LA, 1986.

Craig EV, Crass JR. Sonographic evaluation of the rotator cuff. Proceedings of the Third International Conference on Surgery of the Shoulder. Tokyo, Professional Postgraduate Services, 1985:98.

Crass JR, Craig EV, Feinberg SB. Sonography of the postoperative rotator cuff. AJR 1986; 146:561.

Crass JR, Craig EV, Feinberg SB. Ultrasonography of rotator cuff tears: a review of 500 diagnostic studies. J Clin Ultrasound 1988; 16:313.

Crass JR, Craig EV, Thompson RC, Feinberg SB. Ultrasonography of the rotator cuff: surgical correlation. J Clin Ultrasound 1984; 12:487.

Farrar EL, Matsen FA III, Rogers JV, et al. Dynamic sonographic study of lesions of the rotator cuff. Presented at the American Academy of Orthopaedic Surgeons 50th Annual Meeting, March 1983: 49 (abstract).

Goldman AB, Dines DM, Warren RF. Shoulder arthrography: technique. Diagnosis and clinical correlation. Boston: Little, Brown, 1982.

Hall FM, Rosental DI, Goldberg RP, et al. Morbidity from shoulder arthrography: etiology, incidence, and prevention. AJR 1981; 139:59.

Mack LA, Matsen FA III, Kilcoyne RF. US evaluation of the rotator cuff. Radiology 1985; 157:205.

Mack LA, Nyberg DA, Matsen FA III. Sonographic evaluation of the rotator cuff. Radiol Clin North Am 1988; 26:161.

Mack LA, Nyberg DA, Matsen FA III, et al. Sonography of the postoperative shoulder. AJR 1988; 150:1089.

Mayer V. Ultrasonography of the shoulder. Sonographic exhibit at the American Institute of Ultrasound in Medicine, Dallas, TX, 1977.

Middleton WD, Edelstein G, Reinus WR, et al. Ultrasonography of the rotator cuff: technique and normal anatomy. J Ultrasound Med 1984; 3:549.

Middleton WD, Reinus WR, Melson GL. Pitfalls of rotator cuff sonography. AJR 1986; 146:555.

Middleton WD, Reinus WR, Totty WG, et al. US of the biceps tendon apparatus. Radiology 1985; 157:211.

Middleton WD, Reinus WR, Totty WG, et al. Ultrasonographic evaluation of the rotator cuff and biceps tendon. J Bone Joint Surg 1986; 68A:440.

Neer CS. Anterior acromioplasty for the chronic impingement syndrome in the shoulder. J Bone Joint Surg 1972; 54A:41.

Seltzer SE, Finberg JH, Weissman BN. Arthrosonography technique sonographic anatomy, and pathology. Invest Radiol 1980; 15:19.

Seltzer SE, Finberg HJ, Weissman BN, et al. Arthrosonography: grey-scale ultrasound evaluation of the shoulder. Radiology 1969; 132:467.

MAGNETIC RESONANCE IMAGING OF THE SHOULDER

MICHAEL B. ZLATKIN, M.D., F.R.C.P.(C)
MURRAY K. DALINKA, M.D.

Radiologic evaluation is a necessary adjunct to clinical examination in the patient with shoulder pain. Noninvasive imaging modalities, including plain radiography, radionuclide studies, tomography, ultrasonography, and computed tomography, are often nonspecific. Invasive examinations such as arthrography and conventional and computed arthrotomography may yield a more specific diagnosis but are not without morbidity. Our recent experience with magnetic resonance imaging (MRI) has demonstrated that it can replace many of these techniques and make a precise diagnosis in a noninvasive manner.

TECHNIQUE

The examination is performed with the patient supine in the magnet with a dual surface coil array, anterior and posterior to the shoulder (Fig. 1).

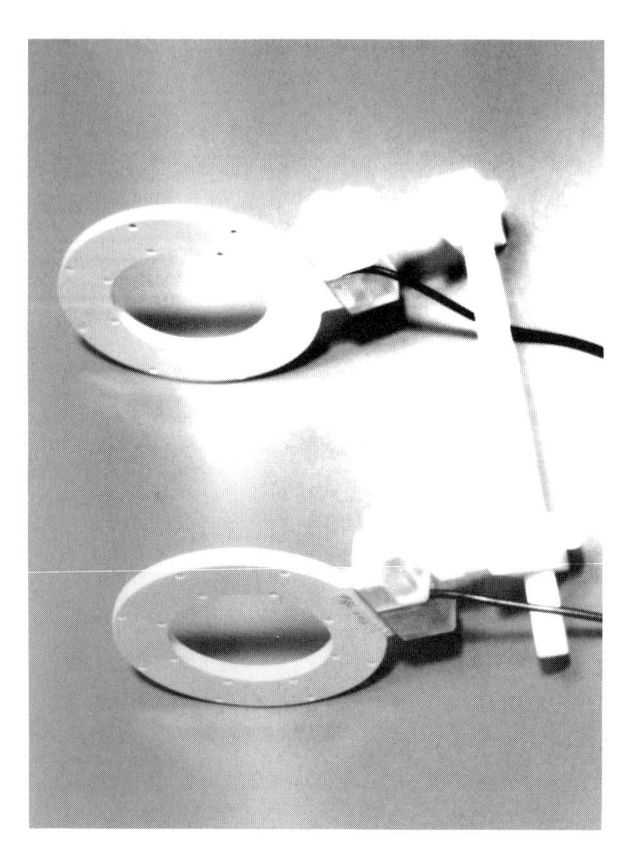

Figure 1 Dual 5½-inch surface coils with adjustable holder used for shoulder imaging.

On the basis of the initial image obtained with a large field of view (40 to 48 cm), the coordinates for determining a field of view centered over the glenohumeral joint are obtained. We routinely take images in three planes: axial, coronal oblique, and sagittal oblique. In patients with rotator cuff tears, the axial images are obtained with 5-mm thickness and are used as a localizer for the subsequent coronal and sagittal oblique images. In patients with suspected shoulder instability, thinner sections (3 mm) are obtained and a separate T2-weighted sequence is performed in order to evaluate the labrum and capsular structures. Planes parallel and perpendicular to the supraspinatus muscle and tendon (coronal and sagittal oblique views) (Fig. 2) are obtained with thin sections and T2-weighting to provide optimal visualization of the rotator cuff and surrounding structures.

Magnetic Resonance Imaging Anatomy

The MRI appearance of the glenohumeral joint has been described. Figure 3 shows images of a normal shoulder in the axial, coronal oblique, and sagittal oblique planes. Subcutaneous fat, intermuscular fat planes, and bone marrow normally have the highest signal on T1-weighted images because of their relatively short T1. Muscles and hyaline articular cartilage have a more intermediate signal intensity. Owing to a relative lack of mobile protons, certain structures have essentially no MR signal and are therefore identified by anatomic location and contrast with surrounding tissues. These structures include cortical bone, the fibrocartilaginous glenoid labrum, the articular capsule, and tendinous and ligamentous structures such as the tendinous insertions of the rotator cuff musculature into the greater tuberosity, and the long head of the biceps as it courses in the bicipital groove.

Axial images demonstrate the relationship between the humeral head and glenoid cavity and are comparable with computed tomographic (CT) images. The articular cartilage and glenoid labrum also are well depicted. The anterior labrum is usually triangular (see Fig. 3*A*), but there normally are considerable variations. The posterior labrum is usually rounded in appearance. The subscapularis muscle and the insertion of its tendon into the lesser tuberosity are well visualized. The long head of the biceps tendon is best seen on axial sections where it appears as a signal void in the bicipital groove. The subscapularis bursa and the capsular structures, including the glenohumeral ligaments, are difficult to identify as distinct structures on T1-weighted images, but may be visualized as separate structures in the presence of joint fluid and T2-weighted images.

The tendons of the rotator cuff muscles are best evaluated on coronal oblique images. As previously stated, this plane is parallel to the supraspinatus

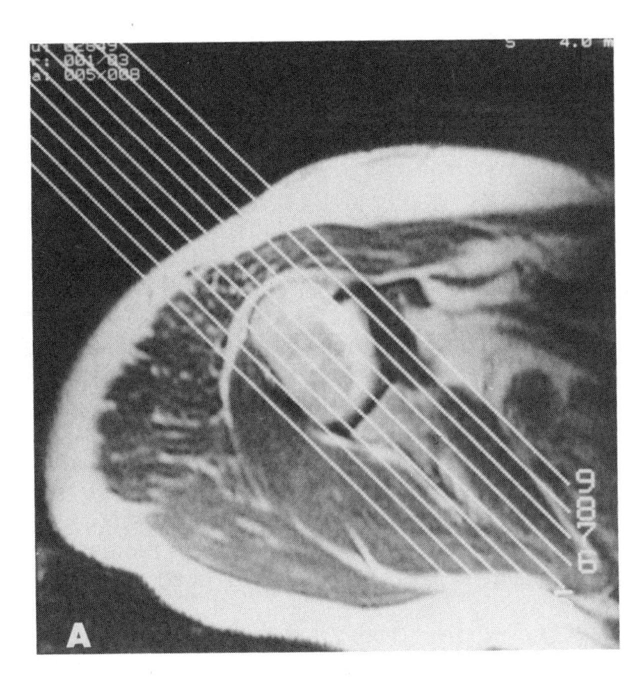

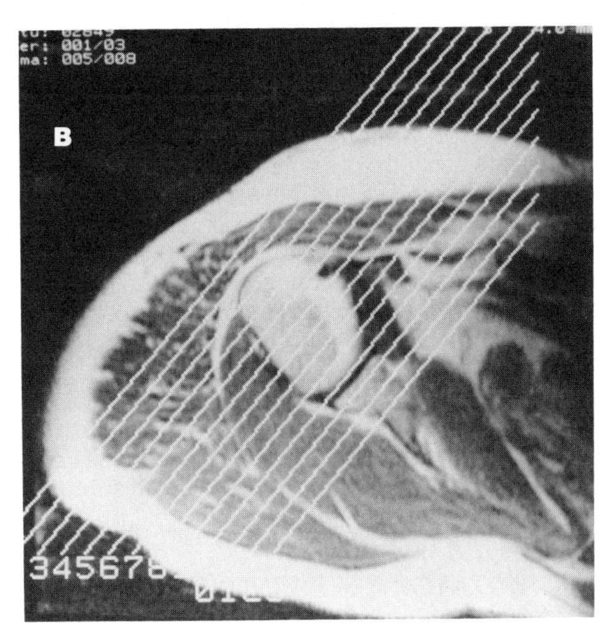

Figure 2 *A,* Axial image with graphic localizer illustrating the imaging plane for coronal oblique images. *B,* Similar image with graphic localizer for the sagittal oblique plane.

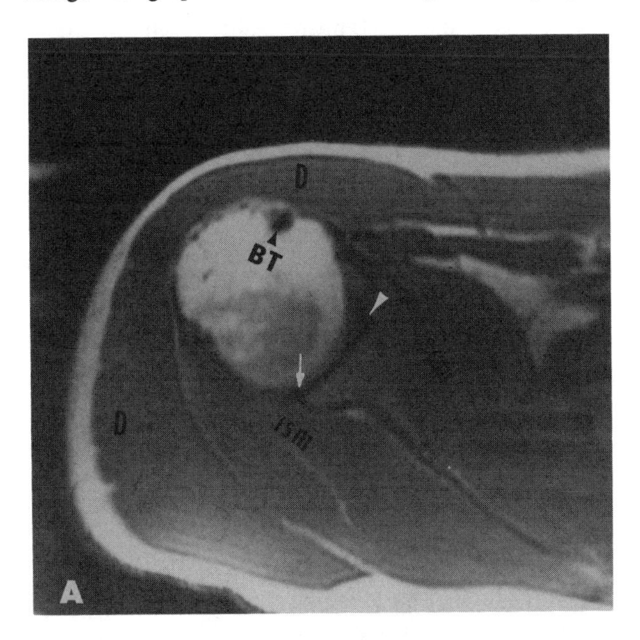

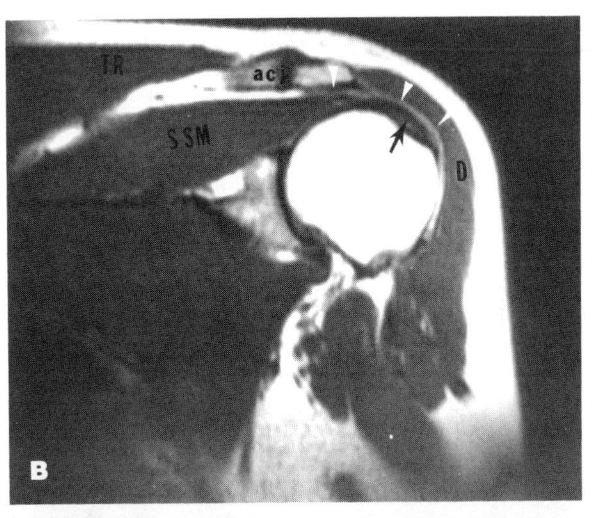

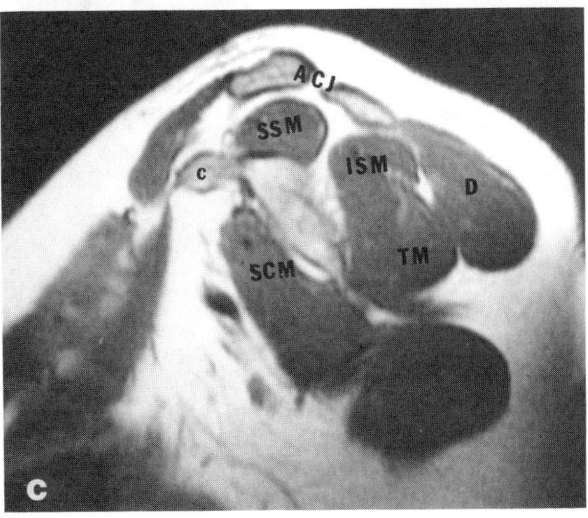

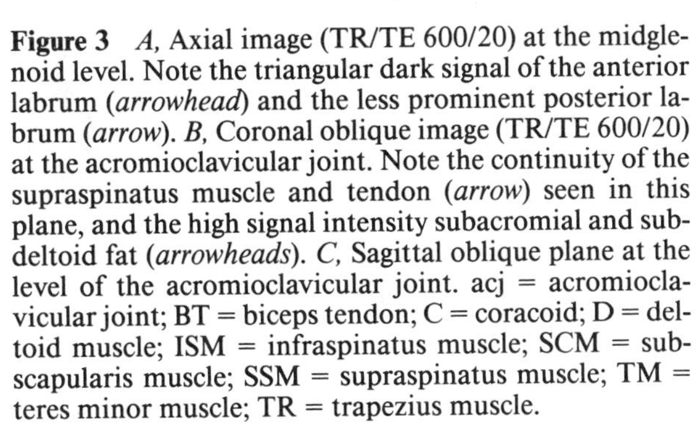

Figure 3 *A,* Axial image (TR/TE 600/20) at the midglenoid level. Note the triangular dark signal of the anterior labrum (*arrowhead*) and the less prominent posterior labrum (*arrow*). *B,* Coronal oblique image (TR/TE 600/20) at the acromioclavicular joint. Note the continuity of the supraspinatus muscle and tendon (*arrow*) seen in this plane, and the high signal intensity subacromial and subdeltoid fat (*arrowheads*). *C,* Sagittal oblique plane at the level of the acromioclavicular joint. acj = acromioclavicular joint; BT = biceps tendon; C = coracoid; D = deltoid muscle; ISM = infraspinatus muscle; SCM = subscapularis muscle; SSM = supraspinatus muscle; TM = teres minor muscle; TR = trapezius muscle.

muscle and tendon, and these structures can be seen in continuity (see Fig. 3*B*). In the normal shoulder the subacromial-subdeltoid bursa represents a potential space and is depicted as a band of high signal intensity corresponding to the abundant fat located within and beneath its synovial lining (see Fig. 3*B*). This bursal complex lies between the rotator cuff tendons and the acromioclavicular joint and deltoid muscle. On the most anterior images, the coracoclavicular and coracohumeral ligaments, the subscapularis muscle, a long head of biceps tendon, and the superior and inferior labrum can also be identified.

The sagittal oblique plane also demonstrates the rotator cuff muscles. The anteroposterior extent of the rotator cuff tendons can be identified. The relationship of the acromion process to the supraspinatus tendon is also depicted.

ROTATOR CUFF ABNORMALITIES

Injuries of the rotator cuff tendons are usually chronic. It is recognized that normal tendons do not tear; 30 percent or more of a tendon must be damaged to produce a substantial reduction in its strength. Therefore, trauma may enlarge a preexisting tear but is rarely the initiating event.

It has been postulated that 95 percent of rotator cuff lesions result from chronic impingement of the supraspinatus tendon against the undersurface of the anterior third of the acromion, the coracoacromial ligament, and the acromioclavicular joint. Injury to the rotator cuff represents a continuum of disease that can be classified into three progressive pathologic stages beginning with edema and hemorrhage (stage I), progressing to inflammation and fibrosis (stage II), and culminating in rotator cuff tears (stage III).

Microangiographic studies have revealed an area of relative avascularity in the supraspinatus tendon 1 cm from the insertion site ("critical zone"); this is where most tendon ruptures occur. Mechanical impingement to this relatively avascular area leads to an inflammatory tendinitis, the first stage in the degenerative process. These reversible inflammatory changes may subsequently involve the acromioclavicular joint, subacromial bursa, and biceps tendon. Continued impingement leads to fibrosis with weakening of the tendon, and further tendinous attrition results in rotator cuff tears. Associated osseous changes, including spur formation about the acromioclavicular joint and the undersurface of the anterior aspect of the acromion, irregularity, sclerosis, and cyst formation in the posterolateral surface of the humeral head, may also occur.

Our experience and that of others indicate that MRI can demonstrate abnormalities in patients with the rotator cuff impingement syndrome. It can reveal tendon abnormalities (tendinitis) as well as rotator cuff tears.

In patients with tendinitis, high signal intensity is seen in the distal tendon and the cuff is intact (Fig. 4). This probably reflects the presence of increased free water within the tendon secondary to edema and inflammation. (This abnormal signal is usually best seen on T1-weighted and proton density images because of better contrast and signal-to-noise on these sequences.) The subdeltoid fat is preserved

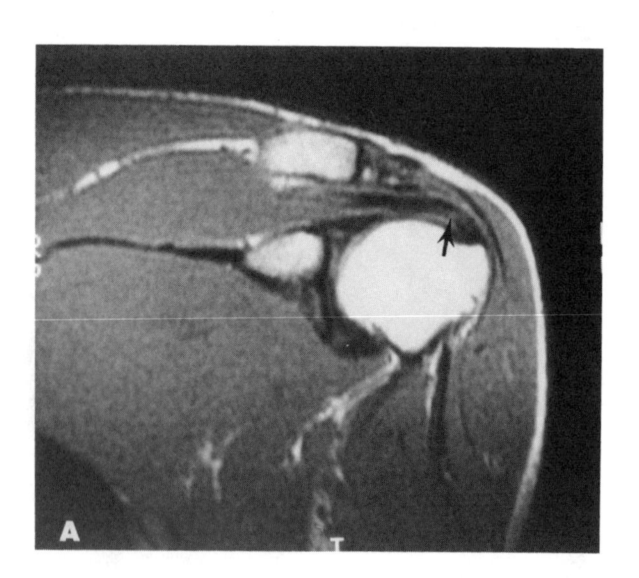

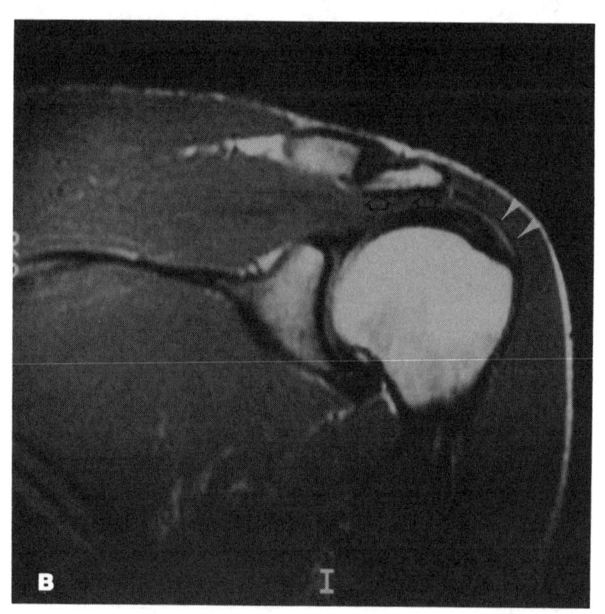

Figure 4 Tendinitis (TR/TE 1000/20). Increased signal intensity is seen in the distal supraspinatus tendon (*A*) (*arrow*), but the tendon is intact, as is the subdeltoid fat (*B*) (*arrowheads*). Note the low-lying acromion, which is narrowing the subacromial space (*B*) (*open arrows*).

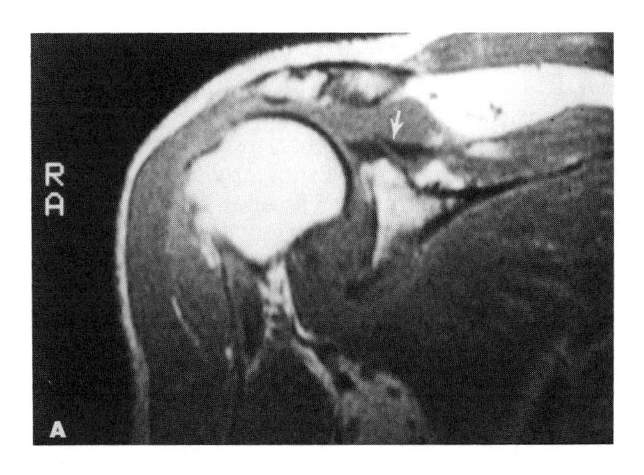

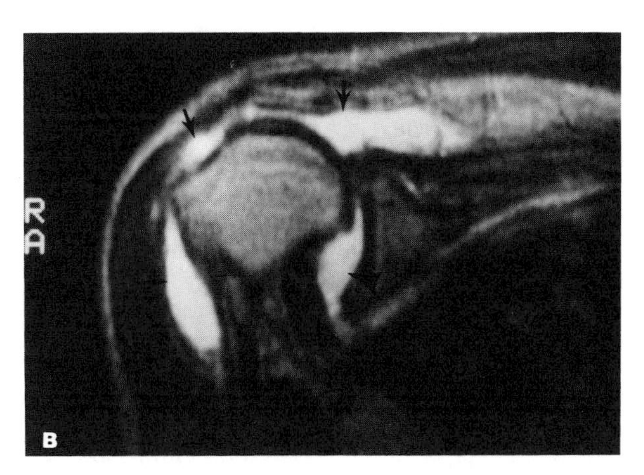

Figure 5 Large rotator cuff tear. *A,* Note the severe atrophy of the supraspinatus muscle, with marked retraction of the supraspinatus tendon (*arrow*) to the superior glenoid margin (TR/TE 1000/20). *B,* High signal intensity fluid (*arrows*) is seen in the subacromial-subdeltoid bursa and within the joint (*arrowhead*) (TR/TE 2500/80).

and no fluid is seen in the subacromial-subdeltoid bursa. In these patients, arthrographic results are normal, but those patients with this abnormality who came to surgery showed inflammation and degenerative changes within the tendon. Bone changes including subacromial spurs, as well as degenerative changes of the acromioclavicular joint and hypertrophy of its capsule, are often seen in these patients. Direct bone impingement on the supraspinatus musculotendinous junction can also be identified.

Small subacromial spurs are characterized by foci of signal void that project from the acromion tip. Large spurs frequently contain marrow and are seen as regions of bright signal continuous with the acromion, which may be surrounded by a rim of signal void representing cortical bone. The ability to image changes within the rotator cuff tendons noninvasively before a complete or partial tear takes place enables a treatment plan to be formulated on the basis of objective criteria.

Complete rotator cuff tears (Figs. 5 and 6) are manifested by loss of the homogeneous signal void or discontinuity of the rotator cuff tendons, usually the supraspinatus. Secondary signs include loss of the subdeltoid fat on T1-weighted and proton den-

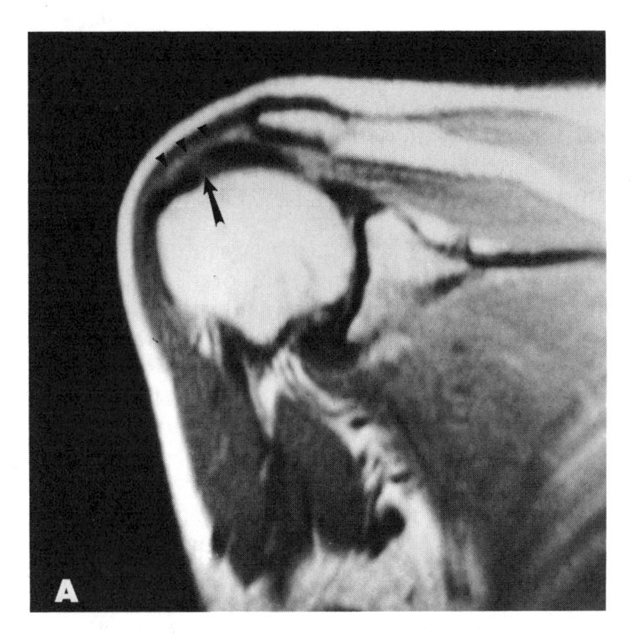

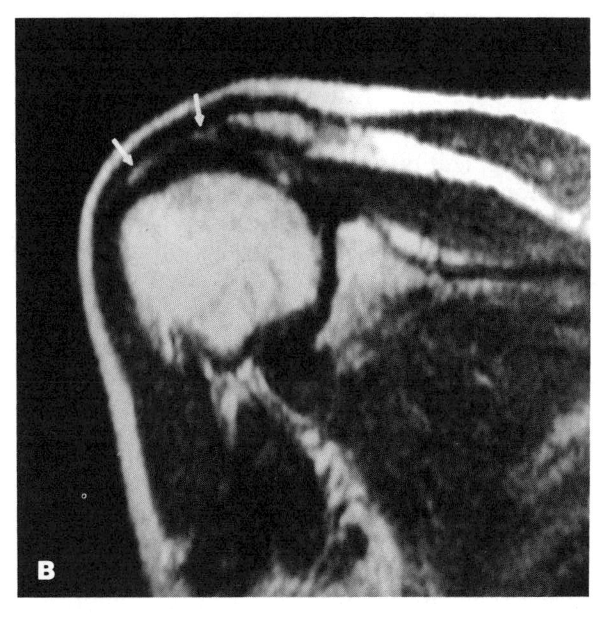

Figure 6 Small rotator cuff tear. *A,* A focus of increased signal intensity is seen within the distal supraspinatus tendon, representing a small tear (*arrow*). The subdeltoid fat signal is almost completely lost (*arrowheads*) (TR/TE 2500/20). *B,* The discontinuity in the supraspinatus tendon is less well seen owing to decreased signal-to-noise on this T2-weighted image (TR/TE 2500/80), but a small amount of high signal intensity fluid is seen in the subdeltoid bursa (*arrows*).

sity images. High signal is identified in the subacromial-subdeltoid bursa on T2-weighted images; this is thought to represent extension of intra-articular fluid through the tear into the subacromial-subdeltoid bursa. In chronic tears, there is often a decrease in muscle bulk and size and the presence of high signal linear bands within the muscle belly, indicative of atrophy. In patients with large tears, there is retraction of the supraspinatus muscle. Zlatkin and colleagues, using the above criteria, diagnosed all 12 surgically or arthrographically confirmed large or moderate-sized rotator cuff tears. Secondary bone changes were seen in five of these patients. The site, size, and extent of these tears, as well as the quality of the residual tendon fibers, can be assessed on the MR images.

Kneeland and co-workers studied 25 patients who had known or suspected tears of the rotator cuff. MRI visualized 20 of the 22 tears that were arthrographically or surgically confirmed. In most cases the tears were identified as a region of increased signal within the cuff on T2-weighted sequences. Kieft and colleagues and others found that the severity of tendon signal changes correlated with the presence of associated rotator cuff tears. The tendons with the most distortion of shape and the greatest amount of increased signal were most likely to have tears. These changes were most evident on T1-weighted images.

The necessity of distinguishing between the severe changes of tendinitis and tendon degeneration, partial tears, and small full-thickness tears in many cases depends on the treating orthopaedic surgeon. The MRI findings in patients with small tears and partial-thickness tears of the rotator cuff are preliminary, as many of these are treated conservatively and little surgical correlation exists. Early results, however, indicate that MRI can detect abnormalities in these patients. We believe that a small full-thickness rotator cuff tear can be diagnosed when a small segment of supraspinatus tendon is replaced by moderate or high signal. Frank discontinuity within the tendon may sometimes be identified. The subdeltoid fat signal is markedly diminished on T1-weighted images. On T2-weighted images the abnormal signal intensity within the tendon may increase, particularly if there is an associated effusion, and increased signal (representing fluid) may be present in the subacromial-subdeltoid bursa.

There are no definitively established criteria to distinguish partial- from full-thickness tears. In the study of Kneeland and colleagues, the MRI appearance of two surgically confirmed partial-thickness tears was similar to that of full-thickness tears. In our limited experience, partial tears of the inferior surface may appear as irregular areas of increased signal, thinning of the undersurface of the tendon, or focal areas of increased signal within the tendon. The subdeltoid fat is usually not preserved in patients with partial rotator cuff tears.

CAPSULAR ABNORMALITIES

The anterior capsular mechanism of the shoulder consists of the synovial membrane, the capsule and glenohumeral ligaments, the labrum, the subscapularis bursa, and the subscapularis muscle and tendon. Lesions of the capsular mechanism are thought to be the most important factor in the development of shoulder instability. Abnormalities of the capsular mechanism and associated structures occur predominantly in patients with a history of recurrent subluxations and dislocations. The spectrum of abnormalities of this mechanism that have been observed clinically and experimentally, in association with recurrent glenohumeral joint subluxations and dislocations, includes capsule and labral tears and detachments, the formation of a large anterior pouch, and laxity of the subscapularis muscle and tendon. Bone defects, particularly the Hill-Sachs lesion, may also be present.

In a laboratory study of cadaveric shoulder specimens subjected to recurrent shoulder subluxations and dislocations, MRI proved capable of demonstrating abnormalities and tears of the glenoid labrum. Three studies have demonstrated the efficacy of conventional MRI in depicting labral pathology. Findings associated with derangement of the labrum include focal or diffusely increased signal, blunting, fraying, and attenuation (Fig. 7*B*).

The normal anterior capsule and glenohumeral ligaments appear as homogeneous dark bands adjacent to, and at times difficult to separate from, the subscapularis tendon. The subscapularis bursa also is usually not seen unless there is an effusion. In the presence of joint fluid, however, these glenohumeral ligaments, as well as other folds of capsular tissue, may be seen as separate structures and should not be confused with pathologic lesions.

Three types of anterior capsule have been described. MRI can define the particular type of capsule, depending on its insertion site: type I inserts into or near the labrum; types II and III insert more broadly along the scapular neck. The posterior capsule inserts directly into the labrum. The type III capsule is thought to be either a predisposing factor for or a sequela of recurrent dislocations. This large "anterior pouch" has been identified with CT arthrography and can be depicted on MRI (Fig. 7*B*), but is best seen in the presence of joint fluid, particularly on T2-weighted images. A distorted appearance of the capsular insertion into the glenoid, with either loss or thickening of the intervening soft tissue layer over the scapular margin, may be seen as well. Seeger and colleagues also found that patients with a history of recurrent dislocations may show evidence of abnormal medium signal intensity in the subscapularis tendon, which these authors believed represented a sign of anterior capsular trauma. Hill-Sachs lesions are identified as large, wedge-shaped defects on the posterolateral surface of the humeral head (Fig. 7*A*).

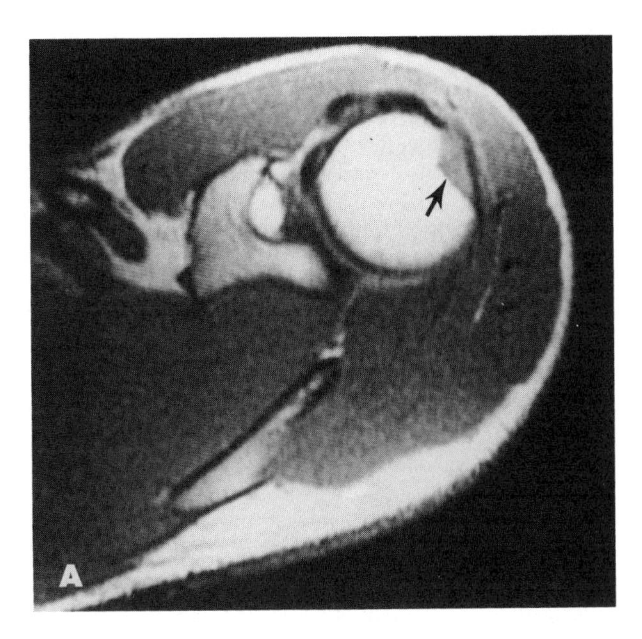

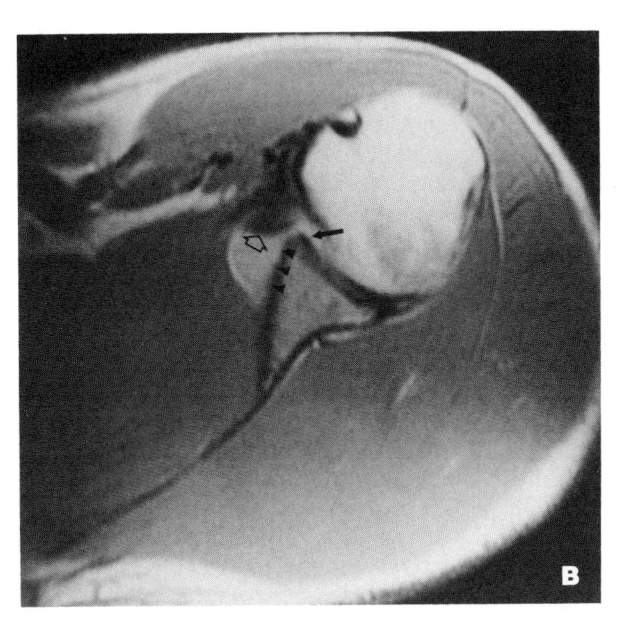

Figure 7 Shoulder instability. *A*, Axial image (TR/TE 600/20) at the superior glenoid level demonstrating a large Hill-Sachs deformity (*arrows*). *B*, Axial image at the midglenoid level (TR/TE 2500/20) showing complete absence of the anterior labrum (*arrow*) with a stripped and anteriorly bowed capsule (*arrowheads*). Note the prominent middle glenohumeral ligament (*open arrow*).

Although at the present time CT arthrography is considered the procedure of choice in patients with a history of recurrent subluxations and dislocations, the ability of MRI to define many of the structural changes seen in patients with clinically significant shoulder instability may eventually allow MRI to replace CT arthrography in studying such patients, since it is noninvasive. This awaits the results of comparative studies of these two modalities.

MISCELLANEOUS ABNORMALITIES

Infectious and Inflammatory Disease

The glenohumeral joint is commonly involved in patients with systemic inflammatory diseases involving the synovium, particularly rheumatoid arthritis (Fig. 8) and ankylosing spondylitis. Loss of articular cartilage and osseous erosions may be visualized with conventional radiography, but MRI may show soft tissue changes and early erosions not seen on conventional radiography. MRI can also depict rotator cuff tears and giant synovial cysts noninvasively. In septic arthritis, MRI can detect intra-articular fluid, abnormal articular cartilage, and associated bone destruction. Localized monoarticular inflammatory diseases such as pigmented villonodular synovitis (PVNS) and synovial osteochondromatosis are easily evaluated. In patients with PVNS, MRI can demonstrate effusions, erosions, and hemosiderin deposition. The pigmented nodules containing hemosiderin have low signal intensity on short and long TR/TE sequences. They are seen best on gradient echo scans because of the paramagnetic effects of hemosiderin. Unfortunately, this is not specific, because hemosiderin deposits, erosions, and effusions can also occur in rheumatoid arthritis and hemophilia.

Trauma

MRI has been helpful in the evaluation of other post-traumatic disorders, including hematomas

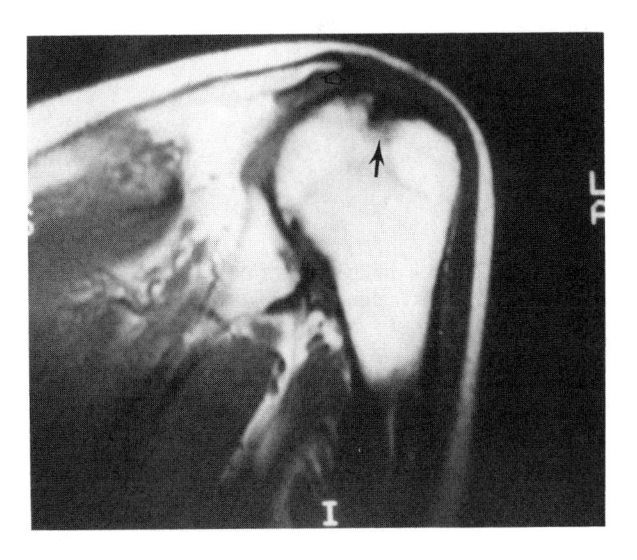

Figure 8 Rheumatoid arthritis. T1-weighted image (TR/TE 600/20) demonstrating humeral head erosion (*arrow*), a narrowed distal clavicle (*open arrow*), marked muscle atrophy, and no visible rotator cuff tendon.

and dislocation of the acromioclavicular joint. In the presence of complicated fractures, or fractures in areas difficult to visualize well with conventional radiography, such as the scapula, the multiplanar capability of MRI can be useful in assessing the extent and location of the abnormalities, and may help to depict involvement of the glenohumeral joint.

Osteonecrosis

MRI has achieved wide clinical acceptance in the early diagnosis of osteonecrosis, since it is more sensitive than plain films or radionuclide imaging. Although we are not aware of specific studies of avascular necrosis in the shoulder, there is no reason to believe that the same findings should not hold true. The appearance of osteonecrosis in the shoulder is similar to that in other joints, with decreased signal intensity at the articular surface in the humeral head due to replacement of fatty marrow (Fig. 9). The addition of high-resolution studies with surface coils can assess the presence of articular collapse and assess the status of the overlying glenohumeral articular cartilage.

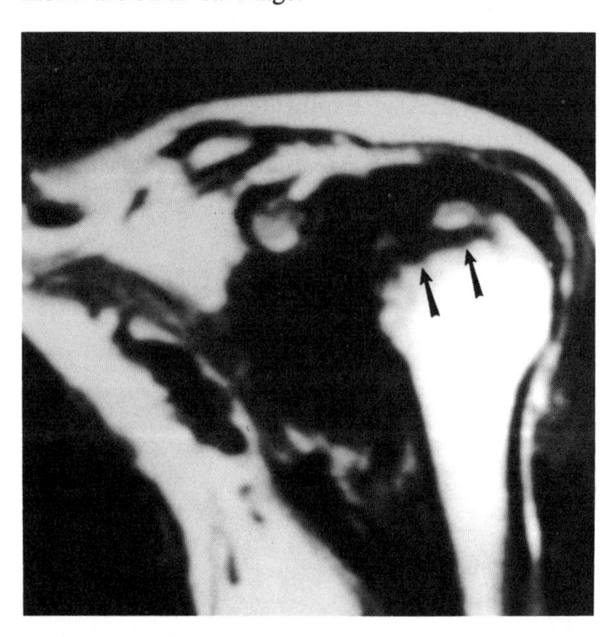

Figure 9 Coronal image performed in the body coil (TR/TE 600/20) revealing a decreased signal in the marrow of the articular surface of the humeral head consistent with avascular necrosis (*arrows*).

Neoplasms

MRI can be used in the staging of tumors about the shoulder, where it can assess the extent of marrow involvement and soft tissue mass and determine the relation of the tumor to the axillary vessels and nerves.

SUGGESTED READING

Cofield RH. Rotator cuff disease of the shoulder. J Bone Joint Surg 1985; 67A:974–979.

Goldman AB, Ghelman B. The double-contrast shoulder arthrogram: a review of 158 studies. Radiology 1978; 127:655–663.

Hall FM, Rosenthal DI, Goldberg RP, Wyshak G. Morbidity from shoulder arthrography: etiology, incidence and prevention. AJR 1981; 136:59–62.

Hoult D, Richards RE. The NMR receiver: a description and analysis of design. Prog NMR Spectroscopy 1978; 12:41–47.

Kieft GJ, Bloem JL, Obermann WR, et al. Normal shoulder: MR imaging. Radiology 1986; 159:741–745.

Kieft GH, Bloem JL, Rozing PM, Oberman WR. Rotator cuff impingement syndrome: MR imaging. Radiology 1988; 166:211–214.

Kieft GH, Bloem JL, Rozing PM, Oberman WR. MR imaging of recurrent anterior dislocations of the shoulder: comparison with CT arthrography. AJR 1988; 150:1083–1087.

Kneeland JB, Middleton WD, Carrera GF, et al. MR imaging of the shoulder: diagnosis of rotator cuff tears. AJR 1987; 149:333–337.

Mink JH, Harris E, Rappaport M. Rotator cuff tears: evaluation using double-contrast shoulder arthrography. Radiology 1985; 157:621–623.

Moseley HG, Overgaard B. The anterior capsular mechanism in recurrent anterior dislocation of the shoulder: morphological and clinical studies with special reference to the glenoid labrum and the glenohumeral ligaments. J Bone Joint Surg 1962; 44B:913–927.

Neer CS III, Craig EV, Fukuda H. Cuff-tear arthropathy. J Bone Joint Surg 1983; 65A:1232–1244.

Rafii M, Firooznia H, Golimbu C, et al. CT arthrography of capsular structures of the shoulder. AJR 1986; 146:361–367.

Rothman RH, Marvel JP, Heppenstall RB. Anatomic considerations in the glenohumeral joints. Orthop Clin North Am 1975; 6:341–352.

Seeger LL, Gold RH, Bassett LW, Ellman HE. Shoulder instability: evaluation with magnetic resonance imaging. Radiology 1988; 166:205–209.

Seeger LL, Gold RH, Bassett LW, Ellman H. Shoulder impingement syndrome: MR findings in 53 shoulders. AJR 1988; 50:343–347.

Zlatkin MB, Bjorkengren AG, Gylys-Morin V, et al. Cross-sectional imaging of the capsular mechanism of the glenohumeral joint. AJR 1988; 150:151–158.

Zlatkin MB, Reicher MA, Kellerhouse LI, et al. The painful shoulder: MR imaging of the glenhumeral joint. J Comput Assist Tomogr 1988; 12:995–1001.

ROTATOR CUFF TEARS

RICHARD J. HAWKINS, M.D.
SANFORD S. KUNKEL, M.D.

The management of rotator cuff tears has been a controversial issue for many years. In the athlete, this pathologic condition presents a unique and challenging problem.

The etiology, pathophysiology, and treatment may depend on the athlete's level of competition. For rotator cuff tears, partial or complete, patients may be divided into three main categories: the recreational athlete, the competitive athlete, and the high-profile athlete who participates in overhead activities such as throwing, tennis, and swimming. The cause and therefore the treatment of these categories may be different. However, there is considerable overlap between each of these levels of participation.

FUNCTIONAL ANATOMY AND PATHOLOGY

Rotator cuff tears may be partial or complete and may be associated with other pathologic conditions such as bicipital and acromioclavicular joint involvement. The classical functional anatomy and pathology relating to complete-thickness rotator cuff tears has been that of impingement, as described by Neer. It is important to recognize other etiologies, in particular that partial and degenerative cuff tears can result from eccentric overload, especially in the presence of loose shoulders and anterior subluxation of the shoulder with secondary impingement.

Impingement

Neer has taught us that the functional arc of elevation of the shoulder is forward, and that impingement occurs predominantly against the anteroinferior edge of the acromion and coracoacromial ligament. Jobe pointed out that in overhead athletic activities, particularly those of high-level throwers and swimmers, impingement also occurs against the lateral acromion. Appreciation of these concepts forms the basis for decompression and in part explains the etiology of rotator cuff tears. Rathbun and Macnab injected micropaque dye into the subclavian artery to demonstrate the vascular compromise of the supraspinatus and biceps tendon. With the arm at the side, the blood supply of the rotator cuff is compromised in the area adjacent to the insertion of the supraspinatus into the greater tuberosity. Authors have described several variations in the shape and geometry of the acromion that may predispose to impingement tendinitis and subsequent rotator cuff tears. These three factors may contribute to the occurrence of impingement and subsequent rotator cuff tears.

Progression of pathology and the impingement process involves an initial tendinitis followed by wear and tear with scarring of the subacromial bursa, resulting in degeneration and partial- and finally complete-thickness rotator cuff tears. Most authors believe that the majority of full-thickness rotator cuff tears are the result of chronic impingement.

Neer classified the impingement process as follows:

Stage I: edema and hemorrhage (at any age).

Stage II: fibrosis and tendinitis (usually in individuals over 25 years of age).

Stage III: degeneration, bone changes, and tendon ruptures (usually in patients over 40 years of age).

A rotator cuff tear in the weekend recreational athlete usually follows the classic impingement process described by Neer. There is often a long history of shoulder pain consistent with impingement tendinitis that results in a rotator cuff tear. The natural history of rotator cuff tears is unknown, and athletes with these injuries have difficulty resuming their sporting activity.

The high-profile competitive athlete with a rotator cuff tear often has a different presentation. The cuff tear can develop over a much shorter time and at a younger age because of repetitive use of the shoulder. With repetitive overhead use such as in swimming and tennis, the musculature stabilizing the scapula may suffer fatigue, leading to a scapular lag. As the arm is brought in the overhead position, the scapula and acromion fail to elevate owing to the muscle fatigue, which leads to a jamming of the greater tuberosity under the anterior and lateral undersurface of the acromion. These patients usually have partial or very small rotator cuff tears.

In both competitive nonthrowing athletes and high-profile athletes who participate in overhead activities, there may be an architectural set-up associated with overuse that results in impingement degeneration and a rotator cuff tear. It is important to establish this etiology in considering the athletic population, because it dictates the choice of treatment.

Eccentric Overload

As in other areas of the body, rotator cuff tendons may be subjected to eccentric overload. With a compromised blood supply and constant overuse of the rotator cuff tendons, substance degenerative tears can result from this mechanism. This is particularly so in high-profile athletes who participate in overhead activities. There may be some overlap relating eccentric overload to impingement tendinitis in many athletes.

Anterior Subluxation and Impingement

The high-profile, overhead-throwing athlete may present with secondary impingement due to anterior instability. With repetitive overhead throwing the shoulder is subjected again to chronic eccentric overload, particularly during the follow-through phase of throwing. Over time this leads to stretching and relaxation of the posterior capsulotendinous structures of the shoulder. Minor anterior subluxation ensues, followed by superior migration of the humeral head, predisposing to a secondary impingement of the cuff structures under the coracoacromial ligament and anterior acromion. Pathology in the cuff is usually limited to partial-thickness tears of a degenerative nature. It is important to understand this mechanism in relation to surgical considerations. The approach for this condition, if surgery is considered, is anterior stabilization without decompression; when impingement is involved, decompression is part of the surgical rationale.

It should be appreciated that the etiology and presentation of degenerative and full-thickness rotator cuff tears in the athlete relate to the population under study. Orthopaedic surgeons who deal with high-profile throwing athletes note a much larger causative incidence of eccentric overload and anterior subluxation, whereas those who handle recreational athletes note a relatively higher incidence of impingement as a causative and initiating factor. It follows, therefore, that the treatment differs.

DIAGNOSIS

Weekend recreational athletes usually present with a prolonged history of shoulder problems, beginning with pain following the inciting activity and continuing with pain so severe that they are unable to compete at the level to which they are accustomed. Symptoms may manifest as minimal or severe aching pain, often worse at night, frequently prohibiting work and sporting activities and sometimes affecting everyday pursuits. Full-thickness rotator cuff tears in these patients show an extremely variable pattern of pain, range of motion, and strength. True weakness is the hallmark of a full-thickness tear, but pain may preclude an accurate assessment of strength. There often is point tenderness over the greater tuberosity and anterior acromion; a painful arc of abduction, maximal at 90 degrees; and often increased pain with resistance at this level. The impingement sign, as described by Neer and Welsh, reproduces the pain and resultant facial expression when the arm is in neutral rotation and forcefully flexed forward by the examiner, jamming the greater tuberosity against the anteroinferior surface of the acromion. Atrophy of the spinati is often present, especially if the cuff tear is long-standing.

The complaints of high-profile competitive athletes often are limited to pain and weakness related to their sporting activity. Classic night pain and pain at rest may be absent. Because of improved conditioning and overall strength of the shoulder, weakness may be extremely difficult to detect. These patients are often younger than weekend recreational athletes, and their cuff tears and symptom complex may develop over a much shorter time. In this setting, the integrity of the rotator cuff is best determined by arthrography, ultrasonography, or arthroscopy.

A rotator cuff tear, especially a partial tear in the high-profile overhead-throwing athlete, can be extremely difficult to diagnose. Complaints are usually limited to pain and fatigue related to the sporting activity. High-level pitchers may complain of pain only after pitching seven or eight innings. Physical findings may be subtle and difficult to appreciate. In these athletes, anterior subluxation may be responsible for the secondary impingement and partial cuff tear. With the patient supine and the arm abducted and externally rotated, upward pressure on the arm may reproduce the symptom complex with increased pain. Posterior pressure then alleviates the discomfort. The classic apprehension sign (fear of the shoulder coming out of joint) is often absent. The impingement sign described by Neer and Welsh may or may not be present.

ASSOCIATED PROBLEMS

Bicipital Tendinitis

Involvement of the biceps tendon is usually part of the impingement process and often is associated with rotator cuff tears. Treatment, whether operative or nonoperative, should be directed toward the rotator cuff. Biceps tendinitis may occur in the absence of the impingement process, especially in throwers.

Acromioclavicular Joint Pathology

In the later stages of impingement, the acromioclavicular joint and supraspinatus outlet may be involved in the same process. Spurring of the undersurface of the acromioclavicular joint or degeneration of the joint itself often accompanies rotator cuff tears. Isolated acromioclavicular joint problems can be handled by injection of local anesthetic into the acromioclavicular joint, resulting in resolution of symptoms. An old acromioclavicular injury may result in pain emanating solely from that joint.

Glenoid Labrum Complex Lesions

Glenoid labrum lesions (e.g., Bankart) have been described, with gross instability of the shoulder. The Bankart lesion can be a small labral detachment or a large, even bucket-handle type of tear. In addition to the complaints of instability, patients may describe a painful catching in the shoulder or a snapping sensation during the throwing motion. An associated history of instability and an apprehension sign are helpful diagnostic clues.

Superior quadrant labral tears have been described in association with eccentric overloading of the biceps tendon and subsequent avulsion of the superior part of the labrum during the follow-through phase of throwing. These lesions have been visualized during arthroscopy in some high-profile throwing athletes. They may be associated with undersurface degenerative tears of the rotator cuff. Debridement has been employed with some success. If impingement is not the cause in these athletes, debridement offers a greater chance of success.

Jobe described changes in the posterior glenoid labrum together with external rotation on the humeral head as the "kissing lesion." This is in association with extreme external rotation, the humeral head abutting against the labrum during the cocking phase of throwing. This is the key arthroscopic change to diagnose anterior instability with secondary impingement as underlying pathology. The approach in these patients is to treat the anterior instability; decompression alone may prove inadequate.

TREATMENT

Treatment depends on the underlying etiology, whether it be impingement related, eccentric overload, or anterior instability with secondary impingement. It also relates to whether the patient is a recreational athlete, a competitive athlete, or an overhead-throwing athlete. Treatment also depends on whether the tear is presumed to be a partial degenerative tear or a complete-thickness rotator cuff tear.

Treatment of the recreational weekend athlete is similar to that of the nonathletic population. A period of rest and avoidance of overhead activity is recommended, in conjunction with nonsteroidal anti-inflammatory medications. Physiotherapy is instituted to maintain range of motion and strength of the shoulder. Patients often respond well to this regimen, but a return to competitive athletics is often difficult. If patients have continuing pain refractory to conservative therapy, operative treatment may be indicated. Surgery is performed primarily for the relief of pain and secondarily for functional improvement. Surgery is never undertaken for the one purpose of return to sports or work, although this is sometimes possible. Surgical treatment of rotator cuff tears in athletes follows the same principles established for the nonathletic population. Adequate decompression, secure rotator cuff repair, and restoration of the deltoid are imperative for success. Partial and small cuff tears (less than 1 cm) are occasionally repaired in a side-to-side or end-to-end fashion. Larger tears should be repaired to a trough in bone.

Treatment of high-profile competitive athletes should be nonoperative whenever possible, especially since most tears in this population are partial and may not be the direct result of impingement. In addition to modification of activities and prescription of medications, patients undergo ultrasonography over the cuff tendons and biceps to increase local blood supply and diminish the inflammatory response. Local steroid injection into the subacromial bursa may temporarily improve the impingement process. Care should be taken to inject the steroid into the subacromial bursa, avoiding the rotator cuff. Collagen necrosis and decreased strength to failure exists in tendons injected with steroid for at least 2 weeks after injection; athletes should therefore be protected from strenuous activity for this period. Local heat before work-outs to increase the blood supply and subsequent flexibility of muscle tendon units is used in conjunction with ice immediately after work-outs to decrease the inflammatory response. Physical therapy emphasizes strengthening of the external rotators and stabilizers of the scapula. External rotation exercises against resistance, and push-ups with the hands together in the midline, strengthen the external rotators and scapular stabilizers, respectively. Athletes can also modify their activity by rotating the trunk during the overhead phase of the shoulder motion.

The purpose of surgery for this group of athletes is to relieve pain unresponsive to nonoperative treatment, functional improvement being a secondary goal. Surgical principles follow those previously mentioned for decompression.

Recently, there has been interest in arthroscopic debridement of partial tears of the undersurface of the rotator cuff. These are frequently associated with superior labral tears and bicipital involvement. In the absence of impingement, this may prove helpful. This operative procedure might apply only to a small, select patient population.

Treatment therefore depends on the underlying etiology. Nonoperative therapy is appropriate. Full-thickness tears generally should be treated surgically. Anterior subluxation requires anterior stabilization. Partial tears may be approached differently, depending on the underlying etiology. We are learning about the use of arthroscopy and its therapeutic applications in the throwing athlete, and long-term studies are required.

RESULTS

Hawkins reported an 86 percent incidence of relief of pain after surgical treatment of rotator cuff tears, regardless of the size of the tear. Most patients believed themselves to be stronger after the operation, but slightly more than half still had demonstrable weakness on follow-up examination. Generally, the smaller the tear, the more likely is a full recovery of strength. Most of the patients in this study were not athletes. Other authors reported satisfactory or excellent relief of pain in 58 to 85 percent of their patients.

Tibone and Jobe reported on 33 athletes surgically treated for the impingement syndrome by anterior acromioplasty; 89 percent were subjectively judged to be improved over the preoperative status. In only 15 of the 35 shoulders operated on (43 percent) was there a return to the same pain-free injury level as in competitive athletics. Only four of 18 athletes involved in pitching and throwing returned to their former preinjury status; these individuals did not have cuff tears.

Tibone and Jobe also described 45 athletes with either a partial or complete tear of the rotator cuff treated by anterior acromioplasty and repair of the tear. Eighty-seven percent of their patients said they were improved, although only 76 percent described a significant reduction of pain postoperatively. Fifty-six percent were rated as having good results that allowed them to return to their former competitive level without significant pain. Forty-one percent who had been involved in pitching and throwing returned to their former competitive status. Only 32 percent of pitchers and throwers who had been active at professional or collegiate level returned to the same competitive level. Of these authors' 45 patients, all but two had small tears that were repaired in a direct side-to-side suturing; these two were repaired to a trough into bone in the greater tuberosity.

Jobe reports that a decompressive procedure may worsen the instability in throwing athletes. Early results of Jobe's recent procedure to stabilize the shoulder in throwing athletes are encouraging. Again, the basis of an understanding of surgical treatment of rotator cuff tears, partial or complete, relates to the underlying cause (i.e., eccentric overload, impingement, or anterior subluxation).

The results of surgical debridement by arthroscopy in high-profile throwers, especially for partial degenerative tears, may be helpful.

REHABILITATION

Postoperative rehabilitation after rotator cuff surgery consists of passive range-of-motion exercises in the first postoperative week. Active range-of-motion exercises are initiated when healing of the cuff is thought to be secure, usually at 6 weeks. Terminal stretching and resistance exercises are added to the program when active range of motion can be performed comfortably, usually 8 weeks after surgery. If there is excessive tension on the repair, the arm is held in an abduction pillow or splint for 4 to 6 weeks. Assisted elevation and abduction above the pillow is begun in the early postoperative period. Emphasis is placed on elevation, external rotation, and internal rotation. A physiotherapy program is continued for a minimum of 1 year postoperatively. Patients must be told that the shoulder will not function comfortably before 6 months have elapsed. Athletes usually are not allowed to resume participation in sports until 6 months postoperatively.

After decompression in a rotator cuff repair, whether partial or complete, in the competitive athlete or high-profile overhead throwing athlete, a prolonged period of rehabilitation and an adequate time for healing are required.

In the high-profile, overhead-throwing athlete, surgical trauma to the anterior musculature of the shoulder is kept to a minimum. The arm is supported in an abduction pillow or splint for 4 to 6 weeks so that scarring between the subscapularis and capsule does not cause a loss of external rotation. Pitchers generally require up to a full year of rehabilitation before they can resume competitive throwing.

Rehabilitation after arthroscopic debridement of the shoulder is fairly rapid, allowing patients to proceed immediately with stretching, active, and resisted exercises in the first weeks after surgery. A period of rest, perhaps weeks or months is still needed before return to the field of competition; this depends on whether the patient is involved in overhead activities or not.

SUGGESTED READING

Andrews JR, Carson WG, McLeod WD. Glenoid labrum tears related to the long head of the biceps. Am J Sports Med 1985; 13:337.

Aoki M, Ishii S, Usui M, Mizuguchi M. The slope of the acromion and rotator cuff impingement. Orthop Trans 1986; 10:228.

Bankart AS. The pathology and treatment of recurrent dislocation of the shoulder joint. Br J Surg 1938; 26:23.

Batemen JE. The shoulder and neck. Philadelphia, WB Saunders, 1972.

Bigliani LU, Morrison DS, Arpil EW. The morphology of the acromion and its relationship to rotator cuff tears. Orthop Trans 1986; 10:228.

Debeyre J, Patte D, Elmelik E. Repair of ruptures of the rotator cuff of the shoulder with a note on advancement of the supraspinatus muscle. J Bone Joint Surg 1949; 47B:436.

Godsil RD, Linscheid RL. Intratendinous defects of the rotator cuff. Clin Orthop 1970; 69:181.

Hawkins RJ, Kennedy JC. The impingement syndrome in athletes. Am J Sports Med 1980; 8:57.

Hawkins RJ, Misamore MD, Hobeika PE. Surgery for full thickness rotator cuff tears. J Bone Joint Surg 1985; 67A:1349.

Heikel HV. Rupture of the rotator cuff of the shoulder: experiences of surgical treatment. Acta Orthop Scand 1968; 39:477.

Jackson DW. Chronic rotator cuff impingement in the throwing athlete. Am J Sports Med 1976; 4:231.

Johansson JE, Barrington TW. Coracoacromial ligament division. Am J Sports Med 1984; 12:138.

Kennedy JC, Willis RB. The effects of local steroid injection on tendons: a biomechanical and microscopic correlative study. Am J Sports Med 1976; 4:11.

McLaughlin HL. Rupture of the rotator cuff. J Bone Joint Surg 1962; 44A:979.

Neer CS. Anterior acromioplasty for chronic impingement syndrome in the shoulder: a preliminary report. J Bone Joint Surg 1972; 54A:41.

Neer CS, Welsh RP. The shoulder in sports. Orthop Clin North Am 1977; 8:583.

Penny JN, Welsh RP. Shoulder impingement syndromes in athletes and their surgical management. Am J Sports Med 1981; 9:11.

Peterson C. Long-term results of rotator cuff repair. In: Bailey JI, Kessel L, eds. Shoulder surgery. Berlin: Springer, 1982.

Rathbun JB, Macnab I. The microvascular pattern of the rotator cuff. J Bone Joint Surg 1970; 52B:540.

Samilson RL, Binder WF. Symptomatic full thickness tears of the rotator cuff: an analysis of 292 shoulders in 276 patients. Orthop Clin North Am 1975; 6:449.

Simon WH. Soft tissue disorders of the shoulder: frozen shoulder, calcific tendinitis, and bicipital tendinitis. Orthop Clin North Am 1975; 6:521.

Tibone JE, Elrod B, Jobe FW, et al. Surgical treatment of tears of the rotator cuff in athletes. J Bone Joint Surg 1986; 68A:887.

Tibone JE, Jobe FW, Kerlin RK, et al. Shoulder impingement syndrome in athletes treated by anterior acromioplasty. Clin Orthop 1985; 198:134.

ANTERIOR GLENOHUMERAL SUBLUXATION/ DISLOCATION: THE BANKART PROCEDURE

CARTER R. ROWE, M.D.

Recurrent instability of the shoulder in an athlete can be a very disabling condition, as the athlete's requirements are strength of the shoulder in all positions of motion, whether in football or ice hockey, which expose the shoulder to maximal body contact, or throwing or racquet sports, in which the need is for rapid and rhythmic coordination of the shoulder. Table 1 lists the different types of shoulder instability. This chapter discusses the traumatic and the transient subluxation (types I and II).

DIAGNOSIS

The diagnosis of a complete traumatic anterior dislocation can be accurately made if there is a subacromial defect, the arm is held in external rotation, and roentgenograms clearly reveal the dislocated head. Diagnosis of a transient subluxation, however, is more difficult, as radiographs do not reveal the diagnosis, but the history and physical findings are consistent. The patient is usually a young adult athlete whose shoulder has been injured by forceful overextension of the arm in elevation, and who on examination shows the typical "apprehension" test results (Fig. 1). Blazina and Satzman first reported

TABLE 1 Types of Shoulder Instability

Types of Shoulder Instability
Traumatic
Complete dislocation
Most common
Subgroup
Transient subluxation ("dead arm" syndrome)
Forceful overextension of arm in elevation and external rotation
Atraumatic
Incurred by functional use of arm
Voluntary
Incurred by muscle control
Involuntary Subluxation
Instability due to chronic laxity of tissues
May be multidirectional

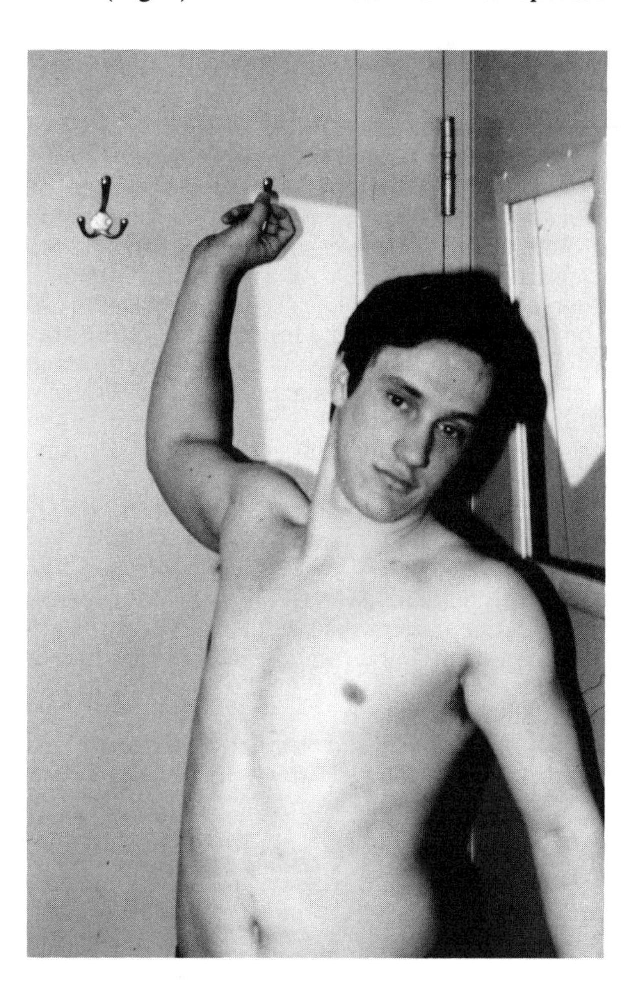

Figure 1 The patient's sudden shoulder pain is reproduced when the arm is in elevation and external rotation in the throwing position. This is referred to as the "apprehension" position.

their experience with transient subluxation of the shoulder in the athlete in 1969. In 1981 Rowe and Zarins identified two types of transient subluxation. In one group, patients were aware of the shoulder momentarily slipping out when the arm was in elevation, such as in throwing or swimming. In the other group, patients were *not* aware of the shoulder slipping out in those motions, but only of a sudden severe pain, which left the shoulder momentarily weak, or "dead." Quarterbacks are unable to throw the "long bomb," baseball players cannot throw out a base runner, and tennis players lose their ace serve. X-ray results are usually normal. Often, patients are confused and depressed, because their problem has not been diagnosed and treatment has not been effective. The "apprehension" test is a consistent physical finding. In this position, the patient's symptoms are reproduced. The arm is elevated and externally rotated, usually in the throwing position. Care must be taken, however, to rule out other conditions such as impingement syndrome, rotator cuff tears, instability of the biceps tendon, or thoracic outlet syndromes, all of which may mimic transient subluxation.

PATHOLOGY

It is generally agreed that there is no one essential lesion in shoulder instability. However, the Bankart lesion (avulsion of the capsule and labrum from the anterior glenoid rim) is the most common causative factor (Table 2). The Bankart lesion is found mostly in complete traumatic dislocation of the shoulder, whereas the lesion in the subluxating shoulder is usually seen in increased laxity or redundancy of the capsule. Damage to the glenoid rim and Hill-Sachs lesions are also more frequently found in complete traumatic dislocation, since added trauma is experienced in this group.

TREATMENT

Many patients wish to know whether there is any treatment other than surgery. This is a logical question. Considering the overall classification of shoulder instabilities (see Table 1), specific resistive exercises are more effective in the atraumatic, voluntary, involuntary, and especially multidirectional groups than in complete traumatic dislocations or traumatic transient subluxations. Of the 50 traumatic transient subluxations in the series of Rowe and Zarins, only 10 responded to exercises; five were graded excellent, three good, and two fair. The remainder were treated surgically.

TABLE 2 Causative Lesions

	Traumatic Complete Dislocations (%)	*Transient Subluxations* (%)
Bankart lesions	85	64
Redundancy of capsule	15	26
Damage to glenoid rim	73	45
Hill-Sachs lesions	77	40

Surgical Treatment

For the athlete who requires maximal strength of the arm in all positions and in forceful contact, we prefer the Bankart procedure for the following reasons:

1. The exposure is anatomic, layer by layer down to the glenoid rim. In this way the various anatomic causative lesions may be identified and corrected. The muscle layers are then returned anatomically to their origins.
2. No muscles are compromised by transplantation. No muscles are traumatized by division or perforation.
3. No metal is used, such as screws and staples, which in contact sports may break or loosen and sometimes travel into the joint or toward the chest wall.
4. The approach is adjustable, so that when a Bankart lesion *is* present, the capsule can be reattached to the entire anterior glenoid rim, where the focus of strength is needed. This also gives more strength than a one-point fixation of reattachment.
5. When a Bankart lesion is *not* present, the cause of the instability is usually a redundant or lax capsule. Since the capsule has been exposed by this procedure, no change in the surgical exposure and no additional incision are necessary. A capsulorrhaphy can be carried out by taking up the laxity of the capsule, and double-breasting the repair along the anterior and inferior glenoid. If the patient also has evidence of multidirectional instability, the posterior capsule can be tightened from this exposure, eliminating the necessity of making a second posterior exposure.
6. Although holes (usually three in the Bankart procedure) are made through the rim of the glenoid (high, mid, and low), the perforations are covered by the smooth capsule, eliminating postoperative traumatic changes of the joint. No traumatic changes have been noted in our follow-up study over a 30-year period.
7. One of the most desirable features of the Bankart procedure is that, in cases of recurrent postoperative dislocations from subsequent injury, the muscle layers are not a mass of scar tissue or in poor condition for reuse, but are preserved and can be safely and effectively used again.

Surgical Technique

For a complete up-to-date review and follow-up of the Bankart procedure, the reader is referred to Rowe's textbook, *The Shoulder.* This chapter discusses the high points and adjustability of the Bankart procedure.

1. The shoulder is exposed through the deltopectoral plane. The deltoid is not removed. The cephalic vein is not ligated.

2. Osteotomy of the coracoid process is optional (Fig. 2). The advantages of osteotomy include less traction on the attached tendons to the coracoid and to the musculocutaneous nerve, and greater exposure of the subscapularis muscles and the joint. The advantages of not osteotomizing the coracoid include earlier use and function of the shoulder, and less chance of nonunion (although we have had only one nonunion in 40 years). In a heavy-muscled football player who wants as early a return of function as possible, one may proceed without osteotomizing the coracoid. However, if better exposure is needed during the surgery, an osteotomy of the coracoid will prove most helpful to the surgeon.

3. We recommend removal of the subscapularis muscle from the anterior and inferior capsule in order to evaluate properly the laxity of the capsule. In this way, if a Bankart lesion is not present, a capsulorrhaphy can easily be performed. As a rule, we ligate the anterior circumflex vessels. This allows better exposure of the axillary fold of the capsule and less oozing during surgery. It also lessens the chance of injury to the axillary nerve, because the nerve is *turned back with the intact muscle.* To substantiate this, we have never encountered injury to the axillary nerve in the past 40 years. One should also avoid cauterizing oozing circumflex vessels, because the axillary nerve might be injured.

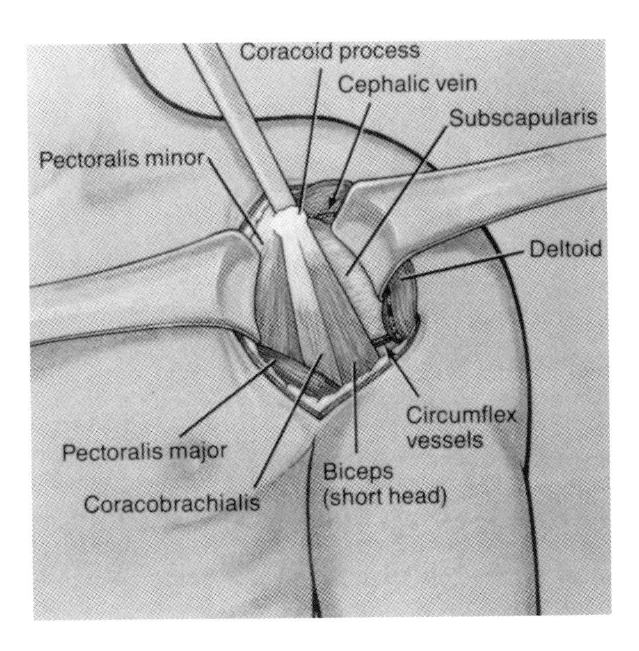

Figure 2 Osteotomy of the coracoid is optional. (From Rowe CR. The shoulder. New York: Churchill Livingstone, 1988: 196. Reproduced by permission of Churchill Livingstone.)

Options

A. Rockwood prefers not to ligate circumflex vessels by leaving the lower portion of the subscapularis attached, and retracting the vessels inferiorly (Fig. 3).

B. Matsen, on the other hand, does not separate the subscapularis muscle from the capsule, but explores the joint by separating the subscapularis attachment from the lesser tuberosity, and working within the joint.

4. With the capsule exposed, its laxity is tested with the arm in complete external rotation. The joint is then opened vertically 0.5 cm lateral to the glenoid rim (Fig. 4). By opening the capsule with the arm in external rotation, maximal external rotation will be obtained postoperatively. The vertical open-

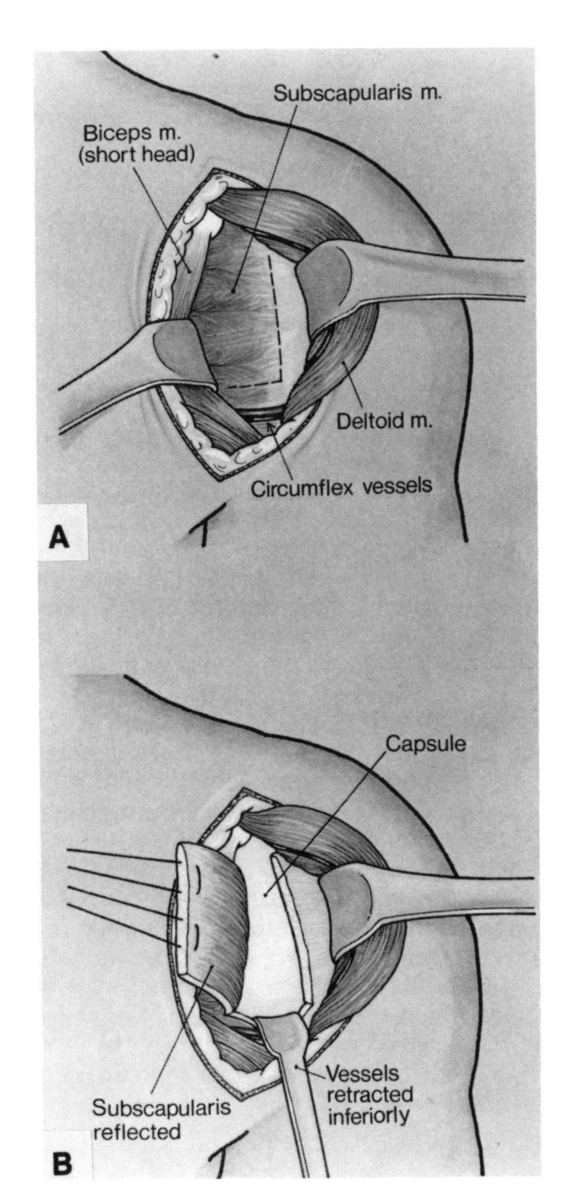

Figure 3 *A, B,* Rockwood retracts the circumflex vessels along with an inferior slip of subscapularis muscle.

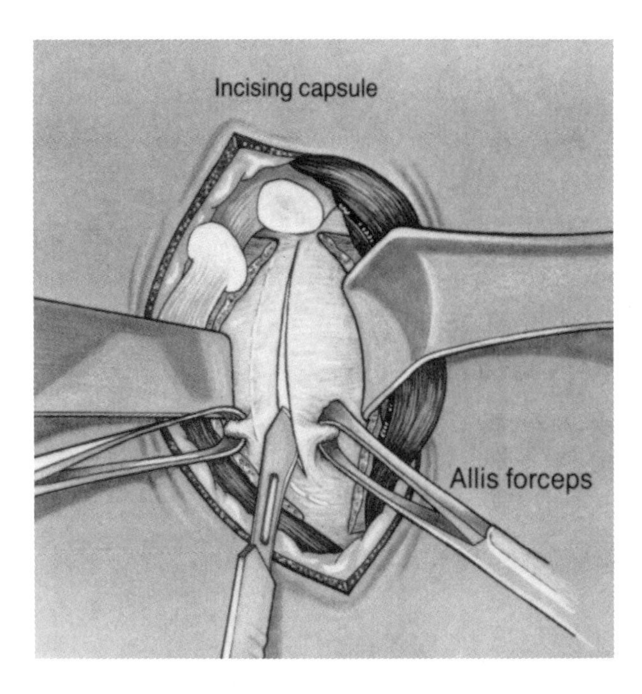

Figure 4 The joint is opened by a vertical incision 0.5 cm lateral to the glenoid rim with the arm in complete external rotation. This ensures maximal return of external rotation. (From Rowe CR. The shoulder. New York: Churchill Livingstone, 1988: 198. Reproduced by permission of Churchill Livingstone.)

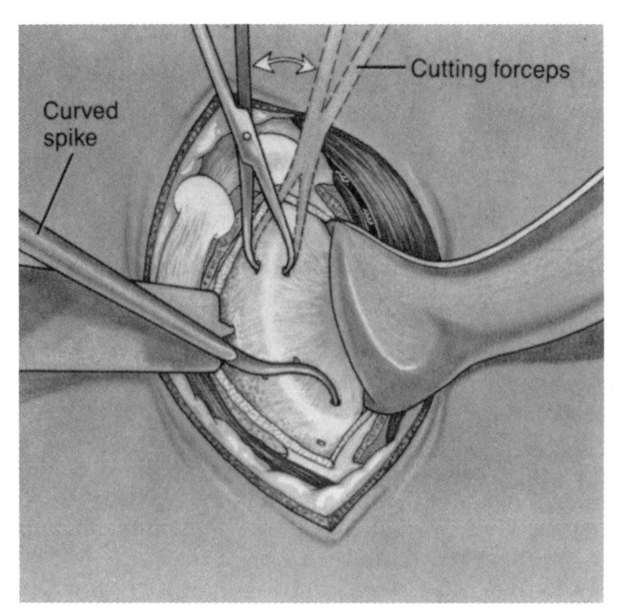

Figure 5 Holes are made through the glenoid rim high, mid, and low with the curved spike and cutting forceps. (From Rowe CR. The shoulder. New York: Churchill Livingstone, 1988: 200. Reproduced by permission of Churchill Livingstone.)

ing of the capsule into the joint is the same for a Bankart procedure as for a capsulorrhaphy. No alteration of the incision is necessary.

5. A special shoulder retractor is necessary to displace the humeral head and provide adequate exposure of the rim and the joint. The glenoid neck should be freshened with a small osteotome. Perforating the cortex of the glenoid neck with a small scaphoid gouge, or drill, facilitates the passage of the curved spike and lessens the chance of breaking or fracturing the anterior glenoid rim.

6. This part of the operation is *easier* with the coracoid osteotomized. Three holes are made through the rim at 10, 8, and 6 o'clock (for a left shoulder) with the curved spike and the cutting forceps (Fig. 5).

7. One's favorite suture is then passed through the holes either with a No. 5 Mayo taper needle or with a barbed hook, and the lateral capsule is sutured to the glenoid rim (Fig. 6A) with overlapping or double-breasting of the medial capsule (Fig. 6B); this gives added strength along the entire glenoid, where it is needed.

8. The muscles are then returned to their original origins.

Capsulorrhaphy

When a Bankart lesion is *not* present, the instability of the joint is due to a redundant or overstretched capsule. Without altering the incision, the capsule can be taken up as necessary and double-breasted along the anterior glenoid rim (Fig. 7). It is best to test the amount of take-up of the capsule to allow at least 35 degrees of external rotation of the arm, before suturing. With 35 degrees of external rotation at the time of closure, the patient will safely regain the remainder of rotation postoperatively. As pointed out previously, in the case of multidirectional instability the posterior capsule can be tightened through the anterior approach by drawing the capsule forward at 7 or 8 o'clock (for a left shoulder).

POSTOPERATIVE REGIMEN

This type of repair is strong enough to allow patients to use the arm as tolerated, immediately after surgery. The sling is omitted, usually on the second day, and the patient is begun on gentle pendulum exercises and encouraged to use the hand and arm within the range of tolerated motion. Forceful use of the arm is discouraged for 3 months, but during this time the patient increases the range of motion of the arm. We have not found specific physical therapy to be indicated. This is the period of healing and motion, not of regaining strength. At 3 months, activities are increased with wall weights, forearm weights, adjusted rowing, and so forth. Elevation of the arm is encouraged in the scapular plane (forward flexion) and not in abduction. By 6 months, with the

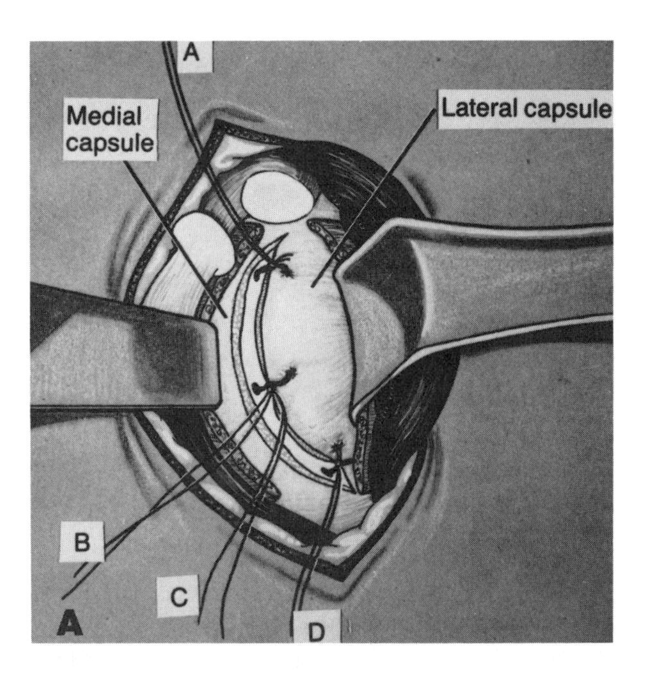

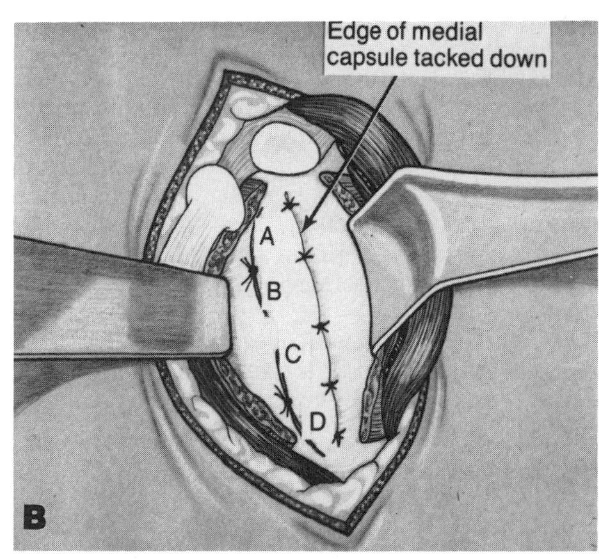

Figure 6 *A,* The lateral capsule is sutured to the anterior glenoid rim through the three holes, and the sutures are passed through the medial capsule flap. *B,* The medial capsule is then double-breasted over the lateral capsule for added strength. (From Rowe CR. The shoulder. New York: Churchill Livingstone, 1988: 201. Reproduced by permission of Churchill Livingstone.)

return of motion and strength, patients are usually able to return to contact sports. Racquet sports may take a while longer for full use in serving. Pitchers must be on a special schedule, also with graduated tossing to throwing on schedule. Full rhythmic body motions, coordinated with the arm motion, are essential.

RESULTS

Our aim with the Bankart procedure is to avoid trauma to the muscle layers at surgery; avoid the use of metal, such as staples and screws; and return all tissues to their natural origins. In this way, complete range of motion with full strength and agility can be obtained. We do not, at any stage, attempt to restrict the functional range of motion, such as external rotation, because the athlete needs as much stable mo-

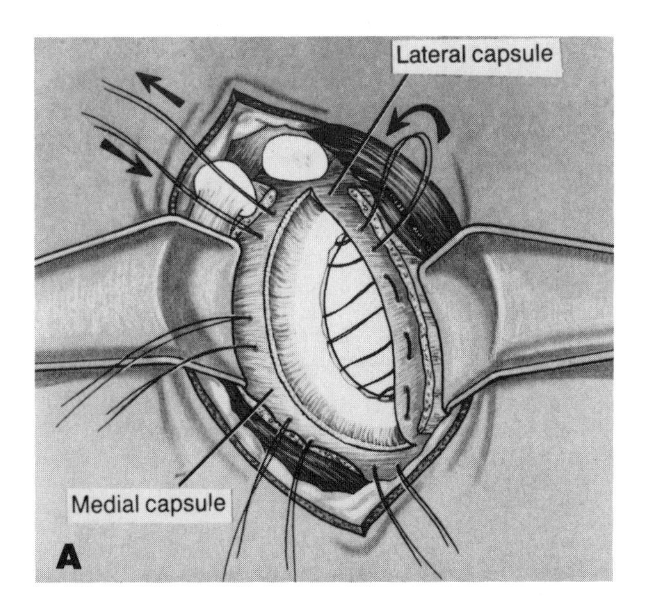

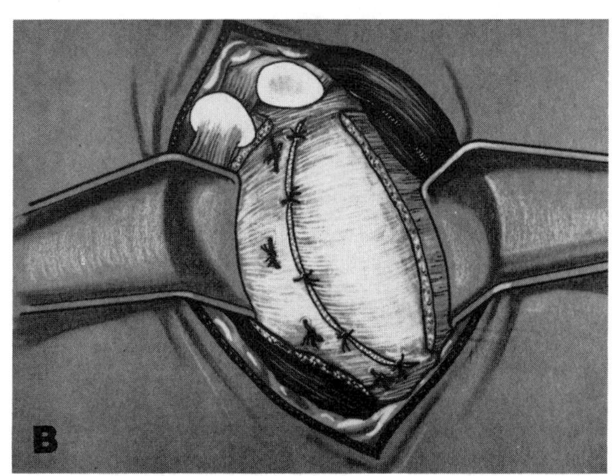

Figure 7 Capsulorrhaphy technique. *A,* When a Bankart lesion is *not* present, the capsule is taken up and double-breasted along the anterior glenoid. The suture is passed under the labrum, out through the lateral capsule, and back under the labrum. *B,* The medial capsule is then double-breasted over the repair, adding extra strength. (From Rowe CR. The shoulder. New York: Churchill Livingstone, 1988: 236. Reproduced by permission of Churchill Livingstone.)

tion as possible, particularly in throwing, serving in tennis, basketball, and swimming free style. For further follow-up results, see Rowe's textbook *The Shoulder.* Seventy percent of our patients regained 100 percent of motion in every phase. Twenty-five percent regained 75 percent of motion, and only 5 percent gained less than this. Our recurrence rate has remained at 3.5 percent up to the present time in college and professional athletes in football, ice hockey, baseball, wrestling, and basketball. Only one patient with a dominant arm and one with a recessive arm failed to return to previous sports activities.

Figure 8 illustrates a college student who had a recurrent dislocation of the right dominant shoulder. At surgery a large Bankart lesion was repaired

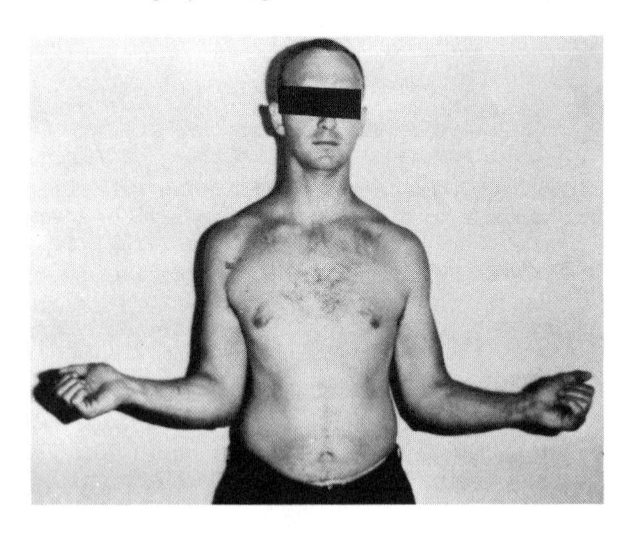

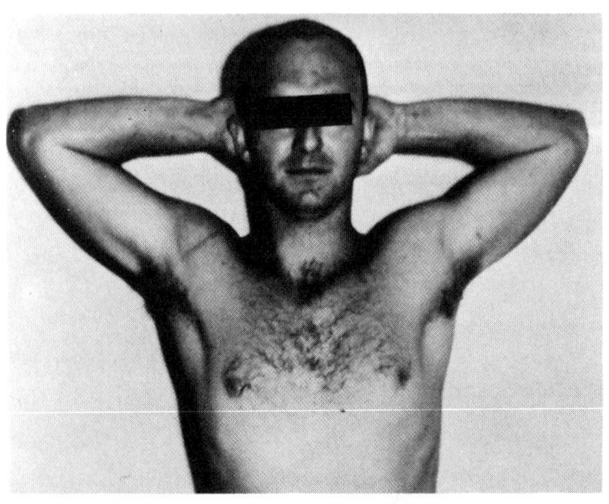

Figure 8 A college student who had a recurrent anterior dislocation of his right shoulder in high school. A Bankart procedure was performed, after which the patient played varsity football as a tight end for 4 years at a large university, ending in a bowl game. The shoulder has been stable for 20 years. (From Rowe CR. The shoulder. New York: Churchill Livingstone, 1988:211. Reproduced by permission of Churchill Livingstone.)

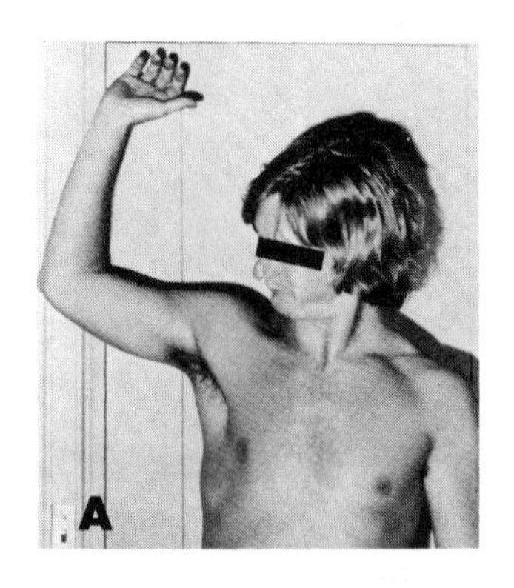

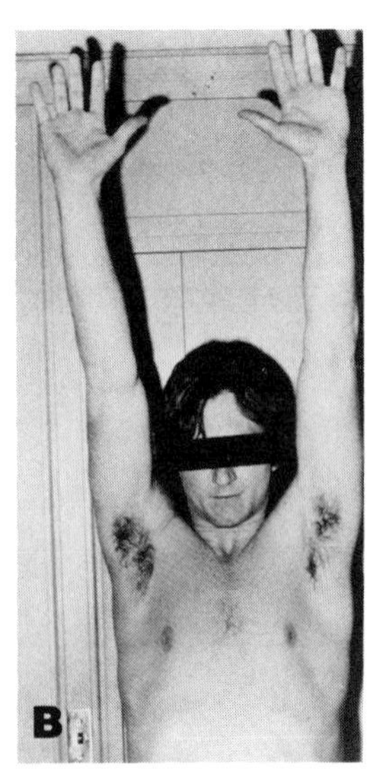

Figure 9 *A,* This college pitcher was disabled for 2 years after excessive pitching. Conservative treatment had been unsuccessful. *B,* At surgery, excessive laxity of the anterior capsule was noted. Eight months after our standard capsulorrhaphy, the patient returned to varsity pitching with full strength and control of his arm. (From Rowe CR. The shoulder. New York: Churchill Livingstone, 1988:243. Reproduced by permission of Churchill Livingstone.)

with a standard Bankart procedure. He played football successfully 4 years for a large university. His shoulder has remained stable for over 20 years.

Figure 9 illustrates a college student who had a "dead arm," due to excessive pitching, that had been unrelieved by conservative treatment. At surgery, the problem involved a redundant overstretched capsule. Our routine capsulorrhaphy was carried out. He returned to successful varsity pitching and basketball 1 year after surgery. He no longer has a "dead arm."

SUGGESTED READING

Blazina ME, Satzman JS. Recurrent anterior subluxation of the shoulder in athletes—a distinct entity. J Bone Joint Surg 1969; 51A:1037.

Cofield RH, Kavanagh BF, Frassica FJ. Anterior shoulder instability instructional course lectures. Am Acad Orthop Surg 1985; 34: 210–226.

Matsen FA. Instructional course on the shoulder. San Francisco: American Academy of Orthopaedic Surgery, 1987.

Neer CS II, Foster CR. Inferior capsular shift for involuntary inferior and multidirectional instability of the shoulder. J Bone Joint Surg 1980; 62A:897–908.

Rockwood CA Jr. Subluxation of the shoulder—the classification, diagnosis, and treatment. Orthop Trans 1979; 4:306.

Rowe CR, Zarins B. Recurrent transient subluxation of the shoulder. J Bone Joint Surg 1981; 63A: 863–872.

Rowe CR, Patel D, Southmayd WW. The Bankart procedure. J Bone Joint Surg 1981; 1:1–16.

Rowe CR. Dislocation of the shoulder. In: The shoulder. New York: Churchill Livingstone, 1988:165.

A MODIFIED BRISTOW-HELFET-MAY PROCEDURE FOR RECURRENT DISLOCATION AND SUBLUXATION OF THE SHOULDER

JOSEPH S. TORG, M.D.

Both recurrent anterior dislocation and recurrent subluxation of the glenohumeral joint are significant if not disabling problems in the athlete. May noted that spontaneous recovery from recurrent dislocation is impossible, and recommended surgery to interrupt the cycle. Among the numerous surgical procedures described are those of Bankart, du Toit, Putti-Platt, and Magnuson and Stack. Helfet and Latarjet reported on conceptually similar but technically different methods. Helfet described placement of the osteotomized coracoid segment and attached conjoined tendon through the subscapularis tendon to the neck of the scapula adjacent to the glenoid rim. It is interesting to note that Helfet attributed this concept to his mentor W. Rowley Bristow, hence the eponym. Four years earlier, Latarjet described a similar procedure in which he completely transected the subscapularis tendon, fixed the coracoid to the scapular neck, and reefed the entire subscapularis tendon anterior to the transplanted coracoid and conjoined tendon. Subsequently, a variety of modifications of the Bristow procedure have been described, although the basic principle of creating a strong anterior buttress to the weak part of the capsule of the shoulder is the same for all of them.

In 1974 we further modified the procedure by directing the osteotomized coracoid and conjoined tendon above and over the superior border of the subscapularis rather than through its substance. The reasons for this modification are threefold. First, approaching the glenohumeral joint and contiguous osseous glenoid cavity superior to, rather than through, the subscapularis tendon and muscle offers extraordinary exposure, thus facilitating accurate and rigid placement of the screw and coracoid segment. Second, use of the entire subscapularis tendon and muscle increases its strength as an anteroinferior musculotendinous sling or buttress. Third, it later became apparent that not placing the coracoid through the subscapularis tendon and muscle markedly simplified salvage in patients who subsequently had recurrences of their dislocation or subluxation.

The purpose of this chapter is to

1. Describe the indications for, technique of, and advantages of our modification of the Bristow-Helfet-May procedure.
2. Analyze the results in 212 shoulders with regard to long-term functional and subjective outcome as well as complications.
3. Determine the effect of the procedure on the muscles that control glenohumeral motion and strength with particular regard to their relationship to overhead throwing.

SURGICAL PROCEDURE

The patient is placed supine on the operating table in a semiseated position. A small roll is positioned under the scapula of the involved side, and the shoulder and upper extremity are draped free. The incision begins 1 cm proximal to the coracoid and is extended 8 cm distally toward the anterior axillary fold (Fig. 1). The deltopectoral groove is easily identified by the fatty streak that runs obliquely across the base of the incision. The dissection then proceeds through the deltopectoral interval, care being taken to identify, protect, and retract the cephalic vein laterally. At the base of the deltopectoral groove the acromial branches of the coracoacromial arterial trunk and accompanying venous structures are identified and ligated.

The coracoid process and the conjoined tendon are then exposed and the medial and lateral borders of the tendon are dissected free from the surrounding fascia for a distance of 6 cm (Fig.2). Care must be taken during the dissection to avoid injury to the musculocutaneous nerve as it courses from medial to lateral into the substance of the coracobrachialis, approximately 4 to 5 cm distal to the coracoid process.

Attention is next turned to the coracoid process. With care not to disrupt the attachment of the conjoined tendon, the coracoacromial ligament, the superior periosteum, and the anterior attachment of the pectoralis major are dissected subperiosteally from the distal 1½ cm of the coracoid process using an electrocautery knife. The distal 1½ cm of the coracoid is then transected with a microsagittal saw or osteotome. It is important to achieve a clean cut at right angles to the long axis of the coracoid process without beveling or splitting the distal segment. The soft tissues are then dissected from the undersurface of the coracoid. With a 3.2-mm drill bit, and starting at the cut surface, a drill hole is made in the long axis of the free coracoid segment (Fig. 3). The glenohumeral fascia and capsular structures are then incised parallel and superior to the superior border of the subscapularis tendon from its insertion into the lesser tuberosity to 3 cm medial to the musculotendinous junction.

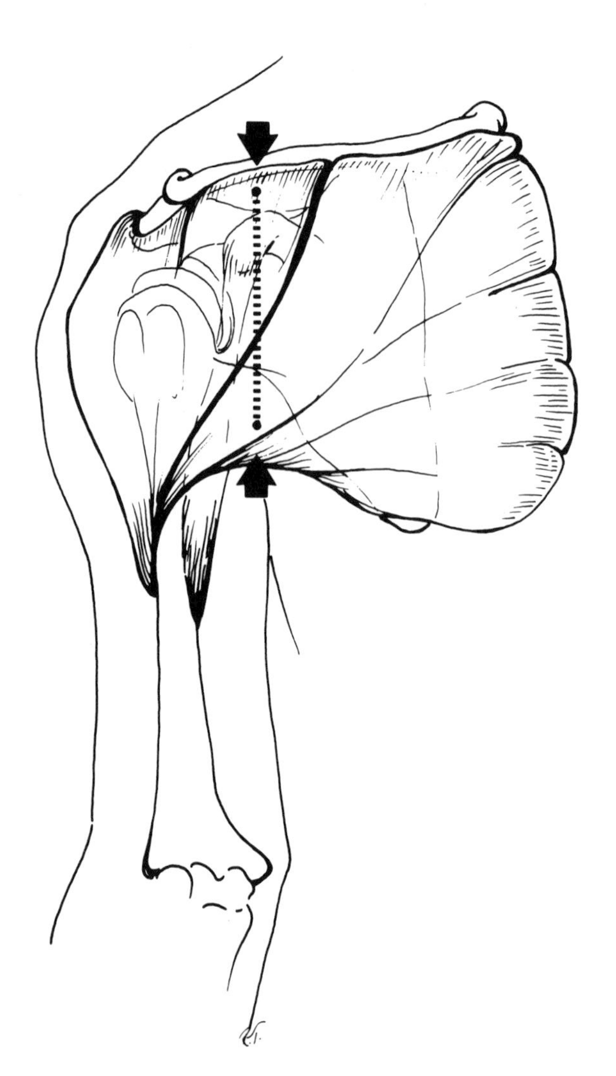

Figure 1 The surgical incision begins 1 cm proximal to the coracoid process and extends 8 cm distally toward the anterior axillary fold. (Republished with permission from Torg JS, et al. A modified Bristow-Heflet-May procedure for recurrent dislocation and subluxation of the shoulder. J Bone Joint Surg 1971; 69-A.)

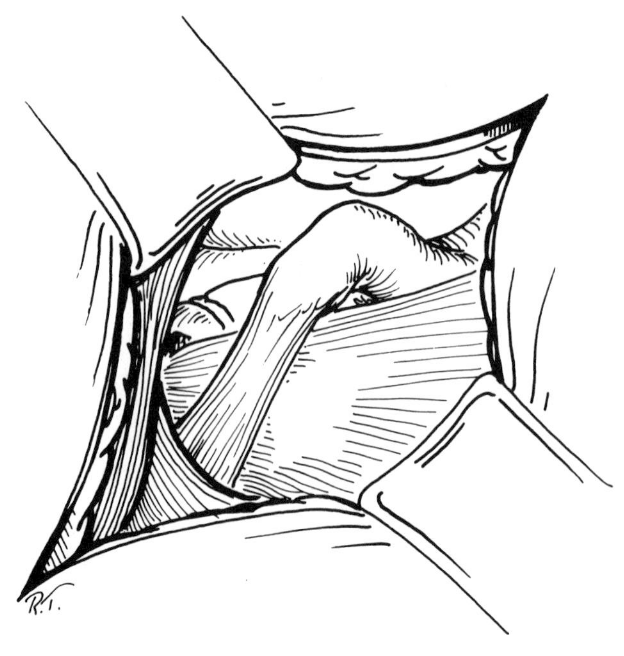

Figure 2 For surgical exposure of the coracoid process and attached conjoined tendon are dissected free from the surrounding fascia. (Republished with permission from Torg JS, et al. A modified Bristow-Heflet-May procedure for recurrent dislocation and subluxation of the shoulder. J Bone Joint Surg 1971; 69-A.)

On entering the glenohumeral joint, the long head of the biceps tendon is identified and protected. The cartilaginous glenoid labrum is excised if it is found to be detached. The anterior part of the osseous glenoid cavity is then denuded of its periosteum, and a site for insertion of the coracoid is selected at a point slightly inferior to the equator rim glenoid. The bed that is to receive the coracoid segment is prepared on the neck of the scapula adjacent to the anterior glenoid rim, and below the equator of the glenoid, by fish-scaling contouring a flat cortical surface with a sharp osteotome. Starting in the center of the bed, a 3.2-mm drill hole is made through the anterior and posterior cortices of the neck of the scapula, and the depth of the drill hole is measured. A 4.5-mm malleolar A0 screw equal in length to the sum of the depth of the drill holes in the coracoid segment and scapular neck is selected. The screw is

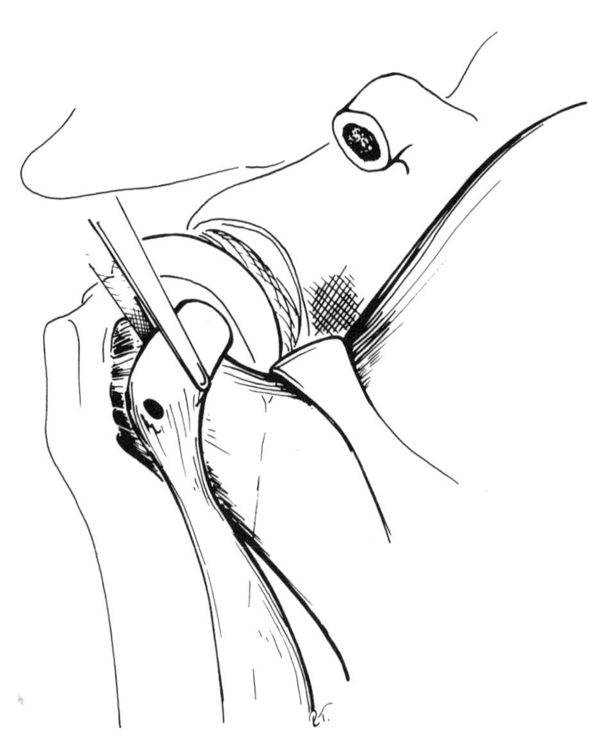

Figure 3 For surgical exposure of the anterior part of the glenoid rim, the distal 1 and 1½ cm of the coracoid process is osteotomized. The coracoid fragment is drilled with a 3.2-mm drill bit. (Republished with permission from Torg JS, et al. A modified Bristow-Heflet-May procedure for recurrent dislocation and subluxation of the shoulder. J Bone Joint Surg 1971; 69-A.)

first placed through the coracoid segment with the subscapularis tendon retracted distally by means of a narrow right-angled retractor. The coracoid segment with the attached conjoined tendon is passed superior to the tendon, and the screw is directed into the drill hole on the scapular neck. Bicortical fixation is required and care should be taken to achieve firm, congruous apposition of the cut surface of the coracoid segment to the prepared bed adjacent to the anterior glenoid rim (Fig. 4).

The wound is then lavaged and the skin and subcutaneous tissues are closed. A compression dressing is applied and the arm is placed in a sling and swathe.

POSTOPERATIVE MANAGEMENT

Postoperative management consists of five phases: (1) complete immobilization (2) limited range-of-motion exercises (3) full range-of-motion and limited isotonic exercises (4) active assisted range-of-motion and variable-resistance isotonic exercises, and (5) return to activities.

During the first 2 postoperative weeks (phase 1) the involved extremity is completely immobilized in a sling and swathe. The patient continues to wear the sling during the third and fourth week (phase 2), but it is removed four times a day for Codman's pendulum and active flexion and abduction range-of-motion exercises to a minimum of 90 degrees. During the fifth and sixth postoperative weeks (phase 3), the sling is worn at night only. At this point there are full, active range-of-motion exercises with light (1- to 2-kg dumbbells) isotonic exercises of the shoulder. These include shoulder flexion and abduction to 90 degrees and extension to 45 degrees. During the seventh and eighth postoperative weeks, emphasis is placed on active external rotation exercises for the humerus, and the weight of the dumbbells is increased to 2 to 4 kg). In addition, isometric internal and external rotation exercises are initiated. During weeks 9 to 12 (phase 4), active assisted external rotation of the humerus is initiated, and variable-resistance isotonic exercises with flexion, abduction, and internal rotation of the shoulder are added. Phase 5 begins in the 12th to 16th weeks with a return to activities that do not involve overhead throwing and striking, and in the 16th to 24th weeks for activities that *do* involve these.

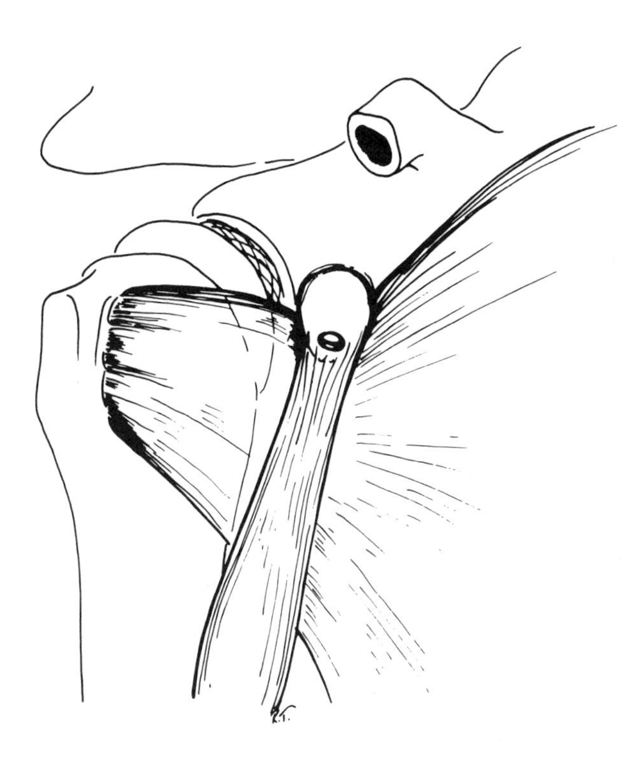

Figure 4 To complete the transfer of the coracoid graft, a 4.5-mm malleolar A0 screw is placed through the coracoid segment. The subscapularis tendon is retracted distally, and the coracoid graft is passed superior to the tendon and fixed to the anterior part of the glenoid rim at a point at or slightly below the equator. Bicortical fixation is essential. Care must be taken to achieve firm, congruous apposition of the graft to the bed. (Republished with permission from Torg JS, et al. A modified Bristow-Heflet-May procedure for recurrent dislocation and subluxation of the shoulder. J Bone Joint Surg 1971; 69-A.)

DISCUSSION

We have reported the results of this modification of the Bristow-Helfet-May procedure in 212 shoulders. The redislocation rate of 3.8 percent and resubluxation rate of 4.7 percent compare favorably with the results of other reported series of Bristow, Magnuson-Stack, Bankart, Putti-Platt, and du Toit procedures.

This modification allows excellent access to the glenohumeral joint and easy identification of the pathologic change without violating the subscapularis muscle and tendon. Use of the entire subscapularis muscle-tendon unit as an anterior restraint provides maximal use of these structures for stability. Placement of the cut surface of the coracoid flush with the prepared bed on the anterior aspect of the neck of the scapula, in as lateral and equatorial a location as possible, is crucial for the success of the procedure. Cancellous bone-to-bone contact is mandatory. Rigid fixation of the coracoid graft to the anterior glenoid rim with a bicortical 4.5-mm malleolar A0 screw allows for early motion of the shoulder.

The eight patients in whom redislocation occurred were operated on during the first phase of this series, suggesting that the learning curve in performing the procedure played a role. Redislocation also appeared to be related to high placement of the coracoid graft, the use of an incorrect screw, and failure to achieve bicortical fixation with the screw. Four of the patients who experienced redislocation and two who had postoperative subluxation underwent repeat surgery. In all six patients no attempt was made to disturb or reimplant the original coracoid graft other than the necessary procedure to remove the screw. A salvage reconstruction was performed by transfer of the subscapularis tendon from its insertion into the lesser tuberosity of the humerus with a 1.0 × 1.3-cm block of bone across the bicipital groove 1 cm distal to the greater tuberosity. The cortical fragment was placed on a prepared cortical bed of similar size and fixed with a cancellous screw and polyethylene washer. On the basis of a review of the charts, it was determined that all six patients did well after the second operation; there was no redislocation or resubluxation after an average of 6 years' follow-up. Thus, it appears that another advantage of this modification of the Bristow procedure is that by not placing the coracoid segment through the subscapularis, a much less technically demanding surgical alternative is available for patients who suffer redislocation or resubluxation.

The average strength in external rotation, internal rotation, and abduction of the shoulders that were operated on failed to match the strength of the shoulders that were not, regardless of which side was dominant. In addition to the deficiencies in strength, limitation of static and dynamic external range of motion was also observed. Halley and Olix and Lombardo and colleagues, using May's modification of the Bristow procedure, reported that the resulting restriction of motion contributes to the inability of the athlete to throw at preinjury level of performance. Only three of 19 athletes in our study whose dominant arm was operated on and who underwent Cybex testing were able to return to their preoperative level. The findings indicate that athletes with only minimal loss of dynamic external rotation were unable to return to the preoperative level of overhead throwing.

Restriction of motion in external rotation may not be the only contributory factor that adversely affects throwing. The strength required for successful completion of the throwing pattern also needs to be considered. The act of throwing, inclusive of the so-called cocking, acceleration, and follow-through phases, is propulsive in nature, and therefore the demands for muscle strength are high. Thus, the act of throwing stresses the elastic capability of the soft tissues that provide control over the glenohumeral joint.

In the cocking phase, vigorous muscular contraction is required to initiate external rotation of the humerus and to achieve the most effective maximally rotated position. A quick changeover is then necessary from the cocking to the acceleration phase, and this is dependent on the timely, synchronous action of the agonistic and antagonistic muscle groups. If there is a limitation of external rotation and deficiencies in strength at the extremes of motion, the propulsive force is compromised and there is a less than effective throwing action. In our clinical study, it has been shown that there is not only a restriction in dynamic range of motion externally, but also a deficiency in strength at the critical areas of motion representing the changeover from the cocking to the acceleration phase. Furthermore, a deficiency in strength was observed throughout the full range of external rotation, which may tend to compromise further the propulsive force generated.

The modification of the Bristow-Helfet-May procedure described here has several distinct technical advantages. First, entry into the joint superior to the proximal margin of the subscapularis and retraction of this muscle inferiorly affords exceptional exposure of the osseous glenoid cavity and cartilaginous labrum, as well as the associated glenohumeral joint. Second, because of this excellent exposure, the technical aspects of the procedure are less demanding than those for comparable procedures. Third, the fact that it is not necessary to violate the integrity of the musculotendinous unit of the subscapularis makes possible more rapid rehabilitation and recovery. The rate of recurrence with this procedure compares favorably with other large series of anterior shoulder reconstructions in the current literature. It is interesting that 120 (92 percent) of the 131 patients who responded to a questionnaire stated that they were able to return to their usual daily activities, and 96 percent were both happy with the results of surgery and were prepared to have the procedure performed again. However, 34 percent continue to experience varying degrees of discomfort and pain. As indicated by other authors, a reconstruction of the glenohumeral joint for recurrent dislocation and subluxation usually results in an inability to return to intensive overhead throwing activities such as pitching a baseball. With regard to the adverse effects on overhead throwing, the data indicate that this is not simply a result of the loss of glenohumeral motion, but also appears to be related to a concomitant loss of strength in the extreme of external rotation and the initiation of internal rotation.

SUGGESTED READING

Bonci CM, Hensal FJ, Torg JS. A preliminary study on the measurement of static and dynamic motion at the glenohumeral joint. Am J Sports Med 1986; 14:12–17.

Braly WG, Tullos HS. A modification of the Bristow procedure for recurrent anterior shoulder dislocation and subluxation. Am J Sports Med 1985; 13:81–86.

Collins HR, Wilde AH. Shoulder instability in athletics. Orthop Clin North Am 1973; 4:759–774.

Halley DK, Olix ML. A review of the Bristow operation for recurrent anterior shoulder dislocation in athletes. Clin Orthop 1975; 106:175–179.

Helfet AJ. Coracoid transplantation for recurring dislocation of the shoulder. J Bone Joint Surg 1958; 40-B:198–292.

Hill JA, Lombardo SJ, Kerlan RK, et al. The modified Bristow-Helfet procedure for recurrent anterior shoulder subluxations and dislocations. Am J Sports Med 1981; 9:283–287.

Hovelius L, Korner L, Lundberg B, et al. The coracoid transfer for recurrent dislocation of the shoulder: technical aspects of the Bristow-Latarjet procedure. J Bone Joint Surg 1983; 65-A:926–934.

Ivey FM Jr, Calhoun JH, Rusche K, et al. Isokinetic testing of shoulder strength: normal values. Arch Phys Med Rehabil 1985; 66:384–386.
Lombardo SJ, Kerlan RK, Jobe FW, et al. The modified Bristow procedure for recurrent dislocation of the shoulder. J Bone Joint Surg 1976; 58-A:256–261.
May VR. A modified Bristow procedure operation for anterior recurrent, dislocation of the shoulder. J Bone Joint Surg 1970; 52-A:1010–1016.

INJURIES TO THE ACROMIOCLAVICULAR JOINT

EDWARD P. FINK, M.D.
R. PETER WELSH, M.B., Ch.B., F.R.C.S.(C), F.A.C.S.

Injuries to the acromioclavicular joint are among the more common disorders of the shoulder. Typically, they are sustained by participants in contact sports or incurred by a fall on the shoulder. Diagnosis of the derangement is seldom difficult or overlooked. Although clinicians have a wealth of experience in caring for patients with this injury, there remains considerable controversy over optimal management. This dilemma derives, in part, from a failure to understand the natural history of the unreduced acromioclavicular dislocation, and a failure to recognize that the clinical results are not always correlated with the radiographic picture. Armed with an understanding of the functional demands of the athlete and a knowledge of the results and complications of operative and nonoperative treatment, the physician may best implement the most suitable course of treatment.

ANATOMIC REVIEW

The acromioclavicular joint is the only articulation between the upper extremity and the axial skeleton. It is a diarthrodial joint, with the articular cartilage of the clavicle and the acromion separated by a fibrocartilage meniscus and lined by a synovial membrane. The acromioclavicular ligaments are thin and weak, encapsulating the joint yet providing little structural stability. It is the contribution of the surrounding soft tissues that helps to maintain the integrity of the joint. The aponeuroses of the anterior deltoid and lateral trapezius blend in with the superior portion of the acromioclavicular ligament to strengthen the articulation. The coracoclavicular ligaments are the primary suspensory ligaments of the upper extremity and help to maintain the anatomic relationships of the acromioclavicular joint by preventing superior migration of the clavicle.

MECHANISM OF INJURY

Injuries to the acromioclavicular joint are usually sustained from a fall resulting in a direct blow to the lateral aspect of the shoulder. There is a sudden forceful depression of the shoulder and the clavicle. The ultimate descent of the clavicle is blocked by the first rib upon which the clavicle impinges. With continuation of the downward force, the shoulder girdle becomes separated from the clavicle, first with the tearing of the acromioclavicular ligaments and then with the disruption of the coracoclavicular ligaments. The trapezius muscle ruptures with descent of the shoulder, while the deltoid may be torn with separation of the acromioclavicular joint and disruption of the muscle's origin on the clavicle. Most acromioclavicular derangements are produced by a direct blow to the shoulder. Much less commonly, a fall onto the outstretched arm forces the humeral head against the undersurface of the acromion, disrupting the acromioclavicular joint and possibly tearing the coracoclavicular ligaments.

CLASSIFICATION OF INJURY

The classification system of acromioclavicular joint injuries is based on the degree of disruption of the ligaments and surrounding soft tissue. In *type I* the acromioclavicular ligaments are stretched, but there is no significant soft tissue disruption and the joint is stable. The acromioclavicular ligaments are torn in *type II* as the force on the shoulder continues inferiorly. The coracoclavicular ligaments are stretched and there is partial tearing of the tendinous attachments of the deltoid and trapezius. The acromioclavicular joint is disrupted and motion occurs in the anteroposterior plane, often with posterior subluxation of the clavicle. Stability in the vertical plane is maintained by the intact coracoclavicular ligaments.

As the force continues the clavicle impinges upon the first rib, causing a complete rupture of both the acromioclavicular and coracoclavicular ligaments. In this *type III* injury the deltoid and trapezius muscles become detached from the distal end of the clavicle and the acromion. A complete acromioclavicular dislocation is produced with superior displacement of the clavicle relative to the acromion.

Severe complete dislocations may be further subclassified into three types, depending on the position of the clavicle. The clavicle in *type IV* is displaced posteriorly into (and occasionally through) and locked within the fibers of the trapezius muscle. The greatest clavicular displacement occurs in type IV injuries as the trapezius muscle is stripped from the lateral clavicle. Along with the inferior subluxation of the shoulder girdle, the clavicle is very prominent and dangerously tenses the skin superiorly; occasionally a *type V* dislocation occurs with the skin actually disrupted. In the rare *type VI* dislocation the clavicle becomes displaced inferiorly beneath the coracoid process and behind the intact biceps and coracobrachialis tendons.

CLINICAL REVIEW

Examination of a suspected acromioclavicular joint injury should be performed with the patient either sitting or standing. The weight of the arm will accentuate an acromioclavicular dislocation. Pain is often localized to the lateral clavicle and acromioclavicular joint. In type II subluxations, clavicular motion may be present in the anteroposterior plane relative to the acromion. In patients with type III dislocations, the clavicle appears prominent superiorly and is freely mobile in both the horizontal and vertical planes. A careful examination of the shoulder may detect coexistent pathology, such as an acute subdeltoid bursitis produced by the fall onto the shoulder.

RADIOGRAPHIC STUDIES

Routine anteroposterior x-ray films of the shoulder may disclose the dislocated acromioclavicular joint. However, this radiograph is exposed for the glenohumeral joint, and often the acromioclavicular joint is underpenetrated. The ideal radiographic views are an anteroposterior view centered over the acromioclavicular joint, directed 15 degrees cephalad, and a lateral view of the acromioclavicular joint. Type I injuries show no radiographic abnormalities, while type II injuries may show only posterior clavicular subluxation, if present, on the lateral x-ray film. In any suspected acromioclavicular injury, stress views of both shoulders should always be obtained to demonstrate the integrity of the coracoclavicular ligament. An increase of the coracoid to clavicle distance of 40 to 50 percent of the normal shoulder is diagnostic of type III acromioclavicular joint dislocation.

MANAGEMENT

Grade I sprains usually involve no treatment dilemmas or complications. Ice may be applied to the injured joint for 24 hours, while a sling provides immobilization for pain relief. Pain diminishes within 7 to 10 days and the sling may then be discarded. Exercises are then implemented and activities may be gradually increased.

Nonoperative treatment for type II acromioclavicular injuries similarly produces good results with minimal complications. Owing to the greater soft tissue disruption, the shoulder needs to be immobilized for 4 to 6 weeks. Gentle range-of-motion exercises may be instituted during this period as pain permits. Gradual return to activities may begin at 4 weeks; overhead arm movements are restricted for 6 weeks. Heavy lifting or contact sports should be avoided for 8 to 12 weeks. The prognosis for complete recovery of strength and motion after types I and II injuries is quite good, and most athletes are able to return to their preinjury level of performance. Close monitoring of rehabilitation and strengthening of the shoulder is essential to ensure a successful outcome.

Considerable controversy surrounds the treatment of acute type III acromioclavicular dislocations. This derives in part from the principles of treatment of other joint dislocations, namely, anatomic reduction and maintenance of the reduction while early protective range-of-motion exercises are instituted. This is true for most joints but the acromioclavicular joint is quite different. The clinical results of no treatment or attempted joint reduction without surgery are often as good as those achieved through operative reduction and fixation of the joint.

The critical issue appears to be whether a complete anatomic reduction is necessary for restoration of normal shoulder function. Studies have shown little correlation between maintenance of a reduction and the clinical result. Patients treated conservatively without surgical attempts at reduction enjoyed more rapid rehabilitation, returned to work and sporting activities more quickly, and were more satisfied with the results of treatment. They had significantly less restriction of shoulder motion or loss of shoulder strength. Even the ability to maintain an anatomic reduction has proved difficult, and late loss of reduction has occurred with both closed and open methods of treatment. Although degenerative changes were seen radiographically in approximately 40 percent of those joints without restoration of an anatomic reduction, there was little correlation between the presence or amount of degenerative changes in the acromioclavicular joint and the patient's complaints of pain in the joint.

Of equal importance in considering treatment is the high incidence of complications from operative reduction of acute acromioclavicular dislocations. Breakage or migration of the metallic devices, failure of fixation, and skin irritation are quite common. Redislocation, infection, prolonged rehabilitation, and further operations to remove retained or fractured fixation devices all compromise the results of operative intervention.

Most individuals with acute type III acromioclavicular dislocation should be managed nonoperatively. A Kenny Howard acromioclavicular strap or similar sling to support the arm should be employed. In this manner a complete reduction is seldom maintained, but the prominence of the lateral clavicle is greatly diminished by more closely approximating the acromioclavicular joint. Immobilization should continue for 4 to 6 weeks, followed by gradual range-of-motion exercises of the shoulder. Contact sports should be avoided for at least 2 months because of the risks of reinjury and redislocation. Sports participation should not be resumed until the return of normal strength and full active range of motion of the shoulder. Closed reduction of types IV, V, and VI should be attempted to convert these injuries into type III. If this is successful, nonoperative treatment can be continued.

Surgery for type III acromioclavicular joint injury should be reserved for specific indications. Irreducible type IV, V, or VI dislocations require open procedures to restore the correct alignment of the clavicle with the acromion. A prominent clavicle in a woman that is cosmetically disfiguring may also warrant operative reduction. Individuals whose job or sports require the shoulder to be in 90 degrees of abduction or flexion may have pain when an unreduced, mobile lateral clavicle impinges on the acromion eccentrically, and may benefit from operative stabilization.

Operative techniques for reduction and stabilization of this joint have included repair or reconstruction of either the acromioclavicular ligament or the coracoclavicular ligament, or both. Many devices have been used to transfix these joints to allow primary or secondary ligament healing. Transfer of the coracoacromial ligament is recommended to rebuild coracoclavicular support. The ligament is left attached at its origin from the coracoid but freed from the acromion and transposed into the lateral end of the clavicle. Maintenance of a reduced acromioclavicular joint, while allowing healing of the acromioclavicular and coracoclavicular ligaments, should be the goal of operative treatment. Good results have consistently been obtained by this technique, which is coupled with debridement of the acromioclavicular joint and stabilization of the clavicle by means of a coracoclavicular screw to allow healing of the coracoclavicular ligament. The screw is removed 6 to 8 weeks after surgery and this is followed by increasing range-of-motion exercises and progressive strengthening of the shoulder. Sporting activities are not allowed for 3 months.

Chronic pain may develop in an acromioclavicular joint that has sustained a type II or III injury. Often this pain becomes manifest within the first 6 months after injury and occurs with activities requiring flexion and abduction of the shoulder. Post-traumatic arthritis may be produced by the subsequent joint incongruity. If the joint is dislocated, pain may arise from the outer clavicle abutting against the acromion whenever the shoulder is placed in abduction or flexion. X-ray films may reveal joint space narrowing and osteophytes indicative of degenerative joint changes. If the joint is adequately reduced and is painful, the outer 1 cm of the clavicle is resected and the joint debrided, preserving the enveloping soft tissues. If the clavicle is clinically dislocated, the outer 1 cm is resected and the prominence beveled before the clavicle is stabilized by placing the acromial attachment of the coracoacromial ligament into the outer end of the clavicle, with tension adjusted to approximate the clavicle more closely to the coracoid process and shoulder girdle. In the late repair, excellent capsular reinforcement can be achieved to further aid stabilization.

Post-traumatic osteolysis of the outer end of the clavicle occurs infrequently after subluxation or dislocation of the acromioclavicular joint. The etiology is unknown, although autonomic nerve dysfunction affecting blood supply to the clavicle is thought to cause resorption of bone from the outer end of the clavicle. Pain and weakness occur with abduction and flexion of the arm. Although symptoms may be self-limiting after 1 year, resection of the outer 1 cm of the clavicle and joint debridement may be required to alleviate the pain and allow restoration of shoulder motion.

In conclusion, late stabilization of acromioclavicular separations is recommended for symptomatic type III dislocations. Simple acromioclavicular resection with beveling and capsuloplasty suffice for type II lesions. Early repair is favored only for the rare types IV, V, and VI disruptions.

ATRAUMATIC OSTEOLYSIS OF THE DISTAL CLAVICLE

BERNARD R. CAHILL, M.D.

According to Strauch, Dupas in 1936 first reported a case of traumatic osteolysis of the distal part of the clavicle. In 1963 Madsen summarized the findings in eight patients of his own and reviewed eight other cases reported in the literature, although he did not review the two patients reported by Stahl. From 1963 through 1982 20 additional cases were reported, making a total of 38 cases described in the world literature. Thirty-four of these 38 patients had a history of acute trauma to the shoulder or acromioclavicular joint.

Atraumatic osteolysis was first reported by Ehricht in 1959 when he described the occurrence of osteolysis of the distal clavicle in an air hammer operator. This report was followed by descriptions of osteolysis in a patient who practiced judo, a delivery man, and a handball player. None of these four patients had a history of injury to the shoulder. In 1982 I reported 46 cases of atraumatic osteolysis, all in males, 45 of whom were weight lifters.

Although pathologic changes in the acromioclavicular joint subsequent to trauma, resulting in osteolysis of the distal part of the clavicle, are common and usually recognized, the same sequence of events in a patient without a history of shoulder trauma continues to be a diagnostic problem for many orthopedists.

The purpose of this chapter is to review the clinical course and findings, radiographic findings, and treatment of atraumatic osteolysis of the distal clavicle (AODC), and to describe the frequent association of this entity with other shoulder conditions producing dysfunction and pain in the athlete.

CASE MATERIAL

Since 1982, when 46 patients with atraumatic osteolysis of the distal clavicle were reported, 67 other patients have been treated by the author. None of these 113 patients had a significant history of injury and none had an acute injury. With the exception of two patients, all were athletes or exercisers.

Strength training exercise as practiced by body builders and competitive weight lifters remains the leading feature of the history of AODC, followed by football and swimming. During the past 20 years, strength training has become an integral part of the training regimen of all sports, and the development of AODC has followed.

Bilateral symptoms are common, representing nearly 20 percent of this series, and joint scintigraphy indicates a 40 percent bilateral involvement of the distal clavicle.

The throwing athlete is no longer immune to AODC. Seven baseball pitchers, four tennis players, and two racquetball players are included in this post-1982 material. Eleven of these athletes had a significant history of strength training.

No cases of AODC in females were reported in 1982. Since then, eight female athletes, all with strength training as a part of their programs, have been treated. Their sports were weight events in track and field (three), volleyball (two), basketball (two), and body building (one).

The average age of patients with AODC reported in 1982 was 23.3 years. This presenting age has dropped to 21 years in the reports from 1982 to 1988 and is presumed to be a result of the cumulative stresses on the acromioclavicular joint generated by earlier entry of the athlete into sports, the addition of strength training, and the intensity of the training programs.

CLINICAL PICTURE

Symptoms begin with a slow onset of pain in the area of the acromioclavicular joint. It is usually described as a dull ache and occurs several hours after the exercise bout. There may be some radiation to the adjacent deltoid muscle or to the superior border of the trapezius. As AODC progresses, the athlete first describes the onset of pain as at the beginning of exercise, and the pain later prevents or interferes with performance.

When strength training is a significant aspect of the training program, the athlete characteristically describes pain at the acromioclavicular joint with bench pressing, dips, or push-ups.

When uncomplicated by other conditions, the range of motion of the glenohumeral joint is normal and muscle atrophy of the shoulder joint has not been noted.

There may be mild prominence of the acromioclavicular joint, although in the common bilateral presentation this may be difficult to evaluate. Tenderness is always present at the acromioclavicular joint. Instability of this joint is not a feature of AODC, but crepitation may be. As AODC progresses, all throwing motions become painful and the activities of daily living may be affected.

RADIOGRAPHIC FINDINGS

Zanca made the most comprehensive radiographic study of the acromioclavicular joint and pointed out the quotidian occurrence of degeneration of that joint, which was usually asymptomatic. He did not compare his data with scintigraphic activity in the acromioclavicular joint.

The radiographic finding in traumatic osteolysis of the distal clavicle, described by Madsen and Levine and colleagues as tapering of the distal part of the clavicle, is not seen in AODC. Murphy and colleagues and Jacobs stated that the earliest radiographic changes of osteolysis after trauma may ensue in 4 weeks. In my experience with AODC, radiographic changes as recorded by standard x-ray techniques are subtle and late manifestations.

These radiographically revealed alterations consist of a loss of subchondral bone detail and microcystic appearances in the subchondral area of the distal clavicle (Figs. 1*A* and 2*B*). Osteoporosis of the lateral third of the clavicle may occur. To evaluate the acromioclavicular joint adequately, the 13-degree cephalad technique as well as joint scintigraphy must be performed. Neither nuclear magnetic resonance nor computed tomographic (CT) scans have been helpful in the diagnosis of AODC.

JOINT SCINTIGRAPHY

Technetium-99m–labeled phosphate scintigraphy is essential to confirm the diagnosis of AODC. Joint scintigraphy demonstrating increased uptake of the radiotracer was positive in one or both shoulders in all 113 patients in this series. It is the sine qua non of AODC.

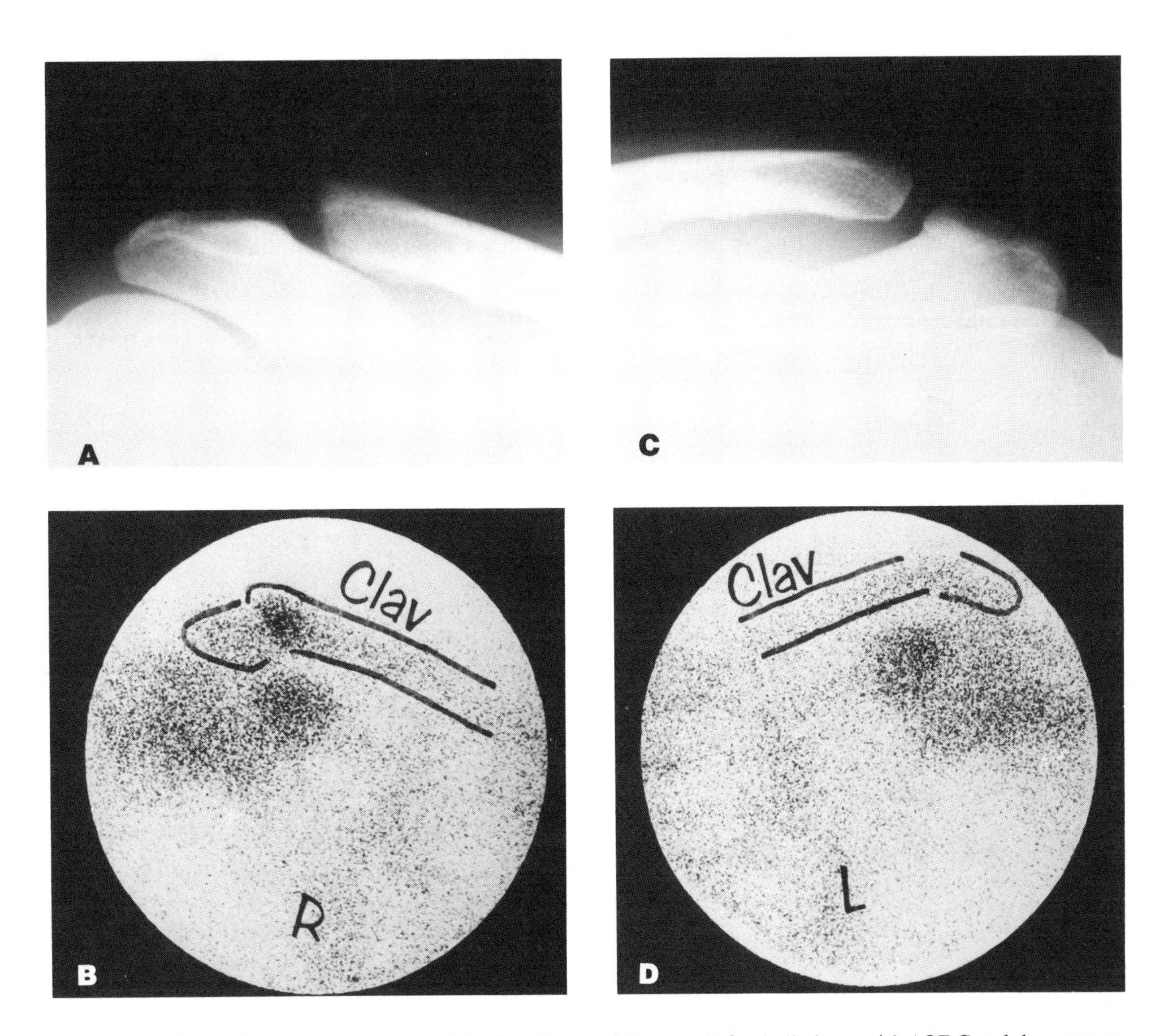

Figure 1 Radiograph of the symptomatic right shoulder of a 17-year-old football player with AODC and the asymptomatic normal left shoulder. *A*, Early microcystic changes and loss of the subchondral line are seen. View taken with the 15-degree cephalad technique. *B*, Scintigram shows that the distal clavicle is involved but not the acromion process. *C*, Radiograph of the asymptomatic left shoulder is normal. Note the intact subchondral line. *D*, Normal joint scintigraphy of the left shoulder.

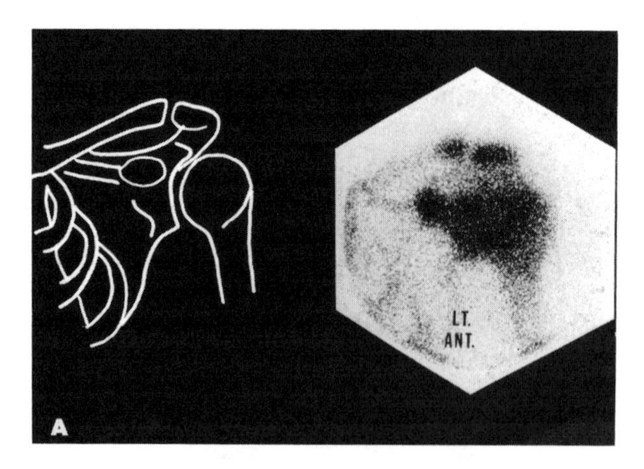

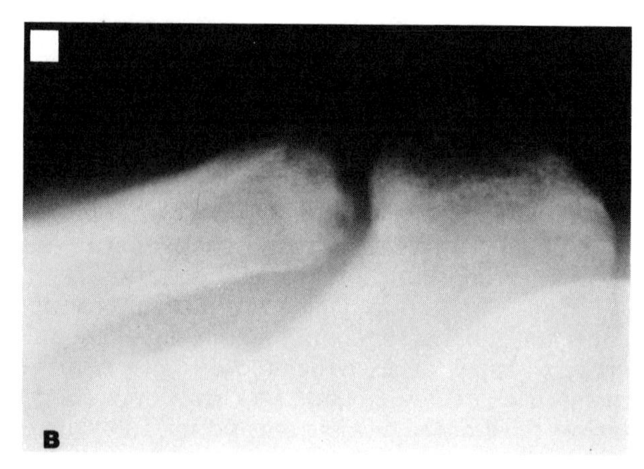

Figure 2 The left shoulder of a college football player. *A*, The asymptomatic left shoulder in 1980. The scintigram shows involvement of both the distal clavicle and the acromion process. *B*, In 1983 the radiograph of the now symptomatic left shoulder shows microcystic changes and loss of the subchondral line. This patient underwent bilateral resections of the distal clavicle, and 14 years after surgery on the right and 5 years after surgery on the left shoulder, considers his shoulders to be normal. (From Cahill BR. Osteolysis of the distal part of the clavicle in male athletes. J Bone Joint Surg 1982; 64A:1053–1058.)

Approximately 50 percent of the patients with AODC will have increased activity scintographic of the adjacent acromion.

Pathologic material from 12 patients operated on was examined microscopically. This material was characterized as representing typical degenerative joint disease. However, there were frequent areas of subchondral microfracture with abundant evidence of healing processes by new bone formation.

Lamont in 1982 reported osteolysis of the distal clavicle and described cystic and erosive changes of the distal clavicle, but not microfractures.

The increased scintigraphic activity seen in patients with AODC is due to increased osteoblastic activity and not to an increased regional blood flow.

The sensitivity of joint scintigraphy in detecting pathology in patients with radiographically normal joints is well known. In 17 percent of patients with asymptomatic, radiographically normal shoulders, scintigraphy was positive. Symptomatic shoulders with normal x-ray results were scintigraphically positive in over 70 percent of the patients.

DIAGNOSIS OF AODC

The diagnosis of AODC must be considered in any athlete or exerciser with pain in the epaulet area (point of shoulder) who also has a history of strength training. The differential diagnosis must consider cervical, glenohumeral, coracoacromial arch, and other sources of shoulder pain. The diagnosis is probable if there is a history of epaulet pain later localizing at the acromioclavicular joint and local tenderness at this joint. Radiography may be contributory to the diagnosis.

The final diagnosis is confirmed only by positive joint scintigraphy of the acromioclavicular joint.

ASSOCIATION OF AODC WITH OTHER SHOULDER SYNDROMES

The cumulative stresses applied to the shoulder joint over an ever-lengthening athletic career and the additional stresses of strength training must eventually become physiologically intolerable to some peculiarly susceptible weak link in some athletes. This physiologic intolerance to cumulative stress is a stress failure syndrome, now poorly termed an "overuse syndrome."

In the shoulder, as with stress failure syndromes elsewhere in the musculoskeletal system, several anatomic areas may become simultaneously or sequentially symptomatic. There may be a cause and effect as in foot dysfunction contributing to patellar stresses and the anterior knee pain syndrome. Alternatively, the stress failure syndrome may be a simultaneous development, as when multiple stress fractures are present in the lower extremity of a runner.

In the shoulder, AODC is frequently associated with the impingement syndrome and glenohumeral instability. It is usually both a contributor to impingement and simultaneously a distinct entity when associated with glenohumeral instability.

Impingement Syndrome

Neer and colleagues pointed out the frequent contribution that the acromioclavicular joint makes to the overall pathology of the impingement syndrome. They further emphasized the importance of resection of the distal clavicle in order to decompress the coracoacromial arch adequately in some patients with impingement. Neer considers the acromioclavicular joint to be an integral part of the arch.

The association of AODC in athletes with the impingement syndrome is probable if there is localized tenderness at the acromioclavicular joint, and this may be confirmed by joint scintigraphy. The latter is not positive in uncomplicated athletic impingement syndromes.

In my series of patients with athletic impingement, the incidence of AODC as demonstrated by positive acromioclavicular joint scintigraphy may be as high as 15 percent.

Therefore all patients with athletic impingement who are potential surgical candidates should undergo a scintigraphic evaluation, and excision of the distal clavicle as a potential adjunctive procedure to standard coracoacromial arch decompression should be considered when scintigraphy is positive.

Glenohumeral Instability

In any athlete with glenohumeral instability, a careful search for shoulder pain during periods of glenohumeral stability is vital. If there is shoulder pain during periods of stability, the clinician should be suspicious of an additional pathologic condition. An additional tocsin of combined pathology is acromioclavicular joint tenderness in the athlete with shoulder instability. If there is a history of pain and acromioclavicular joint tenderness in the absence of pain, joint scintigraphy should be performed and can confirm the association of AODC. In such patients, resection of the distal clavicle should be considered when reconstructing the glenohumeral joint.

There has been no alteration in the rehabilitative pattern or results in eight of my patients with glenohumeral instability and AODC (five with dislocations, three with subluxation) who underwent combined reconstruction and resection of the distal clavicle.

TREATMENT

Conservative treatment of AODC should be directed toward eliminating the most symptom-provocative aspect of the training program. This is usually discovered to be strength training routines. It is often beneficial to eliminate or alter provocative strength training exercises or decrease their intensity. Nonsteroidal anti-inflammatory drugs or intra-articular injections are temporizing and pernicious methods of therapy. They should not be employed in the young athlete.

AODC is inexorably progressive if the implied stresses are not reduced or altered. Since my 1982 report on AODC, it has become increasingly difficult to counsel the athlete to accept a lower level of stress to the shoulder. The reasons are both philosophic and socioeconomic and are a separate topic. As a result, fewer athletes or exercisers are willing to accept conservative recommendations.

The indications for surgical management of AODC are unchanged from my 1982 report and are (1) a confirmed diagnosis of AODC and (2) an unwillingness on the part of the athlete to accept a lower level of performance.

The results of resection of the distal clavicle in patients with AODC in my material are almost always excellent, but I do not share the confidence of Rockwood and Green who describe it as "curative."

Gurd and Mumford, while they both reported resection of the distal clavicle in 1941, were not the discoverers of this procedure. The poor results of this procedure as reported are usually due to the pathologic process the excision was chosen for. Resection of the distal clavicle for acute or chronic acromioclavicular instability has a poor to dismal success rate.

Since 1982, 36 of the 67 AODC patients have undergone resection of the distal clavicles. The results, although still short term, have been good or excellent in 33 patients. I do not hesitate to recommend this procedure to well-motivated mature patients.

SUGGESTED READING

Allen WC. Post-traumatic osteolysis of the distal clavicle. Postgrad Med 1967; 41:A73–A77.

Cahill BR. Osteolysis of the distal part of the clavicle in male athletes. J Bone Joint Surg 1982; 64A:1053–1058.

Dupas J, Badelon P, Dayde G. Aspects radiologiques d'une osteolyse essentielle progressive de la main gauche. J Radiol 1936; 20:383–387.

Ehricht HG. Die Osteolyse im lateralen Claviculaende nach Pressluftschaden. Arch Orthop Unfallchir 1959; 50:576–582.

Gurd F. The treatment of complete dislocation of the outer end of the clavicle: An hitherto undescribed operation. Ann Surg 1941; 113:1094–1098.

Jacobs P. Post-traumatic osteolysis of the outer end of the clavicle. J Bone Joint Surg 1964; 46B:705–707.

Lamont MK. Osteolysis of the outer end of the clavicle. NZ Med J 1982; 95:241–242.

Levine AH, Pais MJ, Schwartz EE. Posttraumatic osteolysis of the distal clavicle with emphasis on early radiologic changes. Am J Roentgenol 1976; 127:781–784.

Madsen B. Osteolysis of the acromial end of the clavicle following trauma. Br J Radiol 1963; 36:822–828.

Mumford E. Acromioclavicular dislocation. J Bone Joint Surg 1941; 23:799–802.

Murphy OB, Bellamy R, Wheeler W, Brower TD. Post-traumatic osteolysis of the distal clavicle. Clin Orthop 1975; 109:108–114.

Neer CS. Impingement lesions. Clin Orthop 1983; 173:70.

Neer CS, Craign E, Fukuda, H. Cuff tear arthropathy. J Bone Joint Surg 1983; 65A:1232.

Rockwood C, Green D. Fractures in adults. 2nd ed. Philadelphia: JB Lippincott, 1984.

Seymore EQ. Osteolysis of the clavicular tip associated with repeated minor trauma to the shoulder. Radiology 1977; 123:56.

Smart MJ. Traumatic osteolysis of the distal ends of the clavicles. J Can Assoc Radiol 1972; 23:264–266.

Stahl F. Considerations on post-traumatic absorption of the outer end of the clavicle.Acta Orthop Scand 1954; 23:9–13.

Strauch W. Posttraumatische Osteolysen des lateralen Klavikulaendes. Radiol Diagn 1970; 11:221–229.

Zanca P. Shoulder pain: involvement of the acromioclavicular joint (analysis of 1,000 cases). Am J Roentgenol 1971; 112:493–506.

ELBOW

OVERUSE INJURY IN THE THROWING SPORTS

FRED L. ALLMAN Jr., M.D.

In the throwing sports, as in other activities, the basic power unit of performance is the musculotendinous unit; therefore, most elbow problems that arise during or as a result of throwing are related to muscular activity. The main offender is a dynamic overload to the musculotendinous unit, which may occur over an extended period as a result of the late effect of microtrauma.

In order to treat properly elbow injuries that result from the act of throwing, it is necessary for the physician, trainer, or coach to have insight into the basic qualities of muscle function and the intricate mechanism of throwing as it relates to the various sports, as well as a working knowledge of the clinical characteristics of each of the various types of injury that may occur.

An understanding of the basic qualities of muscle function is necessary to evaluate these injuries correctly. Clinically, there are three basic qualities of muscle function:

1. Strength: the ability of a muscle to contract.
2. Elasticity: the ability of a muscle to give up contraction and to yield to passive stretch.
3. Coordination: the ability of a muscle to cooperate with other muscles in proper timing and with appropriate power and elasticity.

It is usually possible to explain a deficiency in muscle action as the consequence of one, two, or all three of these basic qualities.

A muscle acts best from an elongated position because the elastic force of the muscle augments its contractile force. A muscle contracts best from its full length; therefore, overuse and overloading lead to fatigue. With fatigue, the muscle relaxes more slowly and more incompletely than normal and enters into a state of temporary myostatic contracture. It is during this period of myostatic contracture that injuries are likely to occur. The resulting injury may be a minor strain to the muscle or tendon, or if repeated over and over again, actual tears may take place in the muscle. Attempts at repair result in fibrosis, and this fibrosis in turn causes a permanent loss of elbow extension.

A basic knowledge of the biomechanics of throwing is essential if these injuries are to be properly understood. The mechanism of throwing has been called intricate and fascinating.

The throwing act consists of four essential steps for proper execution. After the initial stance are the preparatory phase or wind-up, the initial forward action of the arm, and lastly release and follow-through. Injury usually occurs during the forward motion and follow-through phases.

Stresses on the elbow vary according to the various sports. Dr. James Bateman noted that in baseball the most common injury is a tear or partial avulsion of one of the tendon insertions, often the result of medial overload produced by the valgus strain on the elbow.

In football, the wind-up is less than in baseball; the forward fling is shorter, and the follow-through is in a different arc and not as powerful.

Hammer throwing and shot putting place tremendous traction stress on the heavy muscles of the elbow and shoulder because of the momentum of the follow-through and the heavier projectile that is being propelled.

The javelin is released with a powerful extension of the elbow and forcible pronation of the forearm. The pronation is extreme and it is necessary to prevent the whip of the javelin. In the follow-through, the thrower may almost completely turn around.

Studies by the late Jay Bender at Southern Illinois University demonstrated that there may be at least three distinct patterns of throwing. Each pattern can be highly successful within itself; however, the methods of teaching throwing attempt to have a throw made in a more or less standard pattern, which means changing a person's own basic pattern. This not only causes confusion in technique, but also leads to frustration and often injury.

Shands, nearly 50 years ago, showed that trauma to hyaline cartilage produced a definite hyperplasia. The elbow of a pitcher often shows evidence of such hyperplasia. The margins, the tip of the olecranon, and the adjacent surfaces of the condyles of the humerus are constantly traumatized by the act of throwing. The result is a definite osteochondritis with exfoliation of the cartilage, which may produce loose bodies, synovial thickening, or semiattached cartilaginous masses that obstruct and limit the extension of the elbow.

A working classification of injuries involved in the throwing sports may be related to the structure involved, or to the mechanisms described by the late Don Slocum: (1) tension overloads to the inner side of the elbow that is muscular, ligamentous, and capsular; (2) lateral compression injuries—the fractured capitellum, osteochondral fractures, and traumatic arthritis; and (3) injuries to the extensor mechanism—acute traction injuries, disorders resulting from repetitive extensor action, and doorstop action of the olecranon fossa. We would therefore have strains of the flexor muscles and pronator, sprains of the collateral ligament and joint capsule; fractures of the medial epicondyle and of the olecranon (the olecranon fractures representing avulsions), as well as those to the medial epicondyle; and fractures to the radial head and capitellum, being mainly the osteochondritis type of injury.

Tension overload is seen frequently in young players as well as in more experienced players early in the season. Tightness develops on the medial aspect of the involved elbow. The medial muscle mass becomes tense and sore, and there is a temporary loss of extension. If this pitcher is allowed to continue under these conditions (while in a state of myostatic contracture), a more serious injury usually follows as extensive fibrosis results from multiple tearing throughout the muscle with consequent permanent loss of elbow extension.

Although rest, application of ice, gentle massage, anti-inflammatory agents, and other physical modalities are helpful, the main effort in treatment should be directed toward the cause of the condition rather than the resultant effect; i.e., the musculotendinous unit must be slowly and gradually stretched and strengthened to withstand the stress of pitching, without producing an undue overload. Stated in different terms, the treatment of such conditions is aimed at restoration or improvement of the impaired quality of muscle function. If the muscle is weak, it must be strengthened. If the muscle is inelastic, the elasticity must be improved. If the muscle has lost its proper timing and synchronous action, the goal should be to restore proper coordination. The problem may be related to all three qualities: strength, elasticity, and coordination.

It has been said that the great Dizzy Dean was forced to stop pitching because of injuries to his elbow that resulted not from an initial elbow injury, but from altered form while pitching with an injured big toe.

Many ailing pitchers can relate the exact moment of the beginning of their pitching demise, although the demise may be drawn out over a period of years. In many cases, the onset was initiated by pitching too hard, too soon in the season, or too soon after a previous exhausting game. "I felt something pop and the elbow became sore" is often the phrase that pitchers use to explain their first traumatic episode.

Tension overload on the medial aspect of the elbow may ultimately produce traction spurs. These spurs, which initially are asymptomatic, usually become symptomatic in time. They arise from the medial aspect of the ulnar notch and extend proximally. The site of the pain is usually about 1 inch below the medial epicondyle, but the pain may also be located anteriorly over the joint. If the spur is of sufficient length, ulnar nerve symptoms and findings may be noted.

Treatment for early cases without ulnar nerve involvement consists of rest, ice, and (rarely) steroid injection. If symptoms become prolonged, if performance is notably altered, or if there is nerve involvement, surgical excision is indicated.

Tension overload in the Little League age-group most often results in alterations of the medial epicondylar epiphysis. These may take the form of physiologic hypertrophy, minute avulsion, or complete avulsion of the epiphysis. Those avulsions with minimal displacement are best treated symptomatically and with rest. Often the position of the player should be changed from that of a pitcher to that of shortstop or first baseman for the remainder of the season. Avulsions with displacement are best treated by open reduction, with anatomic restoration of the fracture fragments and fixation with suture or pin. Three weeks of immobilization are usually adequate.

Lateral compression injuries are the result of impaction of the head of the radius against the capitellum in the act of throwing. Roughening and degeneration of the cartilage often results from such repeated insults to the articular cartilage. There is perhaps less resistance to this articular damage in the Little Leaguer than in the older player, and certainly the earlier the changes occur, the more guarded is the prognosis.

Again, treatment is symptomatic: initially with rest, ice, anti-inflammatory agents, and (rarely) steroids. Loose bodies should be surgically removed if they interfere with normal joint dynamics and function.

Extension injuries are also a frequent problem in pitchers. Chronic intermittent overload by the extensor mechanism results in hypertrophy of the ulna, the humerus, and the triceps muscle. It also causes a decrease in the size of the olecranon fossa. The tip of the olecranon and the olecranon fossa are the most common sites of osteochondral bodies in professional baseball pitchers.

Treatment is usually conservative, but surgical intervention may be indicated if pain cannot be controlled by more conservative means and especially if the pitcher shows a decline in performance and effectiveness. Two points should be stressed if surgery appears to be indicated. First, do not expect to gain full extension after surgery if there is a limitation of motion before surgery, even if large amounts of debris are removed from the olecranon fossa; second, do not hesitate to remove a generous portion of the olecranon process at the time of surgery. Probably the most gratifying surgery about the elbow is removal of loose bodies from the olecranon fossa.

It should also be noted that the repeated throwing motion in pitchers can result in tears in the ligaments about the elbow. Bleeding, swelling, and eventual calcification and ossification may develop. Continued stress to these areas can result in rupture, either incomplete or complete, in the involved ligament.

Rehabilitation of overuse injuries involving muscles and tendons should always include static stretching after a good warm-up. A progressive resistive exercise (PRE) program should follow. Progressive overload is essential if strength is to be increased. The PRE program should include both concentric and eccentric contractions, with greater emphasis on the latter. As strength increases and symptoms lessen, the speed of contractions can be increased.

In conclusion, it is important to remember the great individual variations in the human species. To my knowledge, there is no way that we can distinguish at an early age those youngsters who are most susceptible to elbow damage as a result of the stress of throwing. Certainly Satchel Paige, even with the best medical advice available, could not have improved his pitching longevity. Phil Neikro, Hoyt Wilhelm, Early Wynn, Gaylord Perry, and Warren Spahn are other classic examples of durability on the mound. However, we are all familiar with other pitchers who have not been nearly so durable and who showed rather pronounced symptoms at a very early age as a result of their stressful occupations.

The danger signals include tightness, soreness, tenderness, swelling, pain, loss of control, and loss of motion. Contraction, fatigue, and weakness are other warning signs.

It is at this stage that the player must be given a careful evaluation by a competent physician who can best make a judgment as to what restrictions or treatment may be indicated.

The vast majority of elbow problems related to throwing can be prevented by a proper conditioning program, in conjunction with more judicious care of the arm before, during, and after competition.

Treatment of the various pathologic conditions about the elbow will never enable athletes to achieve a performance level as high as they might have achieved if the condition had been prevented by proper action instituted at the proper time. Careful analysis of any problem is therefore essential.

ULNAR NEURITIS AND ULNAR COLLATERAL LIGAMENT INSTABILITIES IN OVERARM THROWERS

FRANK W. JOBE, M.D.
JAMES P. BRADLEY, M.D.

Athletes who participate in overarm sports can sustain a host of injuries to the elbow commonly localized to the medial side. Chronic stress is initiated by the repetitious high-velocity nature of these activities, and often predispose the elbow to overuse syndromes. Ulnar neuritis and ulnar collateral ligament compromise in particular are caused by overuse. Many overarm activities (e.g., the baseball pitch, tennis serve, javelin throw, and football pass) require similar movements: rapid forceful extension of the elbow, frequently accompanied by valgus stress and pronation of the forearm (Fig. 1). It is estimated that the range of motion of the elbow exceeds 300 degrees per second during throwing. Also the slight, normal valgus angle of the elbow in extension may predispose the medial aspect of the elbow to overuse injuries. The velocity, power, and repetitiousness of these movements all contribute to the ensuing microtrauma. Thus, overuse is encountered when the body's physiologic ability to heal itself lags behind the microtrauma that is occurring.

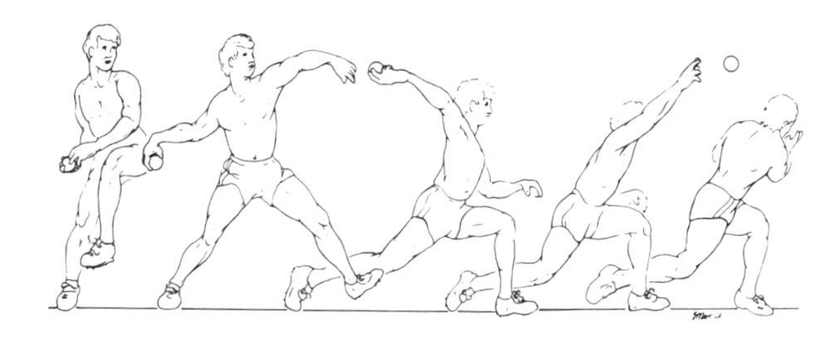

Figure 1 Baseball pitch.

ULNAR NEURITIS

Etiology

In the upper arm the ulnar nerve courses subfascially, anterior to the medial intermuscular septum. At the arcade of Struthers it moves posterior to the septum, passing behind the medial epicondyle with the superior ulnar collateral artery into the cubital tunnel. The boundaries of the tunnel are formed by the posterior band of the medial collateral ligament, the medial edge of the trochlea, the medial epicondylar groove, and the arcuate ligament (which acts as the tendinous arch of the insertion of the two heads of the flexor carpi ulnaris). The nerve continues into the forearm, passing between the humeral and ulnar heads of the flexor carpi ulnaris (FCU) muscle. The ulnar nerve has no branches in the upper arm, but at the elbow there are several small articular branches. Immediately distal to the cubital tunnel the first motor branches emerge to the flexor carpi ulnaris.

During elbow flexion the ulnar nerve elongates an average of 4.7 mm and can be pushed over 7 mm medially by the medial head of the triceps. Cubital tunnel volume is reduced by concomitant stretching of the arcuate ligament and bulging of the posterior portion of the medial collateral ligament. Tightening of the aponeurosis of the flexor carpi ulnaris during flexion may also compress the ulnar nerve. Thus, the proximity of several other mobile structures endangers the mobility of the ulnar nerve.

Entrapment may be caused by pathologic factors (tensile and compressive forces on the medial aspect of the elbow) or physiologic factors (hypertrophy of bone, muscle, or ligament). Entrapment or dislocation of the ulnar nerve, or both, are conditions seen most often in athletes whose arms repeatedly perform a throwing motion that results in valgus stress at the elbow. This group includes baseball pitchers, tennis players, javelin throwers, gymnasts, and football quarterbacks. Biomechanical analysis of arm motion in these athletes reveals three kinds of basic pathologic stresses to the ulnar nerve: compression, friction, and traction. Of course, in any one lesion a combination of these stresses may be present.

Compression of the ulnar nerve may occur in association with several conditions. Physiologic hypertrophy of the medial head of the triceps, anconeous epitrochlearis or flexor carpi ulnaris is occasionally encountered in these top-level athletes. Entrapment of the ulnar nerve beneath a thickened arcuate ligament (the so-called Osborne lesion) is particularly common and may present in conjunction with forearm flexor hypertrophy. Both conditions increase pressure on the underlying nerve. Pechan and Julis demonstrated elevation of intraneural pressures by direct measurement in the ulnar nerve with the wrist extended and the elbow at 90 degrees' physiologic stretch of the nerve, and external compression from the overlying aponeurosis of the flexor carpi ulnaris muscle. Further flexion of the elbow, extension of the wrist, and abduction of the shoulder, such as occurs in the early stages of the overhead pitch, can elevate intraneural pressures to six times that in the relaxed nerve. Intrinsic masses (i.e., ganglion, lipomas) also may compress the nerve.

Friction neuritis commonly results from recurrent subluxation and/or dislocation of the ulnar nerve anterior to the medial epicondyle of the humerus. Childress noted that 16.2 percent of the population demonstrate recurrent dislocation of the ulnar nerve as the elbow moves from complete extension to full flexion. This hypermobility is often secondary to congenital or developmental laxity of the soft tissue constraints that normally hold the nerve in the epicondylar groove. Childress also found that those nerves that incompletely dislocate over the medial epicondyle are more susceptible to direct trauma, whereas those that completely dislocate are more prone to develop friction neuritis.

Traction neuritis may develop when an attenuated or ruptured ulnar collateral ligament allows the medial side of the joint to "open up" excessively, thus placing abnormal stress on the ulnar nerve and creating a valgus deformity. Normally, the ulnar nerve is free to move in the groove both longitudinally and medially. Any restriction of this movement may lead to traction of the nerve during the act of throwing. Repeated microtrauma may lead to inflammation, adhesions, and tethering of the nerve. Further fibrosis may lead to vascular compromise of the nerve. The nerve may also become tethered by fixed flexion deformity, traction spurs, calcific deposits, or an irregular ulnar groove secondary to degenerative changes or an old medial epicondyle separation.

Clinical Presentation

A thorough history, including standard parameters such as duration of symptoms, severity of pain, frequency of pain, neurologic complaints, and aggravating factors, is particularly important in recognizing this type of injury. The chief clinical symptom is pain in the elbow, radiating down the ulnar aspect of the arm into the hand. Numbness and tingling in the ring and little fingers is common. Other symptoms include clumsiness, heaviness, and problems with grasp, especially after throwing. These symptoms may disappear with rest and then recur with return to activity. Painful snapping or popping sensations when the elbow is rapidly flexed and extended, associated with sharp pains radiating into the forearm and hand, are indicative of recurrent dislocation of the ulnar nerve. A history of sudden pain at the elbow without snapping generally indicates subluxation rather than dislocation or entrapment.

The physical examination commonly elicits tenderness to palpation over the ulnar nerve at the elbow, not over the ulnar collateral ligament. Upon palpation the ulnar nerve may feel thickened or "doughy" and can often be subluxed manually. Neurologic abnormalities in regions innervated by the ulnar nerve, including hypoesthesia, interosseous muscle wasting, and dry skin, should be carefully considered. Tinel's sign may be localized to the cubital tunnel behind the medial epicondyle in cubital tunnel entrapment. A Tinel's sign proximal to the medial epicondyle at the intermuscular septum suggests subluxation or dislocation of the ulnar nerve. Weakness of the flexor carpi ulnaris and flexor digitorum profundus is rarely seen because the motor fibers to these muscles lie deepest in the cubital tunnel and are usually uninvolved. However, subtle changes in two-point discrimination over the ring and little fingers and loss of fine intrinsic muscle control may be noted periodically. Evidence of nerve compression lesions at other levels must also be investigated. Cervical rib, thoracic outlet syndrome, superior sulcus tumor, cervical disc protrusion with radiculopathy, compression at Guyon's canal, or compression of the deep branch of the ulnar nerve can all produce symptoms along the ulnar nerve distribution and should be specifically ruled out. A search for intrinsic masses (e.g., ganglion or lipomas) and chronic compartment syndrome of the forearm must also be conducted.

Electromyography usually is not helpful and findings are often inconclusive owing to the intermittent nature of the problem. Neural conduction studies occasionally are negative in milder cases, but a conduction delay across the elbow is the usual finding. A complete roentgenographic series, including a cubital tunnel view, should be performed. Additional symptoms and signs of associated pathologic conditions (e.g., ligamental laxity, loose bodies, degenerative changes, medial epicondylitis of the elbow) should also be investigated, and the condition of the whole joint complex must be considered when decisions are made regarding treatment and rehabilitation.

Treatment

Acute cases of ulnar neuritis, in which symptoms are not yet severe and intrinsic wasting is not present, may respond well to conservative treatment. Rest and ice should be applied and the joint should be immobilized with a splint for 2 to 3 weeks. Anti-inflammatory medications may also be helpful. Steroid injection into the cubital tunnel is not recommended. In most cases surgical intervention is not required. When surgery *is* indicated, submuscular anterior transposition of the ulnar nerve deep to the flexor muscle group provides ample protection from direct and indirect trauma occasioned by throwing. Simple decompression is not sufficient for the long term.

Ulnar Nerve Transfer

A medial incision is made posterior to the medial epicondyle of the elbow, extending approximately 5 cm in either direction from the epicondyle. Special care must be taken to preserve the branches of the medial antebrachial cutaneous nerve during dissection. The fascia of the brachium at the medial edge of the triceps is split and the ulnar nerve is located above the condyle. The dissection is carried proximally to the point where it penetrates the medial intermuscular septum. The ligament of Struthers and the septum are split sufficiently to permit the nerve to be easily displaced anteriorly. The cubital tunnel is unroofed and the nerve, with its accompanying veins, is gently dissected. A Penrose drain is used to retract the nerve. Special care is taken to preserve the articular branches of the ulnar nerve. The fascia between the humeral and ulnar origins of the flexor carpi ulnaris is split so that after anterior transposition there will not be a sharp angulation as it enters the muscle group. Motor nerves to the flexor carpi ulnaris muscle are carefully preserved. After the nerve is completely dissected free, a section of the intermuscular septum is removed to prevent the nerve from impinging when translocated anteriorly. If there is a great deal of scar tissue or hourglass constriction of the nerve, it may be necessary to perform a simple neurolysis. Extensive neurolysis may lead to excessive intraneural fibrosis.

At this point the posterior aspect of the joint may be inspected for loose bodies or osteophytes and treated accordingly. An incision is then made in the superficial flexor-pronator muscle mass, perpendicular to the direction of its fibers and approximately 1 cm from its insertion; this incision is extended proximally to the medial collateral ligament. The top margin of the flexor, in the interval just short of the brachioradialis, is elevated and retracted distally, leaving a carpet of muscle fiber on the ligament to provide a bed of muscle for the nerve. The nerve should then be transposed anteriorly, placed in the flexor muscle fringe, and covered with the muscle belly. To ensure that no entrapment occurs, a small section is cut out of the muscle fascia around the new course of the ulnar nerve. There must be no tethering of the relocated nerve either distally, where it should lie in a bed of muscle, or proximally, where it should lie in a bed of fat. The flexor muscles are reattached to the epicondyle either by direct suture to a soft tissue cuff or through drill holes in the bone. Closure is accomplished with absorbable sutures for the deep structures and 4–0 clear nylon subcuticular sutures for the skin.

Rehabilitation

After closure, the joint should be splinted in 90 degrees of flexion, leaving the wrist free for 10 days. The patient should begin squeezing a sponge or soft ball as soon as comfort permits. Range-of-motion exercises emphasizing extension should begin 2 weeks after surgery. After the patient has regained full range of motion, a gradual strengthening program for the forearm flexors and extensors is instituted. Care must be taken not to neglect the other major muscle groups of the upper extremity during the rehabilitation period; this is especially true for throwing athletes. About 2 months postoperatively, the patient may begin to toss a ball easily, gradually increasing increments of speed and power over the next 3 to 4 months. Return to full activity may be permitted about 6 months after surgery. The earlier in the course of the disease that surgical intervention takes place, the better is the prognosis for a return to full preoperative ability.

ULNAR COLLATERAL LIGAMENT INSTABILITY

Etiology

The anterior portion of the ulnar collateral ligaments is the major stabilizing agent at the elbow (Fig. 2). Injury or laxity of this structure results in instability of the medial aspect of the elbow joint under valgus stress. Injuries to the ulnar collateral ligament in athletes are primarily caused by overuse. Inadequate conditioning, warm-up, and body mechanics can predispose to "microfailures" in the fibers of the ligament as the result of repeated small stresses. If the rate of failure is greater than the rate of repair and reproduction, there will be pain, inflammation, and eventual disruption of the bone-ligament junction. It then takes less stress for the weakened area to be reinjured.

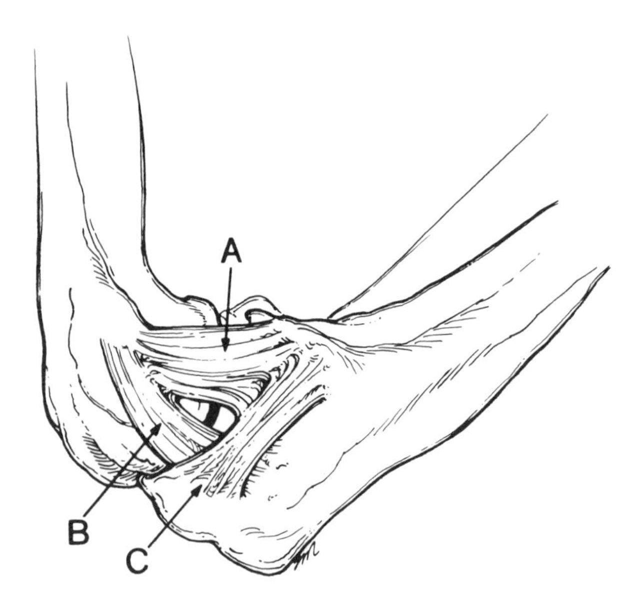

Figure 2 Ulnar collateral ligaments. *A*, Anterior portion; *B*, posterior portion; *C*, oblique portion.

Clinical Presentation

The primary symptom of injury to the medial collateral ligament is pain on the medial aspect of the elbow during throwing. Patients may also exhibit tenderness to palpation and swelling over the ligament medially. Often there is a sensation of the elbow "opening" while throwing, and many patients show a decreased range of motion at the elbow. Ulnar nerve symptoms may become apparent secondary to the unnatural valgus opening during throwing. There is often a single episode of "giving way," which probably represents only the final insult.

Valgus instability at the elbow can be diagnosed clinically by first flexing the patient's arm 20 to 30 degrees to unlock the olecranon from its fossa, then applying a gentle valgus stress. Instability of the joint will allow the medial side of the joint to open. A radiographic gravity stress test of the elbow may confirm the diagnosis. Ulnar collateral instability must be differentiated from forearm flexor muscle rupture. The valgus stress test in the former produces pain and opening, while in the latter resistive flexion of the wrist is painful.

Four stages of the malady have been identified: (1) edema, (2) scarring and dissociation of ligament fibers, (3) calcification, and (4) ossification. Scarring, calcification, and ossification are all stress raisers that focus biomechanical stresses on already weakened areas, thus increasing the likelihood of further damage.

Treatment

If the injury is detected in the early stages, conservative treatment is appropriate. Rest, for a longer time than would ordinarily be recommended, is crucial. Heat and ice should be applied alternately, and injections of lidocaine (Xylocaine) and steroids may be helpful. Injection should be made not into, but on top of the ligament, to bathe it. It is preferable to give no more than three injections, and not more than once a month. If scarring and calcification are present, and if they are accompanied by pain that does not respond to rest, the calcification should be removed and the ligament repaired. If stability of the joint is all that is required, surgery is not necessary; however, if the patient desires to continue participation in a sport requiring throwing or overarm movements, surgery may be required.

Rarely, patients have a history of multiple episodes of pain over the medial elbow while throwing, which initially restricts throwing. However, after a few days to weeks of self-instituted conservative care it will resolve, only to become symptomatic with resumption of throwing. Physical examination elicits pain over the medial elbow with valgus stress associated with snapping along the medial elbow. Instability testing and stress x-ray results are negative. If these patients are unresponsive to 6 months of supervised conservative treatment, open exploration of the ulnar ligaments is indicated.

Surgical reconstruction of the ulnar collateral ligament with a tendon graft is indicated in the following circumstances: (1) acute rupture in throwers; (2) when it is desired to reestablish valgus stability in the presence of symptomatic chronic laxity; (3) after debridement for calcific tendinitis, if there is insufficient viable tissue remaining to effect a primary repair in an athlete; or (4) multiple episodes of recurring pain with throwing after periods of conservative care.

Reconstruction of Unlar Collateral Ligament of Elbow

Using a tourniquet for hemostasis, a standard medial incision is made and carried down through the subcutaneous tissue to the myofascia. Care is taken to protect the median antebrachial cutaneous nerve. An incision is made into the myofascial covering of the origin of the flexor muscle mass, in line with the muscle fibers. The flexor mass is retracted to both sides to expose the anterior oblique portion of the medial collateral ligament.

An incision is made into the ligament, again in line with the fibers, and the ligament is debrided to remove all calcifications. At this juncture the elbow should be flexed 20 to 30 degrees and a valgus stress applied. The medial aspect of the elbow joint should open easily. If sufficient ligamentous tissue remains, a simple primary repair can be effected, but this is the exception and not the rule in throwing athletes. Usually it is necessary to reconstruct the ligament.

If the ligament permits primary repair, the ligament should be debrided and reattached to the periosteum. Slack in the ligament can be tightened by using a figure-of-eight suture on both sides of the longitudinal split, and then testing for snugness. The two halves of the ligament are next approximated and sutured. If the ligament has been torn off its bony insertion, the bone should be rongeured to provide a good base for reattachment. Holes are then drilled in the bone, sutures are passed through the holes, and the ligament is sutured securely to the bone.

If it is necessary to reconstruct the ligament, the flexor muscles should be cut approximately 1 cm distal to the medial epicondyle, leaving a fringe of tendon for reattachment. As the tendon and muscle are reflected distally, a thin carpet of flexor and pronator muscle fibers is left on the medial collateral ligament. This will be used later as a bed for the transposed ulnar nerve, to protect it from scarring. When the muscles are reflected distally, there is excellent exposure of the entire ulnar collateral ligament (Fig. 3).

The ulnar nerve is mobilized from a point 2.5 cm distal to the medial epicondyle to well above the medial epicondyle, and thereafter it is protected with a 6.4-mm Penrose drain. If calcifications or particles of bone are present, they are removed from the ligament and the surrounding soft tissue. Using a slow-speed drill with a drill guide, 3.2-mm holes are drilled in the medial epicondyle and the ulna, corresponding to the points of attachment of the torn ligament (Fig. 4). The holes are placed so that the tendon graft does not rub on either epicondyle or ulnar excrescences. The tendon graft is harvested from either the palmaris, the plantaris, or a 3-mm-wide by 15-cm-long strip of Achilles tendon. The tendon graft is passed through the holes so that it forms a figure of eight and acts as a functional substitute for the anterior oblique portion of the medial collateral ligament (Fig. 5). The graft is pulled taut

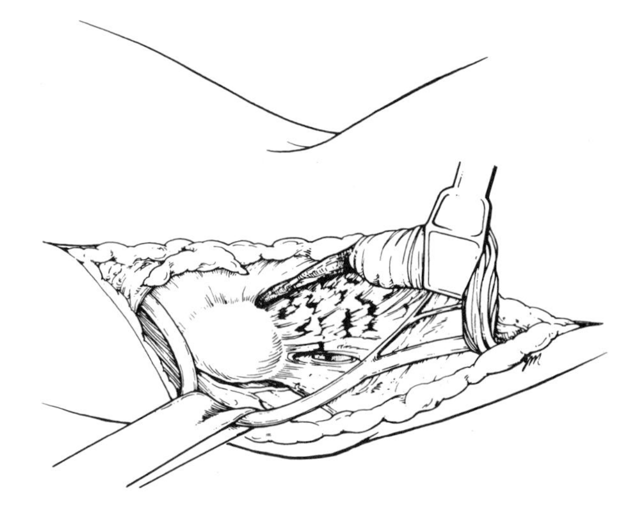

Figure 3 Exposure of the ulnar collateral ligaments.

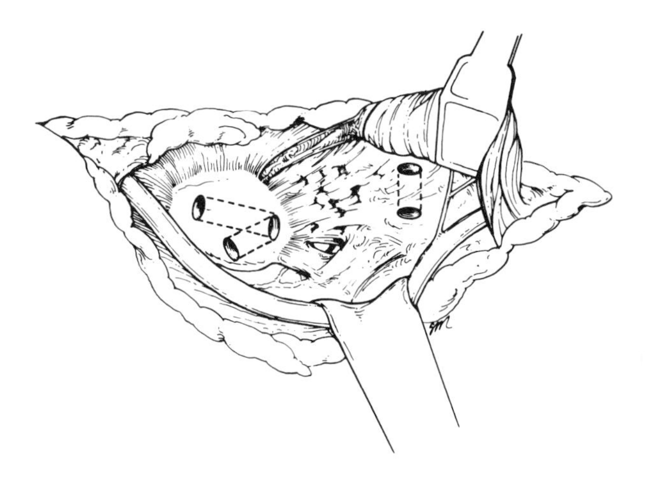

Figure 4 Preparation for the tendon graft.

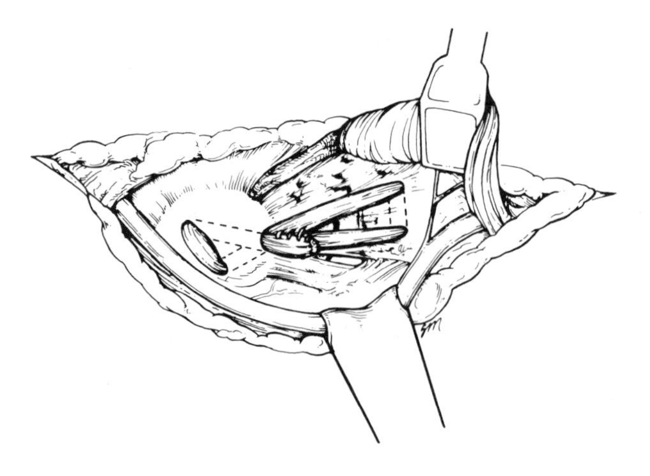

Figure 5 Tendon graft.

and sutured to itself; any remnants of the original ligament are sutured over the graft for added strength. The ulnar nerve is then transposed anteriorly, as previously described, to protect it from damage during and after surgery. The flexor and pronator muscles are reattached over the transferred nerve to the medial epicondyle. The arm is immobilized in a posterior splint with the elbow at 90 degrees of flexion, leaving the wrist free. No brace is used on the arm because the elbow is intrinsically stable.

Rehabilitation

The patient starts the rehabilitation program by squeezing a soft sponge or ball on the first postoperative day or as soon as it is comfortable to do so. Immobilization is discontinued after 2 weeks, at which time gentle passive–active assistive elbow range-of-motion exercises are begun. Passive terminal extension and flexion (i.e., the last 5 to 10 degrees) should be avoided for the first 3 months. Active wrist and shoulder range-of-motion exercises should not be neglected.

Beginning at 1 month, gradually more vigorous muscle-strengthening exercises are performed daily, including flexion, extension, pronation, and supination of the wrist. The patient must also perform range-of-motion and muscle-strengthening exercises for the shoulder, including those that strengthen the rotator cuff, to prevent weakening and contracture of the shoulder.

At 1 to 2 months postoperatively, elbow-strengthening exercises, guarding against terminal extension and flexion, are added to the above regimen. At 3 to 5 months the patient may begin easy tossing of a ball for about 30 to 40 feet (no wind-up) two to three times a week, 10 to 15 minutes per session. The patient must guard against valgus stress and ballistic movements. In 5 to 7 months the program is expanded to include a total body conditioning program. Tossing with wind-up and gradually increasing distances is then initiated. Ice is used after all throwing activities to decrease inflammatory response. At 7 to 12 months a graduated program of range-of-motion exercises, strengthening exercises, total body conditioning, and supervised increased increments of throwing is undertaken.

The described regimen is modified as necessary during the course of treatment to adjust it to the individual patient. Whenever a patient has pain, swelling, or both at the operative site, throwing is discontinued for at least 2 weeks and then gradually resumed. It takes approximately 1 year before a tendon graft and the surrounding tissues regain sufficient strength and endurance to function as a ligament in a throwing athlete. Furthermore, the average time to return to preoperative ability is 18 months for a professional pitcher. Athletes who play other positions require a shorter period of rehabilitation.

SUGGESTED READING

Del Pizzo W, Jobe FW, Norwood L. Ulnar nerve entrapment syndrome in baseball players. Am J Sports Med 1977; 5:182–185.

Jobe FW, Fanton GS. Nerve injuries. In Morrey B, ed. The elbow and its disorders. Philadelphia: WB Saunders, 1985; 497.

Jobe FW, Stark HH, Lombardo SJ. Reconstruction of the ulnar collateral ligament in athletes. J Bone Joint Surg 1986; 68-A:1158–1163.

Morrey BF. Articular and ligamentous contributions to the stability of the elbow joint. Am J Sports Med 1983; 11:315–319.

Schwab GH, Bennett JB, Woods GW, Tullos HS. Biomechanics of elbow instability: the role of the medial collateral ligament. Clin Orthop 1980; 146:42.

Tullos HS, Schwab G, Bennett JB, Woods GW: Factors influencing elbow instability. Instr Course Lect 1981; 30:185–199.

OVERUSE SYNDROMES

C. STEWART WRIGHT, M.D., F.R.C.S.(C)

TENNIS ELBOW

Lateral epicondylitis refers to an overload syndrome affecting the forearm extensor origin at the bone tendon junction. Most authors consider that the extensor carpi radialis brevis (ECRB) is the most responsible tendon. Problems in this area may be the result of a single overload episode such as a poorly hit backhand shot in tennis. Occasionally, local trauma may be the original cause. More commonly, however, it is a cumulative overload against the background of a poorly conditioned extensor mechanism. This underscores the importance of a preseason conditioning program and a pre-exercise warm-up with one of the various types of racquet sports.

The hallmark of this condition is pain at the origin of the extensor tendon, particularly on impact loading. In the chronic state there may be a background of nagging pain exacerbated by activities that use these muscles.

GOLFER'S ELBOW

A similar symptom complex may occur in relation to the medial epicondyle and common flexor origin. As with the lateral side, repeated microtrauma may lead to a mild degenerative reaction with an associated low-grade inflammatory response. Again, the importance of a pre-exercise stretching and strengthening program should be emphasized.

OLECRANON IMPACTION SYNDROME

This third entity involving the elbow is usually seen in the throwing sports. It refers to discomfort centered in the olecranon fossa at full extension of the elbow. It usually presents as an ache that occurs during release of the ball or during some other action that results in full elbow extension or hyperextension. This needs to be differentiated from a triceps tendinitis, which usually shows local tenderness over the insertion of the tendon.

NEUROLOGIC CONDITIONS

Medial epicondylitis should be differentiated from ulnar nerve neuritis. Local sensitivity over the nerve behind the epicondyle and distal sensory complaints usually distinguish the two conditions. Occasionally, the two coexist and may both require treatment.

Lateral epicondylitis may occasionally be confused with a radial nerve entrapment syndrome in the radial tunnel. The area of local tenderness is usually 2 to 3 cm distal to the lateral epicondyle. Clinically, this may present as an ache in the extensor mass with radiation both proximally and distally. Electromyographic (EMG) studies are usually not helpful. Resisted extension of the middle finger with the wrist in neutral (the middle finger test) may reproduce the typical distribution of pain. Pain with resisted wrist extension is more likely to be tennis elbow.

Four potential areas of compression in the radial tunnel are identified in the following locations:

1. By fibrous bands lying anterior to the radial head.
2. By the radial recurrent vessels (the leash of Henry).
3. At the tendinous margin of the extensor carpi radialis brevis.
4. At the arcade of Froshe, a ligamentous band over the deep branch of the nerve at its entrance into the supinator muscle. (This is the most common area of involvement.)

MANAGEMENT

Conservative

Some modification of the athlete's usual activity is required. This may involve a change in racquet head and grip size, string tension, and frequency of activity or may necessitate an evaluation of stroke mechanics. A lesson with the local club professional is often a good starting point.

Local icing, ultrasonography, and deep heat are also useful in the attempt to limit the inflammatory response. Stretching the involved muscle tendon groups is important both before and after exercise. Strengthening exercises are necessary both for conditioning and as part of a rehabilitative program. Flexor muscle bulk may be enhanced by squeezing a soft squash ball or doing wrist curls with light weights. Stretching a firm elastic band by spreading the fingers or doing reverse wrist curls will help to strengthen the extensor musculature.

Nonsteroidal anti-inflammatory agents are most useful in the acute stage of the condition and should probably be used for only 2 to 3 weeks. Steroid injections into the bone tendon junction should be used as a second-line treatment if the nonsteroidal agents fail. A suggested limit of three steroid injections over a 6-month interval should be effective for the vast majority of patients with epicondylitis. Beyond this, surgery should be considered.

Splints and braces designed to dissipate impact load through the forearm musculature may be useful for certain patients. These should not be applied too firmly; they should be positioned over the bulk of the musculature rather than over the point of tenderness. In this manner, they can share the impact load with the musculature.

Surgical

Most patients respond to a combination of conservative measures, but some require surgery.

Lateral epicondylitis is approached through a lateral incision over the epicondyle and radial head. The proximal tendon and extensor origin is exposed and released from the epicondyle. The tendon attachment to the annular ligament is released from the anterior neck of the radius. A portion of the epicondyle is removed with an osteotome and the bed drilled with a 2-mm drill bit. This enhances vascular supply and relieves venous hypertension in the bone. The fascia is then closed and a gentle stretching and strengthening program begun during the first week. Resolution of symptoms usually takes 3 months after surgery. Return to activity should be delayed until full flexibility has been achieved and all pain to local pressure or impact resolved.

Medial epicondylitis is treated in a similar fashion with release of the origin, excision of part of the epicondyle, drilling of the bone bed, and resuturing of the fascia.

In the ulnar impaction syndrome the triceps is split, the tip of the olecranon excised, and the olecranon fossa cleansed of loose body or fibrous tissue. Care is taken to ensure that no bone impingement occurs at full extension of the elbow.

For the radial tunnel syndrome, an anterolateral approach is made (after Henry). The nerve can be identified easily in the interval between the brachialis and the brachioradialis. It can then be traced distally through the potential areas of compression. Both the superficial and deep branches are explored, and care is taken to release the arcade of Froshe adequately, because this is the most common area of compression.

As in the management of other chronic tendonitides, early recognition of the entity and modification of the factors provoking it are the surest way to minimize the disability. Once chronically established, these conditions are difficult to resolve conservatively. The results of surgery are generally very satisfactory, but there may be a protracted period before a return to sporting activities is possible.

SUGGESTED READING

DeHaven KE, Evarts CM. Throwing injuries of the elbow in athletes. Orthop Clin North Am 1973; 4:801.

Eversmann WW. Entrapment and compression neuropathies. In: Green DP, ed. Operative hand surgery. New York: Churchill Livingstone, 1982.

Froimson AI. Tenosynovitis and tennis elbow. In: Green DP, ed. Operative hand surgery. New York: Churchill Livingstone, 1982.

Nirschl RP. The etiology and treatment of tennis elbow. J Sports Med 1974; 2:308.

ARTHROSCOPY OF THE ELBOW

WILLIAM G. CARSON Jr., M.D.

Arthroscopy is most commonly utilized to treat various disorders of the knee; however, it now is also being applied to smaller joints such as the shoulder, the ankle, and even the elbow. Arthroscopic procedures on these smaller joints require meticulous attention to detail, since the arthroscopic instruments must be placed through deeper muscle layers and close to important neurovascular structures. This is unlike the situation in the knee, where instruments pass through a thin retinacular layer only and maintain generous distances from neurovascular structures. Thus, the need for attention to detail when performing surgical procedures such as arthroscopy of the elbow become readily apparent.

INDICATIONS

Arthroscopy of the elbow is a relatively new advancement in the field of arthroscopy, and the indications for its use are still being determined. The following indications appear to be appropriate:

1. Removal of loose bodies.
2. Evaluation and debridement of osteochondritis dissecans of the capitellum.
3. Evaluation and/or debridement of chondral or osteochondral lesions of the radial head.
4. Debridement and lysis of adhesions of post-traumatic origin or arising from certain degenerative processes about the elbow.
5. Partial synovectomy in rheumatoid disease.
6. Partial excision of humeral or olecranal osteophytes.

Contraindications for elbow arthroscopy include bony ankylosis or severe fibrous ankylosis that would prevent the introduction of the arthroscopic instruments into the elbow joint. Further contraindications include certain surgical procedures such as anterior transposition of the ulnar nerve or other procedures that have altered the anatomy around the elbow so that placement of the usual arthroscopic portals might jeopardize the neurovascular structures.

SURGICAL TECHNIQUE

I prefer general anesthesia for elbow arthroscopy as I feel it affords complete relaxation and comfort for the patient. I do not recommend interscalene or axillary block anesthesia as this interferes with the immediate postoperative neurovascular evaluation in the recovery room. A tourniquet is routinely used: care should be taken to use a cuff of the proper size with proper padding, and in most cases to limit tourniquet time to no longer than 2 hours.

The patient is placed on the operating table in the supine position with the affected scapula just to the edge of the operating table, to allow the upper arm and forearm to hang free over the edge of the table. The hand and forearm are placed in a prefabricated forearm gauntlet that is connected to an overhead suspension device so that the elbow is flexed to 90 degrees (Fig. 1). Only enough traction is applied to the arm to allow the arm to suspend and keep the elbow flexed 90 degrees. This position provides excellent access to both the medial and lateral aspects of the elbow, and the forearm may be freely pronated and supinated throughout the surgical procedure. It is important to maintain the elbow in this 90-degree flexed position at all times when examining the anterior structures of the elbow arthroscopically, so as to completely relax the neurovascular structures in the antecubital fossa.

The bony anatomic landmarks are now outlined with a marking pen before the procedure is begun. As there can be a large amount of extravasation of fluid during the arthroscopic procedure, this previous marking allows one to maintain identifiable landmarks throughout the surgery. The bony landmarks that are usually marked are the radial head and the lateral humeral epicondyle on the lateral side of the elbow, and the medial humeral epicondyle on the medial aspect of the elbow. Posteriorly the olecranon is identified.

The three arthroscopic portals used most commonly for elbow arthroscopy include the anterolateral, anteromedial, and posterolateral portals. Before the insertion of the arthroscope into any of the portals, however, the elbow should be maximally distended with fluid through an 18-gauge spinal needle. I prefer to inject this needle into the triangular area over the lateral aspect of the elbow bordered by the radial head, the lateral humeral epicondyle, and the tip of the olecranon. This area is often used to aspirate the elbow for a hemarthrosis, such as

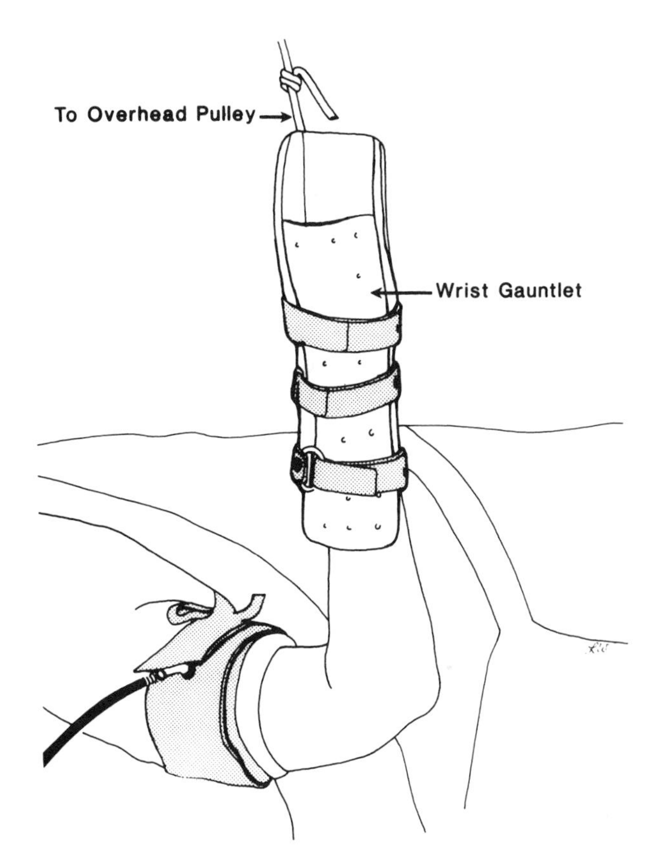

Figure 1 Position of the arm for arthroscopy of the elbow. (Republished with permission from Andrews JR, Carson WG. Arthroscopy of the elbow. Arthroscopy 1985; 1:98.)

would occur with a radial head fracture, and through this area the needle traverses only skin, a thin subcutaneous layer, the anconeus muscle, and the capsule. Thus, with the elbow flexed 90 degrees, the needle is placed into the elbow joint through this area and the elbow maximally distended with the use of a 50-ml syringe connected to an intravenous tubing. Proper placement into the elbow joint is verified by brisk backflow from the needle. Once verification of entry into the elbow is made, the needle is removed and the elbow is left maximally distended. The anterolateral portal is now established.

Anterolateral Portal

The anterolateral portal is the one first used for elbow arthroscopy, primarily for diagnostic purposes. The anteromedial portal is usually established only under direct visualization after the anterolateral portal is already in place. With the elbow flexed 90 degrees and maximally distended with fluid, the 18-gauge spinal needle is now placed 3 cm distal and 2 cm anterior to the lateral humeral epicondyle (Fig. 2); the needle is aimed directly toward the center of the joint. The needle course is just anterior to the radial head, which can be verified by

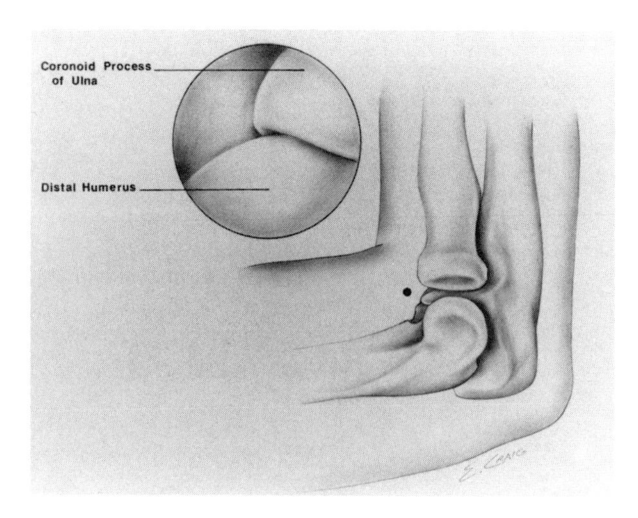

Figure 2 The anterolateral portal is located approximately 3 cm distal and 2 cm anterior to the lateral humeral epicondyle. Arthroscopic anatomy as seen through this portal includes the distal humerus and coronoid process of the ulna. (Republished with permission from Andrews JR, Carson WG. Arthroscopy of the elbow. Arthroscopy 1985; 1:99.)

pronating and supinating the forearm. Verification of entry into the elbow joint is confirmed by free backflow provided by the fluid previously placed into the elbow joint. Once proper needle placement is confirmed and the elbow is maximally distended, the larger arthroscopic instruments can be introduced. At this point a small skin incision is made, taking care to avoid injury to the underlying subcutaneous nerves. The superficial nerves to be avoided during the establishment of the anterolateral portal include the lateral and posterior antebrachial cutaneous nerves. At this point, rather than using the sharp trocar and cannula as is usually the case in the shoulder or the knee, the blunt cannula is used initially. This can often be readily inserted through the subcutaneous fat and the muscles; then, once resistance is noted, the sharp trocar can be inserted to pass through the deeper fascial and capsule layers, and the blunt trocar can be introduced again as the elbow joint is entered. By using the blunt trocar as much as possible, damage to nearby neurovascular structures is minimized, and superficial or deeper nerves may be less injured than with the sharp trocar. Use of the blunt trocar also reduces damage to the articular cartilage in this small joint. As the trocar and cannula system is inserted, great care must be taken to direct the instruments toward the center to the elbow joint as the elbow is kept flexed 90 degrees at all times. Once the elbow capsule is entered, free backflow of fluid will be noted through the cannula, and at this point the arthroscope is inserted and diagnostic arthroscopy begun. Continuous distention of the elbow is maintained by the use of overhead bags of normal saline attached to the arthroscope. Occasionally, more pressure is required to distend the elbow, and an additional inflow can be attached to the arthroscopic sleeve with a 50-ml syringe and intravenous tubing. Suction may be intermittently placed on the arthroscopic sleeve to remove any cloudy fluid or debris.

I use the 4-mm, 30-degree angled arthroscope as I feel this provides optimal visualization of the elbow joint. This is the same arthroscope that is used in larger joints such as the shoulder or knee. The smaller 2.7-mm "needle" arthroscope has been described; however, the difference in diameter between this smaller arthroscope and the larger 4-mm arthroscope is only 1.3 mm. Thus, the rationale of using smaller arthroscopes to avoid injury to neurovascular structures does not appear to be valid.

Intra-articular structures of the elbow that can be visualized from the anterolateral portal are the distal humerus and trochlear ridges as well as the coronoid process of the ulna (see Fig. 2). Flexion and extension of the elbow allows one to see the coronoid process of the elbow, and extension of the elbow provides a better view of the medial and lateral trochlear ridges and the trochlear notch of the distal humerus. By slowly retracting and angling the 30-degree arthroscope toward the radial head, a small portion of this may be seen from the anterolateral portal.

Cadaveric dissections of the arthroscopic portals of the elbow have revealed that during the establishment of the anterolateral portal, the arthroscope passes anterior to the radial head and through the extensor carpi radialis brevis muscle. The arthroscope passes 4 to 7 mm from the radial nerve. Studies have demonstrated that the arthroscope passes within a mean distance of 4 mm from the radial nerve regardless of the flexion or extension of the elbow, with no distention in the capsule with fluid. However, studies have demonstrated that when 35 to 40 ml of fluid is inserted into the elbow capsule, the radial nerve moves an additional 7 mm anteriorly. Thus, maximal distention of the elbow should be maintained at all times when establishing the arthroscopic portals.

Anteromedial Portal

After the anterolateral portal has been established, the anteromedial portal can now be safely established by direct visualization intra-articularly. The anteromedial portal is located approximately 2 cm distal and 2 cm anterior to the medial humeral epicondyle (Fig. 3). With the arthroscope in the anterolateral portal, an 18-gauge spinal needle is inserted at the above-described entry point with the elbow flexed 90 degrees and the elbow maximally distended with fluid. The needle is aimed directly toward the center of the joint. Confirmation of the needle's entry is provided by direct visualization through the arthroscope in the anterolateral portal. The needle passes just anterior to the medial hu-

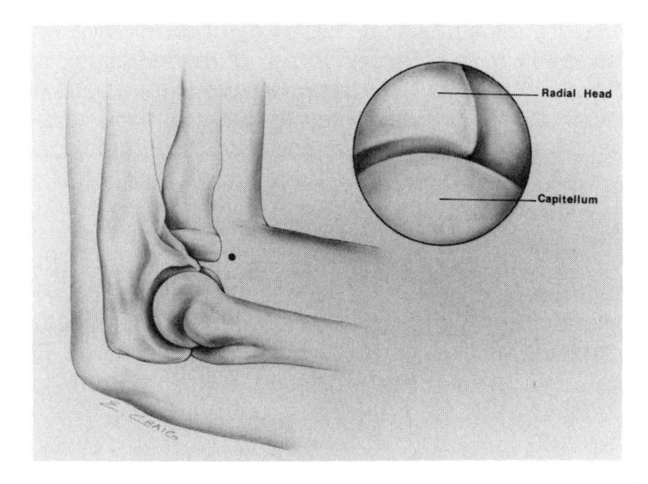

Figure 3 The anteromedial portal is located approximately 2 cm distal and 2 cm anterior to the medial humeral epicondyle. The radial head and capitellum are well visualized from this portal. (Republished with permission from Andrews JR, Carson WG. Arthroscopy of the elbow. Arthroscopy 1985; 1:100.)

meral epicondyle and inferior to the antecubital structures. A small skin incision is made and the arthroscopic cannula and trocar system are introduced. An interchangeable cannula system should be used so that one may freely change from the anterolateral to the anteromedial portal.

The capitellum and radial head are best visualized from the anteromedial portal, with examination of the radial head facilitated by pronation and supination of the forearm. One can occasionally visualize the annular ligament coursing across the radial neck, and by slowly retracting the arthroscope and directing it toward the ulna, the coronoid process is visible through this anteromedial portal.

Most arthroscopic surgical procedures in the elbow are performed for processes located over the lateral aspect of the elbow, such as loose bodies or osteochondritis dissecans of the capitellum. The anteromedial portal provides superior visualization of these structures as compared with the anterolateral portal, and thus it is necessary to be technically proficient at establishing both portals.

Cadaveric dissections have revealed that in establishing the anteromedial portals, the arthroscope enters through the tendinous portion of the pronator teres and penetrates the radial aspect of the flexor digitorum superficialis. As these muscles are penetrated, the median nerve is approximately 1 cm lateral to the arthroscope and the brachial artery is just lateral to the median nerve. As the arthroscope passes deeper and closer to the joint capsule, it comes to within 6 mm of these same neurovascular structures. If 35 to 40 ml of fluid is injected into the elbow, however, the median nerve and brachial artery move 10 mm and 8 mm, respectively, farther anterior from the entering arthroscopic instruments. Thus, again one should keep the elbow in 90 degrees of flexion at all times and provide maximal distention as the arthroscopic instruments are inserted from this anteromedial portal.

Posterolateral Portal

Occasionally a third arthroscopic portal, the posterolateral portal, can be established approximately 3 cm proximal to the tip of the olecranon, just superior and posterior to the lateral humeral epicondyle. This portal is placed just off the lateral border of the triceps muscle (Fig. 4). This portal is established with the elbow in 20 to 30 degrees of flexion, and the 18-gauge spinal needle is directed toward the olecranon fossa. Structures that may be visualized from this portal are the olecranon fossa located over the posterior aspect of the distal humerus and the tip of the olecranon. Flexion and extension of the elbow help to delineate various portions of the distal humerus. Neurovascular structures to be avoided when establishing this portal include the posterior antebrachial cutaneous nerve, which courses over the posterolateral distal humerus, and the ulnar nerve, which lies approximately 2.5 cm medial to the center of the joint.

If a second posterior portal is required for operative procedures, a straight posterior portal may be established under direct visualization 2 cm medial to the previously described posterolateral portal directly through the triceps tendon. This portal is valuable for the removal of loose bodies from the posterior aspect of the elbow, as well as the occasional resection of an impinging olecranal osteophyte.

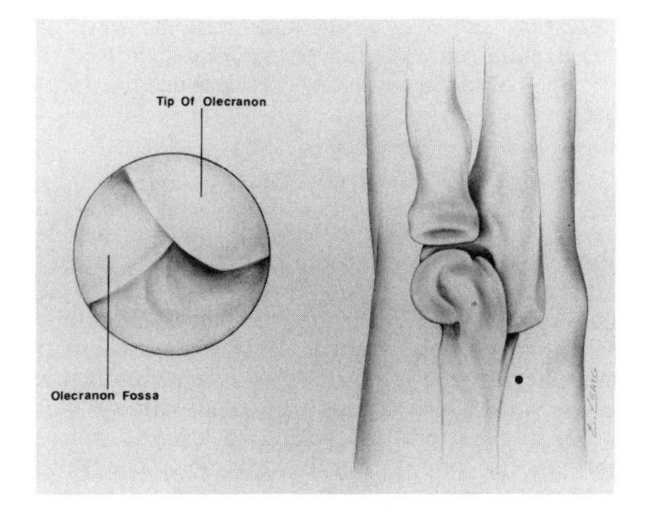

Figure 4 The posterolateral portal is located 3 cm proximal to the tip of the olecranon, just posterior and superior to the lateral epicondyle. This portal is established with the elbow extended to visualize the tip of the olecranon fossa. (Republished with permission from Andrews JR, Carson WG. Arthroscopy of the elbow. Arthroscopy 1985; 1:101.)

Instrumentation

Surgical techniques for arthroscopy of the elbow do not differ significantly from other joints with the exception that greater care is appropriate to avoid causing articular cartilage damage by scuffing of the articular surfaces. The elbow joint has inherent stability and there is less room to maneuver the various instruments in the elbow joint. Arthroscopic instrumentation in the elbow should be slow and deliberate so as not to slip out of the elbow capsule and cause unnecessary reentry of the various cannulas back into the joint. This causes further risk of damage to the articular cartilage, and in addition these repeated passes in and out of the capsule cause fluid extravasation and further risk of neurovascular compromise.

Motorized instruments should be used as much as possible to avoid having to make repeated passes with simple hand-held instruments. All hand-held and motorized instruments should be carefully used within this small joint and should never be wedged between articular surfaces, otherwise breakage could occur. As with arthroscopic surgery of the other joints, the instrument being used should be kept in full visualization at all times.

POSTOPERATIVE ROUTINE

At the completion of the arthroscopic procedure, the joint is thoroughly irrigated to remove all debris. The arthroscopic portals may be either left open or closed with suture material, depending on the preference of the surgeon and the amount of subcutaneous swelling. A soft dressing is applied to the elbow, and in most instances immobilization is not necessary. Active range of motion of the elbow is begun as pain and swelling permit, and then flexibility and strengthening exercises are usually initiated.

COMPLICATIONS

Complications of elbow arthroscopy include the general problems encountered with any arthroscopic procedure: infection, problems related to the use of a tourniquet, instrument breakage, iatrogenic scuffing of articular surfaces, and neurovascular complications. Infection is very infrequent, as it is in the other arthroscopic procedures in various joints, because of the large amount of fluid passed through the joint during the surgical procedure as well as the small incisions required for the arthroscopic instruments. However, neurovascular complications are more of a problem. Multiple complications of elbow arthroscopy have been reported, including a transient low radial nerve palsy, a transient low median nerve palsy, neuroma formation of the medial antebrachial cutaneous nerve, irreparable damage to the ulnar nerve during an attempt at performing abrasion arthroplasty of the elbow, and an injury to the sensory branch of the radial nerve. There have also been reported cases of transient nerve blocks caused by the injection of local anesthetic into the elbow following the arthroscopic procedure; I feel that these should not be injected into the elbow after this surgery, as the medication may leak out of the joint capsule and cause a temporary nerve block. If this anesthetic leaks out of the arthroscopic portals, it may interfere with the assessment of the neurovascular status of the patient postoperatively.

DISCUSSION

Arthroscopy of the elbow is a demanding surgical technique that requires significant attention to detail in order to perform a safe and reproducible surgical procedure. Unlike the knee, where the arthroscopic portals are readily and safely initiated over the anterior aspects of the knee and the most technically difficult part of knee arthroscopy appears to be dealing with the intra-articular pathology, the most demanding part of elbow arthroscopy is the initiation of the arthroscopic portals.

Several technical points warrant further discussion. As previously mentioned, various studies have demonstrated the necessity of maintaining maximal distention of the elbow in order to move neurovascular structures farther away from the arthroscopic instruments, to provide better visualization of the elbow, and to give more room in which to manipulate the various instruments. The distention of the elbow can usually be obtained by using 3-liter bags elevated above the patient, thus allowing gravity to distend the elbow. However, at times additional inflow is required and one can use a 50-ml syringe connected to the arthroscopic cannula to provide further distention manually. I have had no experience with the infusion pump method of distention of the elbow, and feel that this requires further study before its use can be recommended on a routine basis. Because one is trying to maintain maximal distention of the elbow at all times, the extracapsular extravasation can be impressive and needs to be monitored closely. This extracapsular extravasation is most often seen when one has made repeated attempts at establishing the arthroscopic portals, thus making multiple holes in the capsule with resultant fluid leakage. When using an inflow cannula, one needs to be sure that the cannula has an opening at the end only and does not have any "side vents"; if the inflow cannula slips back during the arthroscopic procedure, the side vents will then be outside the joint capsule and fluid will go directly into the subcutaneous tissues.

Because of the obvious risks of damage to nearby neurovascular structures and because fluid extravasation can be significant, it is recommended that the bony landmarks be identified with a marking pen before initiation of the procedure. Thus, the bony landmarks will stay in constant relationship during the arthroscopic procedure and one can maintain proper orientation at all times.

Another technical consideration is the exacting detail required and the actual maneuvering of instruments inside the elbow joint. There is usually a very short distance between the articular surface of the elbow and the joint capsule, and thus it is quite easy to slip out of the capsule when performing elbow arthroscopy. Once the arthroscope does come out of the joint capsule or the cannula slips back, there is further extravasation and one has to reintroduce the arthroscope, with further risk of damage to neurovascular structures or to the articular cartilage. Thus, when performing elbow arthroscopy, one needs to move the arthroscope quite slowly about the elbow, particularly when retracting the arthroscope, and stabilize the cannula sleeve with the opposite hand next to the skin so that one can be sure not to slip out of the elbow joint.

Although elbow arthroscopy involves many technical considerations and the risks of neurovascular injury are real, this procedure has been used effectively to treat various disorders of the elbow and appears to have the best surgical results when extracting simple loose bodies. In addition, certain easily accessible osteophytes about the elbow can be removed. In other instances degenerative processes such as chondroplasties of the articular surface or intra-articular lysis of adhesions can be performed. However, these latter arthroscopic surgical procedures are less rewarding than simply removing a loose body.

SUGGESTED READING

Andrews JR, Carson WG. Arthroscopy of the elbow. Arthroscopy 1985; 1:97–107.

Carson WG, Andrews JR. Arthroscopy of the elbow. In: Zarins B, Andrews J, Carson WG, eds. Injuries to the throwing arm. Philadelphia: WB Saunders, 1985: 221.

Carson WG. Arthroscopy of the elbow. In: Bassett F, ed. American Academy Orthopaedic Surgery Instructional Course Lecture. Vol. 37. St. Louis: C.V. Mosby, 1988:195.

Guhl JF. Arthroscopy and arthroscopic surgery of the elbow. Orthopedics 1985; 8:290–296.

Lynch GJ, Meyers JF, Whipple TL, et al. Neurovascular anatomy and elbow arthroscopy: inherent risks. Arthroscopy 1986; 2:191–197.

VALGUS EXTENSION OVERLOAD IN PITCHING ELBOW

FRANKLIN D. WILSON, M.D.

Pain in the pitching arm is a common problem for baseball players at all levels of participation. It is the purpose of this chapter to emphasize the location of the osteophyte production on the medial aspect of the olecranon as it abuts against the medial aspect of the olecranon fossa. This lesion is underrated, since most emphasis in the past has been on the posterior olecranal osteophyte caused mainly by the extension overload syndrome. The true offending symptomatic lesion is the posteromedial osteophyte as it abuts into the medial margin of the olecranon fossa (Fig. 1). This osteophyte can also create a painful area of chondromalacia on the medial aspect of the olecranon fossa.

Although the lesion has been recognized previously, little attention has been directed to surgical treatment. This lesion may be an isolated phenomenon or may occur with more severe degenerative conditions about the elbow. I believe that this isolated lesion occurs more frequently than is commonly recognized, and emphasize early recognition and aggressive surgical intervention. Bone changes about the elbow can create a major challenge to the orthopaedic surgeon.

ROENTGENOGRAPHIC EVALUATION

Cases demonstrate a posterior osteophyte at the tip of the olecranon process, which is easily seen on routine lateral views. However, identification of the posteromedial osteophyte is difficult. Axial projections at various degrees of flexion may be taken to try to identify this posteromedial osteophyte. I have found that, with the elbow in 110 degrees of flexion and the arm lying on the cassette, the beam should be angled to 45 degrees to the ulna. This gives the best view of the olecranon as it articulates with the trochlea, and it puts the medial aspect of the olecranon in profile. Occasionally I do not see any obvious bony osteophytes, as the lesion can be purely cartilaginous. At the time of surgery, however, I always find exuberant exotosis medially in such cases.

TREATMENT

Conservative Approach

The conservative physical therapy program has two goals: increasing functional strength about the elbow and relieving pain.

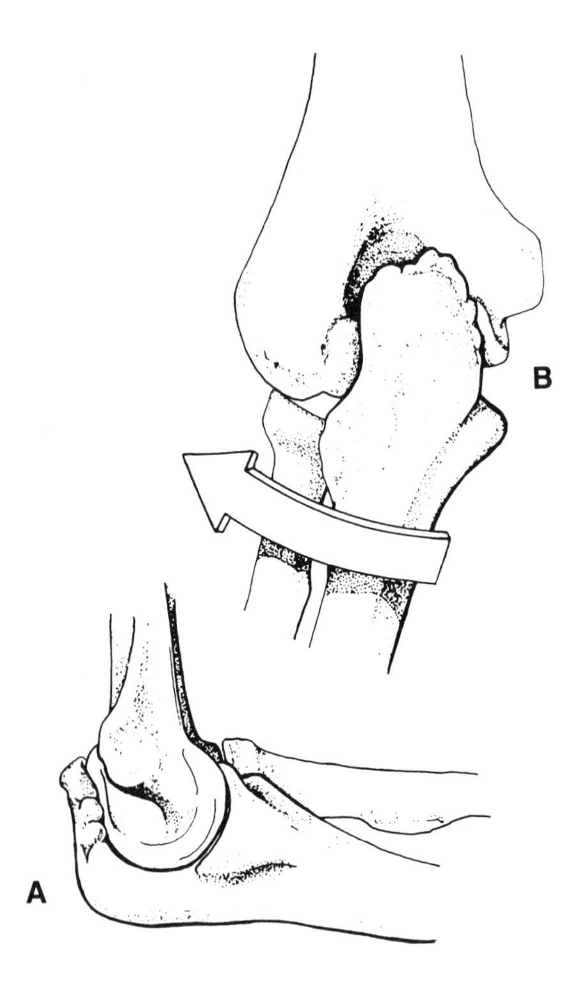

Figure 1 *A,* Side view of elbow showing medial extent of osteophytes around the olecranon. *B,* Posterior aspect of olecranon showing extent of posterior and posteromedial osteophytes as elbow impinges into decranon fossa. Arrow represents direction of dynamic stress and resultant impingement of olecranon process in olecranon fossa. (Republished with permission from Wilson FD, Andrews JR, Blackburn TA, et al. Valgus extension overload in the pitching elbow. Am J Sports Med 1983; 11:83–88.)

With the elbow fully extended and the palm facing upward, the athlete actively extends the wrist and supinates the forearm. He or she assists this with the opposite hand, making sure the thumb is included. The stretch is held for a slow count of 10, released, then repeated 25 times three times a day. In just the opposite way, the extensors are also stretched.

An isotonic regimen of light weights and high repetitions causes less stress about the elbow, yet allows a functional endurance factor. Therefore, the wrist curls are performed in flexion extension of the elbow with the forearm in pronation and supination. A 1-lb hammer or dumbbell is used to start. The weight is increased gradually to 5 lb. Elbow curls from full extension to full flexion are done against gravity, using the opposite hand to support the elbow. The athlete performs elbow extension with the elbow supported overhead as far as possible with the opposite hand. Five sets of 10 repetitions are performed three times a day. The elbow curls and extensions can be performed with 5 lb initially, progressing to 10 lb.

A rope curl-up bar can also be used for both flexors and extensors. A 1-ft-long broomstick with a yard rope attached centrally and a 1½-lb weight at the end can easily be used by having the patient roll up onto the stick. When working the flexors, the palm should be up and the rope curled up on the far side of the bar. For the extensors, the palm should be down and the rope to the far side of the bar. The weight must not be dropped; it should be unrolled slowly. Ten repetitions for the flexors and extensors of the elbow should also be performed.

The athlete should use the therapeutic putty or grip strengtheners frequently throughout the day. Isokinetic programs may be utilized when proper equipment is available, following speeds suggested by Cybex, Inc. (Division of Lumex, Inc., Ronkonkoma, NY). Isometrics may also be used for further strengthening.

Therapeutic modalities include moist heat and ultrasound. Ten percent of hydrocortisone phonophorsed through the skin can be effective. Deep transverse friction massage increases circulation and increases flexibility of the scar. If the athlete continues to throw, ice packs are applied to the elbow after each practice session or game.

If conservative measures prove insufficient to relieve all the symptoms, surgery is recommended. I believe that therapy is beneficial for general overall conditioning and for a satisfactory postoperative result. However, physical therapy has not been curative when there is a posteromedial osteophyte.

Surgical Approach

A straight posterolateral incision starting at the lateral epicondylar ridge at the humerus, extending 5 to 6 cm, is made in all cases. The triceps tendon is identified and sharply elevated off the epicondylar ridge of the humerus; this exposes the posterior compartment of the elbow. The anconeus muscle fibers are elevated off the humerus, allowing visualization of the synovium and the posterolateral aspect of the olecranon process. Various degrees of flexion and extension with varus stress give good visualization of the entire olecranon process, allowing for identification of the pathologic condition. A ¼-inch osteotome is used to make a straight osteotomy of approximately 1 cm of the olecranon process (Fig. 2*A*). When the osteotomy is performed, one should err by going into the normal olecranon process rather than risk leaving any of the posterior osteophyte. Instability is not created by this small osteotomy. The posterior osteophyte is thus removed, allowing exposure to the more important lesion on

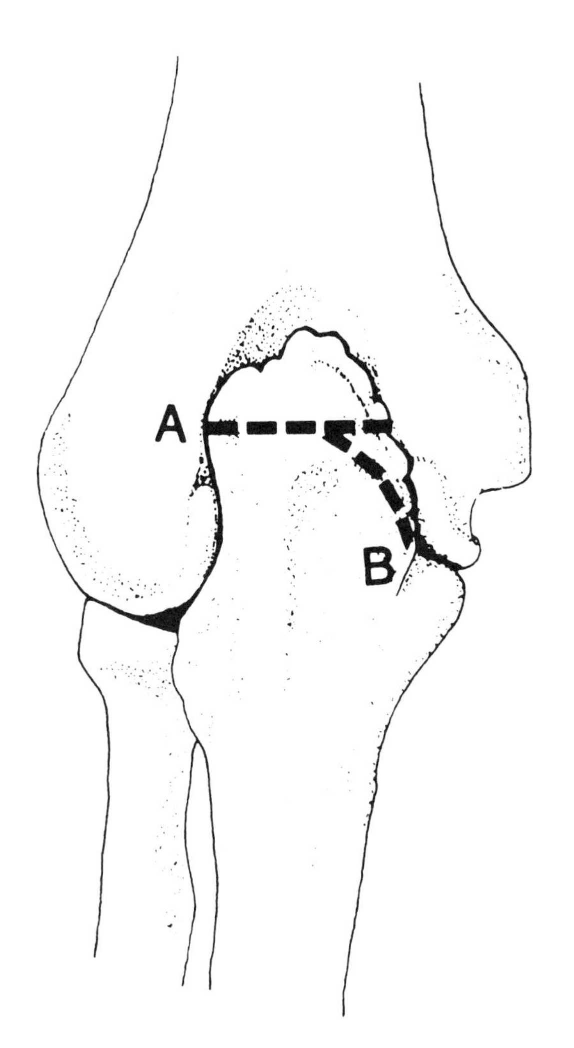

Figure 2 *A,* Posterior view of olecranon—first cut made straight across. *B,* second cut made with curved osteotome. (Republished with permission from Wilson FD, Andrews JR, Blackburn TA, et al. Valgus extension overload in the pitching elbow. Am J Sports Med 1983; 11:83–88.)

the posteromedial aspect of the olecranon. A 1/8- or 1/4-inch curved osteotome can be used to make a curved cut into the posteromedial olecranon (Fig. 2*B*), to remove the offending posteromedial osteophyte. Unless care is taken to make the second cut, the posteromedial lesion can be missed. The medial wall of the olecranon fossa can be visualized once the second osteotomy has been done, and any further offending osteophyte can be rongeured away. Often an area of chondromalacia on this wall is now seen, and enough of the posteromedial olecranal tip must be removed to clear this area and prevent further impingement. Once the area is decompressed in this manner, it requires no further treatment. The ulnar nerve lies more posterior and medial to the osteotomy incisions. Adequate irrigation of the wound is recommended to remove any debris or loose bodies. The triceps is then closed back to the epicondylar ridge of the humerus, and the anconeus is reapproximated with heavy, synthetic, absorbable sutures. Nonabsorbable sutures in the pitcher's elbow may produce postoperative irritations. Because this approach is relatively atraumatic, and because little has been done to cause instability, rapid return of function can be expected.

Flexibility and range-of-motion activities are started at 7 to 10 days. Active and passive assist programs using the opposite hand for assistance are done frequently during the day. The pendulum exercises work very well initially. Mobilization techniques aid in gaining motion. The athlete works into the progressive resistance program as tolerated.

After the pain has been relieved and range of motion completed (approximately 4 to 6 weeks), a long ball-toss program similar to that recommended by Jobe is begun. This starts with the athlete standing in a deep centerfield throwing the ball in a nice, easy over-hand toss so that it stops rolling at second base. This is done for 1 week, at which time the athlete tries to throw to second base on one hop. At the end of the week, the athlete begins to try to toss the entire distance to second base. Throwing time should be limited to take into account the symptoms, and should be no more than 15 minutes a day. The athlete then goes to 30 feet and begins throwing at a little less than half-speed for 15 minutes. After 1 week goes by, or symptoms decrease significantly, he or she advances to 60 feet and throws half-speed. This should be done for approximately 1 week. The athlete then increases throwing speed over the next couple of weeks until he or she is at full strength. It may be necessary to take on-off days with this throwing program. The thrower's progress through this program may be quicker, depending on the pathologic condition.

DISCUSSION

Injuries about the pitching elbow occur in numerous ways, because of the unusual stresses applied to the elbow joint during the pitching maneuver. It is essential to understand the basic aspects of the pitching movement in order to recognize the different areas of stress concentration about the elbow. Slocum deserves credit for outlining the essential steps in the pitching mechanism and the basic overload syndromes. It is often hard to separate the medial tension, lateral compression, and extension overload syndromes. King and colleagues analyzed and divided the throwing mechanism into various phases, including the wind-up or cock phase, the acceleration phase, release, and follow-through. Andrews and associates emphasized these phases and tried to correlate the actual mechanics in the elbow joint with the stress syndromes.

Bennett was the first to recognize that this kind of stress on the elbow could result in "exfoliation of cartilage which could either form loose bodies or cartilaginous masses on the adjacent surfaces of the olecranon and the internal condyle of the humerus." King and colleagues felt that the most common site for these loose bodies or spur formations would be on the posterior aspect of the olecranon process. Before their study, it was thought that this phenomenon was due to the jamming action of the olecranon process into the olecranon fossa; however, cineradiographs taken in the normal pitching elbow have failed to show the olecranon process impinging into the olecranon fossa. King and colleagues believed that a combination of medial elbow stress, cubital valgus, and a narrow bony fossa secondary to hypertrophy was the cause of the impingement of the olecranon process into the medial wall of the olecranon fossa. Indelicato and associates also recognized this problem and related it to the valgus overload during the acceleration phase as well. They also believe that the posterior osteophyte is created by the follow-through mechanism.

I believe that the mechanism of injury in the valgus extension overload syndrome occurs in the early acceleration phase of pitching. In this early phase, excessive valgus stress is applied to the elbow, causing a wedging effect of the olecranon into the olecranon fossa, as shown in Figure 1.

This impingement leads to osteophyte production at the posterior and posteromedial aspect of the olecranon tip, and can cause chondromalacia and loose body formation.

Secondarily, the follow-through phase can cause impingement farther posteriorly and can add stress to this area and further symptoms. However, this syndrome occurs before full extension, because it is known that the olecranon does not impinge posteriorly into the fossa.

In the past, most of the emphasis concerning valgus stress has been centered on the medial stress and tension overload syndromes involving the soft tissues medially. I believe one must be sure that the offending lesion is not the posteromedial osteophyte.

A high index of suspicion and awareness of this entity is necessary when throwers present with the typical pain on pitching that increases early in the game: they frequently complain that they just cannot "let it go." Sometimes they notice a gradual loss of control, causing early release and pitches thrown too high.

An active physical therapy program is always stressed in the conservative management of these patients. Although my experience is that physical therapy is unsuccessful when the pathology lies in the posteromedial osteophyte, I believe that a preoperative therapy program is important for the overall rehabilitation of the patient before and after surgery. Careful analysis of the pitching mechanism should be performed by the coaches, trainers, and physicians. If defects are found, changes should be made early; however, in most cases the pain in the elbow is what causes the disturbance in the pitching movement. If the athlete cannot perform at maximal potential because of the valgus extension overload, surgical correction should not be delayed. However, in our efforts to relieve pain and correct deformity, we should remember what Hugh Tullos has said: "We do not fix baseball players, we only temporarily improve them. If they continue to pitch they will continue to have their problems sooner or later."

SUGGESTED READING

Andrews JR, McCluskey GM, McLeod WD. Musculo-tendinous injuries of the shoulder and elbow in athletes. Schering Symposium. JNATA 1976; 11.

Barnes DA, Tullos HS. An analysis of 100 symptomatic baseball players, Am J Sports Med 1978; 6:62–67.

Bennett GE. Elbow and shoulder lesions of baseball players. Am J Surg 1959; 98:484–492.

Bennett GE. Shoulder and elbow lesions of the professional baseball pitcher. JAMA 1941; 117:510–514.

De Haven KE, Evarts CM. Throwing injuries of the elbow in athletes. Orthop Clin North Am 1973; 4:301–808.

Gartsman GM, Sulco TP, Otis JC. Operative treatment of olecranon fractures. J Bone Joint Surg 1981; 63A:718–721.

Indelicato PA, Jobe FW, Kerlan RK, et al. Correctable elbow lesions in professional baseball players: a review of 25 cases. Am J Sports Med 1979; 7:72–75.

Jones HH, Priest JD, Hayes WC, et al. Humeral hypertrophy in response to exercise. J Bone Joint Surg 1977; 59A:204–208.

King JW, Brelsford HJ, Tullos HS. Analysis of the pitching arm of the professional baseball pitcher. Clin Orthop 1969; 67:116–123.

Slocum DB. Classification of the elbow injuries from baseball players. Am J Sports Med 1978; 6:62–67.

Tullos HS, King JW. Throwing mechanism in sports. Orthop Clin North Am 1973; 4:709–721.

FOREARM, WRIST, AND HAND

TENDON INJURIES IN THE HAND AND WRIST

C. STEWART WRIGHT, M.D., F.R.C.S.(C)

Acute and chronic tendon injuries may occur with many sporting activities, and even minor injuries may be disabling to the athlete. All too often, potentially serious trauma to tendons in the upper extremity is not diagnosed and is passed off as "sprains" or, if diagnosed, is improperly treated, impairing the athlete's performance and causing unnecessary pain. I hope to raise the reader's level of awareness of potential deep structure injury beneath the swollen hand or wrist.

THE WRIST

Flexors

On the flexor surface of the wrist, the tendons most commonly injured are the flexor carpi radialis (FCR) and the flexor carpi ulnaris (FCU). The thumb and digital flexors may also be injured at the wrist, but much less frequently than the wrist flexors. The usual mechanism of injury is a blow against the dorsiflexed wrist (e.g., a fall on the hand or colliding with another player with the arm extended). The FCU is the tendon most often injured, and the patient's complaint is of pain along the volar ulnar aspect of the wrist and upon palpation of the pisiform. Ulnar wrist flexion against resistance produces pain. In all these injuries, a post-traumatic tendinitis must be differentiated from a bone injury, and thus radiographic evaluation is necessary.

An injury to the FCR produces pain on the volar radial aspect of the wrist. There may be pain with flexion and extension of the wrist. Again, FCR tendinitis may mimic fractures of the scaphoid or distal radius.

Acute injuries to the FCU and FCR may also produce volar wrist capsule strains and should be treated with volar wrist splinting. Oral anti-inflammatory agents may reduce inflammation and decrease pain. Steroid and local anesthetic injections seldom are used in acute cases, but are reserved for injuries that do not respond to the initial supportive treatment over 4 to 6 weeks. When injections are given, corticosteroids are used and should be mixed with 1 percent lidocaine (Xylocaine). Care must be taken to ensure that the injection is peritendinous and not intratendinous, intravascular, or intraneural. I do not believe there is a case for more than two or three injections.

When the injections have proved unsuccessful, one must either reconsider the diagnosis or decide whether surgery is appropriate. These injuries should only rarely come to surgery before 6 to 12 months after the traumatic event. The athlete should also have had the benefit of a supervised physical therapy program before surgery is considered. This not only may improve the symptoms, but also gives the physician some idea of how the patient will cooperate postoperatively.

The incision for releasing the FCR should be kept radial to the tendon to avoid injury to the palmar cutaneous branch of the median nerve. At the same time, care is necessary to avoid injury to the radial artery. The thenar muscles are then reflected to expose the scaphoid tubercle and trapezial crest. Portions of these bone prominences are then resected and the FCR is released circumferentially to its insertion. Postoperatively, the patient should begin early wrist motion. With the FCU, tenolysis is necessary, as is removal of part or all of the pisiform.

Extensors

Six extensor compartments are housed on the dorsum of the wrist. Tenosynovitis may involve any of the 12 wrist and digital extensors. As with the flexors of the wrist, the extensor injuries may present as acute tears, repetitive trauma, or repetitive stress (overuse).

The most radial extensor compartment houses the extensor pollicis brevis (EPB) and abductor pollicis longus (APL). At the level of the radial styloid these tendons pass under a ligamentous retinaculum approximately 1 cm in length. A tenosynovitis at this level is referred to as DeQuervain's tenovaginitis, after the man who described the condition in 1895. These patients complain of localized pain over the radial styloid, which may be confused with arthritis of the carpometacarpal joint of the thumb. The so-called Finklestein's test for DeQuervain's disease refers to increased pain at the radial styloid with the ulnar deviation of the wrist after the thumb has been flexed into the palm.

Treatment of this problem should initially include oral anti-inflammatory agents, a splint that immobilizes all three joints of the thumb, heat, and hydrotherapy. The splint is removed for the warm water soaks, but is otherwise worn full time during the acute phase. Local injections of corticosteroid and lidocaine (Xylocaine) may be repeated once or twice. Surgery should be employed when there has been a failure of conservative treatment over 12 to 16 weeks.

A longitudinal incision is recommended, but a horizontal one may be made. The most serious complication is damage to the superficial branches of the radial sensory nerve, which may number one to three. No patient will thank you if you relieve the tendinitis but leave a painful neuroma. The retinaculum is then divided longitudinally and part of it is excised to avoid recurrence. The EPB must be identified as well as the presence of a multiple-tailed APL, which is fairly common. There may be multiple compartments, and it is important to release each and to resect any septa. Bone prominences should be rongeured smooth, and motion should be started within 7 to 10 days postoperatively.

The second extensor compartment contains the extensor carpi radialis longus and brevis (ECRL and ECRB). It is usually possible to delineate the two different tendons inserting at the base of the second and third metacarpals. The acute injuries require splinting and oral anti-inflammatory drugs, followed by steroid injections for patients who do not respond.

Another condition that may be confused with the two previously mentioned is the so-called "intersection syndrome." This occurs on the radial aspect of the wrist, but more proximally than DeQuervain's disease. It occurs at the intersection of the first and second extensor compartment tendons. It has been described in weight lifters, rowers, and canoeists, and has been seen to be associated with hypertrophy of the APL and EPB muscle bellies overlying the tendons of the radial wrist extensors. If conservative means do not resolve the problem, surgical decompression of the sheath of the overlying muscles provides quick relief of symptoms.

The extensor pollicis longus (EPL) is the sole occupant of the third compartment and can become inflamed as it passes around Lister's tubercle on the distal radius. This is an uncommon problem, but when it does occur it requires early surgical decompression because of the possibility of tendon rupture. Surgery should be considered when there is no response to treatment in the first 4 weeks.

Compartment four contains the extensor digitorum communis (EDC) and extensor indicis proprius (EIP), and compartment five contains the extensor digiti minimi (EDM). These tendons all pass underneath the extensor retinaculum and may develop a tenosynovitis at that level. Again, the use of splinting and oral anti-inflammatory preparations is recommended, followed by steroid injection and later by surgical decompression if necessary. If surgery is needed, a portion of retinaculum should be left intact to prevent bowstringing when the wrist is dorsiflexed.

The extensor carpi ulnaris (ECU) is in the last compartment. ECU tendinitis presents with pain on the dorsal ulnar aspect of the wrist and base of the fifth metacarpal. If this condition requires surgical decompression, the dorsal sensory branch of the ulnar nerve must be protected.

DIGITAL TENDONS

Flexors

A tenosynovitis of the digital flexors—flexor digitorum superficialis (FDS), flexor digitorum profundus (FDP), and flexor pollicis longus (FPL)—may present as swelling and tenderness at the metacarpophalangeal (MCP) joint level in the palm. When more severe, this can produce the phenomenon of triggering as the flexor tendon moves through the A1 pulley in flexion and has trouble reentering the flexor sheath with digital extension. Most of these respond favorably to oral anti-inflammatory preparations early in their course, or to corticosteroid injection once triggering begins. For those that do not respond, a trigger-finger release may be carried out under local anesthesia. These are best done through a longitudinal incision in the distal palm, the entire A1 pulley being incised. Care is taken to preserve the A2 pulley, and early motion is started after surgery. In the thumb, the neurovascular bundles are quite volar and the ulnar digital nerve crosses the tendon sheath. These structures must be identified and protected from injury.

Avulsion of the insertion of a flexor profundus tendon (FDP and FPL) is a relatively common injury, especially in athletes. Most occur in the ring digit, but any finger may be involved. It is not uncommon for this injury to be seen late because the significance of the initial injury may not have been recognized. The usual mechanism of injury is an opponent pulling away from a player who has hold of the opponent's jersey or pants. This results in forced extension of the digit while the FDP is maximally contracted, producing avulsion.

These injuries have been divided into three groups. Type 1 is a retraction of the tendon into the palm. This results because of a rupture of the vinculum longus and consequent loss of an important part of the tendon blood supply. No active distal interphalangeal (DIP) joint motion is present, and there is usually a tender lump in the palm where the tendon has retracted. These should be repaired within the first week of injury. The tendon must be threaded back through the tendon sheath and reinserted into the distal phalanx with a pull-out wire.

In type 2, the most common, the tendon retracts to the proximal interphalangeal (PIP) joint level. This occurs because the vinculum is still intact and prevents retraction of the FDP. Once again, there is no active DIP motion and there is pain and swelling at the PIP level. The tendon blood supply is largely intact, and these tendons have been successfully reinserted as long as 8 to 12 weeks after the injury. Ideally, they are repaired during the first week.

Type 3 injuries include avulsion of a large fragment from the base of the distal phalanx. This is usually large enough to catch on the A4 pulley and prevent proximal migration of the tendon. Once again, no active DIP motion is possible. These require open reduction of the displaced fragment along with reinsertion of the flexor tendon.

When these injuries are seen late, many surgeons believe that they are best left alone unless there is a painful lump in the palm or an unstable DIP joint. The tendon stump may be excised and the DIP joint fused if necessary. Depending on the patient's lack of function, a tendon graft or two-stage tendon repair may be considered as an alternative.

Extensors

Extensor tendon injuries in the hand will be considered at three different levels: the DIP, PIP, and MCP joints.

Distal Interphalangeal Joint

At the DIP joint, the so-called mallet finger deformity occurs with avulsion of the extensor tendon at its insertion. This usually happens when the finger is struck end-on by a football, baseball, or basketball. The tendon at this level consists of the conjoined lateral bands and it may be injured in four ways. Type 1 is an avulsion of the tendon from the distal phalanx. Type 2 is associated with a dorsal lip fracture of less than one-third of the articular surface. Type 3 has an associated fracture greater than one-third of the articular surface, and it may render the DIP joint unstable. Type 4 occurs in children, and a Salter I or transepiphyseal injury occurs at the base of the distal phalanx. The type 1 injury is by far the most common.

The vast majority of mallet finger injuries can be successfully treated by conservative means. The DIP joint is splinted in extension or slight hyperextension for 6 weeks full time and then a further 4 to 6 weeks of nighttime splinting. There are good commercially available splints or they may be fabricated on an individual basis by the therapist. The DIP joint is immobilized but the PIP joint remains free. This method of treatment may be successful even if started up to 8 weeks after the injury, provided there is still some inflammatory reaction over the DIP joint. When the associated fracture fragment renders the DIP joint unstable, it may still be possible to do a closed reduction and percutaneous pinning. If this is not successful, an open reduction of the fragment should be carried out. This is done in association with a transarticular Kirschner wire and should have an external splint for 6 weeks to ensure that the K-wire does not break.

Many procedures have been described for repair of the chronic mallet deformity and none has a high success rate. The most reliable operation is a DIP fusion with the joint in 10 to 15 degrees of flexion.

Proximal Interphalangeal Joint

At this level, the central slip is ruptured and there is progressive volar subluxation of the lateral bands. This results in a flexion deformity of the PIP joint because of the unopposed pull of the FDS. Hyperextension of the DIP joint occurs through the pull of the lateral bands and the oblique retinacular ligament, and produces the so-called boutonnière deformity. Initially, the PIP joint may appear only in slight flexion and the injury may be missed. It may be 10 to 21 days before the full-blown deformity develops.

Like mallet finger deformities, most boutonnières may be managed by closed means. This involves splinting the PIP joint in extension, but encouraging flexion of the DIP joint. With the PIP joint splinted, both active and passive exercises are carried out at the DIP joint to help restore normal tendon balance.

Boutonnière deformities discovered late may still be treated by conservative means as late as 8 to 12 weeks after the injury. This may require serial casting or daily monitoring of the splinting to help overcome any PIP flexion contracture that may be present. Chronic deformities at this level are very difficult problems and should be managed by a physician skilled in hand surgery.

Metacarpophalangeal Joint

Injuries to the extensor mechanism at this level usually involve a longitudinal tear of the sagittal band. When this occurs, the extensor tendon is able to sublux or dislocate away from the site of injury. Any digit may be involved, but the middle finger is the most common. Also, the radial side is injured more frequently than the ulnar. Physical examination demonstrates inability to extend the digit fully as well as deviation of the digit away from the side of the injury.

When this injury occurs without extensor subluxation, it may be treated with splinting alone. Otherwise, acute injuries at the MCP joint should be repaired primarily and the joint immobilized for 3 weeks. It is important to ensure that the extensor is centralized over the MCP joint. There is usually sufficient tissue for repair, but if not a portion of juncturae tendinum or a retrograde piece of extensor may be sutured directly into the defect or looped around the lumbrical to realign the extensor mechanism. Any of these latter procedures may be used to correct this injury in its chronic state.

SUGGESTED READING

Doyle JR. Extensor tendons: acute injuries. In: Green DP, ed. Operative hand surgery. New York: Churchill Livingstone, 1982.

Burton RI. Extensor tendons: late reconstruction. In: Green DP, ed. Operative hand surgery. New York: Churchill Livingstone, 1982.

Leddy JP. Flexor tendons: acute injuries. In: Green DP, ed. Operative hand surgery. New York: Churchill Livingstone, 1982.

Schneider LH, Hunter JM. Flexor tendons: late reconstruction. In: Green DP, ed. Operative hand surgery. New York: Churchill Livingstone, 1982.

COACH'S FINGER

FRANK C. McCUE III, M.D.
MICHAEL R. REDLER, M.D.

Injuries to the proximal interphalangeal (PIP) joint of the finger are exceedingly common in athletic competition. The exact frequency of the injury is not completely known, as many are treated on the sideline by the coach, the trainer, or the player himself. Very often, the injured finger is splinted with tape to the adjacent finger and the player is allowed to reenter the game. This sideline treatment may represent the only therapeutic intervention for the injury. The poorly supervised athlete tends to return to competition with unprotected use of the finger long before adequate healing has taken place. The result, 2 to 3 months later, is a painful, stiff and deformed finger that we have previously termed "coach's finger."

The coach's finger problem is further complicated by inadequate diagnosis, lack of x-ray studies, and improper splinting. Proper treatment of injuries to the PIP joint is particularly important because any fixed flexion or extension deformity is extremely disabling. The PIP joint is especially vulnerable to injury because of the relatively long proximal and distal lever arms that transmit lateral and torque stress to this hinge type of joint, which has minimal lateral mobility.

Accurate diagnosis requires a knowledge of the anatomy of the PIP joint and also of the mechanisms of the stress applied in the various injuries. The PIP joint has a range of motion of 0 to 120 degrees in a plane perpendicular to the palm. All the lateral ligaments and the volar plate are thick and strong and, in conjunction with the central slip of the extensor tendon and the volar sheath of the flexor tendons, form a firm soft tissue enclosure. The head of the proximal phalanx is bicondylar. The dorsolateral aspect of the head has a concavity for the proximal attachment of the collateral ligament. As the finger flexes, the ligament glides volarly over a smooth flat area on the head of the phalanx (Fig. 1).

The base of the middle phalanx has a biconcavity with a vertical medial ridge. These concavities articulate with the condyles of the proximal phalanx. The volar lip of the middle phalanx has a roughened area for the thick distal attachment of the volar plate (Fig. 2). The volar plate, with its additional lateral attachments, functions to resist dorsal displacement. The proximal membranous portion of the volar plate attaches to the distal portion of the proximal phalanx. There is a central accordion portion to allow flexion, and lateral thickened attachments to help prevent hyperextension.

The oblique retinacular ligament arises from the flexor tendon sheath about the proximal phalanx, and runs obliquely and distally to insert into the extensor apparatus. It functions as an extensor

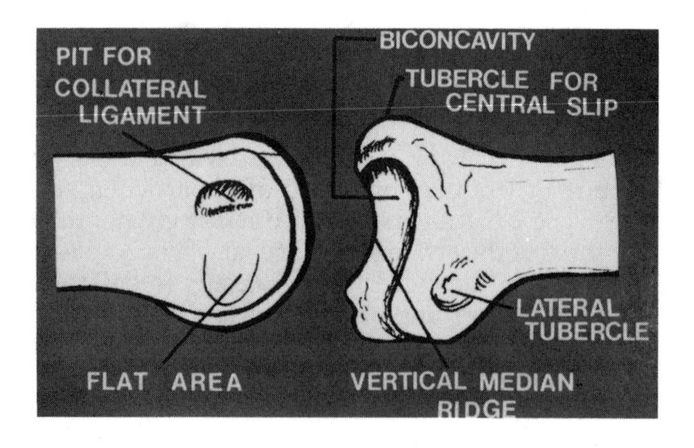

Figure 1 Proximal interphalangeal joint bony anatomy.

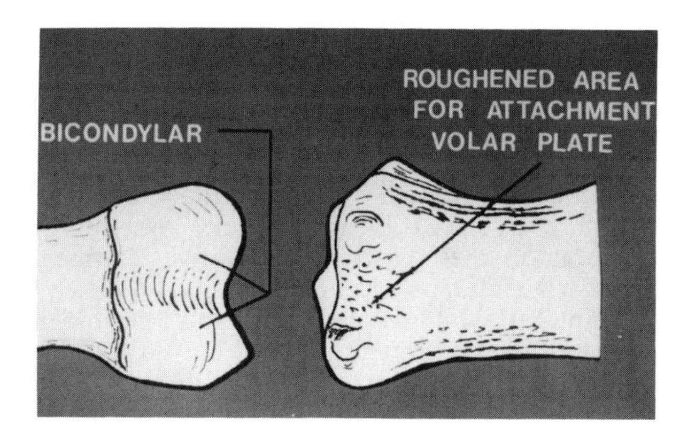

Figure 2 Attachment site of the volar plate.

of the distal interphalangeal (DIP) joint through a tenodesis effect when the PIP joint is flexed. The transverse retinacular ligament lies superficial to the oblique ligament and runs from the flexor tendon sheath to insert on the lateral extensor band. Cleland's ligament arises from the joint capsule deep to the transverse retinacular ligament, and runs dorsal to the neurovascular bundle to insert on the skin. Grayson's thin transparent ligament has an origin off the flexor tendon sheath, and passes volar to the neurovascular bundle.

All these ligaments must move and glide freely to allow proper motion. The volar cul-de-sac must also be free of scar tissue to allow the base of the middle phalanx to glide into the sac during flexion. The synovial pouch that lines this cul-de-sac lies deep to the flexor sheath. Injuries or scarring in any of these regions cause a painful stiff finger that loses much of the necessary motion or stability needed by athletes to compete in their sport.

The coach's finger injuries include collateral ligament injuries, articular fractures, fracture-dislocations, and boutonnière and pseudoboutonnière deformities. We believe that these are all potentially serious injuries. Early recognition and proper treatment is paramount in returning the athlete to competition.

COLLATERAL LIGAMENT INJURIES

Collateral ligament injuries to the PIP joint represent the most common type of coach's finger injury. A swollen, jammed finger is frequently the presenting complaint. The radial and ulnar collateral ligaments are the chief restraints to lateral stress in the initial 20 degrees of flexion. The volar plate aids in lateral stability at this point. The collateral ligament consists of the stronger proper component and a volar accessory component, which may be a factor in flexion contractures with shortening that occurs in the flexed position. The radial side collateral ligament is more commonly injured with avulsion of the proximal attachment. This is usually associated with partial or complete rupture of the volar plate.

The acute injury is often caused by a ball or other dull object striking the extended finger. This is accompanied by pain and localized swelling on the side of the injured ligament. It is important to ascertain whether this injury represents a strain, the more common injury, or a complete disruption of the ligament. Complete rupture creates lateral instability. This can be demonstrated radiographically with stress films or with the finding of a small bone fragment associated with the ligament rupture (Fig. 3). We routinely perform examination under digital nerve block. It is important to remember, however, that too rigorous stress may convert a partial collateral ligament strain into a complete rupture.

The treatment for a mild strain of the collateral ligament consists of splinting the finger in a functional position. The finger is protected until full pain-free motion can be achieved. Protection often consists of molding a polypropylene splint to be used in competition. For a mildly injured finger, we often tape it to the adjacent finger during competition; this provides some support as well as mobility. It must be stressed, however, that taping is not appropriate protection for the acutely injured, swollen, painful finger.

For injuries in which there is joint laxity and incomplete tearing of the ligament, the finger should be splinted in 30 degrees of flexion. Active motion exercises should be started in 10 to 14 days. Protective splinting is continued for at least 3 weeks. Active sports participation is then allowed, with the finger protected with a molded splint. Again, protection is continued until complete pain-free mo-

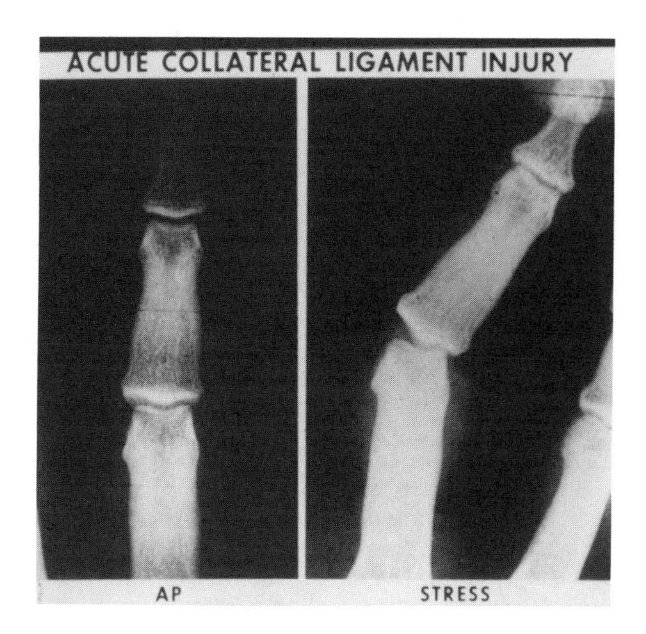

Figure 3 Stress films of a complete tear of the collateral ligament.

tion is possible. Discontinuation of protection too early can lead to further injury, including a complete tearing of the ligament.

Although there is controversy regarding the treatment of complete tears of the collateral ligament of the PIP joint, we believe that optimal treatment of these injuries includes open inspection and repair of the torn ligament. Operative treatment is performed in order to restore stability and decrease subsequent pain, swelling, and functional loss. Nonoperative treatment is prone to leave the patient with a swollen, tender joint that is unstable and susceptible to additional injury, as well as to subsequent degenerative changes.

Acute complete ruptures are approached surgically, using a long midlateral incision. The collateral ligament is exposed by an oblique incision through the transverse retinacular ligament. Most of these ruptures occur from the proximal attachment of the ligament. The acute collateral ligament may be repaired using a Bunnell-type suture of No. 34 wire passed through drill holes in the bone and then tied over a button. In certain cases when an adequate proximal stump remains, a mattress stitch with a nonabsorbable suture may be used. The associated tear of the volar plate is repaired with interrupted absorbable suture. In reconstruction of chronic tears, repair is accomplished by transferring the adjacent sublimis slip to augment the proximal end of the collateral ligament and associated soft tissue. The finger is splinted for 3 weeks, at which point protected motion exercises are employed. Generally, splinting is continued for an additional 5 weeks, or until full pain-free motion is possible.

ARTICULAR FRACTURES

If neglected or improperly treated, fractures of the articular surfaces of the PIP joint have the potential for loss of motion or early degenerative changes. The most common PIP joint fracture involves one condyle of the head of the proximal phalanx. Long and short oblique fractures, T-type fractures, avulsion fractures, comminuted fractures, and fractures of the base of the middle phalanx are also seen.

Stable fractures with minimal disruption of the articular surface and little or no ligamentous instability can be treated nonoperatively. This includes small chip fractures or avulsion fractures. These fractures are splinted with aluminum volar splints lined with moleskin, with the PIP joint in 30 degrees of flexion for approximately 3 weeks. After this initial period, early protected motion is allowed. Splinting is continued during competition and practice until full pain-free motion has been regained.

Indications for open reduction and internal fixation include displaced articular fractures involving more than one-fourth of the articular surface; comminuted or displaced fractures; volar lip fractures, which can cause subsequent subluxation or block flexion; and dorsal avulsion fractures, which include the insertion of the central slip into the base of the middle phalanx. An accurate, anatomic reduction is imperative for maximal return of function and motion of this tight-fitting hinged joint. Reduction may not be possible in massively comminuted fractures; in these cases, nonoperative treatment with early motion is encouraged.

The PIP joint is exposed through a long midlateral incision or through a dorsal curved incision centered at the flexion crease of the PIP joint laterally. The incision should curve in an arc proximally and distally to allow dorsal exposure, which gives optimal visualization of the fragments. The collateral ligament is exposed by making an oblique fiber-splitting incision anterior to the oblique retinacular ligament. The collateral ligament is then divided near its distal attachment. The articular surface is inspected and anatomically reduced. Pinning is done with one or two small, smooth Kirschner wires (Fig. 4). The collateral ligament, joint capsule, and

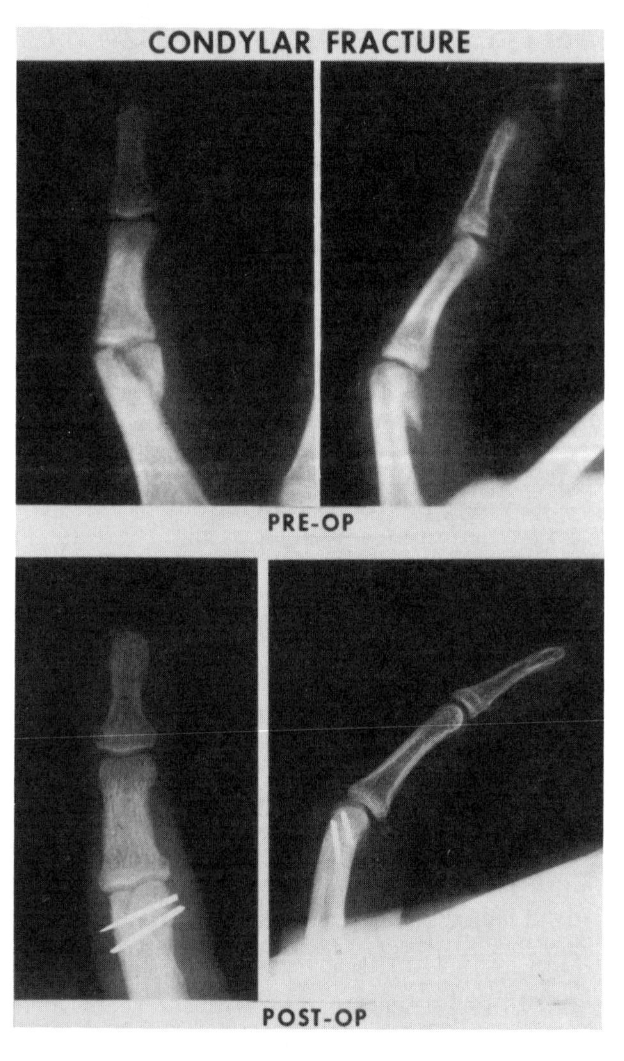

Figure 4 Open reduction and internal fixation of an intra-articular fracture of the proximal interphalangeal joint.

oblique fibers are repaired using 4–0 Tycron sutures.

Postoperatively the finger is splinted in the fashion described for nonoperative treatment. Active isolated motion is initiated 3 weeks after surgery. Return to competition is allowed after 3 to 4 weeks, with a protected molded splint.

FRACTURE-DISLOCATIONS

Hyperextension of the PIP joint, often after a fall, is the most common method of dislocating this joint. The middle phalanx dislocates dorsally, rupturing the volar plate at its distal attachment. This occurs with or without a fracture of the volar lip at the base of the middle phalanx (Fig. 5).

Closed reduction of a dorsal dislocation without a concomitant fracture is usually quite stable. Occasionally, a volar subluxation with avulsion of the central slip of the extensor mechanism occurs. This injury usually requires open reduction, since the head of the proximal phalanx can be entrapped by the lateral band. Postoperatively the finger has to be held in extension to allow for healing of the repaired extensor mechanism.

When a fracture of the volar lip of the middle phalanx does occur, the buttressing effect of this fragment is lost. The volar fragment can vary widely in size and comminution. When the fragment is small enough not to impair stability of the joint, the finger may be splinted in 25 degrees of flexion with an extension block. Early active flexion exercises help prevent the onset of stiffness.

The stability of the joint may not be ascertained from the x-ray film alone. Once closed reduction has been accomplished, examination of the joint, under digital block, is necessary to determine stability. The collateral ligaments must be tested to make certain they are intact and that the injury was not a lateral dislocation. In lateral dislocations, the collateral ligaments and volar plate are both torn. Treatment of these injuries depends on the stability of the joint after reduction. This may be accomplished in conjunction with stress radiography. Instability is an indication for open reduction, as is a large volar lip fragment. The volar lip fragment most often is larger at surgery than it appears on the radiograph.

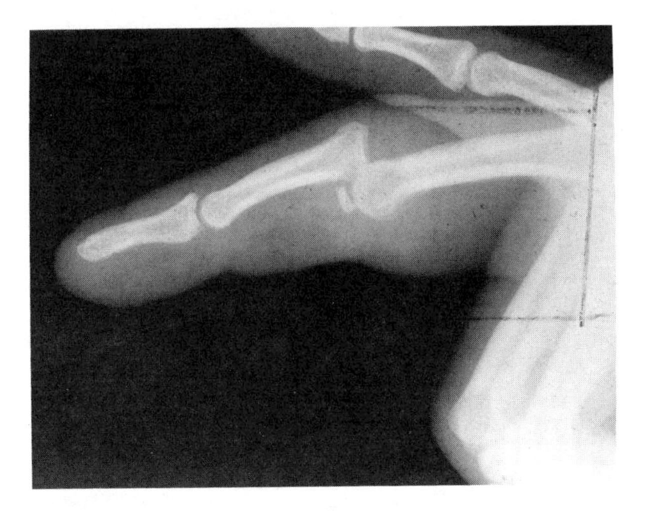

Figure 5 Dorsal dislocation of the proximal interphalangeal joint with a volar lip fracture.

A long midlateral approach is used, and the reticular portion of the fibrous flexor sheath, as well as part of the annular pulley, are excised to allow retraction of the flexor tendons. The volar plate is then detached to give maximal exposure to the volar lip fragments. Single fragments are pinned with a small, smooth K-wire. Multiple comminuted fragments are reduced with a loop of No. 34 wire, which is brought out dorsally and tied over a button. Even fragments that are devoid of soft tissue attachments are pinned when there is no significant evidence of avascular necrosis. A transarticular K-wire is used with the PIP joint flexed to 30 degrees, and the finger is then protected by a splint. Exercise is begun 3 weeks after open reduction, with the finger protected during athletics until complete pain-free motion is possible. In significantly comminuted and unstable fractures with associated dorsal dislocation, treatment by closed means may be best. A posterior flexion block is applied at the angle that prevents dorsal subluxation. When the acute reaction has abated, active flexion under close radiographic control can be carried out. Although the x-ray film may not show an anatomic positioning of the fragment, the functional result often is superior despite joint incongruity. Dorsal protection and early active exercises are also effective treatment in stable volar fractures to allow early return of motion.

BOUTONNIÈRE DEFORMITY

The classic boutonnière deformity consists of hyperextension of the metacarpophalangeal (MCP) joint, flexion of the PIP joint, and hyperextension of the DIP joint. The lesion is a disruption of the central slip from the dorsal lip of the middle phalanx. This disruption is most often due to a closed rupture of the extensor mechanism, and is the second most common closed tendon injury in athletes, after the jersey finger deformity.

The initial injury is usually due to blunt trauma, leaving a buttonhole-like split in the dorsal covering of the middle phalanx. The PIP joint herniates dorsally through the tear in the supporting central slip. The resulting deformity develops over time, especially in fingers in which the diagnosis is not made and that are either not splinted or splinted in flexion.

Early diagnosis is difficult after an acute injury with swelling, because the PIP joint naturally goes into 15 to 30 degrees of flexion. The inability to extend the joint is improperly attributed to pain and swelling, while in reality it is due to disruption of the extensor tendon. If the injury is truly a boutonnière deformity, there will be point tenderness over the dorsal lip of the middle phalanx.

If the finger is incorrectly splinted in flexion, there will be continued separation of the disrupted ends of the central slip and healing will be prevented. The natural course of the untreated boutonnière deformity is flexion of the PIP joint due to unopposed flexors, and contraction of the volarly displaced lateral bands and of the oblique retinacular ligaments.

Any PIP joint injury with an extension lag of more than 30 degrees and tenderness directly over the base of the middle phalanx should be treated as an acute extensor tendon rupture. The PIP joint is immobilized in full extension for at least 6 to 8 weeks, using a splint short enough to allow continued active and passive motion of the DIP joint. Splinting is continued during athletic competition until full pain-free flexion and maximal extension are possible. In injuries with restricted passive extension, correction with a safety pin splint is necessary before surgical reconstruction.

Surgical repair is indicated when an adequate trial of splinting does not control the deformity. Advancement of the central slip with reattachment to the dorsal lip of the middle phalanx is accomplished by direct repair through an S-shaped dorsal skin incision. A transarticular wire across the extended joint is used for 3 weeks in conjunction with an external splint. Additional protective splinting is used for competition until full pain-free motion is possible. Chronic boutonnière deformities have been corrected by a variety of methods, but results are not uniformly predictable.

PSEUDOBOUTONNIÈRE DEFORMITY

A hyperextension injury to the PIP joint can result in a disruption of the volar plate at its thin membranous proximal portion, leading to the formation of a pseudoboutonnière deformity. The volar plate is composed of a thin membranous proximal portion and a thick cartilaginous distal portion attached to the base of the middle phalanx. The volar plate can be injured when an extended finger is hyperextended, as when struck by a baseball, basketball, or football. The patient experiences acute onset of pain and swelling, with point tenderness over the volar aspect of the joint. X-ray films may reveal a small bony avulsion.

A pseudoboutonnière deformity can resemble a true boutonnière deformity, except that there is no disruption of the central slip. The diagnostic features of a pseudoboutonnière deformity include a flexion contracture of the PIP joint that is often resistant to passive flexion, slight hyperextension of the DIP joint, radiologic evidence of calcification at the distal end of the proximal phalanx, and a history

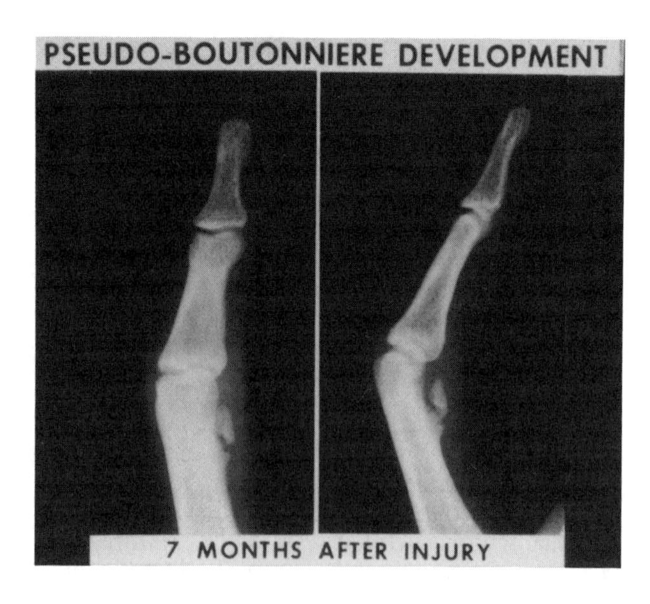

Figure 6 Pseudoboutonnière development with calcification at the distal end of the proximal phalanx.

of a hyperextension or twisting injury to the PIP joint. The little finger seems to be most commonly involved.

Initially after injury the flexion contracture of the PIP joint is less than 30 degrees, but when left untreated it slowly progresses. Radiographic evidence reveals that calcification often develops after 3 to 6 months. Calcification can progress to an osteophyte or a spur with an associated increase in flexion deformity, especially along the radial border (Fig. 6).

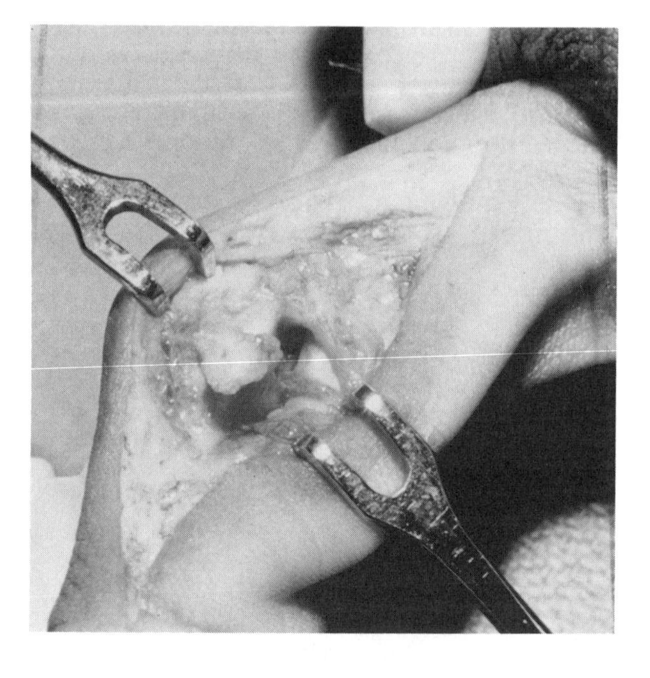

Figure 7 Operative findings in a pseudoboutonnière deformity including scarred volar plate and calcification.

A mild deformity, less than 40 degrees of contracture, usually responds to safety pin splinting, used in conjunction with active and passive range-of-motion finger exercises. The points of pressure of the splint on the volar surface are the base of the distal phalanx and the distal palm. Progressive and continuous traction splinting is applied for 30 to 60 minutes, at least three times a day.

For injuries with a flexion contracture of greater than 45 degrees, surgical correction is usually necessary. Repair is accomplished through a midlateral incision, and consists of release and distal advancement of the scarred proximal volar plate, excision of the bone spur or calcification, and release of the accessory collateral ligament (Fig. 7). The PIP joint is maintained in extension for 3 weeks by use of a transarticular K-wire in conjunction with an external splint.

SUGGESTED READING

McCue FC III, Andrew WF, Oh WY. Athletic injuries of the proximal interphalangeal joint: coach's finger. Contemp Orthop 1981; 6:516–525.

McCue FC III, Andrews JR, Gieck JH. The coach's finger. Sports Med 1974; 2:270–276.

McCue FC III, Hakala MW, Andrews JR, Gieck JH. Fractures and soft tissue injuries of the PIP joint. Contemp Surg 1974; 5:57–64.

McCue FC III, Honner R, Gieck JH, Andrews JR, Hakala M. A pseudo-boutonnière deformity. Hand J Br Soc Surg Hand 1975; 7:166–170.

McCue FC III, Honner R, Johnson MC, Gieck JH. Athletic injuries of the proximal interphalangeal joint requiring surgical treatment. J Bone Joint Surg 1970; 52A:937–956.

Schneider RC, Kennedy JC, Plant ML. Sports injuries: mechanisms, prevention and treatment. Baltimore: Williams & Wilkins, 1985: 743.

FRACTURES AND DISLOCATIONS IN THE HAND AND WRIST

C. STEWART WRIGHT, M.D., F.R.C.S.(C)

Hand and wrist injuries often occur in athletes and may be frustrating for both trainer and physician because of the difficulty of making the diagnosis and obtaining a successful outcome. Acute injuries are usually caused by impact or rotational forces such as a fall on an outstretched hand, which may result in strains, fractures, or dislocations.

THE WRIST

Fractures of the distal radius or wrist usually result from a considerable force, e.g., falling from a height or flying off a speeding vehicle such as a bicycle or motorcycle. Distal radius and ulnar fractures may be extra-articular, the so-called Colles' fracture, or may extend into the joint. In either instance, accurate reduction of the distal radius is important, and if closed reduction fails, operative reduction may be necessary. Fracture-dislocations of the wrist may take the form of volar lip (Barton's fracture) or dorsal lip (reverse Barton's) radius fractures, involving subluxation or dislocation of the carpus. These usually can be easily reduced by closed means, but may need pin fixation to maintain the reduction. A third variation of the wrist fracture-dislocation involves a fracture of the radial styloid (chauffeur's fracture). This also may require pin fixation if closed reduction cannot be maintained with plaster.

Injury to the distal radioulnar joint is usually by a rotational force applied to the forearm through the hand, although impact may also be important. This injury can result in dislocation of the distal ulna dorsally or volarly. The force results in an injury to the triangular fibrocartilage complex, which may take the form of a tear in the articular disc, in the dorsal or volar radioulnar ligaments, or in the ulnar collateral ligament. The joint may appear to be stable on examination, and pain on rotation of the forearm may be the only clue to the injury. Acute injuries with subluxation should be immobilized to maintain proper reduction. Dorsal displacement is stabilized in full supination, and volar subluxation is maintained in neutral position. In both instances, a long arm cast is necessary to maintain the reduced position. A transverse Kirschner wire may occasionally be necessary in addition to the cast.

Finally, one should be alert to an injury that occurs in the adolescent, a Salter type I epiphyseal injury of the distal radius and ulna. Although these appear normal radiographically, there is tenderness just proximal to the radial and ulnar styloids. These injuries can be very painful and may require cast immobilization for 10 to 14 days.

THE HAND

The jammed finger is a common athletic injury, usually caused by an impact force. It may involve any of the digits or the thumb at the carpometacarpal (CMC), metacarpophalangeal (MCP), or interphalangeal (IP) levels.

Carpometacarpal Joint

The CMC joint may sustain a sprain, fracture, dislocation, or fracture-dislocation. These usually require casting until healed; some require open reduction and internal fixation. Bennett's and Rolando's fractures are intra-articular injuries to the CMC joint of the thumb. Accurate anatomic reduction is essential to avoid the sequelae of post-traumatic osteoarthritis. A similar entity occurs at the base of the fifth metacarpal, the so-called baby Bennett's fracture. In this a volar fragment remains intact while the remainder is displaced by the pull of the extensor carpi ulnaris tendon. This injury also should be accurately reduced and stabilized as necessary. Dislocations of the other three CMC joints may be unstable after reduction and may need pin fixation.

Metacarpophalangeal Joint

Dislocations of the MCP joint are most commonly dorsal and caused by hyperextension forces, although they may occur in any direction. "Complex" or "locked" dislocations may be difficult to reduce by closed means or may remain subluxed after attempted reduction. Careful attention must be paid to postreduction roentgenograms for this residual subluxation, the presence of which usually necessitates an open reduction of the joint and freeing of the interposed soft tissues.

Collateral ligament or volar plate injuries of the digital MCP joints may be very slow to heal and require long-term use of "buddy" splinting (adjacent finger strapping). Volar plate injuries often require extension block splinting in addition to the "buddy" taping. This involves the use of a dorsal splint, which blocks extension at a preset angle but still allows for full flexion of the digits. Intra-articular steroids may also be needed to resolve these injuries if they become chronic. In spite of these measures, it may take several months for symptoms to subside. The MCP collateral ligaments most often injured are on the radial side of the index fingers and the ulnar side of the little fingers. Joint instability or a large bone fragment attached to the ligament usually requires surgical repair.

Proximal Interphalangeal (PIP) Joint

Beware of the "swollen" PIP joint. Serious injuries are often missed and therefore not properly treated. One must carefully assess all four sides of the joint and determine the integrity of (1) the volar plate, (2) the radial collateral ligament, (3) the ulnar collateral ligament, and (4) the extensor mechanism. Any or all of these may be disrupted and require specific treatment. Digital block is helpful if pain limits proper examination.

Collateral ligament injuries occasionally occur alone, but are usually associated with an injury to the volar plate secondary to a hyperextension force. The collateral ligament injury can be treated by "buddy" taping to the adjacent finger. Injuries to the volar plate may require the use of extension block splinting for the first 7 to 10 days. Large bone fragments with associated joint instability require surgical repair.

With sufficient force the PIP joint may dislocate, most commonly in a dorsal dislocation. Three variations of this injury include (1) volar plate avulsion from the middle phalanx and a major longitudinal split of the collateral ligaments, (2) fracture-dislocation with a volar fragment from the base of the middle phalanx making up less than 40 percent of the articular surface, and (3) a volar fragment of the middle phalanx greater than 40 percent of the articular surface. The first two can usually be managed by closed reduction followed by extension block splinting. The third variation is usually unstable. Accurate closed reduction is difficult because the volar plate and collateral ligaments are no longer attached to the middle phalanx. This injury generally requires open reduction and reattachment of the fragment with a pull-out wire. If there is considerable comminution of the base of the middle phalanx, a volar plate arthroplasty, as described by Eaton, may be necessary.

Volar dislocations are much less common but may have an associated dorsal lip fracture from the base of the middle phalanx. If this fragment is large and cannot be accurately reduced, open reduction is necessary. In either instance, this injury must be treated with the PIP joint in extension to allow for healing of the extensor apparatus.

Boutonnière deformities are often the result of catching a basketball or softball on the fingertip. They occur at the PIP joint after disruption of the extensor tendon central slip mechanism. This allows volar subluxation of the lateral bands and a flexed posture of the PIP joint. The subluxated lateral bands and oblique retinacular ligament can then produce hyperextension of the DIP joint through their pull. When seen immediately after injury, most boutonnière deformities are passively correctable and can be managed by splinting the PIP joint in extension. The DIP joint is left free, and flexion of this joint is encouraged. It may be necessary to splint the PIP joint full time for 6 to 8 weeks.

An uncommon variation of the boutonnière deformity occurs when a collateral ligament is also torn and becomes trapped inside the PIP joint. The joint then becomes irreducible passively, and requires an open reduction and repair of the collateral ligament.

Distal Interphalangeal (DIP) Joint

At this level the most common injury is the mallet finger deformity that can be caused by catching a hard ball on the tip of a finger. Most of these injuries can be managed by splinting (see the chapter *Tendon Injuries in the Hand and Wrist*). Many athletes are able to continue participation in their sport while wearing the splint.

Dislocations of the DIP joint are usually in a dorsal direction and easily reducible for the most part. The exception to this occurs when the volar plate becomes trapped in the joint, and this may require open reduction. Volar subluxation or dislocation is generally part of an intra-articular mallet finger deformity. Volar displacement is treated with the joint in extension; the dorsal dislocations employ the extension block principle.

Hand Fractures

More than 90 percent of hand fractures seen in the athlete are manageable by nonoperative means. The goal should be early unloaded digital motion (within 7 days). This allows rapid diminution of swelling and prevents intra- and extra-articular adhesions, thus preserving joint mobility. These objectives can be achieved through the use of adjacent finger strapping ("buddy" taping) and extension block splinting, in addition to the early unloaded motion of the digits.

Unloaded motion means avoiding stress on the digit, i.e., avoiding any power grip exercises for the first few weeks.

Hand fractures may be transverse, oblique, or comminuted. Care must be taken to ensure that excessive shortening does not occur, especially in the proximal phalanx; otherwise the extensor mechanism may not function properly. Two other concerns are malrotation and excessive angulation. Rotation can be checked only with the MCP and PIP joints in full flexion, in which position the nail plates should point toward the scaphoid tubercle.

Some angulation is allowed with metacarpal neck fractures (boxer's fractures). In the fourth and fifth metacarpals, 35 to 40 degrees of volar angulation is acceptable because of the mobility of the CMC joints. This is not true of the second and third metacarpals, in which angulations beyond 15 to 20 degrees should be corrected. There is no place for the use of plaster casts with the "90-90" position of the MCP and PIP joints. If this is thought necessary because of instability, I would favor the use of percutaneous pins to obtain stability. The fixation can then be augmented with a gutter splint.

Most phalangeal fractures are stable in flexion and unstable in extension. One must establish a stable arc of motion for the fracture and then allow motion through that range. It may be necessary to anesthetize the digit and examine the fracture stability under anesthesia. If the fracture is stable through a full range of motion, it can be managed with "buddy" taping and early motion. If there is a range of instability, extension block splinting is employed. Weekly roentgenograms should be obtained for the first 3 weeks. The phalangeal fractures that require open reduction are those that are unstable through all ranges of motion, and those with a large intra-articular component that is displaced or unstable. Once stability has been obtained, early unloaded motion should be started.

Thumb Injuries

The most common thumb injury seen in sports clinics is trauma to the ulnar collateral ligament of the MCP joint. This is the so-called gamekeeper's or ski-pole thumb. Most frequently this is caused by a fall on an outstretched hand with hyperabduction of the thumb. Strap bindings on ski poles are probably the most common cause of this injury. Most hand surgeons believe that a complete tear of the ligament should be surgically repaired. Surgery is warranted if there is a large intra-articular fragment attached to the ligament and the piece is significantly displaced. It may also be indicated for late cases of pain and instability of the joint. Strains of this ligament need to be taped during athletics and immobilized with a C splint during the day. This regimen usually suffices when a player cannot take the time away from sports for cast immobilization. A similar injury may occur to the radial collateral ligament, and the principles of treatment are the same as for the ulnar collateral ligament.

Bennett's fracture is an intra-articular injury to the CMC joint of the thumb. A fragment of the volar metacarpal base is held by the volar ligament while the remainder of the thumb is displaced, owing primarily to the pull of the abductor pollicis longus and secondarily to that of the adductor pollicis.

Accurate reduction is important if one is to avoid the problems of osteoarthritis, instability, and late pain in the CMC joint. Failure to obtain an acceptable closed reduction should be an indication for open reduction and internal fixation of the fracture. A K-wire between the first and second metacarpals may be useful to augment the fixation of the fracture. Occasionally one sees a painful nonunion of this fracture, and the ununited fragment can be excised if it is small enough.

Tendon injuries to the thumb are most commonly to the extensor mechanism. Mallet thumb secondary to avulsion of the extensor pollicis longus and boutonnière deformity after central slip injury are treated in a fashion similar to the other digits, with splinting (see the chapter *Tendon Injuries in the Hand and Wrist*). The extensor pollicis longus may rupture secondarily to a fracture of the distal radius when a bony spike is formed around Lister's tubercle. This is usually treated with a tendon transfer employing the extensor indicis proprius as a donor.

Injuries to the nail or nail bed are usually caused by crushing, such as with a football cleat or when it is caught on a piece of equipment. Whenever possible the nail should be retained to use as a splint, even if it has been avulsed. Radiographic evaluation is essential, because this type of bone injury usually constitutes a compound fracture. Lacerations to the nail bed should be carefully repaired with a fine suture, preferably using magnification such as surgical loupes.

SUGGESTED READING

Barton NJ. Intra-articular fractures and fracture-dislocations. In: Bowers WH, ed. The inter-phalangeal joints. New York: Churchill Livingstone, 1987.

DoBuns JH, Linscheid RL. Fractures and dislocations of the wrist. In: Rockwood CA, Green DP, eds. Fractures. Philadelphia: JB Lippincott, 1975.

Eaton RG, Mallerich MM. Volar plate arthroplasty of the proximal interphalangeal joint. J Hand Surg 1980; 5:260.

Green DP, Rowland SA. Fractures and dislocations in the hand. In: Rockwood CA, Green DP, eds. Fractures. Philadelphia: JB Lippincott, 1975.

O'Brien ET. Fractures of the metacarpals and phalanges. In: Green DP, ed. Operative hand surgery. New York: Churchill Livingstone, 1982.

WRIST ARTHROSCOPY

A. LEE OSTERMAN, M.D.
RANDALL CULP, M.D.

While the value of arthroscopy and surgical arthroscopy in the diagnosis and treatment of knee disorders is well accepted, its application to wrist disorders is new and evolving. The anatomic complexity of the wrist, with its eight carpal bones, their intrinsic and extrinsic restraining ligaments surrounded by numerous tendons and neurovascular structures, offer innumerable pathologic possibilities. The proximity of these structures often makes precise diagnosis elusive and chronic wrist pain a diagnostic dilemma. The development of smaller-diameter arthroscopes and more precise instrumentation has made wrist arthroscopy a valuable adjunct not only in the assessment of wrist pain, but also in the treatment of many of its causes.

Physical examination does not always indicate a specific diagnosis. It can, however, provide an index of suspicion. The examiner should search diligently for various clicks and clunks. Table 1 lists the current provocative tests used in examining a wrist. It should be emphasized that, in order for a "click" to be considered pathologic, it should reproduce the patient's pain and should not be present in asymptomatic contralateral wrist. The examination should also include a measurement of grip strength and its quantitation by a Jamar's dynamometer. Grip strength requires a stable, pain-free wrist, and therefore significant wrist disorders will usually weaken grip strength. Finally, well-placed anesthetic injections may help localize and define the anatomic source of the tenderness.

Even if the physical examination seems conclusive, routine four-view studies of the wrist are usually needed. These views may reveal an unsuspected avulsion fracture or static ligamentous deformity. Active studies such as a clenched fist–view or cineradiography may be needed to define a dynamic instability. Triple-phase bone scanning may highlight wrist synovitis or lunate avascular necrosis.

For tears of the triangular fibrocartilage and intrinsic ligament tears, wrist arthrography has become the benchmark. However, radiocarpal arthrography alone may not fully confirm tears of the triangular fibrocartilage. In a study by Roth in which arthroscopy was compared with radiocarpal arthrography in diagnosing perforations of the triangular fibrocartilage, a false-negative arthroscopy rate of 14 percent was found. Furthermore, unlike arthroscopy, arthrography does not allow the determination of the size and type of triangular fibrocartilage complex (TFCC) tear. We are therefore currently performing triple-compartment injections. A radiocarpal injection is followed 1 hour later by injections of the midcarpal and distal radial ulnar joint. This has lowered the false-negative rate to almost zero for tears of the triangular fibrocartilage and the intrinsic ligaments.

Recently we have been using a specialized wrist coil and magnetic resonance imaging (MRI) to define wrist pathology. Its accuracy is extremely high in defining intra-articular fluid, avascular necrosis of the lunate, triangular fibrocartilage tears, and scapholunate tears. It is less accurate in defining lunatotriquetral tears.

None of the abovementioned studies, including MRI, allow visualization of the volar wrist ligaments, or the evaluation of chondral defects of the carpal bones. By allowing direct visualization of the articular surfaces and palpation of the ligaments, wrist arthroscopy approaches these problems directly. Wrist arthroscopy therefore has several advantages over other means of evaluating wrist pathology. It provides direct visualization of cartilage surfaces and ligamentous structures. The exam-

TABLE 1 Provocative Wrist Maneuvers

Test	*Technique*
Radial stress test (for scapholunate stability)	Fingers on Lister's tubercle, thumb on distal scaphoid tuberosity. Causes radial and ulnar deviation of the wrist, both actively and passively.
Shear test (for pisitriquetral problems)	Fingers dorsal to triquetrum, thumb "rocks" or pushes pisiform into triquetrum.
Shuck test (for lunatotriquetral stability)	Fingers dorsal to lunate while thumb is on the pisitriquetral joint. Causes radial and ulnar deviation of the wrist, both actively and passively.
Lunatotriquetral ballottement test (for lunatotriquetral stability)	Fix lunate with thumb and index of one hand, while other hand displaces the triquetrum and pisiform both volarly and dorsally.
Piano-key test (for distal radio-ulnar joint)	Volar-dorsal stability of distal ulnar tested at different rotatory positions.
Triangular fibrocartilage load test (for wrist ulnar deviation)	With passive manipulation of carpus against the ulna will produce painful crepitus.
ECU subluxation test	Examine dorsum of wrist with forearm supinated and ulnar deviation against resistance. A visible and palpable subluxation of the ECU is noted, often with a snap.
Grip strength	The jamar curve from intrinsic to extrinsic grasp should generate a bell shaped curve. A flat-line plot often indicates voluntary submaximal performance.
Rapid exchange grip test	Patient grasps dynomometer strongly at optimal grasp position and is asked to alternate rapidly from one hand to the other. Normally with rapid exchange, grip strength decreases slightly. Voluntary weakness of grip cannot be controlled and often grip strength is elevated.

iner can probe the ligaments and evaluate their tensile strength directly. In intra-articular fractures of the distal radius, the surgeon can confirm the congruency of his reduction, or in scaphoid non-unions, the degree of coexistent arthritic change. Also, wrist arthroscopy can be therapeutic. The surgeon can remove loose bodies, perform synovectomies and chondroplasties, and debride frayed ligaments. If there is damage to the triangular fibrocartilage, he can debride central tears and repair peripheral tears. Finally, he can perform arthroscopic reductions and percutaneous fixation for carpal instabilities. Wrist arthroscopy has been performed at our center for the past 7 years and has been found to be a safe and valuable diagnostic and therapeutic procedure.

BASIC SET-UP AND PORTAL PLACEMENT

The patient is placed supine on the operating table. Either axillary regional block or general anesthesia is administered and a pneumatic tourniquet is applied. The majority of patients undergo operation on an outpatient basis. A sling for weights is placed over the arm. The hand and forearm are prepped and freely draped. The fingers are then placed in sterile finger traps that are suspended from a trapeze connected to the opposite side of the operating table so that there is ample operating space for the surgeon and his assistant. The shoulder is abducted approximately 60 degrees and the elbow is flexed to 90 degrees. If ulnar wrist joint disease is suspected, the small, ring, and long fingers are included in the traps. If a radial wrist disease is predicted, the thumb, and index and long fingers are placed in the trap. A weight of 7 to 12 lb is applied to a hook attached to the sling over the arm to provide a steady countertraction for distraction of the radiocarpal and midcarpal joints. At the beginning of the procedure, the tourniquet is inflated with 250 mm of mercury. The surgeon may be sitting or standing with the monitor, light-source, and video recorder directly opposite on the contralateral side of the patient.

For evaluation of the radiocarpal joint, we prefer a short-barrel (50 to 60 mm) scope with an outside diameter of 2 to 3 mm and an angle of 25 to 30 degrees. For midcarpal and distal radial ulnar joint arthroscopy, the smaller videoscopes measuring 1.5 to 2 mm are more easily maneuvered. A light-weight chip camera is attached to the arthroscope. When the larger radiocarpal scopes are used, irrigation is connected directly to the scope, with the flow maintained by gravity feed. Several instruments are now available to help define and modify wrist joint disease. A small hook-probe is essential for palpating the ligaments and also serves as a reference probe for magnification. Shutt baskets and grasping forceps ranging from 2 to 3 mm are also desirable, and small-diameter shavers with disposable cutting blades and burrs are available.

Arthroscopy is performed from the dorsum of the wrist, and portal sites are defined by the extensor tendons (Fig. 1). There are eight arthroscopic portals: five for the radiocarpal, two for the midcarpal, and one for the distal radial ulnar joints.

It is also important to keep in mind the neurovascular structures on the dorsum of the wrist. These include the deep branch of the radial artery and the superficial dorsal sensory branches of the radial and ulnar nerves. All other major neurovascular structures run on the volar aspect of the wrist; this is the main reason that dorsal portals are used.

The deep branch of the radial artery lies in the anatomic snuffbox entering under the tendons of the first extensor compartment. The superficial radial nerve sweeps across the snuff-box and supplies sensation to the thumb and index and long fingers dorsally. The dorsal branch of the ulnar nerve sweeps dorsally 5 cm proximal to the distal ulna and supplies sensation to the dorsum of small and ring fingers.

It should be emphasized that the portal sites are named for their relationships to the extensor compartments (see Fig. 1). Portal 1-2 lies between the first and second extensor compartments. It is just radial to the extensor carpi radialis longus tendon, distal to the radial styloid, and special care should be taken to avoid the extensor pollicis longus tendon as it turns obliquely across to the thumb. Branches of the superficial radial nerve and dorsal radial artery lie across the entrance of this portal, so care must be taken to spread with a mosquito to the level of the capsule before entering the joint. This portal is used to visualize the scaphoid fossa, radial volar ligaments, and proximal pole of the scaphoid.

Portal 3-4 is the main working portal and the preferred site for the initial examination of the radiocarpal joint. Its central location allows one to examine the radiocarpal joint in both its radial and ulnar aspects. It is located by palpating the radial margin of the extensor digitorum communis tendons and lies 1 cm distal to Lister's tubercle.

Portal 4-5 enters the radiocarpal joint directly over the midportion of the triangular fibrocartilage. It is found by palpating the ulnar side of the extensor digitorum comminus. It is most useful for evaluation of the triangular fibrocartilage, and also serves as a portal for arthroscopic debridement.

Portal 6R (radial to the extensor carpi ulnaris [ECU] ECU) is the main ulnar working portal. Portal 6U (ulnar to the ECU) is useful for joint distension and outflow. Again, care must be taken to spread down to the joint capsule to protect the dorsal ulnar sensory nerve. Through the 6R portal, one has a direct approach to the triangular fibrocartilage as well as good visualization of the ulnaluno and ulnatriquetral ligaments. One also can assess the intrinsic lunatotriquetral ligament.

The radial midcarpal portal (MC) is located just radial to the third metacarpal radial ulnar joint, distal to the proximal carpal row of the scaphocapitate interval. It is palpable as a small depression just radial to the extensor digitorum comminus of the index finger. It is suitable to visualize the articular surfaces of both carpal rows as well as the triscaphe joint. An ulnar midcarpal portal is also available on the ulnar side of the fourth metacarpal, and is a useful portal for shaving and insertion of working instruments.

A final entry portal is present at the distal radial ulnar joint (DRUJ). With the supination of the wrist, the dorsal capsule is relaxed and the scope sheath enters between the TFCC and the head of the ulna. This is useful for visualizing the underside of the triangular fibrocartilage and the articular surface of the ulna. It is not an assessable portal in all patients.

We have found that before initiating the arthroscopic procedure, it is helpful to use a marking pen

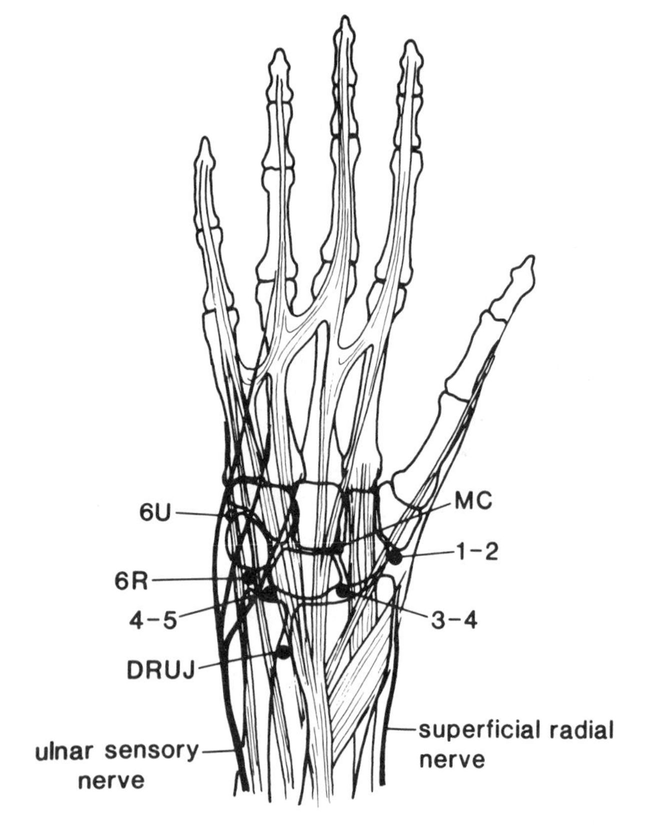

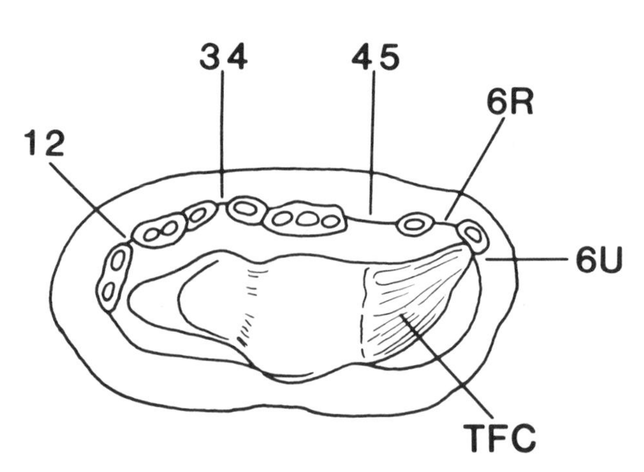

Figure 1 Arthroscopic portals are named for the extensor intervals they define. Care should be taken to avoid the dorsal sensory structures and radial artery.

to mark the Lister's tubercle, the radial and ulnar borders of the extensor digitorum communis, the extensor carpi ulnaris, the extensor pollicis longus, and the radial border of the extensor carpi radialis longus. Once the structures have been distorted by swelling, these landmarks may be more difficult to locate. After the inflation of the tourniquet, a needle is placed in the 3-4 compartment to distend the radiocarpal joint. It should be remembered that the surface of the radius has a volar and proximal tilt, and the needle and arthroscopic sheath should therefore be inserted in this direction. A short, longitudinal skin incision is made with a No. 11 scalpel. Because of the proximity of the extensor tendons, care must be taken not to stab. The wrist joint is entered with the blunt probe.

Postoperatively, a single nylon stitch is used to close each portal incision. The patient's wrist is wrapped in a sterile dressing and immobilized in a volar plaster splint, supporting the wrist and metacarpal phalangeal joints for 1 week unless other arthroscopic procedures have been performed.

VIEWING SEQUENCE

The arthroscopic examination of the wrist should be carried out in an orderly and sequential manner. Intimate familiarity with wrist anatomy is necessary (Figs. 2 and 3).

Inspection of the radiocarpal joint is begun through the 3-4 portal. Immediately upon entering the wrist, the physician will note the synovial fat pad overlying the radioscapholunate ligament (Fig. 4). This not only provides a useful landmark for the underlying ligament, but is directly opposite and intimate with the intrinsic scapholunate ligament and, along with the interfacet ridge, serves as a convenient dividing point between the radial and ulnar sides of the joint.

After this landmark has been identified, the scope is advanced toward the ulnar side of the wrist until the prestyloid recess is seen. A large-gauge needle is then inserted just ulnar to the extensor carpi ulnaris tendon through the 6U portal. The outflow needle can then be observed in the joint.

Next, the 6R portal is established through direct arthroscopic observation just radial to the extensor carpi ulnaris tendon. Aside from palpation, the arthroscopic light itself can provide a guide to establishing this portal. Initially, this portal will be used to insert the probe. The probe will be used as a palpating "finger" to determine the structural integrity and help define both normal and pathologic anatomy. If there is a great deal of active synovitis in the wrist, a small shaver can be inserted through the 6R portal and the joint cleaned of the obscuring synovium before the observation.

Once these portals have been established, the examiner returns to the fat pad overlying the radioscapholunate ligament. As stated previously, this is in intimate contact with the scapholunate intrinsic ligament (see Fig. 4).

When it is intact, the fat pad overlying the radioscapholunate ligament is often indistinguishable from the cartilage of the scaphoid and lunate because of its convex surface. The probe helps distinguish between the articular cartilage and the ligament. When it is disrupted, the probe will pass into the midcarpal joint, and in the case of gross disruption, the scope can easily be passed into the midcarpal joint.

As one advances radially, the scaphoid facet of the radius is obvious, as is the proximal pole of the scaphoid. The radioscaphocapitate ligament is the

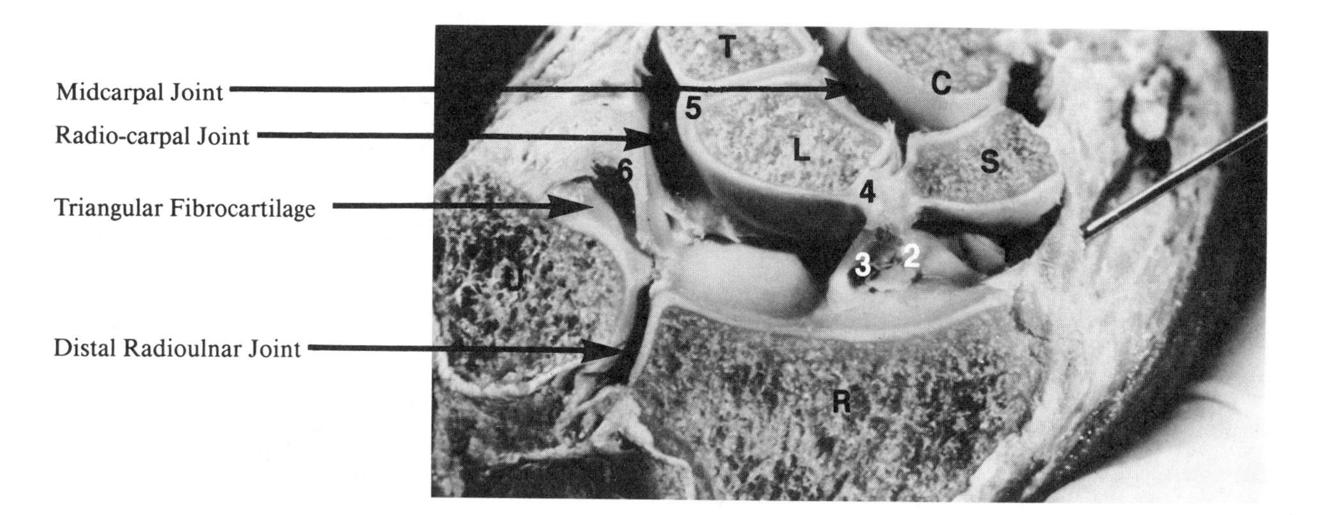

Figure 2 Coronal section of a wrist viewed from the dorsum. R = radius; U = ulna; T = triquetrum, L = lunate, S = scaphoid; C = capitate. 1 = radioscaphocapitate ligament; 2 = radiolunatotriquetral ligament; 3 = fat pad and radioscapholunate ligament; 4 = intrinsic scapholunate ligament; 5 = intrinsic lunatotriquetral ligament; 6 = ulnocarpal ligaments.

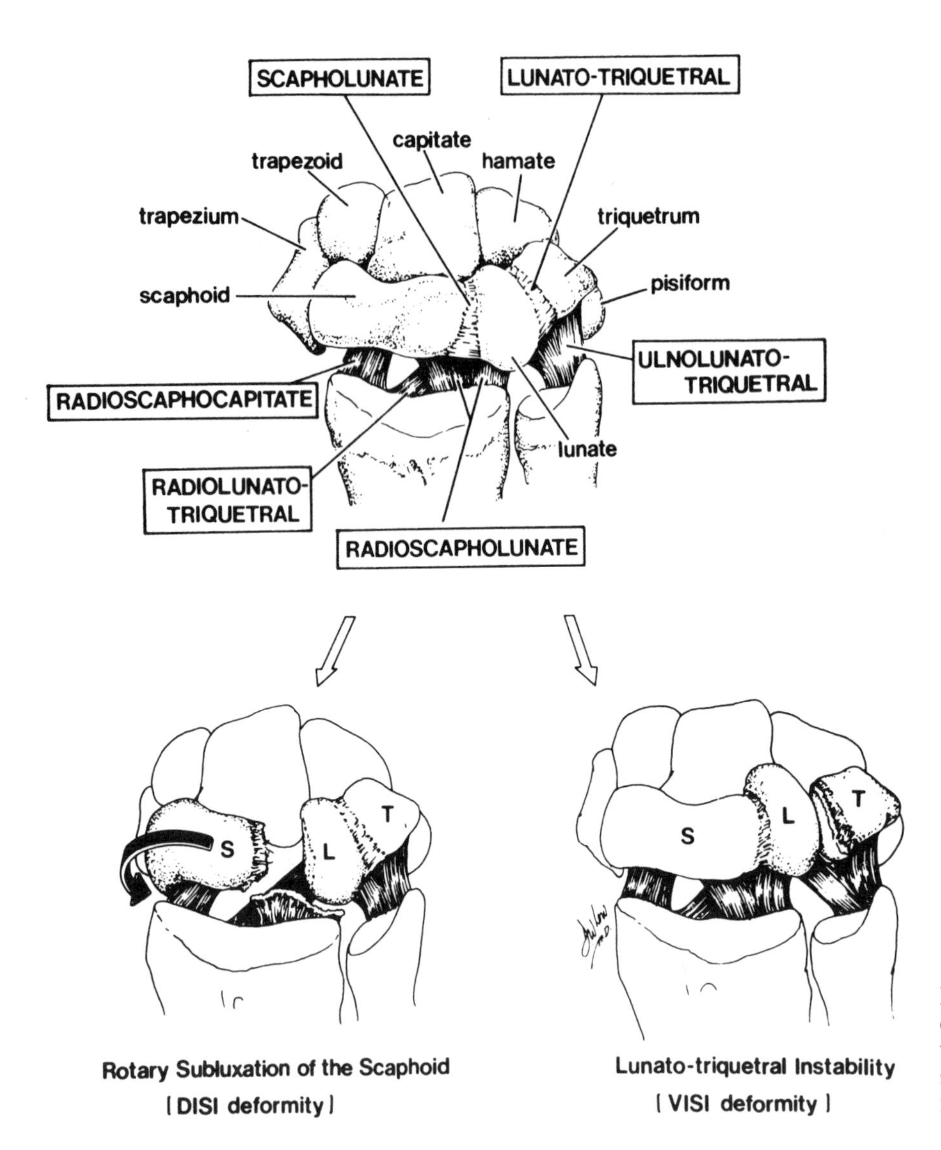

Figure 3 Diagramatic picture of the intrinsic carpal instabilities: rotatory subluxation of the scaphoid and lunatotriquetral instability.

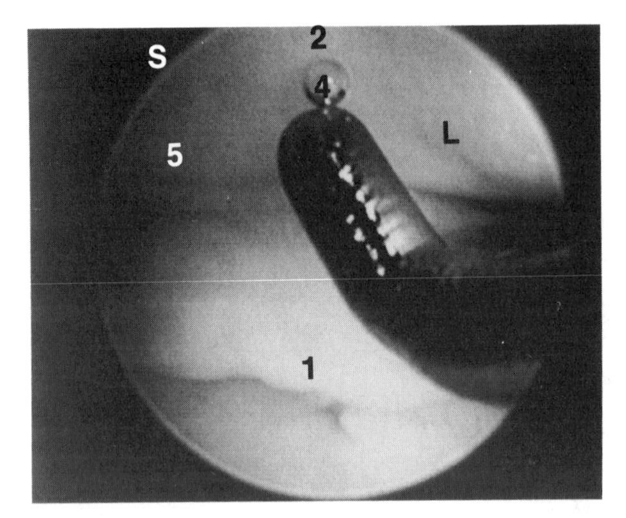

Figure 4 Arthroscopic view on entering the 3-4 portal. 1 = fat pad synovium overlying the radioscapholunate ligament; 2 = intrinsic scapholunate ligament. Prove lies against it and small air bubble (4). S = proximal pole scaphoid; L = lunate.

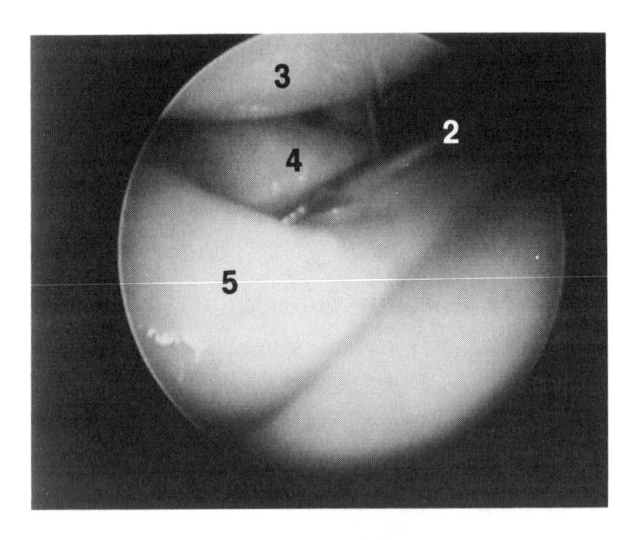

Figure 5 Arthroscopic view from 3-4 portal toward radial side of the wrist. Probe (1) is in the 1-2 portal. 2 = articular surface scaphoid facet of radius. 3 = proximal pole scaphoid; 4 = radioscaphocapitate ligament; 5 = radiolunatotriquetral ligament.

most radial ligament and acts as a fulcrum around which the scaphoid flexes and extends (Fig. 5). Next to it and broader is the radiolunatotriquetral ligament. These fibers are directed from the radius toward the triquetrum. Finally, the radioscapholunate ligament, often called the ligament of Testut, is usually hidden by the fat pad, but can be visualized by moving the fat pad aside with the probe.

Moving ulnar to the fat pad and across the sagittal ridge, one enters the ulnar side of the wrist joint. The lunate facet of the radius and the convex articular surface of the lunate are clearly visualized. One can also visualize the main portions of the triangular fibrocartilage as it originates from the radius and proceeds in an ulnar direction. Here again the probe is helpful in palpating the transition between the radius and the central cartilagenous portion of the triangular fibrocartilage. One can continue to visualize the ulnocarpal ligaments, the lunatotriquetral interval, and the prestyloid recess through the 3-4 portal, but it is most convenient to switch viewing and working portals at this time. The scope is therefore transferred to the 6R portal and the probe to the 3-4 portal. Through the 6R portal, one can fully appreciate the extent of the triangular fibrocartilage as well as the ulnoluno and ulnotriquetral ligaments (Fig. 6). One can visualize the prestyloid recess and the lunatotriquetral ligament. (see Fig. 2).

Midcarpal examination is less frequently performed than radiocarpal examination. Arthroscopy of the midcarpal joint is particularly helpful in evaluating carpal instability since the concave surfaces on the distal aspects of the scaphoid, lunate, and triquetrum provide for more accurate anatomic alignment than do the convex surfaces that are visualized through the radiocarpal portals. Also this view allows visualization of the distal pole of the scaphoid, the scaphoid trapezial area, and the evaluation of the hamate triquetral interface, a common source of early arthritic change. The scope is inserted through the radial midcarpal portal, and the ulnar midcarpal portal is used for outflow and/or probes. The proximal surface of the capitate is a useful source of alignment against which one can visualize the concave surfaces of the scaphoid, lunate, and triquetrum (Fig. 7). Note that the probe can pass freely between the scapholunate and lunatotriquetral joint since on the midcarpal surface of these bones, there is no intrinsic ligament. One can direct the scope radially and observe the scaphotrapezial joint (Fig. 8). One can also observe the volar intercarpal ligaments, such as the triquetro-hamate and deltoid ligaments. Generally, however, the midcarpal joint is an extremely tight joint, and if these structures are easily seen, it implies either significant ligamentous laxity or ligament damage.

Once a thorough examination has been conducted, the examiner can consider certain treatment alternatives. The therapeutic benefits of wrist arthroscopy must be integrated with open surgical procedures in the treatment of wrist disorders. Merely modifying the anatomy by shaving or trimming is not likely to produce a lasting result if a coexisting ligamentous problem is not also addressed. The best therapeutic results occur when arthroscopy can be used in lieu of open procedures with their higher morbidity and achieve a similar result. When this can be done, the patient will have less postoperative pain and an earlier return to function. In the majority of patients, this arthroscopic intervention can be performed on an outpatient basis and in a more economical fashion.

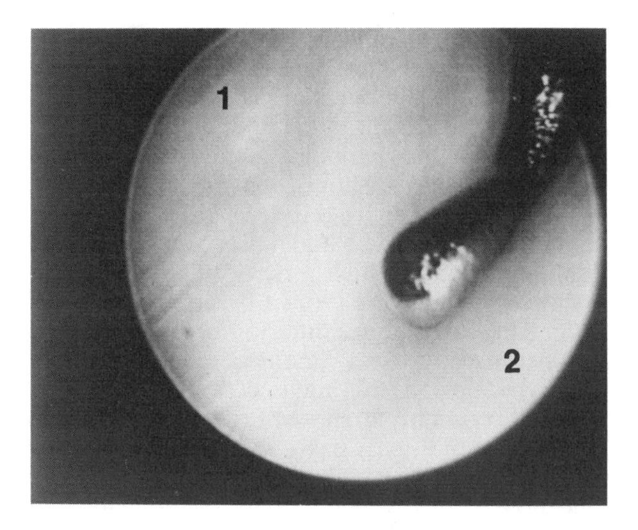

Figure 6 Arthroscopic view of the triangular fibrocartilage and its juncture with the lunate facet of the radius. When the TFCC is intact, the probe may be useful in differentiating the spongy area of the transection from bone. 1 = intact TFCC; 2 = lunate facet of radius.

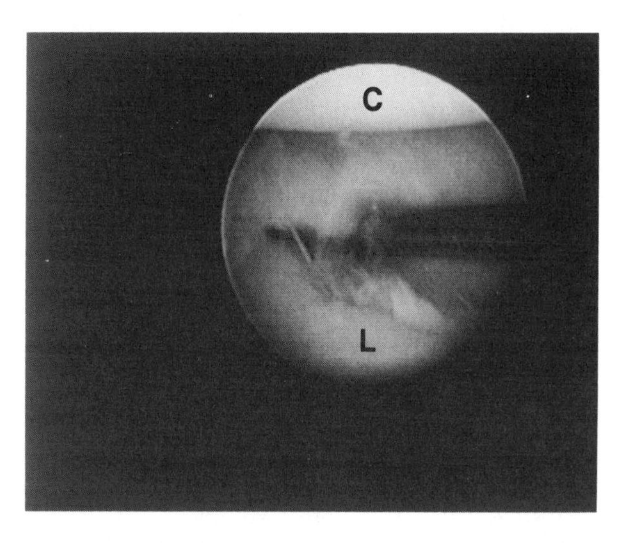

Figure 7 Arthroscopic view of the midcarpal joint. C = capitate; L = lunate distal surface and probe area of tear in volar midcarpal capsule.

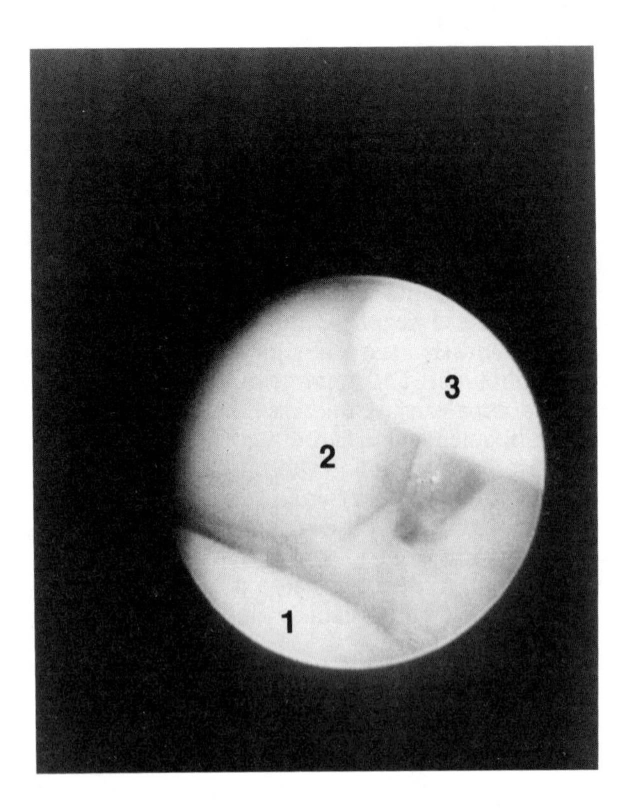

Figure 8 Arthroscopic view of the midcarpal joint. 1 = distal pole scaphoid; 2 = trapezium; 3 = trapezoid.

TRIANGULAR FIBROCARTILAGE LESIONS

The triangular fibrocartilage is a unique structure and differs from the classic knee meniscus. Wrist investigations have clarified its role both as a stabilizer of the distal radial ulnar joint through its volar and dorsal radial ulnar ligaments and as an axial load-bearing role in transmitting forces across the wrist. In a wrist with neutral ulnar variance, approximately 20 percent of the applied load across the wrist is transmitted to the ulna. If less than two-thirds of the central portion of the triangular fibrocartilage is excised, this physiologic load transmission is relatively undisturbed. Excising more than two-thirds of the central portion and disturbing the continuity of the volar and dorsal ligaments as well as the attachments to the base of the ulnar styloid and ulnar carpal ligaments can seriously compromise distal radial ulnar joint stability.

Isolated triangular fibrocartilage perforations are frequently implicated as the cause of chronic wrist pain. Because asymptomatic age-related perforations are common, symptoms related to such perforations are not fully understood and often reflect other mechanical derangements. Although tears or perforations of the central cartilagenous portion will not heal, many will become asymptomatic. Thus most patients should have a trial of conservative treatment involving restriction of activities, splinting, and anti-inflammatories administered either locally or systemically.

Currently the diagnosis of triangular fibrocartilage lesions should be suspected in a patient who has sustained a rotatory injury and presents with pain over the ulnar side of the wrist. Often there is a secondary extensor carpi ulnaris tendonitis, and it is therefore important to rule out instability of the extensor carpi ulnaris tendon. The patient may have symptoms of clicking; this was the case in more than half of our patients, and "catching" or locking was seen in approximately one-fifth. Pain, when present, is usually intermittent and increases with use of the wrist. Ulnar deviation of the wrist with passive manipulation of the carpus against the ulna may reproduce a click or painful crepitus. The clinical diagnosis can be confirmed by radiocarpal and/or distal radial ulnar joint arthrography, and more recently by high-resolution magnetic resonance imaging.

Tears can be classified in two broad categories: traumatic or degenerative. Traumatic tears are usually associated with a defined rotatory event and are more common when the ulnar variance pattern of the wrist is neutral or slightly negative. When the ulnar is long in relationship to the distal radius, the force across the triangular fibrocartilage is increased, and in this situation, attritional lesions of the triangular fibrocartilage are common. Over time, a progressive wear phenomenon occurs with the central cartilagenous portion perforated first, followed by erosions of the lunate, triquetrum, and distal ulna, and in some cases, by lunatotriquetral ligament perforations. In such cases, arthroscopic debridement of the central portion of the triangular fibrocartilage should also include a chondroplasty of the distal ulna. One can shorten the ulna approximately 1 to 4 mm using a burr through the radiocarpal portal. Coexistant lunatotriquetral perforations can be debrided, and in some cases, percutaneously stabilized. Peripheral tears of the triangular fibrocartilage have sufficient vascularity and thus potential for healing. These can be sutured arthroscopically using a pull-out technique. The outcome of such repairs are currently undergoing investigation, and are not in general use.

In 1987, we reported to the American Society for the Surgery of the Hand a prospective series of 50 patients with isolated tears of the triangular fibrocartilage who were treated by arthroscopic debridement. The average duration of symptoms before arthroscopy was 11 months. All patients had failed a trial of splinting and injection. Preoperative physical examination showed that two-thirds had some degree of ulnarly based tendonitis. There was mild limitation of extremes of rotatory motion in one-third. A click could be elicited in 60 percent of the patients. In 70 percent, it was unilateral, and in 29 percent, the click was bilateral. In three-fourths of those patients in whom a click could be elicited, this maneuver reproduced their symptoms.

A radiocarpal arthrogram showing an isolated tear of the triangular fibrocartilage was a criterion for entry in the study. Ulnar variance was positive in 29 percent of the patients, neutral in 39 percent, and negative in 32 percent. It should be emphasized that those wrists with positive ulnar variance were believed to have attritional tears, and in these cases, a resection of the distal portion of the ulnar was also performed. In the majority of patients (96 percent), surgery was performed on an outpatient basis with the patient under regional anesthesia. The operative time averaged 75 minutes (Fig. 9). Follow-up on this series has now exceeded 3 years. Postoperatively, three-fourths of the patients felt that their pain was fully improved, 12 percent continued to have intermittent but milder symptoms, 10 percent felt no change from the preoperative symptoms, and 5 percent experienced worse pain. In those with preoperative clicking and "catching," the clicking resolved within 2 weeks, although in one-fourth, the click remained (but was not painful). Of importance on follow-up, no clinical or radiographic ulnar instability was noted. No infections were noted. A mild extensor tendon derangement was noted in one patient who had a persistent extensor digiti quinti minimi lag of 30 degrees. No unresolved neurovascular problems such as reflex sympathetic dystrophy or neuropraxias occurred. Two patients did have transient dorsal ulnar sensory symptoms which cleared within 3 months. Those patients with injury of a sports-related nature returned to unrestricted activity at an average of 6 weeks. Patients receiving workman's compensation were unable to work for an average of 3.2 months (a range of 1 week to 6.2 months). Patient satisfaction was high, with 88 percent considering the surgery worthwhile. Two of the three patients with bilateral tears had the opposite wrist operated on.

Arthroscopic debridement of an isolated triangular fibrocartilage perforation is not only technically feasible, but in the short-term, is of benefit in reducing symptoms without increasing ulnar instability. It is associated with less morbidity than the other options, which involve either open resection of the triangular fibrocartilage, or procedures addressing the distal ulna. It should be emphasized that if significant positive ulnar variance was noted radiographically or if chondromalacia changes were seen at surgery, a limited resection of the distal ulna was performed (Fig. 10).

OTHER THERAPEUTIC USES FOR WRIST ARTHROSCOPY

Carpal Instability

Instabilities of the scapholunate and lunatotriquetral joint can be treated arthroscopically (see Fig. 3). The torn and frayed ligament and the accompanying synovitis are debrided. An accurate reduction is then performed. The adequacy of the reduction is best visualized by keeping the scope in the midcarpal joint where the concavity of the surface allows more accurate alignment. Particularly in patients with scapholunate instability, the use of joy-stick pins placed percutaneously in the lunate and scaphoid may provide further control in positioning the carpal bones. This technique cannot be used when the deformities are fixed. Once anatomic reduction has been achieved, pins are placed percutaneously across the intercarpal areas. In patients with scapholunate instability, a pin is usually placed

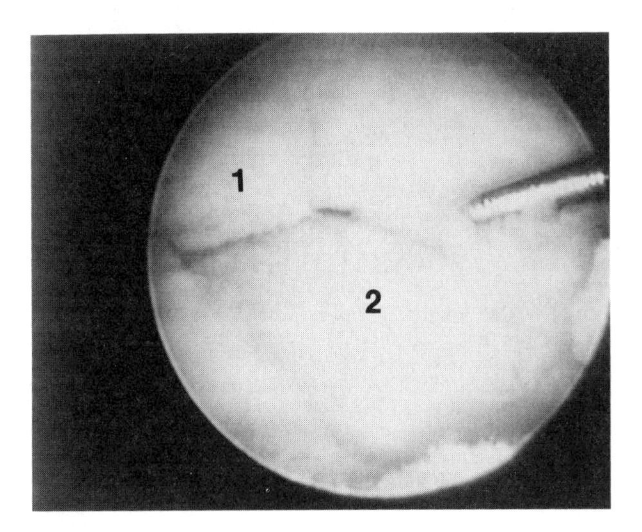

Figure 9 Arthroscopic view of the torn triangular fibrocartilage after debridement. 1 = edge of TFCC tear; 2 = distal ulna.

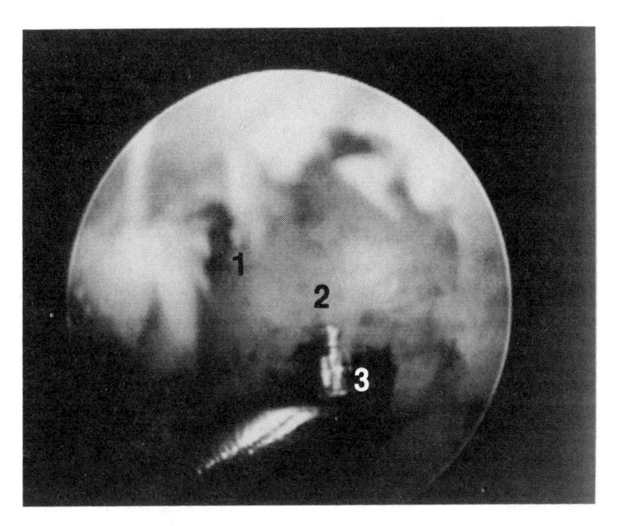

Figure 10 Arthroscopic debridement of chondromalacia distal ulna through a degenerative of the TFCC in a patient with positive ulnar variance. 1 = distal ulna, 2 = edge TFCC; 3 = curette.

across the scapholunate joint and across the scaphocapitate joint. In lunatotriquetral instability, pins are placed across the lunatotriquetral interval. The radiocarpal joint is almost never pinned. The 0.045 Kirschner wires are buried subcutaneously and do not substitute for cast immobilization. At approximately 8 weeks, the pins are removed and motion is begun. The short-term results of these arthroscopic reductions and internal fixations have been rewarding.

Intra-articular Fracture Reduction

Arthroscopy may be beneficial in achieving and confirming congruent reduction of the distal radial or carpal fractures. For example, in certain dye punch fractures of the distal radius, we have applied an external fixation device. The wrist arthroscope is then inserted through the 3-4 portal. Small loose fragments floating free in the joint are removed. Large chondral fragments can be elevated in the position under direct visualization. Subchondral pins are then inserted percutaneously to support the fragments. The external fixator and percutaneous pins are generally left in place for 8 weeks. Certain precautions must be observed in scoping acute injury situations. Currently we keep an Esmarch bandage around the forearm along with elevation of the tourniquet and avoid extravasation of excessive fluid into the soft tissue with its potential for neurovascular compromise. We are also cognizant of the amount of fluid instilled.

Synovectomy and Particulate Body Removal

Through the arthroscope, one can perform a relatively complete synovectomy of the wrist in both the radiocarpal and midcarpal joints. One can also remove foreign bodies or loose bodies arthroscopically.

Chondroplasties

Abrasion arthroplasty and debridement of articular defects in the wrist are similar to those done in the knee, but because it is not a weight-bearing joint, the results are often better. When the chondral lesion is secondary to an underlying ligament derangement, however, the benefit derived is temporary unless the primary problem is addressed.

Carpal Bone Excision

Ectomy surgery of the carpal bones through the scope is also possible. Procedures that we have performed include excision of small proximal pole fragments of the scaphoid, lunate excision in late-stage Kienböck's disease, and proximal row carpectomy. It should be emphasized however that such carpal bone excisions tend to destabilize the wrist, and one should consider the possibility of some type of concurrent carpal stabilization which requires an open procedure.

Modified Darrach Procedures and Radiostyloidectomies

Both of these procedures can be performed arthroscopically. Debridement of the distal ulna has already been addressed in the discussion of triangular fibrocartilage tears associated with ulnar positive variance and chondromalacia of the distal ulna. Approximately 3 to 4 mm can easily be excised. If the triangular fibrocartilage is intact, one must perform an arthroscopic shortening through the distal radial ulnar joint. Although one can observe the distal radial ulnar joint arthroscopically, we have not yet attempted any distal ulna debridements beneath an intact triangular fibrocartilage. In a chronic scaphoid nonunion with degenerative changes, the patient may symptomatically benefit by radiostyloidectomy. When the plain radiographs show early arthritic changes, arthroscopy may allow staging of the amount of change before a definite approach to scaphoid union. If excessive arthritis is present, then a radial radiostyloidectomy can be performed arthroscopically. This should be considered a salvage procedure to be used when achieving scaphoid union would not be likely to improve the patient symptomatically because of the arthritic changes.

COMPLICATIONS

In more than 150 wrist arthroscopies performed to date, the only significant complications have been scarring around an extensor tendon and minor nerve irritations, particularly of the dorsal ulnar sensory nerve. These complications have led us to abandon the 6U portal as a working portal, and it is now used mainly as outflow portal. The potential complications include those relative to anesthesia, equipment failure, neurovascular injuries, infection, reflex sympathetic dystrophy, and iatrogenic cartilage damage.

SUGGESTED READING

Bora FW, Osterman AL, Maitin E, Bednar J. The role of arthroscopy in the treatment of disorders of the wrist. Contemp Orthop 1986; 12:28–36.

Brown DE, Lichtman DN. The evaluation of chronic wrist pain. Clin Orthop 1984; 15:183–191.

Green DP. The sore wrist without a fracture. Instructional Course Lectures. American Academy of Orthopaedic Surgeons 1985; 34:300–313.

Mikic Z. Age changes in the triangular fibrocartilage of the wrist joint. J Anat 1978; 126:367.

North ER, Thomas S. An anatomic guide for arthroscopic visualization of the wrist capsular ligaments. J Hand Surg 1988; 13A:815.

Osterman AL, Bora FW, Maitin EF. Arthroscopic debridement of triangular fibrocartilage tears. Presented at the American Society for Surgery of the Hand; 1987; San Antonio.
Palmer, AK, Werner, WF. Biomechanics of the distal radioulnar joint. Clin Orthop 1984; 187:26.
Palmer AK, Werner, FW. The triangular fibrocartilage complex of the wrist: anatomy and function. J Hand Surg 1981; 6:153–162.
Palmer AK, Werner FW, Glisson RR, Murphy DJ. Partial excision of the triangular fibrocartilage complex. J Hand Surg 1988; 13A:391–394.
Poehling GG. Wrist arthroscopy. In: Illustrated Guide to Small Joint Arthroscopy. Dyonics Company, 1989.
Roth J. Radiocarpal arthroscopy: operative technique. Orthopedics 1988; 11:1309–1313.
Roth JH, Haddad NG. Radiograph arthroscopy and arthrography in the diagnosis of ulnar wrist pain. Arthroscopy 1986; 2:234–243.
Roth JH, Poehling GG, Whipple TL. Arthroscopic surgery of the wrist. Instructional Course Lectures. American Academy of Orthopedic Surgery 1988; 37:183–194.
Viegas SF, Ballantyne G. Attritional lesions of the wrist joint. J Hand Surg 1987; 12A:1025.
Whipple TC, Marotta JJ, Powell JH. Techniques of wrist arthroscopy. Arthroscopy 1986; 2:244-32.

ISOLATED FRACTURE OF THE ULNAR SHAFT

I. W. D. DYMOND, M.B., B.Ch., F.R.C.S. (Ed), F.C.S. (SA) Orth, M.Med.

Isolated fracture of the ulnar shaft is a common injury caused by direct trauma. The fracture occurs most frequently in the distal forearm, where it is known as the "paree fracture." It is an injury often seen in those who practice the martial arts, where the forearm is used in defensive action.

The diagnosis of the fracture itself presents little problem. The difficulty is in establishing

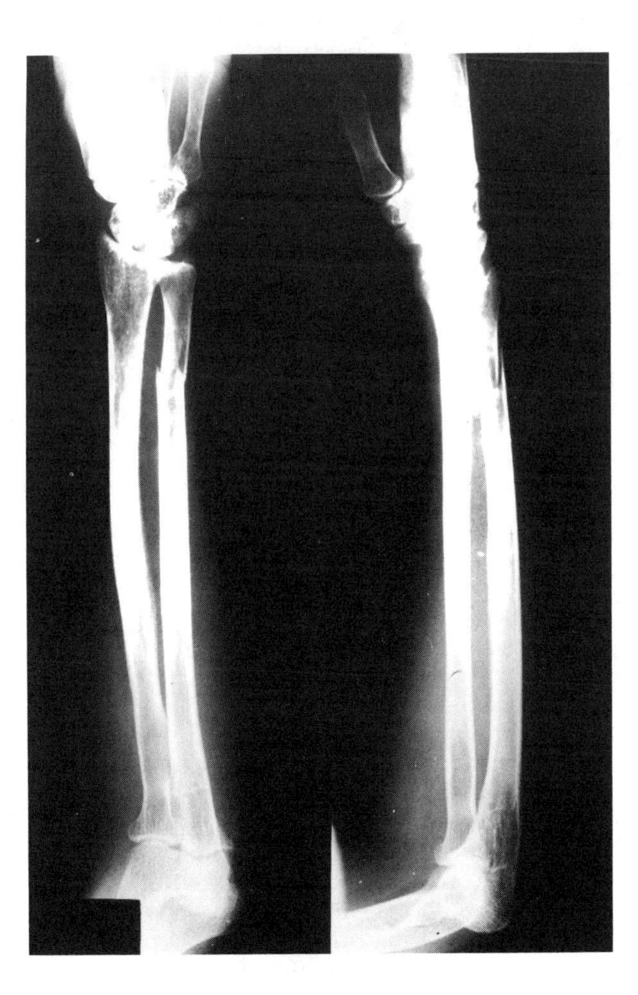

Figure 1 Type I fracture. There is less than 50 percent displacement, which indicates minimal loss of soft tissue integrity.

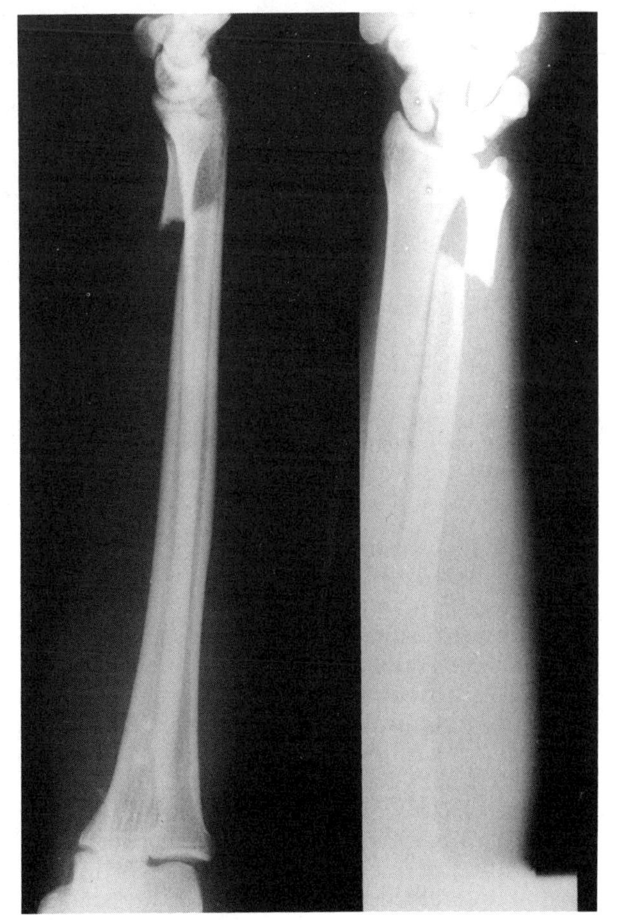

Figure 2 Type II fracture. There is more than 50 percent displacement, indicating disruption of the periosteal sleeve and interosseous membrane.

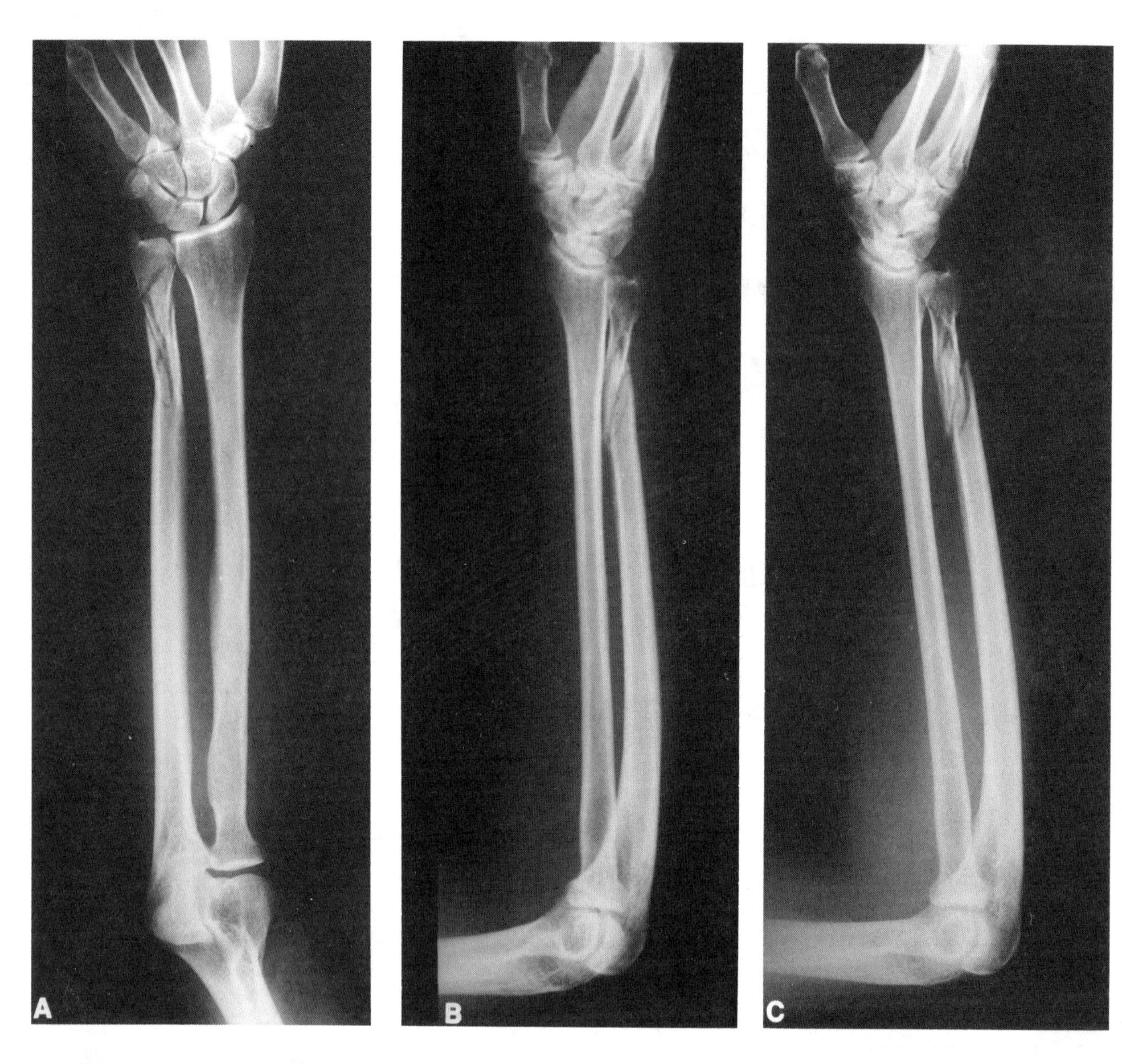

Figure 3 Type I fracture in (*A*) supination, (*B*) neutral, and (*C*) pronation, demonstrating stability of the ulna throughout the range of movement.

whether it is an isolated injury. Two factors that help in making this decision are (1) the mechanism of injury: direct trauma usually results in isolated fractures, whereas indirect or rotatory injuries generally cause complex fractures with involvement of the radiohumeral articulation (Monteggia's fracture), and (2) the location: isolated fractures usually occur in the distal forearm, whereas those that occur proximally are usually complex.

The management of these fractures seems to be simple, yet there is considerable controversy. Immobilization in an above-elbow cast is probably the most frequently used treatment for undisplaced fractures, and open reduction with internal fixation the most common for displaced fractures. Unorthodox methods such as simple bandaging are also known to be used with apparently no adverse results. Modification of the treatment by the patient himself is also not uncommon. Despite these variations in management, the fractures unite with few complications.

According to principles, protection of the fracture and prevention of rotational forces acting upon its fragments require immobilization of the joint above and below the fracture.

Mechanically the ulna participates in flexion and extension of the elbow and wrist, but acts as an immobile support during rotatory movements of the forearm. During pronation and supination of the forearm, the radius rotates around the ulna (the ulna cannot rotate because of its articulation with the trochlea of the humerus). The radius pivots at

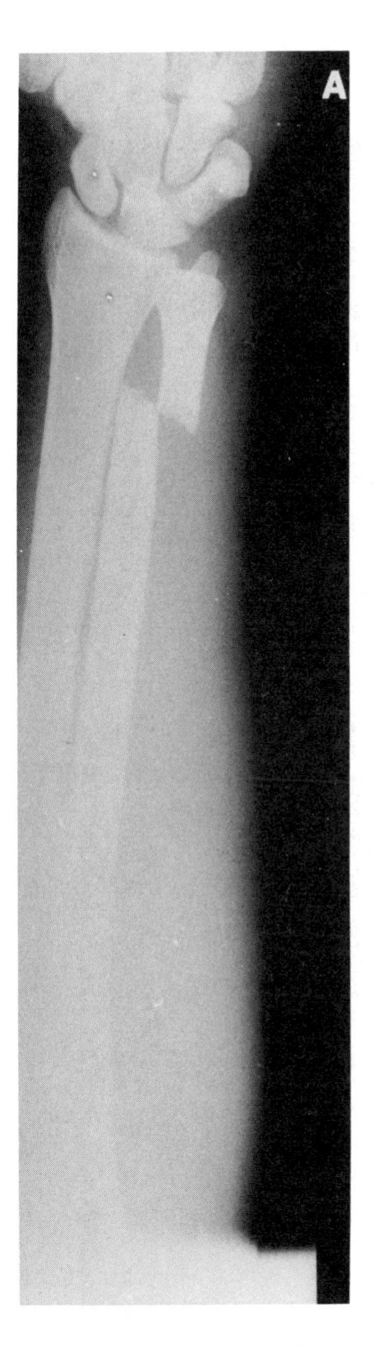

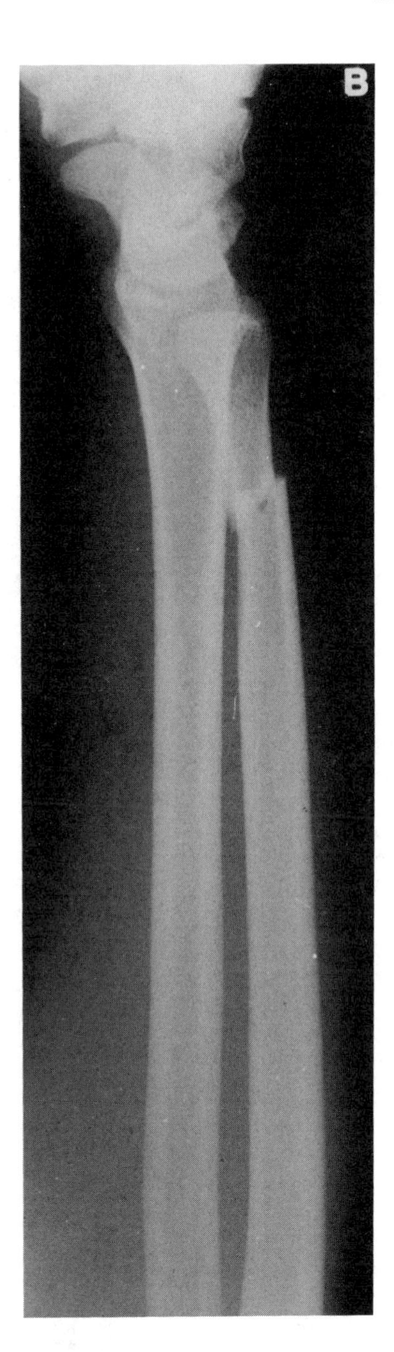

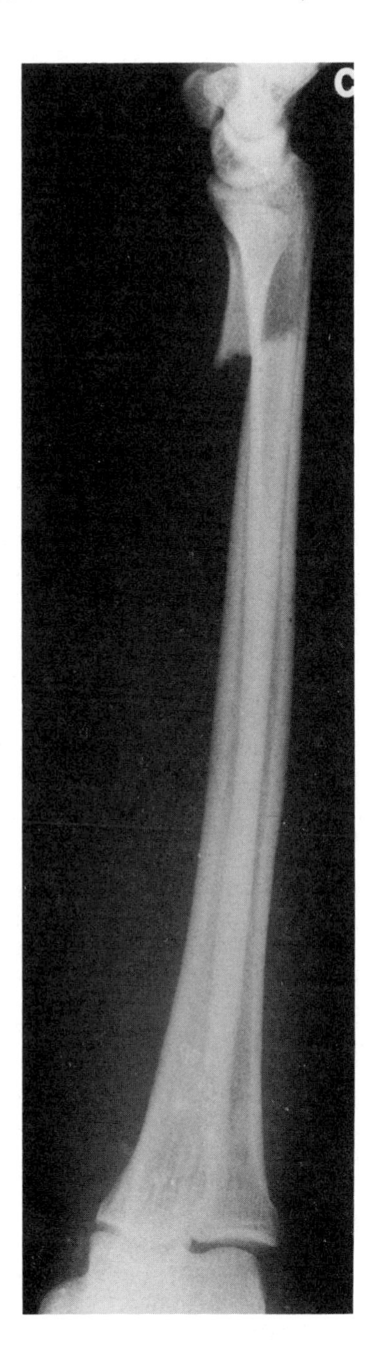

Figure 4 Type II fracture in (*A*) supination, (*B*) neutral, and (*C*) pronation, demonstrating instability of the ulna with movement.

the radiohumeral joint, and hinges at the interosseous membrane and distal radioulnar joint, during these movements. The interosseous membrane not only unites the two forearm bones, but also acts as a restraint to rotational movement of the forearm. Isolated undisplaced fractures behave in a different manner from displaced fractures. This is due to the disruption of the interosseous membrane and periosteal sleeve that occurs with displacement. Experimental studies performed on cadavers revealed that in a fracture that is displaced less than 50 percent of the ulnar diameter, the interosseous membrane is largely intact and the periosteum is minimally disrupted. These fractures are stable throughout a full range of movement. However, in fractures displaced more than 50 percent, marked separation of the interosseous membrane and tearing of the periosteal sleeve occurs. The fracture under these circumstances is unstable during pronation and supination.

From these observations, I classified isolated fractures of the distal ulna into two categories: type

I—fractures with less than 50 percent displacement, which are stable (Fig. 1); and type II—fractures with more than 50 percent displacement, which are unstable (Fig. 2).

Dynamic radiographs taken of acute fractures, under regional anesthesia before immobilization, supported these experimental findings. The injured forearm was rotated from pronation to supination and back again, while the stability of the fracture was observed. In type I fractures no significant displacement occurred, whereas in type II fractures considerable movement at the fracture site took place (Figs. 3 and 4).

These observations were used in a prospective clinical trial in which treatment was determined by the classification described above. Type I fractures in which, because of their less than 50 percent displacement, there was assumed to be a largely intact interosseous membrane and periosteum to help stabilize the fracture, were treated in a below-elbow cast for 6 weeks. During this time the patients were able to continue their daily activities. When the cast was removed, all had a full range of pronation and supination and were generally symptom free. Radiographic union was complete by 9 weeks (Fig. 5).

Patients with type II fractures were assumed to have lost the stabilizing effect of the interosseous membrane and periosteum, and were treated with an above-elbow cast for 6 weeks. Daily activities were severely restricted during this period, and it took 2 to 3 weeks for patients to regain full movement. Radiographic union was complete by 12 weeks.

In my experience, most isolated fractures of the ulna are in the distal half of the bone, are caused by direct trauma, and are less than 50 percent displaced (type I fractures). Treatment consists of a simple below-elbow cast to protect the fracture, since it is inherently stable. This allows considerably more freedom for the activities of daily living than an above-elbow cast.

This simple classification allows for the rational management of ulnar fractures, obviates the unnecessary use of above-elbow casting for fractures that are inherently stable, and identifies accurately those that require additional immobilization.

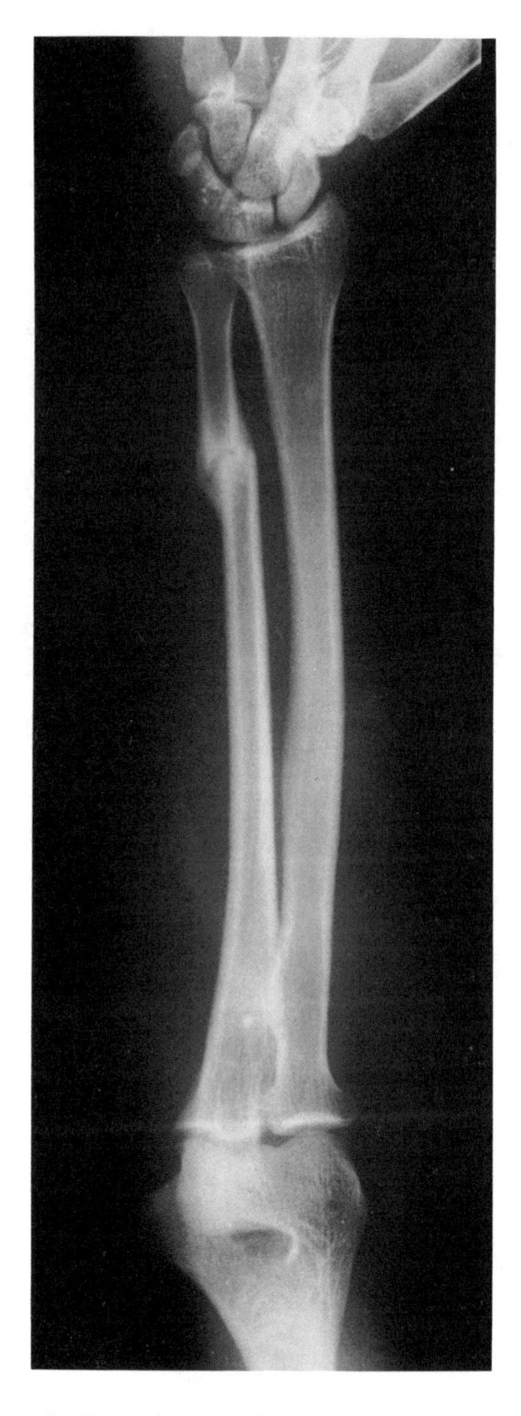

Figure 5 Type I fracture after 6 weeks in a below-elbow cast. The cast was not molded as is done in functional bracing. It was used more for protection than for immobilization.

SUGGESTED READING

Anderson LD. Fractures of the shafts of the radius and ulna. In: Rockwood CA, Green DP, eds. Fractures. Philadelphia: JB Lippincott, 1975; 1:441–485.

Anderson LD, Sisk TD, Tooms RE, Parks WI III. Compression-plate fixation in acute diaphyseal fractures of the radius and ulna. J Bone Joint Surg 1975; 57A:287–297.

Boyd HB, Boals JC. The Monteggia lesion. A review of 159 cases. Clin Orthop 1969; 66:94–100.

Du Toit FP, Grabe RP. Isolated fractures of the ulna shaft. S Afr Med J 1979; 56:21–25.

Dymond IWD. The treatment of isolated fractures of the distal ulna. J Bone Joint Surg 1984; 66B:408–410.

Pollock FH, Pankovich AM, Prieto JJ, Lorenz M. The isolated fracture of the ulna shaft. Treatment without immobilization. J Bone Joint Surg 1983; 65A:339–342.

Sarmiento A, Kinman PB, Murphy RB, Phillips JG. Treatment of ulna fractures by functional bracing. J Bone Joint Surg 1976; 58A:1105–1107.

Watson-Jones R. Fractures and joint injuries. 4th ed. Edinburgh: E & S Livingston, 1952:1.

REHABILITATION

PRINCIPLES OF STRENGTH TRAINING

JOSEPH J. VEGSO, M.S., A.T., C.

Muscular strength is a very important factor in athletic performance. After injury or surgery, a significant portion of the rehabilitation program must be devoted to regaining strength in the muscle groups that have been injured or immobilized. In addition, one must not lose sight of the loss of strength in the other muscle groups that help to support and stabilize the injured joint, or the muscles affected by simple disuse.

In recent years there has been a tremendous increase in the variety of devices available for strengthening muscles. Despite the overabundance and variety of equipment, the basic principles of muscle strengthening have remained unchanged.

Muscle strength is defined as the maximal force that a muscle can exert in a single contraction. Strength can be further defined as being static or dynamic. Static strength is commonly associated with a muscular contraction that does not produce joint movement (i.e., isometric), whereas dynamic strength involves a contraction with associated joint movement. Furthermore, a muscular contraction can be concentric or eccentric in nature.

Concentric muscular contraction is defined as muscle contraction with associated shortening of the muscle and joint movement (e.g., the biceps muscle contracts concentrically as it flexes the elbow). Eccentric muscular contraction is defined as muscle contraction with associated lengthening of the muscle and joint movement (e.g., after a concentric contraction of the biceps muscle, it goes through an eccentric contraction as it controls or resists elbow extension). An important aspect of the eccentric contraction is that a muscle can produce more tension during this phase than during the concentric phase.

There has been and continues to be considerable debate regarding the advantages of eccentric methods of strengthening versus traditional, concentric methods. The advocates of eccentric strengthening methods cite the fact that because a muscle is able to produce more tension eccentrically, a heavier training load will result in a more intense stimulus for greater strength gains.

Research comparing the eccentric method with other methods (concentric-isotonic, isometric, variable resistance, and isokinetics) has not demonstrated a significant advantage. It has shown, however, that eccentric methods of training are as effective in producing gains in strength as the other methods.

ISOMETRIC EXERCISE

Isometric exercise is typically defined as being a muscular contraction without associated movement of the joint or limb on which the muscles act. Simply put, the force a muscle produces is less than or equal to the resistance being applied. The effectiveness of isometric exercise in increasing strength first became popular in the 1950s as a result of the work of Hettinger and Muller. The most recognizable and popular way to exercise a muscle is to contract it for 6 seconds at a minimum of two-thirds maximal effort. The number of repetitions can be varied, depending on the phase of rehabilitation and the condition of the muscle.

There are several considerations for the use of isometric strengthening exercises in a rehabilitation setting. Isometric strengthening is most effective (1) in the very early stages of rehabilitation when joint motion is limited or inadvisable, (2) when the force that a muscle produces is insufficient for the use of weights or other resistance equipment, and (3) for patients with conditions that do not permit strengthening through an isotonic method.

One of the significant limitations of isometric exercise is joint angle specificity. Strength gains are produced at the specific angle of exercise, with minimal carry-over into other angles in the range of motion.

Isometric exercise is an effective method of increasing strength, particularly in a rehabilitation setting. It is convenient and advantageous because it requires minimal equipment and supervision.

ISOTONIC EXERCISE

Isotonic exercise is defined as a strengthening exercise in which the muscle shortens and the joint moves through a range of motion against a constant resistance or weight. This is easily accomplished through the use of a barbell, a sandbag, a weight bench, or other sophisticated equipment such as a universal gym.

As the weight is lifted, the muscle fatigues. Ideally a weight (resistance) is selected that causes the muscle to fatigue within a maximum of six to 10 repetitions. Over time, the muscle adapts and increases in strength. When this occurs, it becomes easier to lift the weight, and additional weight is added to overload the muscles again. This cycle is referred to as "progressive resistance exercise" (PRE). Developed by DeLorme in the 1940s, it is the hallmark of muscle-strengthening programs. Since that time, many variations on the theory have been introduced, but the basic principle has remained unchanged. The amount of weight lifted must be increased progressively in order to increase muscle strength.

Typically, a minimum of three sets of six to 10 repetitions of each exercise are performed during each rehabilitation or exercise session. In many instances, an injured athlete can perform strengthening exercises every day.

When isotonic exercises are used for rehabilitation, it is important to monitor the patient on a regular basis (daily if possible) to ensure that the exercise program is not aggravating the injury. Swelling, discomfort, pain, effusion, and loss of motion are important warning signs that the athlete is not ready for an isotonic strengthening program or is progressing too rapidly.

VARIABLE RESISTANCE

A variation of the isotonic strengthening method that has become popular in recent years is variable resistance exercise. As in isotonics, the joints or muscle groups move through a range of motion against resistance. Unlike isotonics, however, the resistance changes in an attempt to mimic or reproduce the mechanical advantages of the muscle and joint, so that the muscle must work at a near-maximal resistance throughout the range of motion.

In theory, variable resistance exercise should produce strength gains superior to those obtained from constant resistance methods. Unfortunately, objective research has not shown variable resistance training to be more advantageous. Despite the lack of definitive answers, variable resistance equipment has become the most widely used exercise equipment for strength training, thanks in large part to its ease of use and wide availability in health clubs and rehabilitation facilities.

ISOKINETIC EXERCISE

Isokinetic exercise is dynamic in nature, as are the isotonic and variable resistance methods. The aspect of isokinetic exercise that distinguishes it from the other forms of dynamic exercise is maximal accommodating resistance. The equipment provides resistance equivalent to that which the athlete exerts throughout the entire range of motion for every repetition. This is accomplished by controlling the speed at which the exercise is performed, usually through an electrohydraulic system. Typically, the athlete exerts maximal effort on every repetition.

Isokinetics have become the single most popular form of exercise used in rehabilitation today, partly because of the versatility (one piece of equipment can be used for all extremities), multiple exercise potentials (concentric, eccentric, isometric, and isokinetic), and recording and research ability of the equipment. The expense of isokinetic equipment seems to deter very few clinicians from purchasing it.

Like other methods of strength training, isokinetic methods have been scrutinized extensively. Two basic questions remain: what is the optimal training speed, and do strength increases at one particular speed carry over to other speeds? Available data have yet to answer these questions completely. Moderately slow-speed training seems to be more effective than either high-speed or very-slow-speed training for improving strength and carry-over effect.

Without question, isokinetic strengthening techniques will continue to be the most popular method of strengthening for rehabilitation, for the reasons cited and in view of the continuing advances in technology.

MANUAL RESISTANCE

Often overlooked, manual resistance is a very effective method of strengthening muscles in a rehabilitative setting. It requires no equipment, is an excellent method of isolating specific muscles, and can produce isokinetic or near-maximal accommodating resistance. Typically, exercise regimens follow a pattern similar to that of isotonics or isometrics. However, this may vary with the speed of exercise. At faster rates of speed, more repetitions are performed to provide a sufficient workload.

COMMENTS

The best method of strengthening muscles after injury is not easily defined. Factors such as postinjury condition, the availability of equipment, and the knowledge and familiarity of the trainer or therapist with various methods all play an important role in determining the best approach. Therefore, the physician must rely on the basic philosophy of increasing strength along with range of motion, and allow the methods to be dictated by the patient's needs and the equipment available. The most important factor related to the improvement of strength is the intensity of the load. Heavy loads produce the greatest stimulus for strength gain, but maximal loading does not necessarily produce maximal gains. A variety of factors must be considered when selecting the appropriate method of muscle strengthening. For rehabilitation, a combination of methods based on healing time and patient tolerance seems appropriate.

SUGGESTED READING

Atha J. Strengthening muscle. Exerc Sport Sci Rev 1981; 9:1–73.

DeLorme TL, Watkins, AL. Techniques of progressive resistance exercise. Arch Phys Med 1948; 29:263–273.

DeVries HA. Physiology of exercise for physical education and athletics. Dubuque: Brown, 1980.

Fleck SJ, Kraemer WJ. Designing resistance training programs. Champaign, IL: Human Kinetics Books, 1987.

Gettman LR, Pollock ML. Circuit weight training: a critical review of its physiological benefits. The Physician and Sport Medicine 1981; 9:44–60.

Gonyea WJ, Sale D. Physiology of weight-lifting exercise. Arch Phys Med Rehabil 1982; 63:235–237.

Torg JS, Vegso JJ, Torg E. Rehabilitation of athletic injuries: an atlas of therapeutic exercise. Chicago: Year Book Medical Publishers, 1987.

PRINCIPLES OF STRETCHING

JOSEPH J. VEGSO, M.S., A.T.,C.

Flexibility and range of motion are frequently considered synonymous. By definition, however, there are several differences. Flexibility is an integral component of range of motion.

Flexibility most often is defined as the ability of muscles to elongate as a joint or body segment moves through a range of motion. From a physiologic basis, it is a component of physical fitness related to athletic performance. Flexibility can increase through specific exercises or decrease through inactivity and disuse. Flexibility can be body part–specific and sport–specific (e.g., gymnasts require excellent overall flexibility, whereas swimmers need excellent shoulder and upper body flexibility).

Range of motion refers to the movement of a specific joint. This motion is influenced by a variety of factors, including bone congruence, the joint capsule, ligamentous structures, and the flexibility of the muscle-tendon units acting on the joint. In addition, injury, surgery, or immobilization may affect one or more of these structures, thereby reducing or totally restricting range of motion and flexibility.

Full range of motion and flexibility are essential for normal activities of daily living and athletic performance. In many activities such as gymnastics, karate, diving, and ballet, hyperflexibility is the norm for high-level performance. Consequently, most health care professionals, physical educators, and coaches have advocated a regimen of stretching exercises as an integral component of physical conditioning programs and warm-up activities. As a result, attention has been focused on the physiologic basis of stretching and its relationship to injury prevention and athletic performance.

Human contractile tissue is elastic. This elasticity is directly affected by tissue temperature and blood saturation of the muscle. At higher temperatures, contractibility is improved because the internal viscosity of muscle protoplasm is reduced. This phenomenon is reversed when muscle tissue is cooled. It is common in cold weather to hear individuals complain of feeling stiff or that they need more time to warm up. Recent reports also indicate that muscle contracture is more rapid and forceful when the muscle temperature is slightly elevated. This can be attributed to the increase in muscle elasticity and to the increased sensitivity and conductivity rate of the nervous system associated with a temperature increase. In addition to the effects on muscle tissue, joint range of motion is also enhanced at higher temperatures owing to an increase in extensibility of ligaments, tendons, and other connective tissue. As a result of this knowledge and several clinical studies on animals that demonstrated similar increases in flexibility and joint range of motion associated with higher tissue temperature, it has become a common practice for athletes to warm up before stretching.

Typically, a precompetition regimen includes three components: (1) a warm-up period consisting of jogging or moderate calisthenics for 5 to 10 minutes to raise body temperature to a level that produces mild to moderate sweating; (2) a period of generalized stretching, to loosen muscle and joint tissue, progressing to specific stretches to enhance flexibility and range of motion for the particular sport or position; and (3) agility exercises for body coordination and proprioceptive warm-up.

INJURY PREVENTION

Several authors have described flexibility as a component of fitness that is health related rather than performance related. It is difficult to separate the two; an athlete who has a tight muscle group certainly cannot perform at an optimal level without risk of injury. As stated previously, a joint that is unable to move through its full range of motion because of joint capsule or muscle inelasticity is certainly more susceptible to sprains and strains if forced to move beyond its available motion. Loss of flexibility and range of motion in the lower extremities can have a significant effect on normal gait and running patterns, followed by a decrease in performance and conditioning.

When soft tissue temperature increases, several other changes occur in addition to increased elasticity. Muscle contraction tends to be more rapid and forceful with slight rises in temperature. Nerve function is also affected at higher tissue temperatures. The sensitivity of nerve receptors is enhanced and nerve impulse transmission is improved. Theoretically, these changes could improve the athlete's ability to perform complex sensorimotor tasks, thereby reducing the risk of injury.

Early research in the area of flexibility indicated that stretching exercises done on a regular basis may help to improve the tensile strength and elasticity of ligaments and fascia. This concept appears to make sense, in that connective tissue responds to stress by organizing itself along the axis of that stress. Therefore, after injury, stretching can have a significant effect on the healing of connective tissue. As new collagen is formed and placed under stress, it organizes itself in the direction of tension, thereby creating stronger and more elastic tissue and reducing the chance of reinjury.

STRETCH REFLEX MECHANISM

Neurologically, muscle elasticity is controlled by the stretch reflex mechanism. It is a neurophysiologic phenomenon controlling the length-tension relationship within a muscle. Two types of nerve receptors within a muscle respond to changes in muscle length: the muscle spindle and the Golgi tendon organ. The latter also responds to changes in muscle tension.

When a muscle is stretched, the muscle spindle reacts by sending a signal to the spinal cord. In response, the spinal cord informs the muscle that it should contract, thereby resisting the stretch. Secondarily, if the stretch continues for longer than 6 seconds, the Golgi tendon organ reacts to the change in length and tension by signaling the spinal cord. The spinal cord responds by sending a message to the muscle to relax. The coordinated response by both receptors acts as a protective mechanism to allow for controlled extensibility of muscle units.

TYPES OF STRETCHING

Recommendations for a stretching program must be guided by the needs of the individual patient or athlete. After injury or surgery a rehabilitation program may include several types of exercises to regain joint range of motion and maintain or increase muscle flexibility. An athlete should perform routine stretching exercises as part of the warm-up procedure.

Further refinement of the definition of flexibility and range of motion can lead to a clearer understanding of how the therapeutic needs of the patient can be met through the various methods of stretching. There are two types of flexibility: static and dynamic. Static flexibility usually refers to passive movement of a joint. Hence, passive stretching activities are most frequently associated with improving joint range of motion and muscle extensibility after injury or immobilization, whereas dynamic flexibility refers to movement of a joint resulting from active muscle contraction.

These two types of flexibility must be considered when designing a stretching program. In the early phase of rehabilitation, passive range of motion must be developed with the aid of a therapist or athletic trainer. As the athlete recovers and begins to resume athletic activities, more dynamic exercises must be incorporated into the rehabilitation program.

Static Stretching. This is the most popular and safest method of stretching. The techniques used in performing this type of stretching involve moving a joint or muscle to the extreme of comfortable motion and holding the position for a given period, normally 10 to 30 seconds or longer. Several repetitions should be performed (five to 10), depending on the need for improvement.

In therapeutic settings, static stretching should be preceded by the application of a heat modality such as a hydrocollator pack or warm whirlpool. Athletes should perform some type of warm-up activity as described previously before stretching.

Ballistic Stretching. This utilizes repetitive contractions of an agonist muscle or muscles to produce a quick, active stretch of the antagonist muscle(s). An example is a "bouncing" toe-touch exercise to stretch the hamstrings. Although this method of stretching can be effective, it is not widely used for therapeutic purposes because of the potential risk of overstretching. It is, however, widely used as a type of warm-up for multiple muscle groups to simulate specific skill activities such as a golf or baseball swing.

Proprioceptive Neuromuscular Facilitation (PNF). This technique has gained widespread popularity in sports medicine and physical therapy facilities as a versatile way to improve flexibility, range of motion, and proprioception. Several techniques are used in PNF: slow-reversal-hold, contract-relax, and hold-relax. Each involves alternating a muscle contraction with relaxation in order to produce an increase in motion. Typically, the contraction is held for 10 seconds followed by 10 seconds of relaxation (stretch). All three techniques require a partner (therapist or trainer) to assist the athlete.

In the *slow-reversal-hold* technique, the partner passively moves the joint into a position of stretch. The athlete then contracts the antagonist muscles that are to be stretched against the resistance being applied by the partner for 10 seconds. After the 10-second contraction the athlete relaxes the antagonist muscle(s) and actively contracts the agonist muscle as the partner attempts to move the joint further into the range of motion. This sequence is usually repeated three to five times.

The *contract-relax* and *hold-relax* techniques are similar. In both techniques the partner passively moves the joint into a position of stretch. The athlete then contracts the antagonist muscles that are to be stretched against the resistance of the partner. In the contract-relax method the contraction is isotonic; in the hold-relax method it is isometric. After the contraction phase in either method, the partner again passively stretches the antagonist muscles while the athlete relaxes both the antagonist and agonist muscles.

In conclusion, several types of stretching have been proven effective in increasing flexibility and range of motion. However, in terms of safety and injury prevention, the ballistic method has received much less support from the medical community. A variety of factors can influence flexibility: activity, inactivity, the type of injury, immobilization, growth, the type of athletic activity, and tissue temperature. All must be considered when evaluating an individual with poor flexibility.

Finally, it is important to recognize that increasing flexibility is a slow process. Clinicians must emphasize this to help patients avoid the frustrations of slow progress.

SUGGESTED READING

Anderson B. Stretching. Bolinas, CA: Shelter Publications, Inc., 1980.

Lehmann JF, Masock AJ, Warren CG, et al. Effect of therapeutic temperatures on tendon extensibility. Arch Phys Med Rehabil 1970; 51:481–487.

Sapega AA, Quedenfeld TC, Moyer RA, et al. Biophysical factors in range of motion exercises. The Physician and Sports Medicine 1981; 9:57–65.

Sapega AA. Advances in nonsurgical treatment of joint contracture: a biophysical perspective. In: Post Graduate Advances in Sports Medicine, Vol. 3, Lesson 1. Berryville, VA: Forum Medicum Inc., 1988.

Torg JS, Vegso JJ, Torg E. Rehabilitation of athletic injuries: an atlas of therapeutic exercise. Chicago: Year Book Medical Publishers, Inc., 1987.

Index

Note: Page numbers in *italics* indicate illustrations; those followed by t indicate tables.